# BULLETIN

## OF THE NEW YORK ACADEMY OF MEDICINE



Volume 43

1967

THE NEW YORK ACADEMY OF MEDICINE
NEW YORK, N. Y. 10029

SECOND SERIES JANUARY 1967 VOL. 43, NO. 1

# BULLETIN OF THE NEW YORK ACADEMY OF MEDICINE

## *CONTENTS*

**HOWARD REID CRAIG**
**DIRECTOR, THE NEW YORK ACADEMY OF MEDICINE**
**1946-1966**

Howard Reid Craig: An Appreciation
*Robert L. Levy* . . . . . . . . . . . . . . . . . 3

Howard Reid Craig: A Contribution
*John L. Madden* . . . . . . . . . . . . . . . . . 9

The Committee on Public Health: 1946 to the Present
*H. D. Kruse and L. J. Amster* . . . . . . . . . . . . 11

"Our Greatest Material Heritage": The Library, 1946-1966
*Gertrude L. Annan* . . . . . . . . . . . . . . . . 21

The *Bulletin of The New York Academy of Medicine:* 1847-1966
*Paul F. Cranefield* . . . . . . . . . . . . . . . . 33

The Committee on Medical Education: 1946-1966
*Aims C. McGuinness* . . . . . . . . . . . . . . . . 49

The Committee on Special Studies: 1946-1966
*Harry Becker* . . . . . . . . . . . . . . . . . . 70

Financial Management and Building Operation:
The New York Academy of Medicine
*Robert M. Brereton* . . . . . . . . . . . . . . . . 79

AUTHORS ALONE ARE RESPONSIBLE FOR OPINIONS EXPRESSED IN THEIR CONTRIBUTIONS

This issue was prepared under the editorship of
DR. PAUL F. CRANEFIELD
who resigned as of December 31, 1966

*Published monthly by* THE NEW YORK ACADEMY OF MEDICINE
*2 East 103 Street, New York, N. Y. 10029*

SUBSCRIPTION OFFICE: STECHERT-HAFNER, INC., 31 EAST 10th ST., NEW YORK, N. Y. 10003
Annual subscription: United States $10.00, Canada $11.00, all other countries $12.00. Single copies $2.00.
ADVERTISING OFFICE • 421 HUDSON STREET, NEW YORK, N. Y. 10014 • CIrcle 7-7706

SECOND SERIES FEBRUARY 1967 VOL. 43, NO. 2

BULLETIN OF THE NEW YORK ACADEMY OF MEDICINE

# CONTENTS

Memories of Anton Chekhov's Family
*Gregory I. Altschuller* . . . . . . . . . . . . . . . . 87

How to Select the Proper Treatment for the Child with Reflux
*John K. Lattimer* . . . . . . . . . . . . . . . . . 99

Historical Aspects of the Anatomy of the Cardia with Special Reference to Hiatus Hernia
*Gerhart S. Schwarz* . . . . . . . . . . . . . . . . 112

The Action of Streptomycin on Protein Synthesis *In Vitro*
*Sidney Pestka* . . . . . . . . . . . . . . . . . . 126

Presentation of the Fifth Ferdinand C. Valentine Medal and Award to Theodore M. Davis
*John H. McGovern* . . . . . . . . . . . . . . . . 149

Experience in Transurethral Resection
*Theodore M. Davis* . . . . . . . . . . . . . . . . 152

The Clinical Society of the New York Diabetes Association, Inc. Third Annual Prize Essay Contest: Abstracts . . . . . . . . . 167



SAUL JARCHO, *Editor*

*Published monthly by* THE NEW YORK ACADEMY OF MEDICINE
*2 East 103 Street, New York, N. Y. 10029*

SUBSCRIPTION OFFICE: STECHERT-HAFNER, INC., 31 EAST 10th ST., NEW YORK, N. Y. 10003

Annual subscription: United States $10.00, Canada $11.00, all other countries $12.00. Single copies $2.00.

ADVERTISING OFFICE • 421 HUDSON STREET, NEW YORK, N. Y. 10014 • CIrcle 7-7706

# OFFICERS AND STAFF OF THE ACADEMY – 1967

SECOND SERIES MARCH 1967 VOL. 43, NO. 3

BULLETIN OF THE NEW YORK
ACADEMY OF MEDICINE

# CONTENTS

Increased Elastic Tissue in the Dermis: The Dermal Elastoses
*J. Graham Smith, Jr.* . . . . . . . . . . . . . . . . . . 173

Training in Neurological Surgery
*Paul C. Bucy* . . . . . . . . . . . . . . . . . . 186

The Hospital as a Teaching Center
*George H. Humphreys, II* . . . . . . . . . . . . . . 202

Current Efforts in the Municipal Hospitals
*Ray E. Trussell* . . . . . . . . . . . . . . . . . . 211

Health Needs and Programs in Deprived Neighborhoods
*James G. Haughton* . . . . . . . . . . . . . . . . 219

Changing Motor Performance and Personality in Therapeutic Settings
*Manuel D. Zane* . . . . . . . . . . . . . . . . . . 232

The Office of the Medical Examiner of the City of New York
*Committee on Public Health* . . . . . . . . . . . . 241

Avicenna on the Location of Houses . . . . . . . . . . . . . 250

AUTHORS ALONE ARE RESPONSIBLE FOR OPINIONS EXPRESSED IN THEIR CONTRIBUTIONS

SAUL JARCHO, *Editor*

*Published monthly by* THE NEW YORK ACADEMY OF MEDICINE

*2 East 103 Street, New York, N. Y. 10029*

SUBSCRIPTION OFFICE: STECHERT-HAFNER, INC., 31 EAST 10th ST., NEW YORK, N. Y. 10003
ADVERTISING OFFICE • 421 HUDSON STREET, NEW YORK, N. Y. 10014 • CIrcle 7-7706
Annual Subscription United States $10.00. Canada $11.00. All other countries $12.00. Single copies $2.00.

# OFFICERS AND STAFF OF THE ACADEMY – 1967

SECOND SERIES APRIL 1967 VOL. 43, NO. 4

# BULLETIN OF THE NEW YORK ACADEMY OF MEDICINE

CONTENTS

Use of Reticuloendothelial Phagocytic Function as an Index in Shock Therapy
*Burton M. Altura and S. G. Hershey* . . . . . . . . . . 259

Treatment of Pulmonary Embolism with Fibrinolytic Agents
*Eugene E. Cliffton* . . . . . . . . . . . . . . . . . 267

Six Hundred Years of Medicine in Vienna
*Alfred Vogl* . . . . . . . . . . . . . . . . . . 282

Psychopathology of Aggression and Violence
*Gustav Bychowski* . . . . . . . . . . . . . . . . 300

Annual Meeting of The New York Academy of Medicine

Address of the Retiring President
*John L. Madden* . . . . . . . . . . . . . . . . 310

Address of the Incoming President
*Preston A. Wade* . . . . . . . . . . . . . . . . 315

Citation and Presentation of the Academy Plaque to Howard Reid Craig, M.D.
*George Baehr* . . . . . . . . . . . . . . . . . 318

Citation and Presentation of the Academy Medal to Donald D. Van Slyke
*Michael Heidelberger* . . . . . . . . . . . . . . 322

Government and Community Health
*John V. Lindsay* . . . . . . . . . . . . . . . . 325

Ambulance Service in New York City
*Committee on Public Health* . . . . . . . . . . . 336

Scurvy During Magellan's Voyage . . . . . . . . . . . . . 346



SAUL JARCHO, *Editor*

*Published monthly by* THE NEW YORK ACADEMY OF MEDICINE
*2 East 103 Street, New York, N. Y. 10029*

SUBSCRIPTION OFFICE: STECHERT-HAFNER, INC., 31 EAST 10th ST., NEW YORK, N. Y. 10003
Annual subscription: United States $10.00, Canada $11.00, all other countries $12.00. Single copies $2.00.
ADVERTISING OFFICE • 421 HUDSON STREET, NEW YORK, N. Y. 10014 • CIrcle 7-7706

# OFFICERS AND STAFF OF THE ACADEMY – 1967

SECOND SERIES MAY 1967 VOL. 43, NO. 5

BULLETIN OF THE NEW YORK ACADEMY OF MEDICINE

# CONTENTS

Management of Ureteropelvic Obstruction
*Ormond S. Culp* . . . . . . . . . . . . . . . . 355

Meeting of the Career Scientists of the
Health Research Council of City of New York . . . . . . . 378

Health Services: The Impact of New Legislation
*Howard J. Brown* . . . . . . . . . . . . . . . 381

Closing Address
*John V. Lindsay* . . . . . . . . . . . . . . . 388

Abstracts of Presentations by Career Scientists . . . . . . . 392

The Municipal Hospitals of New York City
*Committee on Public Health* . . . . . . . . . . . . 435

Weavers and Computers . . . . . . . . . . . . . . . . 443



SAUL JARCHO, *Editor*

*Published monthly by* THE NEW YORK ACADEMY OF MEDICINE
*2 East 103 Street, New York, N. Y. 10029*

SUBSCRIPTION OFFICE: STECHERT-HAFNER, INC., 31 EAST 10th ST., NEW YORK, N. Y. 10003
ADVERTISING OFFICE • 421 HUDSON STREET, NEW YORK, N. Y. 10014 • CIrcle 7-7706
**Annual Subscription United States $10.00. Canada $11.00. All other countries $12.00. Single copies $2.00.**

# OFFICERS AND STAFF OF THE ACADEMY – 1967

SECOND SERIES JUNE 1967 VOL. 43, NO. 6

# BULLETIN OF THE NEW YORK ACADEMY OF MEDICINE

## CONTENTS

**New York Heart Association Conference on Possibilities and Actualities in the Delivery of Medical Care**

Foreword
*Alfred P. Fishman* . . . . . . . . . . . . . . 449

Municipal Hospitals
*Howard J. Brown* . . . . . . . . . . . . . . 450

Voluntary Hospitals
*Martin Cherkasky* . . . . . . . . . . . . . . 456

Impact of Medicare on Medical Education
*John H. Knowles* . . . . . . . . . . . . . . 463

Prospects of Federal Programs
*John W. Cashman* . . . . . . . . . . . . . . 472

Overview of International Trends in Medical Care
*Stanley W. Olson* . . . . . . . . . . . . . . 479

Regional Medical Programs: A Review
*Robert Q. Marston* . . . . . . . . . . . . . . 490

The Northwest Program
*John R. Hogness* . . . . . . . . . . . . . . 495

Planning and Organization of the Connecticut Regional Medical Program
*E. Richard Weinerman* . . . . . . . . . . . . . . 504

The New York City Story
*James E. McCormack* . . . . . . . . . . . . . . 515

Summation
*George James* . . . . . . . . . . . . . . 522

Medical and Biological Research on Human Beings
*Committee on Public Health* . . . . . . . . . . . . . . 525

Polybius on Medicine and History . . . . . . . . . . . . . . 528

AUTHORS ALONE ARE RESPONSIBLE FOR OPINIONS EXPRESSED IN THEIR CONTRIBUTIONS

SAUL JARCHO, *Editor*

*Published monthly by* THE NEW YORK ACADEMY OF MEDICINE
*2 East 103 Street, New York, N. Y. 10029*

SUBSCRIPTION OFFICE: STECHERT-HAFNER, INC., 31 EAST 10th ST., NEW YORK, N. Y. 10003
Annual subscription: United States $10.00, Canada $11.00, all other countries $12.00. Single copies $2.00.
ADVERTISING OFFICE • 421 HUDSON STREET, NEW YORK, N. Y. 10014 • CIrcle 7-7706

# OFFICERS AND STAFF OF THE ACADEMY – 1967

SECOND SERIES JULY 1967 VOL. 43, NO. 7

BULLETIN OF THE NEW YORK
ACADEMY OF MEDICINE

# CONTENTS

Some Considerations in the Therapy of Pineal Tumors
*Leo M. Davidoff* . . . . . . . . . . . . . . . . . 537

The House of Medicine
*H. D. Kruse* . . . . . . . . . . . . . . . . . 562

Nicholas Romayne: First President of the College of Physicians and Surgeons, New York City
*Byron Stookey* . . . . . . . . . . . . . . . . . 576

The Michael M. Davis Collection of Social and Economic Aspects of Medicine
*Lee Ash* . . . . . . . . . . . . . . . . . 598

The Psychotic Son of Benjamin Rush . . . . . . . . . . . 609

AUTHORS ALONE ARE RESPONSIBLE FOR OPINIONS EXPRESSED IN THEIR CONTRIBUTIONS

SAUL JARCHO, *Editor*

*Published monthly by* THE NEW YORK ACADEMY OF MEDICINE
*2 East 103 Street, New York, N. Y. 10029*

SUBSCRIPTION OFFICE: STECHERT-HAFNER, INC., 31 EAST 10th ST., NEW YORK, N. Y. 10003
ADVERTISING OFFICE • 421 HUDSON STREET, NEW YORK, N. Y. 10014 • CIrcle 7-7706
Annual Subscription United States $10.00. Canada $11.00. All other countries $12.00. Single copies $2.00.

# OFFICERS AND STAFF OF THE ACADEMY – 1967

SECOND SERIES AUGUST 1967 VOL. 43, NO. 8

# BULLETIN OF THE NEW YORK ACADEMY OF MEDICINE

CONTENTS

## CONFERENCE ON BURNS AND FLAME-RETARDANT FABRICS

Opening Remarks
*Paul V. Joliet* . . . . . . . . . . . . . . . . . . 615

Welcoming Remarks
*John L. Madden* . . . . . . . . . . . . . . . . 617

Why Are We Here?
*Richard A. Prindle* . . . . . . . . . . . . . . . 618

Present Status of the Treatment of Burns
*Curtis P. Artz and Dabney R. Yarbrough, III* . . . . . . 627

Statistics and Epidemiology of Burns
*Albert P. Iskrant* . . . . . . . . . . . . . . . . 636

Survey of Fatal Clothing Fires
*Ernest E. Juillerat, Jr.* . . . . . . . . . . . . . 646

Development of Clothing for Protection from Hazardous Thermal Exposure
*R. E. Seaman* . . . . . . . . . . . . . . . . . 649

[CONTINUED ON FOLLOWING PAGE]

AUTHORS ALONE ARE RESPONSIBLE FOR OPINIONS EXPRESSED IN THEIR CONTRIBUTIONS

SAUL JARCHO, *Editor*

*Published monthly by* THE NEW YORK ACADEMY OF MEDICINE
*2 East 103 Street, New York, N. Y. 10029*

SUBSCRIPTION OFFICE: STECHERT-HAFNER, INC., 31 EAST 10th ST., NEW YORK, N. Y. 10003
Annual subscription: United States $10.00, Canada $11.00, all other countries $12.00. Single copies $2.00.
ADVERTISING OFFICE • 421 HUDSON STREET, NEW YORK, N. Y. 10014 • CIrcle 7-7706

CONTENTS (*continued*)

Flame Retardants and Their Application to Textiles
*George L. Drake, Jr.* . . . . . . . . . . . . . . . 656

Pile Fabrics and Their Flammability
*Harry A. Freedman* . . . . . . . . . . . . . . . 663

Application and Development of Flame-Retardant Finishes in Textile Mills
*J. W. Weaver* . . . . . . . . . . . . . . . . 669

Developments in the Cotton Industry
*William M. Segall* . . . . . . . . . . . . . . . 675

Aiding Fabric and Garment Designers in Reducing Fire Hazard
*Herbert J. Wollner* . . . . . . . . . . . . . . . 681

Fiberglas: A True Fire-Safety Fabric
*John F. Ferger* . . . . . . . . . . . . . . . . 685

The Use of Synthetic Modacrylic Fibers
*R. S. Brissette* . . . . . . . . . . . . . . . . 694

Role of the Fire Protection Agency
*Louis Segal* . . . . . . . . . . . . . . . . . 699

The Federal Flammable Fabrics Act
*Henry D. Stringer* . . . . . . . . . . . . . . . 703

U.S. Department of Commerce and the Flammability of Clothing Fabric
*A. F. Robertson* . . . . . . . . . . . . . . . . 706

Controlling the Clothing Fire Problem
*Eugene L. Lehr* . . . . . . . . . . . . . . . . 711

CONTENTS *(concluded)*

Industrial Experience in the Use of Flame-Retardant Fabrics
*Robert S. B. Holmes* . . . . . . . . . . . . . . . . . 716

Flame-Resistant Textiles
*Thomas D. Miles* . . . . . . . . . . . . . . . . . 723

Program Activities of the Division of Accident Prevention, U. S. Public Health Service
*A. F. Schaplowsky* . . . . . . . . . . . . . . . . 727

Merchants' Views on Flame-Retardant Textiles and Injuries from Burns
*P. J. Fynn* . . . . . . . . . . . . . . . . . . 735

Legal Aspects of the Clothing Fire Problem
*Arnold B. Elkind* . . . . . . . . . . . . . . . . 740

Action and Program for the Future
*George F. Crikelair* . . . . . . . . . . . . . . . 749

General Discussion
*William G. Johnson, Herbert J. Wollner, Louis Segal, A. F. Robertson, Albert P. Iskrant, Paul V. Joliet, Joseph R. Palmer, Harry A. Freedman, George L. Drake, Jr., R. Bruce LeBlanc, George S. Buck, Jr., H. C. Hottel, Percy Bugbee, John L. Severance, John Appel, P. J. Fynn, Phil Dykstra, Donald A. Dukelow* . . . . . . . . . . . . . . . 752

---

A Roman Experience with Heat Stroke in 24 B.C. . . . . . . . . 767

# OFFICERS AND STAFF OF THE ACADEMY – 1967

SECOND SERIES SEPTEMBER 1967 VOL. 43, NO. 9

# BULLETIN OF THE NEW YORK ACADEMY OF MEDICINE

## CONTENTS

The Pathology and Pathogenesis of Diabetic Neuropathy
*C. L. Dolman* . . . . . 773

Axons, Schwann Cells, and Diabetic Neuropathy
*Simeon Locke* . . . . . 784

Atherosclerosis: The Facts and the Mysteries
*William Dock* . . . . . 792

Brief Psychotherapy and the Existential Shift
*Jan Ehrenwald* . . . . . 798

The Physiological Significance of Fibrillation Action Potentials
*Joseph Goodgold and Arthur Eberstein* . . . . . 811

Comprehensive Approach to a Child with a Birth Defect
*Myron Winick* . . . . . 819

Factors Affecting the Survival of Patients with Ovarian Carcinoma
*Allan B. Weingold, Sanford Sall, and Martin L. Stone* . . . 829

Health Services in New York City
*Committee on Public Health* . . . . . 843

Homicide by Means of Plague Bacilli . . . . . 850

Officers, Standing and Special Committees of the Academy 1967 . . 852

Officers of the Affiliated Societies and of the Sections 1967 . . . . 856

AUTHORS ALONE ARE RESPONSIBLE FOR OPINIONS EXPRESSED IN THEIR CONTRIBUTIONS

SAUL JARCHO, *Editor*

*Published monthly by* THE NEW YORK ACADEMY OF MEDICINE
*2 East 103 Street, New York, N. Y. 10029*

SUBSCRIPTION OFFICE: STECHERT-HAFNER, INC., 31 EAST 10th ST., NEW YORK, N. Y. 10003
ADVERTISING OFFICE • 421 HUDSON STREET, NEW YORK, N. Y. 10014 • CIrcle 7-7706
Annual Subscription United States $10.00. Canada $11.00. All other countries $12.00. Single copies $2.00.

SECOND SERIES OCTOBER 1967 VOL. 43, NO. 10

BULLETIN OF THE NEW YORK ACADEMY OF MEDICINE

## CONTENTS

A Study of Lee Harvey Oswald: Psychological Capability of Murder
*David Abrahamsen* . . . . . . . . . . . . . . . . . 861

The Problem of Fever of Unknown Origin
*Emanuel Appelbaum* . . . . . . . . . . . . . . . . 889

Granulomatous Colitis: A Panel Discussion . . . . . . . . . . 899

Introductory Remarks
*Henry D. Janowitz* . . . . . . . . . . . . . . . . 900

Clinical Features
*Arthur E. Lindner* . . . . . . . . . . . . . . . . 901

Surgical Treatment
*S. Arthur Localio* . . . . . . . . . . . . . . . . 906

Roentgen Features
*Richard H. Marshak* . . . . . . . . . . . . . . . . 910

A History of the Legal Regulation of Medical Practice in New York State
*John Barry Bardo* . . . . . . . . . . . . . . . . 924

The Longevity of the Ancient Greeks . . . . . . . . . . . 941

AUTHORS ALONE ARE RESPONSIBLE FOR OPINIONS EXPRESSED IN THEIR CONTRIBUTIONS

SAUL JARCHO, *Editor*

*Published monthly by* THE NEW YORK ACADEMY OF MEDICINE
*2 East 103 Street, New York, N. Y. 10029*

SUBSCRIPTION OFFICE: STECHERT-HAFNER, INC., 31 EAST 10th ST., NEW YORK, N. Y. 10003
ADVERTISING OFFICE • 421 HUDSON STREET, NEW YORK, N. Y. 10014 • CIrcle 7-7706
Annual Subscription United States $10.00. Canada $11.00. All other countries $12.00. Single copies $2.00.

# OFFICERS AND STAFF OF THE ACADEMY – 1967

SECOND SERIES NOVEMBER 1967 VOL. 43, NO. 11

# BULLETIN OF THE NEW YORK ACADEMY OF MEDICINE

## CONTENTS

Interactions Between Immunocompetent Cells and Target Cells or Antigens
*John R. David* . . . . . . . . . . . . . . . . 949

Problems in the Development of a TNM System of Staging for Cancer of the Head and Neck
*Joseph Newall* . . . . . . . . . . . . . . . . 959

Therapeutic and Investigational Potential of Heterologous Liver Perfusion
*John C. Norman, William G. Hardison and William V. McDermott, Jr.* . . . . . . . . . . . . 967

The Umbilical Vein in Diseases of the Liver
*Richard E. Kessler* . . . . . . . . . . . . . . . . 977

Implications of Untoward Reactions to Hallucinogens
*Edwin Robbins, Lillian Robbins, William A. Frosch and Marvin Stern* . . . . . . . . . . . . . . . . 985

The Evolution of Gender Identity
*Harry Gershman* . . . . . . . . . . . . . . . . 1000
Discussion – *Natalie Shainess* . . . . . . . . . . . . . 1019
Discussion – *Louis R. Hott* . . . . . . . . . . . . . 1028

Osler's Textbook Revisited . . . . . . . . . . . . . . . . 1034

AUTHORS ALONE ARE RESPONSIBLE FOR OPINIONS EXPRESSED IN THEIR CONTRIBUTIONS

SAUL JARCHO, *Editor*

*Published monthly by* THE NEW YORK ACADEMY OF MEDICINE
*2 East 103 Street, New York, N. Y. 10029*

SUBSCRIPTION OFFICE: STECHERT-HAFNER, INC., 31 EAST 10th ST., NEW YORK, N. Y. 10003
ADVERTISING OFFICE • 421 HUDSON STREET, NEW YORK, N. Y. 10014 • CIrcle 7-7706
Annual Subscription United States $10.00. Canada $11.00. All other countries $12.00. Single copies $2.00.

# OFFICERS AND STAFF OF THE ACADEMY – 1967

SECOND SERIES DECEMBER 1967 VOL. 43, NO. 12

BULLETIN OF THE NEW YORK ACADEMY OF MEDICINE

CONTENTS

## NEW YORK HEART ASSOCIATION CONFERENCE ON MECHANISMS AND MANAGEMENT OF ARRHYTHMIAS

Foreword . . . . . . . . . . . . . . . . . . . . . . 1039

Cardiac Innervation: Anatomic and Pharmacologic Relations
*Thomas N. James* . . . . . . . . . . . . . . . . . 1041

Autonomic Control of Cardiac Rhythm
*Brian F. Hoffman* . . . . . . . . . . . . . . . . . 1087

Experimental Neurogenic Arrhythmias
*Charles H. Hockman, H. Page Mauck, Jr. and Ebbe C. Hoff* . 1097

Clinical Experience with Neurogenic Cardiac Arrhythmias
*Ronald L. Katz* . . . . . . . . . . . . . . . . . 1106

The Electrophysiologic Effects of Beta-Adrenergic Blockade and Cardiac Denervation
*Andrew G. Wallace, Stephen F. Schaal, Tsuneaki Sugimoto, Marvin Rozear and James A. Alexander* . . . . . . . 1119

Phylogenetic Observations on Specialized Cardiac Tissues
*E. Neil Moore* . . . . . . . . . . . . . . . . . 1138

Arrhythmias and Electrolyte Disturbances
*Borys Surawicz* . . . . . . . . . . . . . . . . . 1160

Intracardiac Electrocardiography in Arrhythmia
*Charles E. Kossmann* . . . . . . . . . . . . . . . 1181

New York Heart Association: Abstracts . . . . . . . . . . 1193

General Grant's Headache . . . . . . . . . . . . . . . 1224

Index: Volume 43, 1967 . . . . . . . . . . . . . . . 1229



SAUL JARCHO, *Editor*

*Published monthly by* THE NEW YORK ACADEMY OF MEDICINE
*2 East 103 Street, New York, N. Y. 10029*

SUBSCRIPTION OFFICE: STECHERT-HAFNER, INC., 31 EAST 10th ST., NEW YORK, N. Y. 10003
Annual subscription: United States $10.00, Canada $11.00, all other countries $12.00. Single copies $2.00.
ADVERTISING OFFICE • 421 HUDSON STREET, NEW YORK, N. Y. 10014 • CIrcle 7-7706

# OFFICERS AND STAFF OF THE ACADEMY – 1967

BULLETIN OF
THE NEW YORK ACADEMY
OF MEDICINE

VOL. 43, NO. 1 JANUARY 1967

# HOWARD REID CRAIG

## *An Appreciation*

ROBERT L. LEVY

Past President and Presently Chairman
of the Board of Trustees
The New York Academy of Medicine
New York, N. Y.

MERELY to recount the events in a man's life does not serve adequately to reveal his character or appraise his achievements. Yet, in a brief sketch, this approach must serve as a base, incomplete though the outline may be. On January 1, 1967, Howard Reid Craig will officially retire as Director of The New York Academy of Medicine after having served in this post, with distinction, for 20 years. The occasion is not one for celebration but rather a time to express admiration for one who had a many-faceted career.

Craig was born in New York City on July 15, 1894, and received his preliminary education in the city's public schools. His two sons attended the Trinity School in New York and, as a father, he was impressed by the way it functioned. During the 33 years since then he has maintained an active interest in the school's welfare and growth and is still a member of its board.

As a student at Wesleyan University, Middletown, Conn., he was known to his intimates as "Pinky," a reference to his red hair and a way of distinguishing him from an older boy already known by the nickname of "Red." It is sometimes surprising to hear some of Howard's college classmates hail him in the old familiar way.

He graduated with the degree of A.B. in 1914 and of M.A. in 1915. Rumor has it that his reason for taking a postgraduate year stemmed from his desire to be near a young lady who lived in proximity to the campus. This tale is unconfirmed.

Howard was destined for the ministry, for three uncles were clergymen and his own pastor urged him to follow suit. However, during his postgraduate year at college he obtained a job tending furnace for a doctor in Portland, across the river from Middletown, and this seemingly casual experience altered his plans for a career. The old doctor liked him and took him around with him on his calls. His interest in medicine was aroused and the doctor was obliged to get another furnace tender. Soon afterward Howard entered the Cornell University Medical College, New York City, from which he graduated in 1919.

Throughout his years in college and medical school, Howard worked each summer to earn his way; lack of funds was always a problem. For a time, he played professional basketball. He joined the Musicians' Union at the age of 18 and during one vacation was the pianist in a "combo" in White Lake, N. Y. During part of the summers of 1914, 1915 and 1916 he was superintendent of a Herald-Tribune Fresh Air Camp, attended by 100 children at a time, with a changing population every two weeks. For three summers he tutored three boys of school age, taking them abroad on each occasion.

While at Wesleyan, he played a female role in the Senior Play. He must have done well, for David Belasco offered him a job in one of his productions. Rehearsals were held but the show never opened. Following this disappointing experience, Howard's yearning for a theatrical career appears to have vanished.

Medicine, from graduation on, was his life interest. He interned and was resident, in succession, in Memorial Hospital in 1919, in Bellevue Hospital from 1919 to 1921, and in Babies' Hospital from 1921 to 1922. Serving in Babies' Hospital with Craig were Rustin McIntosh, later professor of pediatrics at Columbia University College of Physicians and Surgeons, and L. Emmet Holt, Jr., now professor of pediatrics at New York University School of Medicine and Director of the Pediatric Service at Bellevue Hospital. Craig himself was appointed

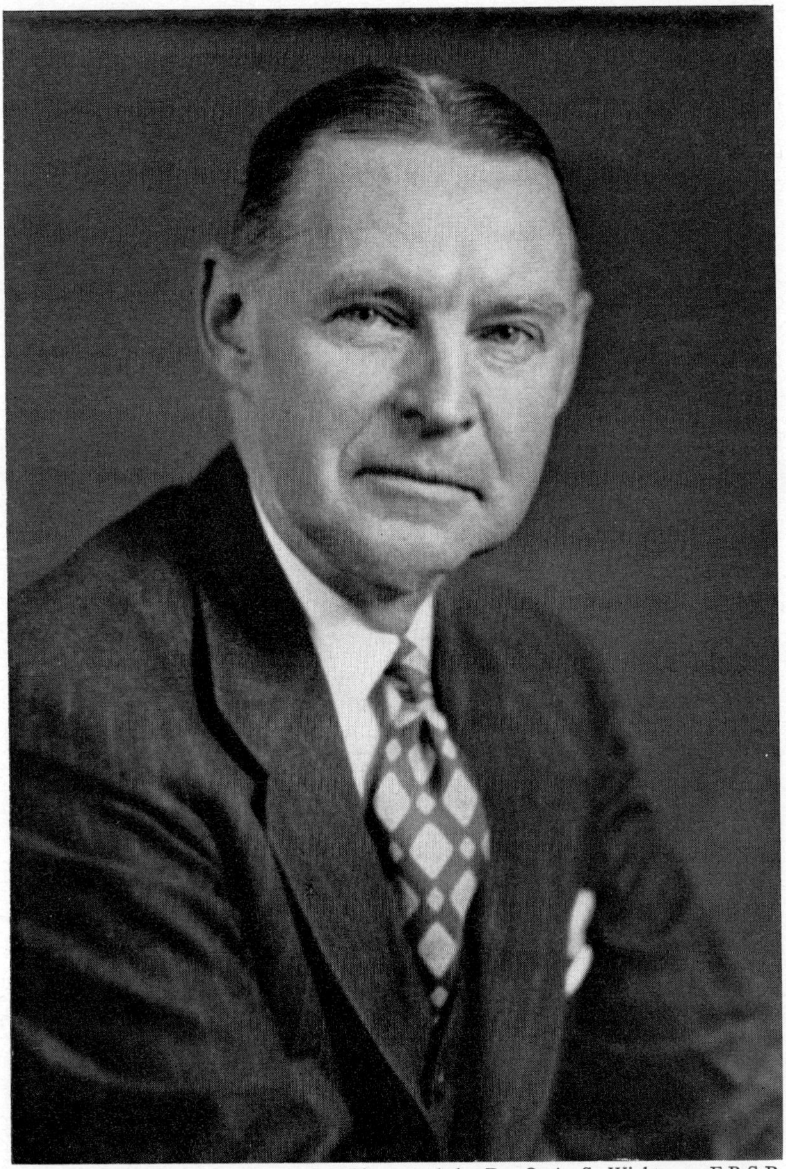

Photograph by Dr. Orrin S. Wightman, F.R.S.P.

HOWARD REID CRAIG

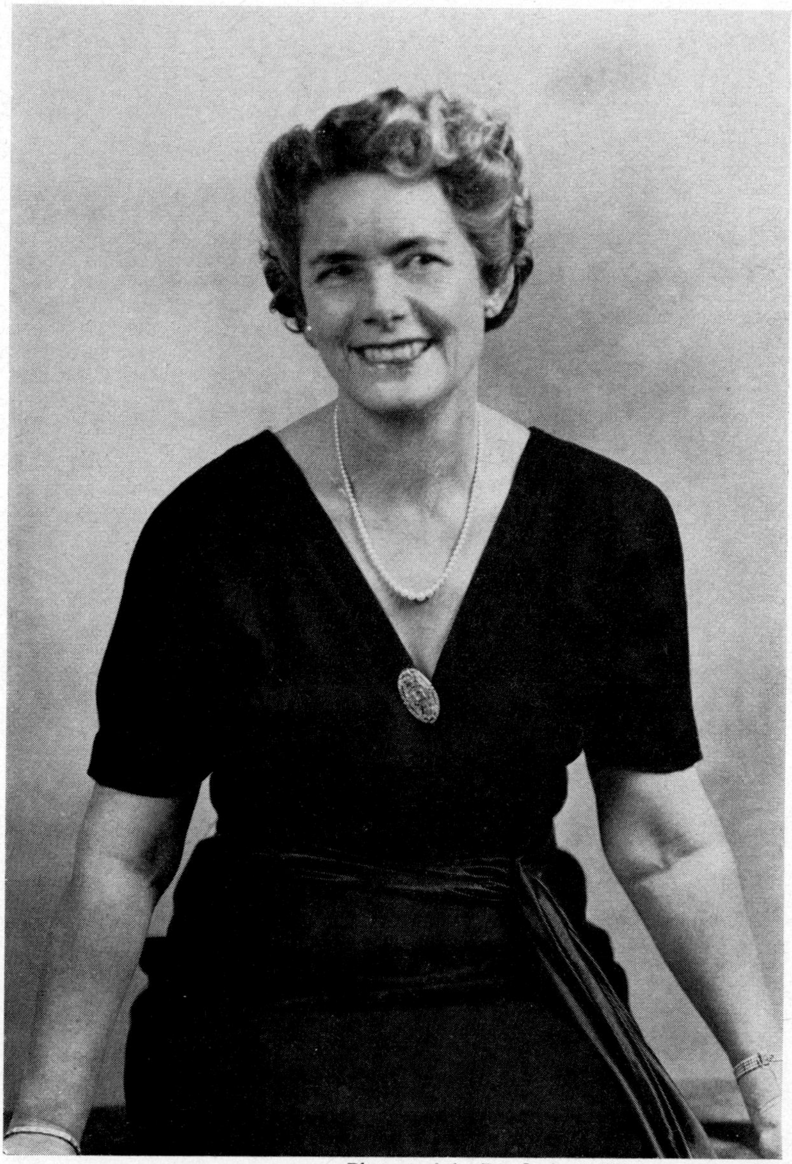

Photograph by Dr. Orrin S. Wightman, F.R.S.P.

AGNES BROWARD CRAIG

associate visiting pediatrician at Babies' and became an associate in pediatrics at the College of Physicians and Surgeons.

In 1922 Craig left academic medicine and entered, as an associate, the office of Dr. Charles Gilmore Kerley, a practicing pediatrician in New York City who had a large following. After remaining with Dr. Kerley for 2 years he opened an office of his own and soon built up a busy practice. In the meantime, he had been courting the charming Agnes Broward, and in 1925 they were married. Their two sons have made successful careers for themselves but showed no inclination to follow in the footsteps of their father.

Dr. Herbert B. Wilcox, who had been Craig's chief at Babies' Hospital, assumed the position of Director of The New York Academy of Medicine after retiring from the chair of pediatrics at the College of Physicians and Surgeons. He knew Howard well and, recognizing his abilities, urged him to become his successor as Director of the Academy.

Howard was then 52 years of age. He had suffered from arthritis for a number of years and the practice of pediatrics made many demands that aggravated the symptoms of this condition. So, in 1946, he took the full-time job that was to occupy him for the next 20 years—a longer term than was completed by any of his predecessors. After a short period in office the arthritis began to ameliorate and eventually disappeared. Perhaps the quieter and more regular life at the Academy played a part in the cure. But Agnes Craig confidently attributes it to the use of her "witches brew," consisting of a combination of lemon, orange, and grapefruit juice, to which she added flowers of sulphur!

Under Craig's tenure of office, the Academy grew in stature and in influence, both local and national and, indeed, international. It became apparent that he was, in every sense of the word, *The Director*. But he also took an active part in many outside activities, of which two may be mentioned as examples. He formed a close relationship between the Academy and the Royal Society of Medicine of London, England. He was the moving spirit in the formation of the Medical Library Center of New York—a depository for little-used medical and other scientific books and pamphlets. The establishment of this type of service has proved to be a boon not only to the Academy but also to the five medical schools in New York City, to the Rockefeller University, and to the Sloan-Kettering Institute. These organizations are partners in the enterprise.

In 1956, following much discussion and deliberation, a Committee of Fellows was appointed to study the Academy's then current status and activities, with respect to future needs and direction of growth, and to make specific recommendations leading to improvement in organization. No exhaustive self-examination had been undertaken since the Academy was founded in 1847. In due time, with the help of a firm of management consultants, an extensive report was issued. As a result of the study many basic changes in organization and practice were made.

Dr. Craig has been much in demand as a consultant in many fields —public health, hospital administration, and research. A fuller account of some of these activities will be given, no doubt, in the tributes of the Academy's executive secretaries, which follow. His retirement will not be complete; he has agreed to serve as consultant to the Academy, on a part-time basis, for 2 years. His familiarity with its affairs will be of great help to his successor and to the Trustees and the Council.

Many honors have been bestowed upon Dr. Craig. Two are worthy of special mention. He is an Honorary Fellow of the Royal Society of Medicine of London and an Honorary Fellow of the National Academy of Medicine of Peru, which awarded him its Gold Medal.

In his "Ode on Solitude," Alexander Pope, an author often quoted but seldom read, devoted two verses to a description of the pleasures of retirement. His sentiments, tersely expressed, seem pertinent to the present situation.

Blest, who can unconcern'dly find
  Hours, days, and years slide soft away,
In health of body, peace of mind,
  Quiet by day.

Sound sleep by night, study and ease,
  Together mixt; sweet recreation;
And Innocence, which most does please
  With meditation.

Pope has been accused more than once of insincerity in his praise of retirement and content. But certainly, Howard Craig will find it possible to formulate a balanced program, in which recreation and meditation, to which may be added a modicum of work, are combined in pleasing proportions. Above all, leisure will afford more time to spend with his devoted family.

# HOWARD REID CRAIG

*A Contribution by*

JOHN L. MADDEN

President
The New York Academy of Medicine
New York, N. Y.

"I DARE do all that may become a man; who dares do more is none." This quotation from Shakespeare exemplifies well the character of Howard Reid Craig, retiring Director of The New York Academy of Medicine.

During the past 2 years as President of the Academy, I have been privileged to be closely associated with Howard Craig in the many and varied activities sponsored by the Academy. It has been most fortunate for me that my term of office coincided with the final 2 of Howard's 20 years of nonpareiled, unselfish, and devoted leadership. This relatively short period of close association has proved a veritable postgraduate course in professional medical administration and human relations. It has been a most profitable experience that I shall always cherish.

What manner of man is Howard Reid Craig? Admittedly this is a most difficult question to answer. I attempt to do so by saying that he is a book. I say that because of his apparent unfathomable depth of knowledge in the many fields of endeavor that are variously related to medicine. He has proved himself a superb administrator, as indicated by the progressive leadership that he has engendered during his tenure of office. He has been gifted with enviable foresight with which he has created progress rather than being stimulated by it. A natural by-product of this talent has been the wisdom to surround himself with the most capable professional personnel available. The selection of each individual member of the team, so to speak, has been on his proved and potential meritorious service. The expertness of his choice is clearly in evidence by a perusal of his administrative staff. His one goal has been the pursuit of excellence, which has gained for The New York Academy of Medicine the respect of the medical profession not only of the local community but of the nation and, yes, of the world at large.

It would be considered a normal reaction for a person who is retiring to ease the burden of work gradually. In relation to Howard Craig the opposite obtains. In fact, it appears to me that his work load has increased rather than lessened. He has organized a committee that has been placed under the aegis of Dr. Robert Levy, a past president of the Academy, to work out plans forthwith relative to an expanded building program for the long-term future needs of the Academy. Similarly, he has been a one-man spearhead in the attempt to unify the seven medical schools within the metropolitan area in their conformity to the various regulatory legislative medical bills enacted by the recent Congress. Despite these and other myriads of activities, the majority being self-propelled, Howard Craig has remained the man—pleasant, efficient, calm, humble, cooperative, and always with the helpful hand extended.

I mentioned previously that our retiring Director of the Academy was a book, and I hastily add that he *is* a book. I personally should consider it a real travesty if Howard were not prevailed upon and duly commissioned to write a book on The New York Academy of Medicine, since a book is long past due, and since no one is better equipped than he to do the job. One may argue that this might prove a Herculean task, but knowing the prospective author and his innate abilities, I am confident that it would prove a labor of love, and a treasure for posterity. My one ardent hope is that this suggested project will come to fruition in the immediate future.

In the retirement of Howard Reid Craig as Director of The New York Academy of Medicine after 20 full years of faithful and devoted service, our sadness is gladdened by the fact that he will remain as a consultant. Accordingly, his wise and mature counsel will be ever available while, hopefully, he is writing *that book*. The close association of Dr. Craig and his most worthy successor, Dr. James E. McCormack, augurs well for the continued preeminence of The New York Academy of Medicine in the years ahead.

In my closing paragraph, I should like to repeat a timeworn phrase, that "behind the success of every man, is an understanding woman." This applies in particular to Howard's good wife, Agnes. My sincere best to them both as well as their two sons, Howard Reid Craig, Jr., and D. Broward Craig and their respective families.

# THE COMMITTEE ON PUBLIC HEALTH: 1946 TO THE PRESENT

H. D. Kruse

Executive Secretary

L. J. Amster

Executive Assistant

Committee on Public Health, The New York Academy of Medicine

If one were looking for an appropriate symbol for the committee on Public Health, he would do well to consider Janus, the god who could see both the past and the future, and the patron of beginnings and endings.

Again and again, throughout the 55 years of its history, the Committee has demonstrated an unique ability to keep both the past and the future in sight even as it continues to devote its undivided attention to problems immediately within its purview.

The genesis of the Committee has been described elsewhere. It came into being in 1911 at the urgent request of the Bureau of Municipal Research, a voluntary agency engaged in studying the problems of the New York City government. At the outset—and for sometime thereafter—the Committee was concerned mainly with such matters as sanitary engineering, control of epidemics, and the budgetary needs of the various departments of the city government that relate to health and hospitals.

Physicians chosen to serve on the Committee were selected then—as now—from the various medical disciplines, but all shared a common and deep-going interest in protecting and improving the public health.

In the course of its history, the Committee's roster has carried the names of many physicians who were or became outstanding leaders in the field of public health, notably: Drs. Hermann M. Biggs, S. S. Goldwater, Haven Emerson, and Harry S. Mustard. In addition, the Committee has enjoyed the distinction of counting among its members a Nobel Laureate, Dr. Dickinson W. Richards, whose work in medicine and physiology won him an award in 1956.

The first chairman of the Committee was Dr. Charles L. Dana. He served for 17 years and was succeeded by Dr. James Alexander Miller, who was chairman from 1929 till 1936, and again from 1942 till 1948. During the interim, the chairman was Dr. George Baehr, who served from 1937 till 1941, and again from 1949 till 1953.

Dr. Baehr was succeeded by Dr. Harry S. Mustard, who served for one year before leaving New York on his retirement as Executive Director of the State Charities Aid Association. The next chairman was Dr. Frederick R. Bailey. He was followed in the office by Dr. Milton J. Goodfriend, who served from 1959 till 1963, when Dr. Bailey was returned to the office. One year later, Dr. Bailey was obliged to resign because of the mounting pressure of his other professional obligations. He was succeeded by Dr. Arthur A. Fischl, the present incumbent.

Long tenure is also a characteristic of the office of Executive Secretary. Dr. Edward H. L. Corwin served in the post for 41 years—from 1911 till his retirement. Dr. H. D. Kruse has been the Executive Secretary since 1952.

With the passage of time, the size of the Committee has grown in order to keep pace with its burgeoning interests. Originally it had 15 members. Currrently it may have as many as 40 members.

A number of the responsibilities set down in the original charge to the Committee on Public Health no longer require its attention—in some instances as a direct consequence of the Committee's efforts. The development of the city's own health and hospital departments, the growth of the U.S. Public Health Service, the World Health Organization, and the proliferation of voluntary health agencies has obviated the need for the Committee to concern itself with matters that formerly engaged its interest.

The objectives and responsibilities of the Committee on Public Health are set forth in the by-laws of The New York Academy of Medicine:

It (the Committee) shall take cognizance of all matters relating to the public health of the community and of any or all matters relating to public or private provision for the care of the sick and policies connected therewith. (In this connection, it should be noted, the Committee is called on frequently to speak for The New York Academy of Medicine.)

It (the Committee) shall keep itself informed on legislation—national, state, and local—that may affect health, the provision for the sick, and the practice of medicine.

An inscription in Latin on the lintel over one of the windows of the Academy building reads: "It is a hard task to give freshness to the old and authority to the new." The record shows that the Committee has tried consistently to direct its energies to the accomplishment of that task.

In 1946 the Committee marked its 35th anniversary in an atmosphere conditioned by the scientific explosion that followed World War II. An earth-shaking volume of new scientific knowledge and new scientific concepts burst upon the world. This had a tremendous effect on every aspect of medicine, including public health. Along with ever greater possibilities, the scientific explosion brought equally great responsibilities.

It was at that point in its history that the Committee joined the entire Fellowship of The New York Academy of Medicine in welcoming the new Director, Dr. Howard Reid Craig. Almost immediately on assuming his new post, Dr. Craig entered into close collaboration with the Committee on Public Health. His interest in the day-to-day work of the Committee and his numerous contributions to the deliberations of various subcommittees have been invaluable.

The first significant collaboration between Dr. Craig and the Committee concerned the planning for the celebration of the Academy's centennial. This event, which took place in 1947, was highlighted by two very successful programs under the Committee's sponsorship—one on public health, the other on hospitals. Each of the programs was carried out in the context of a 3-day institute. It is characteristic of the Committee's approach that in both programs the focus was on future developments rather than on the past.

However, the Committee did not limit its activity in 1946 to the planning for the centennial. In a report summarizing the Committee's work during that year, there are references in more or less detail to 17 topics and slighter references to 20 other topics.

It is interesting, from the present perspective, to see what subjects engaged the Committee's attention 20 years ago. Among them were: alcoholism; birth control; care of laboratory animals; the shortage of nurses; the procurement, distribution, and utilization of human blood; misuse of barbiturates; and aid for the physically handicapped.

Some of these subjects have a familiar ring. Indeed, it is not surprising to find the incumbent Executive Secretary of the Committee noting, as he did recently, that: "For the Committee, each year is a time of both sowing and reaping. . . . Furthermore, as often as not, the harvest does not come in the same calendar year as the sowing. Sometimes there is a lag of many years before the Committee may see that its views are beginning to prevail. . . ."

The past year, for example, provided a bountiful harvest for the Committee. Several of these developments were the culmination of 35 to 40 years of effort by the Committee.

Forty years ago, the Committee on Public Health evinced deep concern about the problem of drug addiction. It pointed out that the punitive attitude that characterized the approach of the Federal Bureau of Narcotics was self-defeating. The Committee noted particularly that withdrawal was only the first of many steps in the treatment of the disease, that psychiatric care and environmental factors were essential in dealing with the problem.

In 1951 and again in 1952, the Committee sponsored several conferences on drug addiction among adolescents, a problem that was growing to considerable proportions. In 1955, the Committee issued its first report on drug addiction and presented a comprehensive program to deal with the problem. In fact, the Committee was the first medical body in the country to develop such a program and stood alone for many years in advocating the position that the addict is a sick person and that addiction is a disease. Because several of the key recommendations it made were misinterpreted, the Committee issued a second report on drug addiction in 1963. But confusion and misinterpretation still persisted, and the Committee was prompted to issue a third report in 1965.

Now, after 40 years, the Committee can see signs of a serious effort to control the drug addiction epidemic. Both federal and state officials have shown a sincere desire to grapple with the problem. At the local level, more facilities are being made available and more addicts are under treatment. New York State and California, two states with large addict populations, are attempting to implement programs that seek to place all addicts under medical supervision.

The Committee has recorded another achievement in the area involving the misuse and abuse of barbiturates. It became concerned as far back as 1920 over the increasing illicit trade, accidental deaths, and near-deaths associated with these drugs. Repeatedly—in 1929, 1943, 1956

—the Committee recommended stricter control of the distribution and retail sale of barbiturates by tighter state and local laws. Such laws were enacted.

Then, in 1964, the Committee noted three adverse developments. Two other therapeutic agents, tranquilizers and amphetamines—as well as barbiturates—were being misused on a large scale. In a major report on the subject, the Committee stressed the need for federal legislation to control the distribution of these drugs every step of the way from the producer to the consumer.

Federal legislation designed to control distribution of stimulating and depressant drugs from the manufacturer to the retail drug store was enacted in 1965.

In 1946 the Committee studied for the second time the problems involved in the operation of birth-control clinics in New York City. Having previously recommended the continuation of contraceptive clinics already in existence, the 1946 report urged recognition of medically indicated contraception as an integral part of preventive medicine. Eighteen years later, the Committee was requested by the Commissioner of Hospitals to submit a statement specifying the medical indications for contraceptive counseling. The pronouncements in this document have become the authoritative guide in municipal hospitals and are used also in other areas. In the past year, the governor of New York State signed a bill revising the State Penal Code to permit the sale, distribution, and possession of contraceptive articles to persons over 16 years of age.

The Committee had been in existence 8 years when it began its fight against venereal disease. In 1923, it recommended that a Wassermann test be obligatory in every obstetrical case. For many years, the Committee sponsored a session on venereal disease at the Annual Social Hygiene Conference. It had an active and continuing concern with the problem.

In 1964, the nation again experienced a resurgence of venereal disease. The U.S. Public Health Service mounted a major campaign to combat the spread of venereal disease. A program based on epidemiological principles was instituted. Organized teams of trained workers were sent out to interview contacts and arrange for testing them. However, the workers reported two insurmountable obstacles. About 80 per cent of the cases were seen initially by private practitioners. Many of these cases were not reported and, in too many instances, the physicians did not permit their patients to be interviewed.

In its study of the problem the Committee noted that it was ironic that an epidemic was raging for which there was effective treatment. The difficulty lay in finding the infected persons early enough to give them treatment and so stop the spread of disease.

A key to the problem, the report observed, was the private practitioner. His lack of cooperation, the Committee suggested, could block effectively any efforts to control the spread of the disease. The private physician, the Committee stated, has a paramount responsibility to public health that transcends all other considerations. This report provided the main theme at a subsequent national conference sponsored by the Venereal Disease Branch of the U.S. Public Health Service.

But the cooperation of the private practitioner was not sufficient by itself, the Committee soon realized. If the campaign to eradicate venereal disease by 1972—a goal set by the Public Health Service—were to be achieved, it would be necessary to make the public aware of the epidemic and to enlist its support.

Thus, the Committee thought it essential to prepare a second report on venereal disease in which it urged an intensive program designed to carry the message throughout the country. The effectiveness of the second report became apparent quickly when the Committee began to receive requests for the document from every section of the nation. Soon the campaign derived added stimulus as the various media of information began to carry the story of the war against venereal disease.

In studying the resurgence of venereal disease, the Committee noted that the problem involved a large element of homosexuality. This problem, viewed in conjunction with spiraling illegitimacy, perinatal mortality, and the vast commerce in salacious literature, induced the Committee to explore the matter of health education.

On the basis of the evidence it assembled, the Committee concluded that health education is in a sorry state in our country, despite the nation's admitted superiority in technics of mass communication.

The report on health education is one of the most sought-after documents ever published by the Committee. Health educators, public health professionals, and many others have shown great interest in and general agreement with the Committee's findings and recommendations for upgrading health education throughout the nation.

The *Bulletin of The New York Academy of Medicine* for July 1966 published a major report by the Committee on Public Health on the subject of air pollution and health. This report is perhaps the most comprehensive treatment ever accorded the subject. But it is not the first time the Committee has considered the problem. For, incredible as it may seem, the Committee's earliest work on air pollution goes back 40 years. In 1926, the Committee published the findings of a 6-year study of the concentration of carbon monoxide in various parts of the city under different climatic conditions. The report suggested that some means should be found to convert carbon monoxide to carbon dioxide.

Five years later, the Committee issued a second report describing various pollutants and their sources and pointed out how these substances were injurious to health.

In 1948 a serious episode of air pollution in Donora, Pa., claimed 20 lives and caused severe illness among 43 per cent of the inhabitants of the surrounding area. This episode called attention to the hazards of air pollution and stimulated the New York City Council to propose a Bureau of Smoke Control in the Department of Housing and Buildings. The Committee on Public Health supported this move, so far as it concerned smoke alone, but urged that the Department of Health retain its authority to deal with noxious fumes. The city government accepted the recommendation, but difficulties encountered in setting up the administrative organization prompted the establishment in 1952 of an independent Department of Air Pollution Control. Dr. Leonard Greenburg, a physician, was appointed Commissioner of Air Pollution Control.

The Committee made another investigation of the enigma of air pollution in 1958 at the request of Governor W. Averell Harriman. In its report the Committee urged that in view of the vagueness of current knowledge of health effects, it was necessary to carry a full-scale program of research to determine the precise relationship between air pollution and cardiopulmonary diseases.

The Committee's latest report on Air Pollution and Health forms an important section of the omnibus report prepared by the special task force created by Mayor John V. Lindsay.

Another aspect of community health that the Committee has studied for a long time involves the problems surrounding the clinical testing of drugs to determine their efficacy and safety. In 1962 the Committee studied the problems in considerable depth, reviewed the literature, interviewed clinical investigators, pharmacologists, drug manufacturers, and others in the field. Since that time it has made several efforts to gain acceptance for an entire series of recommendations designed to improve the quality of clinical testing.

In view of its long history of concern with blood supply for transfusion purposes, the Committee often has been asked to advise on problems incidental to this matter. In 1948 the Committee lent its influence to bring about the establishment of transfusion clinics in city hospitals for patients with Mediterranean anemia and sickle cell anemia. From time to time, also, the City Department of Health asked advice about the control of blood donors and blood banks. In 1954 the Department of Health made a thorough revision of the Sanitary Code section on blood and plasma banks. The Committee scrutinized this document carefully and made several suggestions for clarification and safety measures.

In 1956 many blood banks had been established, both in hospitals and as independent agencies. But there was no organized relationship among them. Reports indicated many deficiencies and irregularities. A group of agencies, acting as an ad hoc committee, asked the Committee on Public Health to make an exhaustive survey and to offer recommendations for improvement in all phases of blood handling.

The final report, prepared under the direction of Dr. H. D. Kruse, Executive Secretary of the Committee, was published in 1958. It contained 60 recommendations highlighting the basic needs that had to be met in order to overhaul the entire operation of blood handling in the city.

Within a year, the Community Blood Council was established with a membership comprising almost all the agencies handling or using blood, and work was begun on carrying out the other recommendations.

For many years the Committee had been critical of the ruling that gave the New York State Department of Welfare jurisdiction over hospitals. It was the Committee's view that whatever justification there may have been once for this assignment of power, this was no longer the case. Two developments pointed up the pressing need of bringing the hospitals under control of the Health Department of the State: hospitals have been used to greater purpose in the past decade; and there appeared the prospect that hospitals would be used even more in the immediate future in line with benefits provided by the recent federal legislation.

Thus, the Committee urged that the authority over hospitals be transferred from the State Welfare to the Health Department. Finally, in 1965, the State Legislature enacted a law effectuating this change of authority.

The Committee on Public Health pioneered in the area of alcoholism. In cooperation with the Research Council on Problems of Alcohol, the Committee conducted a survey of treatment facilities in New York City that was completed in 1946.

The gist of the information assembled was that there was no organized effort to deal constructively with this social blight. In an independent report the Committee on Public Health recommended multiple approaches that could be carried out as conditions permitted.

In 1947 the Committee joined with the Research Council to sponsor a conference at The New York Academy of Medicine, which led to the development of a comprehensive program designed to deal with the problem of alcoholism and the alcoholic.

In the following year, the Committee arranged a conference aimed at reconciling divergent views of the several groups interested in doing something constructive about alcoholism. In 1952 the New York State Legislature enacted a law along the lines recommended by the Committee and the Association of the Bar of New York City. Under this law, alcoholism was made a primary responsibility of the State Mental Commission. A small sum of money was set aside to establish a clinic in Syracuse and another in the Home Term Court in New York City. But these two clinics were discontinued after a brief time.

Two years later, when the program on alcoholism appeared to be lagging, the State Mental Health Commission asked the Committee on Public Health to organize a conference in order to find a new approach to alcoholism as a medical problem. Directed specifically toward physicians, the conference brought together four different views on the causation of alcoholism: the organic, the psychodynamic, the behavioristic, and the sociologic.

In 1959 the Interdepartmental Health Resources Board of New York State, which held primary responsibility for the state's program on alcoholism, reviewed the state's progress toward amelioration of this problem. It was noted that many of the operations in force at that time reflected the recommendations made by the Committee on Public Health in its early reports.

A signal contribution by the Interdepartmental Health Resources Board to education on alcoholism was a booklet, *Problem Drinking and Alcoholism*, edited by Dr. H. D. Kruse, the Committee's Executive Secretary. The booklet was published in 1957 under the auspices of the Advisory Committee on Alcoholism of the Board.

More recently, the Committee undertook a study of the tortuous, labyrinthine issues in medical assistance to the aged. On one point, the Committee had no doubt: illness should not impoverish a person. It stressed the view that the ratio of medical cost to the person's resources should be the proper basis for determining eligibility under the law. The fact that the newly enacted Title 19 reflects this formula is a source of great satisfaction to the Committee.

Also, the Committee cautioned against neglecting the provisions of the Kerr-Mills Law in the midst of the enthusiasm over the proposed Medicare legislation. It pointed out that any realistic Medicare program was unlikely to provide unlimited benefits. Hence, when benefits under the new law were exhausted, Kerr-Mills would be available to serve as a backstop. That its view in this connection is being noted is a further source of pleasure to the Committee.

It has been observed that there is nothing so powerful as an idea whose time has come. From this point of view, an important lesson may be drawn from the Committee's experience during the past two decades: achievement often is a matter of perseverance.

The realization that the end of one year also marks the beginning of another obliges one to think of what lies ahead. All the signs point to a period of unprecedented challenge and opportunity in the coming years. Certainly, there is no dearth of problems awaiting the Committee's attention.

In looking back over the past—more particularly the past 20 years—the Committee on Public Health is mindful of the work shared and the goals achieved during Dr. Craig's tenure as Director of the Academy. At the same time that it salutes Dr. Craig, the Committee looks ahead to the future with confidence that it will continue to serve effectively in improving the community health.

# "OUR GREATEST MATERIAL HERITAGE"

## THE LIBRARY
## 1946-1966

GERTRUDE L. ANNAN

Librarian, The New York Academy of Medicine
New York, N. Y.

In these words Dr. Craig referred to the Library in 1956: "It is my conviction that regardless of demand or operational problems or cost or competition, the Library, as our greatest material heritage and treasure, must be maintained at full strength and full effectiveness." Such a view expressed by the Director of the Academy assured the vigorous support necessary to maintain the Library during his administration, a period critical in the survival of medical society libraries and in the burgeoning demands of the scientific community.

When Dr. Craig assumed office in late 1946 on the eve of the Academy's centenary, the Library had been under the skilled and scholarly direction of Dr. Archibald Malloch for more than 20 years. Under his guidance the Library moved from dingy quarters in the old building to the magnificence of the new, and was transformed from a poorly staffed collection to a departmentalized modern library operation with a well-trained corps of librarians. Dr. Malloch's illness in 1948 led to his resignation in 1949, and his place was taken by Janet Doe, who had long served with distinction as Assistant Librarian. Her high purposes are clearly reflected in the annual report of 1950, and deserve a wide audience in 1966 as well. "The possession of an outstanding accumulation of the scientific literature brings with it a certain moral obligation to see that its resources are accessible to all who need them. It has extended its general services as far as seems justifiable on a free basis; it has developed various special services, most of them free, but some unavoidably on a paid non-profit basis. Further, it has believed wholeheartedly in the practice of mutual help among libraries as the surest way to advance the interests of all. By assistance to and from each other, the ability of all libraries to give better service has been increased."

## Services

In this same report is an account of a survey made of the collection and the effectiveness of its services. It is of particular interest to read that: "Its lending services are, and are intended to be, of minor importance, being restricted to Fellows, Subscribers, and non-profit libraries outside New York City; its prime function is the provision of literature for reference within its walls where readers who come there can reasonably expect to find it." Yet such was the dramatic change in the use of the Library that in only 2 years the annual report indicates a new trend already revolutionizing the functions of the Library. In the Library report for 1951-1952, we find that "The great expansion of our photoduplication work in recent years has made much more correspondence necessary. The output of photostats is sevenfold what it was in 1931, entailing, in addition to seven times the labor of mechanical reproduction, seven times as much work by the reference assistants in getting out the material and in identifying the incorrect references. This large increase is undoubtedly one of the explanations for the fewer number of readers today: an article is now read in photostat or microfilm at the office or laboratory instead of our reading-rooms and perhaps by a number of individuals. . . . Another cause of fewer readers has been the tenfold increase in the number of library subscribers: 22 in 1931 have become 244 in 1951. Many of these send messengers to borrow books instead of coming in person, and thus no reader registers. Further, the much greater number of telephone calls probably means that inquirers have found it simpler and quicker to get their information that way."

Another reason cited was the improvement in the smaller medical libraries. "This does not mean that the need for the Academy's resources is lessening; rather it indicates a change in emphasis. A constantly higher proportion of out-of-the-way material is sought here."

This new trend, however, had more significance than was realized, for it represented a change in library use that would intensify in the years ahead. Photocopy requests have more than tripled; interlibrary loans have soared nearly 10 times. The busy physican and scientist prefers to have the literature brought to him in his office, hospital, school, or laboratory. Improvement in the smaller libraries has brought more requests for the literature, not less, and funds available for research and education have meant the establishment of many new libraries with the resultant increase in demands upon the resources of the established ones.

Funds pouring into these facilities have rarely provided enough for library support, and the strain is felt in all our institutions. Telephone requests, too, reflect the need for time-saving methods, and they emphasize the use of the Library staff in serving those not coming in person. Furthermore, teletype and telefacsimile systems will soon greatly facilitate and increase the transmission of our materials. In 1964 interlibrary loans went from here to 40 states and Canada, with the heaviest use in New York State, where a total of 7,460 items were sent to other libraries. New Jersey was second with 2,234. During the same year photocopy of our texts went to 39 states and 22 foreign countries. It is of interest to note that 70 per cent of the loans went to hospitals and medical schools, but the greatest users of photocopy were commercial firms, accounting for 62 per cent.

The readers who now come to the Library represent a changing order, too. In 1947 the largest group, 44 per cent, were physicians who were not Fellows. Today this figure has dropped to 17 per cent, explaining somewhat the increase in lending to other libraries. Happily, the percentage of Fellows has risen from a low 6 per cent in 1947 to 13 in 1963, with an additional 7 per cent of Fellows' representatives. A major increase has been in student use, students other than medical, nursing, or dental advancing from 7 to 21.5. As these young people will be the scientists of tomorrow, the Library's responsibility to the community covers all phases, and contributes substantially to education in both science and medicine, as well as to research and industry. The emphasis is service to this area, but through interlibrary loans and photocopy, its resources are shared with libraries throughout this country.

One service discontinued in this period was the Bibliographical Department, which for a fee compiled bibliographies, made translations from various languages, performed editorial chores, and carried on a current awareness service, citing each month references to articles on specified subjects appearing in the literature. Originally planned for the purpose of supplying Fellows and other physicians with services not elsewhere available, the department had become almost entirely a service for representatives of commercials firms, who could easily find free-lance workers expert in filling these needs. It seemed prudent to abolish the department and maintain a file with names of translators, bibliographers, editorial assistants, typists, and others skilled in preparing manuscripts for publication, so that any required help could be obtained.

For a time the current references service continued, but the obvious handicap of delaying current foreign journals from reaching the shelves for our readers' use led to its discontinuation in 1957. Today commercial firms use data-processing techniques for extremely effective current awareness programs of their own.

## Building Facilities

The Academy does not want a static library, but the frightening proliferation of publications has caused acute and painful space problems for all dynamic collections. In 1953 several additions were made to the Library to ease the situation. A balcony built in the Current Periodicals' Reading Room was designed to fit well into the decor and provide desperately required working space for the staff of that department. Stacks were installed on five floors at the eastern end of the building, formerly used for the museum and other purposes. One floor was also made available for Library staff requirements. Of the five stack floors, one with a locked grill has meant that the Rare Book Room's overflowing additions could be safely housed. During the building of the area the staff worked hard in the old stacks, segregating the 18th-century volumes for the Rare Book Room's collection, the 19th-century volumes and those from 1901-1929 for the new stacks, and those published between 1930 and 1950 for the 9th floor of the old stacks. This left one whole floor for the more current monographic literature in the newly adopted classification of the National Library of Medicine. The purpose of the new shelving was to permit growth of the collection for 25 years, but such has been the outpouring of the world's presses that within 3 years it was evident that other means of expansion must be provided. Other libraries were facing this same problem, and in 1957 the Library Committee invited several New York medical librarians to discuss the possibility of a cooperative venture. In March 1958 a meeting was held at the Academy of administrators and librarians. As a result, in January 1964, the Medical Library Center of New York came into being with Dr. Craig as the Chairman of the Board. Dr. Craig spared no effort in raising funds for the establishment of this important service. Already the Library has cleared its shelves of 1600 bound volumes and 100,000 foreign theses, and our crowded stacks are once more in reasonable order. The volumes sent to the Center mean no loss to the Academy's research collection, as they are chiefly runs of journals of pharmacy, nursing, or library science. Also, they and the theses are available on 24 hours' notice for use within the Library through the Center's delivery service, which daily stops at the participating libraries to pick up and deliver volumes going from one collection to another. In 1965, 14,000 volumes were carried.

The current reference collection, which must be easily available for both readers and staff, has far outgrown shelving convenient to the main area of use, a prime requisite for this material. New means of photo reproduction and data processing have brought a flood of important reference tools to shelves that cannot expand to accommodate them. Staff to process and service the collection has increased from 48 to 54 since 1947, with resultant crowding. The area containing the rare book and history of medicine collections became inadequate for both staff and volumes. Three additional small rooms on the mezzanine were requisitioned for staff, archives, and stack shelving. Valuable gifts and purchases of early material added to the many histories, and important reference tools overflowed the limited space, so that weeding was necessary to transfer many to other quarters, especially to the locked stack floor assigned to the department. Filling some of this stack area were boxes of museum materials packed away when the museum was turned to other purposes. The advent of the Medical Library Center temporarily solved this particular problem, for the transfer of foreign theses released a basement room that now houses this interesting collection. Unfortunately, the lack of a display area or a curator to make this a vital instrument in the study of the history of medicine greatly curtails its use and discourages important donations.

## Collections

The effectiveness of a library cannot be judged solely by the size of its collections, but yearly additions do indicate somewhat the vigor of continuing operations. Despite a policy of regular weeding of inappropriate materials, the Library has developed in 20 years from 252,000 bound volumes and 149,000 pamphlets to 360,000 bound volumes and 165,000 pamphlets. In 1946, 1,652 journals were received regularly and, in 1965, 4,330. This seemingly substantial increase does not reflect in any way a maintenance of the same percentage of the published literature, for the number of journals published throughout the world in the postwar years has proliferated at an alarming rate. More alarming, however, is the staggering proliferation in subscription costs. Today the Library, vainly endeavoring to stay within its budget, must cautiously consider acquisitions that would have been automatically ordered a decade ago. In 1964, $13,000 above the budgeted amount was spent and, in 1965, $7,000. Curtailments have been made, but costs rise more quickly than predicted. Current subscriptions in 1946 came to only $4,629; in 1965 to $41,562. Such costs daunt the most generous library supporter. Yet it is especially necessary for a collection to maintain its important current journal subscriptions in an era when data processing has accelerated indexing in depth of an ever-growing number of journals. That the number of our journal subscriptions has not much more than doubled during a period when their cost has climbed tenfold makes the outlook for the future of some concern.

For the scientist the most recent literature is all-important, and efforts must be continued to acquire and process it as rapidly as possible, so that its dissemination may be prompt. Yet the value of a research library depends upon its total resources: current books, journals, indexes, reference tools, and also the literature of the past, ancient and more recent. The Academy Library has been fortunate in its builders, who have understood the need for preserving the material of medical history. Preeminent in understanding its value was the true "father" of the Library, Samuel Smith Purple, whose contributions did not fall within the time period of the last 20 years, but whose influence upon the growth and development of our collections still firmly prevails. Dr. Malloch, too, was a medical historian, and his untiring interest was responsible for the materialization in 1933 of the Rare Book Room that now bears his name.

The year 1946, the first of Dr. Craig's administration, saw also the inauguration of an association of enormous significance in the growth of our collections. Through the efforts of Dr. Alfred M. Hellman and Dr. Frederic D. Zeman, the Friends of the Rare Book Room was established, and it is no coincidence that in the years that followed, not only were gifts of value and importance acquired through the efforts of the Friends, but collections of richness and variety came in unprecedented numbers. These and other gifts purchased or inspired by the Friends have been well described in the little publication, *Academy Bookman*, which twice a year provides information about these exciting acquisitions and about the activities of the members of the Friends and the staff of the library.

The first president of the Friends was the late Dr. Fenwick Beekman, whose own splendid collection came to us several years later. Undoubtedly, as president of the New York Historical Society in 1948, his influence was felt in the decision by that Society to present to us, jointly with the Brooklyn Museum, the famous Edwin Smith surgical papyrus, one of the earliest texts known relating to medicine. The first issue of the *Academy Bookman* in the spring of 1948 appropriately begins with an article by Dr. Claude E. Heaton, "Samuel Smith Purple, 1822-1900," an account of one of our greatest benefactors written by another. Dr. Heaton served for 23 years on the Library Committee, and the issues of the *Bookman* list many treasured items from his collection. Many are of New York medical interest, the field in which Dr. Heaton made important contributions. Other names appear frequently as donors in these early issues: Dr. Hellman, whose magnificent copies showed his judgment as a bookman; Dr. Reginald Burbank, who collected books reflecting his own specialty of joint diseases; Mr. Arthur Houghton, generous and knowledgeable benefactor of many libraries; Mr. Lee Ash, editor, bookman and friend of all libraries. These and other individuals added appreciably to the gifts acquired through use of the funds the Friends annually make available to fill gaps on our shelves at a time when the ever more expensive and elusive material becomes available. Our modest budgetary funds would not permit continuing support for our outstanding collection. As readers of book-dealers' catalogs and auction records know, scientific literature has skyrocketed in price as more and more desirable copies are deposited in libraries with fewer coming again to the market. Our debt to all the members of the Friends is great, to those who have continued their financial support, to those who have served as officers, and to Dr. Hellman and Dr. Zeman who planned this valuable resource. Special mention should be made of Mrs. Hellman's annual donation in memory of her late husband.

Later issues of the *Bookman*, 1956-1965, show volumes from the Library of Dr. Karl Vogel of more than usual interest. In 1956 our collection of early contributions to naval medicine was greatly enriched by both major and out-of-the way books from his shelves. One of his most exciting and valuable treasures came in 1965, Benvenuto Cellini's *Autobiography*, first edition, 1728. The astonishing variety of collections offered to us from 1957 to 1965 have been described in "Embarrassment of Riches," 1965, this *Bulletin,* vol. 41, pp. 1117-24, so they need not be repeated here except to draw attention to their variety: the Neinken collection of public health broadsides, 16th to 19th centuries; the Robert L. Levy library of classics in cardiology; the Hunterian collection of Dr. Beekman with other outstanding texts indicating his wide interests; the Hayes Martin collection of medical prints; more than 200 signed photographs of medical friends of the late Paul B. Hoeber; the fine group of works by Francesco Redi and his scientific contemporaries assembled by Rufus Cole; the Treves bequest of pharmacy jars and silver; the albums containing medical stamps from Dr. Peter Denker. For the prospective museum of the future are promised exquisite manikins, including 22 Chinese doctor dolls, from Jerome P. Webster, and the William Shehadi collection of x-ray tubes. Abner I. Weisman's rich treasures of the pre-Columbian medical sculpture also await such a home.

One collection mentioned as a future donation as early as 1960 has now arrived, the Michael M. Davis library on economic and social aspects of medical care. Anyone studying the movements that led to Medicare must have recourse to this extraordinary material, which includes published and unpublished records of the most important development in health care in the United States.

## Archives

The importance of preserving an institution's own records has been particularly emphasized by industry and government, and today there are archivists trained in methods for caring for such materials. The Academy, stimulated long ago by the wisdom of Dr. Purple, is rich in the documents of its history. In 1957 a half-time position of archivist was authorized, and through the imaginative efforts of Bettina Thrall in that position records and information from all of the Academy's offices have been assembled and analyzed. Housed separately, but in overflowing quarters, the Archives require much more space for appropriate care. Archives of other organizations, particularly of local New York medical societies have come to the Library for safekeeping. Some national organizations have asked for permission to deposit their papers here; in one instance an international association. Such records are of prime historical interest, and in the future, when room is provided, a substantial archival program can be established. Already an informal group exists, the Medical Archivists of New York, whose purpose is to encourage local medical facilities to ensure the preservations of their records.

## Preservation

Concern has long been felt in libraries about the chances of survival of many volumes emanating from the 1860's to the present. Poor paper and the effects of storage in centrally heated rooms have resulted in crumbling leaves. In 1947, when Philip Van Ingen compiled the Academy's history, he had bound, at his own expense, the only known copies of some the Academy's official publications. Ten years later the leaves, pulled from the binding, were ready to crumble to dust on handling. Now, fortunately, treatment by the Barrow method of deacidification and lamination, has restored these same volumes so that they may be used without anxiety. The Library budget each year includes the sum of $1,000 for rehabilitation by this method, and items are carefully selected.

## Publications

By 1947 the History of Medicine series of the Library Publication Committee consisted of seven titles. No. 8, issued in 1949, was Dr. Van Ingen's centennial history of the Academy. In the next 10 years there were 4 additions to the series. Then new arrangements made with the Hafner Publishing Company of this city proved stimulating and fruitful. From the publication of the handsome 3-volume English edition of Morgagni, through 11 paperback facsimiles of classics and several hard-cover volumes, the series has now reached No. 29, with others in preparation. No. 27 is of particular interest, as it brings together the contributions by Fielding H. Garrison, originally published regularly in the Academy *Bulletin*, 1925-1935.

The *Academy Bookman*, previously mentioned, was brought into being through the interest of Frederic D. Zeman, who served as editor for its first decade. In 1956 a small brochure, *Your Library, What Every Fellow Should Know*, was compiled to ensure that Fellows are aware of their library privileges. A copy goes to each new Fellow.

## Library Committee

Library literature has many articles discussing the function and value of a library committee. Many are doubtful if such a committee is advantageous. In the minds of those who have been Librarians of the Academy there has been no such question. The minutes of this Committee over the years show informed and interested support of the Librarian in coping with the needs and problems of this ever expanding and costly department of the Academy. When Dr. Craig became Director of the Academy he had been on the Library Committee for several years and had been its chairman from 1942 to 1946. Claude Heaton was his successor, 1947-1950, and was followed by Samuel W. Lambert, Jr., 1951-1957, William C. White, 1958-1961, and Bronson S. Ray, 1962 to the present time. The Library has benefitted greatly from their guidance and the Librarians have had wholehearted appreciation of their continuing interest and active support. The Book Selection Subcommittee under Saul Jarcho's chairmanship is called upon often for judgment, especially in areas peripheral to medicine in this period of interdisciplinary orientation. Dr. Jarcho's 20 years on the committee and his readiness to respond to cries for assistance, have led to frequent dependence upon his knowedgeable advice. The Subcommittee on Administration has been long chaired by the Library's good friend, Samuel W. Lambert, Jr., who has patiently and vocally supported the Librarian's annual burden of the budget. The House Subcommittee, whose chairman is Hilton H. Stothers, is seldom called upon, but any building plans for the future will be under its guidance. A new subcommittee has the role of advising on matters relating to new mechanical aids and will be increasingly consulted. Edgar Bick, a former president of the Friends of Rare Book Room, is its chairman.

## Technical Progress

Perhaps the most satisfying progress is the elimination of backlogs. In each department discouraging piles of work waiting for attention clogged offices and shelves and threatened to overwhelm the staff. Extra help at times, and heroic action by the staff cleared the basement and made it a usable area. Extra funds and help brought up to date acquisitions files far too cumbersome for efficient management, and a reorganization of procedures was introduced to speed the receipt of current materials. A cataloger was added to the staff for the sole purpose of processing an accumulated backlog of thousands of volumes coming in various donations. Unbelievably, hundreds of bound pamphlet volumes from the New York Public Library piled on floors, tables, and shelves, gradually disappeared and were properly cared for by the new cataloger, Mrs. Helen Bayne Cherami, who went on to complete the cataloging of Dr. Beekman's Hunterian collection and to attack the mounting arrears of miscellaneous historical papers in the Rare Book Department.

To avoid the arduous typing of catalog cards and the necessary proofreading, an IBM system was installed capable of being adapted later to other functions. Its first use has been limited to typing cards and the monthly accessions list. Among new photocopying equipment acquired to answer the needs of our clientele is a new microfilm camera and a Polaroid camera that can supply color prints and transparencies as well as black and white photographs. A reader-printer makes it possible to get copy from small portions of films. The 914 Xerox gets the most constant usage and, hopefully, in the future the large and expensive Copyflo machine will be obtained to enable us to provide full-size copy from microfilms, easing the heavy use of Xerox.

## Technological Problems

Large budgetary increases for libraries in the past 20 years seldom represent realistic figures for development. Instead, no matter how generous, they are often a disappointing minimum necessary to cover expenses for another year without hope of expansion or maintenance on a desired level. If the Academy Library is to maintain its position as a resource collection, additional funds will be required. Government funds through the Medical Library Assistance Act should offer some assistance, but the needs are great and we must look to other sources for financial help. Acquisitions and staff needs predominate, and proper quarters to house both for effective service. The high cost of data processing must be considered. Prompt dissemination of information is a library's first responsibility, and should funds be supplied for free photocopying in lieu of interlibrary loans, the deluge will be immediate. A study under the direction of the Academy and funded by the Health Research Council of New York resulted in a provocative analysis, *Interlibrary Request and Loan Transactions among Medical Libraries of the Greater New York Area*, by Lee Ash and Vernon Bruette, New York, 1966. The heavy use of the Academy's collections reported here would have been very much greater were it not for our lending restrictions and high charges for photocopy. Expansion of this important service is impossible without similar expansion of staff and facilities. Obviously, for acquisitions, processing, and dissemination, a well-trained staff and efficient housing are essential.

These 20 years have seen vast changes in library practices and administration, and the Academy Library must adapt to them, so that the great collections brought together here during the past century will continue to attract the support needed for both maintenance and progress. Our "greatest material heritage" must have sustenance, as the next 20 years will show.

# THE BULLETIN OF THE NEW YORK ACADEMY OF MEDICINE 1847-1966

PAUL F. CRANEFIELD

Executive Secretary
Committee on Publications and Medical Information
The New York Academy of Medicine
New York, N. Y.

ONE of the first actions of The New York Academy of Medicine was to provide for publication of its proceedings in a periodical known as the *Transactions of The New York Academy of Medicine.*[1] The *Transactions* was mentioned in the original by-laws of the Academy, which were adopted at its first formal meeting on January 6, 1847. The Academy has published, with longer and shorter interruptions, either a *Transactions* or a *Bulletin* ever since. In all there were three publications prior to the present *Bulletin*, namely the *Transactions*, series 1; the *Bulletin*, series 1, and the *Transactions*, series 2. The present *Bulletin* (series 2) has been published monthly since 1925.

The general pattern of the founding and survival of medical periodicals in the earlier period of medicine in the United States is of some interest in relation to the history of the Academy's publications. Myrl Ebert, in her bibliography of early medical periodicals in the United States,[2] lists the *Transactions of The New York Academy of Medicine* as the 219th medical periodical to appear in the country (of these 219, none dates back into the colonial period). But of these 219 periodicals fewer than a dozen survive at the present time, so that the Academy's journal may be reckoned as among the 10 oldest medical periodicals in the United States. A few of the older periodicals were also the publications of societies, including the *Transactions of the College of Physicians of Philadelphia* and the *Proceedings of the Connecticut State Medical Society* (both of which survive today under different titles). Our oldest general medical publication is the *New England Journal of Medicine*, a periodical founded in 1812. *The American Journal of the Medical Sciences* is the continuation of a periodical founded in 1818. The Medical Society of the State of New York and the New York

County Medical Society began publication in periodical form as long ago as 1806. The journal most nearly the same age as the Academy's periodicals is *The American Journal of Psychiatry*, founded in 1844 as *The American Journal of Insanity*.

The Academy's publications have appeared in different series and somewhat irregularly; the longest interruption of publication was from 1901 to 1925. Each publication will be discussed in some detail below, but a quick survey of the whole series is of some interest. The initial publication, as already stated, was the *Transactions of The New York Academy of Medicine*, which appeared in three volumes. Although 1847 is always given as the date of the first part of the first volume, it appears that it was not actually printed until 1851. The last part of volume 3 appeared in 1872. The second periodical published by the Academy was not a successor to the *Transactions* but appeared parallel with it. That was the *Bulletin of The New York Academy of Medicine*, which appeared in four volumes, the first volume being published in parts from 1860 to 1862. The fourth volume appeared in 1872. This first *Bulletin* was succeeded by a new series of *Transactions*. The *Transactions of The New York Academy of Medicine*, second series, appeared in 13 volumes. Volume 1 was published in 1874, and volume 13 was published in parts during the years 1898-1901. The Academy's current publication, the *Bulletin of The New York Academy of Medicine*, second series, began publication with volume 1, No. 1, in March 1925. It is still in existence and has appeared monthly since that time, and is now in volume 43 (1967).

### *Transactions of The New York Academy of Medicine*, 1851-1872

We have seen that the Academy voted at its first meeting in 1847 to establish a means of publishing its proceedings. However it was not anticipated that a volume should be published until enough material accumulated to make it worthwhile and, in July 1850, the Committee on Publications was still waiting to have enough material to make a volume of 350 pages. In April 1851 it was decided to print all material on hand as volume 1, part 1; it actually appeared in June 1851. Its 165 pages foreshadowed the future of the Academy's publications in that they contained articles on the history of medicine, on public health, and on clinical medicine. The first article, Pliny Earle's "Historical Sketch of the Institutions for the Insane in the United States of America," remains to this day an important source of historical information. The second article represents one of the Academy's permanent and major interests: its concern with public health. The title of this paper by Augustus K. Gardner is "Report of a Committee Appointed by The Academy of Medicine upon the Comparative Value of Milk Formed from the Slop of Distilleries and Other Food." This report is most unsettling, and it makes us grateful for the progress we have made. The pressing problems of public health that surround us today at least do not include those of children fed on milk obtained from cows shut in stables and fed exclusively on distillery slops. Volume 1 of the *Transactions* concluded in 1857 with two long papers by Charles E. Isaacs that are of considerable importance in the history of our knowledge of the kidney. These papers are entitled "Researches into the Structure and Physiology of the Kidney" and "On the Function of the Malpighian Bodies of the Kidney." They are cited in the Garrison and Morton list of classic contributions to medicine (Nos. 1233 and 1234) with the following note: "Isaacs confirmed and corrected the findings of Bowman; he introduced dye experiments in the structure of the kidney, from which he drew the important conclusion that the Malpighian bodies are the most important agency in the secretion of urine."[3] The *Transactions* continued through its three-volume career as a place for the publication of long and important articles on clinical and scientific subjects. Many of these articles are of historical importance, and they still make interesting reading.

### *Bulletin of The New York Academy of Medicine*, 1860-1872

The *Transactions* was a distinguished publication, but it never managed to stay up to date. Long delays intervened between the delivery of papers at the Academy and their appearance in the *Transactions.* Moreover the *Transactions* was reserved for rather long formal papers and did not contain any account of the other proceedings of the Academy. It was therefore decided to initiate a second publication to bring out more ephemeral material and to provide for the more rapid publication of at least some of the formal papers delivered at the Academy. The first attempt at this sort of bulletin was the publication of the proceedings of the Academy in *The New York Journal of Medicine.* Two rather brief reports of Academy meetings appeared in that journal in 1860 but the Academy was not satisfied with this form of publication and founded its own *Bulletin.* The first 29 pages of the *Bulletin* reprinted the proceedings that had already appeared in *The New York Journal of Medicine.* This new *Bulletin* was very different from the *Transactions* and, when the first volume had been completed, a preface was affixed to it that included the following statement: "The *Bulletin of The New York Academy of Medicine* was established for the purpose of presenting to its members and to the profession at large, a record of its current proceedings and of the discussion at its meetings, and also to furnish a receptacle for papers not assigned a place in the *Transactions* of the Academy, the only previously recognized medium for their appearance." This paragraph exactly describes the contents of the *Bulletin.* Papers presented at the Academy were presented in summary, and a rather full report was given of the discussion after each paper. In addition a certain amount of Academy business was reported in the *Bulletin,* which also carried obituaries of Fellows of the Academy, in some cases including an account of their last illness and of the postmortem findings!

The *Bulletin* for 1865 records that on April 19 the Academy unanimously adopted the following resolution:

> *Whereas,* Our Nation has been bereaved by the sudden and violent death of its Chief Magistrate at the hands of an unprincipled assassin:
>
> *Resolved,* That in common with our fellow-citizens of every class, the members of this Academy mourn over the loss which our Country has sustained.
>
> *Resolved,* That we cherish with grateful hearts the memory of the virtuous life of our late President, and the remembrance of the distinguished services which he has rendered to the Nation in the trying times in which he was called to preside over our destinies.
>
> *Resolved,* That we regard with abhorrence the wicked and brutal violence which has deprived the country of his valuable services, and which has cast a gloom over every loyal house and heart thoroughout the land.

After some discussion the Academy decided not to send a copy of this resolution to the family of President Abraham Lincoln on the grounds that if all societies were to send such resolutions it would simply be a burden to the family to receive them. Dr. John Robert Vankleek then added: "This Nation mourns, as no Nation ever mourned before, and the occasion for, and the depth and universality of the grief has never before had a parallel in the history of the world! It is certain that no twenty millions of people were ever before swayed to such an extent by an emotion of grief springing as this did from a single source."

The *Bulletin* continued to appear in much its original style up to its demise in 1872. Fairly long papers were published occasionally without discussion but, in general, a rather short report of the main paper presented at any meeting was followed by a rather careful report of the discussion that followed it. In 1872 the first series of the *Transactions* and the first series of the *Bulletin* both came to an end. On the last page of the last volume of the *Bulletin* we find the following:

> With this number, the publication of the "Bulletin" of the N. Y. Academy of Medicine ceases, and, by a change in the By-laws, the work will henceforth be continued under the title of "Transactions." The Committee on Publication regret exceedingly the delay in the appearance of this number; but, from circumstances, it has been unavoidable. They hope in future, to issue the "Transactions" with greater punctuality.

Thus the first series of the *Transactions* and of the *Bulletin* came to an end, and the stage was set for a second series of *Transactions.*

*Transactions of The New York Academy of Medicine*, 1874-1901

In many respects the early volumes of the second series of the *Transactions* more nearly resembled the *Bulletin* than did the first series of *Transactions.* It continued to publish short reports of papers presented before the Academy and transcripts of the discussion of those papers. It also carried information about business transacted at Academy meetings. Like its predecessor, the second series of the *Transactions* was plagued by a great deal of irregularity in publication. For example, 5 years elapsed between the publication of the final part of volume 2 in 1876 and the publication of the first part of volume 3 in 1881. The *Transactions* seemed finally to get on a regular basis in 1890, and a volume appeared every year from 1890 to 1895. But the last volume, dated 1896-1901, represented not only a break in the regularity of publication but the end of the second series of the *Transactions.* The history of the Academy does not clearly show why these interruptions and delays occurred but it is obvious that the cost of publishing was a factor. Another factor, probably of great importance, was the fact that the editorial work and operation of all of the first three periodicals of the Academy was the responsibility of voluntary committees of Fellows whose other duties were undoubtedly pressing.

The second series of the *Transactions* maintained the general policy that is in force even today: papers on clinical and scientific subjects delivered at the Academy; reports of Academy studies, especially in the field of public health; and articles on the history of medicine with special reference to the history of medicine in New York City and New York State make up nearly all of the publication. As the years passed, the *Transactions* returned increasingly to the publication of a few selected long papers. Among the authors whose names are still familiar to us were John C. Dalton, Austin Flint, Samuel S. Purple, Gurdon Buck, E. C. Seguin, Frank H. Hamilton, Abraham Jacobi, Bernard Sachs, Simon Baruch, George M. Sternberg, Charles McBurney, Charles L. Dana, Hermann M. Biggs, E. L. Trudeau, Henry Koplik, John S. Billings, S. Weir Mitchell, J. B. Murphy, and Christian A. Herter. The final volume of the *Transactions* was devoted to reporting the celebration of the 50th anniversary of the founding of the Academy. This gala affair, held at Carnegie Hall, New York, N. Y., was marked by an address to the Academy by President Grover Cleveland.

### *Bulletin of The New York Academy of Medicine*, 1925-1937

The second series of the *Bulletin* of The New York Academy of Medicine resumed publication in 1925. The first article in the first issue was an editorial briefly reviewing the history of the Academy's publications and outlining policies that govern the *Bulletin* through 1937. That editorial stated in part:

> The *Bulletin* will be partly educational and partly informative. Lectures, discussions and papers presented at Academy meetings will form a considerable part of the contents of each number. Activities of the Committees will be presented from time to time in the form of papers and reports. The trustees and officers of the Academy will use the *Bulletin* as the official medium for presenting their reports and recommendations. Announcements of forthcoming meetings and programs and other items of current interest will be made from month to month.

Thus the second series of the *Bulletin* adopted a policy very similar to that of the first series of the *Bulletin* and to the second series of the

*Transactions:* scholarly articles were intermingled with reports of Academy business, announcements, and the like. The policy of assigning responsibility for the conduct of the *Bulletin* to a committee of the Fellows was continued, and there was no editor, although the director of the Academy was responsible for the editorship in a general way. The initial publications committee consisted of Drs. Charles L. Dana, Fenwick Beekman, Samuel A. Brown, Charles A. Elsberg, E. Livingston Hunt, Albert R. Lamb, Frederic E. Sondern, and George B. Wallace. The *Bulletin* was guaranteed a high level of competence by the fact that Fielding H. Garrison was retained as consulting librarian to the Academy and contributed monthly articles on historical subjects. This arrangement lasted for 11 years although, when the stringencies of the depression made it impossible for the Academy to pay Garrison the salary he had been receiving as consulting librarian, he was paid a lesser salary for the sole duty of writing an editorial or historical article for the *Bulletin* each month. Some of Garrison's most important contributions appeared in the *Bulletin* as the result of this arrangement, and, similarly, some of the most important articles in the *Bulletin* were those by Garrison. The first article in this series appeared in April 1925; the last in March 1935. A bibliography of these articles appeared in the *Bulletin* after Garrison's death. The Library Publication Committee and the Hafner Publishing Company have recently published a volume which gathers together the bulk of those articles.[4]

The *Bulletin* became a regular monthly publication with the inception of the second series and has appeared without interruption ever since (the September and October issues, however, were omitted until 1928). It is hardly practicable to review its contents, since they are so extensive. Nevertheless a few remarks may be of interest. Readers unfamiliar with the history of cardiac surgery will be surprised to find an article in May 1925 on cardiac surgery. In it Dr. Samuel A. Levine reviewed the attempts made by himself, Dr. Elliott C. Cutler, and Dr. Claude S. Beck for the surgical relief of mitral stenosis. Another article on the same subject by Dr. Beck appears in the same issue with reports of five cases of the surgical treatment of mitral stenosis (with a mortality of 80 per cent). Those early efforts at mitral valvulotomy, although technically unsatisfactory, were eminently rational. The criteria for operation and the goals of the operation were exactly what they are today. In August 1927 the *Bulletin* contained an interesting symposium, *The Evolution of Mind*, with articles by Frederick Tilney, William A. White, and Henry Fairfield Osborn. The year 1928 began with the publication of a distinguished annual address by John Dewey entitled "Body and Mind." Both of these contributions suggest that the Academy was open to lectures from persons of broad non-medical interests, and it is especially interesting to note that Osborn, who was very famous indeed by 1927, opened his lecture by remarking that when he first came to the city of New York in 1885, he had been invited to give the Cartwright Lectures at the Academy and had devoted one of them to the subject "The Contemporary Evolution of Man." A supplement to the January 1928 issue contains an excellent 50-page symposium in memory of Lister that included a catalogue of an exhibit and articles by Archibald Malloch and Fielding Garrison. The last two issues of 1928 and the first issue of 1929 were devoted to that oldest of medical specialties which is, as Erwin H. Ackerknecht has pointed out, perpetually being rediscovered as a new specialty: the medical problems of aging. The first issue of 1929 opens with another distinguished Anniversary Discourse: "What Medicine Can Do for the Law," by Benjamin Cardozo, who was at that time chief justice of the Court of Appeals. In October 1933 there appeared a symposium celebrating the centennial of the publication of William Beaumont's *Experiments and Observations on the Gastric Juice and Physiology of Digestion.* In addition to a number of excellent articles this symposium was illustrated by a reproduction of a daguerreotype of Beaumont that had never been previously published. This daguerreotype was given to the Academy by Dr. Irving Pardee, who had obtained it from a descendant of Beaumont's brother, Abel Beaumont. The August 1934 *Bulletin* carried an obituary of Marie Curie, who had been elected an honorary Fellow of The New York Academy of Medicine in 1930 and who may have been the only non-physician ever to become an honorary Fellow of the Academy.

The involvement of the Academy in problems of social and economic aspects of medicine began to be reflected in the depression years. The Anniversary Discourse for 1934, published in February 1935, was a hard-hitting lecture by Mayor Fiorello H. La Guardia, in which he made it clear that if no one else would take care of the medical needs of the people of the city of New York the municipality would do so. This paper was followed by an anonymous article entitled "The Doctor and the State," in which the author stated, among other things, "It is with a sense of shame that we recall that when Dr. Hermann Biggs wished to make a real advancement of the public health interests he was opposed by The New York Academy of Medicine. . . ." In September 1935 there was an article by Thomas Parran, Jr., entitled "Public Responsibility for Public and Personal Health: The Biggs Health Center Plan of 1920 in Retrospect," while in December 1935 there appeared, as the Anniversary Discourse of 1935, "Aspects of a Philosophy of Government in a Sick World," by Walter Lippmann.

December 1937, with the appearance of the last number of volume 13, saw the end of the *Bulletin* in the format in which it had appeared since 1925. Although there was no interruption of publication, the *Bulletin*, when it appeared in January 1938, had a completely new format and new editorial policies.[5]

### *Bulletin of The New York Academy of Medicine*, 1938-1966

From the initial decision of the Academy to issue a scholarly periodical in 1847 until the middle of the 1930's the Academy's publications did not have an editor* nor did they have a regularly constituted editorial board. For much of the late 1920's and early 1930's the *Bulletin* was under the direction of the Committee on Medical Education. In 1934 an editorial board was appointed to take over the responsibility of conducting the affairs of the *Bulletin* but that board met only once and apparently disbanded. In January 1936, however, another editorial board met for the first time and it did indeed assume responsibility for the *Bulletin*. The chairman of the new Editorial Board, Dr. Jerome P. Webster, continued as chairman until 1961, when he was succeeded by Dr. Charles Kossmann, who has been chairman since that time.

In addition to Dr. Webster the original editorial board consisted of Drs. Alfred E. Cohn, Eugene F. Dubois, Robert F. Loeb, H. Burton Logie, Archibald Malloch, Karl Vogel, John A. Hartwell, and Frederick P. Reynolds. This board immediately turned itself into a hard-working group, meeting monthly for prolonged and serious discussions about the *Bulletin*. One of the first problems to come before the board was that of the acceptability of advertising. The *Bulletin* had had no hard and fast policy on this matter, and it had been criticized for carrying advertising that some of the Fellows considered improper in a publication of

*In the *Transactions*, second series, the name of George Thomas Jackson appears as editor, and also, for some years, as Librarian. I have been unable to find any further information about his role or duties in this connection.

the Academy. The problem was not an easy one to resolve for two reasons. The advertising at that time paid a very substantial part of the cost of printing the *Bulletin* and it was predicted (correctly) that new and more restrictive policies would result in a serious loss of income. Thus no policy could be adopted without the assurance that other sources of revenue would become available to the publication. The second problem, less serious, concerned contracts with advertisers. Since the *Bulletin* had made contracts on an annual basis it was felt that even those advertisements that it might regard as unacceptable could not be dropped until the expiration of whatever contract covered them. The Edtiorial Board was convinced that a new policy was needed, and it persuaded the Council of the Academy to meet whatever loss might result from the fall in advertising revenues. As a result, in January 1937, the *Bulletin of The New York Academy of Medicine* carried the following announcement on page 10:

> It is announced that after the expiration of present contracts, advertisements for medical products will be accepted by the Council on Pharmacy and Chemistry or the Council on Physical Therapy of the American Medical Association.
>
> Advertisements for medical products not considered by the councils of the American Medical Association will be accepted only with the approval of the Editorial Board.
>
> Advertisements for non-medical products will be accepted if advertisements are in conformity with the type approved by the Editorial Board.

While studying the problem of acceptable advertising, the Board was also actively concerned with the format of the *Bulletin*, which had remained essentially unchanged since the appearance of the second series of the *Bulletin* in 1925. It appointed a subcommittee on format under the chairmanship of Dr. Alfred E. Cohn. It is unfortunate that the minutes of the Editorial Board do not record the names of the other members of that subcommittee or contain any records of their deliberations, which evidently were careful and detailed. The subcommittee eventually decided to place the designing of the new format in the hands of Mr. David Silve, a noted typographer of the period. His recommendations resulted in a total revision of the appearance of the *Bulletin*, since the new *Bulletin* was to have a different page size, a different cover, and a new typeface. The *Bulletin* made its first appearance in its new format in January 1938, and no major changes have been made since that time apart from the introduction of a new cover. The new cover, which first appeared in January 1965, was designed for the Academy by Gilda Kuhlman (Mrs. Roy Kuhlman) of New York. It permits the names of the articles and of their authors to appear on the cover, it emphasizes the words New York Academy of Medicine instead of emphasizing the word *Bulletin*, and it is in accord with recent trends in the design of covers for scientific periodicals. It retains the traditional orange color by which the publication has become so widely known and so readily identifiable. During 1965 a few minor changes in the internal format of the *Bulletin* were made. The interested reader can identify them by comparing a copy of the January 1965 *Bulletin* with that for January 1966. In general, however, the internal design of the publication remains unchanged and is a tribute both to its original designer and to its original Editorial Board and its subcommittee on format.

A sidelight on the format of the *Bulletin* concerns the seal with the head of Hippocrates. That seal, which still appears in one form or another on the cover of the *Grey Folder*, on the Academy *News Notes*, and on the first page of each *Bulletin*, was designed by Dr. R. L. Dickinson, as was the decorative border that appeared on the cover of the *Bulletin* from 1938 through 1964. Dr. Dickinson designed three versions of the seal, and each has been used at various times on the various Academy publications. The present seal, which bears the name of the Academy in English, is a descendant of much earlier devices used by the Academy. Some sort of device bearing the head of Hippocrates can be found on nearly every Academy publication or diploma since 1847. Two earlier versions can still be seen on the Fellowship diplomas. One is printed in black on the diploma while another can be seen impressed into the red seal near the lower left hand corner of the diploma. Dr. Dickinson's version of this seal has many advantages, not the least of which is the use of English in giving the name of the Academy. The seal printed on the diplomas bears the doubly cryptic initials N. E. A. M., which represent the name of the Academy in Latin. Unfortunately a raging controversy over how the Academy's name should be translated into Latin has never been settled. The one point on which all agree is that the order of the words must be A. M. N. E., not N. E. A. M. To avoid dispute I shall merely remark that A. M. stand for Academia

Medicinae while N. E. stand for New York in Latin (*Novum Eboracum*). The difficulty in translation comes in the combining of the words and in giving them their proper case. At least one form of the Latin name of the Academy apparently really means The New Academy of Medicine of York. When the Latin inscriptions for the Academy building were selected in the 1920's, consultation with many scholars and professors produced many irreconcilable suggestions as to the proper translation, but what was finally carved on the west side of the building is *Academia Medicinae Nova Eboracensis.* Dr. Dickinson may have suspected that few Fellows in 1938 read Latin or he may have wished to avoid the delicate problem of how to render the Academy's name in Latin, but in any event he was undoubtedly wise on composing his version of the seal in sticking to English.

The appearance of the *Bulletin* in its new format was paralleled by new policies on content. The publication's policies today are very nearly those established for the *Bulletin* of January 1938. The major emphasis is on substantial and scholarly articles based upon lectures delivered at the Academy. Minor details of Academy business are excluded, the annual report of the Academy is excluded, and nothing of a "house organ" character is included apart from the proceedings of the Annual Meeting, namely the Presidential Address, the Anniversary Discourse, and the presentation of the Academy Plaque and Medal. Deaths of Fellows, names of new Fellows, and brief summaries of the section meetings appeared in the *Bulletin* in 1938 but those are now found in the Academy News-Notes. In editorial policy, advertising policy, and format the present *Bulletin* is essentially the creature of its original editorial board and, as such, is a tribute to the long and thoughtful planning to which the members of the board devoted nearly 2 years.

As mentioned above, the first editor of the *Bulletin* was not appointed until 1937, 90 years after the Academy was formed, and he undertook to publish a scholarly journal. That editor, Dr. Mahlon Ashford, continued to edit the *Bulletin* until 1951 when he was succeeded, at the beginning of 1952, by Dr. Robert L. Craig, who maintained the distinguished standards set by Dr. Ashford and the original editorial board until his retirement in 1963, when he was succeeded by Paul F. Cranefield. Dr. Cranefield was succeeded as editor by Dr. Saul Jarcho on January 1, 1967.

## THE PRINTING AND PUBLISHING OF THE *Bulletin*

Throughout most of the early course of the Academy's publications the responsibility for the production of the journal was in the hands of various firms, including William Wood and D. Appleton. Since 1928 the second series of the *Bulletin* has been published by a single firm, that founded and still headed by Mr. Charles C. Morchand. The high standards of printing and design, the obtaining of acceptable advertising, and the efficient and accurate printing and production of the *Bulletin* all testify to its incalculable debt to Mr. Morchand's professional ability and his devotion to the Academy and its publications. In recognition of these contributions the Academy conferred its Plaque upon Mr. Morchand in January 1958 with the following citation:

> In 1924, a young man, recently out of college, had set himself up on a small scale in the printing business on West 49th Street. His first job was to go out and solicit business. This he did by the laborious but effective method of just going from office to office in the business sections with a pack of samples in his hand, getting any order he could, large or small. In the course of these perambulations he reached the old Academy of Medicine building on West 43rd Street. The story runs that when he told the person at the entrance desk the purpose of his visit, he was told to sit down in the corridor. After an interminable wait, a tall, dignified and rather impressive gentleman entered the front door, and, passing by, asked the young man if there was anything he could do for him. The gentleman was Dr. Linsly R. Williams, the first full-time Director of the Academy and the day was his first on his new job. The result of the meeting of these two men was a small order for the printing of some cards. Thus began an association between the young man and the Academy which has endured for thirty-three years.
>
> In 1926, he undertook the publication of what everyone knows as the "Grey Folder," which has become almost an institution in itself and has grown with the years from an eight page pamphlet to its present size of twenty-four pages. Up to 1928, the Academy *Bulletin* had been published by an out-of-town firm and difficulties had arisen in connection with deadlines, publication dates and the problems of mail communication. So in 1928 our energetic young man took over the publication of the *Bulletin*. The *Bulletin* of that period was a modest production, drab in format and not too enlivening between its covers. It was in great part a house organ. In 1937, the Editorial Board decided on drastic changes. In these deliberations, our young man played an important role, displaying not only a rare knowledge of the intricacies of type, paper and printing, but as well that rarer quality, an artistic sense. Thus, in 1938, came into being the present format of the Academy *Bulletin* of which we all are proud. There has been no change in this format in twenty years and I hope there will be no change for many years to come. It is known and recognized, not only in this country but also abroad, as an example of the printer's art at its best. In addition to the production of the Grey Folder and the *Bulletin,* our

friend has acted as advertising manager, an onerous, taxing and oft-times unpleasant task.

But, more important than the mere recital of facts and dates, has been the spirit of friendly cooperation and help, day in and day out, over thirty-three years that has characterized the association of the Academy with Mr. Charles C. Morchand. No task has been too great or too small. Every problem has been met with vigorous energy, high competence, and a cheerfulness that has endeared him to every member of the Academy staff. As the years have gone on, the relationship of the Academy to Charles C. Morchand has been not merely a business one, or that of publisher to client, but much rather, one of friendship, confidence and trust. He has become a real part of the Academy. Such relationships are rare, indeed.

## The Present Status of the *Bulletin* and Its Future Role

The *Bulletin of The New York Academy of Medicine* has come to occupy an unusual place among medical publications. One of the oldest medical journals in the United States, it is now one of the few publications of international circulation that still publishes articles on every aspect of medicine. It publishes both articles and abstracts reporting recent and often recondite advances from scientific laboratories; it publishes articles reporting the results of clinical research, reviews of clinical problems, and reports of new approaches to therapy. It publishes articles in the field of medical history, reports of detailed studies of problems in the field of public health, studies on problems in medical education, and articles dealing with all aspects of the social and economic side of medicine. And in spite of the belief of some potential contributors that their articles would receive a wider audience by publication in an appropriate specialty journal, author after author has found that publication of an article in the *Bulletin* yields far more requests for reprints than does publication in any specialty journal.

It seems, therefore, that the *Bulletin* is widely read in spite of the eclectic and diverse nature of its articles, and one must wonder whether, perhaps, the publication might be read so widely precisely because of that diversity. The nonspecialized medical periodical is far rarer than it once was, and the *Bulletin* is very nearly the last nonspecialized monthly medical periodical in the world. The eclectic quality of the *Bulletin* derives from the fact that it draws upon the activities of the Academy for its articles, and the Academy is open to all aspects of medicine through its sections and committees.

The strength and importance of the *Bulletin* is thus not the result of its own virtues but of the virtues of the Academy, and its future role is entirely tied to the future of the Academy. The *Bulletin* has a second less obvious source of strength that also derives from the Academy. It is subsidized, and it is sufficiently subsidized to be virtually independent of any need to please either advertisers or subscribers. This virtue could become a defect were the *Bulletin* ever to ignore the needs and interests of its readers, but that danger is minimized by the way in which the *Bulletin* draws for its articles upon the activities of the Academy, which are constantly determined by the interests of the medical profession as represented in its Fellowship. If there has been little occasion in this brief history of the *Bulletin* to make reference to its history during the period when Howard Reid Craig was director of the Academy, it is because no fundamental changes in the *Bulletin* occurred during that period. The *Bulletin* enjoyed in that period something of far greater value than it could have derived from any such changes: it has enjoyed the unfailing support of its policies of independence, and it has enjoyed unfailing financial support from the resources of the Academy. More than that, as the public voice of the Academy, everything it has published has reflected Dr. Craig's skill in maintaining and advancing the role of the Academy in addressing itself to problems of vital interest to the medical profession.

The future of the *Bulletin* is thus at one with the future of the Academy. While the Academy remains strong, active, independent, and concerned with every aspect of medicine, the *Bulletin* will reflect these interests and that independence. The Academy, with a tradition of 120 years of independence and of commitment to the problems of medicine, is clearly ready for another century of service to medicine; and thus the future of the *Bulletin* as a forceful voice seems assured.

*APPENDIX*

The original Editorial Board of the *Bulletin* that met on March 9, 1934 apparently never met again. It included: John A. Hartwell, who presided, Bernard Sachs, Frederick P. Reynolds, Henry A. Riley, Bernard S. Oppenheimer, and George B. Wallace. Members of the board since 1936 have included: Jerome P. Webster, Karl Vogel, Eugene H. Pool, Alfred E. Cohn, Eugene F. Dubois, Robert F. Loeb, H. Burton Logie, Archibald Malloch, Mahlon Ashford, who was appointed editor in 1937, Philip Van Ingen, Walter W. Palmer, David P. Barr, William Dock, John G. Kidd, Janet Doe, Lelia Charlton Knox, Louis

M. Rousselot, Robert L. Craig, appointed editor in 1952, Margaret Bevans, Gertrude L. Annan, Charles E. Kossmann, Charles A. Ragan, Ralph W. Gause, and Paul F. Cranefield, appointed secretary and editor in 1963.

## *NOTES AND REFERENCES*


1. Much of the material on the earlier history of the Academy's publications has been obtained from the publications themselves or from Van Ingen, P. *The New York Academy of Medicine, Its First Hundred Years.* New York, Columbia Univ. Press, 1949.
2. Ebert, M. Rise and development of the American Medical Periodical 1797-1850. *Bull. Med. Libr. Assn. 40*:243-76, 1952.
3. Morton, L. T. *Garrison and Morton's Medical Bibliography.* London, Grafton, 1954, 2d ed., p. 109.
4. Garrison, F. H. *Contributions to the History of Medicine from the Bulletin of The New York Academy of Medicine 1925-1935.* New York, Hafner, 1966.
5. Much of the material on the history of the *Bulletin* since 1936 is based upon the minutes of the editorial board on file in the office of the editor of the *Bulletin.*
6. Craig, H. R. Citation and Presentation of the Academy Plaque to Mr. Charles C. Morchand, *Bull. N. Y. Acad. Med. 34*:239-241, 1958.

# THE COMMITTEE ON MEDICAL EDUCATION 1946-1966

Aims C. McGuinness

Executive Secretary, Committee on Medical Education
The New York Academy of Medicine
New York, N. Y.

Howard Reid Craig first met with the Committee on Medical Education as Director of the Academy on January 9, 1947, the beginning of the Academy's Centennial year.

This was at a critical period in medical education. The undergraduate medical schools were just beginning to realign their curricula, which had been disrupted so seriously during the years of World War II. Internships and residencies were being reorganized, and the demand for specialty training and for short refresher courses on the part of thousands of physicians returning from active duty with the armed services still was at peak level.

All programs of postgraduate education at the Academy were being attended by large audiences. The time was ripe for a review of the education of the physician at all levels, as well as the Academy's role in medical education. As its special contribution to the Academy's Centennial Celebration, the Committee on Medical Education arranged the three-day Institute on Medical Education held in April of that year. A group of nationally distinguished educators discussed virtually every phase of the education of a physician starting with the responsibility of the secondary school and concluding with the continuing education of the practitioner. The proceedings of the Institute were edited by Dr. Mahlon Ashford, then Executive Secretary of the Committee, and were later published in book form by the Commonwealth Fund.[1] A rereading of these proceedings 20 years later reveals them to have been remarkably prophetic in terms of what occurred in the succeeding two decades, as well as in terms of many problems still unsolved. Following the Institute, Dr. Condict W. Cutler, the 1947 Chairman of the Committee on Medical Education, appointed subcommittees to review the suggestions coming from the Institute, and subcommittees later were appointed on undergraduate, graduate, and postgraduate medical education. As might be expected the Institute and the reports emanating from the three subcommittees served as spring boards for many of the activities of the Committee on Medical Education in subsequent years. Highlights of the Committee's activities during the 20 years of Howard Reid Craig's directorship, as well as some of the related activities of the Academy's Sections and its Office of Medical Education will be reviewed in the pages that follow. Before getting to these, however, it seems appropriate to turn briefly to the earlier history of the Committee.

The beginning of the Committee on Medical Education dates back to 1912 when the Society for the Advancement of Clinical Study in New York was organized. This Society undertook to establish a Bureau of Clinical Information in the Academy of Medicine building, then on West 43rd Street, and began publication of a daily bulletin of surgical clinics. In 1919 the New York Association for Medical Education was organized. During the following few years the Association published several bulletins setting forth in some detail opportunities for postgraduate medical study that were offered in New York City. The Association also made a study of the requirements for the training of specialists and published outlines of a number of comprehensive courses leading to qualification for special practice in the clinical branches. The Association concluded its activities as a separate organization in 1924 when it merged with the Society for the Advancement of Clinical Study to form the Committee on Medical Education of The New York Academy of Medicine. Among the early activities of the new Committee were: the continuation of the Bureau of Clinical Information, maintenance of a continuous survey of opportunities for postgraduate education; the planning and arrangement of programs for the Academy's Stated Meetings and other special meetings, and the provision of assistance to Section officers in planning programs for the Academy's several Sections.

The Friday Afternoon Lecture series was inaugurated in 1925 and the Graduate Fortnight in 1927. In the latter year, the Committee assumed responsibility for the editorial direction of the Academy's monthly *Bulletin*. In addition to these continuing responsibilities the Committee from the beginning considered and took action on a number of special problems related to medical education. Among the earlier ones were a 5-year study of the training of specialists, and a preliminary study of problems of internship that culminated in the formation in 1934 of The New York Committee on the Study of Hospital Internships and Residencies, which will be referred to later in more detail. This was a joint effort of the Academy and the five New York medical schools.

As already mentioned, following the 1947 Institute, subcommittees were appointed to consider the Committee's activities in the fields of undergraduate, graduate, and postgraduate education. While these particular subcommittees served for only a year or so, activities of the Committee on Medical Education in these three areas during the directorship of Howard Reid Craig will be discussed in some detail.

## Undergraduate Medical Education

Although throughout its history the Academy has had a broad and continuing interest in undergraduate medical education, and had made a somewhat extensive analysis of some of its problems prior to the Flexner Report in 1910, its specific approaches to the undergraduate curriculum have been infrequent. At the end of 1948 a subcommittee chaired by Dr. William Dock made a number of recommendations based in part upon analysis of questionnaires submitted to a group of recent medical graduates. At the meeting at which these recommendations were presented, it was reported that the American Medical Association and the Association of American Medical Colleges were about to institute a joint survey of medical education to begin on January 1, 1949, and to continue for 3 years under the direction of Dr. John E. Deitrick. In view of the very comprehensive nature of the proposed AMA-AAMC Study, it was voted to table the report and the recommendations of the subcommittee. Again, in 1964, after many expressions of dissatisfaction with the then current status of undergraduate medical education, it was voted to recommend to the Council that the Academy embark on a long-range study of medical education from the beginning of medical school through the residency. To date this recommendation has not been implemented for a number of reasons, but in large measure because of recognition of the greatly increased attention being given to the problems and goals of undergraduate medical education by the individual schools themselves, as well as by the Association of American Medical Colleges and the latter's Coggeshall Committee in particular, and because of the pending report of the Citizens Commission on Graduate Medical Education, chaired by John S. Millis, Ph.D., President of Western Reserve University, Cleveland, Ohio.

## Graduate Medical Education

### *Internships and Residencies*

Graduate medical education, including chiefly the internship and the residency, has received considerable attention from the Committee in the past 20 years. As already mentioned, the Committee on Medical Education played a major role in the establishment of the New York Committee on the Study of Hospital Internships and Residencies in 1934. Although this was a joint undertaking of the Academy and the City's five medical schools, the original New York Committee of 12 members included Dr. John A. Hartwell, Director of the Academy, and six other members of the Committee on Medical Education: Dr. Carl Eggers, chairman, and Drs. William S. Ladd, Joseph F. McCarthy, Bernard S. Oppenheimer, Willard C. Rappleye, and John Wycoff. Dr. Wycoff was the first chairman of the New York Committee.

The New York Committee was extremely active in its early years and, in 1938, it published an extensive report[2] of an intensive study of New York City internships and residencies conducted under the direction of Dr. Jean A. Curran, its Executive Secretary. The New York Committee became active again for the 10 years following World War II. It finally was dissolved in 1965. Among those members of the Committee on Medical Education who were particularly active with the New York Committee in later years, and who served as chairmen of the New York Committee, were Drs. Clarence E. de la Chapelle, James E. McCormack, and George G. Reader. Dr. Reader was its last chairman.

From 1947 to 1949 there was considerable discussion of internships and residencies in the Committee on Medical Education, particularly those in the nonuniversity affiliated hospitals including those of the Department of Hospitals of the City of New York. Stress was laid on the success resulting from the experiment of installing full-time compensated instructors in medical education at St. Vincent's and Roosevelt Hospitals under grants from the Commonwealth Fund, and it is reported that by 1950 such forerunners of today's directors of medical education were to be found in many of the city's voluntary hospitals. After much discussion of the length and content of the internship, the Committee on Medical Education in 1949 adopted a resolution recommending a 2-year program, although many of the Committee decried rapid rotation through a multitude of specialty services. Considerable concern also was expressed in regard to the manner of placement of interns, there then being many more internships than graduates to fill them. Many hospitals entering the initial national placement program were necessarily disappointed, but the plan appeared to have definite advantages over earlier haphazard systems of recruitment and appointment.

### *Shortage of House Staff in New York State Mental Hospitals*

In 1950 Dr. B. S. Oppenheimer first brought to the attention of the Committee the serious shortage of residents in New York State Mental hospitals, which was thought to be due in measure to the isolation of many of these hospitals and to their poor training programs. Dr. Oppenheimer subsequently became chairman of a subcommittee that studied the problem over the next 4 years, working with the close cooperation and collaboration of Dr. Newton Bigelow, then State Commissioner for Mental Hospitals. Part of the program developed to upgrade the teaching programs in the State Hospitals was to send in visiting teams to meet with the resident and attending staffs of the hospitals, and two such teams actually began their visits in 1952 under the direction of Dr. M. Ralph Kaufman. The program ultimately had to be abandoned, however, as the Commissioner was unable to secure the necessary funds for its support. This was most unfortunate, as a questionnaire sent out by the subcommittee had elicited a willingness to participate on the part of about 300 psychiatrists.

### *The Effect of Hospital and Medical Fee Insurance on Residency Training Programs*

In the spring of 1959, Dr. Harold A. Zintel first opened a discussion of the effect of hospital and medical fee insurance on resident teaching programs in voluntary hospitals. Dr. Zintel subsequently became chairman of a subcommittee that concluded that serious problems did exist in many hospitals with regard to the decreasing number of ward patients available for teaching and in regard also to the means of providing adequate financial support for residency training programs. The subcommittee recommendations, later approved by the parent Committee and by the Council, were to the effect that the collection of professional fees derived from insurance sources for ward service to ward patients be allowed with appropriate safeguards, that these fees be placed in a separate fund to be used for educational purposes only, and that they should be administered by the professional staffs of services with approved residency training programs. It was recommended further that this be appropriately publicized after consideration by the Liaison Committee of the Medical Society of the County of New York and the Academy. It was not until December 28, 1960, however, that a joint meeting was held of the Ad Hoc Committee on Hospital-Physician Relations of the Medical Society of the County of New York, which had been studying the problem for some time, and a corresponding Ad Hoc Committee of the Committee on Medical Education of The New York Academy of Medicine. Representing the Medical Society were Drs. C. Joseph Delaney, chairman, George Himler, William B. Rawls, and Bernard J. Pisani; representing the Academy were Drs. Peter Marshall Murray, chairman, Marsh McCall, John L. Pool, and Aims C. McGuinness. At this meeting agreement was reached on minor changes in language, but to all intents and purposes the Academy's recommendations were left unchanged and a resolution was adopted by the Comitia Minora of the Medical Society on April 10, 1961, which again resembled closely the joint resolution of the Academy-Society Ad Hoc Committees. At its May 1961 meeting, by a vote of 141 to 119, the Society adopted the resolution of the Comitia Minora, but a parliamentary motion "to reconsider and spread upon the minutes" was made immediately after the report of the favorable vote, and the matter thus was held over until the next business meeting, which was held in November 1961. By that time the opposing forces had mustered considerable strength, and the resolution went down to defeat in a secret ballot by a vote of 318 to 198. Had the resolution passed, it would have been a first step, albeit an important one. Implementation would have necessitated the passage of similar resolutions by the other 16 county medical societies in the United Medical Service-Blue Shield Greater New York Area.

### *Foreign Medical Graduates*

The Committee first became concerned with foreign medical education when, in 1952, it was requested by the Municipal Civil Service Commission to "evaluate the foreign internships of foreign graduates who were candidates for vacancies in the medical services in the City departments." After looking into the matter, the Committee concluded this was not feasible, but because of the large number of foreign graduates coming into New York City the Committee developed a continuing interest in them that remains to the present. At the Committee's meeting on March 12, 1953, Dr. Joseph C. Hinsey brought out the fact that there was a growing demand for a national commission on accreditation to replace the then existing method of evaluating foreign medical schools, a method that had been established by the American Medical Association. It was suggested at this meeting that all foreign graduates might be required to take the examinations of the National Board of Medical Examiners "to serve as a criterion of their fitness." Needless to say, the Committee followed closely and with great interest the developments that led to the establishment in 1956 of the Educational Council for Foreign Medical Graduates (ECFMG). Since 1959, the Committee has had a close liaison with the ECFMG through the Executive Secretary who has been a trustee of the ECFMG since 1957 and is its present president. Currently the Committee is concerned with the educational experience foreign medical graduates are receiving in hospitals not affiliated with medical schools.

### *Postgraduate Medical Education*

Postgraduate medical education long has been a major activity of the Academy and has been carried on both through the activities of the Committee on Medical Education and those of the Academy's clinical Sections. Here will be reviewed the postgraduate activities of the Committee on Medical Education that for many years comprised the major work of the Committee and its subcommittees.

It will be recalled that a Friday afternoon lecture series was inaugurated in 1925, and the Graduate Fortnight in 1927. The Fortnight consisted of a 2-week program of lectures, seminars, and scientific exhibits at the Academy, as well as concurrent special clinics in a number of the New York hospitals. Beginning in 1927, the Committee assumed responsibility for arranging the scientific programs for the Academy's

Stated Meetings. In addition, for a number of years the Committee arranged an annual series of clinical research meetings.

Attendance at the Committee's scientific meetings, particularly the 20 Friday Afternoon Lectures and the Annual Graduate Fortnight, was excellent in the period immediately following World War II. Beginning about 1950, however, attendance began to fall off. In 1952 the Friday Afternoon Lectures were replaced by six Monthly Panel Meetings on Therapeutics, on the first Friday afternoon of the months November through April. Also, since opportunities for presenting the results of clinical research were offered by the Federated Societies and other special societies as well as by the Academy's Sections, there no longer was need for the Clinical Research Meetings.

In 1957, the Graduate Fortnight was changed to a 1-week program entitled the Postgraduate Week, and the Stated Meeting programs to be arranged by the Committee were reduced to three—November, December, and April. Also in 1957 a special subcommittee was appointed consisting of Dr. Ludwig W. Eichna, chairman, Dr. E. Hugh Luckey, and Dr. Rustin McIntosh to study and make recommendations concerning the Committee's programs. It was concluded that the rise of the large medical centers, the increase in the number and quality of educational programs in hospitals—sometimes but not always under pressure from the various national accrediting bodies—all had served to surfeit the practitioner with meetings and make inordinate demands on his time. A three-pronged approach was suggested to reach general practitioners, specialists, and the basic research groups. For the general practitioner it was recommended that if and when the opportunity was presented, programs should be offered on open-circuit television. In 1958, a subcommittee under the chairmanship of Dr. Louis J. Soffer suggested that for general practitioners there be courses to familiarize them with basic concepts and to bring them abreast of present trends and developments, as well as courses to stress clinical application and therapy. It was felt that the Section programs were in best position to meet the needs of the specialists. With respect to the research group, plans were developed for an initial conference on electrolyte and fluid metabolism to be held outside New York City, but the necessary funds were not forthcoming. In the fall of 1958, however, the Subcommittee on Programs for General Practitioners, under the chairmanship of Dr. George G. Reader, conducted an extremely successful course on practical applications of fluid and electrolyte balance. In the fall of 1960 a weekly Tuesday evening program was inaugurated entitled the Correlated Clinical Science Course. This was somewhat in line with the recommendations of the Soffer Committee in 1958, except that instead of being a course or a series of courses of several sessions each, it ran throughout the academic year. The course was eminently successful. It drew very substantial audiences in its first 2 years, and was attracting fairly good though smaller audiences in January 1963, when the program was transferred to open-circuit television. The latter program will be discussed in another section.

To return once more briefly to the Monthly Panel Meetings and the Postgraduate Weeks: despite the successful efforts by the Committee in arranging splendid programs, interest and attendance continued to lag. Therefore, the panels were discontinued in 1960 and the Postgraduate Week after the 1961 session.

## Special Programs

### *Psychiatry for Practitioners*

In 1945, when military medical officers began returning to civilian life, Dr. Thomas A. C. Rennie first raised before the Committee the need of all physicians for a better understanding of psychiatric problems. Dr. Rennie was to repeat his concern many times in the years ahead, but it was not until 1954 that the Committee expressed itself formally in favor of the Academy's conducting a 2-week course open to all practicing physicians, the course to be designed to emphasize early detection of incipient mental illness. The implementation of this recommendation, however, was not approved by the Council.

In January 1959 the Subcommittee on Programs for General Practitioners, chaired by Dr. George G. Reader, recommended application to the National Institute of Mental Health for a grant in support of a course of seminars in psychiatry for the general practitioner under the "General Practitioner Education Project" of the American Psychiatric Association. The course was to be cosponsored by the New York County Chapter of the American Academy of General Practice, which was represented on the Subcommittee by Dr. Joseph A. Pincus, then president of the Chapter. Also on the Subcommittee, by invitation, was Dr. Manuel D. Zane, psychiatrist-internist of New York Medical College, who subsequently became course director.

The recommendation of the Subcommittee was approved by the Academy, and the grant application received favorable action by the Public Health Service. The first course, consisting of eight weekly sessions, began on February 29, 1960, with an enrollment of 88 physician students who worked with a group of six instructors under the leadership of Dr. Zane.

This course was considered a great success by both students and instructors, but all wished it had been longer. The course therefore was extended to fourteen consecutive weekly sessions the following year, and this format continued until 1965. Since the beginning of the 1965-1966 academic year, the course has been divided into two seven-week sessions—a fall session and a spring session.

A very successful section on emotional and psychiatric problems in pediatric practice was added in 1963.

In the fall of 1966 a section was added on emotional and psychiatric problems in obstetrics and gynecology.

Fifty-three physician students are enrolled in the current course, which continues under the leadership of Dr. Zane, now Associate Attending Psychiatrist at Montefiore Hospital.

### Television at The New York Academy of Medicine

At the 22nd Annual Graduate Fortnight in October 1949, a demonstration of the radiologic examination of the gastrointestinal tract conducted by Dr. Ross Golden at the Presbyterian Hospital was shown by closed-circuit television to an audience at the Academy. The closed-circuit telecast was conducted by the Radio Corporation of America in collaboration with E. R. Squibb and Sons, Inc. On the Monday, Wednesday, and Thursday mornings of each of the two weeks of the October 1950 Graduate Fortnight, a televised program of surgical operations was conducted at St. Clare's Hospital, with surgeons from several hospitals participating. The operative clinics, followed in each case by dry clinics and panel discussions, were transmitted by closed-circuit color television from one of St. Clare's operating rooms to a basement conference room in the hospital where the monitors for viewing the programs were located. The Allen B. DuMont Laboratories provided the equipment and the technical operation of the demonstration of the DuMont telecolor chain. The operative clinics and scientific programs were arranged by Dr. John L. Madden.

At the January 11, 1951, meeting of the Committee, Dr. Howard Reid Craig reported that the Academy had sent a letter to the Federal Communications Commission requesting that body to consider allocating 20 per cent of its channels for educational purposes and, at the same meeting, Dr. Alfred Angrist proposed that the Committee take action in support of the reservation on national television channels of space specifically for medical education. In January 1952, Dr. Angrist was appointed chairman of an interim subcommittee on television, and in April of that year it was voted to recommend to Governor Thomas E. Dewey that he appoint to his recently appointed Committee on Educational Television a person familiar with problems of medical education.

Virtually the entire meeting of the Committee on Medical Education on December 11, 1952, was devoted to the subject of television. Dr. Alfred Goldsmith, consultant to RCA-Victor, and Mr. Seymour N. Siegel, Director of Radio Station WNYC and President of the National Association of Educational Broadcasters, spoke on technical and historical aspects of television, and the status of educational television in New York State. An important role was forecast for television in medical education. Following this enthusiastic meeting, a subcommittee was appointed, also chaired by Dr. Angrist, to investigate and study further the use of television in medical education.

In January 1953 Dr. Angrist presented the Academy's case before the public hearing of the Temporary State Commission on the Use of Television for Educational Purposes. The report of this Commission, however, opposed the use of state funds for educational television. In the spring of 1953, Dr. Angrist became one of a group of New York educators who formed the Metropolitan New York Committee on Television, which ultimately led to the establishment several years later of the Metropolitan Educational Television Association (META). At the October 1953 Graduate Fortnight open-circuit scrambled image television was first utilized for medical educational purposes in a special program that originated at station WOR and was decoded on special receivers at the Academy. The program demonstrated the technique of sternal bone marrow puncture.

Four years then elapsed until the fall of 1957, when a subcommittee under the chairmanship of Dr. E. Hugh Luckey proposed a specific project for the production of six 1-hour programs that were to be broadcast from station WPIX and followed by an evaluation. Unfortunately the funds required for the project were not forthcoming and it had to be abandoned. Finally the great opportunity arrived! On November 1, 1962, the New York City Municipal Broadcasting System acquired UHF (ultra-high frequency) Channel 31, and began operation of WNYC-TV. On November 8th, Mr. Seymour N. Siegel, its Director, offered to televise the Academy's Tuesday evening Correlated Clinical Science Seminars, also on Tuesday evenings, and at the prime hour of nine to ten. The Correlated Clinical Science Seminars were switched to the Televised Clinical Science Seminars on January 7, 1963. As of the end of December 1966, the program will have been on the air 201 of the preceding 208 consecutive weeks. WNYC-TV has contributed all the studio time as well as the telecasts. Eleven foundations and other organizations, including the Public Health Service, have contributed more than $100,000 to the production and study costs of this first demonstration of open-circuit (not scrambled) television as a medium of continuation medical education in a large metropolitan area.

An audience survey conducted in the winter of 1964 in collaboration with Herbert Menzel, Ph.D., and associates of the Bureau of Applied Social Research of Columbia University revealed that 923 or 13 per cent of the practicing internists and general practitioners in New York City and 12 surrounding counties had viewed at least one program in the preceding 6 months, and that the average viewer had watched 8. Another audience survey is planned for February 1967.

## Fellowships of the Committee on Medical Education

### *The Bowen-Brooks Scholarships*

In 1930, Mrs. Elizabeth Cochran Bowen, widow of Harry S. Bowen, with a gift of $2,000, initiated a scholarship in memory of her son, Alexander Cochran Bowen, to provide an opportunity for 1 year or more of foreign study for selected graduates of the public charity hospitals of New York City. It ultimately was made clear that the donor wished the award to be limited to men, although the first scholarship, awarded in 1930, went to Dr. Helen J. Rogers of Bellevue Hospital for studies in England and in Holland.

Mrs. Bowen continued the contribution for the single award annually until the death of Dr. Harlow Brooks in 1936, when she added an equal amount for a scholarship in his memory. Mrs. Bowen died in

1941, and in her will she bequeathed $100,000 to the Academy, the income from which was to be used to continue the scholarships, henceforth to be known as the Bowen-Brooks Scholarships.

The awards are made by the Committee on Medical Education on recommendation of the Subcommittee on Awards, originally the Subcommittee on the Bowen Scholarship. After the initial award to Dr. Rogers, two scholarships were awarded each year through 1941. During World War II the program was suspended; then, from 1945 through 1954, small grants were made annually to from two to six young physicians to assist them in pursuing studies interrupted by military service. In 1955 it was voted to return to a single scholarship for foreign travel. As the annual income from the fund by then was insufficient, however, to provide a stipend adequate to provide transportation and support for a year of study abroad, the Committee voted in 1956 to make the award on a biennial basis. The 1966 Bowen-Brooks Scholarship carrying a stipend of $5,200, was awarded to Dr. James J. Coyne of the Columbia-Presbyterian Hospital for studies in England in the field of cardiology.

### *The Glorney-Raisbeck Fellowship*

The Glorney-Raisbeck Fellowship in the Medical Sciences was established in October 1959 by the Glorney Foundation in honor of Dr. Milton J. Raisbeck, who had been physician to the late Miss Ethel Glorney, who created the Foundation prior to her death in 1957. Dr. Raisbeck, vice-chairman of the Committee on Medical Education since 1961, and a member of the Committee since 1943, also is chairman of the Subcommittee on Awards.

The Glorney-Raisbeck Fellowship is open to physicians from the New York area and adjacent states for one year of research or study in any field of medicine or its allied sciences. The first award, made in 1961, went to Dr. Richard R. Warner of the Mount Sinai Hospital for studies in gastroenterology. The 1966 award, carrying a stipend of $7,500 went to Dr. William H. Fleming of the Columbia-Presbyterian Hospital for studies in cardiac physiology.

### Other Activities of the Committee

While this brief historical account opened with descriptions in some detail of a number of the Committee's special activities in the fields of undergraduate, graduate, and postgraduate education, it might have been more appropriate at the outset to suggest that perhaps the Committee's most important function over the years has been to provide for a group of New York's leading medical educators and practitioners a forum in which to exchange views and opinions on current happenings and problems in medicine and medical education. On many occasions throughout the past 20 years, special guests have been invited to participate in these discussions. At other times, the Committee has concerned itself with matters of special interest to one or more of its members. Examples of some of these activities are recounted here.

Of concern to all members of the Committee over the years has been the continuing education of neighborhood physicians without hospital affiliation. In late 1947, a letter was addressed to the medical boards of 60 hospitals asking, among other things, whether these boards felt that the general practitioners in the areas of the hospitals should be invited and encouraged to attend conferences and ward rounds. Less than one third of the hospitals responded. The Committee concluded that because of lack of time on the part of hospital attending staffs, of marked hospital specialization, and in some instances lack of general interest on the part of practitioners, it did not seem advisable to extend the practice materially at the time.

Eleven years later, in 1958, the Subcommittee on Educational Facilities for Physicians without Hospital Affiliations addressed a questionnaire to all nonspecialist physicians who had graduated in medicine since 1920 and were listed in the New York State Medical Directory as having offices in the Borough of Queens. Queens was selected because of the small number of hospitals—voluntary and municipal—in the county. Questionnaires also were addressed to the 12 hospitals asking if they would be interested in helping establish programs for neighborhood physicians. Replies were received from 160, or 20.8 per cent of the 800 physicians to whom questionnaires had been addressed. Of these 160, only 44 proved to have no affiliations and, of these, 13 specifically refused. Six of the 12 hospitals indicated willingness to cooperate by establishing programs.

In the spring of 1954, the Committee became concerned with the New York State Education Law, particularly with the so-called Brydges Amendment of 1953 (repealed in 1966) which, among other stipulations, required foreign graduates on immigrant visas to have temporary certificates stating they were eligible to take the State Board Examinations if they were to serve in voluntary hospitals but exempted them from this requirement if they were to serve in state and municipal hospitals. One of the most disturbing facts about this amendment was that it removed all educational requirements for appointment to internship. It was not even necessary for a foreign graduate to provide evidence that he had a medical degree. A subcommittee studied this situation, reported back to the parent Committee, and formal resolutions were adopted and sent to New York State government officials and legislators in 1955.

In 1959 the Committee was considering, in collaboration with the Committee on Public Health, the educational and training programs for intern and resident staffs of municipal hospitals. Although no action was taken, it was the consensus that a full-time person should be employed as director of medical education in each of these hospitals, and that other full-time physicians should be employed in each major department in the hope that more well-trained staff members would be attracted to the institutions. Once more in 1963, the Committee addressed itself briefly to the question as to what the Academy might do to enhance the teaching for house staff and attending staff in voluntary and city hospitals not affiliated with universities.

In 1964, a subcommittee chaired by Dr. Alfred Angrist assisted Herbert Menzel, Ph.D., and associates of the Bureau of Applied Social Research of Columbia University in the development of an instrument to be used in a study of physicians' information levels as affected by milieu, contact with colleagues, and current awareness activities. The instrument or interview questionnaire was adapted from that used the same year in the intensive study of the Academy's television program. The Physicians' Information Study, supported by a grant to Columbia University from the Public Health Service, was conducted in 1965; it involved interviews with 413 physicians in Michigan, Ohio, and Pennsylvania. Analysis of the findings still is incomplete.

## The Academy's Sections

The Academy's Sections long have played an important role in its educational activities; and their scientific meetings, now perhaps more than ever before, form the bulwark of the Academy's postgraduate programs. It is for this reason that brief consideration of Section activities is included in this article, even though responsibility for the Sections is not a function of the Committee on Medical Education, but rather of the Committee on Sections. This Committee is composed of the current chairmen and secretaries of the several Sections, and is chaired by one of the three vice-presidents of the Academy elected to the position by the Council each year at its January meeting. Both committees since 1924 have been served by the same executive secretary.

There were 11 sections in 1947: Dermatology and Syphilology; Genito-Urinary Surgery (now Urology); Historical and Cultural Medicine (now Historical Medicine); Medicine; Neurology and Psychiatry; Obstetrics and Gynecology; Ophthalmology; Orthopedic Surgery; Otolaryngology; Pediatrics; and Surgery. The Section on Microbiology (now Micro- and Molecular Biology) was added in 1948; Anesthesiology and Resuscitation, and Occupational Medicine, in 1961; Physical Medicine and Rehabilitation in 1965; and Plastic and Reconstructive Surgery in 1966.

In 1947 the Sections generally were holding eight scientific meetings a year which, like other scientific meetings at the Academy in those days, were extremely well attended. For a few Sections some decrease in attendance began in the early 1950's, but 1966 finds the majority of the Sections strong, although most now limit their meetings to about five each academic year because of competition and conflict with other societies, particularly the national specialty societies.

Particularly noteworthy among the Section activities have been the 12 published symposia of the Section on Microbiology and the 2 published symposia of the Section on Anesthesiology and Resuscitation. These have included:

*Section on Microbiology*

*Diagnosis of Viral and Rickettsial Infections*, Frank L. Horsfall, Jr., editor (1949); *Evaluation of Chemotherapeutic Agents*, Colin M. MacLeod, editor (1950); *The Pathogenesis and Pathology of Viral Diseases*, John G. Kidd, editor (1950); *Parasitic Infections in Man*, Harry Most, editor (1951); *Nature and Significance of the Antibody Response*, A. M. Pappenheimer, Jr., editor (1953); *The Effect of ACTH and Cortisone upon Infection and Resistance*, Gregory Shwartzman, editor (1953); *Streptococcal Infections*, Maclyn McCarty, editor (1954); *Cellular Metabolism and Infections*, Efraim

Racker, editor (1954); *Cellular and Humoral Aspects of the Hypersensitive States*, H. Sherwood Lawrence, editor (1959); *Viral Infections in Infancy and Childhood*, Harry M. Rose, editor (1960); *Fungi and Fungous Diseases*, Gilbert Dalldorf, editor (1961); *The Pathology of Laboratory Animals*, William E. Ribelin and John R. McCoy, editors (1965)—the latter in collaboration with the New York Pathological Society.

*Section on Anesthesiology and Resuscitation*

*Uptake and Distribution of Anesthetic Agents*, E. M. Papper and Richard J. Kitz, editors (1962); *Effects of Anesthetics on the Circulation*, Henry L. Price and Peter J. Cohen, editors (1963); both in collaboration with the National Research Council of the National Academy of Sciences.

The Section on Occupational Medicine in 1966 sponsored a conference at the Princeton Inn, Princeton, N. J., on "The Future of Medicine in Industry" that promises to serve as an important take-off point for future deliberations on the direction of this relatively new but very important specialty. The Ferdinand C. Valentine Medal and Award and the Fellowships of the Section on Urology, created under a bequest from this prominent urologist who died in 1907, have done much to bring the programs of the Section on Urology into the national picture. The first Valentine Medal was awarded in 1962 to Dr. Charles B. Huggins who, 4 years later, in 1966, was to receive the Nobel Prize in Medicine and Physiology in recognition of his discoveries concerning the hormonal treatment of cancer of the prostate. The succeeding medalists have been Dr. Meredith F. Campbell (1963), Dr. Harry Goldblatt (1964), Dr. Moses Swick (1965), and Dr. Theodore McCann Davis in 1966. The Ferdinand C. Valentine Fellowship program was inaugurated in 1964 with awards to Dr. Irving M. Bush of the Sloan-Kettering Institute, Memorial Hospital, and to Dr. Amir S. Girgis, Francis Delafield Hospital, Columbia University College of Physicians and Surgeons.

Again, as stated at the outset, the Sections, strong in 1947 and, with several exceptions, perhaps even stronger in 1966, now constitute the Academy's principal educational program, one that involves more Fellows than any of its other activities.

## The Office of Medical Education

The Office of Medical Education, formerly known as the Bureau of Medical Education, is the administrative center of the Academy's educational activities. It was formed, together with the Committee on Medical Education, in 1924 to continue many of the functions initiated by the Society for the Advancement of Clinical Study and the New York Association for Medical Education. Supervision of the Bureau's activities was the responsibility of Dr. Frederick P. Reynolds, who became Assistant Secretary of the Academy in 1924 after his retirement from a distinguished career in the Army Medical Department; in 1931 he became Medical Secretary of the Committee on Medical Education. As already mentioned, the Bureau had responsibility for maintenance of up-to-date information on opportunities for postgraduate education, the planning and arrangement of programs for the Academy's Stated Meetings and other special meetings, and the provision of assistance to Section officers in planning their scientific programs.

At the end of 1936 Dr. Reynolds retired after 12 years of service to the Academy and was succeeded by Dr. Mahlon Ashford, also a recently retired Army Medical Department officer with a distinguished record. Dr. Ashford was named Executive Secretary of the Committee on Medical Education on January 1, 1937 and, a month later, became the first editor of the *Bulletin of The New York Academy of Medicine.* Responsibility for editorial management of the *Bulletin* had been vested in the Committee on Medical Education in 1927, but was transferred to an editorial board in 1936, a year before Dr. Ashford assumed office.

Dr. Mahlon Ashford served the Committee, the *Bulletin,* and the Office of Medical Education for 15 years, retiring in 1951 when he was succeeded by Dr. Robert L. Craig, a New York obstetrician and gynecologist, a younger brother of Howard Reid Craig. On November 1, 1959, Dr. Robert Craig became Executive Secretary of the newly activated Committee on Publications and Medical Information, and Dr. Aims C. McGuinness became Executive Secretary of the Committee on Medical Education. Dr. McGuinness had resigned as of that date from the post of Special Assistant (Health and Medical) to the Secretary of Health, Education, and Welfare, a position he had occupied the 3 preceding years. He served as Executive Secretary of the Committee on Medical Education through 1966.

When Dr. Howard Reid Craig came on the scene in January 1947, the Office of Medical Education was a very busy place. In the preceding 12 months it had given assistance to 1,578 demobilized veterans, to 161 United States civilians, and to 232 foreign physicians, chiefly from South America. In addition to providing the administrative implementation of the activities of the Committee on Medical Education, the Bureau of Medical Education, as already indicated, advised and assisted physicians from all parts of the world in respect to opportunities for graduate and postgraduate medical education. Although the Bureau never conducted an official physician placement service, it maintained a list of available opportunities for physicians seeking practice opportunities. The Bureau assisted the Academy Sections in arrangements for their programs, and arranged special meetings for the Academy. In addition to its responsibility for publication of the monthly *Bulletin*, the then semimonthly program schedule and other Academy reports, the Bureau published the *Daily Surgical Bulletin*, a *Bulletin of Medical Clinics* open to visiting physicians, a *Bulletin of Surgical Clinics* (nonoperative) open to visiting physicians, and a *Bulletin of Pathological Clinics, Conferences and Rounds*. The semimonthly program schedule, familiarly known as the *Grey Folder*, became a monthly publication in 1949. On recommendation of the Committee on Medical Education, the publication of the daily medical and surgical bulletins was discontinued in 1952 and, instead, the Bureau began the preparation annually of a list of regularly scheduled rounds, conferences, and clinics open to visiting physicians. In 1963, however, this list was discontinued. Otherwise the activities of the Bureau remained essentially the same until 1959, when responsibility for the *Bulletin* and the *Grey Folder* was transferred to the new Committee on Publications and Medical Information.

Since the reorganization in 1959, the Office of the Committee on Medical Education, known now as the Office of Medical Education, has devoted an increasing amount of its effort in support of the activities of the Sections and has absorbed much of the clerical work formerly handled by the personal secretaries of the several Section officers. The staff of the Office of Medical Education has been responsible for the administrative aspects of such special programs as the 1963-1966 television study, and it took an active part in the actual conduct of the 1963 and 1964 audience surveys. In October 1962, under a grant from the Health Research Council of the City of New York, the Office began the publication of the *Calendar of Seminars in the Basic Medical Sciences*, now entering its fifth year. The *Calendar*, published monthly from September through June, lists, primarily for the New York Medical research community, seminars and other meetings of interest to that group. The Office also handles the administrative details connected with the Annual Course on Emotional and Psychiatric Problems in Medical Practice, the Televised Clinical Science Seminars, and other special conferences and educational programs. The Office still is an important information point on matters concerning both postgraduate and undergraduate medical education, and still welcomes many visitors from home and abroad.

In concluding these brief remarks concerning the Office of Medical Education, special mention should be made of certain key members of the secretarial staff without whose hard work and loyal support over the years the work of the Committee and of the Sections could never have been accomplished: Miss Grace Johnson, 1924 to 1945; Mrs. Angelica Anthony, 1946 to 1953; Miss Diane Joffe, 1935 to 1961; Mrs. Clara G. Binswanger, 1951 to 1960; and Mrs. Una Ryan Bodden, 1953 to the present.

ACKNOWLEDGMENT

Most of the material in this account of the educational activities of The New York Academy of Medicine during the 20-year period of Dr. Howard Reid Craig's directorship derives from the Minutes of the Committee on Medical Education and from other material in the files of the Office of Medical Education. Additional information was contributed by several members of the Committee and Academy Staff, but special appreciation is expressed here for the guidance and assistance given the author by Dr. James E. McCormack and Mrs. Una Ryan Bodden.

REFERENCES

1. Ashford, M., ed. *Trends in Medical Education.* New York, Commonwealth Fund, 1949.
2. Curran, J. A. *Internships and Residencies,* Report by the New York Committee. New York, Commonwealth Fund, 1938.

*APPENDIX*

# CHAIRMEN
# COMMITTEE ON MEDICAL EDUCATION

1924-1966

| | |
|---|---|
| 1924-26 | Charles N. Dowd |
| 1927 | James F. McKernon |
| 1928-32 | Nellis B. Foster |
| 1933-34 | Harlow Brooks |
| 1935-40 | Carl Eggers |
| 1941-42 | Arthur F. Chace |
| 1943-45 | Bernard S. Oppenheimer |
| 1946-47 | Condict W. Cutler, Jr. |
| 1948-50 | Paul Reznikoff |
| 1951-52 | Ross Golden |
| 1953-54 | Franklin M. Hanger |
| 1955-56 | Irving S. Wright |
| 1957-58 | Louis J. Soffer |
| 1959-60 | John L. Madden |
| 1961-64 | James E. McCormack |
| 1965-66 | M. Ralph Kaufman |

# THE COMMITTEE ON SPECIAL STUDIES

## 1946-1966

Harry Becker

Executive Secretary, Committee on Special Studies
The New York Academy of Medicine
New York, N. Y.

When Howard Reid Craig took office as Director of The New York Academy of Medicine on October 1, 1946, the Committee on Medicine and the Changing Order, with Malcolm Goodrich as chairman, was completing its studies and was beginning to prepare its final report. The numerous publications issued under the auspices of this special project committee, which was a special activity of the Committee on Medical Information, were landmarks in the efforts of the Academy to relate medical care planning to current social and economic thinking. This concern with the social and economic environment in which medical care is provided has characterized the Committee on Medical Information from its inception under Iago Galdston, its Executive Secretary, until the present day. Today, however, the Committee operates under the name of the Committee on Special Studies—the name it assumed in 1960.

The Committee on Medical Information was established in 1939. Its purposes were to foster public education concerning health matters; to furnish advice to the mass media on medicine; to answer requests from the public, interested groups, and the medical profession; to advise physicians on press relations; to conduct lectures to the laity; to conduct conferences on topics of interest to persons in public health and related areas; to conduct special studies on health or health education and related subjects; and to publish reports.

In the past 20 years, although details of the Committee's operations have changed and its perspectives may have been altered somewhat, the basic concern is the same, whether the instruments are analyses, consultations, conferences, studies, special projects, lectures, publications, or participation in planning and evaluating various community health care activities: to seek continually an understanding of the new social and economic frontiers of health care. The approach adopted by the Committee to achieve these goals has been described as multidisciplinary and interdisciplinary.

Without the support and encouragement of members of the profession who take time out of busy practices to participate in the affairs of the Committee these broad concerns would never have developed. The Committee has been especially fortunate in its distinguished chairmen during the past 20 years: Harold R. Mixsell, Frank J. McGowan, Donald B. Armstrong, Arthur M. Master, and Norton S. Brown.

Dr. Mixsell was chairman of the Committee from 1940 to 1949. Under his leadership the Committee grew in prestige, influence, and scope of service to the community. During his 10-year term of office the Committee instituted the Eastern States Health Education Conference, held such pioneering conferences as the Institute of Social Medicine and the Conference on Law, Medicine, and the Unstable Family. The Committee continued to sponsor the *Lectures to the Laity*, begun in 1935, and held an annual Press and Radio Dinner for persons working as reporters and writers on health subjects. The *Lectures to the Laity*, planned under a committee headed by Harold Brown Keyes, were broadcast over Radio Station WNYC for a number of years. These lectures and conferences were the basis for an outstanding series of publications.

One of the most distinguished symposia ever held at the Academy, the Institute on Social Medicine, was held in March of 1947 under the auspices of the Committee on Medical Information and the special Committee on Medicine and the Changing Order. Outstanding authorities on the history of medicine and specialists in epidemiology, nutrition, and psychiatry participated in the symposium. The publication based on this conference was widely reviewed and used throughout the world.

During the early 1950's the Committee continued its work with representatives of the public. It received thousands of phone calls yearly from the general public and the press. The Committee brought before the public in this period new information on such matters as cortisone and antihistamine therapies, diabetes, and cardiology. It pioneered in developing relationships with the ministry, and a series of conferences were held on Ministry and Medicine in Human Relationships that were chaired by Frank Fremont-Smith in 1950 and 1952. The purpose of these meetings was to review the historical roles of the ministry and medicine and to develop ways in which physicians and ministers might work together in the patients' interest and to strengthen the role and interrelationships of the two professions.

Particularly active in the work of the Committee at that time were William Shephard of the Metropolitan Life Insurance Company, Lester J. Evans of the Commonwealth Fund, Willard C. Rappleye, Charles Glenn King, Paul Klemperer, and Orrin Sage Wightman. Harold Brown Keyes and Edward Tolstoi took primary responsibility for selecting subjects for the *Lectures to the Laity*. Norton S. Brown, before he became chairman of the Committee in 1961, was chairman of the subcommittee responsible for the broadcasting arrangements for the lectures and for the special programs for the medical profession. Some of the lectures were rebroadcast by the Voice of America and the British Broadcasting Corporation.

Donald B. Armstrong succeeded Dr. Mixsell as chairman of the Committee in 1949 and served for 2 years. In 1951 Frank McGowan became chairman, Arthur M. Master taking over as chairman of the Executive Committee.

In March 1953 the Committee conducted the first of its Institutes on Medical History. Others were held in 1955, 1958, and 1961. The purpose of these Institutes on Medical History, in the words of Dr. Galdston, was "to inquire whether medical history can effectively serve to illuminate current problems and issues in medicine."

At the first conference on medical history, in 1953, dealing with The Utility and Value of Medical History, such historians as Owsei Temkin, George Rosen, Erwin H. Ackerknecht, and Gregory Zilboorg sought to illuminate the role of medical history in present-day society.

In 1955 the second Institute, on The Impact of the Antibiotics on Medicine and Society, a symposium was conducted on the effects of antibiotics on medicine, society, and industry. At this meeting Lynn Thorndike, Selman A. Waksman, John F. Fulton, and many others took an active role.

The third Institute, in 1958, a Conference on Nutrition, dealt with its subject in an anthropological and historical framework. It discussed anthropological knowledge of man's food practices, the influence of food on culture and civilization, the history of the theory of nutrition, nutrition and the industrial revolution, and the modern science of nutrition. The interdisciplinary approach of this meeting was brought out by the participation of historian Karl Wittfogel, explorer Vilhjalmur Stefansson, agriculturist Henry A. Wallace, and Charles Glenn King of The Nutrition Foundation, among others.

The fame of the Institute on Medical History became so widespread that in March 1953 the Committee received a letter from the Impartial Chairman of the Transit Industry asking advice on "whether our men who had a history of coronary disease are able to operate a bus without undue hazard to the riding public." The communication had been forwarded to the Committee in the mistaken belief that the Institute on Medical History dealt with medical case histories.

Among other outstanding meetings during the 1950's were the Institutes on Panic and Morale held in 1951 and 1954.

The two conferences on Panic and Morale were conducted at Arden House, Harriman, N. Y., under the cosponsorship of the Josiah Macy, Jr., Foundation. Professor Hans Zetterberg, of Columbia University, was the research associate. The conference, conducted in an informal manner, stressed sociological and psychological aspects of morale. M. Ralph Kaufman was the chairman of the conferences. The publication based on this Conference was one of the most popular produced by the Committee.

Other noteworthy meetings arranged by the Committee were the anniversary celebrations of great figures in medicine. In 1954 there was a meeting commemorating the 1,000th anniversary of the Arab physician Avicenna. The same year the celebration of the 100th anniversary of the birth of Paul Ehrlich took place. And in 1956 the 100th anniversary of the birth of Sigmund Freud was celebrated at the Academy. Under the chairmanship of Thomas Peightal, a subcommittee arranged a distinguished program at which Paul Lemkau, Roy Grinker, Kenneth Appel, Paul H. Hoch, Gregory Zilboorg, Clyde Kluckhohn, H. Houston Merritt, M. Ralph Kaufman, and Iago Galdston spoke.

In 1955 the Executive Committee voted to recommend that the Committee on Special Studies undertake a series of studies to examine the direction in which medicine was moving. A committee headed by Norton S. Brown undertook this project, which was financed by a grant from the Commonwealth Fund. The deliberations of this special committee, in which about 16 physicians and invited guests participated, centered around the following topics: 1) The Economics of Medical Practice, 2) The Rendering of Medical Service, 3) The Increasing Power and Influence of Labor Unions in the Field of Health Services, 4) The Crucial Role of the Medicinal Industries, 5) The Role of Technology in the Practice of Medicine, 6) The Changing Demographic Spectrum, and 7) The Challenge of Unobstructed Leisure.

The over-all theme for this project was *Whither Medicine?* The work of the Committee extended over a period of three years. Many distinguished leaders in the field of medicine, industry and the social sciences appeared before the group. The members of the committee were Norton S. Brown, Duncan W. Clark, Paul Fejos, M. Ralph Kaufman, Charles G. King, Iago Galdston, Robert S. Morison, Thomas C. Peightal, Herbert Pollack, William P. Shepard, William C. Spring, Jr., and Arthur M. Master. Duncan Clark served as recording secretary for the study.

Among those who spoke at the special dinner meetings were George A. Wolf, the Right Hon. Lord Cohen of Birkenhead, England, Stanhope Bayne-Jones, Ray E. Trussell, Odin W. Anderson, Michael M. Davis, Talcott Parsons, Willard C. Rappleye, Sir George Pickering, James P. Dixon, and Thomas McKeown.

This series of seminars comprised an invaluable educational experience for the participants and many of the special papers were published. This project helped set the stage for subsequent meetings of the Committee on Social Policy for Health Care, initiated about 7 years later.

In 1956 Dr. Master took over as chairman of the Committee after serving as acting chairman from June 1955 to September 1956 during the illness of Dr. McGowan. Under his leadership the Committee conducted its third Institute on Medical History and an Institute on Medicine and Anthropology, as well as the anniversary celebration in honor of Sigmund Freud. A 1959 survey of the Academy recommended that the press and public relations activities of the Committee be transferred to another of the Academy's standing committees. It was also recommended that the name of the Committee be changed to the Committee on Special Studies to reflect more fully the Committee's changing program emphasis.

The fourth Institute on Social and Historical Medicine was conducted in 1961. This Institute on Medicine and Anthropology was supported by grants from the National Institutes of Health, the Wenner-Gren Foundation, and the Ickleheimer Fund. Participants included Paul Fejos, Marston Bates, Sol Tax, René J. Dubos, Jurgen Ruesch, and William Caudill.

Iago Galdston, Executive Secretary of the Committee, retired in 1962, after 34 years of distinguished service to the Academy and the Committee. Under his leadership the Committee's reputation for pioneering studies on the economic and social aspects of health care was established. The Committee, as a source for medical information on and for understanding of contemporary economics and social issues, had become widely recognized. In this same year Norton S. Brown, chairman of the Committee, appointed a Subcommittee on Procedure to review the operation and functions of the Committee. This Subcommittee recommended that "the committee continue the special projects, institutes, conferences and lectures as have been traditionally established" and that the Committee continue to undertake analyses and to advise groups on a national as well as on a local basis.

In November 1962 Harry Becker became Executive Secretary of the Committee. Mr. Becker had had varied experience as Vice-President of Program Planning and Research for the Blue Cross Association, Associate Director of the Commission on Financing Hospital Care, and work in the fields of medical care and welfare administration, and his assignment gave the Committee an opportunity to look ahead and help formulate goals and programs for the improvement of health care for all people.

In conformity with the guidelines of the Subcommittee on Procedure, the Committee on Special Studies has conducted in the past few years a series of health conferences on topics that have been national in scope: *The Expanding Role of Ambulatory Services in Hospitals and Health Departments (1964); Closing the Gaps in the Availability and Accessibility of Health Services (1965);* and *New Directions in Public Policy for Health Care (1966).*

The words "Eastern States" have been removed from the name of these annual health conferences of the Academy in keeping with the fact that national audiences participated in them. More than 600 persons attended the 1966 Conference. The proceedings, now published as regular volumes of the *Bulletin*, which has a circulation of about 5,000, are now being purchased by members of the health and related professions. The total annual circulation of these annual Conference proceedings is 10,000.

The untimely death of Harold Jacobziner of The New York City Health Department, chairman of the subcommittee planning these annual health conferences, deprived the Committee of his enthusiastic leadership. His dedication to these conferences was largely responsible for their success. Milton Terris is now chairman of the subcommittee on the annual health conferences. He brings to this task a rich background of experience in public health and medical care research, teaching, and administration.

Recognizing the need for a national study of social policy for health care, the Ford Foundation in 1963 made a grant to the Academy to establish, through its Committee on Special Studies, a Committee on Social Policy for Health Care, which conducted a series of monthly seminars through 1965 and 1966 on the organization and financing of health services. Distinguished leaders in health care, public health, industry, labor, education, and in other professions were invited to participate in the work of this Committee. Background papers were prepared by Senator Eugene J. McCarthy of Minnesota, Seymour E. Harris, Eveline M. Burns, Eli Ginzberg, Brian Abel-Smith, and John H. Knowles. These papers have appeared separately in past issues of the *Bulletin*. At the end of their deliberations the Committee adopted a "Policy Statement on the Role of Government Tax Funds in the Problems of Health Care." The Trustees and Council of the Academy studied the statement and adopted it on May 26, 1965, essentially as formulated by the initial study group (see *Bulletin of The New York Academy of Medicine* of July 1965, pp. 795-796). This policy statement was the basis for a front page article in *The New York Times*, and the text was published in the *Congressional Record*. Requests for over 10,000 copies of this policy statement have been received and it is being used extensively throughout the country in teaching and in public statements.

The Ford Foundation has made another grant to the Academy for a new series of such seminars on social policy for health care. The Executive Secretary of the Committee on Special Studies will continue to serve as Secretary of this special Committee on Social Policy for Health Care. The topics for the 1967-1968 seminars are listed in an Appendix at the end of this article.

In 1964-1965 the National Institute of Mental Health entered into contracts with the Academy to conduct a Cost Analysis Study of the Community Mental Health Centers and to study the impact of new legislative developments on sources of support for community mental health programs. These studies have been directed by Marvin Lieberman, a Career Scientist of the Health Research Council, working with the Committee staff.

The Committee on Special Studies has continued to be called on in recent years for consultation and advice by such agencies as committees of Congress and the State Legislature, the Public Health Service, the National Institute of Mental Health, the Social Security Administration, the State Departments of Health and Welfare, and the New York City Departments of Health, Hospitals, and Welfare. In addition, numerous public groups representing consumer organizations, health, welfare, industry, and labor have made inquiries on a variety of issues.

From time to time the Committee sponsors seminar sessions on timely subjects. One such meeting was held at the Academy in the spring of 1966, at which George Wyman, State Commissioner of Social Welfare, and Hollis Ingraham, State Commissioner of Health, met with members of the Committee on Special Studies as well as with invited members of the community, to discuss policy issues in the implementation of Title 19 in New York State. During hte summer of 1966 another special seminar was arranged for persons in the health field on ambulatory care.

In all these efforts the Committee and its Executive Secretary have been the beneficiaries of the wise counsel, helpful encouragement, and generous assistance of Howard Reid Craig.

## *APPENDIX*

## Social Policy for Health Care Seminars: 1966-1967

### I

### National Goals

The New Dimensions of National Social Policy Goals for Health and Welfare: Implications for Implementation.

### II

### The Technological Base for Today's Health Care Programs

Changing Patterns of Disease: New Techniques for Prevention, Detection, and Treatment.

## III

### Current Deficits

1) What are Today's Problems and Dilemmas in Current Health Care Programs?

2) What are Today's Deficits–including Health Manpower Problems–in the Health Care Sector?

## IV

### Economic Measurements

1) Economic Analyses for Evaluating Effectiveness of Proposed Programs for Expanding Health Services.

2) Measuring the Impact of Medical Services on the Health Status of the Population.

## V

### The Urban Crisis

1) The Emerging Urban Requirements for Restructuring the Delivery of Social Services: Problems of Planning, Financing, Intergovernmental and Public-Private Sector Relationships.

2) Restructuring Urban Organization for Delivery of Health Services: Planning for the Changing Roles and Relationships, Organization and Financing.

3) The Neighborhood Health Center Model.

## VI

### Implications of Patterns of Operation of Current Programs

1) A Look at the National Social Insurance Programs for the Aged.

2) A Look at the Federal Grant-in-Aid Welfare Programs.

3) A Look at the Public Health Service Grant-in-Aid Programs.

4) A Look at the Poverty and Related Programs.

## VII

### New Program Requirements To Achieve Today's Emerging Social Goals

# FINANCIAL MANAGEMENT AND BUILDING OPERATION: THE NEW YORK ACADEMY OF MEDICINE

ROBERT M. BRERETON

Business Manager
The New York Academy of Medicine
New York, N. Y.

OVER the past 20 years, from 1946 to 1966, annual expenditures for operating the Academy have risen from $358,000 to $1,097,000. This increase in costs is attributable to a great extent to the strong inflationary forces that existed during this period. To a somewhat lesser degree but still of considerable importance were the increased costs involved in maintaining a sound competitive position in respect to personnel salaries. Severe shortages developed in the personnel market, particularly in New York City. This was due to the large business expansion that followed World War II. The shortage of personnel, felt most acutely in the secretarial, clerical, and professional librarian areas, meant that salaries in general increased; and the Academy, in order to maintain an adequate and properly qualified staff, had to meet the rising market rate. Since salaries represent a major share of the total expense of any service organization—in this case 70 per cent—the increase in over-all salary costs was substantial. The problem of meeting these costs remains a severe one today. Qualified personnel remain in short supply. In order to minimize the problem and still remain in as competitive a position as possible a program of extended fringe benefits was recently put into effect. Previously the chief fringe benefit had been an annuity progam to which the employer still contributes 10 per cent of each full-time individual's salary. This amount is placed in a special fund from which the employee receives an annuity upon retirement. Participation in the social security program has also been provided, as well as a small amount of group life insurance. These benefits remain in effect, but have been extended to include health insurance coverage of both the basic and the major medical types. The basic coverage is without cost to the employee, and the major medical is on a cost-sharing basis. With the great increase in the cost of medical care these benefits represent attracive inducements to employment at the Academy. Also,

TABLE I

| *Departmental Expense* | *1946* *Per cent* | *1965* *Per cent* |
|---|---|---|
| Administration | 19.8 | 16.9 |
| Building and plant | 15.3 | 14.2 |
| Library | 37.5 | 42.4 |
| Medical Education | 5.6 | 5.1 |
| Public Health | 6.6 | 6.1 |
| Special Studies | 5.8 | 6.2 |
| Publications and Medical Information | 9.4 | 9.1 |
| | 100.0 | 100.0 |

the group life insurance program has been extended to permit male employees to participate on a contributory basis, the employer, however, paying most of the costs of subscribing to an amount of insurance equal to the individual's annual salary.

Another factor seriously affecting rising costs has been an increase in the prices paid for books and periodicals. The increase in this category of expense has been felt over a broad area, not only in the cost of medical publications but in almost all types of publications.

A breakdown of the operating costs of the various departments for the years 1946 and 1965 is shown in Table I. As may be seen from this table a larger proportion of the total expense was attributable to the Library and, to a lesser extent, to the Committee on Special Studies in 1965 than was the case in 1946.

The sources from which the Academy derived its income is shown in Table II, which clearly indicates that income from investments is still the major source of income. In fact such income is even more important now than it was in 1946 when, as this table indicates, income from investments was 44 per cent of the total. It is now almost 70 per cent. This increase has been due to two important factors. First, there was an increase in endowment through bequests from Fellows; the Academy has been most fortunate in this respect. Second, there was an increase as a result of the farsighted investment in common stocks of sound companies that participated in the growth of the national economy. Were it not for these substantial increases in income the Academy

TABLE II

| *Sources of Income* | *1946 Per cent* | *1965 Per cent* |
|---|---|---|
| Investment income | 44.0 | 69.7 |
| Fellows' dues | 20.9 | 10.3 |
| *Bulletin* advertising | 7.8 | 2.2 |
| Room assessments | 7.0 | 6.6 |
| Photoduplication | 4.7 | 3.9 |
| Library subscriptions | 0.6 | 1.7 |
| Other | 15.0 | 5.6 |
| | 100.0 | 100.0 |

could not have continued to grow. Another major source of income, almost 21 per cent in 1946, was Fellows' dues. As may be seen from Table II, this source has dropped in proportion to total income, but it remains the second most important source. With the exception of Library subscriptions, all other income categories now represent a smaller proportion of total income than they did in 1964.

In order to provide practical operating guidelines it has been customary to prepare annual budgets for both income and expenditure. The expense budget is initially prepared by the various department heads, reviewed by the director, and then presented to the Budget Committee. Final approval rests with the Trustees and the Council. In recent years monthly reports have been forwarded to the department heads to help them keep within the approved budget. These reports show how the actual expense for any given month and for any cumulative period within the year compares with the amount budgeted for that period.

As already mentioned, the greatest proportionate share of income is derived from investments. Table III shows how the endowed funds were invested in 1946 and in 1965, the percentages shown being based on market values. It is interesting to note from this table that in 1946 two thirds of the investments were in fixed-income securities and one in common stocks. By 1965 the relationship was changed considerably, 75 per cent of the total investments now being in common stocks and 25 per cent in fixed-income securities. This change reflects to a great extent the excellent growth made by the companies in which the Academy had

TABLE III

| *Investment of Funds* | *1946 Per cent* | *1965 Per cent* |
|---|---|---|
| U.S. Government bonds | 18.3 | 3.2 |
| Corporate stocks | 8.3 | 16.2 |
| Preferred stocks | 14.9 | 3.1 |
| Common stocks | 33.3 | 74.6 |
| Mortgages | 23.7 | 1.0 |
| Savings accounts | 1.5 | 1.9 |
| | 100.0 | 100.0 |

invested. Were the foregoing comparisons to be predicated upon the actual cost of securities, then the relationship for 1946 would remain approximately the same, whereas that for 1965 would be close to 50 per cent each for both fixed-income securities and common stocks.

The Trustees over the years have followed a sound investment policy in that securities purchased were of institutional investment quality. However, as may be seen from Table III, the type of securities in which investment was made has changed, as in the case of other educational organizations. Generally speaking, investment in corporate bonds and common stocks has increased and investment in real estate mortgages has decreased.

## BUILDING OPERATION

In 1946 the Academy building was 20 years old. Indications were already present that the Library would require additional space. An architectural firm was engaged to study the requirements. A drive was activated to raise the necessary funds and, shortly thereafter, alterations were begun. An area at the far easterly end of the building was converted into five floors of stacks and one floor of work space for library purposes. In addition a balcony was erected over part of the periodicals area to provide more space there. Lighting in the reading room was improved. The last phase of this program was the demolition of two tenement buildings to the east, providing an area that was made into a small parking lot for cars of employees. The total cost of the program was $370,000.

The next major building change, which took place in 1956, involved the renovation of the Presidents' Gallery. This included the application of wood paneling to the walls, the installation of new lighting fixtures, acoustical treatment, and improvement in the heating and ventilation of the area. The cost of this alteration amounted to $26,000. This area now provides a very attractive setting for most of the dinner meetings held at the Academy.

Since 1957 several other projects have been carried out. A survey of the electrical wiring was made, and it was found that the supply of electric current to the building was no longer adequate to carry the demands placed upon it. It was decided to double the supply of electric current and to distribute the additional amount throughout the building. It then became possible to bring general lighting up to present-day standards and to install some badly needed air conditioning. In order to improve the effectiveness of meetings held at the Academy, public address systems were installed in meeting rooms that had none, and defective systems were replaced in other rooms. All slide and film projection equipment was replaced. It was necessary also to replace a sizable amount of office furniture and equipment which, due to long use, was beyond repair. This replacement of equipment and redecoration of office areas maintained personnel morale at a high level, and replacement personnel of high caliber was attracted to the organization. To safeguard the library collection adequately an automatic fire alarm was installed. Any extraordinary, sudden rise in temperature in any area of the Library will now activate the alarm. To keep pace with changes in the building code, major alterations were made in the heating plant, particularly in terms of automatic safety controls. The exterior of the building also received repairs of a major nature, including the repointing of stonework and the repainting of window frames and other metal surfaces, and waterproofing was done where required.

Two major changes were effected on the operational side. The first was to contract with an outside commercial organization for cleaning the building. Previously the Academy had employed its own personnel for this activity. It was felt that it would be more economical and would produce better results to have an outside contractor perform these services. This expectation proved correct beyond question. The second operational change was similar to the first but in a different area. The operation of the cafeteria, as well as the serving of dinners prior to evening meetings, had been contracted out to individuals. With the relatively rapid turnover of persons employed in this service, quality suffered to a great extent. It was felt advisable to place this activity in the hands of a truly competent catering concern that could consistently maintain high quality of service and adequate personnel coverage. This was done, and the resulting improvements that had been anticipated were effected at a minimal increase in costs.

In concluding this description of the major changes and improvements made in the financial management and operation of the building during the past 20 years, mention should be made of the retirement in 1959 of Arthur E. Eberle. Mr. Eberle retired after almost 30 years of service to the Academy. He was succeeded by Robert M. Brereton, business manager.

Perhaps a few words should be said about the future. As in the past, continued close control of expenditures must be maintained. Present sources of income are merely sufficient to maintain the existing level of activity. They do not permit of any major expansion of activity. Yet such expansion will no doubt take place in the future as it has in the past. This is only normal for an organization such as the Academy. However, new sources of funding must be found to finance any increased program. These sources conceivably could include contributions to the endowment. It is only because of such generous past contributions that it has been possible to offset the large increase in expense mentioned earlier. Another source of funds that could provide the necessary financing of new projects would be grants from foundations or governmental bodies. Many other organizations have been aided by these sources in the financing of special projects.

The building that houses our activities is now 40 years old. It is normal in the case of a building of this age for maintenance and repairs to become more extensive and correspondingly more costly. As time goes on these problems will become more acute, and they will include such major items as replacement of the entire heating plant, including the steam lines and their returns; replacement of the hot and cold water lines; and, last but not least, replacement of the elevators. With such costly repairs as these certain to occur in the not too distant future, perhaps it would be more practical to think in terms of new building.

BULLETIN OF
THE NEW YORK ACADEMY
OF MEDICINE

VOL. 43, NO. 2 FEBRUARY 1967

# MEMORIES OF ANTON CHEKHOV'S FAMILY*

GREGORY I. ALTSCHULLER

I DON'T remember Chekhov. I saw him, I was often in his house, but as a child, and my memory does not retain his image. I spent many hours in his house, in fact, many days. When I got measles, it was thought only natural that I should be moved to the Chekhovs' to keep me away from my brothers; and there, in a big guest room downstairs, with a famous portrait of Pushkin on the wall behind my bed, I spent more than a month under the stern but kind supervision of Chekhov's sister, Maria Pavlovna. My sister also went promptly to the Chekhovs when, in her turn, she got German measles. The big downstairs guest room must have been occupied, because she slept on the sofa behind Chekhov's desk.

The first thing I remember vividly is the day my father brought us a book written by Chekhov.

"Children, Anton Pavlovich sends you this book."

The book, a wonderful dog story, I kept through all the years of

*This article is based upon a speech given by Dr. Gregory Altschuller in Russian in 1960, on the 100th anniversary of the birth of Chekhov. Several years before that, Dr. Altschuller presented the library of The New York Academy of Medicine with a group of photographs of Leo Tolstoy and Anton Chekhov, with copies of letters from Chekhov, all of which originally belonged to Dr. Altschuller's father, Dr. Isaac N. Altschuller, who was the physician of both Chekhov and Tolstoy. The fact that the Academy possesses these letters and photographs is little known, and Dr. Altschuller has kindly consented to the publication of this article and some of the photographs to call attention to this interesting collection. A version of this article in Russian appeared in *Novoye Russkoye Slovo*, New York, N. Y., February 21, 1960.

my émigré life, and it is now in the possession of my children and my grandchildren.

I knew so well the world Chekhov lived in during the last years of his life. Not the great world of literature, theater, and worldwide fame, but the small world of a little provincial town, the now-famous Yalta, and the still smaller circle of the Chekhov family, which was so infinitely close and dear to my father and, through him, to me.

My father met Chekhov in Yalta in the winter of 1898. Both had come to the Crimea after many months in Nice, France. Both suffered from pulmonary tuberculosis. They had never met in France, but in Yalta they not only met but for many weeks shared a room while they looked for an apartment. Chekhov's family was still far away in the north; my mother, with the children, still lived in Torzok, where my father was a country physician. Both Chekhov and my father were lost and lonely in Yalta. Thus began a close friendship between the well-known and ailing writer and the young doctor. Soon after that, my father became Chekhov's physician, and this relationship of physician and friend lasted to the end of Chekhov's life. Among the letters I sent to Moscow I found the first of his to my father: "Bring, young colleague, your little stethoscope and laryngoscope."

There were many letters. Most of them disappeared and were lost during the stormy years of 1905 and 1906, when my father's house was searched by police agents. The letters that remained—those that I sent back to Moscow where they belong—were friendly and warm, with occasional bitter complaints about failing health, cough, and fever. They were all written by Chekhov from Moscow on trips he made there from Yalta.

The end came in the summer of 1904.

"I shall be back in Yalta in August," wrote Chekhov to my father in May of that year, 5 weeks before his death. He died in Germany, taken there by his wife.

This last trip, almost an abduction of the dying man from his beloved Moscow, was the last act of a silent drama that took place in the last years of Chekhov's life. Now that no one who took part in this drama is alive, one can talk about it more freely. All those years my father was not only Chekhov's physician, but he fought a losing battle with the selfishness and misdirected sense of duty and devotion of the woman who had become Chekhov's wife.

In this desperate struggle for his friend's life, my father had only one ally—Maria Pavlovna, Chekhov's only sister. Maria Pavlovna knew what my father thought about the circumstances surrounding Chekhov that were draining out of a very sick man the last drops of strength and life. Probably it was these years of sorrow and helpless anger that brought Chekhov's sister and his physician-friend, my father, together for the rest of their lives.

As I grew, I couldn't but feel and accept the admiration and love for Chekhov that prevailed in our house. Not only my family but the whole town was full of memories of the great writer. There were still many around who could say, "When he said to me . . ." or "Oh, how he laughed when he heard this story." The townspeople were all a bit proud of the fact that he had chosen to stay and live with them in our Yalta, that he was always ready to share with them their little troubles and worries, whether it was in the local medical council (he was naturally appointed a member, being himself a doctor), on the teacher's council of the then young and struggling local girls' high school, or in many other local welfare and charity agencies that took care of the ever-growing number of penniless tuberculosis patients. Chekhov never refused his help, doing in our town the same inconspicuous, patient work that took so much of his time and strength in Moscow, Lopasna, and Melichovo. No wonder that a money order came once to Yalta carrying this address: To Anton Chekhov, who takes care of the needy sick people in Yalta.

He had friends everywhere. I knew many of them. There was S. Bonier, an aging lonely woman always in love with literature and writers. She was in Chekhov's house almost daily, helping him find money and rooms for poor sick students who asked him for help. Well-dressed and well-groomed, with a ruddy complexion, all the rest of her life she lived for the memories of her acquaintance with Chekhov. He called her in one of his letters "a red rooster with a white comb."

Then there was S. J. Elpatevsky, also a physician and a writer like Chekhov himself. Elpatevsky, old doctor Orlov, and my father were the three friends who persuaded Chekhov to settle in Yalta and to build a home there. Elpatevsky was a popular writer of stories, and Chekhov used to say about him that "his stories are pretty good, but he cannot mention in them the word 'love'—his wife does not let him—and what kind of a good story can it be without love?"

I remember the very eccentric and very rich widow, O. M. Soloviev, the owner of a resort called Sook-Soo. Chekhov wrote once of her in desperation, "O. M. came and for four hours blabbed God knows what—how could I write after that?"

There was the strict, solemn principal of the girls' high school, V. K. Kharkeevich, whom Chekhov respected and liked for her clear honest mind. There were many others; the whole town was full of such friends. They never talked much about Chekhov; they recalled a word, a smile, a nod of the head, as when one speaks of someone very dear to you who died not so long ago and is still with you. They knew in their hearts that Chekhov abhorred flowery words and solemn expressions of admiration.

There was a bench on the quay near the bookstore of Isaak S. Sinani. It was a small bookstore indeed, but it always had the latest big-town novels and one could hear there the latest gossip about artists, musicians, and writers. On that bench Chekhov used to sit, observe the crowd passing by, and chat with Sinani, with whom he grew very friendly. As the years went by, the little bookshop got smaller and poorer. A new bookstore squeezed it slowly out of existence, but the famous bench remained on the quay, and people would stop and look and say to each other, "This bench . . . Chekhov used to sit here so often. . . ."

He was remembered in those days of my youth not only by writers, doctors, and others of the local intelligentsia; he was remembered by his neighbor, an illiterate Tartar, who would only shake his head in silent respect, by local shopkeepers, and by our *isvoshchiks*, the hack drivers. Everyone knew him. "Take an *isvoshchik* and tell him 'To Chekhov' "—wrote Anton Pavlovich once to his sister—"he will say to you 'To Chekhov? Oh, to our *reader*.' Why reader? I know not. That's the way I am known here in Yalta."

Chekhov's house was on the outskirts of the town, near a muddy little river or, rather, a brook. It was a desolate place when Chekhov bought it: there was a dusty old road above it, and a deserted Moslem cemetery between the lot and the brook. Chekhov built a house there, very quaint and modern and cozy, with a balcony and a little closed veranda and a little well-planned garden around the house. In a faraway corner of the garden, with a view of the Black Sea and Yalta, stood a bench. Chekhov used to sit there alone, deep in thought, when he could escape from the endless stream of friends and visitors.

This house, now a museum, has remained exactly as it was the day the tragic news of Chekhov's untimely death reached his sister. The leaf of the calendar, bearing the date, was never turned; a sheet of white paper and his pen remained on the desk. Behind the desk was a little niche with the soft cozy sofa on which my sister had slept. On the walls hung pictures of famous people and photographs of friends. In a little bedroom stood a simple bed and a night table. Nothing was changed; it was as if the house were forever waiting for the homecoming of its lost owner.

At the time I got measles and stayed at Chekhov's house, his mother, Evgenia Yakovlevna, was already very old; after an operation, the nature of which remained unknown to me, she had become weak and childish. She lived upstairs, in a neat, light room, under the loving care of her daughter.

Chekhov's mother had been the only bright spot in his childhood. His father was a stern and morose man, religious to the point of hypocrisy, owner of a small general store in Taganrog. In this store he sold eggs and needles, olive oil and kerosene, smoked fish and cheap tea, and thousands of other items that could be found in any third-rate general store in a small provincial town in Russia in those days. He forced his two older sons, still young boys, to sit in the store till late at night, teaching them how to sell and supervise and how to keep accounts. When they brought bad marks from school, he whipped them without mercy. "I had no childhood," Chekhov used to say years later. But his mother was kind and loving and, in her limited way, she tried to help the children get away from the store to obtain an education. She was dominated by her husband and rarely argued with him. Only once, when he told the children to quit school and to work the whole day in the store, she rebelled. "Don't do it, Pavel Egorovitch!" she cried. "I will complain about you to God." The children remained in school.

I knew her when she was already old and in ill health. When I had recovered from measles but for some reason had to stay with the Chekhovs for a few more weeks, I spent many hours with her, relieving Maria Pavlovna and giving her a little much-needed freedom. We got friendly and chummy, the old sick woman and the very young boy, and I listened to her talk for hours about "Antosha," whom she thought of as her little boy and whom she expected any moment to enter the room and tell her stories about school and people and books.

Sometimes I played an innocent trick on the old lady—Maria Pavlovna taught us these little jokes—and I would whisper to her, "I think that Michail Mikhailovitch is coming to the house." Mikhailovitch was the chief of the local police and Evgenia Yakovlevna had been told that he was madly in love with her and could not live without seeing her. And the old lady would blush and fix her hair and patiently wait for the visitor who never appeared.

On another occasion, when she would ask time and again, "Where is Masha, where is Masha?" I would tell her, "Masha is strolling on the quay with the hussar." Then Evgenia Yakovlevna would smile happily and ask no more questions. She probably still hoped to see her only daughter happily married.

Jokes and laughter and good-natured teasing were always in Chekhov's home. Everyone in it loved laughter and jokes, and they used words they coined themselves, Chekhov's words, which remained forever in this little house, like a spirit of the master who used to sit and look at everyone with a little smile and with a twinkle in his sad eyes.

However, already as a boy and then later as a grown man, I felt, in this house and in the new house built by Chekhov's sister on the shore of the Black Sea, not only grief for a beloved brother but a strange tense relationship between his widow and his only sister.

They were so very different. Maria Pavlovna, then in her early forties, a former teacher who understood and loved youth, was without a trace of sentimentality. She was clever, not a talkative woman, had a good sense of humor, and was an amateur painter who also tried her hand at sculpture. In many ways she reminded one of her famous brother. She probably once met a man with whom she fell in love and with whom she could have found her happiness. She somehow missed her chance. There were people who knew with certainty, who whispered his name, but who could be sure? Maria Pavlovna, like her brother Anton, shared her most intimate feelings and thoughts with no one. And for the rest of her life, she knew only one real love—her brother Anton.

And then there was Olga Knipper-Chekhov, clever, too, but in a different way, a talented actress given to a big-town ironic smile instead of good-natured Chekhovian jokes, widow of the famous author of *The Cherry Orchard*, who now visited Yalta only in the spare time of her busy life in Moscow.

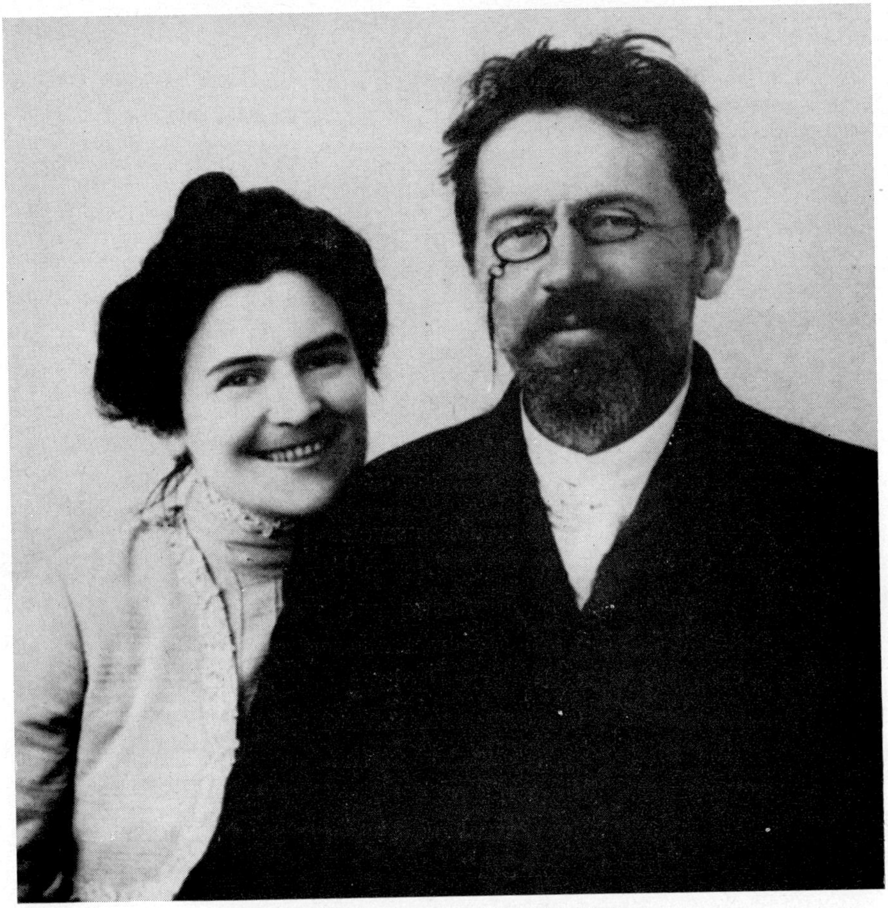

Anton Chekhov and his wife Olga Knipper.

There was no love between the two women and no trust. Both lived a long life and died at the age of 90. But I felt as a boy, from a few overheard words, from courteous smiles on their faces, and perhaps from what I heard from my father, that their uneasy relationship never changed. The difficulty may have been simply the jealousy of a sister for a woman who had taken away her brother; maybe it was a feeling that if Olga Leonardovna had not entered the Chekhov's family circle, Anton Pavlovitch could have lived longer, weak and ailing, but still able to create his beautiful plays and stories.

On the other hand, Olga Leonardovna could probably never forget that she had been unwanted by those close to Chekhov, that for years she was a stranger and an intruder, and that Anton Pavlovich shared his most intimate thoughts and plans not with her, his wife, but with his sister.

Maria Pavlovna wrote about all this to her brother only once:

> Dear Antosha, allow me to tell you what I think of your marriage. The wedding ceremony to me is something terrible. If someone loves you, he will not desert you. . . . You can say that from me to your Knipshitz. . . . One has to think first of all about the state of your health. Don't think, for God's sake, that I am egoistic; you always were for me the closest and dearest one. I don't want anything else for you than to be happy and healthy. . . . But, God alive, how terrible it will be to live in Yalta even two months without you.
>
> If you don't answer this letter soon, it will hurt me terribly. Give my regards to "her."

And then later, after she read his answer:

> Forgive me for not being able to keep my feelings to myself. I thought you would understand and forgive me. This was the first time that I opened my heart. I regret it. . . .

Many years passed, and Maria Pavlovna touched upon this subject again, this time in a letter to my father. In 1924 the letters written by Chekhov to his wife were published for the first time. Maria Pavlovna wrote to my father: "I haven't read these letters. I don't even have the book. I think it is very tactful of Olga not to give me those letters to read. It would be too painful."

It would have been painful indeed. Chekhov knew of the silent struggle that took place around him, and he suffered, being helpless to change anything.

> Olga, dear . . . I'll tell you one thing: have patience and don't say a word only for one year, for one year only. And then everything will be clear to you. Whatever anyone may tell you, whatever you might imagine, keep mum, keep mum. . . .

He wrote this in 1901; three years later he died.

Nowhere, neither in the little house on the outskirts of Yalta nor in Maria Pavlovna's bright and sunny house on the seashore, did I feel so much the real world of Chekhov as in Moscow, where I used to visit her in the intimacy of her little apartment. She was always surrounded by youth on those evenings, and she was free from grief and worries, and would exchange jokes with us and laugh at us, using

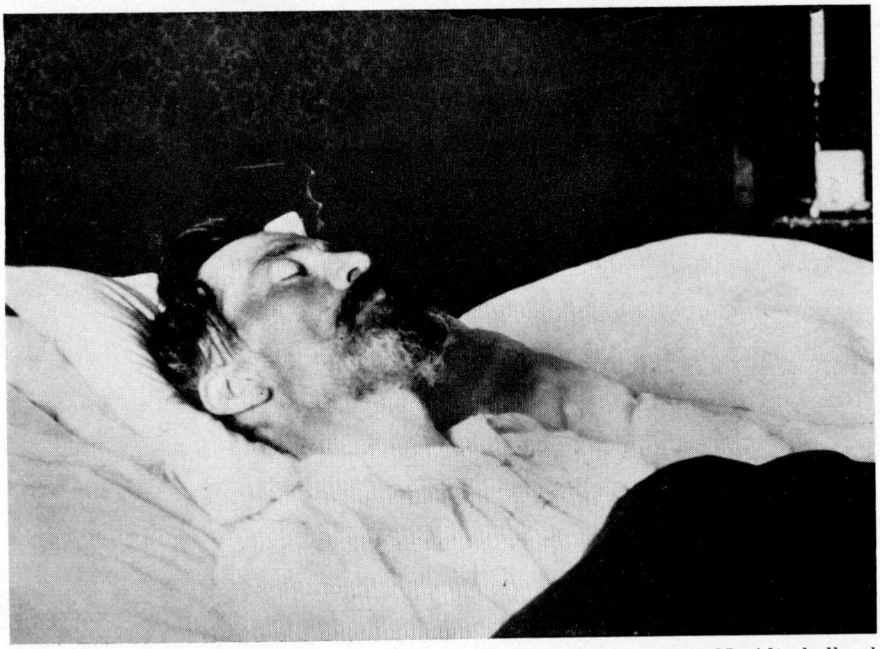

Anton Chekhov on his deathbed. From a photograph given to Dr. I. N. Altschuller by Olga Knipper.

favorite words of Chekhov. Michael Chekhov, a nephew, who died a few years ago in Hollywood, would be there, too. Maria Pavlovna was very attached to him. Many years later she wrote to my father: "When you see Misha, the actor, give him a kiss from me–I miss him so much." Michael, then Misha to us, when asked by Maria Pavlovna, would stage little scenes created on the spur of the moment. He was helped by his cousin, Volodia Chekhov, a very young lawyer. And all of those present would look and laugh and admire Misha, a great actor, the idol of Moscow.

And then came the upheaval. The year was 1918. The Chekhovs stayed in Moscow; we were in Yalta. In 1920 we left Russia. Never again did I meet any members of the Chekhov family.

In the 1920's my father was living in Berlin. There he saw Olga Leonardovna in 1929, when the Moscow Art Theatre went abroad, 25 years after Chekhov's death. Time had changed many things that had been so painful to my father during the last few years of the life of Anton Pavlovich. Olga Leonardovna was now friendly and gracious and seemed glad to meet my father again. They talked about Maria Pavlovna, about the Moscow Art Theatre, about herself. Not a word was said about the great writer. She was now a famous actress, beloved by Moscow; she was now Olga Leonardovna Knipper-Chekhova, not the widow of Chekhov.

Soon after, my father got a letter from Maria Pavlovna, who had stayed in the country. Many letters followed. Life was not easy in those days in the Soviet Union.

> "Our house in Yalta is called now the Chekhov Museum," she wrote. "I am taking care of the museum. I see visitors, talk about the life and work of my brother. . . . I am terribly tired, so tired that sometimes I could cry aloud. . . . Eight thousand people visited the house this year."

She was busy with reports, the budget, the office, clerks, repairs on the house after the earthquake of 1922. ("What a terrible thing is an earthquake . . . the walls cracked and sagged, all have to be repaired.") Work, work, work.

> My dear faraway friend, you say that my handwriting has changed. No wonder. Day in and day out I write official reports—quite an exercise.
>
> Was I really so bad before, that I have to change in order to be better?
>
> Life is austere and hard here now; we also will live better.

Maria Pavlovna always insisted that my father publish his memories of her brother:

> You must do it. . . . And please, I implore you, don't get sick. We have to see each other; there are so many things we have to talk about. Dear friend, please keep well and don't die. It will be one more reason for me to cry. . . .

And always the same refrain:

> Tired, terribly tired, right now I have a terrible headache. I wish I could phone Dr. Altschuller. But he is gone far away.

She always wrote a few words about my brothers, my sister, and me; she had known us as children: "The visitors always ask me about the photograph of your four children that is hanging on the wall in Anton Pavlovich's study."

She worked hard and she was terribly tired, but she took enormous pride and satisfaction in her work. She aged, got weaker, but never ceased to work to keep alive the memory of her brother. In a preface to a little booklet published in 1949, she wrote, "I am 87 years old and

I can say I am happy. I fulfilled what I wanted to do."

Maria Pavlovna's correspondence with my father ended abruptly in 1930. In 1943 my father died in New York City. For 25 years not a word reached me from the Chekhovs. And then, in the hot summer of 1954, when Chekhov's widow was almost 90, I got a few short lines from a friend in Paris: "Olga Leonardovna, before returning to Moscow, asked me to give you her last greetings."

Perhaps the note was not a coincidence. It was 50 years after the death of Chekhov.

## *THREE LETTERS FROM ANTON CHEKHOV TO DR. I. N. ALTSCHULLER*

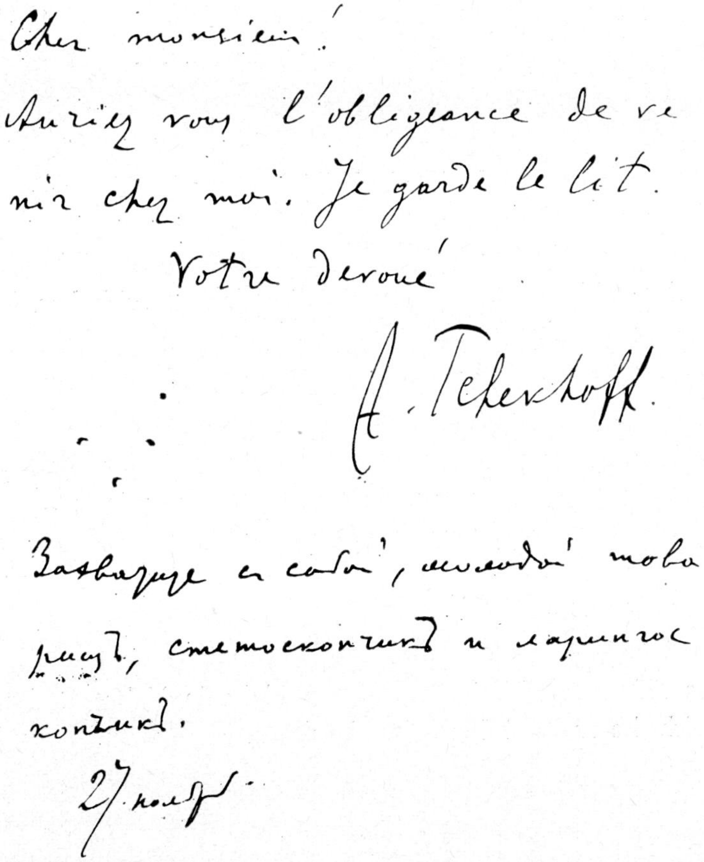

Cher monsieur!
Auriez vous l'obligeance de venir chez moi. Je garde le lit.
Votre dévoué
A. Tchekhoff.

The first letter from Chekhov to Dr. I. N. Altschuller. Translation on page 98.

*Cher monsieur.* *November 27, 1898*

*Auriez vous l' obligeance de venir chez moi. Je garde le lit.*

*Votre devoué*

A. Chekhov

Take with you, young colleague, your stethoscope and laryngoscope.

Dear doctor, *April 24, 1899*

I am still waiting for a letter from you about Korobova: how is her condition of health?

When I arrived in Moscow it was cold and snowing. Then it got warmer and now it is cold again. I did not like the apartment in Moscow and I had to move to another one. Endless stream of visitors, endless talks and on the second day of the Holidays from sheer fatigue I hardly could move and felt as a lifeless corpse.

Yesterday I was at Fedorova for supper which lasted till 2 o'clock in the morning. This I did to spite you. . . .

Write me about your health and how you feel. Also about my Crimean property and whether Nikolaj Makarych did not grab it during my absence.

Keep well and happy, regards to your wife and children. In June I shall arrive with my sister and I shall visit you with her.

And now goodby and don't forget me.

Your

A. Chekhov

Dear Isaac Naumovich, *May 26, 1904*

Since the day I arrive in Moscow I am lying in bed, day and night, did not get dressed once. Diarrhea stopped, now I suffer from constipation. The day before yesterday I took ill with some kind of an infection, in the afternoon my temperature went up and I could not sleep all night. My cough is getting better. June 3rd we are going abroad to Schwarzwald, in August I will be in Yalta. O, how I am fed up with the enemas! I am already allowed coffee and I am drinking it with pleasure. But eggs and soft bread are still forbidden.

I heartily shake your hand. I am lying now on a sofa and having nothing better to do I am cursing all day long Ostroumov and Schchurovsky.* What a pleasure!

Your A. Chekhov

Today was the first night that I slept well.

*Professors of internal medicine.

# HOW TO SELECT THE PROPER TREATMENT FOR THE CHILD WITH REFLUX*

JOHN K. LATTIMER

Professor of Urology
Columbia University College of Physicians and Surgeons
Squier Urological Clinic and The Babies Hospital
Bird S. Coler Hospital
New York, N. Y.

PART of my assignment for this paper on ureteral reflux and bladder outlet obstruction was to answer the question "Do children ever outgrow ureteral reflux?" There is no doubt in my mind that the answer to this question is "Yes." I believe that a proportion of children with reflux do get over it without any treatment whatsoever, although the proportion must be small.

The difficulty in arriving at an accurate proportion lies in the matter of how strictly we interpret the question. Talking about reflux is almost like talking about sin. We know we are against it, but there are so many different types of each and so many different degrees of severity of each type that the type and degree of severity must be clearly stated before a clear answer can be given about the probability of cure for each particular patient. The problem comes down to the question of "How to select the proper treatment for each child with reflux." A chart of the various categories and causes of reflux is included here for orientation, even though the discussion of the various types is not in the same order as those listed in Chart A.

It seems entirely possible that some defect of the ureterovesical junction, even if slight, may be necessary before any of the other factors will cause reflux. The defect may be so slight that it would not cause reflux by itself until infection or some increase in pressure occurs, for any of the reasons listed in Chart A.

## REFLUX DUE TO INFECTION

It is well known that some patients, when the bladder becomes infected, either from the kidneys or the urethra, will begin to have

*Presented at a meeting of the Section on Urology at The New York Academy of Medicine, January 19, 1966.

Chart A.—CLASSIFICATION OF CAUSES OF REFLUX

1) *Defects of ureterovesical junctions*
   a) short tunnel (roof) due to incomplete muscle layer development
   b) weak trigone, leaving orifice *slack*
   c) ureter too near portal of entry through bladder wall, as near a diverticulum
   d) defective orifice (as in exstrophy or after operative failure)

2) *Factors that increase bladder pressure*
   A) Strictures of urethra
      1) meatus (common)
      3) urethral valves (rare)
      2) distal urethral ring (infrequent)
      4) bladder neck contracture (rare)
      5) traumatic stricture (rare)
   B) Children who hold urine too long
   C) Neurogenic bladder with sphincter that will not relax
   D) Prostatism (adults)

3) *Infection*
   Can aggravate any of the other factors, and reflux may then occur

reflux. This reflux may occur on only one side, and it may go only part way or all the way up the ureter. It usually occurs only at high pressures and after a considerable volume has accumulated in the bladder. It is presumed to be due to a stiffening of the tissues around the normally pliable tunnel where the ureter enters the bladder obliquely, and it tends to disappear as the infection clears and normal flexibility of the tissues returns, permitting the layers to fall together more easily, thus preventing reflux. It is this type of reflux, one might anticipate, that would cease spontaneously when the infection cleared; also, the growth of the child would assist, since a small urethra might be a contributing factor and, as the child grew, the capacity of the urethra to permit the outflow of urine more easily would improve as the third power of the radius of the urethra. Thus, even a tiny improvement in the size of the child's urethra might produce an inordinately great improvement in the ease with which the urine escaped, thus achieving lower bladder pressure during voiding. This type of reflux might also be superimposed upon any of the other types discussed here.

## Reflux Due to Bladder Outlet Obstruction and High Bladder Pressures

There is also no doubt that a substantial proportion of patients with bladder outlet obstruction and resultant high bladder pressures during voiding will eventually begin to have reflux, first on one side and then on both. At first this reflux occurs only at high pressures and with large volumes in the bladder, but later, as the ureterovesical valve is stretched further, the reflux begins to occur at lower pressures and lower volumes on one and then on both sides.

Examples of this can be seen in a certain proportion of men with large prostate glands that are obstructing the bladder outlet. Eventually they begin to suffer reflux, first on one side and then on the other, and the reflux, which is only at high pressures at first, later occurs at lower pressures as the ureters dilate at the ureterovesical junctions.

Neurogenic bladders probably begin to produce reflux on this same basis of elevated bladder pressures. For example, children with meningomyeloceles are usually born with ureters of normal caliber, with good peristalsis. Because the urinary sphincter does not relax at the time the detrusor contracts or the child presses to void, the resultant high bladder pressures eventually break down the ureterovesical valves and permit reflux to occur at successively lower pressures and lower volumes until severely decompensated, dilated ureters are eventually seen. Even such reflux from neurogenic bladders may sometimes be reversed by relatively conservative measures that lower the pressure in the bladder during voiding, by lowering the resistance of the bladder outlet by some type of resection or revision. This is especially true if the neurological lesion is not complete. Recurrence of the obstructing hypertrophy of the neurogenic bladder neck is frequent, however, and must be watched for in such cases.

## Reflux Due to Defective Ureterovesical Valves

A defective ureterovesical valve, which causes the ureter to enter the bladder in an end-to-side fashion, with no oblique tunnel, will always permit free reflux, even at low bladder pressures and low bladder volumes. The most obvious example of this is in exstrophy of the urinary bladder, where the ureters meet the bladder at right angles, rather than with an oblique tunnel, and can be seen even to prolapse in and out through the bladder wall in the child with unrepaired exstrophy, projecting 1 or 2 cm. above the surface of the bladder like long mobile stalks. When these bladders are replaced into the abdomen, these ureters have no valve at all at their lower end, and free reflux at low pressures is the rule.

Other children are born with a partially defective valve, in the form of a short tunnel through the bladder wall, even though it still may be slightly oblique. These children may have reflux only when high pressures in the bladder occur, or during infection. At other times, the valves may be just long enough to be competent. All degrees of this defect probably exist, accounting for the differences in pressures at which patients have reflux. It has been pointed out in several studies that children with reflux ordinarily have an increased distance from the bladder outlet to the ureteral orifice, possibly due to the fact that the distal portion of the roof of the long oblique tunnel is missing in these children, due to congenital deficiency. F. Douglas Stephens of Melbourne, Australia, believes that these short tunnels may mature and grow longer as time goes on, providing still another means by which some children may "outgrow" their reflux.[1]

## Weak Trigone

Still another defect that may permit reflux may be a weak trigonal musculature, which does not keep the distal ureter stretched tightly in the direction of the bladder outlet during diastole. Emil A. Tanagho and his associates[2, 3] believe this may be congenital, whereas others think it may be caused by infection. In any case, inspection of the trigone with the cystoscope may reveal a flaccid or hypoplastic trigonal muscle that may be contributing to the reflux. Advancement of such an orifice may cure the reflux. The possibility that a weak trigone may mature and improve with age does also exist, but is difficult to prove.

## Congenital Deficiency May Always be Present

There is certainly a good possibility that some degree of congenital deficiency of the ureterovesical valve may be present in almost all patients with reflux except possibly in those with neurogenic bladders.

## How to Distinguish Among the Various Types and Causes

Reflux due primarily to infection will ordinarily not be accompanied by greatly dilated ureters. The reflux may go only halfway to the kidneys, and it may come as a surprise in what appears to be a normal tract. Such a patient might be treated empirically for his infection on the basis of the urine culture and drug susceptibility studies. Repeat cystograms may show that the reflux has disappeared. This type of reflux will usually be found to occur only at high pressures and with large volumes of urine in the bladder. The orifices may appear relatively normal through the cystoscope, or may be wider than usual and slightly farther from the bladder neck than usual. Sometimes reflux will occur in a ureter only when infection is superimposed upon a slight shortening of the ureteral tunnel. It seems entirely possible that in those patients where the bladder pressure on voiding rises only moderately, due to a partial obstruction of the bladder outlet either by a meatal stricture, a distal urethral stricture, or an enlarged prostate, the normal ureteral vesical valve would not break down and permit reflux, whereas a partially deficient valve, with a short roof over its tunnel, would break down when the pressure became high enough, and permit reflux. Likewise, a normal, long tunnel would not permit reflux even when stiffened by infection, whereas a short tunnel when stiffened by infection might permit reflux.

In clinical practice, this group of patients with only moderate increases in voiding pressures, if any, are the largest group found, and it is certainly reasonable to assume that partial deficiencies of the uterovesical valves might be more common than complete deficiencies.

At the other end of the scale, partial deficiencies of the ureterovesical valve and partial obstructions of the urethra would be more likely to occur than extreme obstructions of the urethra, as with a neurogenic bladder which is, after all, relatively rare, or with obstructing congenital urethral valves, which are very rare. Thus, the statistical likelihood of this combination of events fits the pattern suggested above, in that partial deficiency of the ureterovesical valves might be expected most likely to occur. This pattern might underlie the vast majority of patients with reflux and mild infection or in conjunction with a slight increase in voiding pressures due to a moderate stricture of the bladder outlet. If the pressures are not very high and the tunnels not too short, simple correction of the infection will bring about a cessation of the reflux. Sometimes it will be necessary to correct two of the factors: namely, the infection and the narrowing of the bladder outlet by simple dilations of the bladder outlet, whereupon the reflux will cease even though the tunnels may still be shorter than normal.

Certainly infection can combine with either of the other factors:

namely, increased bladder pressure or congenital shortness of the ureterovesical tunnel, to bring about reflux. Thus the cure of infection is an important facet of the treatment, in any case.

## Congenitally Short Tunnels

This congenital defect in the ureterovesical valve, permitting reflux at certain pressures, depending upon the extent of the defect, can be discerned through the cystoscope by measuring the distance from the bladder neck to the orifice, by placing the tip of the ureteral catheter at the orifice, and by reading the centimeter marks on the catheter between the orifice and the bladder neck. A further test may be to insert the tip of the catheter into the orifice and lift up on the orifice so that the length of the portion of the tunnel just under the urothelium can be observed and measured. The third factor is the size and shape of the actual orifice. Whereas the normal orifice is a longitudinal slit in the axis of the ureter, the shorter tunnels begin to have a more rounded cross-section, looking first oval, then like a crescent lying transversely across the axis of the ureter, like the mouth of a tunnel. The roof of the tunnel becomes higher and higher as the shorter tunnels are encountered, until the ureter with no tunnel at all looks like a large black hole through which the lumen of the ureter can be clearly seen with the cystoscope. The shorter the tunnel, the larger the opening into the ureter, and the greater the ease with which the fluid can flow back into the ureter at lower and lower bladder pressures and lower and lower bladder volumes.

*Bladder outlet obstruction.* This is best studied by instrumentation, supplemented by specialized urethrograms, bladder pressure measurements, and urine flow rates. The degree of obstruction may range from a slight narrowing of the meatus, which is probably the most common, and will respond to meatotomy, to a contraction of a fibrotic ring just inside the meatus (which may respond to meatotomy, internal urethrotomy, or a simple overdistension) to actual atresia of the urethra, which is fortunately rare and may respond to internal urethrotomy with the Otis urethrotome, or to actual contracture of the bladder neck, which ordinarily will cause the most severe obstructions and may require Y-V or other operative widening procedures. It is my opinion that the possibility of inadvertent perforation of the bladder neck in female children should argue against the use of the electric resectoscope on the bladder neck in these patients, except in rare circumstances.

Bladders that are neurogenic because of *complete* neurologic lesions are usually best treated by diversion, as by ileal conduit or with cutaneous ureterostomy of one ureter, the other ureter being implanted into the side of the first, in cases where the ureters are already dilated, thickened, and have a substantial blood supply. Children with *partial* neurogenic bladders may be successfully treated by operations to diminish the bladder outlet resistance, although it is difficult to achieve exactly the right balance between the possibility of incontinence and the possibility of gradual recurrence of obstruction.

*Selection of proper treatment.* It is apparent from the above discussion that the selection of the proper treatment depends upon diagnostic tests to determine, first, the type of lesion responsible for the reflux, and then to find how severe the reflux is as determined by measuring the pressure at which the reflux occurs. This can be done most accurately by filling the bladder gradually at increasing pressures and volumes, the child's ureters being observed continuously under the cinefluoroscope, so that the instant reflux occurs on each side the pressure and volume can thus be read. However, the pressure and volume can also be measured in a simpler way. This is to fill the child's bladder slowly with contrast medium (mixed with antibacterial medications) with the reservoir of contrast medium held first at a height of 5 cm. above the pubis. When the fluid stops running in, another minute can be allowed for reflux to occur, and an x-ray film can be taken of the kidneys, ureters, and bladder. If reflux is present on either side, it can be assumed that the reflux occurred at less than 5 cm. water pressure. On the other hand, if no reflux has occurred at that pressure, the reservoir can be raised to 10 cm. and another film taken to see if reflux has occurred at medium pressure. If not, the reservoir can be raised to 15, 20, and then 50 cm. to see if reflux will occur at those higher pressures. The volume of contrast medium required to achieve each of these pressures should also be measured, since ureters that permit reflux at very low volumes and very low pressures are the most severely decompensated of all, and are the most likely to require operative intervention.

The pressure at which the reflux occurs will determine how serious the reflux is and whether or not operation is likely to be necessary, regardless of the cause of reflux. A child with low-pressure reflux is very likely to need operative correction of the reflux sooner or later, even though some of these children will surprise one by having sterile urine and no symptoms, with a minimum of chemotherapy and treatment, subsequent to the dilation of their bladder outlets. Thus, we feel that almost every child should have a brief trial of conservative therapy, even though the probability of operative therapy must be recognized in those with low-pressure reflux. On the other hand, if the child has high-pressure reflux, which occurs only when the bladder is greatly distended by a large volume of fluid, then the likelihood that operative intervention will be required is very slight, and a concentrated effort for success through conservative therapy, such as dilations or urethrotomy, plus chemotherapy, should be pursued.

Pressures in the bladder can be measured either with a tiny No. 6 infant feeding tube inserted through the urethra, or through a suprapubic needle puncture, or by a tiny radio set that floats in the bladder and radios out the pressures without the interference of wires or tubes running through the bladder wall or urethra. These radiotelemeters are not practical for routine use, however, but are helpful for demonstrating that either of the other methods is satisfactory. Certainly the suprapubic puncture is satisfactory, and when the child is so large that the urethral tube does not partially obstruct the bladder outlet, thus interfering with flow rate measurements, it too appears to be satisfactory.

Urine flow rates can be accurately measured by having the patient void into a cylinder that has a strain gauge in the bottom that can detect instantaneous variations and fluctuations in the flow rate. Flow rates can also be measured by flowmeters that weigh the volume of urine passed and record it on a moving strip. The use of static flowmeters such as the Drake flowmeter or the stopwatch and cylinder method give rough approximations of the flow rate but are useless for the next step, namely the calculation of bladder outlet resistance.

*Bladder outlet resistance.* This parameter can be measured by dividing the bladder pressure by the square of the flow rate plus a factor. This utilizes the principle of Ohm's law, allows for the turbulent nature of the urine flow in the urethra, and results in a figure that is reasonably consistent from one patient to the next when factors such as a patient's nervousness or an inadequate volume of urine have been eliminated. Multiple tests should be done until a consistent reading is obtained at some consistent hour of the day, perhaps 10 or 11 in the morning. The patient should be given fluids so that volumes of 300 cc. at a time are obtained in adults, with correspondingly smaller amounts for the smaller children. Below the age of 4 years it is difficult to obtain cooperation from any child for these delicate measurements, unfortunately. It is necessary to measure the flow rate and the bladder pressure at exactly the same instant, when the flow rate is maximal; otherwise the measurement is not valid. This is the reason why the stopwatch and cylinder technique is not suitable for this calculation, since this method measures the total void, including the times when the rate of flow is slow at the beginning and end of the micturition. Those who state that this measurement is not accurate have not had the advantage of seeing how valuable it can be when done correctly.

The usefulness of this measurement becomes obvious when elevated bladder outlet resistance values are obtained in little girls admitted routinely to the service because of recurring urinary tract infections. If their elevated values fall immediately towards normal after simple dilation of the bladder outlet, then one can presume that one is on the right track and one can continue conservative therapy with assurance. On the other hand, if simple dilations do *not* improve the bladder resistance figure, then one may assume that more drastic measures such as operative widening of the bladder outlet may be necessary.

There is certainly much room for improvement and for better testing methods in this field, but the methods now available do provide considerable information for determining not only what type of lesion is present but also how severe it is and what the likelihood is that drastic operative intervention will soon be necessary. Measurements of the success of conservative treatment are also possible by these means.

*Locating the point of bladder outlet obstruction.* The bougie-à-boule will locate meatal strictures, intraurethral strictures, and bladder neck contractures, although the contractures of the bladder neck are the most difficult to evaluate. They are difficult to evaluate through the cystoscope, and they may appear unduly alarming by urethrograms, even when taken by special techniques. For example, one sometimes sees what appears to be a contracture of the bladder neck followed by a carrot-shaped dilation of the urethra, ending in a narrowing at the meatus. It is common on the voiding urethrogram. In some cases a simple meatotomy will cure this situation entirely. If it does not, it still may be necessary to do a widening operation such as the Y-V plasty

CHART B.—ORDER OF DIAGNOSTIC PROCEDURES

1) Intravenous pyelogram, including ureteral compression for the first 10 minutes, and also a postvoiding plate. Do prone plate if hydronephrotic pelvis is seen on early plates. Look for enlarged bladder and trabeculation. Wide or irregular ureters indicate possible reflux.

2) Measure flow rate before any instrumentation is done. Volume must be large in order to be accurate. Use the best flowmeter available to you whether Drake, Kaufman, cylinder-and-stopwatch, strain-gauge, or electromagnetic. Repeat test until patient is familiar with apparatus and until he reports he is voiding normally. If equipment is available for pressure-flow studies, measure bladder outlet resistance at this time. Repeat if there is doubt the patient is doing his best. Measure detrusor pressure if equipment is available.

3) Cystogram with voiding urethrogram and triple-voiding (void 3 times at 5-minute intervals) taking a film between each. Do 30-min. delayed film to see if reflux has occurred. Include in all cystograms 5 cc. of floating lipiodol, as well as antibacterial additives, to the solution of contrast medium. Do 24-hour plates to see if floating lipiodol has completely disappeared.

4) If reflux is seen on the cystogram, do a pressure study with the cystogram reservoir placed first 5 cm. above the pubis, then 10, 15, 20, then finally 50 cm., taking a film after the fluid stops running in, at each new level of pressure. Note the pressure and volume at which the reflux occurs.

5) Under anesthesia, calibrate the urethra with *bougie-à-boule* to note where the narrowest point is, and whether there is more than one narrow point in the urethra. Determine at what point, if at any, the *bougie-à-boule* hangs in the stricture.

6) Inspect interior of bladder and urethra with a McCarthy panendoscope, looking for fine or coarse trabeculation and cellules as the bladder distends, noting whether cystitis exists. Note whether the trigone has a firm ridge of muscle between the orifices and the bladder neck. Measure the distance from bladder neck to trigone with a calibrated ureteral catheter. Pick up the orifice and determine the length of the tunnel under the urothelium. Note the appearance of the orifice, whether it is a slit, an oval, a crescent, or a golf hole. Give the patient indigo carmine and notice if the ureteral peristalsis is vigorous or flaccid.

7) Do radioactive renogram if one kidney function is depressed, as well as differential PSP, osmolality, specific gravity, and other renal function tests as indicated.

If a neurogenic bladder is suspected, do Lapides tests, sphincteric reflexes, electromyography of the sphincter to see if it relaxes as the detrusor contracts, and do detrusor pressure determinations. Test hot and cold sensation in the bladder.

on the bladder neck. Repeated testing after each treatment will reveal whether the operation has been successful. The presence of trabeculation of the bladder is one of the most dependable signs of bladder outlet obstruction and, in general, the coarser the trabeculation, the more severe the obstruction. On the other hand, the mere presence of trabeculation does not mean that conservative treatment may not suffice. If the urethra is dilated to a large enough size, in the range of 32 to 38 French, either with sounds or the urethrotome, even in young girls, the trabeculation may slowly disappear as normal bladder pressures are resumed. Hypertrophy of the detrusor may be such that it will continue to force urine out violently through the widened urethra, thus leading to some temporary incontinence or episodes of urgency incontinence whenever the bladder becomes filled and the child does not answer the call. The detrusor pressure can also be measured, using modifications of the above techniques.

*Neurogenic bladders can be detected.* Not only does the ordinary cystometrogram help to detect neurogenic bladders, but determinations of whether the temperature detection sense is present or absent, and measurements of the detrusor contraction and sphincter contraction either simultaneously, as in the neurogenic bladder, or reciprocally, as in the normal bladder, can be detected by electromyographic techniques. In children, since the commonest cause of neurogenic bladder is meningomyelocele, differential diagnosis does not pose a great problem. The diagnosis of neurogenic bladder is ordinarily quite obvious because of the large meningomyelocele present.

## Studies Suggesting That Some Reflux Stops Without Treatment

Dr. Roger Baker and his associates[4] did cystograms on 150 adults and 555 pediatric patients, all with bladder neck or urethral obstruction, and they observed that a large proportion of the children had reflux while a large proportion of the adults did not. From this he suggested that the reflux was cured spontaneously in 75 per cent of the children. However, because he did not observe the same cases from childhood into adulthood, this conclusion cannot be easily defended. A doctor who generally avoids instrumentation and depends largely upon chemotherapy for treatment of children, many of whom must have reflux, is Dr. Alexander J. Michie of Philadelphia, Pa. Here again, however, the lack of complete documentation, which can be obtained only by repeated instrumentation and testing, permits no real figures, in my opinion, as to the efficacy of noninstrumental treatment. It should be made clear that these patients had no instrumental treatment, and they should not be confused with a similar group of patients who underwent "conservative" treatment at the hands of our own group; these patients received vigorous dilation or local urethral incision (categorized as conservative treatment rather than operative treatment), and were greatly improved thereby. Drs. Robert Lich, Jr.,[5] and Robert A. Garrett[6] also report that substantial proportions of their patients responded to conservative treatment of reflux.

## Summary

Reflux is due to several factors, for example congenital shortness of the ureterovesical valve, which may be so severe as to permit reflux by itself, or, if partial, may permit reflux only when infection or increased bladder pressures *are* superimposed upon the weak valve. Partial stricture of the bladder outlet or meatus is probably the commonest cause of such increased pressures. Severe increases in pressure, as in the neurogenic bladder, may break down even a normal ureterovesical tunnel-valve.

The precise nature of the cause of the obstruction can be fairly well determined by present diagnostic methods, even though better methods are under development and will be welcome.

Regardless of the cause of the reflux, an indication of its severity and the likelihood that it will respond to conservative treatment can be obtained by measuring the pressure at which the reflux occurs. Patients who have reflux at low pressures are more likely to require operative treatment, whereas those with reflux only at high pressures are more likely to respond to conservative treatment.

Research is providing more and more information on both the causes and on technical improvements in therapy, and while the reflux and bladder neck problem is not yet entirely under control, it is far better understood and far better treated today, thanks to the efforts of many men present on this occasion, than it was even 5 years ago.

With regard to the question of whether a child can "outgrow" reflux, there are certainly three possible anatomical areas that might improve as the child grows older, thus tipping the scales in a favorable direction, if the reflux has been only slight and the defect of marginal importance in the first place. These three areas are, first, the roof of the ureteral orifice "tunnel," which may grow longer and firmer as the child grows older. The second is the "weak" trigone that may be present in some children with reflux and fails to stretch the ureter down toward the bladder neck (which helps to shut off reflux); if the trigone grows stronger with maturity, the reflux, if marginal, may cease. The third area in which growth may help is in the radius of the urethra, where even tiny increases improve the capacity of the urethra by the third power of the radius. A fourth feature that might be correlated with growth is the improved ability of the child to take care of herself by emptying the bladder more frequently, using triple voiding to get it completely empty, by avoiding tub baths or contaminated swimming pools, and by using better personal hygiene of the area of the urethra to avoid external contamination.

The fact that another valve in the body, located at the junction between the esophagus and the stomach, stops reflux in almost every "burping" newborn infant, does lend credence to the view that our natural values may mature with age.

It is my belief that very small degrees of high-pressure reflux, like very small degrees of sin, may be overcome spontaneously in a few patients, but that in a very *large* group of patients moderate reflux can be overcome by moderate treatment. Also, that a relatively small group requires operative treatment for severe low-pressure reflux and obstruction. These various groups even now can be distinguished from one another by thorough testing.

*REFERENCES*

1. Stephens, F. D. and Lenaghan, D. Anatomical basis and dynamics of vesicoureteral reflux, *J. Urol. 87*:669-80, 1962.
2. Tanagho, E. A. and Hutch, J. A. Primary reflux, *J. Urol. 93*:2, 158-164, 1965.
3. Tanagho, E. A., Hutch, J. A., Meyers, F. H. and Rambo, O. N., Jr. Primary vesicoureteral reflux: experimental studies of its etiology, *J. Urol. 93*:2, 165-76, 1965.
4. Baker, R., Maxted, W., McCrystal, H. and Kelly, T. Unpredictable results associated with treatment of 133 children with ureterovesical reflux, *J. Urol. 94*: 5, 362-75, 1965.
5. Lich, Robert, Jr. Personal communication, 1965.
6. Garrett, R. A. Antireflux surgery in children, *J.A.M.A. 195*:124-26, 1966.

# HISTORICAL ASPECTS OF THE ANATOMY OF THE CARDIA WITH SPECIAL REFERENCE TO HIATUS HERNIA*

GERHART S. SCHWARZ

Radiology Service, Bird S. Coler Memorial Hospital and Home
Department of Radiology, New York Medical College Center for Chronic Disease
New York, N. Y.

INTEREST in the anatomy of the cardia as it relates to hiatus hernia was closely related in past centuries to human rumination. Human rumination or merycism seemed to captivate the imagination of physicians of previous times, and it was their desire to find an anatomic explanation for it, modeled on the four stomachs of the herbivorous split-hoofed animals. Figure 1 depicts the textbook description of the digestive apparatus of the cow with its four pouches: the rumen, the reticulum, the omasum, and the abomasum. This apparatus is by no means confined to cattle but is found also in camels, llamas, giraffes, deer, antelopes, sheep, and goats. Birds possess three stomachs: the crop, the prostomach, and the main stomach.

In 1838 Arnold described stomachs recovered from three ruminating individuals possessing a bulbar expansion at the top, separated from the stomach proper by a furrow or sulcus that later became known as Arnold's furrow and that we today apparently regard as the incisura cardiaca. He called the bulbar expansion above the stomach *Vormagen* (forestomach) and likened it to the rumen or paunch of the cow.

The incisura cardiaca, i.e., the angle formed by esophagus and stomach came soon under scrutiny because it was thought to hold the secret of gastroesophageal reflux, obviously a prime requisite for rumination. A. von Gubaroff, a Russian, investigated the animal kingdom, measuring the angle of the incisura in different species according to a formula developed by Smirnoff, and he concluded that the horse cannot vomit because it possesses the smallest angle, i.e., the deepest incisura.

In 1857 Luschka described the stomach of a 35-year-old ruminating

*Presented at a meeting of the Pirquet Society of Clinical Medicine at The New York Academy of Medicine, February 9, 1966.

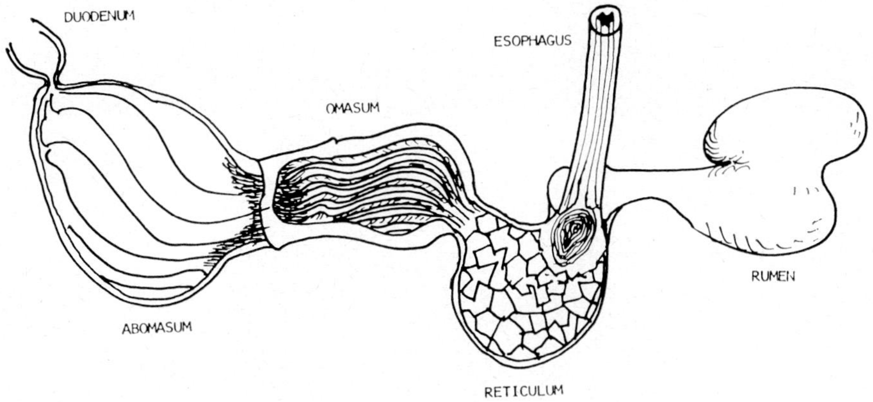


Fig. 1. Digestive apparatus of the cow.

woman with two expansions above the cardia, declaring he had found a true *Vormagen* in the upper of the two, whereas the lower one was merely an antrum cardiacum that had been mistaken by Arnold to be the former. Since then the term antrum cardiacum or cardiac antrum likewise has become an accepted term that has found its way into the official nomenclature of anatomy. Hyrtl in 1879 was the last one to list human rumination caused by a *Vormagen* as an entity, calling it a "*curiosum anatomicum rarissimum.*" The term itself fell into disrepute by the turn of the century, only to be resurrected in 1965 by J. D. Hollowell. However, the controversy lingered on, and the true anatomy of the cardia was yet to be explained.

P. Poirier and A. Charpy in successive editions of their textbook of anatomy described the lower esophagus as possessing a *fuseau broncho-diaphragmatique*, i.e., a spindle extending from the left main bronchus to the diaphragm and an *entonnoir infradiaphragmatique* or *terminal*, i.e., a terminal funnel, the latter of which seemed to coincide with Luschka's antrum cardiacum. In 1883 Laimer, a pathologist at the University of Graz, Austria, examined 60 cadavers and noted that the narrowest point of the esophagus lay invariably above the diaphragm. He published a table of the measurements on each case that permits the modern reader to construct his own distribution curve.

In 1898 Mehnert proposed the enteromere theory, according to which the esophagus was basically a string of pearls that developed from

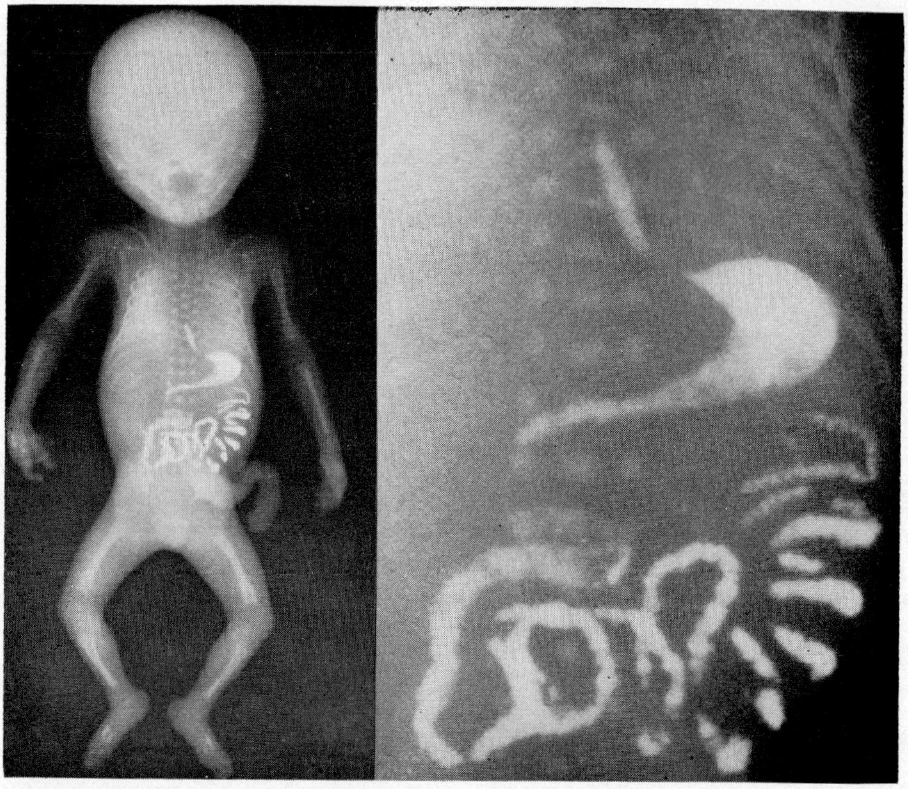

Fig. 2. Phrenic ampulla in a 3.5-month-old fetus; author's radiograph of a preparation by Dr. Edith Potter.

12 separate bubbles corresponding to the 12 thoracic segments. Enteromere No. 11 was equated by him to the *Vormagen*, enteromere No. 12 to the cardiac antrum. However, in the same year Otto Zusch countered this theory with the argument that there is no evidence of a segmental innervation of the esophagus, hence there could not be a segmental development of this organ. Finally, Hasse and Strecker in 1905, having been prompted by their late teacher, William His, Sr., used the term phrenic ampulla to describe a normal fusiform expansion of the lowermost thoracic esophagus, and this term has been accepted by anatomists. The authors state in their paper: "Although absent at birth, the phrenic ampulla forms in infancy." To dispute a minor point of their argument, I herewith submit the radiograph of a 4½-month-old fetus in which contrast material outlines a fusiform

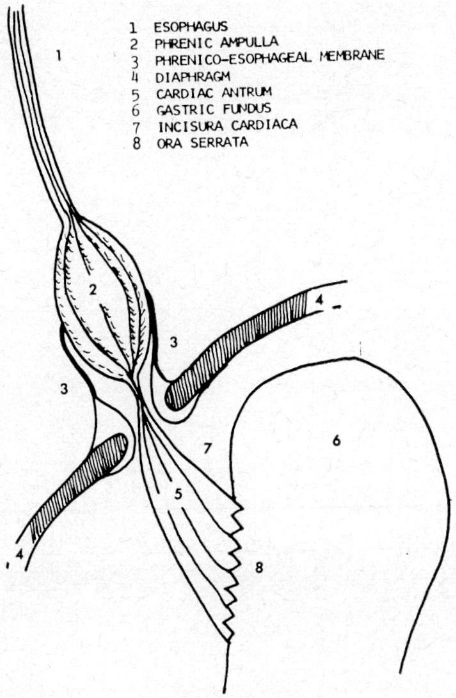


Fig. 3. Gastroesophageal junction in humans; majority view of anatomists.

expansion of the lower esophagus quite in keeping with the phrenic ampulla (Figure 2). Whatever the time of natural appearance of the phrenic ampulla is in a given individual, the year 1905 marks the official debut of the term phrenic ampulla in international anatomical circles. A majority viewpoint began to crystallize now among anatomists regarding the cardia, shown in Figure 3. A routine radiograph of the barium-filled cardia seems to support this diagram at least in part (Figure 4).

It took another 21 years, however, before radiologists began to take note of its existence, though successive editions of D. J. Cunningham Jr.'s *Anatomy* mentioned the existence of a phrenic ampulla as a normal anatomic structure, at least since 1912. Reich, in Vienna in 1926, was the first radiologist to demonstrate the phrenic ampulla radiographically and to correlate its contrast-filled image to a longitudinal section of a frozen cadaver. He and Hitzenberger also made paraffin casts of stomachs, demonstrating the cardiac antrum by this method as well as by radiography. They were inclined to consider the cardiac antrum to be

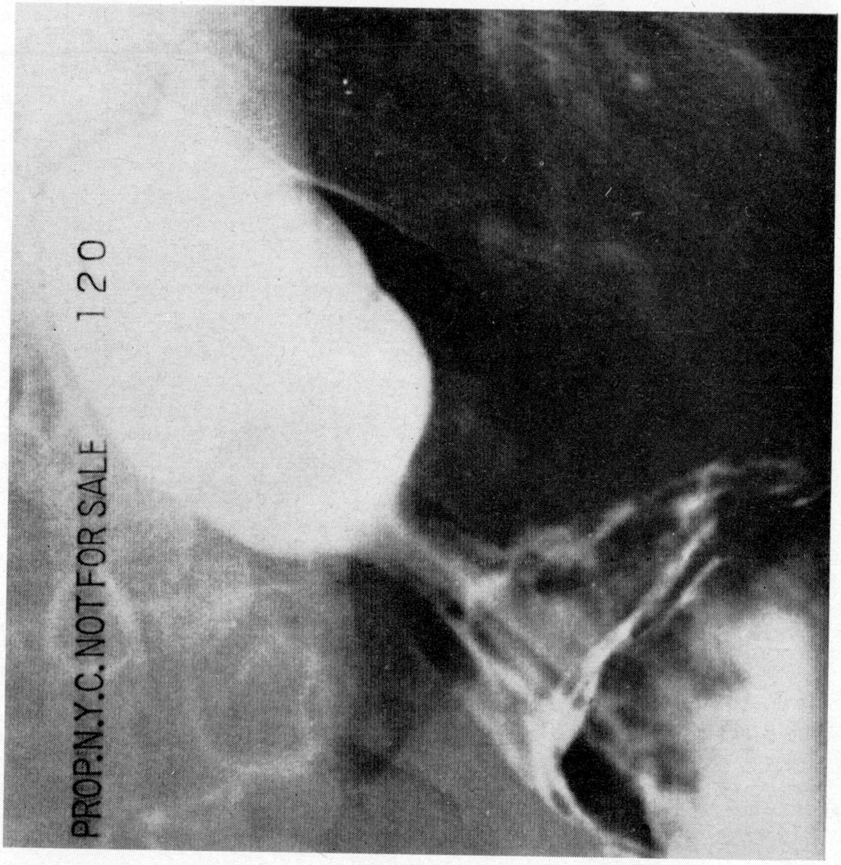


Fig. 4. Simultaneous demonstration of phrenic ampulla and cardiac antrum, the former filled with barium, the latter containing air. The barium-coated walls of the cardiac antrum suggest a border line between stomach and esophagus. This radiograph seems to refute the unitarian view held by a minority of anatomists and radiologists, according to which only a single "cardioesophageal vestibule" exists.

part of the stomach rather than the abdominal portion of the esophagus.

One might wonder what the radiologists had been doing between the turn of the century and 1926 when they first demonstrated the phrenic ampulla and the cardiac antrum. This in itself is fascinating history. W. B. Cannon and R. Moser in Boston were the first to study the anatomy and physiology of the cardia by means of contrast material. They made patients swallow capsules filled with bismuth. Bismuth was considered so poisonous at that time that they attached the capsules to strings that permitted them to pull the capsules out soon after they had passed the cardia. They noted that the capsules indeed were temporarily

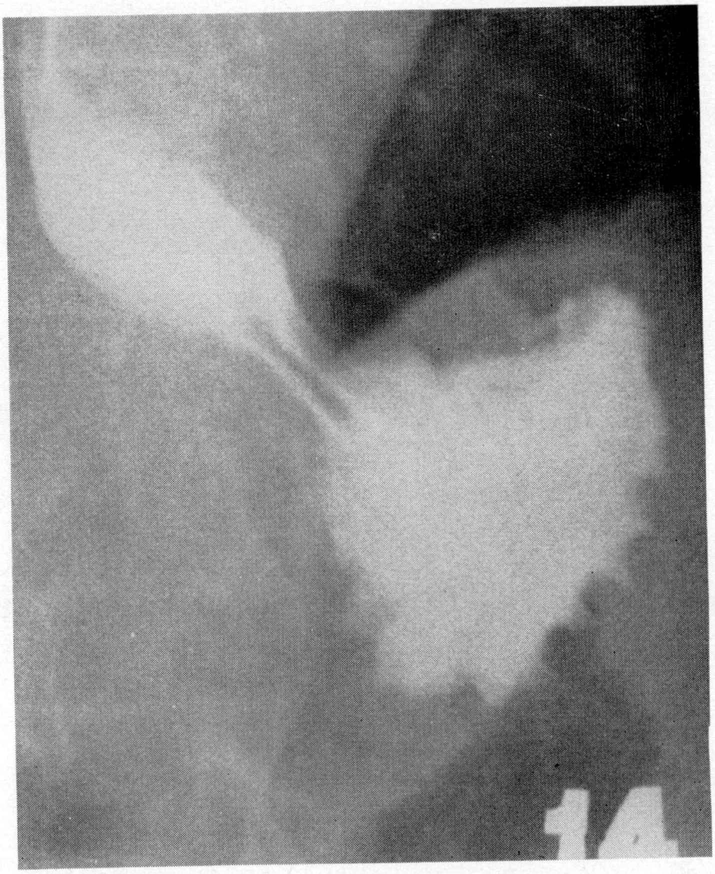

Fig. 5. Barium-filled funnel-shaped cardiac antrum, a zigzag border line is suggested here.

arrested immediately above the cardia. In 1899 Moriz Benedikt repeated the experiment with a mercury-filled bougie. In 1900 the United States radiologist Hirsch diagnosed the first hiatus hernia by means of x rays and a mercury-filled balloon. In 1904 Eppinger diagnosed the first hiatus hernia in a live patient, a diagnosis proved by autopsy, and it is interesting to note that he made his diagnosis first on the basis of auscultation and used x rays only to support his clinical judgment. In 1930, Markus Hajek, the otolaryngologist, described a special fluoroscope that permitted viewing the cardiac antrum to better advantage. With the ordinary fluoroscope or spotfilm device, the radiologist will miss the cardiac antrum because it is collapsed when the patient stands upright and is obscured by the gastric fundus when the patient lies

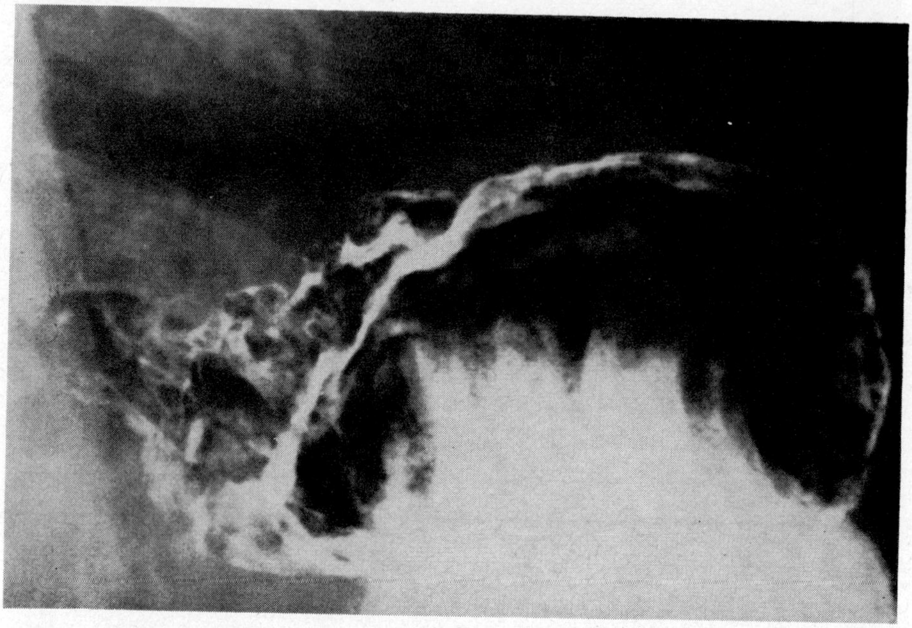

Fig. 6. Cardiac antrum, double contrast study, i.e., its wall coated with barium, its lumen filled with air.

supine. Hajek's machine permitted one to angle the x-ray tube toward the patient's head. In 1942 Dr. F. E. Templeton introduced me to the radiographic demonstration of the phrenic ampulla and showed me the existence of a ringlike indentation around its equator. Under his guidance, I exhibited such radiographs at the meeting of the American Roentgen Ray Society at Chicago, in 1942. Moreover, in his book *X-Ray Examination of the Stomach*, which appeared in 1944, he published two radiographs of a phrenic ampulla possessing an annular indentation. In 1953 Schatzki described a ring bisecting the phrenic ampulla that he thought to be pathological. It now bears his name and Schatzki ring is now considered a disease, while Templeton and I had heretofore considered it a normal anatomical structure frequently demonstrable in asyptomatic patients.

All these considerations did not seem to clarify the diagnosis of hiatus hernia since even a definition of this entity was lacking. At first it seemed simple to make the existence of a hiatus hernia dependent on the location of the border between esophagus and stomach. If it lay above the diaphragm the diagnosis of hernia appeared justified since

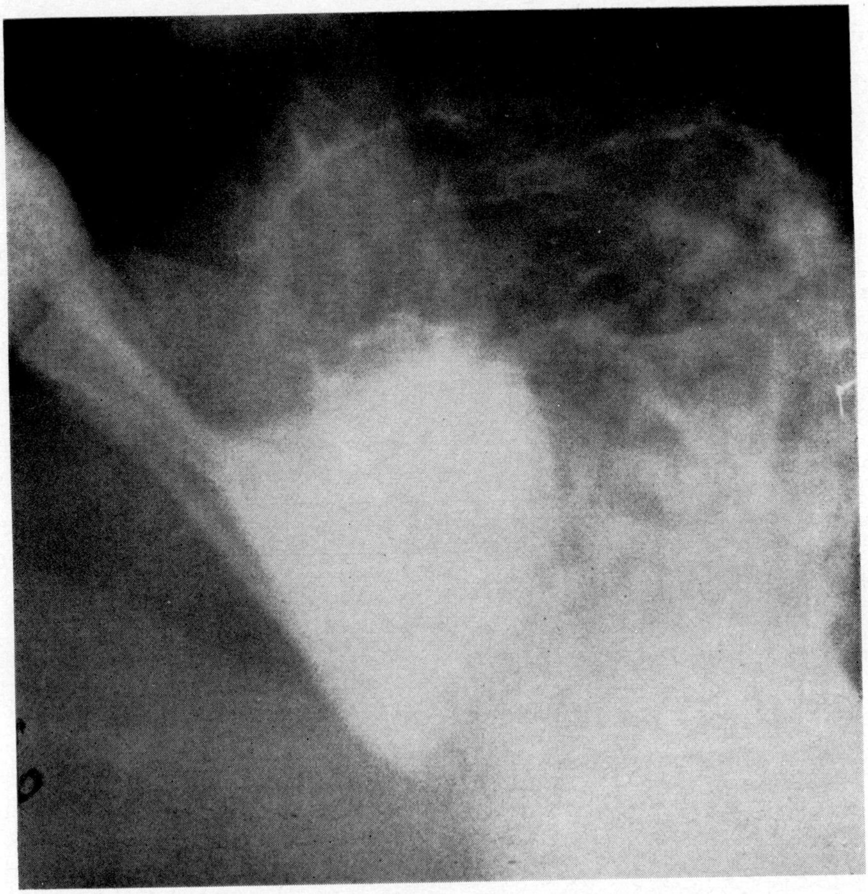

Fig. 7. Barium-filled funnel-shaped cardiac antrum without zigzag line. The gastric fundus is visible here through barium coating.

this would imply that indeed part of the stomach had been pulled into the thoracic cavity, unless—of course—this border line would *normally* reside in the chest. The question now crystallized into the need of first determining and locating the normal border line between esophagus and stomach. The older anatomists mentioned earlier, and also F. Magendie, described a distinct circular zigzag line marking the border between esophageal and gastric mucosa and named it ora serrata, nowadays frequently referred to as Z-line. They made it coincide with Arnold's furrow and the incisura cardiaca.

As early as 1841 Theile described a phrenicoesophageal membrane that arose from the diaphragm and inserted into the esophagus a few

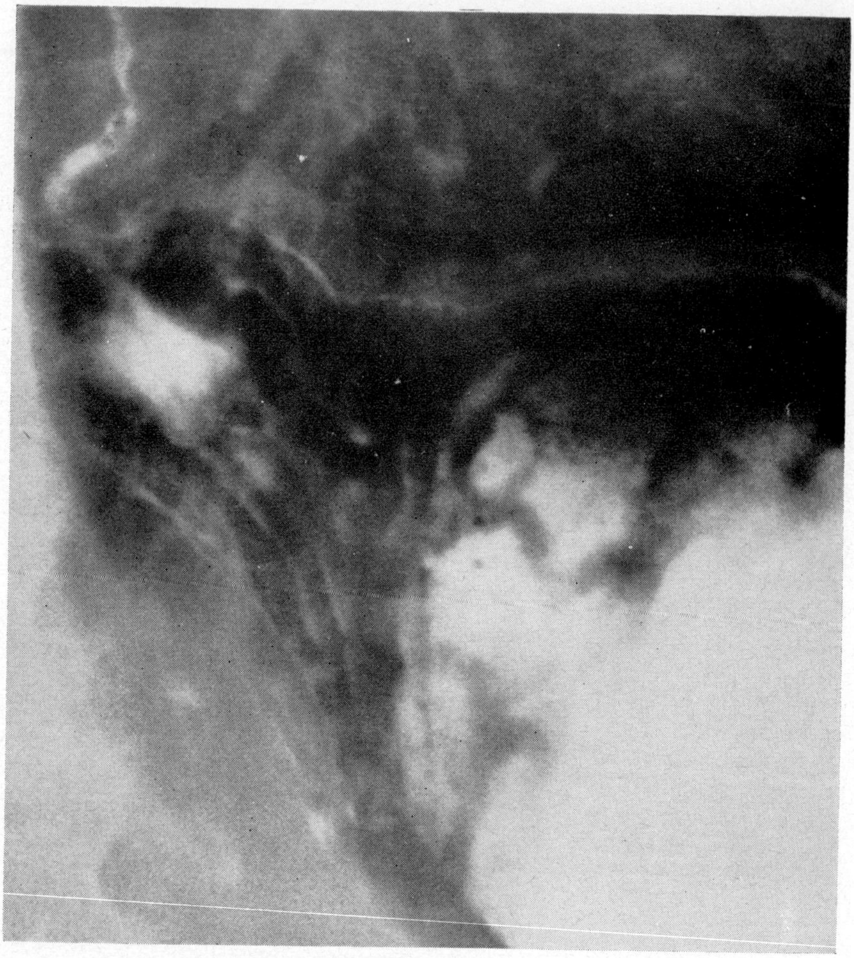

Fig. 8. Cardiac antrum during the act of belching.

centimeters above the hiatus. Hyrtl elaborated on it in 1844 and called it phrenoesophageal ligament. The anatomist von Hayek stated in 1933 that this membrane inserts below the phrenic ampulla. In 1942 Templeton and I suspected that it may insert into the convexity of the phrenic ampulla and possibly coincide with the esophageal ring but we could not prove it. In 1956 Gary, as an associate of Schatzki, published in the *New England Journal of Medicine* a single case that came to autopsy; in it a Schatzki ring coincided with the mucosa border line. The photograph of the specimen is not convincing, however. In the early 1950's Sir Stanford Cade implanted silver clips into the esophagus through an

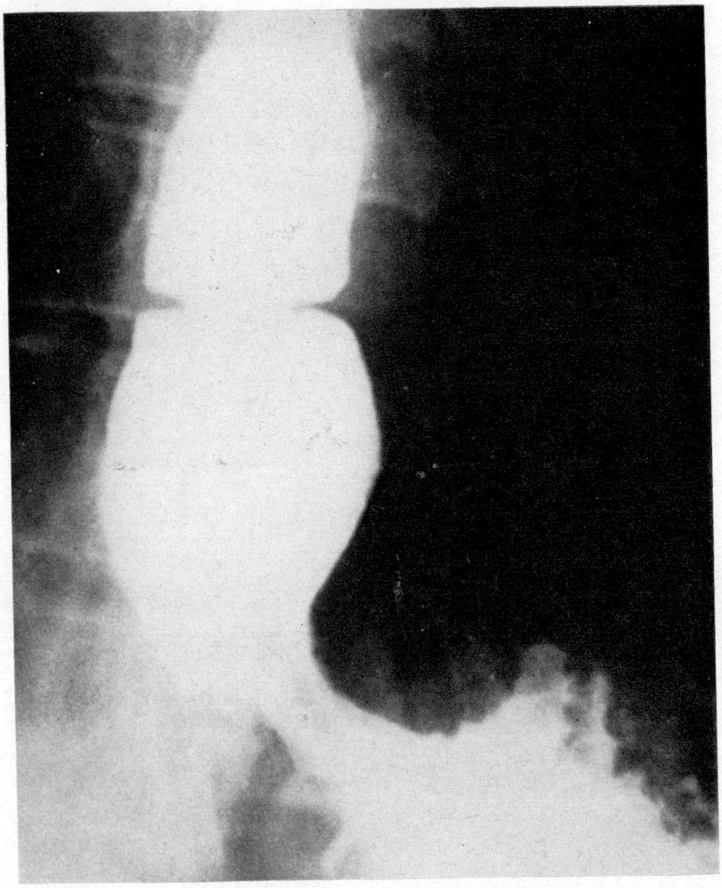

Fig. 9. Lower esophageal ring, transsecting the phrenic ampulla in an asymptomatic patient.

esophagoscope for the purpose of marking the mucosa border line. His radiologist reported then that these clips seemed to lie above the diaphragm. A similar approach is being taken currently by Dr. Charles Flood at the Columbia Presbyterian Medical Center, New York, N. Y., by introducing the endoscope down to the visible mucosa border line and then asking the radiologist to fluoroscope with the scope in place.

Obviously, if the mucosa border line indeed lies *normally* above the diaphragmatic hiatus, an additional element of confusion is introduced. Moreover, this difficulty is doubly compounded by a condition called "gastric-lined esophagus." It is being diagnosed with increasing frequency by some radiologists who consider it pathological. It is said

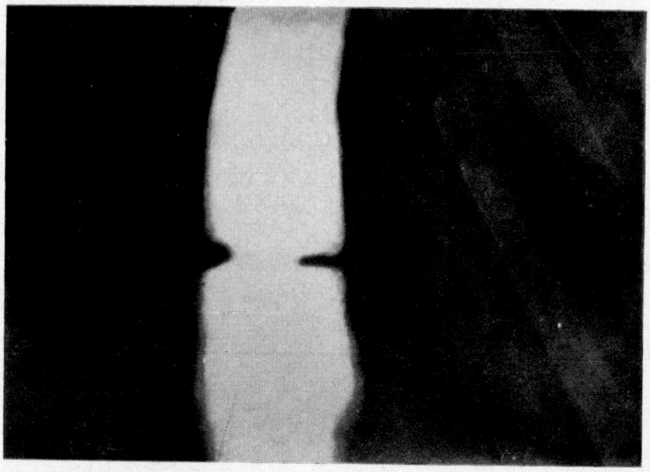

Fig. 10. Lower esophageal ring in an asymptomatic patient who did not exhibit a phrenic ampulla.

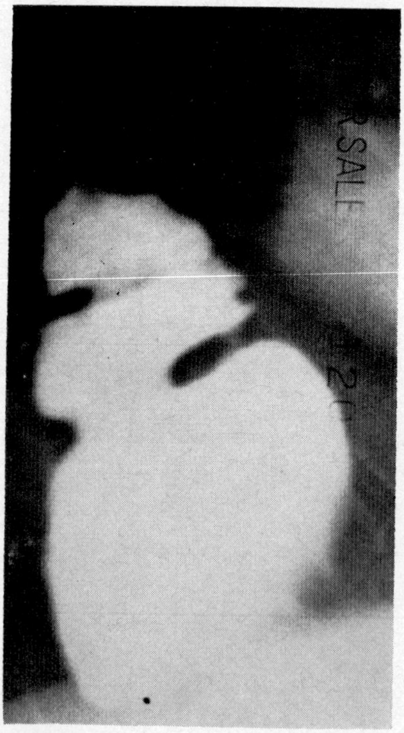

Fig. 11. Phrenic ampulla with two lower esophageal rings.

to be conducive to esophageal ulcers without gastroesophageal reflux as it occurs as an undesirable complication in some of the hiatus herniae. To moderate these opposing views, in regard to the location of the normal mucosa border line, one must quote Schaffer, who had been my teacher as chairman of the Department of Histology of the University of Vienna. In successive editions of his textbook of histology, he stated in the 1930's that there is an intermingling of gastric and esophageal epithelium near the gastroesophageal junction with the creation of gastric mucosa islands within the esophagus, so that one cannot truly speak of a distinct border between the two organs. Had the *Medical Tribune and Medical News* been aware of this, it could have saved itself considerable effort when on January 19, 1966, it printed a report headed: "Sharp Questions are Raised: Gastric Lining in Esophagus not Rare but 'Unrecognized.' "

It seems, then, that in the year of 1966 we have not come any closer to the solution. Radiographs of the cardiac antrum that I took suggest the existence of an ora serrata coincident with Arnold's furrow, in agreement with the older anatomists, but I cannot prove that the structure in question is indeed the mucosal border line (Figures 5 and 6). It is not always present (Figures 7 and 8).

An equal uncertainty exists at the present time about the significance of the lower esophageal ring. I for one believe that it is usually normal, for one can demonstrate its presence in about 80 per cent of asymptomatic patients by inducing the patient to swallow a very large bolus and to perform an extreme Valsalva test in Trendelenburg's position or by applying mild abdominal compression, or by having the patient cough vehemently (see Figures 9 and 10). In one instance, I have recently seen two esophageal rings, one on top of the other, separated by a distance of approximately 0.5 cm. (Figure 11). The frequency with which the lower esophageal ring can be observed in asymptomatic patients casts doubt also upon the theory that a visible ring constitutes a hiatus hernia, though some authors believe that indeed the presence of such a ring within the thoracic cavity is incontrovertible proof of diaphragmatic hernia. To illustrate the current disagreement, it is well to quote two papers, both of which appeared in December 1960 in two highly respected journals. In a paper entitled "The Lower Esophagus," published in the *American Journal of Roentgenology, Radium Therapy and Nuclear Medicine*, Walter S. Keyting *et al.*, under their subheading "Summary and Conclusions," state: "We unreservedly support the concept that the ring is the cardio-esophageal junction and that, therefore, when this ring is above the diaphragm, it indicates a hiatus hernia"; whereas Lauran D. Harris *et al.* in a paper entitled "Relation of the Lower Esophageal Ring to the Esophagogastric Junction," published in the *New England Journal of Medicine*, state under an identical subheading "The lower esophageal ring cannot be relied upon to mark the esophagogastric junction."

CHRONOLOGICAL TABLE

| | | | |
|---|---|---|---|
| Arnold, F. | 1838 | *Eppinger, H. | 1904 |
| Theile, F. W. | 1841 | Hasse, C. and Strecker, F. | 1905 |
| *Hyrtl, J. | 1844 | *Reich, L. | 1926 |
| Luschka, H. | 1857 | *Hajek, M. | 1930 |
| *Hyrtl, J. | 1879 | *Schaffer, J. | 1930 |
| *Laimer, E. | 1883 | *Hayek, H. von | 1933 |
| Gubaroff, A. von | 1886 | Templeton, F. E. | 1942 |
| Smirnoff, P. | 1886 | Cade, S. | ca. 1950 |
| Mehnert, E. | 1898 | Schatzki, R. | 1953 |
| Zusch, O. | 1898 | Gary, J. E. | 1956 |
| Cannon, W. B. and Moser, A. | 1898 | Keyting, W. S. *et al.* | 1960 |
| *Benedikt, M. | 1899 | Harris, L. D. *et al.* | 1960 |
| Hirsch, I. Seth | 1900 | | |

To summarize the historical events that contribute to our present knowledge or ignorance of the roentgen anatomy of the cardia, one might refer to the Table in which most of the authors quoted in this paper are listed in chronological sequence. Those preceded by an asterisk belong to the Graz—Vienna—Prague orbit, as is proper to point out to members of this society. Dr. Leo Reich is not only alive and well as a practicing radiologist in Arizona, but is also an active member of this society.

## *BIBLIOGRAPHY*

Arnold, R. *Untersuchungen im Gebiete der Anatomie und Physiologie.* Zurich, Hoehr, 1838.

Barret, N. R. Chronic peptic ulcer of the oesophagus and "oesophagitis," *Brit. J. Surg. 38*:175-82, 1950.

Cannon, W. B. and Moser, A. Movements of food in the esophagus, *Amer. J. Physiol. 1*:435-44, 1898. (As quoted by F. E. Templeton: see below.)

Cauthorne, R. T. *et al.* Study of patients with lower esophageal ring by simultaneous cineradiography and manometry, *Gastroenterology 49*:6, 632-40, 1965.

Cohen, B. R. *et al.* Correlation of manometric, oesophagoscopic and radiological findings in the columnar-lined gullet, *J. Brit. Soc. Gastroenterology 4*:406-12, 1963.

Eppinger, H. Beitrag zur Roentgendiagnostik und pathologischen Anatomie

einer Hernia diaphragmatica (vera) paraoesophagea. *Z. Heilkunde, Abt. Innere Med.* *25*:364-77, 1904.
Gary, J. E., Schatzki, R. and McMahon, H. E. Pathology of the lower esophageal ring, *N. Eng. J. Med.* *259*:1-8, 1958.
Gubaroff, A. von. Ueber den Verschluss des menschlichen Magens an der Kardia, *Arch. Anat. Physiol., Anat. Abt.* 1886, p. 395.
Hasse, C. and Strecker, F. Der menschliche Magen. *Arch. Anat. Physiol., Anat. Abt.* 1905, pp. 33-54.
Harris, L. D. *et al.* Relation of the lower esophageal ring to the esophagogastric junction, *New Eng. J. Med.* *263*:24, 1232-35, 1960.
Hayek, H. von. Die Kardia und der Hiatus oesophageus des Zwerchfells, *Z. Anat. Entw.* *100*:218, 1933.
His, W. Studien an gehärteten Leichen über Form und Lagerung des menschlichen Magens, *Arch. Anat. Physiol., Anat. Abt.* 1903, p. 345.
Hollowell, J. G. *et al.* Rumination and growth failure in male fraternal twin, *Pediatrics* *36*:565-71, 1965.
Hyrtl, J. *Lehrbuch der Anatomie des Menschen,* vol. 5, 14th ed. Vienna, Braumüller, 1878.
Ingelfinger, F. J. and Kramer, P. Dysphagia produced by contractile ring in lower esophagus, *Gastroenterology* *23*:419-30, 1953.
Jutras, A. *et al.* Etude radiologique de l'oesophage para-diaphragmatique et du cardia. Rapports, VIIe Congr. de Méd. electrorad. de Langue Fr., Paris, 1949, *J. Radiol. Elect.* *30*:373-414, 1949.
Keyting, W. S. *et al.* Lower esophagus, *Amer. J. Roentgen.* *84*:6, 1070-75, 1960.
Laimer, E. Beitrag zur Anatomie des Oesophagus, *Med. Jahrb.*, Vienna, 1883, 333-88.
Lerche, W. *The Esophagus and Pharynx in Action.* Springfield, Ill., Thomas, 1950.
Luschka, H. Das Antrum cardiacum des menschlichen Magens, *Virchow's Arch. Path. Anat.* *11*:427-33, 1857.
Mehnert, E. Ueber die klinische Bedeutung des Oesophagus und Aortenvariationen, *Arch. klin. Chir.* *58*:183-252, 1899.
Palmer, E. D. Attempt to localize normal esophagogastric junction, *Radiology* *60*: 825-31, 1953.
Pernkopf, E. Die Entwicklung des Vorderdarmes insbesondere des Magens der Wiederkäuer: Eine vergleichend-embryologische Studie, *Z. ges. Anat.* (Abt. 1) *94*: 490-622, 1931. (As quoted by H. Plenk.)
Poirier, P. and Charpy, A. *Abrégé d'anatomie.* Paris, Masson, 1908.
Reich, L. Ueber die Lokalisation der Kardia, *Mitt. Grenzg. Med. Chir.* *40*:481-503, 1927.
Reich, L. and Hitzenberger, K. Studien über die Form und Lage des Magens an der Hand von Ausgüssen mit einer rasch erstarrenden Masse. *Wien. Arch. inn. Med.* *9*:187, 1924.
Schatzki, R. and Gary, J. E. Dysphagia due to a diaphragm-like narrowing in the lower esophagus, *Amer. J. Roentgen.* *70*: 911-22, 1953.
Schaffer, J. *Lehrbuch der Histologie und Histogenese.* Vienna, Berlin, Urban, Schwarzenberg, 1933.
Schwarz, G. S. Scientific exhibit, the Phrenic Ampulla, *Amer. J. Roentgen.* *48*:4, 548, 1942.
Seaman, W. B. and Wylie, R. H. Observations on the nature of the stricture in Barret's esophagus (Allison and Johnstone's anomaly), *Radiology* *87*:30-32, 1966.
Smirnoff, P. As quoted by A. von Gubaroff (see above).
Templeton, F. E. *X-ray Examination of the Stomach.* Chicago, Univ. of Chicago Press, 1944, 1964.
Wolf, B. S. Gastroesophageal vestibule on roentgen examination: differentiation from the phrenic ampulla and minimal hiatal herniation, *J. Mount Sinai Hosp.* *25*:2, 167-200, 1958.
Anon. Gastric lining in esophagus not rare but "unrecognized," *Med. Tribune* *7*:9 (Jan. 19), 1966.
Anon. Pinpointing the "ring" in dysphagia. *Med. World News* *7*:12, 46, 1966.

# THE ACTION OF STREPTOMYCIN ON PROTEIN SYNTHESIS *IN VITRO**

SIDNEY PESTKA

National Heart Institute, National Institutes of Health
Bethesda, Md., 20014

STREPTOMYCIN produces numerous effects on bacteria prior to its ultimate destruction of cells sensitive to the antibiotic. In *Escherichia coli* cells Dubin, Hancock, and Davis[1] reported that the antibiotic produces an acceleration of potassium efflux together with an immediate stimulation of RNA** synthesis. This is shortly followed by a loss of viability and inhibition of protein synthesis with subsequent further gross changes as the cell degenerates.[1] Using polyauxotrophic mutant strains of streptomycin-sensitive *E. coli* with requirements for thymine, uracil, adenine, histidine, or arginine, Stern and Cohen[2] have demonstrated an immediate inhibition and subsequent stimulation of RNA synthesis by streptomycin. In their study, the stimulatory phase of RNA synthesis correlated with the loss of viability of streptomycin-sensitive *E. coli.*

It was early established by Fitzgerald, Bernheim, and Fitzgerald[3] that streptomycin inhibited protein biosynthesis in bacteria sensitive to the antibiotic, and many studies have subsequently confirmed these findings.[3-8] In streptomycin-dependent *E. coli* strains, Spotts[9] demonstrated that the synthesis of various enzymes was inhibited from O to 95 per cent when these strains were deprived of the antibiotic. These studies demonstrated that streptomycin could inhibit protein biosynthesis. These inhibitions were not seen in cells resistant to the antibiotic.

Another mode of action of streptomycin on protein biosynthesis was suggested by studies of streptomycin-dependent suppression.[10-13]

*Presented as part of a symposium on *Mode of Action of Penicillin and Streptomycin,* held at a meeting of the Section on Micro- and Molecular Biology, The New York Academy of Medicine, December 13, 1965.

**The following abbreviations are used: RNA, ribonucleic acid; A, C, G, U, and I, the bases adenine, cytosine, guanine, uracil, and hypoxanthine, also the corresponding nucleosides or nucleotides; in the case of polynucleotides, poly U refers to polyuridylic acid, poly A to polyadenylic acid, poly C to polycytidylic acid, and poly I to polyinosinic acid; sRNA, transfer or soluble ribonucleic acid; mRNA, messenger ribonucleic acid; Phe-sRNA, phenylalanyl-transfer ribonucleic acid, Ileu-sRNA, isoleucyl-transfer ribonucleic acid, etc. In the shorthand writing of oligonucleotides, as in UpUpUpC, the letter *p* to the left of the nucleoside initial indicates a 5′-phosphate; the letter *p* to the right, a 3′-phosphate; oligonucleotides are sometimes written as a series of letters without the phosphates to designate sequence with simplicity as UUC. One $A_{260}$ unit is the amount of material that in 1 ml. would yield a value of one for the absorbancy of 260 m*u* measured in a cuvette with a path length of 1 cm. SM in the tables and figures represents streptomycin.

Gorini, Gundersen, and Berger[10] described a new class of auxotrophic mutants of *E. coli* whose arginine requirement could be satisfied partially by streptomycin. Gorini and Kataja[11] showed that this phenomenon of "conditional-streptomycin-dependence" was not limited to the arginine pathway, but occurred also in many other types of auxotrophic mutants. Biochemical studies of conditional-streptomycin-dependent arginine mutants[10,11] showed that in the presence of streptomycin the missing enzyme of the arginine pathway (ornithine transcarbamylase) was synthesized to a slight extent. Since there was evidence that mutations of the streptomycin locus influence ribosomal structure,[14-16] Gorini and Kataja[11] suggested that streptomycin could influence the accuracy of reading of the genetic code during the translation of messenger RNA codons into the primary amino acid sequence of proteins. In addition to streptomycin-dependent suppression, other effects of streptomycin on regulatory systems have been described in streptomycin-dependent *E. Coli.*[17,18]

In *E. coli,* genetic analysis has shown that sensitivity, dependence, and single-step resistance to a high concentration of streptomycin are determined by multiple alleles at a single genetic locus.[19-21] From these and other studies, Spotts and Stanier[22] aptly predicted that the ribosome would be the common site of these alterations in streptomycin-sensitive, -dependent, and -resistant bacteria. They suggested that in streptomycin-sensitive cells, streptomycin prevents the attachment of mRNA to ribosomes; in streptomycin-dependent cells, it is required for mRNA attachment; and in streptomycin-resistant cells, mRNA attachment to ribosomes is unaffected by the presence of the antibiotic.

Despite the vast number of studies on the influence of streptomycin on cellular metabolism *in vivo* and *in vitro*, the precise mechanism by which the antibiotic performs its lethal act remains an enigma. Whether or not the effect of streptomycin on RNA synthesis, protein synthesis, or another system is the primary lethal event, it has been possible to study and to elucidate *in vitro* the effects on protein synthesis. It is the purpose of this paper to review and examine the effects of streptomycin on protein biosynthesis *in vitro*.

## Outline of Protein Biosynthesis

Protein biosynthesis in cell-free extracts occurs via the steps outlined in the following three reactions:

$$\text{Amino Acid} + \text{sRNA} + \text{ATP} \underset{\text{Enzymes}}{\overset{\text{Mg}^{++}}{\rightleftharpoons}} \text{Aminoacyl-sRNA} + \text{AMP} + \text{PP}_i \qquad (1)$$

$$\begin{array}{c}\text{Aminoacyl-sRNA}\\ + \\ \text{Ribosomes} \\ + \\ \text{sRNA}\end{array} \overset{\text{Mg}^{++},\ \text{K}^{+}}{\rightleftharpoons} \left[\begin{array}{c}\text{Aminoacyl-sRNA}\\ | \\ \text{Ribosomes} \\ | \\ \text{mRNA}\end{array}\right] \qquad (2)$$

$$\left[\begin{array}{c}\text{Aminoacyl-sRNA}\\ | \\ \text{Ribosomes} \\ | \\ \text{mRNA}\end{array}\right] \underset{\substack{\text{Polymerization}\\ \text{Enzymes}}}{\xrightarrow{\text{GTP, Mg}^{++},\ \text{K}^{+}}} \begin{array}{c}\text{Ribosomes} + \text{mRNA}\\ + \text{sRNA} \\ + \text{Polypeptides}\end{array} \qquad (3)$$

The first reaction represents the formation of a specific aminoacyl-sRNA.[23-27] The formation of aminoacyl-sRNA is not influenced by streptomycin at manyfold the concentration at which protein synthesis is markedly inhibited *in vivo* and *in vitro*.[7,16,28,29] Reaction 2 represents the specific binding of aminoacyl-sRNA to ribosomes in response to an oligo- or polynucleotide template.[30-34] This second reaction is the codon recognition process in protein biosynthesis whereby an aminoacyl-sRNA molecule is matched to its specific template codon. It occurs not only with 70 S ribosomes, but also with purified 30 S subunits.[35-38] Reaction 3 represents the sequential addition of amino acids into a polypeptide chain subsequent to matching of aminoacyl-sRNA species to template codons along the mRNA chain and requires the polymerization enzymes.[39-42] Although the codon recognition step 2 can occur with 30 S ribosomes alone, the polymerization reaction 3 requires 50 S subunits also.[38,43]

## Ribosomal Localization of Streptomycin-Sensitivity, -Resistance, and -Dependence

Using a cell-free amino acid incorporating system from mycobacteria, Erdös and Ullmann[44] showed that protein synthesis in cell-free extracts from streptomycin-sensitive bacteria was inhibited by streptomycin; however, protein synthesis in the extracts from streptomycin-resistant bacteria was insensitive to inhibition by the antibiotic. Using all possible combinations of supernatant and ribosomes from streptomycin-sensitive and -resistant *E. coli* strains, several laboratories[14-16] localized the streptomycin-sensitive site to the ribosomes. Similarly, using various combinations of 50 and 30 S subunits from streptomycin-sensitive and -resistant *E. coli* strains, Davies[45] and Cox, White, and Flaks[46] showed that the streptomycin-sensitive site resided on the 30 S subunit of the 70 S ribosome. Davies[45] also demonstrated that streptomycin did not interfere with the binding of $^{14}C$-poly U to streptomycin-sensitive ribosomes even though poly U-directed polyphenylalanine formation was markedly inhibited by the antibiotic. This demonstrated that streptomycin did not prevent this polynucleotide template (mRNA) from binding to the ribosome. The streptomycin effect was therefore localized somewhere between codon recognition and amino acid polymerization. Furthermore, Cox *et al.*[46] showed that 50 and 30 S subunits from streptomycin-dependent and -resistant *E. coli* strains behaved similarly with respect to $^{14}C$-phenylalanine incorporation into protein in the presence of a poly U template: streptomycin did not inhibit the $^{14}C$-phenylalanine incorporation into protein when ribosomes from a streptomycin-dependent strain were employed; in addition, no *in vitro* dependence on exogenous streptomycin was demonstrated for the $^{14}C$-phenylalanine incorporation.

## Miscoding During Protein Synthesis: Stimulation by Streptomycin

Although poly U predominantly stimulates the incorporation of phenylalanine into protein in cell-free extracts, under various conditions poly U can stimulate substantial amounts of leucine, isoleucine, or other amino acids into protein.[47-56] Alterations in the concentration of magnesium ions,[47, 49-52] *p*H,[55] temperature of the reaction,[49, 50] presence of organic solvents[56] or ratio of sRNA to ribosomes[53, 55, 56] can influence miscoding. Such nonspecific effects on coding occur regardless of the streptomycin phenotype of the *E. coli* strain from which the cell-free extracts are prepared. Studying protein synthesis in cell-free extracts from streptomycin-sensitive *E. coli* strains, however, Davies, Gilbert, and Gorini,[51] and Knippenberg, Classen, Grijm-Vos, Veldstra, and

Bosch[52] showed that streptomycin (and also other aminoglycoside antibiotics) can stimulate miscoding. Specifically, in the presence of poly U, streptomycin stimulates leucine, isoleucine, serine, and tyrosine incorporation into protein, using cell-free extracts from streptomycin-sensitive *E. coli* strains. Miscoding stimulated by streptomycin was small or negligible with cell-free extracts prepared from a streptomycin-resistant strain. Several groups[58, 59] presented evidence that, in the presence of streptomycin, miscoded amino acids incorporated into protein appeared to substitute for the proper amino acid in its position in the peptide chain.

Davies, Gorini, and Davis[53] surveyed the effect of seven aminoglycoside antibiotics on the coding specificity of the homopolymers poly U, poly A, poly C, and poly I. They found that the spectrum of misreading varied markedly with the antibiotic as well as with the polynucleotide template.

After studying the effect of the aminoglycoside antibiotics on polypeptide synthesis stimulated by polynucleotides of alternating nucleotide sequence, Davies, Jones, and Khorana[60] came to several conclusions concerning the nature of the misreading process. They found that the coding changes produced by streptomycin are highly specific, whereas those produced by neomycin are very extensive. Namely, alternating poly $(UC)_n$, which directed the incorporation of serine (UCU) and leucine (CUC), in the presence of streptomycin also stimulated the incorporation of phenylalanine (UUU, UUC), proline (CCC, CCU, CCA, CCG), and a slight amount of histidine (CAU, CAC). In the presence of neomycin, nine additional amino acids were incorporated into protein using the same poly $(UC)_n$ template: phenylalanine, proline, and histidine as well as arginine (CGC, CGU, CGA, CGG), isoleucine (AUU, AUC, AUA), threonine (ACU, ACC, ACA, ACG), glutamine (CAA, CAG), tyrosine (UAU, UAC), and cysteine (UGU, UGC). Their data support the conclusions that streptomycin stimulates the misreading of the 5′-terminal and internal positions of a trinucleotide codon, of only one base at a time, and of pyrimidines more frequently than purines. Neomycin, however, produces the streptomycin-coding errors as well as misreading of the 3′-terminal nucleosides and sometimes two bases of a codon at one time. In addition, it appears that reading frame shifts need not be invoked to explain any of the antibiotic-induced misreading phenomena and that the miscoding stimulated by streptomy-

TABLE I.—EFFECT OF STREPTOMYCIN ON BINDING OF $^{14}$C-AMINOACYL-sRNA's TO RIBOSOMES IN PRESENCE OF TRINUCLEOTIDES

| $^{14}$C-Aminoacyl-sRNA | Trinucleotide | μμMoles $^{14}$C-aminoacyl-sRNA bound to Ribosomes: Sensitive ribosomes —SM | +SM | Δμμ Moles | Resistant ribosomes —SM | +SM | Δμμ Moles |
|---|---|---|---|---|---|---|---|
| $^{14}$C-Phe-sRNA | None | 0.20 | 0.16 | —0.04 | 0.37 | 0.35 | —0.02 |
| | UpUpU | 0.58 | 0.33 | —0.25 | 0.68 | 0.70 | +0.02 |
| | UpUpC | 0.74 | 0.43 | —0.31 | 0.85 | 0.88 | +0.03 |
| $^{14}$C-Lys-sRNA | None | 0.32 | 0.32 | 0.00 | 0.49 | 0.57 | +0.08 |
| | ApApA | 1.07 | 1.29 | +0.22 | 1.25 | 1.28 | +0.03 |
| | pApApA | 1.26 | 1.64 | +0.38 | 1.50 | 1.53 | +0.03 |
| $^{14}$C-Pro-sRNA | None | 0.07 | 0.09 | +0.02 | 0.08 | 0.08 | 0.00 |
| | pCpCpC | 0.21 | 0.30 | +0.09 | 0.26 | 0.25 | —0.01 |

Each reaction mixture of 0.05 ml. contained the following: 0.03 *M* magnesium acetate; 0.05 *M* potassium acetate; 0.1 *M* Tris acetate, *p*H 7.2; 1.1 $A_{260}$ units of ribosomes from streptomycin-sensitive cells, 1.2 $A_{260}$ units of resistant ribosomes; 2 × $10^{-5}$ *M* streptomycin where indicated; 4.5 μμmoles $^{14}$C-Phe-sRNA (0.11 $A_{260}$ unit); 8.1 μμmoles $^{14}$C-Lys-sRNA (0.42 $A_{260}$ unit); 3.1 μμmoles $^{14}$C-Pro-sRNA (0.47 $A_{260}$ unit); 5.0 mμmoles UpUpU, 3.4 mμmoles UpUpC, 2.1 mμmoles ApApA, 2.1 mμmoles pApApA and 3.9 mμmoles pCpCpC. Incubations were carried out for 15 min. at 24°C. Assays were performed as previously described.[34] The Δμμmoles represents the difference between the binding of $^{14}$C-aminoacyl-sRNA in the presence and absence of SM.

cin of a specific base in a codon is to some extent dependent on the adjacent nucleotides. Thus, for example, it appears that a U between a 5′-and a 3′-terminal G in a codon is protected from misreading in the case of alternating poly $(UG)_n$. It should also be noted that in the case of the alternating copolymers poly $(AC)_n$ and poly $(AG)_n$ streptomycin produced no miscoding, but only inhibition of the amino acid incorporation stimulated by these templates.

## Localization of the Site of Action of Streptomycin on Protein Synthesis to the Recognition Process

Although streptomycin was shown to influence protein synthesis by cell-free extracts of cells, the specific reaction (i.e., 2 or 3) that was affected by streptomycin remained uncertain. Pestka, Marshall, and Nirenberg,[57] Pestka,[61] and Kaji and Kaji[62] showed that the recognition process was the step in protein biosynthesis that was influenced by the antibiotic. The data of Table I show that in response to trinucleotide templates the specific binding of aminoacyl-sRNA to ribosomes from streptomycin-sensitive cells is altered by streptomycin. The binding of

TABLE II.—EFFECT OF STREPTOMYCIN ON SPECIFICITY OF CODON RECOGNITION

| *¹⁴C-Aminoacyl-sRNA* | *Polynucleotide* | *μμMoles ¹⁴C-aminoacyl-sRNA bound to ribosomes* Sensitive ribosomes —SM | +SM | ΔμμMoles | Resistant ribosomes —SM | +SM | ΔμμMoles |
|---|---|---|---|---|---|---|---|
| ¹⁴C-Phe-sRNA | None | 0.64 | 0.52 | —0.12 | 1.15 | 1.11 | —0.04 |
| | Poly U | 9.38 | 9.37 | —0.01 | 10.1 | 10.3 | +0.20 |
| ¹⁴C-Ileu-sRNA | None | 0.14 | 0.12 | —0.02 | 0.14 | 0.14 | 0.00 |
| | Poly U | 1.22 | 2.94 | +1.72 | 1.03 | 1.05 | +0.02 |
| ¹⁴C-Leu-sRNA | None | 0.54 | 0.65 | +0.11 | 1.26 | 1.30 | +0.04 |
| | Poly U | 0.49 | 0.81 | +0.32 | 1.17 | 1.18 | +0.01 |
| ¹⁴C-Val-sRNA | None | 0.38 | 0.37 | —0.01 | 0.49 | 0.45 | —0.04 |
| | Poly U | 0.42 | 0.41 | —0.01 | 0.46 | 0.46 | 0.00 |
| ¹⁴C-Ser-sRNA | None | 1.52 | 1.53 | +0.01 | 1.79 | 1.68 | —0.11 |
| | Poly U | 1.36 | 1.83 | +0.47 | 1.54 | 1.49 | —0.05 |
| ¹⁴C-Pro-sRNA | None | 0.15 | 0.19 | +0.04 | 0.16 | 0.16 | 0.00 |
| | Poly U | 0.12 | 0.15 | +0.03 | 0.12 | 0.11 | —0.01 |

Each reaction mixture contained the components indicated in the legend of Table I in addition to the following: 2.2 $A_{260}$ units of ribosomes from streptomycin-sensitive *E. coli*, 2.4 $A_{260}$ units of ribosomes from the resistant strain; 16.0 μμmoles ¹⁴C-Phe-sRNA (0.44 $A_{260}$ unit); 18.4 μμmoles ¹⁴C-Ileu-sRNA (0.40 $A_{260}$ unit); 21.5 μμmoles ¹⁴C-Leu-sRNA (0.41 $A_{260}$ unit); 20 μμmoles ¹⁴C-Val-sRNA (.40 $A_{260}$ unit); 51 μμmoles ¹⁴C-Ser-sRNA (2.1 $A_{260}$ units); 4.6 μμmoles ¹⁴C-Pro-sRNA (0.70 $A_{260}$ unit); and poly U, 32 mμmoles base residues, where specified. The Δμμmoles represents the difference between the binding of ¹⁴C-aminoacyl-sRNA in the presence and absence of SM. Incubations were carried out for 20 min. at 24° C.

¹⁴C-Phe-sRNA in response to UpUpU or UpUpC is inhibited by streptomycin; the binding of ¹⁴C-Lys-sRNA in response to ApApA or pApApA is stimulated by streptomycin; and the binding of ¹⁴C-Pro-sRNA in response to pCpCpC is slightly stimulated by the antibiotic. Ribosomes prepared from a streptomycin-resistant *E. coli* strain showed little or no effects. These studies were carried out at 0.03 *M* $Mg^{++}$. When ¹⁴C-Lys-sRNA binding to ribosomes in response to pApApA was studied at 0.02 *M* $Mg^{++}$, streptomycin inhibited ¹⁴C-Lys-sRNA binding.[28]

The effect of streptomycin on template specificity is shown in Table II. In the presence of streptomycin and a poly U template ¹⁴C-Ileu-, ¹⁴C-Leu-, and ¹⁴C-Ser-sRNA were stimulated to bind to ribosomes prepared from a streptomycin-sensitive *E. coli* strain. Ribosomes from a streptomycin-resistant *E. coli* strain showed little or no effects. Figure 1 shows that a concentration of approximately 1 streptomycin molecule

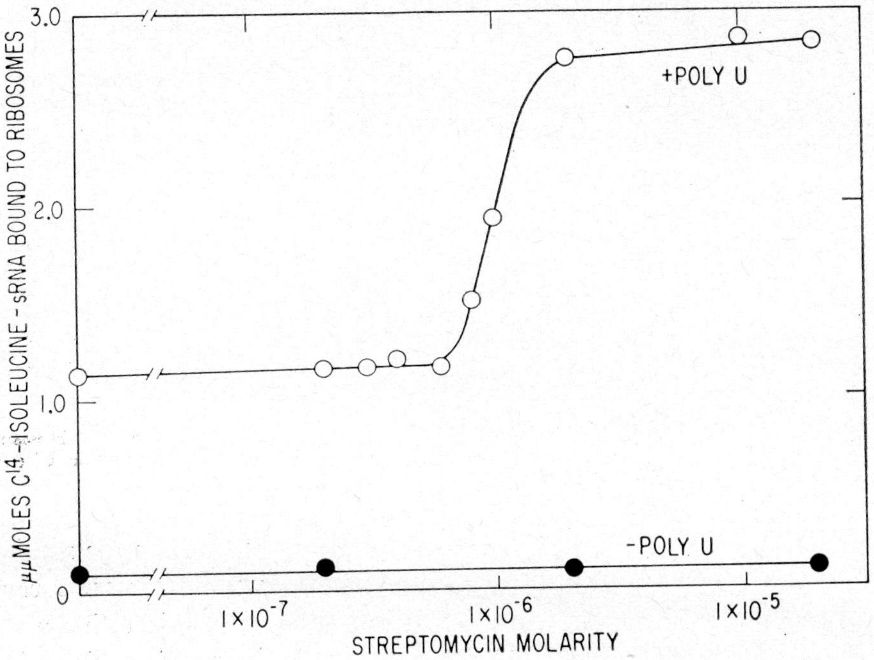


Fig. 1. The stimulation of poly U-dependent $^{14}$C-Ileu-sRNA binding to ribosomes as a function of streptomycin concentration. Reaction mixtures were similar to those described in the legend of Table II. Ribosomes from streptomycin-sensitive *E. coli* were used.

per ribosome was sufficient to produce the stimulation of binding of $^{14}$C-Ileu-sRNA to ribosomes in response to a poly U template. Furthermore, the data of Table III show that the stimulation of miscoding of $^{14}$C-Ileu-sRNA by streptomycin appears to be a function of template chain length: UpUpU, pUpUpU and $(pU)_4$ did not stimulate any binding of $^{14}$C-Ileu-sRNA to ribosomes in the presence of streptomycin; $(pU)_6$ probably did and $(pU)_{12}$ as well as poly U did stimulate the binding of $^{14}$C-Ileu-sRNA to ribosomes in the presence of streptomycin. It thus appears that, indeed, neighboring nucleotides can influence codon recognition as was recently also shown by Davies, Jones, and Khorana.[60]

A hypothesis of miscoding where there occurs a replacement of one amino acid by another appears inadequate to explain all the effects of streptomycin on codon recognition during protein biosynthesis. Such a hypothesis of misreading in the presence of streptomycin would predict that the sum of the inhibitions of all the amino acids would equal the sum of all the amino acid stimulations. The data of Knippenberg *et al.*[52] and Davies *et al.*[53] do not fit this prediction. Whether there is a

TABLE III.—EFFECT OF CHAIN LENGTH ON THE $^{14}$C-ILEU-sRNA AMBIGUITY

| *Oligo U* | *μμMoles $^{14}$C-Ileu-sRNA bound to ribosomes* —*SM* | +*SM* | Δ*μμMoles* |
|---|---|---|---|
| None | 0.08 | 0.12 | +0.04 |
| UpUpU | 0.10 | 0.10 | 0.00 |
| pUpUpU | 0.10 | 0.13 | +0.03 |
| $(pU)_4$ | 0.09 | 0.11 | +0.02 |
| $(pU)_6$ | 0.08 | 0.16 | +0.08 |
| $(pU)_{12}$ | 0.09 | 0.24 | +0.15 |
| Poly U | 0.66 | 2.12 | +1.46 |

Reaction mixtures were similar to those described in the legend of Table II. Ribosomes were from streptomycin-sensitive *E. coli* cells, and 15 mμmoles of base residues of each template were used where specified.

net stimulation or inhibition of protein synthesis depends on the specific oligo- or polyribonucleotide template, the magnesium concentration, and several other factors.[51-53, 57, 60-62] It should be emphasized, however, that ribosomes prepared from streptomycin-resistant *E. coli* strains, although relatively insensitive to inhibitions and stimulations of protein synthesis and codon recognition produced by streptomycin, show reproducible persistent slight effects in the presence of streptomycin.[51, 52, 57, 61, 63] In fact, Anderson, Gorini, and Breckenridge[64] also have recently shown that streptomycin stimulated miscoding with ribosomes prepared from some streptomycin-resistant *E. coli* strains; and they demonstrated that there was a correlation between the ability of the ribosomes to miscode in the presence of streptomycin *in vitro* and the ability of streptomycin to correct or substitute for an arginine requirement (ornithine transcarbamylase defect) *in vivo*. Specifically, if streptomycin could correct the arginine requirement *in vivo*, then *in vitro* streptomycin stimulated miscoding with ribosomes isolated from these strains. In those streptomycin-resistant strains whose arginine requirement could not be corrected by streptomycin *in vivo*, then *in vitro* the antibiotic did not stimulate any detectable miscoding with ribosomes isolated from these *E. coli* strains.

## Effect of Ribosomal Dissociation on Streptomycin Action

When 70 S ribosomes are dissociated into subunits before studying the binding of aminoacyl-sRNA in response to poly U, this binding

TABLE IV.—EFFECT OF DISSOCIATION ON $^{14}$C-PHENYLALANINE-sRNA BINDING TO RIBOSOMES IN PRESENCE AND ABSENCE OF STREPTOMYCIN

| | | *μμMoles $^{14}$C-phenylalanine-sRNA bound to ribosomes* | | | | | |
|---|---|---|---|---|---|---|---|
| | | *Sensitive ribosomes* | | | *Resistant ribosomes* | | |
| *Treatment of ribosomes* | *Polynucleotide* | *—SM* | *+SM* | *ΔμμMoles* | *—SM* | *+SM* | *ΔμμMoles* |
| Nondissociated | None | 0.09 | 0.06 | —0.03 | 0.24 | 0.22 | —0.02 |
| Nondissociated | Poly U | 3.73 | 3.61 | —0.12 | 4.24 | 4.54 | +0.30 |
| Reassociated | None | 0.09 | 0.15 | +0.06 | 0.27 | 0.29 | +0.02 |
| Reassociated | Poly U | 5.67 | 2.91 | —2.76 | 5.75 | 5.67 | —0.08 |

Each reaction mixture contained the components indicated in legend of Table I except for the following: 0.02 *M* magnesium acetate; 18.5 mμmoles of base residues of poly U where specified; 8.8 μμmoles $^{14}$C-Phe-sRNA (0.22 $A_{260}$ unit). The Δμμmoles represents the difference between the binding of $^{14}$C-Phe-sRNA in the presence and absence of streptomycin. Nondissociated ribosomes (in 0.014 *M* $Mg^{++}$) are 70 S ribosomes which have never been exposed to a magnesium concentration below 0.014 *M* $Mg^{++}$. Reassociated ribosomes are 70 S ribosomes which have been dissociated into 50 and 30 S subunits by dialysis against 1 x $10^{-4}$ *M* $Mg^{++}$ and then reassociated to 70 S ribosomes by addition of magnesium to 0.01 *M* or greater.

differs from that observed using ribosomes that have never been dissociated into subunits.[63] The data of Table IV show that the binding of $^{14}$C-Phe-sRNA in the presence of poly U to reassociated* ribosomes from streptomycin-sensitive cells is inhibited by streptomycin, whereas the same binding to nondissociated* ribosomes is unaltered by the antibiotic. In contrast, the binding of $^{14}$C-Ileu-sRNA in response to poly U is decreased in the presence or absence of streptomycin if ribosomes are first dissociated (Table V). These results suggest that there may be different sites for inhibition of protein synthesis and for miscoding. Davies, Jones, and Khorana[60] came to similar conclusions in their studies on the effect of streptomycin on the incorporation of amino acids into protein directed by polynucleotides of alternating base sequence. Supporting the hypothesis that inhibition and miscoding of protein synthesis are produced by different mechanisms, Davies, Anderson, and Davis[65] established that the antibiotic spectinomycin could inhibit protein synthesis *in vivo* and *in vitro*, but produced no detectable miscoding *in vitro*. Furthermore, spectinomycin is bacteriostatic rather than bactericidal, as is streptomycin, suggesting that miscoding may be related to

*Nondissociated ribosomes refer to 70 S ribosomes from *E. coli* that have been prepared and stored in 0.014 *M* magnesium acetate so that they have never been dissociated into subunits during preparation. Reassociated ribosomes refer to 70 S ribosomes dissociated into 30 and 50 S subunits by dialysis against 1 × $10^{-4}$ *M* magnesium acetate and then reassociated to 70 S ribosomes by raising the magnesium concentration to 0.01 *M* or higher. As used in this paper, the word "ribosomes" refers to nondissociated 70 S ribosomes unless otherwise specified.

TABLE V.—EFFECT OF STREPTOMYCIN AND DISSOCIATION OF RIBOSOMES ON BINDING OF $^{14}$C-ISOLEUCINE-sRNA TO RIBOSOMES

| *Treatment of ribosomes* | *Polynucleotide* | *μμMoles $^{14}$C-Ileu-sRNA bound to ribosomes* — *Sensitive ribosomes* —SM | +SM | Δμμ*Moles* | *Resistant ribosomes* —SM | +SM | Δμμ*Moles* |
|---|---|---|---|---|---|---|---|
| Nondissociated | None | 0.14 | 0.12 | —0.02 | 0.14 | 0.14 | 0.00 |
| Nondissociated | Poly U | 1.22 | 2.94 | +1.72 | 1.03 | 1.05 | +0.02 |
| Reassociated | None | 0.12 | 0.16 | +0.04 | 0.14 | 0.14 | 0.00 |
| Reassociated | Poly U | 0.98 | 1.20 | +0.22 | 0.58 | 0.50 | —0.08 |

The reaction mixtures were similar to those described in the legend of Table II, with minor modifications. Nondissociated and reassociated ribosomes were prepared as described in the legend of Table IV.

the lethal event.

Herzog[66] observed a relationship between streptomycin action and ribosomal dissociation. He found that after exposing streptomycin-sensitive *E. coli* cells to the antibiotic, 70 S ribosomes isolated from these cells did not dissociate as readily as ribosomes from cells not exposed to streptomycin. In control experiments he showed that exposure of isolated ribosomes to streptomycin did not alter their ability to dissociate and, furthermore, that the dissociation of ribosomes isolated from a streptomycin-resistant *E. coli* strain was not influenced by treating the cells with streptomycin. In addition, he demonstrated that chloramphenicol blocks this effect of streptomycin on ribosomal dissociation and, since chloramphenicol also blocks the lethal action of streptomycin, he suggested that this "sticking effect" might be related to the lethal action of the antibiotic. This observation may be related to the fact that nondissociated ribosomes miscode better than reassociated ribosomes (Table V). If ribosomal dissociation were obstructed by streptomycin, it might be expected that there would be more miscoding. Thus, if the miscoding phenomenon were the lethal event, the "sticking effect" might well be related to the lethal action of streptomycin.

In addition, when the binding of $^{14}$C-Phe-sRNA to isolated 30 S ribosomal subunits in response to poly U is examined as a function of magnesium concentration as shown in Figure 2, streptomycin was found to inhibit this binding at magnesium concentrations less than 0.03 *M*. Thus it is clear from this curve that streptomycin can influence the recognition process which occurs on the 30 S ribosome alone. So far,

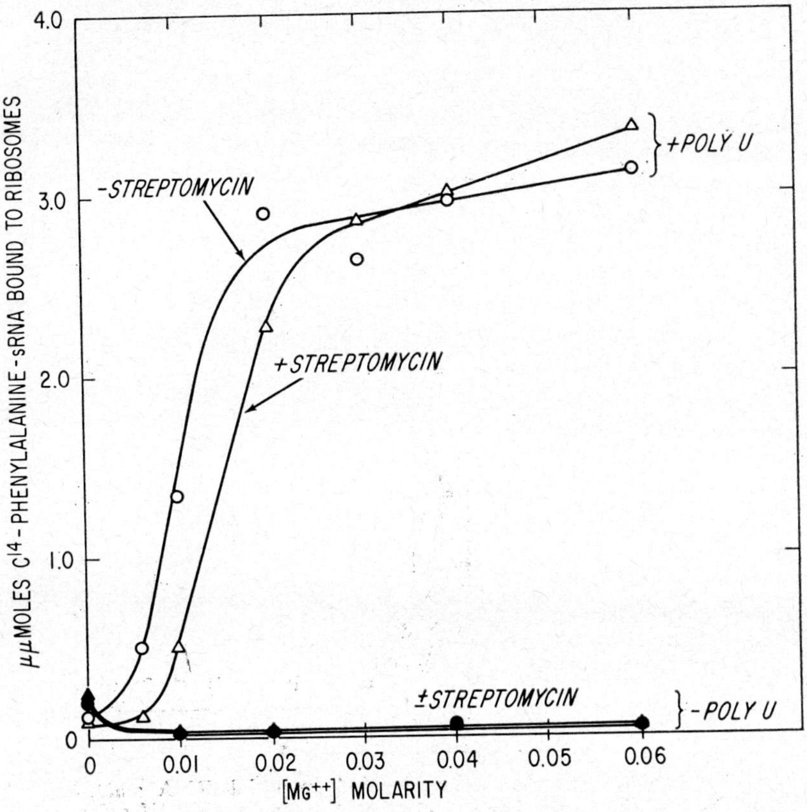


Fig. 2. The effect of magnesium concentration and streptomycin on the $^{14}$C-Phe-sRNA binding to 30 S ribosomes. The binding of $^{14}$C-Phe-sRNA to purified 30 S subunits was determined as described in the legend of Table II, with the exception of the following: 18 mμmoles of base residues of poly U where indicated; 8.8 μμmoles of $^{14}$C-Phe-sRNA (0.22 $A_{260}$ unit); 0.27 $A_{260}$ unit of 30 S ribosomes from streptomycin-sensitive *E. coli*.

however, no miscoding has been demonstrated using 30 S subunits alone. Perhaps 50 S subunits have a role in miscoding.

## Effect of Streptomycin on Polydeoxyribonucleotides and Other Templates

In recent experiments McCarthy and Holland[67] showed that in the presence of streptomycin or similar antibiotics denatured DNA could serve as a direct template for protein synthesis in cell-free *E. coli* extracts. Similarly, it was found that in the presence of neomycin denatured ribosomal and soluble ribonucleic acids could serve as templates for amino acid incorporation into protein in cell-free extracts.[68] Under

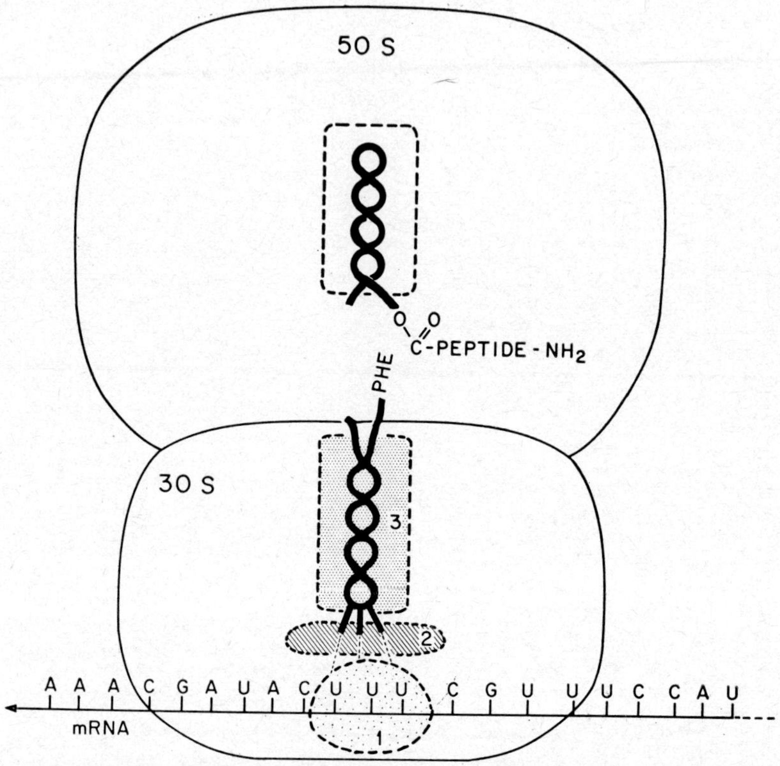


Fig. 3. This diagram represents aminoacyl-sRNA, peptidyl-sRNA and mRNA bound to a 70 S ribosome. Phenylalanyl-sRNA is shown matched to a UUU codon on the 30 S ribosome. Although the site for binding of aminoacyl-sRNA is shown on the 30 S subunit and the site for binding of peptidyl-sRNA on the 50 S subunit, it is possible that aminoacyl- and peptidyl-sRNA each overlap the two subunits. In fact, the precise number of binding sites for the various types of sRNA's and the specific relationship between them remains to be clarified.

usual conditions of *in vitro* protein synthesis in cell-free extracts, polydeoxyribonucleotides do not serve as templates for amino acid incorporation into polypeptides[67, 69] or for codon recognition.[34] By permitting polydeoxyribonucleotides to serve as templates streptomycin, neomycin and kanamycin clearly alter the structural requirements for the template in protein synthesis. In this case, the antibotics make the 2′-hydroxyl group of polyribonucleotides unnecessary as a template requirement whereas it was apparently necessary in their absence. In addition, in the absence of neomycin native ribosomal ribonucleic acid is a poor template for protein synthesis in cell-free extracts dependent on synthetic polynucleotides.[48, 67] Neomycin, however, permits native ribosomal ribonucleic acid with substantial secondary structure to serve as a tem-

TABLE VI.—EFFECT OF STREPTOMYCIN AND OLIGOAMINES ON $^3$H-PHE-sRNA BINDING TO RIBOSOMES

| *Addition* | *μμMoles $^3$H-Phe-sRNA bound to ribosomes* —*Streptomycin* | +*Streptomycin* |
|---|---|---|
| None | 0.06 | 0.08 |
| Putrescine and spermidine | 0.66 | 0.67 |

Reactions carried out were similar to those described in the legend of Table II, with the exception of the following: 0.01 *M* magnesium acetate; 0.05 *M* Tris acetate, *p*H 7.2; 0.013 *M* putrescine and 0.002 *M* spermidine where indicated; 1.5 $A_{260}$ units of reassociated ribosomes from streptomycin-sensitive *E. coli;* 1.9 μμmoles of $^3$H-Phe-sRNA (0.058 $A_{260}$ unit). No template was added to these reaction mixtures.

plate for protein synthesis. Usually template secondary structure inhibits amino acid incorporation into proteins in cell-free extracts.[70] Thus, during protein synthesis the aminoglycoside antibiotics presumably cause substantial perturbation to the ribosome-template structure thus permitting as templates structures that ordinarily do not serve this function.

## Some Recent Experiments to Localize Further the Action of Streptomycin

Although the action of streptomycin on protein biosynthesis has been localized to the recognition process,[57, 61, 62] a more precise definition of its action has not been delineated. The diagram (Figure 3) indicates that aminoacyl-sRNA and template both bind to the 30 S ribosomal subunit.[35-38, 71] The aminoacyl-sRNA that binds to the 30 S subunit is that molecule involved in the recognition step. In fact, there may be two sites for aminoacyl-sRNA on the 30 S subunit.[38] The 50 S subunit probably contains the site for the sRNA molecule bearing the nascent protein chain.[72] However, the total number of sRNA molecules on the 30 and 50 S subunits and the precise relationship between them is not clear at present. Since it has been established that streptomycin acts on the 30 S ribosomal subunit,[45, 46] the antibiotic could interfere with the process of codon recognition by reacting with the aminoacyl-sRNA site (site 3), by influencing the codon attachment site (site 1) or by interfering with the aminoacyl-sRNA-codon interaction (site 2).

The data of Table VI indicate that streptomycin does not influence the oligoamine-stimulated binding of aminoacyl-sRNA to ribosomes

TABLE VII—EFFECT OF STREPTOMYCIN AND OLIGONUCLEOTIDES ON BINDING OF $^{14}$C-PHE-sRNA TO RIBOSOMES

| *Oligonucleotide* | *μμMoles $^{14}$C-Phe-sRNA bound to ribosomes* −SM | +SM | ΔμμMoles |
|---|---|---|---|
| None | 0.21 | 0.19 | −0.02 |
| UpUpU | 0.85 | 0.55 | −0.30 |
| UpUpUp | 0.68 | 0.48 | −0.20 |
| pUpUpU | 1.27 | 1.96 | +0.69 |

Reactions were carried out as described in the legend of Table I, with the following exception: 8.5 μμmoles of $^{14}$C-Phe-sRNA (0.31 $A_{260}$ unit); approximately 0.25 $A_{260}$ unit of trinucleotides, where indicated. Ribosomes used were prepared from streptomycin-sensitive *E. coli*.

in the absence of a template. The results are similar with reassociated or nondissociated ribosomes. It is apparent that in the absence of any added template, the addition of oligoamines stimulates substantial $^{3}$H-Phe-sRNA to bind to ribosomes. Streptomycin does not influence this oligoamine-stimulated binding. In addition, it should be noted that the oligoamines cannot inhibit or prevent the streptomycin inhibition of Phe-sRNA binding to reassociated ribosomes in response to poly U (data not shown). These results suggest that a template may be necessary to mediate the streptomycin effect and that streptomycin does not act directly on the aminoacyl-sRNA binding site (site 3).

Table VII presents data indicating that alterations on the template influence the effect of streptomycin on $^{14}$C-Phe-sRNA binding to ribosomes. Streptomycin inhibits the binding of $^{14}$C-Phe-sRNA to ribosomes directed by UpUpU or UpUpUp templates with a 3′-terminal or no terminal phosphate. On the other hand, the presence of a 5′-terminal phosphate reverses the streptomycin inhibition of $^{14}$C-Phe-sRNA binding to ribosomes in response to pUpUpU. In fact, the data of Table VII show that streptomycin stimulates the binding of $^{14}$C-Phe-sRNA in response to pUpUpU. This possibly suggests that streptomycin may interact with the codon site (site 1) and that the presence of a 5′-terminal phosphate can significantly alter this interaction. This possible interaction of streptomycin with the 5′-terminal end of a trinucleotide codon may be related to the fact that streptomycin appears predominantly to produce miscoding of the 5′-terminal or internal base of a codon.

Furthermore, the data of Table VIII show that streptomycin can

TABLE VIII—EFFECT OF STREPTOMYCIN ON $^{3}$H-OLIGONUCLEOTIDE AND $^{14}$C-PHE-sRNA BINDING TO RIBOSOMES

| | | *μμMoles bound to ribosomes* | | | |
|---|---|---|---|---|---|
| | | *$^{3}$H-oligonucleotide* | | *$^{14}$C-Phe-sRNA* | |
| *Oligonucleotide* | *sRNA* | *−SM* | *+SM* | *−SM* | *+SM* |
| None | $^{14}$C-Phe-sRNA | — | — | 0.56 | 0.43 |
| $^{3}$H-UUC | None | 0.42 | 0.36 | — | — |
| $^{3}$H-UUC | $^{14}$C-Phe-sRNA | 1.24 | 0.87 | 1.40 | 0.95 |
| $^{3}$H-UUUC | None | 1.29 | 1.05 | — | — |
| $^{3}$H-UUUC | $^{14}$C-Phe-sRNA | 3.17 | 2.39 | 1.51 | 1.17 |

Reactions were carried out as described in the legend of Table I, with minor modifications. The ribosomes used were from streptomycin-sensitive *E. coli.* Data taken from Hatfield and Nirenberg.[75]

influence the binding of templates as well as aminoacyl-sRNA to ribosomes. Hatfield[73, 74] and Hatfield and Nirenberg[75] have shown that tri- and oligonucleotide templates and aminoacyl-sRNA require the presence of each other for their maximal binding to ribosomes. As may be seen in Table VIII, the data show that streptomycin can inhibit the binding of $^{3}$H-UpUpC and $^{3}$H-UpUpUpC as well as the binding of $^{14}$C-Phe-sRNA stimulated by these templates. The data do not distinguish whether streptomycin acts primarily on the binding of the template or the aminoacyl-sRNA, for the binding of one is dependent on the binding of the other. In any case, it appears possible that streptomycin may act directly on the binding of the template.

The effect of streptomycin on the binding of aminoacyl-sRNA's and on the incorporation of amino acids into protein appears to be a function of the template rather than the amino acid or aminoacyl-sRNA. Specifically, phenylalanine incorporation can be inhibited by streptomycin if the template is poly U,[14, 15] but is stimulated if the template is alternating poly $(UC)_n$.[60] On the contrary, serine and leucine incorporation is stimulated by streptomycin if the template is poly U,[51-53] but is inhibited by the antibiotic if the template is alternating poly $(UC)_n$.[60] Other examples can be given of streptomycin having different effects on the incorporation of a given amino acid depending on the polynucleotide template. These results further serve to support the hypothesis that streptomycin does not act directly on the binding of aminoacyl-sRNA to ribosomes, but probably on the template itself. It may distort the codon itself or it may alter the over-all interaction

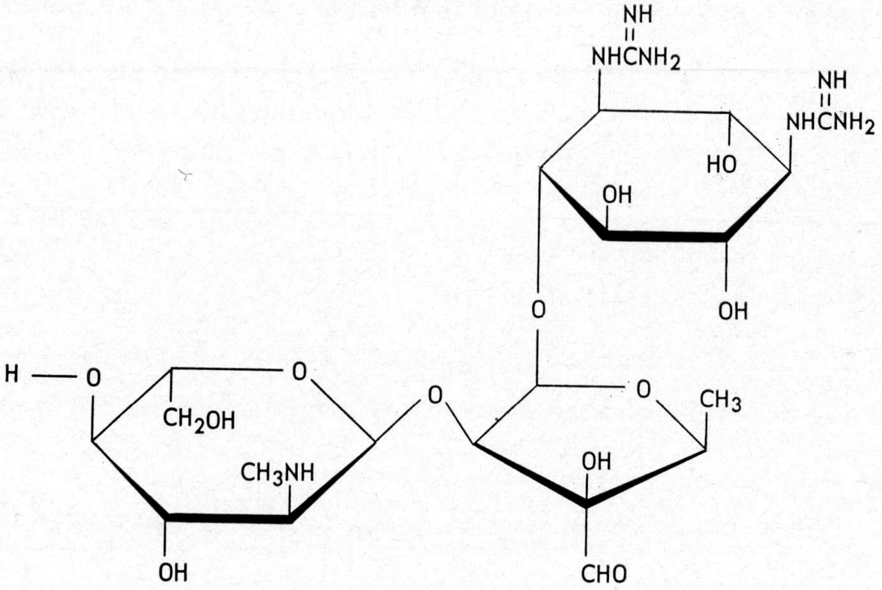


STREPTOMYCIN

Fig. 4. The structure is taken from Rinehart.[77]

of the codon and the aminoacyl-sRNA which occurs on the 30 S ribosome during the recognition process.

## STRUCTURAL REQUIREMENTS OF STREPTOMYCIN ACTION

Various modifications of the streptomycin[76] molecule (Figure 4) can be made without destroying its antibiotic activity. The aldehyde group can be converted to a hydroxyl group (dihydrostreptomycin) without altering its antibiotic action. Also, after the addition of mannose to the 4-hydroxyl of the *N*-methyl-L-glucosamine moiety (mannosidostreptomycin) or the conversion of the methyl group of streptose to a hydroxymethyl group (hydroxystreptomycin), the molecule retains its antibiotic activity.[76] These structural changes do not alter the net positive charge of the molecule. On the other hand, two structural derivatives in which the net positive charge is altered (dideguanyldihydrostreptomycin and monocarbobenzyloxy-dihydrostreptomycin) are both devoid of biological activity *in vivo*.[76] Correspondingly, upon removal of the guanido groups of dihydrostreptomycin, there is a loss of activity on aminoacyl-sRNA binding to ribosomes with respect to inhibition, stimulation, or miscoding of aminoacyl-sRNA binding.[28]

## Some Miscellaneous Comments on Streptomycin-Resistance and -Sensitivity

It should be noted that not all forms of streptomycin-resistance reside in the ribosomal structure. Some *E. coli* strains with a "multiple drug resistance" episome are resistant to several antibiotics because of reduced permeability for them.[78] In fact, although the organism is resistant to streptomycin *in vivo*, in cell-free extracts from an *E. coli* strain containing this episome phenylalanine incorporation in response to poly U is inhibited by streptomycin similar to cell-free extracts from streptomycin-sensitive *E. coli* strains.[79] This and other evidence support the claims that drug resistance in these strains carrying the episomal resistance factor is due to reduced permeability for the antibiotics to which they are resistant, and not to any ribosomal changes.

Mammalian cells and cell-free extracts appear to be relatively resistant to the action of streptomycin.[29, 80, 81] The concentration of streptomycin necessary to kill mammalian cells is 1000-fold the concentration that kills sensitive *E. coli* cells.[80] Mammalian ribosomes are, therefore, probably inherently resistant to the antibiotic. Although sensitivity and resistance to streptomycin have been reported in mammalian cells,[80, 81] this phenomenon appears to be a function of the presence or absence of cysteine in the growth medium. Furthermore, mammalian cells that are sensitive to streptomycin are unaffected by dihydrostreptomycin.[81] Since streptomycin and dihydrostreptomycin affect *in vivo* and *in vitro* bacterial systems similarly, the action of these antibiotics on mammalian and bacterial cells appears to be inherently different. On the other hand Krueger[82] has suggested that streptomycin stimulates the formation of antibody with altered serological specificity in a manner similar to its effect on protein synthesis in bacterial extracts. However, the precise nature of this altered antibody remains to be elucidated.

## Conclusions and Comments

In this paper, the effects of streptomycin on *in vitro* protein synthesis have been discussed. The antibiotic produces various effects on polynucleotide-directed amino acid incorporation depending on both the specific polynucleotide template and the amino acid. From data presented and other studies, it appears that a molecule of streptomycin bound to the 30 S subunit of a streptomycin-sensitive cell interacts with the ribosome-template structure, thus altering the interaction between the template codon and its matching aminoacyl-sRNA. In this way the antibiotic produces inhibitions, stimulations, or misreadings during protein biosynthesis. The specific effects that the antibiotic produces on codon recognition *in vitro* are a function of the template as well as of the state of the ribosomes. It appears that the misreading phenomena can be explained by assuming that streptomycin causes one base of a trinucleotide codon (most often a 5′- or internal base) to be misread. This misreading is not random; on the contrary, it is quite specific.

Protein synthesis and codon recognition with ribosomes from streptomycin-resistant *E. coli* strains (single-step resistance) are unaffected or only slightly influenced by the antibiotic. In contrast, these cell-free assays (of protein synthesis and codon recognition) employing ribosomes from streptomycin-sensitive *E. coli* strains are highly sensitive to the presence of the antibiotic at a level close to one molecule of streptomycin per ribosome. Although the correlation of *in vivo* and *in vitro* sensitivity and resistance to the antibiotic is excellent, the specific nature of the lethal event is not clear. Mere inhibition or stimulation of protein synthesis cannot account for its bacteriocidal action. For example, chloramphenicol, which inhibits protein synthesis *in vivo* and *in vitro* is bacteriostatic. Nevertheless, the stimulation of miscoding by the antibiotic remains a plausible hypothesis for its lethal effects. It remains to be demonstrated, however, whether inactive or lethal proteins containing miscoded amino acids accumulate as the cells are killed by streptomycin.

In any case, because *in vivo* and *in vitro* protein synthesis (in intact cells and in cell-free extracts from streptomycin-sensitive *E. coli* cells respectively) is very sensitive to streptomycin, it is probable that protein synthesis is closely related to the lethal event if, indeed, the effect of streptomycin on protein synthesis is not the lethal event itself. The close correlation of *in vivo* sensitivity and *in vitro* ribosomal sensitivity makes it likely that the effect of streptomycin on the recognition process during protein synthesis is a necessary part of its lethal action.

ACKNOWLEDGMENTS

I should like to thank the following for their contributions: Dr. Dolph Hatfield, for permission to present his experimental data (Table VIII) prior to publication; Dr. Fritz Rottman, for preparations of

$(Up)_3$ and $(pU)_3$; Drs. J. Davies, D. S. Jones, and H. G. Khorana, for permitting me to quote from their manuscript prior to publication; Dr. W. J. Polglase, for a generous sample of dideguanyldihydrostreptomycin; and Dr. Marshall Nirenberg, in whose laboratory this work was done.

*REFERENCES*

1. Dubin, D. T., Hancock, R. and Davis, B. D. Sequence of some effects of streptomycin in *E. coli, Biochim. Biophys. Acta 74*:476-89, 1963.
2. Stern, J. L. and Cohen, S. S. Lethality and the stimulation of RNA synthesis by streptomycin, *Proc. Nat. Acad. Sci. U.S.A. 51*:859-65, 1964.
3. Fitzgerald, R. J., Bernheim, F. and Fitzgerald, D. B. The inhibition by streptomycin of adaptive enzyme formation in mycobacteria, *J. Biol. Chem. 175*:195-200, 1948.
4. Erdös, T. and Ullmann, A. Effect of streptomycin on the incorporation of tyrosine labelled with carbon-14 into protein of Mycobacterium cell fractions *in vivo, Nature 185*:100-01, 1960.
5. Hahn, F. E. and Ciak, J. Studies on the mode of action of streptomycin. I. Inhibition of bacterial protein synthesis by streptomycin, *Bact. Proc. 59*:131, 1959.
6. Roote, S. M. and Polglase, W. J. Effect of dihydrostreptomycin on the formation of adaptive enzymes by a strain of *E. coli, Canad. J. Biochem. Physiol. 33*: 792-96, 1955.
7. Eaton, N. R. and Caffrey, R. Effect of dihydrostreptomycin on *E. coli, J. Bacteriol. 81*:918-23, 1961.
8. Anand, N. and Davis, B. D. Damage by streptomycin to the cell membrane of *E. coli, Nature 185*:22-23, 1960.
9. Spotts, C. R. Physiological and biochemical studies on streptomycin dependence in *E. coli, J. Gen. Microbiol. 28*:347-65, 1962.
10. Gorini, L., Gundersen, W. and Burger, M. Genetics of regulation of enzyme synthesis in the arginine biosynthetic pathway of *E. coli, Cold Spring Harbor Symp. Quant. Biol. 26*:173-82, 1961.
11. Gorini, L. and Kataja, E. Phenotypic repair by streptomycin of defective genotypes in *E. coli, Proc. Nat. Acad. Sci. U.S.A. 51*:487-93, 1964.
12. Lederberg, E. M., Cavalli-Sforza, L. and Lederberg, J. Interaction of streptomycin and a suppressor for galactose fermentation in *E. coli* K-12, *Proc. Nat Acad. Sci. U.S.A. 51*:678-82, 1964.
13. Valentine, R. C. and Zinder, N. D. Phenotypic repair of RNA-bacteriophage mutants by streptomycin, *Science 144*:1458-59, 1964.
14. Speyer, J. F., Lengyel, P. and Basilio, C. Ribosomal localization of streptomycin sensitivity, *Proc. Nat. Acad. Sci. U.S.A. 48*:684-86, 1962.
15. Flaks, J. G., Cox, E. C., Witting, M. L. and White, J. R. Polypeptide synthesis with ribosomes from streptomycin-resistant and dependent *E. coli, Biochem. Biophys. Res. Comm. 7*:390-93, 1962.
16. Mager, J., Benedict, M. and Artman, M. Common site of action for polyamines and streptomycin, *Biochim. Biophys. Acta 62*:202-04, 1962.
17. Polglase, W. J. Insensitivity to valine of streptomycin-dependent *E. coli* K-12, *Molec. Pharmacol. 1*:109-12, 1965.
18. Bragg, P. D. and Polglase, W. J. Biosynthesis of valine in streptomycin-dependent *E. coli, J. Bact. 89*:1158-59, 1965.
19. Newcombe, H. B. and Nyholm, M. H. Inheritance of streptomycin resistance and dependence in crosses of *E. coli, Genetics 35*:603-11, 1950.
20. Lennox, E. S. Transduction of linked genetic characters of the host by bacteriophage Pl., *Virology 1*:190-206, 1955.
21. Hashimoto, K. Streptomycin resistance in *E. coli* analyzed by transduction, *Genetics 45*:49-62, 1960.
22. Spotts, C. R. and Stanier, R. Y. Mechanism of streptomycin action on bac-

teria: A unitary hypothesis, *Nature 192:* 633-37, 1961.
23. Weiss, S. B., Acs, G. and Lipmann, F. Amino acid incorporation in pigeon pancreas fractions, *Proc. Nat. Acad. Sci. U.S.A. 44:*189-96, 1958.
24. Schweet, R. S., Bovard, F. C., Allen, E. and Glassman, E. Incorporation of amino acids into RNA, *Proc. Nat. Acad. Sci. U.S.A. 44:*173-77, 1958.
25. Berg, P. and Ofengand, E. J. Enzymatic mechanism for linking amino acids to RNA, *Proc. Nat. Acad. Sci. U.S.A. 44:*78-86, 1958.
26. Hoagland, M. B., Stephenson, M. L., Scott, J. F., Hecht, L. I. and Zamecnik, P. C. A soluble ribonucleic acid intermediate in protein synthesis, *J. Biol. Chem. 231:*241-57, 1958.
27. Holley, R. W. An alanine-dependent, ribonuclease-inhibited conversion of AMP to ATP, and its possible relationship to protein synthesis, *J. Amer. Chem. Soc. 79:*658-62, 1957. (Note correction: *79:*6579, 1957.)
28. Pestka, S. Unpublished observations.
29. Nishimura, T., Tanaka, N. and Umezawa, H. Selective toxicity of kanamycin and streptomycin, *J. Antibiot.,* Ser. A., *17:*238-45, 1964.
30. Arlinghaus, R., Favelukes, G. and Schweet, R. A ribosome-bound intermediate in polypeptide synthesis, *Biochem. Biophys. Res. Comm. 11:*92-96, 1963.
31. Nakamoto, T., Conway, T. W., Allende, J. E., Spyrides, G. J. and Lipmann, F. Formation of peptide bonds: I. Peptide formation from aminoacyl-sRNA. *Cold Spring Harbor Symp. Quant. Biol. 28:* 227-31, 1963.
32. Spyrides, G. J. Effect of univalent cations on the binding of sRNA to the template-ribosome complex, *Proc. Nat. Acad. Sci. U.S.A. 51:*1220-26, 1964.
33. Kaji, A. and Kaji, H. Specific interaction of soluble RNA with polyribonucleic acid induced polysomes, *Biochem. Biophys. Res. Comm. 13:*186-92, 1963.
34. Nirenberg, M. and Leder, P. RNA codewords and protein synthesis: Effect of trinucleotides upon the binding of sRNA to ribosomes, *Science 145:*1399-1407, 1964.
35. Matthaei, H., Amelunxen, F., Eckert, K. and Heller, G. Mechanism of protein biosynthesis. I. Binding of messenger-RNA and aminoacyl-sRNA to ribosomes, *Ber. Bunsengesell. 68:*735-42, 1964.
36. Suzuka, I., Kaji, H. and Kaji, A. Binding of specific sRNA to 30 S subunits—comparison with the binding to 70 S ribosomes, *Biochem. Biophys. Res. Comm. 21:*187-93, 1965.
37. Pestka, S. RNA codewords and protein synthesis: Formation of sRNA-30 S ribosome-template complexes. *Fed. Proc. 25:*781, 1966.
38. Pestka, S. and Nirenberg, M. Regulatory mechanisms and protein synthesis. Codon recognition on 30 S ribosomes, *J. Molec. Biol. 21:*145-171, 1966.
39. Nathans, D. and Lipmann, F. Amino acid transfer from aminoacyl-sRNA to protein on ribosomes of *E. coli, Proc. Nat. Acad. Sci. U.S.A. 47:*497-504, 1961.
40. Bishop, J. O. and Schweet, R. S. Participation of two enzyme fractions in the transfer of amino acids from aminoacyl-sRNA to reticulocyte ribosomes, *Biochim. Biophys. Acta 54:*617-19, 1961.
41. Fessenden, J. M. and Moldave, K. Studies on aminoacyl transfer from soluble ribonucleic acid to ribosomes: Resolution of two soluble transferring activities, *J. Biol. Chem. 238:*1479-84, 1963.
42. Conway, T. W. On the role of ammonium or potassium ion in amino acid polymerization, *Proc. Nat. Acad. Sci. U.S.A. 51:*1216-20, 1964.
43. Gilbert, W. Polypeptide synthesis in *E. coli.* I. Ribosomes and the active complex, *J. Molec. Biol. 6:*374-88, 1963.
44. Erdös, T. and Ullmann, A. Effect of streptomycin on the incorporation of amino-acids labelled with carbon-14 into ribonucleic acid and protein in a cell-free system of a Mycobacterium, *Nature 183:*618-19, 1959.
45. Davies, J. E. Studies on the ribosomes of streptomycin-sensitive and resistant strains of *E. coli, Proc. Nat. Acad. Sci. U.S.A. 51:*659-64, 1964.
46. Cox, E. C., White, J. R. and Flaks, J.

G. Streptomycin action and the ribosome, *Proc. Nat. Acad. Sci. U.S.A. 51:* 703-09, 1964.

47. Gonano, F. and von Ehrenstein, G. An isoleucine acceptor sRNA from *E. coli* transferring isoleucine into polypeptide in response to polyuridylic acid, *Fed. Proc. 23*:478, 1964.

48. Matthaei, J. H., Jones, O. W., Martin, R. G. and Nirenberg, M. W. Characteristics and composition of RNA coding units, *Proc. Nat. Acad. Sci. U.S.A. 48:* 666-77, 1962.

49. Szer, W. and Ochoa, S. Complexing ability and coding properties of synthetic polynucleotides, *J. Molec. Biol. 8*:823-34, 1964.

50. Friedman, S. M. and Weinstein, I. B. Lack of fidelity in the translation of synthetic polyribonucleotides, *Proc. Nat. Acad. Sci. U.S.A. 52*:988-96, 1964.

51. Davies, J., Gilbert, W., and Gorini, L. Streptomycin, suppression, and the code. *Proc. Nat. Acad. Sci. U.S.A. 51*:883-90, 1964.

52. Van Knippenberg, P. H., Van Ravenswaay Claasen, J. C., Grijm-Vos, M., Veldstra, H. and Bosch, L. Stimulation and inhibition of polypeptide synthesis by streptomycin in ribosomal systems of *E. coli,* programmed with various messengers, *Biochim. Biophys. Acta 95*:461-473, 1965.

53. Davies, J., Gorini, L. and Davis, B. D. Misreading of RNA codewords induced by aminoglycoside antibiotics, *Molec. Pharmacol. 1*:93-106, 1965.

54. Bretscher, M. S. and Grunberg-Manago, M. Polyribonucleotide-directed protein synthesis using an *E. coli* cell-free system, *Nature 195*:283-84, 1962.

55. Grunberg-Manago, M. and Dondon, J. Influence of pH and sRNA concentration on coding ambiguities, *Biochem. Biophys. Res. Comm. 18*:517-22, 1965.

56. So, A. G., Bodley, J. W. and Davie, E. W. Influence of environment on the specificity of polynucleotide-dependent amino acid incorporation into polypeptide, *Biochemistry 3*:1977-82, 1964.

57. Pestka, S., Marshall, R. and Nirenberg, M. RNA codewords and protein synthesis. V. Effect of streptomycin on the formation of ribosome-sRNA complexes, *Proc. Nat. Acad. Sci. U.S.A. 53*:639-46, 1965.

58. Schwartz, J. H. Effect of streptomycin on the biosynthesis of the coat protein of coliphage $F_2$ by extracts of *E. coli, Proc. Nat. Acad. Sci. U.S.A. 53*:1133-40, 1965.

59. Old, D. and Gorini, L. Amino acid changes provoked by streptomycin in a polypeptide synthesized *in vitro, Science 150*:1290-92, 1965.

60. Davies, J., Jones, D. S. and Khorana, H. G. Further study of misreading of codons induced by streptomycin and neomycin using ribopolynucleotides containing two nucleotides in alternating sequence as templates, *J. Molec. Biol. 18*:48-57, 1966.

61. Pestka, S. RNA codewords and protein synthesis: Effect of streptomycin on formation of sRNA-ribosome-RNA codon complexes, *Fed. Proc. 24*:408, 1965.

62. Kaji, H. and Kaji, A. Specific binding of sRNA to ribosomes: Effect of streptomycin, *Proc. Nat. Acad. Sci. U.S.A. 54*:213-19, 1965.

63. Pestka, S. Studies on the formation of transfer ribonucleic acid-ribosome complexes I. Effect of streptomycin and ribosomal dissociation on $^{14}$C-aminoacyl transfer ribonucleic acid binding to ribosomes, *J. Biol. Chem. 241*:367-72, 1966.

64. Anderson, W. F., Gorini, L. and Breckenridge, L. Role of ribosomes in streptomycin-activated suppression, *Proc. Nat. Acad. Sci. U.S.A. 54*:1076-83, 1965.

65. Davies, J., Anderson, P. and Davis, B. D. Inhibition of protein synthesis by spectinomycin, *Science 149*:1096-98, 1965.

66. Herzog, A. Effect of streptomycin on the dissociation of *Escherichia coli* 70 S ribosomes, *Biochem. Biophys. Res. Comm. 15*:172-76, 1964.

67. McCarthy, B. J. and Holland, J. J. Denatured DNA as a direct template for *in vitro* protein synthesis, *Proc. Nat. Acad. Sci. U.S.A. 54*:880-86, 1965.

68. Holland, J. J., Buck, C. A. and McCarthy, B. J. Stimulation of protein synthesis *in vitro* by partially degraded

ribosomal ribonucleic acid and transfer ribonucleic acid, *Biochemistry 5*:358-65, 1966.

69. Nirenberg, M. W. and Matthaei, J. H. Dependence of cell-free protein synthesis in *E. coli* upon naturally occurring or synthetic polyribonucleotides, *Proc. Nat. Acad. Sci. U.S.A. 47*:1588-1602, 1961.

70. Singer, M. F., Jones, O. W. and Nirenberg, M. W. Effect of secondary structure on the template activity of polyribonucleotides, *Proc. Nat. Acad. Sci. U.S.A. 49*:392-99, 1963.

71. Takanami, M. and Okamoto, T. Interaction of ribosomes and synthetic polyribonucleotides, *J. Molec. Biol. 7*:323-33, 1963.

72. Gilbert, W. Polypeptide synthesis in *Escherichia coli.* II. Polypeptide chain and sRNA, *J. Molec. Biol. 6*:389-403, 1963.

73. Hatfield, D. RNA codewords and protein synthesis: Binding of trinucleotide codewords to ribosomes, *Fed. Proc. 24*: 409, 1965.

74. Hatfield, D. RNA codewords and protein synthesis: Characteristics of $^{3}$H-oligonucleotide binding to ribosomes, *Fed. Proc. 25*:776, 1966.

75. Hatfield, D. and Nirenberg, M. Characteristics of oligonucleotide binding to ribosomes. To be published.

76. Polglase, W. J. Contribution of the cationic groups of dihydrostreptomycin to biological activity, *Nature 206*:298-99, 1965.

77. Rinehart, K. L. *The Neomycins and Related Antibiotics.* New York, Wiley, 1964.

78. Watanabe, T. Infective heredity of multiple drug resistance in bacteria, *Baceriol. Rev. 27*:87-115, 1963.

79. Rosenkranz, H. S. Basis of streptomycin-resistance in *Escherichia coli* with a "multiple drug resistance" episome, *Biochim. Biophys. Acta 80*:342-45, 1964.

80. Metzgar, D. P. and Moskowitz, M. Studies on the effect of streptomycin on mammalian cells in culture: I. Isolation of resistant strains, *Exp. Cell. Res. 30*: 379-87, 1963.

81. Moskowitz, M. and Kelker, N. Aminoacid control of streptomycin action on mammalian cells, *Nature 205*:476-77, 1965.

82. Krueger, R. G. Effect of streptomycin on antibody synthesis *in vitro, Proc. Nat. Acad. Sci. U.S.A. 54*:144-52, 1965.

PRESENTATION OF

# THE FIFTH FERDINAND C. VALENTINE MEDAL AND AWARD TO THEODORE M. DAVIS*

JOHN H. MCGOVERN

Chairman, Section on Urology
The New York Academy of Medicine
New York, N. Y.

DR. THEODORE MCCANN DAVIS was born on December 23rd, 1889, in Greenville, S. C., where he still resides. After preliminary education in that city, he attended Furman University, worked for a while in electrical engineering, and ultimately chose medicine as a career. In 1914 he was graduated with highest honors from the School of Medicine of the University of Maryland, receiving the Faculty Gold Medal. The next year he served as resident surgeon in the University Hospital. He then became assistant and later associate to Dr. W. C. Black of Greenville, S. C. As early as 1920 he began to limit his practice to urology. Dr. Davis became interested in transurethral surgery, a technique known for a number of years but never perfected. During the next five years he studied intensively the early work of Bottini,[1] Freudenberg,[2] Young,[3] and Caulk,[4] and later the work of Stern.[5, 6, 7] Ultimately Dr. Davis perfected an electromagnetic switch permitting instantaneous change from cutting to coagulating current for prostatic resection. This required modification and major innovations in instruments and allied equipment. Dr. Davis used this equipment to remove all the adenomatous portion of the prostate, not merely to carve a channel through it; this appears to have been a new conception among those considering transurethral removals. He reported the results of 246 cases at the 1931 AMA Convention in Philadelphia, Pa.[8] The original paper had the effect of a bombshell on the urologic world–some for, most against! Undaunted by the unfavorable comments[9] on his work, Dr. Davis continued to strive to improve the instrument and his technique. In 1935 he published the results of the operation in 748 cases.[10]

*Presented at a meeting of the Section on Urology, The New York Academy of Medicine, March 16, 1966.

Dr. Davis' ability was recognized by Reinhold Wappler, an electrical wizard and the famous founder of the American Cystoscope Makers, Inc.[11] In a letter dated April 27, 1931, to Dr. A. J. Crowell of the Crowell Urological Clinic in Charlotte, S. C., where Dr. Davis commuted to do part of his work, Mr. Wappler stated, "I hope to be permitted in a small way to carry out my commission of executing the mechanical details of Dr. Davis' epoch-making technique of prostatic resection. Perhaps it is the way of providence that I failed to recognize, at an early date, the advent of genius." Mr. Wappler blamed Dr. Davis' "modesty."

The operation, although then relatively safe and simple in the hands of Dr. Davis and less traumatic to the patient than an open procedure, could not be duplicated when attempted by untrained surgeons. Indeed, for surgeons not familiar with endoscopy the Davis operation was impossible—for the others it was still difficult! Also, electrical manufacturers deluged surgeons with literature on the efficacy of their particular equipment and the simplicity and safety of the operation. This led to many unfortunate results. Hence, the procedure did not achieve prompt popularity. However, time and open-minded, hard-working urologists proved that Dr. Davis' work was the basis for the final acceptance of transurethral resection as a legitimate surgical procedure. In fact, transurethral prostatectomy is a strictly urologic technique—one of the justifications for the separate speciality.

In 1937 Dr. Davis suffered a severe attack of coronary occlusion and retired from active medical life.

Dr. Davis has been honored by many offices and by membership in many learned societies. He has long been a member of the Greenville South Carolina Medical Society and served as its president in 1919. He was a member of the staff of the Greenville County Hospital and president in 1922, and for many years chief of the Urology Service. He was president of the staff of St. Francis Hospital, Greenville, in 1923. He is a member of the American Medical Association, the American Association of Genito-Urinary Surgeons, the Southern Medical Association, and is a Fellow of the American College of Surgeons. Among other learned societies, he has a membership in the Société Internationale D'Urologie and is a charter member of, and a diplomate of the American Board of Urology. He is an honorary member of the Hollywood, Florida, Academy of Medicine, and has published numerous articles on prostatic resection.

On March 14, 1965, at a Symposium on Transurethral Surgery of the Southeastern Section of the American Urological Association, a Certificate of Merit was awarded him on the basis of his outstanding pioneer work and his many contributions to the development of transurethral surgery.

The Medical Alumni Association of the University of Maryland on June 3, 1965, recognized Dr. Davis' contribution to the field of urology, and gave him its highest honor, the Alumni Honor Award and Gold Key "for important contributions to medicine and for distinguished service to mankind."

Somewhat belatedly and, therefore, with exceptional enthusiasm and esteem, the Section on Urology of The New York Academy of Medicine recognizes the monumental contribution of Dr. Theodore McCann Davis to the specialty of urology and, more important, to the welfare of man, by presenting him with its Valentine Award for 1966.

*REFERENCES*

1. Bottini, E. *La galvano-caustica nella pratica chirurgica.* Novara, F. Merati, 1873, 125 pp.
2. Freudenberg, A. *Ein modificierter Bottini'scher Incisor.* Leipzig, 1897, 5 pp. Freudenberg, A. *Ein modificierter Cauterisator prostatae zur Bottini'schen Operation.* Berlin, 1899, 5 pp.
3. Young, H. H. *Practice of Urology.* Philadelphia, Saunders, 1926.
4. Caulk, R. Obstructive lesions of the prostate, *J.A.M.A.* *94*:375, 1930.
5. Stern, M. Paper read before Section on Urology of The New York Academy of Medicine, Jan. 20, 1926.
6. Stern, M. Resection of obstructions at vesical orifice by means of new cystoscopic instrument employing a cutting current capable of operation in water medium, *Phys. Ther.* *44*:439, 1926.
7. Stern, M. Resection of obstructions at vesical orifices; new instruments and new methods, *J.A.M.A.* *87*:1726-29, 1926.
8. Davis, T. M. Prostate operation. Prospects of the patient with prostatic disease in prostatectomy vs. resection, *J.A.M.A.* *97*:1674-79, 1931.
9. Discussion on prostatectomy. (Section on Urology, 82nd annual session, A.M.A., Philadelphia, June 10, 1931.) *J.A.M.A.* *97*:1775-77, 1931.
10. Davis, T. M. Transurethral prostatic resection with report of 748 cases, *Southern Med. J.* *28*:693-700, 1935.
11. Letter in the files of The New York Academy of Medicine.

# EXPERIENCE IN TRANSURETHRAL RESECTION*

*The Fifth Ferdinand C. Valentine Memorial Lecture*

THEODORE M. DAVIS

Greenville, S. C.

I AM deeply touched by the great honor conferred upon me as recipient of the 1966 Ferdinand C. Valentine award in recognition of my work and contributions to transurethral surgery. In doing this work I followed the trail blazed by Maximilian Stern, one of the Academy's own members; where the trail ended I found it necessary to hew my own pathway to the summit of success.

It was in 1926 that Dr. Stern introduced his ingenious instrument for removing obstructions at the vesical orifice. He called this instrument the resectoscope. A generator of high-frequency current that would activate a loop electrode under water to section tissue he called the resectotherm.

Dr. Stern called his method of resection a minor operation that permitted the removal, electrically, of any number of pieces of tissue obstructing the vesical orifice, and he claimed that the current sectioned tissue without hemorrhage.

Intrigued by Dr. Stern's description of his operation, I made several appointments with him in the hope of observing him perform one of his operations, but each appointment was canceled for one reason or another a few days before I was ready to leave Greenville, S. C., for New York City.

I mentioned this to a friend, P. A. Jensen of the Kronenberg X Ray Co., Baltimore, Md.; this firm represented throughout the southeastern states the Wappler Electric Co., Inc., of New York City, which had constructed Dr. Stern's equipment. A short time later I received an invitation from the Wappler company to come to New York, assuring me that it would obtain for me an opportunity of watching Dr. Stern operate.

*Presented at a meeting of the Section on Urology, The New York Academy of Medicine, March 16, 1966.

I thus finally witnessed an operation performed by Dr. Stern on a patient having a small median lobe. From this patient Dr. Stern removed a number of pieces of tissue from the obstruction, each piece 2 mm. in diameter and 1 cm. in length. Despite the claim made for bloodless procedure, there was a moderate amount of hemorrhage, for which there was no provision for control other than an indwelling catheter.

I then attempted to place an order with the Wappler Electric Co. for a duplicate of the equipment it had made for Dr. Stern, but I found that they could not comply without Dr. Stern's approbation. While waiting for this necessary approval I visited the office of the Chas. R. Bard Co., Inc., also in New York City, where I met and talked with E. L. Outwin, president of the company. I asked Mr. Outwin if the firm could make for me a double-channel catheter with a bag near the tip, one channel opening into the bag to permit its dilation with a measured quantity of water. It was my impression that when such a balloon was filled it could be drawn into the vesical orifice to act as a tourniquet controlling any hemorrage. I was informed later it was impossible to obtain satisfactory bags.[1]

Dr. Stern failed to approve my order for the resectoscope, stating that he was "not entirely satisfied with the equipment and would probably approve at a later date."

Returning to Greenville, I again contacted my friend Mr. Jensen, who promised to see what he could do. His company succeeded in having the Wappler Electric Co. ship me the equipment on a loan basis, as its contract with Dr. Stern did not preclude loaning it.

Figure 1 shows the resectoscope, consisting of a sheath with a five-eighths-inch fenestra near the beak, an obturator, a right-angled vision telescope, and the working parts, which consisted of a direct-vision telescope, a light carrier, a water conduit, and a loop electrode.

Figure 2 shows the resectotherm generator.

Elated over having received the equipment, I sectioned beef hearts with it until I was thoroughly familiar with the actions of the instrument.

The first operation I attempted with it, on a patient with a small median lobe, was in my office. (Later events proved how fortunate this was; had it been in a hospital, my experience would no doubt have parallelled that of others who had employed this equipment; a cystostomy would have been necessary to control the bleeding.)

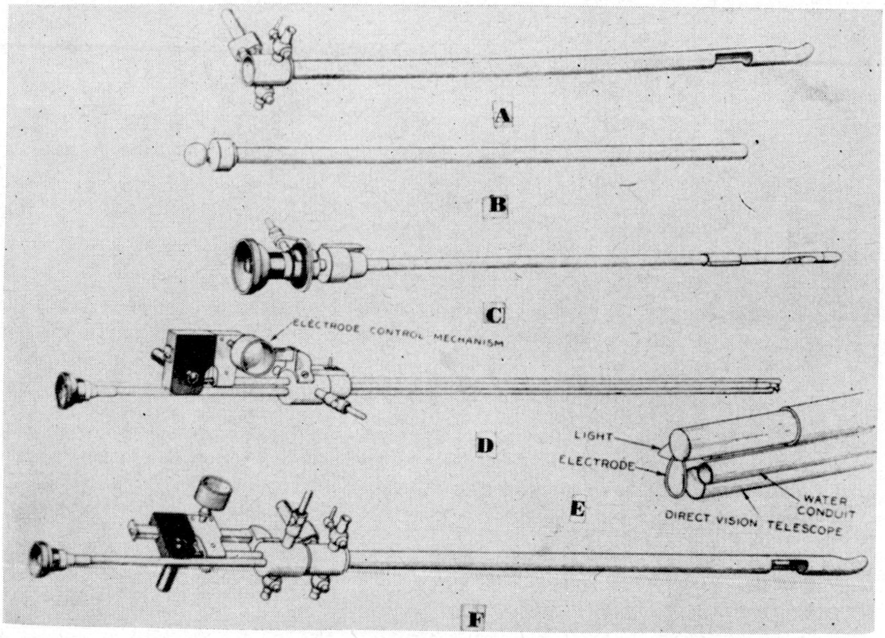


Fig. 1. Stern resectoscope. *A, B,* sheath and obturator; *C,* examining telescope; *D,* working parts, consisting of direct vision telescope, water conduit, light carrier, and cutting loop; *E,* end of working parts enlarged; *F,* instrument assembled with electrode or loop in fenestra moving toward its distal end. Reproduced by permission of the *Journal of the American Medical Association.*

Employing sacral anesthesia, I injected 20 cc. of a 2 per cent solution of Novocaine into the sacral canal and 2 cc. into each sacral foramen. Everything went well until about five sections had been made. Then an artery was sectioned, and it looked, through the magnification of the telescope, as though the aorta itself had been perforated. Inasmuch as the current was supposed to section tissue without hemorrhage, attempts to control the bleeding by application of the current were made but without avail.

A diathermy generator was on a nearby table, and the thought occurred to me that application of the current through the loop electrode might control the bleeding. I disconnected the resectotherm wires and connected the diathermy current wires to the loop, but pressing the foot switch put the loop electrode out of business!

The patient was bleeding profusely, the operator was sweating even more. What to do? It occurred to me that if this were a bladder tumor a convex Brown-Buerger cystoscope and Bugbee fulgurating electrode

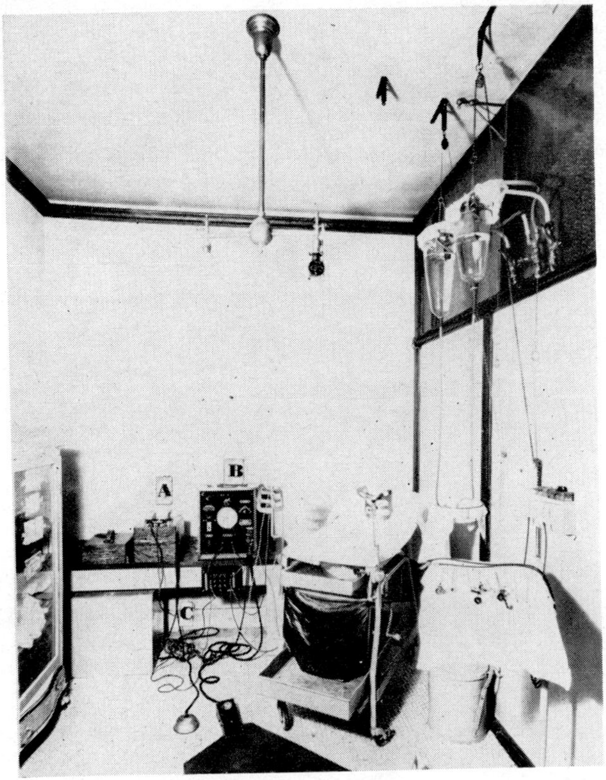


Fig. 2. Generators in resection operating room, office of the author in Greenville, S. C., 1927. *A*, Stern teletherm; *B*, diathermy; *C*, manual-controlled switch below diathermy generator. Reproduced by permission of the *Journal of the American Medical Association.*

would be used. Putting the thought into action, I removed the resectoscope and introduced a Brown-Buerger cystoscope into the bladder. Inserting the Bugbee electrode, the bleeder was readily discernible. I placed the electrode in contact with the bleeder and applied the current, obtaining immediate control of the hemorrhage. The sigh of relief that went up from the operator may well be imagined, and he felt that he was master of any bleeding in the future.

A new loop was placed in the working parts of the instrument and the operation was completed, tissues being sectioned until bleeding interfered with clear vision, when the cystoscope was employed again to control the hemorrhages. Repeating these procedures, about 4 g. of tissue was removed in 2 hours.

The method was employed for several months. Meanwhile I de-

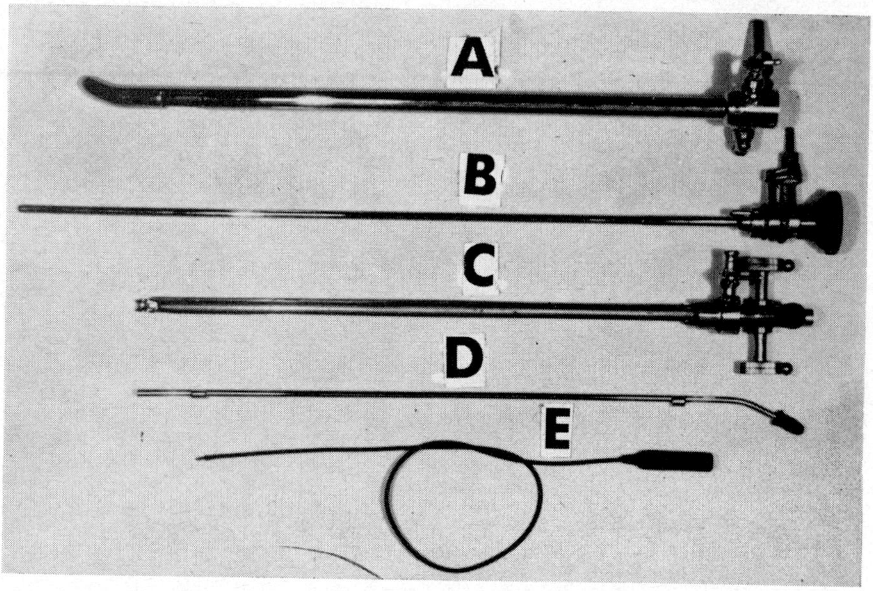


Fig. 3. Earliest interchangeable electrode used in resection to control hemorrhage, with working parts: *A,* resectoscope sheath; *B,* right-angled telescope with light carrier; *C,* deflecting mechanism; *D,* cannula to admit Bugbee electrode; *E,* Bugbee electrode.

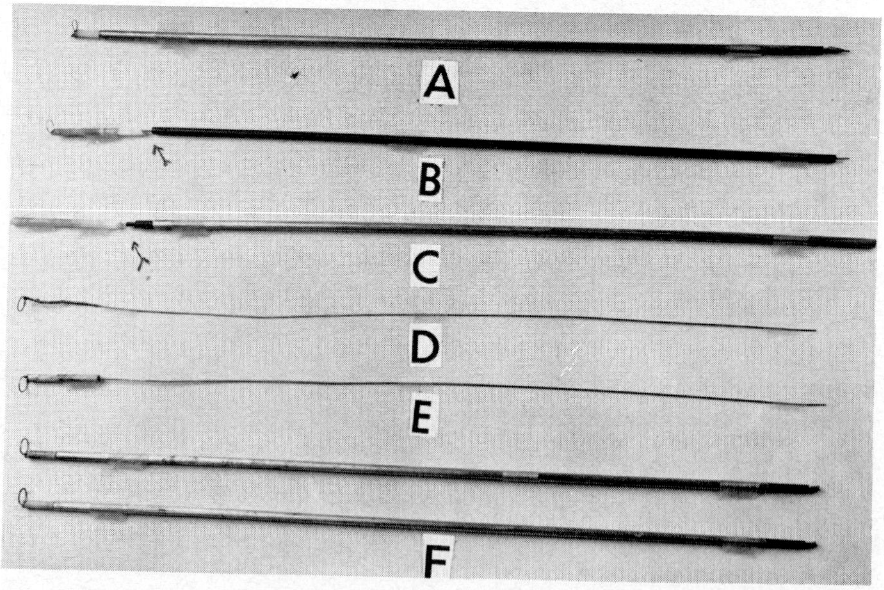


Fig. 4. Stern electrode, *A,* showing original loop. *B,* defect in electrode: quartz tube and hard rubber insulator abuts forming a noninsulated joint that was shorted by the diathermy current. *C,* telescoping hard rubber into quartz, which corrected the defect; *D,* silver tubing employed to join loop to wire, bent for stability; *E,* silver tubing pushed into the quartz; *F,* complete improved loops that permitted both currents to be employed.

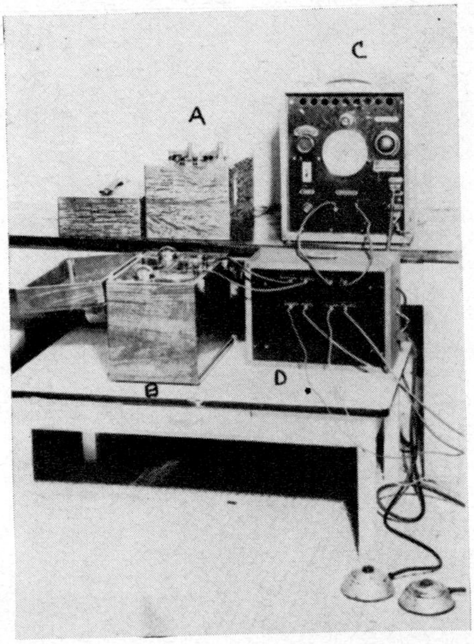


Fig. 5. *A*, Stern resectotherm; *B*, improved generator; *C*, diathermy generator; *D*, electromagnetic switch for instantaneous use of either of the two currents. All machines are activated by foot switches and the magnetic switch.

signed an instrument whose parts could be interchanged with those of the resectoscope for control of hemorrhage.

Figure 3 shows this instrument, which consists of a right-angled telescope with a light carrier, a deflecting mechanism, and a tubular conduit that permits the tip of the Bugbee electrode to be near the fenestra when the working parts of the instrument are interchanged. Tissue is sectioned until hemorrhage interferes with clear vision. The working parts are then replaced with those of the coagulating instrument, and diathermy current is employed to control any hemorrhage. Using this equipment, I was able to remove 12 g. of tissue on one occasion in 2 hours.

Early in 1928 I began experimenting in loop construction. Dissecting the original loop, a defect was located and a method of correcting it was developed.

Figure 4 shows the original Stern loop, the defect in it, the method used to correct it, and the improvement in its construction. The new loop permitted use of the cutting current to section tissue and of the diathermy current to control hemorrhage. *This happy development*

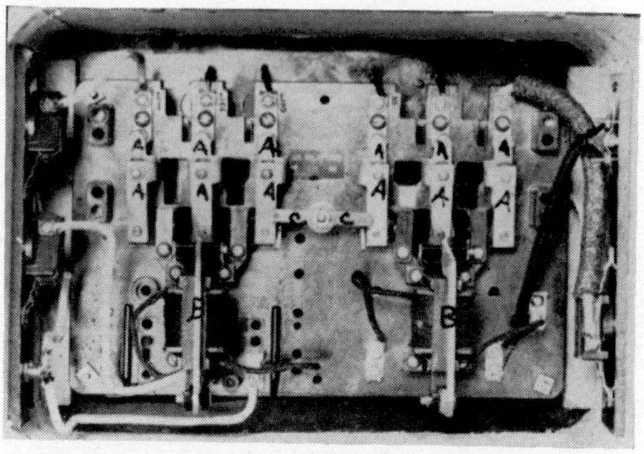

Fig. 6. Interior of electromagnetic switch.

*marked the advent of modern resection.*

As the wires from either generator had to be changed with each change of currents, I designed and built a double-throw, triple-pole switch, permitting the interchange of currents by manipulating the switch by hand. Figure 2 shows the manual switch.

Attempts to use larger loops of larger wire were restricted by the resectotherm generator, which was not powerful enough to activate them. In fact, most of my operations had to be done on Sundays in order to have sufficient voltage to activate the resectotherm generator properly. Following suggestions and diagrams that I made, the Wappler Electric Co. produced a generator that had ample power.

Figure 5 shows this improved generator, also the electromagnetic switch I made in 1928. This switch permits the instant interchange of the two currents by means of two foot switches. It is said that all modern generators used for this purpose employ this method of changing currents.

Figure 6 shows the interior of this electromagnetic switch.

In 1928 I made experiments in sheath construction. The elongated beak of the original Stern sheath was removed, and a tube size 28F was found to be the most suitable. A seven eighths-inch fenestra with a depth one half the diameter of the sheath was adopted. The working parts were modified to permit longer excursions of the loop, and larger lamps were used for more illumination.

Difficulty was experienced with the tendency of the more powerful currents to arc to the objective end of the telescope, cracking or discoloring the lens; this interfered with clear vision. The difficulty was

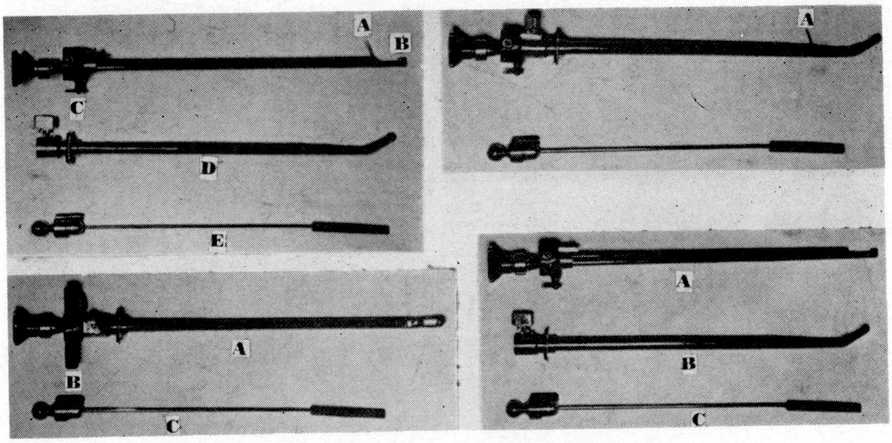


Fig. 7. *Upper left:* components of retrograde fulgurating cystoscope made by the author. *A, B, C,* top retrograde lens telescope with electrode (*A*) elevated; *B,* retrograde telescope objective lens; *C,* insulated mechanism for operating electrode, also electrical connection of the instrument; *D,* sheath; *E,* obturator. *Upper right:* cystoscope assembled with electrode (*A*) elevated. *Lower left: A,* cystoscope assembled with electrode depressed; *B,* insulated mechanism to control electrode, also electrical connection to generator; *C,* obturator. *Lower right: A,* working parts with electrode depressed; *B,* sheath; *C,* obturator.

solved by using lenses of quartz made for me in Germany by Reinhold H. Wappler.

On April 19, 1928, I presented a paper at a meeting of the South Carolina Medical Association.[2] Prostatic resection was received with much skepticism. In this paper I described the first balloon catheter I had made and used in 1927.

In a paper I read before a meeting of the Southern Medical Association in Asheville, N. C., November 12 to 15, 1928, I described the first use of a 15 per cent solution of caroid powder to dissolve a mucus ball in the urinary bladder.[3]

A letter I wrote to the president and secretary of the Section on Urology of the American Medical Association, asking for a place on the program of the Association's meeting to be held in Detroit, Mich., in 1930, remained unanswered. (The doctors addressed visited me at the Crowell Clinic of Urology and Dermatology in Charlotte, N. C., in 1931, following my establishment there.)

Late in 1930, Dr. A. J. Crowell, after watching operations at my clinic in Greenville, thought it would be of mutual benefit to us if I were to join the Crowell Clinic in Charlotte, N. C. After several meetings between us it was agreed that I should do so without, however, giving up my office in Greenville.

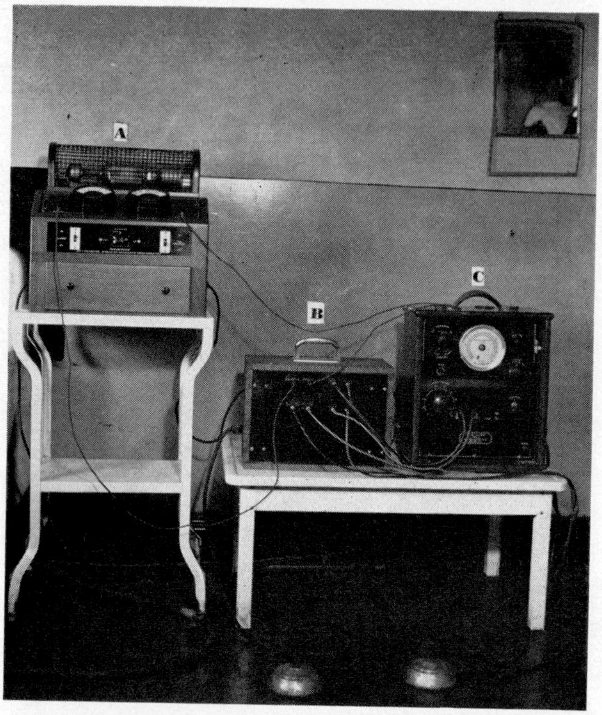


Fig. 8. *A,* Comprex generator, modified for use with *B,* electromagnetic switch; *C,* diathermy generator. Reproduced by permission of the *Southern Medical Journal.*

On January 1, 1931, announcements were mailed out stating that I had become a member of the Crowell Clinic of Urology and Dermatology as chief of the Department of Prostatic Resection and Operative Cystoscopy. Immediately we were invited to present papers and to show motion pictures of resections at meetings all over the United States; and for a number of years thereafter there were always several physicians attending our clinic from various parts of the United States and from some foreign countries as well.

I retain the warmest affection for Dr. Crowell, whose vision paralleled mine in helping to put resection on the medical map.

Figure 7 shows a retrograde fulgurating cystoscope that I made in my Greenville office shop. A description of it was published in the *Journal of Urology* in September 1931.[4]

I had never met Reinhold H. Wappler in person, as he had always been away from his office when I visited New York City and, on learning that he was to attend the meeting of the Tennessee State Medical

Society in Knoxville, Tenn., in April 1931, I met him there. He saw the motion pictures of resection and seemed much impressed by them.

Returning to Greenville, I received a telephone call from Mr. Wappler requesting an appointment to visit me in Greenville. He came and stayed 2 days, went with me to Charlotte for 3 days, and we then went to Durham, N. C., to attend a meeting of the North Carolina State Medical Society. As he did not have a reservation we shared a room during our stay. We discussed several new types of resectoscopes and I made several sketches for him to take back to New York City.

Mr. Wappler, whose son Fred had developed a generating machine to be used in resections, desired to bring this generator to Charlotte for me to try out; he wanted my opinion of its currents. At the same time he was to bring with him the several new resectoscopes we had discussed. The Wapplers arrived several days prior to a meeting of the American Urological Association, Inc., to be held at Memphis, Tenn., in May 1931. They brought with them a generator called the Comprex, but not any of the new resectoscopes, explaining that it had been impossible to obtain the necessary Bakelite tubing on such short notice.

Figure 8 shows the Comprex generator, which I later modified, as I have described, to allow the use of the diathermy current.

There were 11 cases to be operated on in Charlotte in 2 days before we left for Memphis, and we used the Comprex generator. The cutting current we used in the first operation was the best I had used up to that time; however the coagulating current left everything to be desired (the method employed to produce the coagulating current was to reduce the plate voltage, thereby reducing the output of the tube). This coagulating current, being of the same frequency as the cutting current, did not coagulate rapidly enough to control hemorrhage. It was necessary to revert to my usual equipment to complete each operation in which the Comprex generator was used. I supposed that these demonstrations had convinced the Wapplers that the coagulating current of the Comprex was insufficient to control hemorrhage rapidly.

We entrained for Memphis, where we arrived after a most pleasant trip. I read a paper before the meeting and showed motion pictures of a resection, the first ever shown before a national meeting. The operation of resection was again received with much skepticism.

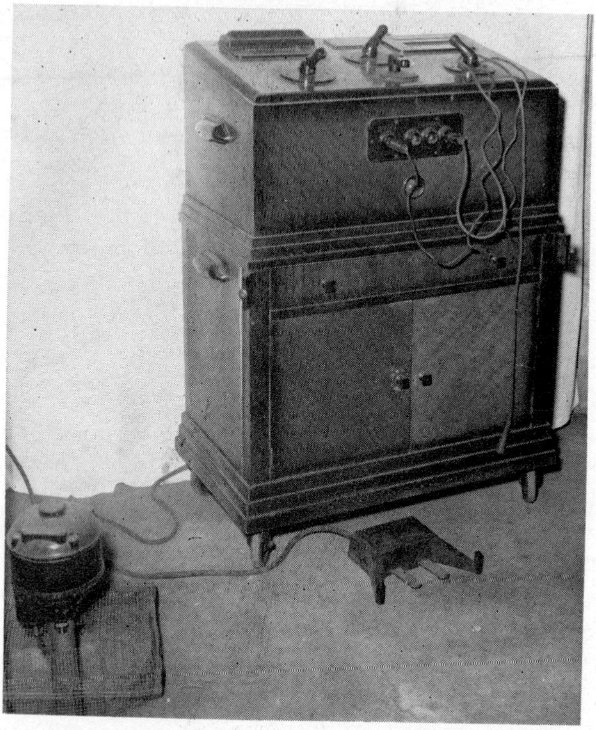

Fig. 9. Davis-Bovie generator developed for resection by the author and the Liebel Flarsheim Co., Cincinnati, Ohio.

Imagine my surprise when Dr. Joseph F. McCarthy of New York, N.Y., showed the Comprex generator as the McCarthy generator, making the claim that it had the best cutting and coagulating currents of any generator (which may have been true in that this was the only generator presumed to have both currents). In my discussion I found it necessary to disagree with the claim that this generator had a satisfactory coagulating current. Since that time the Wapplers deemed it wise or otherwise to discontinue all contact with me.

On June 10, 1931, I read a paper on resection before the Urological Section of the American Medical Association at a meeting held in Philadelphia, Pa.[5] I also showed the films on resection.

Shortly after this, G. H. Liebel of the Liebel Flarsheim Co., of Cincinnati, Ohio, came to Greenville to ask me to join him in developing a suitable generator for resections. Starting with the Bovie unit, which had an excellent spark gap, we designed and tested several models from which, finally, a unit was developed that became known as the Davis-Bovie generator. It produced a high-frequency current to section tissue and a moderate-frequency highly damped current to control hemorrhage rapidly. The currents were interchangeable by means of an electromagnetic switch. In my earliest experimental operations I had been delighted to be able to remove several grams of tissue. Improvements in the resectoscope and in the generating currents, and also the additional experience I had gained now permitted me to remove almost an entire prostate gland. The removal of 100 g. was a common occurrence. In one operation 155 g. of tissue had been removed in 1 hour and 25 minutes.

On October 20, 1931, I presented a paper entitled "Transurethral Prostatectomy" at a meeting of the Seventh District Medical Society held at Albemarle, N.C. The technique I described is as follows. Sectioning is usually begun in the right lateral lobe, starting at the vertical orifice and making longitudinal sections to the level of the verumontanum with maximum excursions of the loop. Sectioning is repeated in the same location until the capsule is reached. The lateral lobe can be peeled away, more or less, from the so-called capsule and the entire lobe removed. The same procedure is employed on the left lateral lobe and the median lobe is removed, all hemorrhage being controlled prior to inserting the urethral catheter.

Recognition of the capsule must be acquired by experience. Tissue near the capsule is more pliable; the capsular tissue is fibrous, differing from the more dense prostatic tissue. Sectioning into the capsular tissues, one will enter a venous plexus. This hemorrhage is difficult to control, as this areolar tissue does not coagulate sufficiently to hold a good coagulum. At times a small amount of bleeding may have to be tolerated. The bleeding usually ceases after the retention catheter is *in situ* and manipulations have ceased (a Foley catheter may be used).

It has become the custom to remove all obstructive tissue before crushing any calculus, as this permits better visibility of the bladder, all bleeding being controlled before inserting the retention catheter. The Ellick evacuator greatly facilitates removal of all sections of tissue from the bladder as well as fragments of any crushed calculus. This evacuator is also useful in removing blood clots.

About 20 per cent of the enlarged prostates were of a cancerous nature. A few of these were in the earliest stages and thought to be ideal for Young's operation. Several were referred to Dr. Hugh H. Young for this radical operation, and one of these patients lived for 20 years afterward.

It was noticed during operations on cancerous malignancies that there were two distinct types of tissue: in one the sectioned tissue was rather smooth, dense, and of a whitish color; in the other type there were numerous nestlike structures, and within the nests were cauliflowerlike growths. From my observations of both types I came to believe that in the first type metastasis was much slower and that most of the patients with this type lived on 5 to 8 years; patients showing the second type did not live longer than 2 years.

In cancerous malignancies we removed as much obstructive tissue as was practicable and slightly coagulated the entire sectioned areas. Deep x-ray therapy was employed in all these cases, and radon seed was implanted in the remaining tissue. Evaluation of these latter procedures remains problematical.

All operations performed in Greenville were done in my office with one exception: a man shown in the 1929 films voiding 2½ years after the operation. All operations performed in Charlotte were done in offices of the Crowell Clinic.

Each patient in Greenville was examined by an internist who was present during the operation. In Charlotte the patients were examined by the clinic staff. Every patient received the necessary preliminary treatment, and any patient with large residuals or retention was given the necessary decompression along with treatment of any physical infirmity.

Each of the first 18 patients operated on was allowed to return to his home wearing a retention catheter. One of them was plowing his garden the next morning when I called, even though he was wearing his retention catheter. The 18th patient, a prominent citizen, was operated on in the afternoon and allowed to return home. When I called that evening he was not at home, as he had gone visiting. The next morning, on my way to the hospital, whom should I see on the corner of a main street but this same happy patient. I insisted on taking him home and that he stay there and remain quiet for a few days.

Thereafter every patient, following his operation in the office, was sent to the hospital in a taxi or in his own car until, one day, a patient was kept waiting in the receiving room for more than an hour and fainted; he was immediately put to bed. From that time on every patient, following his operation in the office, was sent to the hospital, and any patient undergoing treatment in a hospital was brought to the office for his operation and then returned to the hospital in an ambulance.

The operation of resection was made possible only by untiring persistence in developing an instrument that in its original form was not practicable into one that would really do what it was intended to do.

The Davis technique of transurethral resection is the employment of a high-frequency current to section tissue and of a highly damped diathermy current to control hemorrhage. This is the technique used by most urologists today.

With the equipment described, 1,231 patients in Charlotte, N.C., were operated on with a mortality of 7 (as we were being severely criticized we included any fatality that occurred among these patients within 3 months after operation). In Greenville, S.C., 812 operations were performed with a mortality of 1: a patient who refused to consume either water or food during the month that he lived after his operation.

The complications we encountered are listed below.

| | *No.* | *Description* |
|---|---|---|
| Accidents | 1 | Rupture of a diverticulum during a preliminary cystoscopy in a violent coughing spell. Immediate cystoscopy with drainage. Later, prostatectomy with complete recovery. |
| Hemorrhage | 0 | Immediate postoperative. |
| | 10 | Postoperative from 10 days to 2 months, readily controlled by evacuating the blood clots and coagulating the bleeding vessel. |
| Ejaculate, intravesical | 12 | |
| Incontinence, permanent | 2 | |
| Epididymitis | 15 | Preoperative |
| | 23 | Postoperative |
| Pyelitis | 1 | |
| Hemorrhagic nephritis | 1 | |
| Phlebitis, right leg | 1 | |
| Bronchopneumonia | 1 | |
| Uremia | 1 | |

*REFERENCES ON FOLLOWING PAGE*

*REFERENCES*

1. Outwin, E. L. Development of the modern catheter, *Amer. Surg. Trade Ass. J.*, June 1955.
2. Davis, T. M. Resection of obstruction at the vesical orifice with the Stern resectoscope, *J. S. Carolina Med. Ass. 24*:274-279, 1928.
3. Davis, T. M. Resection of prostate gland obstructions with Stern's resectoscope equipment, *Southern Med. J. 22*: 528-534, 1929.
4. Davis, T. M. New cystoscope for retrograde fulguration, *J. Urol. 26*:491-496, 1931.
5. Davis, T. M. Prostate operation, *J.A.M.A. 97*:1674-79 and 1775-1777, 1931.
6. Davis, T. M. Transurethral prostatectomy. Unpublished.

# THE CLINICAL SOCIETY OF THE NEW YORK DIABETES ASSOCIATION, INC.

THIRD ANNUAL PRIZE ESSAY CONTEST

Held at The New York Academy of Medicine, May 19, 1966

## *Effects of Diazoxide Administration on Plasma Glucose, Insulin, and Lipids in von Gierke's Disease*

GABRIEL SPERGEL

Fellow in Diabetes and Endocrinology
Clinical Metabolic Research Unit, The Jewish Hospital of Brooklyn
Brooklyn, N. Y.

Diazoxide, a nondiuretic thiazide, has been noted to cause hyperglycemia and has been used therapeutically in the treatment of the hypoglycemia associated with leucine sensitivity and insulinomata.

The mechanisms by which this drug induces hyperglycemia were studied during the treatment of a 12-year-old boy with type 1 glycogen storage disease and marked hyperlipemia.

1) Inhibition of the plasma immunoassayable insulin response to administered glucose was shown, as well as an increase of 30 to 70 mg./100 ml. in postprandial plasma glucose levels. Oral glucose tolerance decreased during treatment with diazoxide. These changes in plasma glucose were not due to glycogenolysis, by virtue of the enzymatic defect present in this patient.

2) During treatment, skin xanthomata disappeared although plasma triglycerides rose. Serum cholesterol was unchanged while plasma-free fatty acids initially rose but subsequently spontaneously declined.

3) Analysis of serial oral glucose tolerance tests suggests that diazoxide inhibits hepatic glucose uptake, as part of its hyperglycemic action.

# *Reevaluation of the Role of Calcium in Corticotropin-Induced Lipolysis* in Vitro

MELVYN KLEIN

Fourth-Year Medical Student
State University of New York Downstate Medical Center
Brooklyn, N. Y.

The calcium-dependent nature of corticotropin (ACTH)-induced lipolysis *in vitro,* shown by Engel *et al.,* was reinvestigated. Epididymal fat tissue from fasted Wister rats was incubated in Krebs-Ringer bicarbonate buffer. Incubated tissues and media were then analyzed for free fatty acid (FFA) release. The three hypotheses were examined, and the results of these investigations were:

1) *Calcium could reduce glucose entry into fat tissue and, by diminishing triglyceride synthesis, facilitate net lipolysis.* In the presence of 1 mg./ml. ethylenediamine tetra-acetate (EDTA) and 2 gm./100 ml. albumin, the lipolytic response to 1 μg./ml. ACTH was found to be dependent on the presence of added calcium, irrespective of the presence or absence of glucose in the medium.

2) *The lipolytic system activated by ACTH could require calcium to function.* EDTA suppressed ACTH-activated lipolysis only in the presence of albumin: in its absence, EDTA was wholly without liposuppressive effect.

3) *Primary ACTH receptor sites might contain calcium whereas, under EDTA blockade, less specific sites (for example, sulfhydryl groups), could permit ACTH attachment to fat tissue.* In the presence of EDTA, inhibition of ACTH-induced lipolysis was logarithmically related to albumin concentration in the incubation media. Sulfhydryl-group blockade proved ineffective in inhibiting ACTH-activated lipolysis in the absence of albumin. Several high molecular weight polypeptides and carbohydrate polymers were substituted for albumin in the presence and absence of EDTA, but had no liposuppressive effect.

These experiments suggest that the role of calcium in ACTH-activated lipolysis is to permit or facilitate ACTH attachment to adipose tissue.

# *Effects of Induced Hypokalemia on Carbohydrate Metabolism, Free Fatty Acids, Tissue Potassium, and Glycogen in the Rat*

PHILIP SCHMIDT,* GABRIEL SPERGEL,* AND ALAN G. STERN**

The Jewish Hospital of Brooklyn
Brooklyn, N. Y.

The relationship between the potassium ion and carbohydrate metabolism has been the object of renewed interest. An animal study was undertaken to correlate changes in plasma glucose, free fatty acids, and tissue glycogen with alterations in plasma and tissue potassium.

Forty-two male Wistar rats were divided into three groups and fed a low potassium diet for 2 weeks.

Group I: controls, saline injected for 7 days, diet supplemented with potassium.

Group II: DOCA injected for 7 days, no potassium supplementation.

Group III: Same as II but with potassium supplementation.

One week after the last injection, fasting animals were anesthetized and heart blood drawn for potassium, glucose, and FFA. An intracardiac injection of glucose (1 g./kg.) was given and tail blood sampled for glucose at 5-minute intervals for 30 minutes. Two hours after glucose injection, heart blood was again collected for potassium, glucose, and FFA, the animal sacrificed, and tissue (muscle, liver, and epididymal fat pad) obtained for potassium and glycogen determinations.

1) Profound hypokalemia was established in Group II while normal serum potassium was maintained in Groups I and III.

2) Significantly, adipose tissue and liver showed no loss of potassium despite marked decreases in both plasma and muscle potassium in Group II.

3) Potassium depletion did not produce a significant change in glucose disappearance rate. Fasting and 2-hour glucose values, however, were significantly elevated in potassium-depleted animals.

4) Liver and muscle glycogen was significantly increased in the potassium-depleted animals.

5) Plasma FFA (fasting and postglucose) were unaffected by potassium depletion.

*Fellow in Diabetes and Endocrinology, Clinical Metabolic Research Unit.
**Intern in Medicine.

## TELEVISED CLINICAL SCIENCE SEMINARS

Tuesday Evenings, 8:30-9:30 P.M.

STATION WNYC—TV UHF—CHANNEL 31

**February 7, 1967**

### SERUM ENZYMES — DIAGNOSIS OF CLINICAL DISEASE STATES

C. HILMON CASTLE
Associate Professor of Medicine
University of Utah College of Medicine

GERALD T. PERKOFF
Professor of Medicine
Washington University School of Medicine
Chief, Medical Service
St. Louis City Hospital

### USE OF ESOPHAGEAL MOBILITY TESTS IN CLINICAL DIAGNOSIS

C. HILMON CASTLE
Associate Professor of Medicine
University of Utah College of Medicine

FRANZ J. INGELFINGER
First Conrad Wesselhoeft Professor of Medicine
Boston University School of Medicine

EDWIN ENGLERT, JR.
Associate Professor of Medicine
University of Utah College of Medicine

**February 14, 1967**

### CUTANEOUS DISEASES RELATED TO SUNLIGHT EXPOSURE

RUDOLF L. BAER
Professor and Chairman
Department of Dermatology
New York University School of Medicine

LEONARD C. HARBER
Associate Professor of Dermatology
New York University School of Medicine

ALFRED W. KOPF
Professor of Dermatology
New York University School of Medicine

**February 28, 1967**

### CORONARY ARTERY DISEASE

CHARLES E. KOSSMANN
Professor of Medicine
New York University School of Medicine

TIMOTHY J. REGAN
Associate Professor of Medicine
New Jersey College of Medicine and Dentistry

FRANK C. SPENCER
Professor and Chairman
Department of Surgery
New York University School of Medicine

---

## Eighth Annual Program on EMOTIONAL AND PSYCHIATRIC PROBLEMS IN MEDICAL PRACTICE

**Spring Series: Starting March 13, 1967**

**FEE: $10.00**

Courses will be offered on problems encountered in the practice of medicine, pediatrics, and obstetrics and gynecology. Each course will consist of seven weekly, small-group, one and one-half hour sessions.

*For further information Office of Medical Education*

THE NEW YORK ACADEMY OF MEDICINE
2 East 103 Street, New York, N. Y. 10029

BULLETIN OF
THE NEW YORK ACADEMY
OF MEDICINE

VOL. 43, NO. 3 MARCH 1967

# INCREASED ELASTIC TISSUE IN THE DERMIS: THE DERMAL ELASTOSES*

J. GRAHAM SMITH, JR.

Division of Dermatology, Department of Medicine
and the Center for the Study of Aging,
Duke University Medical Center, Durham, N. C.

## INTRODUCTION

ELASTIC fibers and collagenous fibers are morphologic entities made up primarily of the fibrous proteins elastin and collagen respectively. Elastic tissue stains in various connective tissue diseases have demonstrated increased amounts of elastic fibers in the dermis. The increased elastic tissue staining has been referred to as elastosis and these dermal disorders as the *dermal elastoses* (Smith, 1963; Smith *et al.*, 1966). It is proper to question the specificity of elastic tissue staining and, as a result, other morphologic, physical, and chemical criteria have been applied to ascertain if the fibers taking elastic tissue stains in these dermal disorders represent true elastic fibers or altered collagen. Before reviewing these criteria in relation to the dermal elastoses, the properties of elastic fibers and collagen will be considered briefly. There is no longer any question that elastic tissue and collagen are different and that elastic tissue is not derived from collagen, as indicated in exten-

*The *Fifth Howard Fox Memorial Lecture,* presented at a meeting of the Section on Dermatology and Syphilology at The New York Academy of Medicine, April 5, 1966. The studies described in this paper were supported in part by N.I.H. grants 5T1 AM 5335, AM 05812, and AM 07583, and by a grant from The Proctor & Gamble Co., Cincinnati, Ohio.

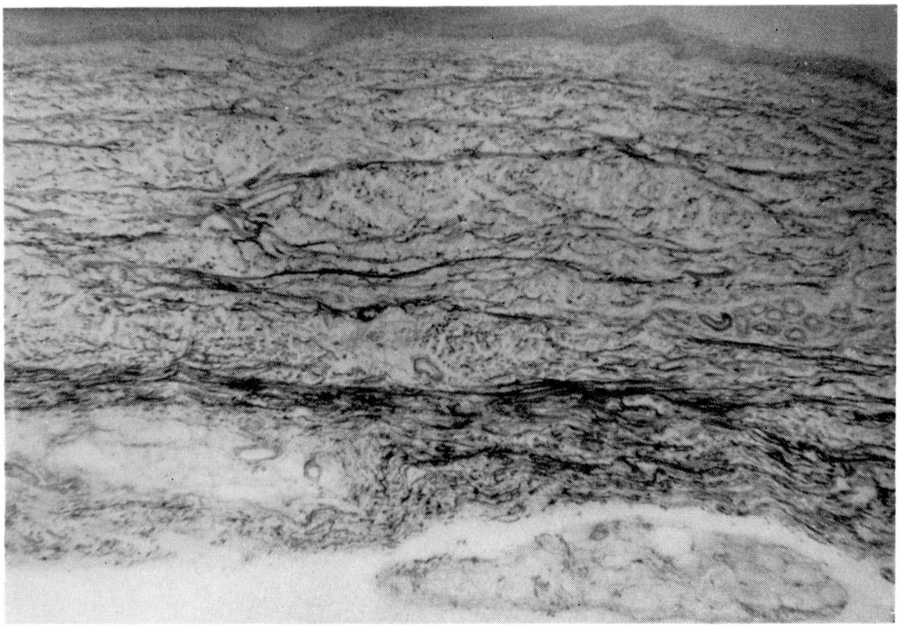

Orcein stain of human skin, ×400. Note alternation of linear and "chopped-up" elastic fibers and parallelism between the elastic and collagen fibers.

sive reviews of elastic tissue and collagen (Ayer, 1964; Lansing, 1959; Partridge, 1962; Harrington and von Hippel, 1961; Jackson, 1964).

## *Morphology*

In the light microscope, the fibers of elastic tissue appear delicate, straight, and freely branching; collagen fibers are coarse and wavy. Elastic fibers are invariably associated with collagen and lie parallel to the collagen fibers. The orthogonal grid pattern seen in amphibia also occurs in human skin when sections are oriented parallel or perpendicular to wrinkle lines although it is less striking (see accompanying figure). The predominant orientation of the fibers is parallel to the wrinkle lines (Holmstrand *et al.*, 1961). Collagen fibers and elastic fibers in the upper dermis are much finer and more delicate than those in the lower dermis close to the subcutaneous fat.

Elastic fibers viewed in the electron microscope appear amorphous but, after limited digestion with elastase, they seem to be made up of smaller fibrils (Lansing *et al.*, 1952). Collagen fibers are characterized by periodicity in the range of 700 Å in the natural, undried state

(Quigley and Hjørting-Hansen, 1962). Periodicity of elastic fibers has not been observed.

*Physical Properties*

Elastic fibers are refractile while collagen fibers are birefringent (Felsher, 1961). A characteristic x-ray diffraction pattern is seen with collagen (Harrington and von Hippel, 1961) but not with elastic tissue (Partridge, 1958). Elastic tissue is fluorescent, and the fluorescence increases with aging (La Bella and Lindsay, 1963) while collagen fluoresces poorly (Felsher, 1961). Both the tensile strength and Young's modulus of elasticity of elastic tissue are less than those of collagen (Hass, 1942*a*; Burton, 1954; Harkness, 1961). Elastic tissue will also stretch up to 100 per cent of its original length before breaking, while collagen will stretch only 50 per cent before breaking (Burton, 1954). Acids, bases, and certain salts swell collagen, and temperatures of 60 to 70° C. shrink it down to three quarters of its original length, while elastic tissue is much more resistant to swelling and shrinkage under these conditions (Felsher, 1961).

The cross-link in the elastin protein molecule that is probably primarily related to its elasticity is through two polyfunctional amino acids, desmosine and isodesmosine (Thomas *et al.*, 1963) whose precursor is lysine (Miller *et al.*, 1964). Lysinonorleucine may also represent a cross-linking agent in elastin (Franzblau *et al.*, 1965). Collagen, however, forms both intra- and intermolecular cross-links that increase with age (Verzar, 1964). Copper is required for normal elastin synthesis, and both copper deficiency and penicillamine inhibit the formation of desmosine and isodesmosine from lysine (Miller *et al.*, 1965). Penicillamine also decreases collagen synthesis in induced granulomas and produces a marked increase in soluble collagen, *i.e.*, a decrease in cross-linking (Nimni and Bavetta, 1965).

Elastin and collagen may be separated because of their differences in solubility. Collagen is solubilized by 23 *N* formic acid at 45° C. for 72 hours (Hass, 1942*b*), autoclaving at 50 lb. for 4 hours or 25 lb. for 6 hours (Lowry *et al.*, 1941), and 0.1 *N* sodium hydroxide at 98° for 45 minutes (Lansing, 1954), leaving a residue of elastin. Varying amounts of elastin are dissolved by these operations and products are obtained that differ in their properties and morphology (Gotte and Serafini-Fracassini, 1963). Immature and newly synthesized collagen is more soluble and thus more easily extracted than older collagen (Jackson and Bentley, 1960), and this is true also for newly synthesized elastin. Extracted immature soluble collagen can be quantitated by measurement of hydroxyproline and, only recently, means of measuring immature soluble elastin have been developed utilizing hemagglutination (Jackson *et al.*, 1966).

## *Chemical Properties*

Orcein, Weigert's resorcin fuchsin, aldehyde fuchsin, Verhoeff's, and orcinol new fuchsin stain elastin selectively but not specifically. Acid fuchsin in the van Gieson, aniline blue in Masson's trichrome stain, and luxol fast blue stain collagen (Fullmer, 1962; Hale, Cromartie, and Dobson, 1960). Various *in vitro* manipulations such as methylation to block elastic tissue staining and acetylation and benzoylation of collagen to cause it to take elastic tissue stains suggest possible mechanisms for connective-tissue staining but probably have no *in vivo* significance.

Elastin and collagen are digested by few enzymes. Elastin is digested only by pancreatic and bacterial elastase (Mandl, 1961*a*), by pepsin (Fisher *et al.*, 1960), and by the plant enzymes papain, ficin, and bromelin (Thomas and Partridge, 1960). Undenatured collagen is digested only by clostridial, amphibian, and mammalian collagenases (Eisen and Gross, 1965; Mandl, 1961*a*; Woods and Nichols, 1965*a*, *b*). Neither is digested by crystalline trypsin, chymotrypsin, cathepsin, or testicular hyaluronidase (Thomas and Partridge, 1960). Denatured collagen, however, is susceptible to many proteolytic enzymes such as pepsin, papain, and trypsin. This restricted susceptibility to enzymes of these proteins in their undenatured state allows ready differentiation of elastic tissue and of undenatured and denatured collagen in histochemical studies (Finlayson *et al.*, 1966).

Purified elastin from a variety of mammalian tissues has a constant amino acid composition (Ayer, 1964; Partridge, 1962) and is readily differentiated from collagen from any source. Collagen and elastin contain nearly equivalent amounts of glycine and proline, but collagen contains three or four times as much acidic and basic amino acids and approximately ten times as much as hydroxyproline. Collagen also contains aspartic acid, glutamic acid, lysine, and arginine with little or no tyrosine. Elastin, contains large amounts of tryrosine and valine.

The amino acid sequences of elastin and collagen are quite different. Pro-gly dipeptides are frequent in bacterial elastase digests of elastin (Mandl, 1961*b*) but are infrequent in collagen. Gly-pro, hypro-gly, gly-pro-ala, and gly-pro-hypro are, however, common in digests of collagen (Harrington and von Hippel, 1961; Gallop and Seifter, 1962). Elastin is made up of randomly coiled peptide chains lying parallel to the long dimension of the fiber and held together by cross-links through a chromophoric nucleus formed by the condensation of four lysines making up desmosine and isodesmosine (Miller *et al.*, 1965). *Alpha*-chains in the collagen molecule are cross-linked near the *N*-terminal end of the molecule by condensation products formed by two lysyl residues (Bornstein *et al.*, 1966).

## Elastinlike Fibers

The terms elacin, collacin, and collastin were invented by Unna (1896) to describe the various morphologic staining elements he observed in actinic elastosis termed by him senile degeneration of the skin. A little over a quarter of a century later, Kissmeyer and With (1922) reported that "Unna has now abandoned this classification, nor does he mention it in his *Biochemie der Haut*, published in 1913. Unna also has personally emphasized to one of us (Kissmeyer) that he no longer attaches much importance to these distinctions in the degenerated elastin."

Later, however, a number of other workers studied elastinlike fibers and proposed that "elastin" or manufactured elastin might be formed from collagen with so-called "moth-eaten fibers" as an intermediate (Burton *et al.*, 1955; Keech *et al.*, 1956). They produced this "elastin" by extracting collagen with alkaline borate buffers, phthalate buffer, phthalate buffer with sodium metaperiodate at *p*H 5, ultrasonic radiation, collagenase, and other enzymes. The peptides extracted by these treatments were rich in hydroxyproline and arginine but had little valine. The residues had morphologic and tinctorial properties similar to elastin and were more resistant to solubilization in boiling water and acetic acid than normal collagen. These residues differed in amino acid composition significantly from true elastin, having lesser amounts of alanine, valine, proline, and greater amounts of arginine, lysine, hydroxyproline and of aspartic and glutamic acid (Hall, 1961). Fullmer and Lillie (1957) were not able to demonstrate elastic tissue staining of collagen extracted with phthalate and borate buffers according to Keech's (1954) methods. Grant (1965) has also produced elastinlike fibers by treating collagen with glutaraldehyde and autoclaving. However, there is no evidence that such artificially produced fibers occur in any *in vivo* situation, and it is unlikely that these artifacts represent a method for synthesis of elastin (Partridge, 1958; Lansing, 1959; Ayer, 1964).

## The Dermal Elastoses

These morphologic, physical, and chemical properties of elastic tissue and collagen serve as a basis from which the specificity of elastic tissue staining in a number of dermal disorders may be evaluated. Some of these disorders have been studied extensively biochemically and some only with elastic tissue stains and the light microscope. Those that are associated with increased dermal elastic tissue staining have been classified as follows:

I) Primary
  - A) Localized
    - 1) Elastoma
    - 2) Elastosis perforans serpiginosa
  - B) Systemic
    - 1) Pseudoxanthoma elasticum
    - 2) Cutis hyperelastica (Ehlers-Danlos syndrome)
    - 3) Werner's syndrome
    - 4) Osteogenesis imperfecta
    - 5) Epidermolysis bullosa acquisita with elastosis and primary amyloidosis

II) Secondary
  - A) Localized
    - 1) Actinic elastosis
    - 2) Erythema ab igne
    - 3) Submucous fibrosis of the palate
  - B) Systemic
    - 1) Chronic acidosis
    - 2) Chronic hypercorticism

### *Elastoma*

This is a group of benign dermal connective tissue tumors associated with increased amounts of elastic tissue seen in the light microscope. Included are nevus elasticus and nevus elasticus vascularis (Staricco and Mehregan, 1961), elastotic connective tissue nevi frequently associated with tuberous sclerosis (Rocha and Winkelmann, 1962), juvenile elastoma (Weidman, Anderson, and Ayres, 1933), and the elastoma reported by Smith and Waisman (1960). Stimmermann and Stout (1962) have also reported a tumor associated with increased elastic tissue staining, elastofibroma dorsi, which forms beneath the dermis in the subscapular space under the latissimus dorsi muscle.

Intradermal, compound, and blue nevi (Mehregan and Staricco, 1962), and the nevus of Ota (Mishima and Mevorah, 1961) have been reported in association with elastosis; however, it is not clear whether this represents actinic elastosis.

### *Elastosis Perforans Serpiginosa*

The dermal elastosis occurring in this disorder has the morphological characteristics of elastic tissue in the light and electron microscope (Cohen and Hashimoto, 1960), the staining characteristics of true elastic tissue, and the fibers are digested by elastase (Hashimoto and Hill, 1960).

### *Pseudoxanthoma Elasticum*

Although the fibers taking the elastic tissue stains in pseudoxanthoma elasticum appear curled upon themselves, their appearance in both the light and electron microscope is that of true elastic tissue (Moran and Lansing, 1958; Fisher *et al.*, 1958; Sams *et al.*, 1962). The fibers are refractile and fluoresce (Fisher *et al.*, 1958). Elastic tissue isolated by extraction with hot alkali from the involved skin of one patient with pseudoxanthoma elasticum was increased to 6.3 mg./100 mg. dry weight of dermis as compared with 10 controls having 2.4 $\pm$ 0.7 mg. elastin/100 mg. dry weight dermis (Smith *et al.*, 1962*a*). These elastic fibers take the elastic tissue stains (Moran and Lansing, 1958; Fisher *et al.*, 1958) and are digested by elastase (Findlay, 1954; Moran and Lansing, 1958) and pepsin, but not by crystalline trypsin (Fisher *et al.*, 1958). The amino acid composition of the fibers isolated from hot alkali is quite similar to normal human dermal elastin isolated in the same manner and to bovine ligamentum nuchae elastin isolated by autoclaving (Smith *et al.*, 1962*b*). Collagen is reduced in amount but apparently not abnormal (Smith *et al.*, 1962*b*).

### *Cutis Hyperelastica (Ehlers-Danlos Syndrome)*

Most histologic investigations of this disorder have demonstrated dermal elastosis (McKusick, 1960) and recent careful studies have also confirmed the increase in elastic tissue using the light and electron microscope (Hult *et al.*, 1964; Wechsler and Fisher, 1964). The elastic fibers stain with a variety of the elastic tissue stains, are fluorescent, and are digested by elastase and pepsin (Wechsler and Fisher, 1964). Using hot alkali to extract elastin from skin involved with cutis hyperelastica, however, no increase in elastic tissue was found (Varadi and Hall, 1965), and no abnormality in the amino acid composition of cutis hyperelastica elastin as compared with normal dermal elastin was found. Although there does appear to be a relative increase in elastic tissue histologically, it is probable that the primary defect in this disorder is in the collagen.

### *Werner's Syndrome*

Using histologic methods, R. C. Smith *et al.* (1955) found an increase in dermal elastic tissue suggestive of the changes seen in pseudoxanthoma elasticum. Recent studies of the skin from two patients with Werner's syndrome made available by the late S. W. Becker, Sr., and M. Tannenbaum did not show elastosis (Smith and Finlayson, 1964). Further study of this disease is required.

### *Osteogenesis Imperfecta*

Histological elastosis was found in the dermis of nine patients with osteogenesis imperfecta but none in eight normal family members of these patients by Stadil (1961). This observation has been confirmed in one patient by Sams and Smith (1964*a*) who used orcein, aldehyde fuchsin, and Verhoeff's stains. An increase in argyrophilic fibers with absence of mature normal collagen has also been reported (Follis, 1953) and it is probable that there is a defect of collagen in this disorder associated with the increased elastic tissue staining.

### *Epidermolysis Bullosa Acquisita*

A 74-year-old patient with bullous and hemorrhagic lesions of the axillae, inguinal folds, elbows, knees, palms, and soles and with elastosis histologically throughout the dermis in the involved areas but not in the uninvolved skin, has recently been reported (Sams and Smith, 1964*b*). Elastic tissue isolated with hot alkali revealed a threefold increase in the involved areas but with an amino acid composition that differed considerably from normal human dermal elastin.

### *Actinic (Senile) Elastosis*

Underneath a small "Grenz" zone of connective tissue that is normal in appearance (Gillman *et al.*, 1955), there are in the upper part of the dermis thick, curled, clumped, and amorphous staining elastic fibers. These stain with the classic elastic tissue stains and under the electron microscope have the appearance of elastic tissue (Lansing *et al.*, 1953; Banfield and Brindley, 1963).

Felsher (1961) has studied these fibers extensively using physical techniques, and he has found that they are refractile and fluorescent. In swelling agents they do not become translucent as collagen does and they resist swelling and dissolution in acids, salts, and bases, as true elastic tissue does.

Using hot alkali extraction, Smith *et al.* (1962*a*) found an increase in elastic tissue in actinic elastosis as compared with unexposed control skin. The elastic tissue in actinic elastosis is digested by elastase (Lansing *et al.*, 1953; Findlay, 1954; Loewi *et al.*, 1960). Loewi *et al.* (1960) also showed that these fibers were not digested by collagenase or crystalline trypsin. If they represented collagen, they should be digested by collagenase whether denatured or not; if they represented denatured collagen, they should be digested by crystalline trypsin. Felsher (1961) showed that the elastic fibers from actinic elastosis had a much lower hydroxyproline content than collagen. Elastin isolated with hot alkali from actinic elastosis had an amino acid composition similar to normal human dermal elastin and bovine ligamentum nuchae elastin but quite dissimilar from collagen (Smith *et al.*, 1963). Elastosis has been produced experimentally in animals with ultraviolet light (Sams *et al.*, 1964*c*). Decreased total collagen with an increase in soluble collagen in actinic elastosis has been reported (Smith *et al.*, 1962*a*).

### *Erythema ab Igne*

The elastotic fibers in the upper dermis in this condition stain with orcein, Verhoeff's, and aldehyde fuchsin and have the morphologic characteristics of true elastic fibers (Finlayson *et al.*, 1966). They are digested by elastase but not by collagenase or crystalline trypsin, and are refractile and fluorescent.

### *Submucous Fibrosis of Palate*

Elastic fibers are increased, stain with elastic tissue stains, and have an amorphous elastic tissuelike appearance in the electron microscope in submucous fibrosis of the palate (Sirsat and Khanolkar, 1962). The fibers are digested, however, by elastase, trypsin, and collagenase. Without knowledge of the purity of the enzymes used, these studies are difficult to interpret.

### *Chronic Acidosis*

Patients with metabolic or respiratory acidosis of nine months' duration or longer have elastosis in their connective tissue throughout the body (Finlayson *et al.*, 1964*a*). Histologically, the fibers stain with classic elastic tissue stains and are digested by elastase but not by collagenase or trypsin. This disorder has been produced experimentally in animals, and an increase in elastic tissue, with an amino acid composition similar to that of true elastin, has been demonstrated (Finlayson and Smith, 1964). The fibers are refractile and fluoresce.

### *Chronic Hypercorticism*

Patients on long-term corticosteroid therapy demonstrate atrophy of the skin associated with increased elastosis throughout their connective tissue. These fibers have the morphologic appearance of true elastic tissue and stain with classic elastic tissue stains (Finlayson *et al.*, 1964*b*). They are refractile and fluoresce. It is probable that the increase in elastic tissue is relative and due to decreased amounts of collagen present.

## Discussion

Modern morphological, biophysical, and biochemical methodology make possible differentiation between elastic tissue and collagenous tissue. Despite reservations concerning the specificity of elastic tissue stains, it is noteworthy that in all the disorders thus far studied by other techniques the high degree of specificity of elastic-tissue staining has been confirmed. It is obvious that more work needs to be done in a number of the dermal elastoses to prove that these disorders are associated with increased amounts of true elastic tissue; however, the intensive studies already carried out in elastosis perforans serpiginosa, pseudoxanthoma elasticum, actinic elastosis, erythema ab igne, and chronic acidosis suggest that the specificity of these stains will be confirmed in future studies also. It is entirely probable in certain of these diseases, especially cutis hyperelastica and osteogenesis imperfecta, that biomolecular abnormalities of collagen will be demonstrated in association with the increase in elastic tissue. It is also probable that the alterations in disorders such as chronic acidosis and chronic hypercorticism in large measure are due to a relative deficiency of collagen rather than to an increase in elastic tissue. In any case, a syndrome of systemic elastosis can be suggested based on the common denominator of the hemorrhagic phenomena, bone lesions, and poor wound healing prominent in most of the systemic elastoses. The potential usefulness of such drugs as penicillamine to decrease cross-linking of elastin and collagen suggests that biomolecular therapy of connective tissue diseases is not an unreasonable possibility in the future.

## Summary

Elastic tissue is different morphologically, physically, and chemically from collagen and, although it is invariably associated with collagen, is not derived from collagen.

Emphasis is placed on dermal disorders associated with increased elastic tissue to draw attention to these fibers, which also play an important role in connective tissue disease.

Elastic tissue stains appear to be quite specific and, in those elastoses studied extensively by other techniques, abnormal increases in elastic tissue have been confirmed. There is no evidence as yet to suggest that the material that stains with elastic tissue stains represents a degraded or abnormal collagen.

Experimental methods available for production of increased elastic tissue in the dermis such as ultraviolet rays and chronic acidosis should aid the study of the synthesis of this fibrous protein.

*REFERENCES*


Ayer, J. P. *Int. Rev. Connect. Tissue Res. 2*:33, 1964.

Banfield, W. G. and Brindley, D. C. *J. Invest. Derm. 41*:9, 1963.

Bornstein, P., Kang, A. H. and Piez, K. A. *Proc. Natl. Acad. Sci. U.S.A. 55*:417, 1966.

Burton, A. C. *Physiol. Rev. 34*:619, 1954.

Burton, D., Hall, D. A., Keech, M. K., Reed, R., Saxl, H., Tunbridge, R. E. and Wood, M. J. *Nature 176*:966, 1955.

Cohen, A. S. and Hashimoto, K. J. *Invest. Derm. 37*:15, 1960.

Cooper, D. R. and Davidson, R. J. *Biochem. J. 97*:139, 1965.

Eisen, A. Z. and Gross, J. *Develop. Biol. 12*:408, 1965.

Felsher, Z. *J. Invest. Derm. 37*:163, 1961.

Finlayson, G. R., Smith, J. G., Jr. *Fed. Proc. 23*:235, 1964.

Finlayson, G. R., Smith, J. G., Jr. and Moore, M. J. *J.A.M.A. 187*:659, 1964*a*.

Finlayson, G. R., Lund, H. and Smith, J. G., Jr. Unpublished observations, 1964*b*.

Finlayson, G. R., Sams, W. M., Jr. and Smith, J. G., Jr. *J. Invest. Derm. 46*:104, 1966.

Findlay, G. H. *Brit. J. Derm. 66*:16, 1954.

Fisher, E. R., Rodnan, G. P. and Lansing, A. I. *Amer. J. Path. 34*:977, 1958.

Fisher, E. R., Rosenthal, T. B. and Lansing, A. I. *J. Histochem. Cytochem. 8*:102, 1960.

Follis, R. H., Jr. *Bull. Hopkins Hosp. 93*: 225, 1953.

Franzblau, C., Sinex, F. M., Faris, B. and Lampidis, R. *Biochem. Biophys. Res. Comm. 21*:575, 1965.

Fullmer, H. M. *J. Dent. Res. 41*:223, 1962.

Fullmer, H. M. and Lillie, R. D. *J. Histochem. Cytochem. 5*:11, 1957.

Gallop, P. M. and Seifter, S. In: *Collagen.* N. Ramanathan, ed. New York, Interscience, 1962, pp. 249-61.

Gillman, T., Penn, J., Bronks, D. and Roux, M. *Arch. Path. 59*:733, 1955.

Gotte, L., Serafini-Fracassini, A. *J. Atheroscler. Res. 3*:247, 1963.

Gotte, L., Serafini-Fracassini, A. and Moret, V. *J. Atheroscler. Res. 3*:244, 1963.

Grant, R. A. *Biochem. J. 97*:5c, 1965.

Hale, D. M., Cromartie, W. J. and Dobson, R. L. *J. Invest. Derm. 35*:293, 1960.

Hall, D. A. *The Chemistry of Connective Tissue.* Springfield, Thomas, 1961, 110 pp.

Harkness, R. D. *Biol. Rev. 36*:399, 1961.

Harrington, W. F. and von Hippel, P. H. *Advances Protein Chem. 16*:1, 1961.

Hashimoto, K. and Hill, W. R. *J. Invest. Derm. 35*:7, 1960.

Hass, G. M. *Arch. Path. 34*:971, 1942*a*.

Hass, G. M. *Ibid.*, 807, 1942*b*.

Holmstrand, K., Longacre, J. J. and de Stefano, G. A. *Plast. Reconstr. Surg. 27*: 597, 1961.

Hult, A. M., Goltz, R. W. and Midtgaard, K. *Acta Dermatovener.* (Stockh.) *44*:415, 1964.

Jackson, S. F. In: *The Cell, Biochemistry, Physiology, Morphology.* J. Brachet and A. E. Mirsky, eds. New York, Academic Press, 1964, vol. 6, pp. 387-520.

Jackson, D. S. and Bentley, J. P. *J. Biophys. Biochem. Cytol. 7*:37, 1960.

Jackson, D. S., Sandberg, L. S. and Cleary, E. G. *Biochem. J. 98*:13*p*, 1966.

Keech, M. K. *Yale J. Biol. Med. 26*:295, 1954.

Keech, M. K., Reed, R. and Wood, M. J. *J. Path. Bact. 71*:477, 1956.

Kissmeyer, A. and With, C. *Brit. J. Derm. 34*:175, 1922.

LaBella, F. S. and Lindsay, W. G. *J. Geront. 18*:111, 1963.

Lansing, A. I. In: *Ciba Foundation Colloquia on Aging.* Boston, Little, Brown, 1954, vol. 1, pp. 88-103.

Lansing, A. I. *The Arterial Wall.* Baltimore, Williams, Wilkins, 1959, pp. 136-60.

Lansing, A. I., Rosenthal, T. B., Alex, M. and Dempsey, E. W. *Anat. Rec. 114*:555, 1952.

Lansing, A. I., Cooper, Z. K. and Rosenthal, T. B. *Anat. Rec. 115*:340, 1953.

Loewi, G., Glynn, L. E. and Dorling, J. *J. Path. Bact. 80*:1, 1960.

Lowry, O. H., Gilligan, D. R. and Katersky, E. M. *J. Biol. Chem. 139*:795, 1941.

McKusick, V. A. *Heritable Disorders of Connective Tissue.* 2d ed. St. Louis, Mosby, 1960, 333 pp.

Mandl, I. *Advances Enzym. 23*:163, 1961*a*.

Mandl, I. Abstract 2.104 in: *Fifth International Congress of Biochemistry, Moscow 1961*. New York, Macmillan, 1963, vol. 9, p. 100.

Mehregan, A. H. and Staricco, R. G. *J. Invest. Derm. 38*:271, 1962.

Miller, E. J., Martin, G. R. and Piez, K. A. *Biochem. Biophys. Res. Comm. 17*:248, 1964.

Miller, E. J., Martin, G. R., Mecca, C. E. and Piez, K. A. *J. Biol. Chem. 240*:3623, 1965.

Mishima, Y. and Mevorah, B. *J. Invest. Derm. 36*:133, 1961.

Moran, T. J. and Lansing, A. I. *Arch. Path. 65*:688, 1958.

New York Heart Association. *Connective Tissue: Intercellular Macromolecules*. Boston, Little, Brown, 1964, 260 pp.

Nimni, M. E. and Bavetta, L. A. *Science 150*:905, 1965.

Partridge, S. M. In: *Recent Advances in Gelatin and Glue Research*. G. Stainsby, ed. New York, Pergamon, 1958, pp. 255-56.

Partridge, S. M. *Advances Prot. Chem. 17*: 227, 1962.

Quigley, M. B. and Hjørting-Hansen, E. *Acta Odont. Scand. 20*:359, 1962.

Rocha, G. and Winkelmann, R. K. *Arch. Derm. 85*:722, 1962.

Sams, W. M., Jr., Smith, J. G., Jr. and Davidson, E. A. *J. Histochem. Cytochem. 10*:710, 1962.

Sams, W. M., Jr. and Smith, J. G., Jr. Unpublished observations, 1964*a*.

Sams, W. M., Jr. and Smith, J. G., Jr. *Arch. Derm. 90*:137, 1964*b*.

Sams, W. M., Jr., Smith, J. G., Jr. and Burk, P. G. *J. Invest. Derm. 43*:467, 1964*c*.

Sams, W. M., Jr. and Smith, J. G., Jr. In: *Advances in Biology of the Skin*. W. Montagna, ed. New York, Macmillan, 1965, vol. 6, chap. 12, p. 199.

Sirsat, S. M. and Khanolkar, V. R. In: *Collagen*. N. Ramanthan, ed. New York, Interscience, 1962, p. 327.

Smith, A. D. and Waisman, M. *Arch. Derm. 81*:249, 1960.

Smith, R. C., Winer, L. H. and Martel, S. *Arch. Derm. 71*:197, 1955.

Smith, J. G., Jr. *Arch. Derm. 88*:382, 1963.

Smith, J. G., Jr. and Finlayson, G. R. Unpublished observations, 1964.

Smith, J. G., Jr., Davidson, E. A. and Clark, R. D. *Nature 195*:716, 1962*a*.

Smith, J. G., Jr., Sams, W. M., Jr., Davidson, E. A. and Clark, R. D. *Arch. Derm. 86*:741, 1962*b*.

Smith, J. G., Jr., Davidson, E. A., Sams, W. M., Jr. and Clark, R. D. *J. Invest. Derm. 39*:347, 1962*c*.

Smith, J. G., Jr., Davidson, E. A. and Hill, R. L. *Nature 197*:1108, 1963.

Smith, J. R., Jr., Sams, W. M., Jr. and Finlayson, G. R. In: *Modern Trends in Dermatology*. R. M. B. MacKenna, ed. London, Butterworths, 1966, p. 110.

Stadil, P. *Danish Med. Bull. 8*:131, 1961.

Staricco, R. G. and Mehregan, A. H. *Arch. Derm. 84*:943, 1961.

Stimmerman, G. N. and Stout, A. P. *Amer. J. Clin. Path. 37*:499, 1962.

Thomas, J. and Partridge, S. M. *Biochem. J. 74*:600, 1960.

Thomas, J., Elsden, D. F. and Partridge, S. M. *Nature 200*:651, 1963.

Unna, P. G. *Histopathology of Diseases of the Skin*, N. Walker, tr. New York, Macmillan, 1896, p. 976.

Varadi, D. P. and Hall, D. A. *Nature 208*: 1224, 1965.

Verzar, F. *Int. Rev. Connect. Tissue Res. 2*: 243, 1964.

Wechsler, H. L. and Fisher, E. R. *Arch. Path. 77*:613, 1964.

Weidman, F. D., Anderson, N. P. and Ayres, S., Jr. *Arch. Derm.* (Chicago) *28*:182, 1933.

Woods, J. F. and Nichols, G., Jr. *J. Cell Biology 26*:747, 1965*a*.

Woods, J. F. and Nichols, G., Jr. *Nature 208*:1325, 1965*b*.

# TRAINING IN NEUROLOGICAL SURGERY

*The Charles A. Elsberg Memorial Lecture**

PAUL C. BUCY

Professor of Surgery in charge of Neurological Surgery
Northwestern University Medical School
Chicago, Ill.

THE future of neurological surgery is, in large measure, dependent upon the nature and quality of our training programs. Only by the selection of outstanding trainees and by the maintenance of outstanding training programs can we hope to see neurological surgery continue as the vigorous, progressive, valuable medical specialty that it was in the pioneer days of Charles Elsberg, Harvey Cushing, Charles Frazier, Victor Horsley, and Walter Dandy. But we can no more be content to limit our training programs to the lines that our predecessors developed than we could be satisfied with the diagnostic and therapeutic procedures of the 1920's. In those days a bright young man with or without some experience in general surgery could spend a year with one of these pioneers and go on to become one of the outstanding neurological surgeons of the world. Many did as has been shown by Percival Bailey, Kenneth McKenzie, Sir Hugh Cairns, Clovis Vincent, Max Peet, and Alfred Adson. Today more is required.

The basic essential is unchanged. Whether the trainee will become one who limits his work to the clinical practice of neurological surgery, or whether he will direct a clinic, or become a teacher of his specialty, or an investigator, he must first of all be an accomplished neurological surgeon. There seem to be times when we lose sight of this. There is no substitute for hours, days, and years spent with patients in historical inquiry, in examination and in diagnosis, at the side of a master neurological surgeon at the operating table and, finally, in those tests of fire when, under proper supervision, the trainee takes the scalpel in his own hand. Training in general surgery and in clinical neurology, conference after fatiguing conference, and years in the laboratory can

*Presented at a meeting of the New York Society of Neurosurgery at The New York Academy of Medicine, May 17, 1966.

never take the place of adequate training in clinical neurological surgery. There are many investigations in human neuroanatomy and neurophysiology which can be made only by or with the cooperation of the neurological surgeon, but research in these fields requires that the neurological surgeon concerned be a skillful and knowledgeable surgeon as well as an investigator. The same is true of the teacher in this specialty. This is not to deny the importance of training in the ancillary fields. In fact, with the development of our specialty in an increasingly complex fashion, training in basic and clinical neurology and in research techniques has become of steadily increasing importance.

It would seem obvious that if training in neurological surgery is to remain at a high level, if the field of neurological surgery is to retain a spirit of progressive vigor, the direction of our training programs must be held tightly in the hands of the neurosurgeons. This is not as simple as it may seem. With the extension into the field of agencies such as the American Board of Neurological Surgery, the Council on Medical Education and Hospitals of the American Medical Association, the American College of Surgeons, and the National Institutes of Health, there have developed varying degrees of dictation as to how our residency training programs should be organized and conducted. All of these agencies act with the best of intentions—*as they see them*. But not all are fully informed and conversant with the problems of neurological surgery. And often their prime interest is different from that of the neurological surgeon. Nor are such influences confined to agencies outside the walls of our own institutions. Deans, heads of departments of general surgery, neurology and radiology, committees on curriculum and on interns and residents may each exert influence on our training programs. I do not contend that all these influences are bad or unwanted. I wish only to remind you that they do exist and that, accordingly, the director of each training program must decide for himself what he wishes to achieve and the course that he wishes to follow. He must then be prepared to accept those recommendations which will strengthen his program, must be prepared to adjust to those he can not resist, and to oppose those which are patently undesirable. Progress is not the product of a committee or of a dictator. Progress comes—if it comes at all—from the individual and often from an individual who is a nonconformist. Governmental and most other control is headed in the opposite direction. The creed of such control is to conform—to conform to the dictates of the group—of the administration. Conform or else—or else you don't get the approval or the money.

Of all these outside agencies, that child of our own creation, the American Board of Neurological Surgery, is obviously the best informed and the most directly concerned with the best interests of our specialty. Yet even here accomplishment leaves something to be desired. When, as is true today, one third of the candidates for certification by the Board fail to receive the Board's approval, something is wrong. All these candidates have completed training in programs which have been examined and have been approved by the Board. Either these examinations are not adequate for the purpose, or candidates are being selected improperly, or the training programs are not living up to the high standards expected of them. Ideally all candidates who have completed approved courses of training should pass the examinations and be certified by the Board. Perhaps this ideal is too much to expect in our everyday world, but that one-third are failures is too much.

Unquestionably the Board is doing what it thinks best to improve the training of the neurosurgeon, but at times its actions must be questioned. It says, "The trainee must have a year of training in general surgery." Why? Presumably in order that he may be trained in the principles of surgery, whatever that may mean. The Board says literally that the "general surgeon" is more capable of giving that training than the neurological surgeon—an assumption which I hope and believe is not true. There is no such thing as a "general surgeon" and there has not been for a long, long time, fortunately. Those surgeons who assert their superiority under the title of "general" are belly and neck surgeons. And for the most part the year spent by the trainee in general surgery is a year spent learning to take out appendices and repair hernias—a year spent largely in learning how to tie knots in a string.

For years we have been increasing the period of training for our specialty and have devoted no consideration to conserving the all too few active years of our trainees. We are devoting what we know to be the most active, thoughtful and productive period of the lives of these men to training. Seldom do they have time to think and to experiment. When they complete their training, in their mid-thirties, they are married and have families. And of these you will recall that Sir Francis Bacon said 400 years ago, "He that hath a wife hath given hostages to fortune; for they are impediments to great enterprises, either of virtue or mischief." Most of our trainees also have debts. Is it surprising that they find it necessary to devote the next years of their lives intensely to making a living? How many promising investigators who might have contributed great things to the field of neurological surgery—and it badly needs such contributions—have we discouraged and snuffed out by the rigidity of the long years of training which we require? That these early years are often the most original, the most productive, is easily demonstrable. To take examples known to every one of us: Percival Bailey's *Classification of the Tumors of the Glioma Group* was published when he was 34 years old, and Earl Walker's *The Primate Thalamus* when he was 31. In both instances the work that preceded the appearance of these classics was done when they were even younger and in both instances this work was possible because these scientists were trained in a liberal permissive atmosphere, with no rigid requirements as to how a man must be trained to become a neurological surgeon.

In other respects too our Board has developed questionable requirements. Training in general surgery is not acceptable unless it is obtained within the confines of North America. General surgical training obtained as a surgical intern is quite acceptable, but identical training obtained in the same institution as a rotating intern is not acceptable. Training in clinical neurology or basic neurological science is acceptable, and presumably of value as training, only if it is obtained after the trainee decides to become a neurological surgeon and has arranged with the director of a program for his training.

It is time that we stopped to give thought not to a set of rules to which everyone must conform but to how we can aid intelligent young men to obtain adequate training to become neurological surgeons in the shortest time. We must provide for those unusual people, the Baileys and the Walkers, and give them every opportunity to make the contributions of which they are capable. It is inexcusable to require them to spend a year in training under those "belly" surgeons who have little of value to teach them that a neurological surgeon should be able to provide, or to require them to undergo the same training twice simply because the time and the manner in which it was obtained does not fit some predetermined rule. I realize that the rules contain loopholes through which they can be circumvented. But these are not enough. Our trainees must be *encouraged* to vary their training, to follow unusual interests, not merely *permitted* to do so on occasion.

There can be no question of the devotion, the sincerity and the integrity of the members of the Board, and I make that statement as one of the founding members of the Board and one who served as an officer and member for 8 years. Compassion for the applicants and tolerance for differences of opinion have always characterized its members. Nor do I wish to imply that the Board has not been greatly concerned with these problems. Over the past several years the Board has devoted much time and effort in learning where the difficulties lie. I urge that they persist in these efforts, and I hope that with the sympathetic help of their neurosurgical colleagues they will ultimately arrive at a solution.

The Council on Medical Education and Hospitals has played a much more subsidiary role. It has spent time, money and effort to assist the Board in evaluating residency training programs but it has left the final decision as to the acceptance or rejection of a given program to the Board. The Council has established no requirements beyond those that apply to residency training programs in other fields of medicine or surgery. The American College of Surgery has played an even lesser part.

The position of the National Institute of Neurological Diseases and Blindness (NINDB) of the U. S. Public Health Service is quite different. Here, too, I speak as one who has been associated with that Institute in one capacity or another for the past 10 years. Since its formation the Institute has been concerned primarily with research. Subsequently, it also became concerned with the training of investigators and teachers as it concluded that its research aims could not be achieved unless the number of investigators and teachers of investigators was increased. More recently it has also concerned itself with the training of practitioners in certain special fields, notably neurology, because of a belief that there was a great need for more practicing doctors in this field. More by accident than by design, NINDB has also supported the training of practitioners in otolaryngology and ophthalmology. All this time, however, it has consistently refused to admit that it is its purpose to train practitioners and has continued to declare that its purposes in training are limited to the training of investigators and teachers. In the field of neurological surgery, where it has supported very few training programs, it has not yet deviated from its expressed intent.

In the past the specialty of neurological surgery has expressed its disapproval of the participation of the federal government in medicine, by official notice to the National Institute of Neurological Diseases and Blindness that it did not approve of federal support for neurosurgical training programs regardless of whether they were concerned with the training of men who would devote themselves to clinical practice or who would become teachers and investigators. During all this time it should be noted, however, that research projects conducted by neurosurgeons have always sought and have been given financial support by the Institute, and many individual neurological surgeons have served this governmental agency loyally and well in various capacities, as consultants and as members of study sections and review committees. Five years ago a neurological surgeon was for the first time appointed to the Advisory Council of the National Institute of Neurological Diseases and Blindness after the Society of Neurological Surgeons notified the NINDB that it wished to cooperate more fully with it. Since then the participation of neurological surgeons in the activities of NINDB has steadily increased. The number of neurological surgeons on the training review committees has been doubled from two to four. Eight neurosurgical programs have been supported as training centers for teachers and investigators. This number was to be increased to 14 on July 1, 1966.

In my opinion, the expansion of participation by neurosurgeons in the activities of NINDB and the increased support of neurosurgical training programs by the Institute have been both advantageous and desirable. I am also convinced that further expansion is desirable but this is a matter to which we must give serious thought and one that we must view critically. There are people who believe that all residency training should be supported by the federal government and there are undoubtedly forces pushing toward that end. This is not surprising. There is, unfortunately, a general trend to turn to the federal government for support in all fields. With the obvious expansion of the government's interest in medicine—in the investigation and treatment of cerebrovascular and cardiovascular diseases, of mental retardation, of the paralyzed and handicapped child, of the veteran and of the aged—it finds that it needs an ever increasing number of medical specialists. Naturally it turns to its own agency—the National Institutes of Health—to fill those needs. Hospitals that get support for the training of residents in psychiatry, neurology, neurological surgery, otolaryngology, or ophthalmology, and hospitals that see their fellow hospitals receive such support are inclined also to seek similar support from the National Institutes of Health in those and several other medical fields. At the present time practically all residency programs—other than those supported by the Institute—are supported by the hospitalized patients. Many sensible people look upon this as grossly unfair and unwise. Why should these people already burdened with heavy expenses of an illness bear the added burden of advanced medical education? Would it not be more fair and better over-all that this cost be shared equitably by the public through federal taxation? This is an attractive idea, as are most plans to have the federal government take over the support of things, but it carries with it serious disadvantages which are so great that I think we should vigorously oppose federal support of post-graduate medical education except in well-defined special situations.

Let us look first at the apparent inequity in the present method of supporting residency training programs, that is, by the hospitalized patient. This is not as unfair as it may seem at first glance. There can be no doubt that the medical care of patients is improved by the mere existence of a residency training program in a hospital. The patient benefits by the fact that the resident is there, just as he benefits by the fact that the hospital employs nurses, maids, janitors, and elevator operators for whom he must also pay. The patient benefits perhaps even more from the fact that the residents are being trained in the hospital where he is being treated. The presence of residents stimulates the attending neurological surgeon to give his best efforts to the problems at hand, and they often teach him almost as much as he teaches them. As a result the best neurosurgical care is given in the hospitals with residency training programs. Furthermore, at the present time about 75 per cent of all hospitalized patients have some form of hospital insurance. As a result the expenses of the hospitals, including the support of residency programs, is much more evenly distributed than it would seem at first glance. One may well question whether federal taxation would provide any fairer distribution of costs, or less expense to the public.

Even more important than the question of the equitable distribution of costs is the fact that the support of all residency training programs by the federal government would carry with it very grave disadvantages. The most serious of these would be that the neurological surgeon would lose control of the training programs to individuals less informed regarding the needs of the field. Despite the fact that the administration of the National Institute of Neurological Diseases and Blindness has leaned over backward to avoid dictating to individual institutions, the fact still remains that the agency that controls the purse strings has the obligation to see that the money entrusted to it is properly spent. This it does in the light of its own opinions and determinations as to what constitutes proper utilization of funds. Its decisions in this regard may or may not be in accord with the opinion of the neurological surgeon in charge of a program or with the opinions of neurological surgeons in general as to what constitutes a good neurosurgical residency training program. The possibility of differences of opinion in this regard are inherent in the organization of any governmental agency. The administrator of the National Institute of Neurological Diseases and Blindness is likely to have been trained in one of the medical disciplines of that Institute. That is, he will probably be a neurologist, a neurosurgeon, an ophthalmologist, or an otolaryngologist. It would be impossible for him to be competent in all of these fields. He has and will continue to gather about him a large group of consultants and advisors in many related disciplines and he will be guided by their opinions and advice. The opinion of a neurologist, or an ophthalmologist, or a neuropathologist as to what should constitute an acceptable neurosurgical training program may be far different from yours and mine. And again let me emphasize that to place the control of our residency training programs in these hands will remove it from ours.

Perhaps even more serious is the centralization of control. Good training programs will vary in their organization from director to director, from institution to institution, and from one part of the country to another. The National Institute of Neurological Diseases and Blindness has tried to recognize both the necessity and desirability of such variation, but this is not easy. With any centralized control the simplest course is always to establish some rigid requirements for those programs that are to be supported and then require that everyone conform. In spite of the Institute's efforts to avoid such regimentation the forces in this direction are strong and will increase. It is to the credit of Richard Masland, present director of NINDB, that he has consistently resisted these forces that press toward uniformity. He has recognized that no one man or group of men has the superior wisdom to know what is best, and that experimentation and variation in different programs are desirable. However, as Dr. Masland will not always be the director of NINDB, we can not afford to place the control of training in neurological surgery in unknown hands.

Federal support of residency training has another very serious disadvantage. It may be withdrawn on a moment's notice and for a variety of reasons. Should this happen the neurological surgeon in charge of the training program will likely find himself without resources to fall back upon. This is not mere conjecture. It has happened in the past and it will happen in the future. Removal of such support may be restricted to an individual program and for a variety of reasons. The program may not measure up in some minor or major way to the preconceived requirements of the federal agency concerned. There may be a change in directorship of the residency training program. There may develop some other real or supposed deficiency in the program. Even more serious, however, is the fact that the President of the United States or one of his many associates may decide that the money allocated to medical training programs can be better used to support an antipoverty program, for example, or is needed to finance a war. Congress may fail to appropriate adequate funds for the support of training programs. This happened recently when enough funds were appropriated to continue support of programs already accepted but not enough to support programs not already receiving federal aid regardless of their quality or their need. Neurology continued to be well supported insofar as training programs were concerned, whereas neurological surgery, which had only a few programs approved for support, could not expand. Whether it was desirable for more neurosurgical programs to be supported by federal funds is another matter, but had we been working in a situation in which we looked to the federal government for our only support we would have found ourselves in serious trouble.

I realize my position here may be confusing to some of my hearers and I shall restate it in other terms. I am opposed to the support of clinical neurosurgical training from federal funds. I am in favor of such support for the training of neurosurgical residents in the basic neurological sciences and research. I am also in favor of the support of such residents during their training in clinical neurology, on the same basis that applies to medical neurological residents. Such training is important in enabling them to meet the many medical neurological problems that face them because of the lack of a sufficient number of adequately trained neurologists in this country. To this end, as well as in the interests of the support of research in which neurological surgeons do and should take an active part, the neurological surgeons of this country must continue to demonstrate their interest in the National Institute of Neurological Diseases and Blindness. They must insist upon adequate representation on its Advisory Council and on its various review committees, and must willingly accept their obligation to serve that Institute when called upon to do so.

Our concern today with training in neurological surgery is by no means restricted to the influence of outside agencies. Of even greater importance is the organization and control of our training programs by ourselves.

The first and perhaps the most important obligation we have is the proper selection of trainees, and this is not easy. Mistakes will always be made. We must utilize every means to insure that the men selected for training in neurological surgery will make good neurosurgeons. There can be no doubt that an outstanding man can become a good neurological surgeon even with training in an inferior program, but the best training program in the world can not make a good neurosurgeon of an inferior man. All too frequently men are accepted as trainees because the program needs another man and not because the man presents evidence of his ability and integrity. I am convinced that this is one of the more important reasons for the high percentage of failures before the American Board of Neurological Surgery. Those who are directors of residency training programs must have the courage and determination—it takes courage and determination—to remove a man from a program when he has demonstrated that he is not a suitable trainee. His deficiencies may lie in various directions. He may not be as intelligent as was originally thought when he was selected. He may not have the capacity to become a neurosurgeon in spite of adequate intelligence. He may lack the moral fiber which is essential to the members of this specialty. Regardless of the reason, when one is convinced that the man is not suitable, he should be removed regardless of the effect upon the program itself. This is one of the most difficult responsibilities that any training director will encounter.

What must our training programs include? As I have already stated, there must be adequate training to insure that the man will become a competent neurological surgeon. This is the first and the most outstanding requirement. It is not enough for the program to include an adequate number and variety of cases. It is not enough for the resident to have a large number of patients upon whom he himself may operate. Were these the requirements, our large charity hospitals would have the best training programs–they seldom do. If this were the case, Harvey Cushing would not have been the world's greatest trainer of neurological surgeons. The first requirement of any training program is that it be directed by an outstanding neurological surgeon who is intensely interested in his patients and in his residents. There is no substitute for the teacher. Surprisingly enough the outstanding teacher and director is not always the world's greatest technical surgeon, but he must be a competent one. He must train his men by his example. He must train them in neurological diagnosis. He must develop their judgment. He must show them how to operate. He must lead them in postoperative care. And he must develop in them a philosophy of medicine and its responsibilities that extends far beyond the confines of the neurosurgical operation. This means that he must devote time, thought, and care to the responsibilities he has assumed. In my opinion the director who sees his trainees for an hour once a day, or who makes rounds with them once a week is not fulfilling his obligations.

Because the direction of a residency training program is a time-consuming job the opinion has developed in some quarters that it should be a full-time job. With this I should agree if it means that the neurosurgeon should confine his efforts to one institution and devote all of his time to the direction of the training program, to teaching, research, and the care of his patients. However, all too frequently the term "full-time" does not refer at all to how the man spends his time but to how he is paid. All too frequently "full-time" is taken to mean that the man is to be paid only by salary and not by his private patients. In many instances this is only a subterfuge intended to make the neurosurgeon support the residency training program, the hospital itself, and even other less productive members of the faculty of the medical school. From years of experience under both systems–full-time salaried and private practice–I am convinced that in general the fully salaried plan is the least satisfactory. Part salary and part private practice, or complete self-support ordinarily results in a better, more well-rounded residency training program that is fairer to the neurosurgeon. However, the neurosurgeon should be free to elect which of these plans he desires. A full-time salaried position should not be forced upon him. His competence as the director of the training program should be judged on the basis of his performance and not on how he is paid. In my opinion, the trend of medical schools and also of the National Institutes of Health to force full-time salaried positions on the directors of residency training programs will result in poorer programs, not better ones.

How training in clinical neurological surgery is to be attained will and should vary from one center to another. It will depend upon the director and the members of his attending staff. It will depend upon the nature and location of his hospital. No rigid requirements in this matter should be established, only minimal requirements. There are certain levels that must be reached, but the director should be left free to experiment as he thinks best and to adjust his program to the local situation, and to the trainee. No perfect program of training has yet been designed, nor is it likely to be.

We have spoken of the proper selection of trainees. There is another aspect of this serious problem that I would touch upon here: that is, the foreign trainee. In my opinion we here in the United States have a responsibility to the rest of the world. It is not confined to us. It extends to our colleagues in Europe and elsewhere, but I am concerned about ourselves. Medicine knows no national boundaries. It knows no color or creed. True physicians are interested in the welfare of mankind. In the past we have benefited and we are still benefiting from training in other lands and from the experience of other peoples. Many of us have been received with open arms for training in England, Germany, Scandinavia, France and elsewhere. We have the obligation to repay that debt by training men from other countries where such training is so badly needed, and there are many such places. We should be as rigid in our requirements of these foreign trainees as we are with our own men and, in addition, we should impose upon them certain other requirements. It is impossible to give adequate training in neurological surgery without the trainee having intimate contact with the patients. It is essential, therefore, that he have a good command of the English language. We must insist that these foreign trainees complete the same long course in training that we require of young men in the United States. In various countries throughout the world I have seen men who have had a 1-year or even only a 6-months' experience in an otherwise adequate training center. When such a man returns to his country he seldom does credit to his teachers and often brings criticism upon the country where he has been trained and upon neurological surgery in general. I will not accept as a trainee any man who does not agree to complete a 5-year course of training. We should insist that the trainee we accept from a foreign country be regarded highly by his teachers and colleagues at home. We should have evidence of this high regard by assurances that this is a man they want back in their country—a man they need—and that they have a hospital and/or a medical school in which he will be accepted and where he can work. Last, we must have the assurance from the man concerned that he will return to his home once his training is complete. Some directors of training programs have endeavored to implement this last requirement by not giving the man a training adequate to permit him to take the examinations of the American Board of Neurological Surgery. I think this is wrong. Such a man is entitled to this certificate of his training and competence. It is important to him and to the institutions that have endorsed him and promised him a place in which to work.

Beyond adequate training in clinical neurological surgery, what else should our programs provide? Should we require training in basic neurological science and in research? Certainly, circumstances vary greatly in this regard. If by training in the basic sciences, one merely means that the trainee should repeat the courses in neuroanatomy and neurophysiology given in the preclinical years of our medical schools, I should not agree. Little is gained by having a man needlessly repeat a course. A course of instruction given by a nonclinician is often disappointing so far as the training of a neurosurgeon is concerned. Neuroanatomy and neurophysiology should be taught to the resident as it applies to the neurosurgical patient. This is not easy but it is an end to be sought. If possible, the instruction in these basic subjects should be given by or in collaboration with neurological surgeons and should be oriented toward existing clinical problems with which the resident is familiar.

There should be a definite period of training in neuropathology, and again it should be correlated as closely as possible with the clinical cases with which the resident is familiar. This training in pathology should not be limited, however, to neurosurgical problems. The trainee should become familiar with the pathology of neurological disease in general. He can not hope to be an adequate neurological surgeon without such knowledge.

In my opinion, the neurosurgical resident should have training in and experience with medical neurology. Without such knowledge he can not deal adequately with the diagnostic and therapeutic problems that will confront him. Unfortunately, adequate training in clinical neurology suited to the neurosurgical resident is not easy to obtain. On occasion the medical neurologist is a biased individual who is not even a good diagnostician in his own field. Too frequently patients are carried year after year in the neurological clinic with the diagnosis of multiple sclerosis, or cerebral vascular disease, when the spinal cord tumor or brain tumor responsible should be recognized and removed. Medical neurology has made great strides in recent years but not all neurologists or neurological centers are aware of these advances. On the other hand, the neurological surgeon should not delegate all the instruction of the resident in diagnostic neurology to his medical neurologist colleague. Differential diagnosis is as much a part of neurological surgery as it is a part of medical neurology and it is not just a matter of air, Pantopaque, Hypaque, and radioactive isotopes. The competent neurological surgeon, and particularly the neurosurgical teacher, must be familiar with nonsurgical neurological disease. Instruction in differential diagnosis should be an every day occurrence in the neurosurgical wards. Furthermore, the necessity for familiarity with medical neurological disorders is not limited to the differential diagnosis of neurosurgical cases. Unfortunately, in many parts of the United States no competent medical neurologist is available and the local medical profession understandably turns to the neurological surgeon for help. He will be faced with this responsibility whether he wants it or not, and he should be prepared to meet it.

What about research? Many men in training in neurological surgery are not particularly interested in research and, lacking such interest, they are not likely ever to engage effectively in research. In my opinion, those men who plan to engage in teaching and who will be associated with academic centers should be interested in research and should be required to have research experience. All others will benefit to some extent by such training. Fortunately, neurological surgery is still a rapidly advancing specialty, but not all change is advance and not all research is good. The man who has had personal experience in research will be better able to evaluate the investigations and the conclusions of others, even though he may never again personally engage in such pursuits. The importance of research experience to the field of neurological surgery can hardly be overestimated. There is still much to be learned about the nervous system, and much that we need to know about the nervous system of man that can be learned only from man. In many instances, the active participation of a neurological surgeon in the investigation of man is imperative. He will contribute much more to any investigation if he is himself a competent investigator rather than if he is just a pair of skilled hands.

One of the trouble spots in neurosurgery and in neurosurgical training has been the subject of neuroradiology. In foreign countries where neurological surgery is concentrated in a few large clinics and where the individual patient is not always of as much concern to the attending physician or surgeon as he is here, it has become common practice to place all radiological diagnostic procedures exclusively in the hands of the neuroradiologist. In my opinion, close cooperation between the neurosurgeon and the radiologist is essential to the operation of a neurosurgical center, but to take neuroradiological procedures completely out of the hands of the neurosurgeon is highly undesirable. This is particularly true in a training center. Many men, once they have completed their training, will settle in cities where there is no neuroradiologist. If they have not been well trained in these diagnostic procedures, they will not be competent neurosurgeons. Even in larger centers where neuroradiologists are available, the neurosurgeons can not and should not be relieved of this responsibility. The patient has chosen the neurosurgeon as his physician and the responsibilities associated with this relationship can not and should not be delegated. In spite of all precautions myelography, pneumoencephalography, ventriculography, and angiography are attended with risks not commonly encountered in other radiological diagnostic procedures. The decision as to what tests should be done, when and how they should be performed, when to stop any given diagnostic procedure in mid-flight must rest with the surgeon in charge. The selection of patients is his, and the evaluation of the findings must be made in the light of other information about the patient that the radiologist does not have. The neuroradiologist has much to contribute to neurological surgery, but it is in the field of radiological techniques and in the evaluation of radiological studies in other fields. He should not be overlooked or pushed aside, but he must not be allowed to "take over."

And now we have come full circle. We are back where we started: that is, to the basic concept that neurosurgical training, if it is to be adequate and if neurological surgery is to advance, must be kept in the hands of the neurological surgeon. He must personally design and participate in the training program. The responsibility is his, and his alone. He can not allow it to slip into other hands. Whether we shall produce more Elsbergs, or Cushings, or Dandys is not really open to question if we remain in charge of our own ship.

# THE HOSPITAL AS A TEACHING CENTER

*The Third Godfrey Nurse Lecture**

GEORGE H. HUMPHREYS, II

Valentine Mott Professor of Surgery
Columbia University College of Physicians and Surgeons
New York, N. Y.

IN considering any one aspect of a hospital, we must first ask ourselves an apparently simple question. What is a hospital? The answer is not as simple as it seems. A hospital is many things, depending on who is looking at it. The people who establish and support it, the group of patients whose needs it serves, the doctors who work in it, and the university that affiliates with it, all see it through different eyes. Each judges it by his own separate standards. There is, in consequence of these differing views, a broad area for differences of opinion or even for acrimony when differing needs conflict on priorities, or when decisions based on the criteria of one group appear to hamper or disregard the needs of another. Since we are now entering a period of change, in which traditional values and relationships must increasingly be revised to fit new circumstances, it is perhaps worthwhile to stand back for a few minutes from the sometimes controversial aspects of our immediate problems and review a few basic premises. If these can be seen clearly and correctly, it should help us to recognize where we must adjust our thinking and adapt our actions to the changing role of the hospital.

We must consider two groups of people: 1) the community and the medical profession, and 2) two institutions created by, serving, and being served by these people—the hospital and the university. Each of these four is related in its own way to each of the other three. Let us first take a quick look at the hospital through the eyes of each, and then explore the relation of each to the others in this context.

Historically, hospitals developed from hostels or hospices conducted by religious orders for the care of weary travelers, needy paupers, the

*Presented under the auspices of the Department of Surgery of the Harlem Hospital Center, New York, N. Y., at The New York Academy of Medicine, April 6, 1966.

crippled, and the sick. To a basic humanitarian motive to help the poor and suffering was added, later, a desire on the part of communities to protect themselves by isolating the diseased and to provide alms for those unable to care for themselves. Provision of care for responsible members of the community came much later, and with it motives of financial or political gain that clouded the perhaps purer charitable basis of the earlier hospitals. A loss in purity of motive, however, was often a gain in quality of care.

We seem to be entering the last phase of this transition in the way the community views its hospital, and remnants of the older view still confuse many issues. But it is increasingly clear, now, that the nation as a whole expects its hospitals not merely to offer charity to the needy, but to provide an ever ready source of medical care to all, with equal standards of care for all, and without the need of gratitude for charity on the part of any of those receiving care. The community has now charged its agents, the hospital trustees, hospital commissioners, public health officials, and federal agencies with this new theme in their traditional responsibility.

To the medical profession the hospital has a different aspect. True, the doctor, like the community he serves, has humanitarian instincts that find outlet in charitable service in the hospital. The philanthropist gives money; the doctor gives service. But many practicing doctors in any community may have no time or opportunity for such service, and in the proportion that the hospital improves its facilities for patient care it may appear to them as a competitor. In particular, as the hospital shifts from providing philanthropically, by private donation or public tax, the means for doctors to donate their services to the needy, to an institution established by the public treasury for the service of everyone, the relationship of the hospital to the outside practitioner needs revision.

The staff doctor, on the other hand, may consider the hospital his workshop, a place in which, and a means whereby, to earn his living. He tends to assume that it can best serve the community by making things efficient for him rather than for the patient. He may forget that as he is no longer expected to give his services as charity, so he cannot now expect the patient to yield gratefully to his convenience. Even more, for the doctor, the hospital is a continuing school—a place in which to learn, to gain experience, and to improve his understanding of disease. Here he can best develop new treatments by comparing methods under controlled conditions or by investigating the causes or phenomena of disease by the accumulation of data.

Finally, the doctor thinks of the hospital as a place to teach. The precious Hippocratic obligation to pass on hard-earned knowledge and skill is not confined to academic medical teachers, it is a deep and widespread professional need. Teaching of clinical medicine can never completely separate itself from an apprentice period, and each doctor, having assisted and learned from his predecessors, has the obligation and the desire to be assisted by, and to teach, his successors. This is still best done in a hospital service.

The university views the hospital in relation to its own teaching obligations. It must attract a faculty of scientists, and it must construct laboratories for their research and teaching, as well as the classrooms, libraries, and other facilities for the student's basic instruction. But clinical teaching requires a hospital. Here is the living text the medical student needs, and here also is a willing, often self-supporting, group of teachers. Furthermore here is a source for clinical study and investigation; here a basic university need, the obligation to increase knowledge, can be fulfilled.

The hospital is changing, in the view of the community, from its traditional aspect as a charitable community obligation to a service facility supported by and serving all equally, as fulfilling a common right. It may appear as a competitor to some practitioners, or as a workshop to its own staff, though it should be neither. But it serves all the profession as a classroom and a laboratory, and as such it may also serve and be served by the university.

Back of the hospital stands the relationship between doctors and the people they serve. This relationship is best when it is most free. A doctor recognizes his obligation to serve those patients he feels best qualified to treat. The patient is free to request advice and care from the doctor of his choice. No patient should be obliged to accept care from a doctor in whom he lacks confidence, and no doctor should be obliged to care for a patient under unsatisfactory conditions. On the other hand, the doctor's obligation to care for patients who choose him is limited only by his ability to serve them well. It is not limited by the social, geographic, or economic circumstances of the patient, but it may be limited by his competence to care for the presenting problem, by the pressure on him of other commitments, or by his ability to command an appropriate facility for treatment. As a responsible member of the community, a doctor may take part in community hospital activity, but he has no professional obligation to support the hospital directly: his professional obligation is solely to his patients.

A hospital, then, is created by the community to provide the doctors of its choice with facilities for the care of those patients it wishes to serve. The community, whether church, charity, or city, determines both the conditions in the hospital and the composition of its staff. This is not a function or prerogative of the medical profession. But the profession is ready, and indeed anxious, to provide the community with standards and, through the mechanism of accreditation, to inform the community of professional approval. The community determines what local obligation the hospital is to serve. The type of service will be determined, in turn, by the local need. Primarily this need will usually be patient care, often modified in respect to certain categorical problems such as chronic care or mental illness. Or a hospital may be created to deal with a special problem, such as cancer. The need may be specific geographically or it may be determined by other criteria, such as teaching and research, which have no geographic limitation nor regional obligation.

It is the obligation of the community to supply the facilities for the doctors it has chosen to do the work it has asked them to do. But it is not the obligation of the community, through the hospital, to supply professional medical care directly. This is the obligation of the profession. When care is given by the hospital without charge as a charity to the patient, the doctor should do the same and may have to accept less than optimal conditions. With care now demanded as a "right" backed by citizen taxation, the community has also obligated itself to provide adequately both facilities and reimbursement for the doctors who have accepted that responsibility. But no doctor can be commanded by his community to serve in its hospital if he considers the conditions unsatisfactory, nor can any doctor demand staff appointment in the community's hospital except by community choice.

The relationship of the hospital to the doctors, therefore, is a partnership. Neither is the other's master; neither is the other's servant. Each serves the other and, together, both serve the community. The hospitals cannot serve their patients without doctors; doctors, on the other hand, can care for patients without need of a hospital, though the services they can really render well in this way are becoming progressively more restricted. The doctor serves best when he is not an employee of the hospital, and hospital management is best when its manager is not employed by the doctors. Both should be employees of the community. The method of payment is not important as long as it is perfectly clear to the employer—that is to the community—just what he is paying for each component of the service he receives. He may pay the hospital and the doctor separately and directly, either from his own resources or with help from insurance. He may pay them together by contract or taxation, but he still should know how much he is paying and to whom and for which service. Only in that way can the community judge costs, and seek to modify them if need be.

It follows that the hospital not only should not employ doctors, but also that it has no obligation to furnish its staff with a livelihood. Unless it is a proprietary hospital, its basic function is not to provide a workshop for the doctor. Rather, it should provide for the patient's needs and should make it convenient for the doctor to meet his obligations in providing care. Neither is it the doctor's obligation to supply the hospital with the facilities he needs. The community must distinguish its obligations to the hospital from its obligations to the doctors, but it must support them both equally and without confusion.

Facilities for teaching and research may be supplied by hospitals, especially those with university affiliation, as a means of attracting and holding professional personnel. This, however, is also not a primary hospital obligation. If the community wishes university participation, it may build facilities or make research grants directly, or may assist the university to do so. The university, on the other hand, has a duty to support the teaching and research activities of its staff, since this is not a hospital obligation. In the long run the hospital will attract to work in it doctors in numbers and competence in proportion to its ability to supply adequate facilities for their primary needs. When it does so, the doctor's ability to render the best quality of care of which he is capable, the experience he gains in doing it, and his opportunities to pass on his knowledge and skill to younger men are his chief incentive and reward.

Leaving hospitals and doctors for a moment, let us look at the university and its relations to the community. The university's primary function, as its name implies, is universal rather than local. Its purpose is to gather, store, transmit, and add to knowledge of every kind. Though it may be locally supported by philanthropy or taxation, as is the hospital, unlike the latter it will be effective in its mission in proportion to its freedom from parochial demands. Direct or indirect tax support is a recognition by the community of local benefits. Though incidental to the university's main purpose, such benefits are nonetheless real. Many people from porters to professors are directly employed, and many more indirectly. The presence of distinguished scholars and able leaders in all professions not only gives cultural depth to the community but also provides it with a pool of experts who may be called upon for advice or direct service. Yet it should not be forgotten that direct community service rendered by its members is not a function of the university as an institution. Rather it is the obligation of the university to remain aloof from local issues. The "ivory tower" removes its occupants from ground-level controversy and puts them in a position of greater perspective. It is their obligation from this position to observe, comment, advise if asked, and even shout warnings when not asked, but not to take direct part in rendering service except as it may serve their primary academic function. This local irresponsibility of the university is an often misunderstood source of friction even among its own members.

In this respect the relation of the medical profession to the university is unique. Law can be taught, even by the case method, without need of university participation in actual court action. Journalism can be taught without competing with the publishing business. Architecture can be taught without actual construction of buildings, and even business administration can be taught without running a corporation or factory. But medicine cannot be taught without actually treating patients. Service is a necessary and inseparable part of clinical teaching. And if it is to serve as a teaching example, the service rendered must be exemplary.

Thus it becomes a university obligation, when its medical teachers enter the arena of hospital patient care, to see to it that the community provides them with the means to demonstrate the best care possible. By the same token it is the obligation of the university to be highly selective in its choice of staff teachers. "Good enough" is not sufficient.

It is the most sacred obligation of all for the university to insure not only that, in educating physicians, it is serving its primary function of passing on to a new generation the wisdom of the past and adding new knowledge to it, but also that it is constantly demonstrating to them and to the practicing profession, in a daily life-and-death struggle, the best application of that wisdom.

It is only natural, if the medical school is at all successful in this purpose, that demands will come to it from the community to extend services more widely. The secondary and incidental community gain will be mistaken for a primary university obligation. But this is the responsibility of the practicing profession, not of the university. It is sufficient, indeed it is all that it can possibly do, for the university to recognize its obligation to support the profession in this responsibility. It must perpetuate the profession by providing young men with basic scientific education, by teaching them current medical knowledge and training them in skills, and by providing the means to advance knowledge through research. It must either support its clinical teachers, or see to it that they have the means to support themselves and, at the same time, that they are provided with facilities to teach while rendering exemplary care. It should also, to a greater extent than it has done in the past, bring support to the practicing profession by making more easily available to it the benefits of its advancing knowledge.

If there is a lag, as is commonly thought, between "ivory tower" knowledge and "blood and guts" application, it is a joint fault of the university and the profession. Traditionally the initiative to "keep up" has been left to the practitioner; the university has been satisfied with offering, in a not too accessible way, the means for him to do so. If the response has been meager and both have been disappointed, the community has been even more disillusioned. This effect can be corrected only by real effort on both sides. It now seems possible that the means will become available. But the need for effort must be understood, it cannot be legislated. The first step in establishing such a working relationship is a clear appreciation on the part of community, profession, and university of the different but interlocking objectives and obligations of each.

These interlocking objectives come to a focus in the hospital when it becomes a teaching center. Ideally, the community will make certain that such a hospital is equipped not only to provide its staff with the means to give the best and latest in diagnosis and treatment but also will create there facilities for the university to teach its students, investigate disease, and bring to the practicing profession the benefits of its studies. The profession will supply the university with selected teachers and investigators, who will discharge their community service obligation for patient care as an inseparable part of their teaching, training, and research functions. The major service load, however, will be carried by the practicing profession, which will be adequately supported by the community and reinforced by the teaching, training, and investigative skills of its university members. The university will arrange with the community for adequate facilities and support for its hospital staff to teach and study disease as well as care for patients, and it will provide the practicing profession, and through it the community, with new doctors, new methods, and new insight into illness. Though details of procedure will require constant adjustment, there can be no conflict in basic objectives once the functions, the needs, the limitations of responsibility, and the obligations of each element are understood.

How, finally, do these generalities apply to Harlem Hospital? Here there is real regional service need, too long inadequately supported by the community but now coming into its own. Generous tax support is an expression by the city as a whole of awakened interest and responsibility for all citizens. This is expressed by the new building rising beside the old, and by the enlistment of university interest and staffing support. This interest is genuine. It is not a mere token or charity service to a local regional need, however real and serious that need may be. It is, rather, that the university also has a need that Harlem Hospital can supply. For the need to come to grips with the problem of establishing good medical care "across the board" to previously deprived people is the most vital sociomedical question of our time. Here the university has a magnificent opportunity to make a major contribution, local in immediate effect but universal in application. In this effort, it must have and must be able to rely on the support of the profession, not only of the teaching staff it will enlist but also of the practicing profession of the community. It will in turn support their local and personal interests in improving the care they can give to their patients.

This opportunity coincides fortuitously and, we hope, fortunately, with a national awakening in the same direction. Federal support may now be added to that of the city to make of this hospital a model regional center. Thus a true partnership of mutual interest should be possible, each element helped by and supporting the other. City, state, and nation will gain their objective of extending to all, without onus of charity, the care that only the profession can give. Through the profession the university can both assist and gain its own objectives, not only of teaching and adding to knowledge but also of devising methods to diffuse more widely than ever before the benefits of that knowledge. The profession will in turn come closer to fulfillment of its deepest need, to care for all to its best ability, to improve its own skill and experience, and to pass on what it has gained to its successors. If we can work together successfully toward this goal in a spirit of mutual self-interest and common ideals the Harlem Hospital will be a teaching center of which we can be proud.

This will not happen overnight. A heritage of neglect in structure, facilities, and organization must be surmounted. Without losing sight of the lessons of the past, the stalwart veterans who have held the line so long must be reinforced by fresh forces bringing new methods, devising new solutions to problems old and new. There is no place, now, for petty jealousy, small-minded jockeying for position, power plays, or personal prestige. We stand together or we fall apart. Destructive action in any area is destructive to all; constructive action anywhere will help everywhere. Our task is too big to be surmounted in the context of the past. We must see the big objective, and all of us—practitioners and professors, municipal and university administrators and, above all, the representatives of the community, city, state, and nation—must work together to achieve, here, this possible model for the future. We must recognize that, in the words of Pogo, the comic-strip opossum from Okeefenokee: "We have met the enemy and they are *US!*"

# CURRENT EFFORTS IN THE MUNICIPAL HOSPITALS*

RAY E. TRUSSELL

Director
Columbia University School of Public Health and Administrative Medicine
New York, N. Y.

THE topic of health care for people in deprived areas is one that is certainly a pertinent topic in New York City today. Despite strenuous efforts we have not completed the job by any stretch of the imagination.

When Dr. Alonzo S. Yerby was announced as my successor as Commissioner of Hospitals, we spent about 5 hours together, at which time I gave him a single-spaced, several-page checklist of things that I did not get done, including some sticky problems, some of which you still read about. Today, as reported by the *New York Times*, the nurses were threatening to resign. Dr. Arthur Bushel says he has it all rigged. Any nurse who leaves the Department of Hospitals has a guaranteed job with the Department of Health.

The Department of Hospitals, which is my favorite subject, has had many problems in the last several years. I should like to go over some of the highlights of what was done to improve care, what is being done, and talk a little bit more specifically about the Harlem Hospital as a prototype of an institution trying to meet many needs in a deprived area.

We all recall that back in the late 1950's the municipal hospital system was a two-phase system—six hospitals staffed by medical schools that were getting along reasonably well, medically doing quite well—and 16 hospitals that were in varying stages of deterioration.

The worst of these was Gouverneur Hospital. This was the year, you will recall, that the American Medical Association said that an accredited hospital that used an intern or a resident who had not passed the screening examination given by the Educational Council for Foreign Medical Graduates, Evanston, Ill., to take care of patients would lose its accreditation.

*Presented as part of a panel on *Health Problems and Programs in Deprived Areas in New York City*, sponsored by the Public Health Association of New York City and held at The New York Academy of Medicine, February 17, 1966.

I met the administrator of Gouverneur for the first time and began to sympathize with him because I knew the place had lost its accreditation, affiliation, and training approvals. He said, "I have no problems, I have 35 interns and residents. I'm not accredited, I don't have to worry." What he had done was to import 35 doctors who had flunked the examination.

This is the level of care that the city of New York was providing for only one deprived area of the city. We succeeded, with the mayor's assistance, and the assistance of a couple of labor union committees, plus some expert medical advice, in getting the place closed up, and that was the first step.

From then on, we set out to try to put the unaffiliated hospitals on a competitive basis, and leave the city system on, at least, a level with the old-time affiliated hospitals that were staffed by medical schools. We did this by a series of contractual agreements between the city of New York and various medical schools, or voluntary teaching hospitals, whereby they would staff the municipal hospitals professionally. These affiliations were worked out at various periods of time over a 4-year period. They have been consummated with a variety of institutions of varying size, sponsorship, and strength. They have to be judged in point of perspective in time. One affiliation has just started on a planning basis and can hardly be called an affiliation as yet; others are more than 4 years old. Today, of these original 16 unaffiliated hospitals, 2 are closed. One is the Gouverneur inpatient service. The institution is affiliated, on the other hand, with Beth Israel Hospital for ambulatory care. Most of you know about the work that Howard Brown has done with the Gouverneur Clinic, on the lower East Side. The excellent program there has created much interest and community satisfaction.

The other place we closed was the Riverside Narcotic Hospital as a treatment center for adolescents because it was close to being a 100 per cent failure. There was no reason to continue something that was of no value whatsoever. Narcotic addiction was moved to a research status. There now is an apparent breakthrough in the Methadone Maintenance Program, which started at the Rockefeller Institute, and now is centered in Manhattan General Hospital. The second such unit just opened at Harlem Hospital as a first expansion of the program into a general municipal hospital.

In the Bronx, Montefiore Hospital is staffing Morrisania, and they have built a program there to the point where they have matched 100 per cent, 2 years in a row, in the intern matching plan. The Lincoln Hospital is largely staffed by the Albert Einstein College of Medicine. This was a hospital that was in very deep trouble—now the quality of care and the availability of care have greatly improved. The building is obsolete and there is money in the capital budget to replace it.

Fordham Hospital is affiliated with Misericordia Hospital and, of course, the Bronx Municipal Center is staffed by the Albert Einstein College of Medicine.

In Queens, there are two affiliations—there are really four. Elmhurst is affiliated with Mt. Sinai Hospital and they will both end up ultimately being affiliated with the Mt. Sinai Medical School. Queens General is affiliated with Long Island Jewish Hospital, the Hillside Psychiatric Hospital, and Mary Immaculate Hospital.

In Brooklyn, the Maimonides Hospital is staffing Coney Island, and the Brooklyn Hospital is staffing the Cumberland Unit. The Brooklyn Jewish Hospital is staffing Greenpoint.

And the State University of New York Downstate Medical Center, of course, has a tremendous complex known as Kings County Hospital, something of a size that should never have been built.

In Manhattan, there are three medical schools in Bellevue. Of course, the Sloan-Kettering Memorial Hospital complex handles the Ewing Hospital, and Columbia University has Harlem Hospital and Delafield Cancer Research Hospital. The only unaffiliated hospital at the present time is Sydenham in Manhattan.

On Welfare Island, we have New York University handling Goldwater Memorial, and the New York Medical College handling Bird S. Coler.

These contracts do nothing more than to put the unaffiliated city hospital on the same footing with the previously affiliated city hospital, but at city expense instead of university expense. Administratively, the relationships are identical; all are subject to the policies of the Commissioner of Hospitals, the rules and regulations of the department. All are administered by city administrators who are accountable to the commissioner. But the professional staffing is a service purchased by the city from the voluntary system. This was necessary because the job was not getting done under the combination of city civil service and the voluntary attending doctor system.

Other cities around the United States are all beginning to take a hard look at what has happened here, because they see another possible solution to some of their problems. And contractual relationships solve many problems. You get out of the bind of that monstrous complex known as the Career and Salary plan, where everybody is related to everybody else. Yet inflation in salary levels and shortages of personnel have far outreached the potential of the Career and Salary plan, to solve the problems of New York City's hospitals. Witness our current nursing shortage as an example.

I come to Harlem Hospital as an example of one center trying to do a job in a deprived area. Columbia University, over a period of about 3½ years, has assumed a series of contracts for various departments at Harlem until, today, our university has the responsibility for the total professional staffing at the Harlem Hospital Center. Each of the major department heads at Harlem is a member of the faculty at Columbia University, and Columbia has the responsibility for recruiting, assigning, and direction of staffs at the center. Some of these contracts are 3½ years old; some of them have hardly begun.

Each of these contracts not only provides for ample personnel in the various departments, recruited in line with the university employment practices, but they also provide for a one-shot updating of equipment, so that we are getting rid of obsolete equipment, outdated chemicals, and so on. New equipment is arriving continuously at the Harlem Hospital Center, as it is at all the newly affiliated hospitals.

We are at a point now where Dr. Yerby's primary concern with the medical staffing of hospitals is with the large centers, which I deliberately had to neglect, in the interest of putting out the bonfires, or correcting the deteriorated situation in the unaffiliated institutions. But even before I left I had started to write certain contracts for the centers—for example, the Medical Records Room at Bellevue was so bad that the hospital was put on 1-year probation by the Joint Commission of Accreditation; so we contracted the Records Room to New York University and things are getting straightened out.

The Department is now working on other contracts with certain centers, trying to strengthen services.

The Department, the Board of Hospitals, and I were grossly misinterpreted at times as to our intent with these contracts. Our effort has been to redistribute the medical manpower and the technical manpower around the city, which was concentrated in the large teaching centers, both voluntary and municipal. There was, for example, a terrible shortage of good patient care in Harlem Hospital, yet it was surrounded by Presbyterian, St. Luke's, and Mt. Sinai. This required organization and financing to overcome.

The financing in the last 4½ years turned out to be not so much of a problem. In fact, the department's budget, as I recall, went up about $125 million in 4 years and, currently, the cost of the affiliation contracts in effect this year is in the area of $70 million. That is an input of close to $60 million in people, and the rest is for various kinds of services and emergency purchases of supplies and equipment, and that sort of thing. In the meantime, the departmental collections went from $35 million to $95 million.

This has made a radical difference in many ways. It has improved the medical staffing of these institutions; it also has created severe shortages in certain places because of the competition for manpower; it has created an inflationary pressure on salaries paid to doctors. Today a young doctor can leave his residency and earn a salary that is four times the amount a professor received when I went to medical school.

At Harlem, Columbia not only has responsibilities for the various medical services, the inpatient and outpatient emergency room, and home care. We also have responsibility for the Records Room—the records librarian is a member of our faculty now; for social service—the New York School of Social Work, which is Columbia University's School of Social Work—has taken over the staffing of social service at Harlem Hospital as part of our contract responsibility, and by July 1, 1967, we shall have a budget of $1 million for social service in this community of great need, which is probably the biggest social service budget of any hospital in the world. It certainly is a service that is desperately needed, and it is being very ably organized by Dr. Maurice Russell, who was on the Harlem Hospital staff, and who has been made an associate professor at Columbia. He is recruiting social workers over the next 2½ years to staff this center adequately in terms of its responsibilities to the community—social service not only for inpatients but for clinics, for the emergency room, for home care, and for in-community activities.

In addition to trying to render services to that particular part of the city—and we are a long way from being perfect in our efforts—we are concentrating right now on trying to improve the organization and direction of the clinics. The resources are now available, financially, and what we are now doing is recruiting people to help improve the clinic organization, direction and staffing. For example, you run into interesting things, such as people having an appointment system, but they are all told to come at the same time.

Finally, there will be a built-in, permanent evaluation part of the program, which to me is one of the most exciting aspects of the entire relationship.

The Department of Hospitals, to go back to its concern with people in deprived areas, and as a matter of fact, its responsibilities for medical care for certain segments of an entire community, has done some other things in the last few years. The Board of Hospitals consists of five physicians and five laymen appointed by the mayor for staggered terms of 5 years each. They have some clearly stated responsibilities in the City Charter, including the establishment and promotion of the highest possible standards of care in institutions that the Department operates, in institutions that the Department licenses (and that comprises 36 proprietary hospitals and 86 proprietary nursing homes) and any institution with which the city does business. The city purchases care from the voluntary system to the extent of about $70 million a year.

Under a new state law which says the city has to pay the full state rate, the price tag for additional payments to the voluntary system is about $15 million for this year. For years the city has been underpaying our best hospitals, and even overpaying some of the smallest hospitals in the voluntary system. This inequity is now being corrected.

Throughout the past several years' efforts the emphasis has been on improving the quality of care for all people. As examples of what I am talking about, I should like to conclude this opening statement with a simple listing of what has been done to improve standards in New York City, reflecting problems of, particularly, urban areas.*

### Accreditation

1) The city will not pay for care in a voluntary hospital that is not accredited by the Joint Commission.

2) The Board of Hospitals adopted a regulation that unaccredited proprietary hospitals would be given 3 years in which to

*This summary is excerpted from remarks made at the White House Conference on Health held in Washington, D.C., November 3 and 4, 1965.

become accredited as a condition of continued licensure. At the time this occurred 13 of 33 proprietary hospitals were accredited. Today, every proprietary hospital in New York City is accredited.

### Additional Over-all Standards

1) *Municipal Hospitals.* As indicated earlier, the Department of Hosptials has been substantially reorganized through contractual affiliations between medical schools or voluntary hospitals and previously unaffiliated municipal hospitals. Four years ago there were six affiliated municipal hospitals. Today, 18 are fully affiliated, one is in the process, and one probably will be within a few years. The cost of these new affiliations this year is about $70 million. This approach to upgrading care has been tested by a taxpayers' suit and upheld.

2) *Proprietary Nursing Homes.* With the help of a very large expert committee working for almost a year, a revised code for licensure and supervision of proprietary nursing homes was adopted by the Board of Hospitals. This has been described before a Senate Committee as the most stringent code in America. In fact, after its adoption, about 30 substandard nursing homes either were closed, closed voluntarily, or converted to hotels for senior citizens. Contrary to dire predictions, new nursing homes are still being built in New York City.

3) *Proprietary Hospitals.* With the help of a very large expert committee, working for well over a year and against great opposition, the Board of Hospitals adopted a revised code for purposes of licensure and supervision of proprietary hospitals, of which there are 36 with about 25 per cent of the private care beds in the city. As examples of pertinent requirements, one can cite that:

It is now illegal for an unqualified obstetrician to handle a complicated obstetrical problem in a proprietary hospital, including the performance of cesarean operations.

It is now illegal for any physician other than a qualified specialist to perform major surgery in a proprietary hospital.

Needless to say, this matter is now in the courts, and to date has been upheld.

4) *Voluntary Hospitals.* The city, acting through the Inter-Departmental Health Council, has most recently promulgated stand-

ards to be observed by voluntary hospitals caring for patients paid for by the city. The main thrust of these standards is that patients must be cared for on services approved for residency training or by qualified specialists. In addition, children are not to be cared for on an unapproved pediatric service under any circumstances, except in dire emergency.

5) *Medical Care in Proprietary Nursing Homes.* The Health and Welfare Departments have taken major steps to correct demonstrated substandard medical care in proprietary nursing homes by contracting with voluntary hospitals, group practice plans, and a medical school to provide medical care for public assistance recipients, thus replacing a highly unsatisfactory welfare panel physician system.

### Categorical Standards

Through the Inter-Departmental Health Council, consisting of the Commissioners of Health, Hospitals, Mental Health Services, and Welfare, expert committees of nongovernmental professionals recommend standards for patients with special problems. After adoption, the city first interprets, then reviews existing practices, then implements the standards or criteria. For example:

1) The city will pay for the care of amputees in only 14 approved amputee services.

2) The city is just now beginning to implement a program of limiting payments to voluntary hospitals for the care of patients with cancer to institutions that have *(a)* a full 4-year approved program for residency training in internal medicine and obstetrics and gynecology; *(b)* approved program in radiology, including radiation, or a level of service acceptable to members of the expert committee or an organized transfer arrangement; and *(c)* a full-time board-certified pathologist qualified in tissue diagnosis or a fully accredited training program in pathology.

Time precludes citing more examples; I shall close by pointing out that in New York City government has turned to all that is good in the voluntary systems to discharge the public responsibility. This series of combinations of voluntary resources, governmental responsibility and authority, and channeling of public funds offer some lessons that can well be studied.

# HEALTH NEEDS AND PROGRAMS IN DEPRIVED NEIGHBORHOODS*

JAMES G. HAUGHTON

Executive Director of Medical Care Services, New York City Department of Health
Medical Welfare Administrator, New York City Department of Welfare
Coordinator of Welfare Services, New York City Department of Hospitals
New York, N. Y.

ONE of the first rules of public speaking is that the speaker should not apologize to his audience for being unprepared to discuss the subject before him. Because, after all, if he is unprepared to speak on the subject, why should his audience listen? I came prepared to apologize to you for discussing this subject, not because I felt that I was unprepared, but because I was not really enthusiastic about it. It seemed to me that volumes have been written about the health needs of the poor and that the subject has been talked to death.

But from what I see of the large group of people here on this occasion I am prepared to withdraw that apology. Apparently, either you have not heard about the needs of the poor or you are ready to listen to the same story again.

On October 9, 1964, Dr. George James, former Health Commissioner of this city, in speaking to a general session of the 92nd Annual Meeting of the American Public Health Association, stated that—I quote—"Poverty is the third leading cause of death in New York City." In telling how he arrived at this conclusion, Dr. James pointed out that he had taken 5 of the 10 leading causes of death, and had compared Flushing, a middle class area about 97.5 per cent white, with the Bedford district of Brooklyn, which is a poor section, roughly one third white, the rest Negro and Puerto Rican. The causes of death that Dr. James compared were the cardiovascular renal group, cancer, diabetes, the pneumonia-influenza group, and accidents. These causes were chosen because they are conditions for which death rates tend to vary less between the comfortable and the poor areas of the city. In each case, in Bedford, the death rates were higher than for the city of New York as a whole, and lower in Flushing than for the city

*Presented as part of a panel on *Health Problems and Programs in Deprived Areas in New York City,* sponsored by The Public Health Association of New York City and held at The New York Academy of Medicine, February 17, 1966.

Table I.—COMPARISON OF POPULATION, BIRTHRATE, PREMATURITY, PRENATAL CARE, DEATH RATE, INFANT MORTALITY BY HEALTH CENTER DISTRICT, NEW YORK CITY, 1964

| *Health district* | *Population* | *Birthrate* | *Pre-maturity* | *Late or no prenatal care* | *Death rate* | *Infant mortality* |
|---|---|---|---|---|---|---|
| *Manhattan* | | | | | | |
| Central Harlem | 227,000 | 23.7 | 17.3 | 40.7 | 13.0 | 41.8 |
| Kips Bay | 217,000 | 11.3 | 8.4 | 12.3 | 13.4 | 24.6 |
| *Bronx* | | | | | | |
| Morrisania | 258,000 | 26.8 | 12.7 | 39.6 | 9.9 | 37.3 |
| Westchester | 270,000 | 17.9 | 7.7 | 15.2 | 10.1 | 18.2 |
| *Brooklyn* | | | | | | |
| Bedford | 281,000 | 27.2 | 15.2 | 45.8 | 10.4 | 41.9 |
| Bay Ridge | 283,000 | 18.3 | 7.0 | 8.4 | 10.8 | 19.1 |
| *Queens* | | | | | | |
| Jamaica East | 305,000 | 20.7 | 10.6 | 23.8 | 9.3 | 28.0 |
| Maspeth-Forest Hills | 293,000 | 16.1 | 6.4 | 8.5 | 10.4 | 13.8 |

as a whole. Dr. James, therefore, concluded that if the city as a whole could maintain its health level at the level of Flushing's it would save about 13,000 lives a year. And since 13,000 deaths rank third on our list of causes of death in New York City, and since poverty is the underlying difference between these two districts, therefore poverty is the third leading cause of death.

On October 10, 1964, the local press reacted to Dr. James' speech in a variety of ways, but the reaction that caught my fancy appeared in the Long Island *Star Journal.* Over an article giving a full factual report of the speech was the following caption (I quote): "Come to Flushing and Live Longer."

Am I being oversensitive, or do I detect a note of flippancy in this caption? And if it is flippancy regarding the fact of 13,000 preventable deaths, is it perhaps a reflection of our apparent acceptance of these disparities in health indices between the poor and the affluent? We certainly cannot call it a lack of science or technical know-how necessary to reproduce Flushing's record, because we do reproduce it in Kips Bay, in Westchester, and in Forest Hills.

Let us look at some of the evidence. In Table I we have chosen two districts from each of the four major boroughs of the city—one affluent, one poverty-striken. And we have compared certain health indices in each of these pairs of districts.

You will notice that in each borough we have chosen districts of comparable size. Look first at the birthrate column. You will see that in every case the birthrate is considerably higher in the lower income area than it is in the affluent area. I wonder whether this suggests to us something about the availability of family-planning resources in these districts?

Look now at the death rate, and you will see that in every instance there is very little difference, hardly any, in fact, in the death rates between these districts.

Let us now look at the remaining three columns: Prematurity, Prenatal Care, and Infant Mortality—all areas in which prevention is possible and in which we have the technical know-how to intervene. We find that in every instance the index is higher in the deprived area than it is in the affluent area.

Why are these comparisons the same in all of these boroughs when these indices are compared? We have already agreed that we do have the technical knowledge to intervene in these situations. The city administration recently asked all city departments, including those providing health services, to find ways of effecting a 10 per cent reduction in budget. The Congress has been discussing President Lyndon B. Johnson's budget in terms of "guns and butter," suggesting that this great nation, which is spending hundreds of millions of dollars on moon probes, cannot support the Vietnamese conflict and at the same time spend a mere $1.5 billion on the antipoverty program.

But what will it ultimately profit this nation to put a man on the moon while children die of rat bites in Harlem, tuberculosis in Bedford, malnutrition in Brownsville, and perhaps of all three in some parts of the Bronx? It would seem that if some congressional legislators had their way, the poor would pay for the war in Vietnam, in terms of continuing deprivation and suffering. This dialogue concerning "guns and butter" reflects a system of values that stresses the development of natural resources while ignoring our appalling waste of human resources.

It may well be that one major question that this generation must

TABLE II.—PERCENTAGE OF BIRTHS AND PERCENTAGE OF INFANT DEATHS BY COLOR, NEW YORK CITY 1954 AND 1964

| | *1954* | | | *1964* | | |
|---|---|---|---|---|---|---|
| | *Per cent births* | *Per cent infant deaths* | *I.M. rate* | *Per cent births* | *Per cent infant deaths* | *I.M. rate* |
| White | 74 | 63 | 20.2 | 60 | 45 | 20.1 |
| Nonwhite | 15 | 24 | 37.2 | 25 | 38 | 41.0 |
| Puerto Rican | 11 | 13 | 28.8 | 15 | 17 | 29.6 |

answer is whether we shall be known as the generation that put a man on the moon, or the generation that solved the major problems of poverty and that erased the health differences between economic strata by raising them all to a higher level of health.

As we look closely at the data we have collected over the years, we find that even in situations where there has been improvement, the improvement tends to be less in districts that are economically and culturally deprived. Table III shows comparable statistics for puerperal mortality by color. Notice that the 1954 puerperal mortality rate among whites in New York City was 3; while among nonwhites it was 17.7. In 1964 we see that there has been a 50 per cent decrease in puerperal mortality among whites but, even though the nonwhite index has improved, this decrease is only 30 per cent.

TABLE III.—PUERPERAL MORTALITY RATE BY COLOR, NEW YORK CITY 1954 AND 1964

| | *1954* | *1964* | *Difference* |
|---|---|---|---|
| White | 3.0 | 1.5 | 50% |
| Nonwhite | 17.7 | 12.5 | 30% |
| Puerto Rican | 8.3 | 2.8 | 67% |

Table II shows the percentage of births and the percentage of infant deaths, again a comparison between 1954 and 1964. As we look at this, we note that while for some parts of the population the rates have improved, for other parts of the population they have actually become worse in spite of all of our technical knowledge. Note the percentage of infant deaths and the infant mortality rate among whites in 1954 as compared to 1964. You will see that while the percentage of births has

TABLE IV.—NUMBER OF NEW ACTIVE TUBERCULOSIS CASES REPORTED: COMPARISON OF CERTAIN HEALTH DISTRICTS, 1953 AND 1965

| *Health District* | *1953* | *1965* | *% Change* |
|---|---|---|---|
| *Manhattan* | | | |
| Central Harlem | 917 | 452 | —51 |
| Kips Bay-Yorkville | 154 | 46 | —70 |
| *Bronx* | | | |
| Tremont | 129 | 111 | —14 |
| Fordham-Riverdale | 85 | 50 | —41 |
| *Brooklyn* | | | |
| Bedford | 386 | 349 | —10 |
| Bay Ridge | 99 | 47 | —53 |
| *Queens* | | | |
| Jamaica East | 178 | 153 | —14 |
| Flushing | 137 | 62 | —55 |

increased, the percentage of infant deaths has decreased; and the infant mortality rate has decreased slightly. But now look at the nonwhite population. You find that the percentage of births has increased; the percentage of infant deaths has increased; and the infant mortality rate has increased considerably despite our improved knowledge and technology.

In Table IV, we compare newly reported cases of tuberculosis reported in 1953 with those reported in 1965. Again, we have taken two districts from each of the boroughs and compared statistics on them: in each case statistics on an affluent district with those on a relatively poor district. We find that throughout the city there have been improvements. But notice the disparity in the change. In central Harlem, the number of newly reported cases has decreased 51 per cent; but in Kips Bay it has decreased 70 per cent. In Tremont, the Bronx, there was a decrease of 14 per cent; but in Fordham-Riverdale, 41 per cent. In Bedford, there was a decrease of 10 per cent as compared to 53 per cent in Bay Ridge. In Queens, Jamaica has decreased only 14 per cent, but Flushing has decreased 55 per cent.

We see, then, that not only have some of these statistics worsened among the poor, but even when they have improved, the improvement has lagged. We could go on and on with these comparisons, but I think the point is amply made.

What are we doing about this? Happily, here in New York City, efforts have been made toward improving the conditions indicated by these statistics as we have seen them.

One of the first steps, perhaps, was the appointment of the task force that Dr. Ray E. Trussell previously mentioned. One of the recommendations of that task force was that a Bureau of Medical Services be established in the New York City Health Department to plan medical care activities for that department. Another was that the Division of Medical Care Services, in the New York City Welfare Department, then a part of the Bureau of Public Assistance, be removed from that bureau and made an independent bureau. A third recommendation was that a physician trained and experienced in medical care administration be assigned as director of the bureau established in the Health Department, and that this same physician be assigned as director of Medical Care Services in the Welfare Department. You will recognize this decision as a landmark, for since 1952 the American Public Health Association and the American Public Welfare Association have issued joint statements periodically extolling the virtues of health and welfare coordination and affiliation in providing for the health needs of the poor. But until then this had been merely lip service. And this was the first time that two major departments, those of Health and Welfare, had implemented such a recommendation. And so in 1960, Dr. Alonzo S. Yerby was appointed to this dual position and served in it, as you all know, until recently, when he became Commissioner of Hospitals.

Dr. Yerby addressed himself to the problems of health care for the poor in New York City, especially those on public assistance, from three points of view. One, he looked at the services of the Welfare Department and tried to identify those in which administrative streamlining would tend to improve the service; two, he set about to develop standards for some of the programs; and, three, he began to look about for demonstration projects that would set up service programs to provide services to people on public assistance.

In some of the administrative streamlining, we have been able to reduce steps in providing care from eight or nine steps to two steps in some situations. In our hearing-aid program, for example, we were able to improve the standards by insisting that we would not accept recommendations for hearing aids from hearing and speech centers, other than those approved in the program for handicapped children.

Among the demonstration projects, there have been several. Some of them you know about, and others you may not know in detail. Perhaps the first major service-oriented demonstration was the Health Insurance Program (HIP) that began in 1962. In that program, the Department of Welfare purchased a package of ambulatory care services for about 13,000 people in the old age assistance and medical assistance categories. This particular group of recipients was chosen for administrative reasons. Approximately 1,600 of these 13,000 persons were residing in nursing homes, and so HIP set out to establish a program that would meet the needs of both of these populations: the ambulatory and those in the nursing homes. This program in the community has been relatively successful. About two thirds of those who are enrolled have been utilizing the services well; another one third have not utilized them, or have utilized them poorly. We are taking steps to identify those who do not utilize them and to try to stimulate utilization.

Perhaps the most successful part of the HIP experience is the experience in the nursing homes, in which each group related to nursing homes has established a staff of physicians who take full responsibility for the medical care of the residents of these homes; and I must pause here to describe to you the prevailing system before this program began in the nursing homes.

As a welfare recipient was admitted to a private nursing home, a Welfare Department panel physician who was a private physician in the community, was assigned to that patient. It would be his responsibility to visit this patient at least once a month, as mandated by the Nursing Home Code, or more often if the patient's medical needs required. He would be notified each month that it was time for his visit, and if there was an emergency between these visits he would be called by the Department to make the visit.

However, very often, the physician responsible for this patient would not be available for emergency calls, so another physician would make the visit, and this physician would know very little (or nothing) about the care the patient had been receiving because many of the panel physicians did not keep records. There was, therefore, a complete lack of continuity in this kind of care, and we felt that some change was necessary.

Under the HIP Program, the physicians make daily visits to the nursing home, take care of any acute situations that exist, provide on-going care for those who need continuous supervision, and check those who are not ill at least once a month, to make sure that no problems develop. All the facilities of the group's centers are available to these residents–their diagnostic services, their specialists, consultation–all the package of services available to any HIP enrollee. We have had many letters from members of the families of these persons who say to us, "Thank you for starting this program." Just last week, I received such a letter in which a member of the family told us of the kind of service that had been provided to her relative in one of these nursing homes under HIP supervision, naming the doctors who had provided the care, and thanking them and the department for having established the program.

There have been some good by-products of this program other than medical care, and these relate to nursing care and staff morale. Nurses have written to us to say, "We now feel like professionals again, because we are working in a professional milieu as nurses who have physicians to whom we can relate, of whom we can ask questions, on whom we can call when necessary. We can now plan a nursing program because the doctor comes on schedule and we get all our orders at once." There is now less turnover in the staff, both at the nursing level and at the nurses' aides level.

A second program began in the same year, this one relating specifically to the nursing home. It was Dr. Yerby's feeling that the best way to provide medical supervision in a nursing home would be to have a hospital near the nursing home supervise the care. Dr. Yerby worked at this for over a year, and finally convinced a hospital to try this. In September 1962, the Lutheran Medical Center of Brooklyn agreed to attempt to provide this kind of service to the 100 patients in a nursing home about eight blocks from the hospital. The program began in October 1962. The hospital established a staff, including medical residents, who made rounds in the hospital daily. This program has been directed by one of the attending physicians of the hospital who supervises residents on their rounds and in their provision of medical services. The nursing program is also supervised by this physician. When these patients need hospitalization, they are hospitalized at that hospital. This has had important results.

In addition to the fact that the medical care has improved consider-

TABLE V.—PRIVATE NURSING HOMES BY CAPACITY, WELFARE CENSUS, AND MEDICAL COVERAGE, NEW YORK CITY, 1966

| *Size of home* | *No. of homes* | *Capacity* | *No. homes with D.W. census* | *D.W. census 1/1/66* | *% of D.W. census* | *D.W. census as % of capacity* | *No. homes under med. supvr.* | *D.W. census in such homes* | *Census as % of D.W. census* |
|---|---|---|---|---|---|---|---|---|---|
| TOTAL | 86 | 8788 | 73 | 6193 | 100 | 70 | 45 | 5227 | 86 |
| Under 50 capacity | 25 | 919 | 18 | 454 | 7.3 | 50 | 10 | 326 | 71 |
| 50-99 capacity | 29 | 2019 | 23 | 991 | 16 | 49 | 11 | 565 | 57 |
| 100-199 capacity | 22 | 3117 | 22 | 2096 | 33.8 | 67 | 14 | 1684 | 75 |
| 200-299 capacity | 6 | 1478 | 6 | 1417 | 22.8 | 95 | 6 | 1417 | 100 |
| Over 300 capacity | 4 | 1255 | 4 | 1235 | 20.0 | 98 | 4 | 1235 | 100 |

ably, and the nursing care as well, there has been a considerable decrease in the length of hospital stay of these patients. Previous to this program, the length of stay for welfare patients in that hospital averaged 32 days. At the end of the first year of this program, the average length of stay for this nursing home population was 12 days; the reason, of course, being that the same staff provided the care in both institutions and it was possible to discharge patients more rapidly since the same physician would follow up the care in the nursing home. This has been one of our most successful programs and, as a result of its successes, we have been able to encourage other hospitals to participate. We now have 12 private nursing homes under the supervision of voluntary hospitals.

One other approach to care in the nursing home involved the organization of physicians in private practice within a community into a team that would function in the nursing home in much the same way that the HIP group, or the staff from the hospital, would operate in a large nursing home. This has been attempted in Rockaway. It has worked successfully. We have recently been able to tie this program, with transfer agreements, to the Coney Island Hospital, so that there is now some hospital affiliation for this program also.

Table V shows the nursing home situation in New York City as it exists today, both in relation to existing private nursing homes, and the Department of Welfare's activities in this area. You can see that there are now 86 licensed private nursing homes, with about 8,700 beds. And you can see the breakdown in terms of capacity of these homes. You will notice that in New York City almost 8,000 of the 8,700 beds are in homes with capacities of over 50. You will notice also that the Welfare Department places patients in about 73 of these nursing homes. They occupy about 6,200 beds, which represent about 70 per cent of the total private nursing home capacity of the city. But, actually, in the 73 homes in which we do place patients, we occupy more than 80 per cent of those beds.

You will note further that of the 73 homes in which we have patients, 45 now have supervised programs for about 5,200 of our patients. Consequently 86 per cent of our welfare nursing home population is now under supervision of one of the three kinds of programs I have described, and these patients are receiving well-organized, well-supervised, and coordinated medical services. We have almost 1,000 patients outside of supervised programs, but they are scattered in about 28 smaller homes, in each of which we have 10, 20, or 30 patients, and it is very difficult to design a program that can provide for such groups. But we are still thinking about it and are trying to figure out some way of providing for them.

Let us now turn to some of the Health Department's recent activities in the way of improving health services for people in deprived areas. The Health Department's activities have been based on its position in regard to providing service. This position is that the function of the Health Department should not be to provide services in competition with other treatment agencies, nor to duplicate such services, but rather to fill the gaps.

And so, in order to fill a gap about three years ago, when considering utilization of the Children's Receiving Clinic at Kings County Hospital, we found severe overcrowding there: more than 100,000 visits were being made a year. We found also that a large number of these children came from the Bedford-Stuyvesant district, and we decided that perhaps we might relieve the pressure on Kings County Hospital if we established a pediatric program at the Bedford Health Center. We tried at that time to get one of the local community hospitals to staff and supervise this program for us, but we were unsuccessful. We therefore began the program as a Health Department activity. Last year about 80,000 visits, perhaps more, were made to the Bedford Pediatric Clinic. In the meantime, we began to recognize that we should try to provide more than just a pediatric program, because the adult population in that area has serious medical needs.

We therefore began to plan for the expansion of the Bedford program. We realized that very often a health agency designs a program, puts it into a community, and then sits back and waits for the community to come and use it, and that sometimes this does not happen. We applied for and received a planning contract from the Public Health Service to develop a health program for a deprived community in a large city.

Miss Naomi Weiss, who is with us today, took on the responsibility of not only preparing the Bedford community for an expansion of the services at the Bedford Health Center, but also for finding out what the Bedford community thought it needed in terms of medical services. To our knowledge, this was the first time that a health agency had gone out and talked to a community and then tried to design a program that seemed to fit its needs. Of course, it was necessary for us to provide some leadership, because when Miss Weiss went out to that community, she found that it's leaders felt that they needed an addiction program, an alcoholism program, a family-planning program, and a whole list of other programs, and that they wanted a building for each one.

Actually, if we had started to provide these services by putting up a building for each one, we should have had to raze about half of Bedford. And, incidentally, I think that what that reflected was the way that organized medicine has provided care for this population. We have conditioned people to feel that they should get little bits and pieces of care, in different places, and that in order to get care, they must have a program for each service.

At least we had identified the services that they felt they needed, and then we set about to try to convince them that there was a better way of providing that package than the way they had proposed. As some of you probably know, we were able to convince them of this. We designed a program that we submitted to the city; the budget was approved and a contract was signed in January 1966 with the St. John's Hospital, a local voluntary hospital about six blocks from the Bedford

Health Center. This hospital will supervise the medical program; it is providing the staff and the medical supervision. The health officer of this district will have administrative responsibility for the program. The medical staff will be responsible to him, and a Joint Policy Committee has been established that will set policy for this program, determine priorities, and screen applicants for positions in the program.

In keeping with the Health Department's policy with regard to providing services, the program that Dr. Vaughan C. Mason mentioned briefly—the prenatal program—was begun. Here, again, it was felt that there was a need for filling the gap in these services. A program of prenatal clinics in the Health Department centers, supervised by local voluntary hospitals, was established about two years ago; it has been functioning well. I recently heard someone say that Dr. Mason's program at the Riverside Health Center is perhaps the best one in the city. There are now nine such programs in the five boroughs of the city, all functioning in the district health centers; the deliveries take place in the local voluntary hospital supervising the program. I have been told that the return for postpartum care has been excellent, especially since these programs provide an entire spectrum of maternal health service, including family planning.

As we have developed these programs, we have come face to face with two issues. One is, what is really the role of an official health agency? Should we try to provide service or should we, rather, provide the leadership and the funds by which existing voluntary treatment agencies can provide the service? In some instances we have purchased; in other areas we have provided the services ourselves when no other resources were available. But this is an issue about which there may be strong argument on both sides.

The second issue is whether or not we should continue to design services for the poor. It has been my observation that whenever services are designed for the poor, sooner or later they become poor services, for a variety of reasons, not the least of which is the pressure of mere numbers. Dr. Howard Brown's program at the Gouverneur Ambulatory Care Unit, for example, is in danger of reaching this point. If the demand for service is very great, the staff may become so harassed that the quality of the program may decline. Dr. Brown, of course, is taking steps to see that this does not happen. But this is the tendency.

Also, when budgets begin to be cut, very often it is the budgets related to the poor that are cut, simply because the poor do not have loud voices; or, often, they do not have strong advocates. And so the question that must at some time be answered is whether, perhaps, we should not try to design services for all the population, in which the only difference between patients would be: Who pays for the service? If the patient is one who requires the government to pay for the service, then he should use the service and the government should pay. If he is a patient who has health insurance, then he should use the service, and health insurance can pay; and if he is a person who can pay for it from his own resources, why should he not do so? The service should be so attractive that he might want to use it. Of course, I realize that this kind of thinking would put us into a collision course with organized medicine, and with the principle that the patient should have free choice of physician. But perhaps it is time for organized medicine to realize that while the idea of free choice of physician is democratic, the thesis that perhaps the patient should not only have free choice of physician but also free choice of system is also democratic. Why must a person who has money and can pay his way go into the fee-for-service market if he does not wish to do so? He should have the freedom to use a group practice program or a publicly sponsored program if one of them is attractive enough and he wishes to use it and pay for it.

These are issues that must be considered, and I am sure that, in time, solutions for them will be found.

In conclusion, I should like to cite a quotation that I first heard used by Dr. Yerby, one I like so much that I have used it many times since. It is taken from a book entitled *Tropical Africa* by G. H. T. Kimble, describing conditions there. The author says: "It is bad enough that a man should be ignorant, for this cuts him off from the commerce of men's minds. It is perhaps worse that a man should be poor, for this condemns him to a life of stint and scheming in which there is no time for dreams and no respite from weariness. But what surely is worse is that a man should be unwell, for this prevents his doing anything much about either his poverty or his ignorance." It would behoove us not to dampen the effect of the war on poverty by failing to provide the means by which the poor can cease to be unwell.

*ACKNOWLEDGMENT*

Data cited in the tables accompanying this article are drawn primarily from *Summary of Vital Statistics 1964*, published by the Department of Health of the City of New York, New York, N. Y.

# CHANGING MOTOR PERFORMANCE AND PERSONALITY IN THERAPEUTIC SETTINGS*

MANUEL D. ZANE

Associate Attending Psychiatrist
Consultant to the Division of Rehabilitation Medicine
Montefiore Hospital and Medical Center
Bronx, N. Y.

In rehabilitation medicine, nonmedical professionals do most of the concrete work. It is they who observe the patient's changing performance under varying circumstances and discover, empirically, the conditions needed to improve his function. If we are to suit better our rehabilitation programs to the individual, I believe that physicians responsible for prescribing the program must begin to study and conceptualize, in terms compatible with neurophysiologic models, what goes on in the actual therapeutic situation.

As a psychiatrist concerned with rehabilitation problems (particularly in the physically handicapped) for 15 years, I have veered from trying to affect behavior by identifying presumed psychologic mechanisms to studying and conceptualizing motor performance *as it changes in the therapeutic situation.* By this approach I have come to comprehend the obvious: that changing motor function (like all behavior) depends upon the ceaseless interplay of social, biologic, and psychologic factors.[1] Here, "social" refers to stimuli originating from one or more persons, "biologic" from bodily changes–anatomic or physiologic–and "psychologic" from thoughts, feelings, and images. My hypothesis, in accord with contemporary neurophysiologic findings,[2, 3] is that performance changes as the organism, affected by changing internal and external conditions, shifts attention among varying social, biologic, and psychologic factors. Presumably, each shift in attention excites new patterns of response and influences behavior.** The personality (i.e., the person's involuntary, characteristic ways of reacting to the bodily

*Presented as part of a symposium on *Changing Motor Performance and Personality* at a combined meeting of the Section on Physical Medicine and Rehabilitation with the New York Society of Physical Medicine and Rehabilitation, held at The New York Academy of Medicine, January 5, 1966.

**Adrian[3] states "the operations of the brain seem to be related to particular fields of sensory information which vary from moment to moment with the shift of our attention."

effects of stress) as a major internal, and the therapist's activity as a major external condition affects the focus of attention, the sensory input and the action produced. This simple but basic concept, relating varying performance to sensory input, is also championed and supported by Dr. Belmont and his colleagues.[4]*

By use of clinical vignettes and edited tape-recorded material, demarcating *small sections of changing behavior,* I shall attempt to demonstrate in the natural therapeutic setting some of the effects of personality upon motor performance. All three of the cases selected exhibited hysterical and phobic reactions to stress. "Hysterical" refers to an involuntary tendency to overreact massively, and "phobic" to a tendency to avoid automatically a situation harboring an excessively disturbing stimulus. Other ways of reacting to stress, such as schizoid, obsessive, compulsive, paranoid, etc., some of which I have dealt with elsewhere,[5] will not be considered here.

## Case Material

A. The first patient was a 35-year-old woman with postpoliomyelitis paraparesis of 6 years' duration. She came to me for psychotherapy in December 1958, to overcome her morbid fear of standing alone. Two years earlier she had completed a year's rehabilitation elsewhere without learning to stand alone. She ambulated with a Lofstrand crutch while holding on to her husband. He had to carry her up steps.

After examination, the consulting physiatrist anticipated unassisted crutch ambulation and step-climbing with knees bent. A rehabilitation program was then prescribed, consisting of physical therapy twice and psychotherapy once weekly. At times, to study her responses to our program, I had her try to stand in my office. On the first occasion she became upset and shaky and refused to go on, stating, "I feel I really don't want to walk." Then, at my urging, she did try—first to stand with me holding her, then alone, and finally to take a step. I have broken down these few events into stimulus (S) and response (R) sequences and have noted some of the associated changes in performance (italicized) in bodily (B) and in psychologic (P) reactions.

S-1—"Stand alone."

R-1—Pictured herself falling (P), appearing awkward (P), and get-

*Rehabilitation medicine, concerned with improving function in the disabled, may thus be said to achieve its goals by introducing a series of stimuli—in the form of graded tasks and therapeutic approaches—to which the individual, under the circumstances existing at that time, attends and reacts more effectively.

ting hurt (P). As she *started to arise* she began to shake (B), felt panicky (P), *resumed her seat* and *refused to go on.*

S-2—"Stand. I'll hold your arm."

R-2—*Arose;* no shaking (B); no fear (P).

S-3—"Stand alone. I'll be near to protect you."

R-3—*Stood;* no shaking (B); felt slightly uneasy (P).

S-4—"Take a step alone."

R-4—Anticipated falling (P); became shaky (B); felt afraid (P); *did not move.*

## Comments

Here we see that disturbing thoughts, feelings, and images arising in anticipation of and during her efforts were associated with decline and with inhibition of motor functioning. Usually, when the task was not too great, physical or verbal contact with the therapist reduced such psychologic responses and was followed by better performance. She was helped to see the relationship of some of her psychologic responses and her performance and was encouraged to make efforts in our presence. Initially, with people supporting her on all sides, and then gradually by herself, she managed to ambulate alone within five weeks.

During a tape-recorded session I tried to learn her view of what, for 6 years, had blocked her and also her view of what had now helped her progress. I asked:

*Band No. 1*

Dr.: How come you didn't try to learn every day by yourself to walk to the bathroom?

Pt.: Why? Fear. Pure, unadulterated fear. Fear of what will happen if I try and fail, and frustration because it takes so long. By the time you start to get anywhere you get disgusted.

I observed that she had made excellent progress. She replied:

*Band No. 2*

Pt.: Actually, yes.

Dr.: What makes it possible for you to do this?

Pt.: I don't know. How did I go up the steps with the knee bent? I certainly didn't become very strong in the past couple of weeks from a few treatments. I've wanted to try on a step maybe an inch high and I couldn't do it. I just couldn't. Now why suddenly can I do it?

*Comment.* My observations in the office suggested that, in the past also, involuntary reactions that had conflicted with her efforts to stand alone or walk had led to motor instability, automatic tendencies to withdraw, loss of confidence, hypersensitivity to others, and "poor motivation." Apparently, she made no progress until she was involved in a stepwise program geared to her individual ways of reacting (elucidated by observations of the therapist *and* patient).

B. In the next two cases, to conserve space, identification of the stimulus and response aspects of the patients' reactions will not be attempted.

Much greater understanding of how psychologic factors change and affect motor performance may be gleaned from our second case, a 34-year-old psychiatric patient who was in his third year of psychotherapy. A minor problem was his fear of snakes—even pictures of snakes disturbed him.

To study his responses to a known stressful stimulus I handed him a book on reptiles with illustrations in color[6] and said:

*Band No. 3*

Dr.: Do you think you can open up a page at random?

Pt.: I can do it—I can try it.

He turned some pages. Then suddenly he *threw the book down* and exclaimed:

*Band No. 4*

Pt.: Jesus Christ!

Dr.: What happened?

Pt.: Soon as I saw all these coiled snakes here I got very upset. Whew! That was a big one (laughs). Wow! That was a shocker.

Dr.: What was the shocker?

Pt.: The coiling. The first thing that struck me was the coiling.

Dr.: Which one?

Pt.: This one (points).

Dr.: Now you touched that just now . . . how come?

Pt.: 'Cause you're holding it. You're with me and you were asking me questions. Now if I was alone in the room and you weren't here, my mind would pick this up and this thing here . . . it might even move a little bit. Not coming towards me necessarily but just creeping around on the floor and as I'm telling you this now. . . . It's upsetting. I feel it. (His hands were moist and his heart was palpitating rapidly.)

Then he asked:

*Band No. 5*

Pt.: Shall I turn the page again? . . . I'm fearful of doing it again. If I get to it I'm better off. I don't know what it is . . . the idea of turning the page is something that's going to be very repulsive to me or hideous or fearful, frightful.

Dr.: Do you expect the same kind of shock you had before?

Pt.: I feel it's like this, Dr. Zane, it's like I've built in my head . . . put notches in my nerves upstairs. . . . I've built a conditioned pattern . . . so when I see this snake it's not only the snake that stirs me but the whole thing goes on fire and I react. . . . I just become distorted.

Dr.: What does that mean?

Pt.: It means that it brings back every experience I suffered as a child with a snake. It brings back all the experiences I've seen. I remember as a child looking at *Life* magazine and seeing snakes. I remember burying a small dead snake. I see a snake in school crawling on a table. It recalls all these memories very quickly (snaps fingers). The whole thing falls right in, everything I . . . not everything . . . but most of the outstanding features I've witnessed and suffered as a child and as an adolescent comes into focus when I go into the snake book business or when we talk about it.

Dr.: All this comes back. For the second you're living not just one dread. . . .

Pt.: Very good point. . . . I'm living all the dreads all over again. That's why my fear is exaggerated. Now, as you bring this in, for example, as I'm talking to you now, I'm seeing a snake that somebody brought in to me while I was in junior high school . . . crawling on the table. A big black snake . . . harmless . . . but I'm feeling the fear that I had when I saw that black snake on the table. There is no black snake on the table now. That was when I was a child but the feeling is so damn strong. . . .

*Comment.* His remarkable communicative ability revealed an inner world of involuntarily interacting physical and mental reactions that multiplied in lightning fashion, dominated his perceptions, disturbed his organism, and disrupted his performance in the task. External stimuli, arising from the therapist, apparently inhibited this riotous expansion of internal stimuli and permitted him to perform remarkably better with the picture than he did only a few moments earlier. Performance changed as his attention shifted from internal and external stimuli that had such radically opposed bodily effects.

C. The third patient was a 65-year-old woman who was admitted to the Division of Rehabilitation Medicine at Montefiore Hospital, New York, N. Y., in October 1965, several weeks after she had had a myocardial infarction complicated by a right-sided hemiparesis.

She gave a history of claustrophobia and other oppressive fears prior to her present illness. On the ward she was a serious problem. She screamed and demanded immediate attention when she became uncomfortable. At such times she became short of breath, felt pressure in her chest, and was afraid that something terrible would happen. When confronted with new or difficult tasks, she usually refused to try and said, "I can't." Her ways of reacting to stress (WRS) disturbed almost everyone. However, the staff slowly learned to recognize and to cope better with her obstructive, involuntary WRS. Slowly she progressed in dressing, in balancing, and in walking.

This tape shows how her performance changed in different tasks with different staff members under varied conditions.

In the gym on November 11, 1965, the therapist cried:

*Band No. 6*

Therapist: Wheel yourself over!

Pt.: I can't.

Therapist: Is that true?

Pt.: I can do it but it's very hard.

In the parallel bars the therapist urged:

*Band No. 7*

Therapist: Pull, pull! One more step!

Pt.: I'll be going over.

Therapist: You're not going anywhere. Come on!

Dr.: Are you doing it?

Pt.: Yeh. . . .

Dr.: You just said before you can't do it.

Pt.: Sometimes I can't.

To explore further the effect upon her behavior of personality and what the therapist did, I asked her occupational therapist in the noisy gym:

*Band No. 8*

Dr.: In your experience with her, is this the kind of thing you see?

O.T.: Yes, I find she's negative about most things. You have to talk with her . . . maybe change the subject for a while and go back to it and she'll do it. You have to explain the task first . . . very fully because she wants to know everything so she's not afraid of it. Once you've explained it, you have to go right into it because she becomes fearful and claims she can't do it. So you have to start right away.

I asked her to be more specific.

*Band No. 9*

Therapist: Take something she didn't have to learn like buttons and snaps. She claimed she couldn't do it.

Dr.: (to paitent) I want you to hear.

Pt.: I'm listening.

Dr.: She is telling me that in the beginning even with buttons and snaps . . .

Pt.: I always say, "I can't do it."

Dr.: Why?

Pt.: Because that's me.

Dr.: Let me ask you a question. You just walked down here. It that right?

Pt.: Yeh.

Dr.: What was your reaction?

Pt.: I feel grateful that I'm able to do it. You know . . . that they are helping me.

Finally we hear the patient responding characteristically to a request, this time from a physician:

*Band No. 10*

Pt.: All of a sudden they want me to take a skull x ray. Why the skull? What's with the skull?

Dr.: Because sometimes when you have pain here, there might be something in the skull which may indicate you have this particular disease.

Pt.: Now I definitely won't go down there. Oh boy! you sure said something to me now.

Dr. Z.: What did he say?

Pt.: "A disease." My daughter explained it to me another way. . . .

Dr. Z.: What did she say?

Pt.: To see if I had a blood clot there.

Dr. Z.: Same thing.

Pt.: Where has the skull to do with the brain?

Dr.: Sometimes we may not find the reason in the skull, but we look for it.

Pt.: Oh boy! All right. I'm going down for it so don't question me. Lookit, I don't want to know the results of it. I'm a frantic person. I'm a frightened person. I don't want to know. If I have to die, let me die with it.

*Comment.* Her stereotyped "I can't" reflected her automatic expectation that she would fail to function adequately and would feel unbearably bad under the new conditions. Therapists had to work around such obstructive reactions and introduce stimuli in such a way as to evoke a desired reaction and inhibit the disabling, internal train of events. Thus, by directing her attention to their appropriate actions and words, they kept her excessive reactions to the thought of "going over" and to the word "disease" from mushrooming and creating panic and uncontrollable disorganization.

## Discussion

These cases demonstrated that personality reactions affected mental and bodily functioning and so influenced changes in motor performance. In addition, as these patients focused inwards, an accelerating process, based on the continuous, expanding interplay of biologic and psychologic factors, began and led swiftly toward an incontrollable disorganizing process. When the attention was shifted either by removal from the offending situation or by introduction by the therapist of other stimuli to which the patient reacted effectively (i.e., achieved what he was trying to do), the disorganization usually stopped and performance improved.[7] Appropriate programming for such patients necessitated awareness of these constantly changing mental processes, which are of such critical significance for understanding human behavior.[8]

Finally, it seems probable that in addition to improving the physician's participation in and understanding of the rehabilitation process, such *naturalistic observations of sequential changes in performance*[9] hold great promise, particularly when combined with multiple physiologic measurements, for fruitful investigation of the relationships of behavior, structure, mental operations, and social influences.

## SUMMARY

Small sections of changing motor behavior from three patients in therapeutic settings were presented by use of tape-recordings. The material demonstrated that personality affected motor performance. In these patients, growing disorganization, panic, and deterioration of performance accompanied conflicting reactions generated automatically by attention to increasingly opposed psychologic and biologic objectives. Presumably, the therapist's successful activities altered the sensory input and evoked a more integrated response by shifting attention to objectives that were more realizable and compatible.

### *REFERENCES*

1. Zane, M. D. Psychotherapy and changes in motor behavior, *Compr. Psychiat. 7:* 46-56, 1966.
2. Hernandez-Peon, R. Psychiatric implications of neurophysiologic research, *Bull. Menninger Clin. 28:*165-185, 1964.
3. Adrian, E. D. The physiologic basis of perception. In: *Brain Mechanisms and Consciousness,* a symposium. Springfield, Ill., Thomas, 1954, p. 238.
4*a*. Birch, H. G., Belmont, I. and Karp, E. The relation of single stimulus threshold to extinction in double simultaneous stimulation, *Cortex 1:*19-39, 1964.
*b*. Belmont, I. Relation of afferent changes to motor performance in the rehabilitation of cerebrally damaged patients, *Bull. N.Y. Acad. Med. 42:*918-22, 1966.
5. Zane, M. D. Psychiatric problems in acute stroke, *New York J. Med. 66:* 2001-04, 1966.
6. Zim, H. S. and Smith, H. *Reptiles and Amphibians.* New York, Golden Press, 1953.
7. Zane, M. D. Therapeutic process and behavior—as observed in physical rehabilitation, *Amer. J. Psychiat. 119:* 246-250, 1962.
8. Herrick, C. J. *The Evolution of Human Nature.* New York, Harper, Torchbook ed., 1961, p. 25.
9. Butler, J. M., Rice, L. N. and Wagstaff, A. K. On the naturalistic definition of variables: an analogue of clinical analysis. In: *Research in Psychotherapy.* Strupp, H. H. and Luborsky, L., eds. Amer. Psychol. Assoc. vii, 1962, p. 180.

# THE OFFICE OF THE MEDICAL EXAMINER OF THE CITY OF NEW YORK*

REPORT BY THE
COMMITTEE ON PUBLIC HEALTH
THE NEW YORK ACADEMY OF MEDICINE

THE interest of the Committee on Public Health and its predecessor committee in the operation of the medical examiner system in New York City covers a period of 60 years. The present Committee began its study in 1912 of the system for investigating criminal, suspicious, accidental, or unexplained deaths.

It was the Committee's view that any death that may have legal implications should be investigated immediately and properly. In criminal cases the determination of the cause of death may involve the fixing of guilt, while in civil cases it is a factor in the payment of death claims or damages. Thus, the Committee believed, it is essential that all deaths of a violent, accidental, or suspicious nature—a significant percentage of all deaths in New York City—should be investigated promptly by competent persons of good character who would be thoroughly trained for their duties.

Before 1918 the determination of the cause of death was the responsibility of a county coroner, usually an obscure politician who was elected by the voters. Generally, the coroner was assisted by a physician appointed by the board of coroners. This physician, more often than not, lacked special qualifications for the position he held.

In addition, there was no machinery for the prompt and efficient medical examination of deaths coming within the coroner's jurisdiction. The coroner's physician was not required to be on the case immediately, and this made it possible for interested persons to intervene for their own purposes. Special medical examination and testimony could be obtained only by the written consent of the District Attorney and a Justice of the Supreme Court. The law as to who was to determine the necessity for autopsy was ambiguous.

In 1915, the Committee on Public Health played a key role in the reform of the prevailing system. The Committee was instrumental in drawing up and aiding in the passage of a bill that abolished the coroner's office in New York City as of January 1, 1918, and established the Office of the Chief Medical Examiner. Since that time, the Committee has been in the forefront of the movement to strengthen the operation of the present system.

From the beginning the Committee on Public Health envisioned a larger role for the Office of the Chief Medical Examiner. It was thought that adequate medico-legal facilities for New York City should include an Institute of Forensic Medicine. Such an institute is now a reality, and the Committee takes special pride in having played a part in bringing the plan to fruition.

*Approved by the Executive Committee of the Committee on Public Health, October 31, 1966. Approved by the Committee on Public Health, November 7, 1966.

In more recent years, the Committee has endeavored to enhance the quality of the services of the Office of the Medical Examiner by encouraging harmonious relationships between that facility and other agencies that may become involved when death occurs in a hospital. In 1950 the Committee issued a carefully prepared *Autopsy Manual* with a chart in the form of a plaque to be hung on the walls of autopsy rooms. The *Manual* and the chart were distributed to hospitals with a letter indicating the need to acquaint new interns and other hospital personnel with procedures at the time of death. Many hospitals in New York City and elsewhere requested copies of the *Manual* for each new class of interns and residents and the booklet has gone through several editions since its initial publication.

A very important section of the *Autopsy Manual* defines a medical examiner's case and outlines the procedures to be followed when a person dies in a hospital ". . . from criminal violence; by casualty; by suicide; suddenly when in apparent health; when unattended by a physician; or in any suspicious or unusual manner. . . ." Accordingly, a responsible agent of the hospital must report the case promptly to the Office of the Chief Medical Examiner in the borough in which the death has occurred.

Once a case has been accepted as a Medical Examiner's case, its status never changes except on decision of the Medical Examiner, the *Manual* points out. The present laws and regulations concerning Medical Examiner's cases provide that the Medical Examiner will certify the cause of death in all Medical Examiner's cases.

In 1959 Dr. Milton Helpern, Chief Medical Examiner, prompted a survey of the agency by the City Administrator. One consequence of the survey was the partial centralization of the structure of the Office of the Chief Medical Examiner. Borough offices in Brooklyn, Queens, and The Bronx were closed. Dispatching and record-keeping functions of the three borough offices were transferred to a central office in Manhattan. Postmortem examinations and autopsies continued to be performed in morgue facilities in the several boroughs.

In December 1965, just at the close of the previous administration in New York City, there appeared a report of the results of a survey made to determine what further steps might be taken in order to improve the organization of the Office of the Chief Medical Examiner. In a letter accompanying the report, Dr. John Connorton, erstwhile Deputy Mayor, indicated that he had conducted the survey at the request of Dr. Milton Helpern, Chief Medical Examiner.

Because it describes the present situation in some detail, the Committee on Public Health believes it would be helpful to quote from the Connorton report at length:

> During the reporting year ending June 30, 1964, a total of 30,249 cases were reported to the medical examiner for investigation. This number includes 2,847 cremations and 4,045 "No Cases," where investigation has shown that no further action is required by the Office of the Chief Medical Examiner. While these two categories do not always result in elaborate examinations, procedures require a report from the field medical examiner as in all other cases.

On the subject of Medical Examiner Field Response, the Connorton survey shows that, "generally speaking, field visits are either not being made at all or are being made after considerable lapse of time. Study of a sample of some 300 medical examiner cases covering the period from June 1963 through June 1964 indicates that delays of four to six hours, between time of notification and time of arrival on the scene, are not unusual. Intervals as long as eight hours have been reported. In

60 per cent of the reports studied arrival time was not recorded by the field medical examiner—in 34 per cent not even the *date* of arrival was recorded. In only 15 per cent of all cases reviewed was full information available regarding the time of notification of the field medical examiner and his arrival on the scene." Further:

> If he does not visit the scene, the medical examiner must order the body to be brought into the morgue, if any doubt exists as to the cause of death. Information which he should gather in the field must be sought subsequently. As a result, some of the medical examiners have made unauthorized use of the clerical staff, which may include typists and stenographers, to telephone the police and others for needed information with which to fill out their reports.

The survey notes that the procedure followed by some field medical examiners is undesirable for several reasons:

> 1) Observations made by others at the scene are not those of trained medical examiners. Opportunities to question certain witnesses may be lost. The completeness of the information obtained over the telephone is limited to the ability of the clerical personnel to ask questions sufficient for filling out a form. Such questions obviously lack the breadth and depth necessary to establish or confirm essential facts related to the death.
>
> 2) The time the clerical personnel must spend in making telephone inquiries to complete the medical examiner's report results in damage to other activities. As one conspicuous result, the number of untranscribed cases continues to rise at a fast rate.
>
> 3) Bodies are ordered unnecessarily into the morgue and released to families only after examination. These could have been released immediately if the medical examiner had visited the scene. The families might have been saved some additional delays and emotional stress—perhaps some needless expense. The City would have been saved the cost of transporting the body unnecessarily.
>
> The unduly delayed visit also is unsatisfactory because opportunities may be lost to make immediate and essential observations concerning the condition of the body and circumstances surrounding the death.

Dr. Connorton's survey describes the procedures followed in reporting field investigations:

> Handwritten reports of field investigations are prepared by medical examiners. Reports of examinations made in the morgue are dictated to stenographers. Reports of autopsies are dictated to recording equipment in Manhattan. In the other boroughs, a stenographer is present to take the report. The field reports are made part of the case record in their hand-written state. The other reports are transcribed. The chief medical examiner is required to deliver to the appropriate district attorney copies of all records relating to every death in which, in the judgment of the medical examiner, there is any suspicion of criminality. Such records are not open to public inspection. Requests for copies of reports of other cases are received from insurance companies, lawyers, government agencies and others.
>
> Priority in transcribing records is given to cases of criminality. The "requested" cases receive next consideration. At the end of 1963, there were over 1,100 requests for cases not yet transcribed. But this figure is miniscule compared to the total of 27,000 cases, in all, which were awaiting transcription at that time.

In recent years, use of modern recording devices has brought changes in legal definitions of required record keeping. The Corporation Counsel has given his opinion that filing of reports in the form of voice dictation of autopsies and examinations conducted by the medical examiner is not in conflict with the requirements of the Charter or Administrative Code.

Because of delays in providing copies of "requested" cases, many individuals seeking information go to the Office of the Chief Medical Examiner to review the case record and make their own notes. Clerks are available to locate the record and return it to the files after it has been read. No charge is made for this service.

In the matter of autopsies, the survey says that "the Office of the Chief Medical Examiner offers generally excellent medical examiner services to the City of New York. The Chief Medical Examiner has steadily moved toward reducing the incidence or possibility of error but standards of performance are not uniformly high. In no other borough is the level of performance consistently as high as in Manhattan." Moreover:

> Lack of proper supervision in a borough office may sometimes permit hasty, superficial autopsy performance. Limited experience may also lead to errors. The medical examiner may not recognize an unusual condition or lack someone with greater experience to consult.
>
> X-ray equipment, highly important to the work of the medical examiner, is available only in Manhattan. Installation of such equipment, with trained operators, is not economically justifiable in the borough offices.

In the light of its findings, the survey by Dr. Connorton recommends greater centralization of the operation of the Office of the Chief Medical Examiner and indicates the following specific steps to implement the recommendation:

> *A.* All services of the Office of the Chief Medical Examiner should be centralized at its Manhattan office. The consolidation of services is essential to permit the Chief Medical Examiner to utilize to the utmost the professional capabilities within the organization as well as the modern resources and technical equipment of the new Manhattan headquarters building. Better supervision, closer review, and increased availability of experienced professional consultation will result from centralization.
>
> *B.* To advance the professional potential of the medical examiners through training, research, and consultation as well as to promote higher quality of professional services, the Office of the Chief Medical Examiner should be reorganized with the duties and responsibilities of the Deputy Chiefs clearly specified.
>
> *C.* To assure proper transcription of necessary reports, priorities for transcribing case records should be established by the Chief Medical Exmainer.
>
> *D.* Fees for providing information on case records should be adjusted to cover transcribing costs. The fees should include a charge for examination of records in the Chief Medical Examiner's Office.

The Committee on Public Health believes that the survey by Dr. Connorton fails to deal with a number of questions that are pertinent to a serious review of the operation of the Office of Chief Medical Examiner.

Among these questions are the following:

1) How many Assistant Medical Examiners are qualified pathologists certified by the American Board of Pathology?

2) In as much as the medical examiners' responsibilities concern medicolegal matters, how many members of the Office of Chief Medical Examiner are certified in the subspecialty of forensic pathology?

3) What percentage of cases referred to the medical examiner are autopsied in New York City?

4) How many cases are studied microscopically? How many are studied toxicologically, bacteriologically, and virally?

5) How thorough is the record-keeping? It would be revealing to evaluate the quality of performance in the recording of findings from a random selection of records from all the boroughs. How far behind now are the records on autopsy cases from reaching completion in typed form?

6) How many full-time medical examiners are there? Most assistant medical examiners do not consider themselves engaged in a career service. What has been done to make the position a career service?

7) How many assistant medical examiners have appointments on medical school faculties? Why aren't there more affiliations with medical schools?

8) How many assistant medical examiners are teaching, thus using the invaluable material that clears through the Office of the Chief Medical Examiner to advance medical education?

9) How many research projects are now under way in the Office of the Chief Medical Examiner? How many assistant medical examiners are doing research? How much of the research space is being used currently by medical examiners?

10) How much training in forensic pathology is being made available to fellows and residents in the medical schools and other departments of pathology in New York City?

11) Why does not the Office of the Chief Medical Examiner make use of the abundant talent in pathology that is available in the voluntary hospitals of New York City? Such pathologists could be appointed assistant medical examiners and upon assignment by the Chief Medical Examiner, would handle those cases originating in their hospitals, specifically those cases in which the hospital is not a potential litigant. The hospital pathologist would be responsible for the quality and thoroughness of the autopsy and be required to file a full report of these cases promptly with the Office of the Chief Medical Examiner. This would avoid delay for all concerned and help solve the problem of overlapping jurisdiction which presently causes much friction and ill-will.

12) Why does not the Office of the Chief Medical Examiner give serious consideration to the creation of one central office for the reporting and certification of all deaths?

13) Why cannot the present statute be amended so that it will not require that a qualified medical examiner—a physician or pathologist—visit each and every scene of death immediately upon the report of a case? This requirement is not being met adequately in any case.

In the opinion of the Committee on Public Health, these are questions that require serious study. But the report by Dr. Connorton has failed to take any of them into account.

And whereas Dr. Connorton's report presents one view of the problem, there is a directly opposite point of view which has been brought to the Committee's attention. At the heart of this opposing view is the belief that decentralization, together with other changes, not greater centralization, is the way to achieve improved services, greater economy, and a higher level of efficiency in the medical examiner system.

A number of persons familiar with the functions of the Office of the Medical Examiner have suggested that a plan of decentralization should be designed to strengthen the borough offices of the medical examiner.

The present policy of centralizing all services in Manhattan is creating a number of very serious problems, according to the proponents of decentralization:

1) Histologic studies, often an important part of the examination, take many weeks before the slides are returned.

2) In the matter of toxicological studies, organs are left standing around for 24 to 48 hours (or longer) before being taken to the central office in Manhattan. Much of this time, tissues are not refrigerated. Further, the results of the procedures that are performed are not made available for a period that may extend from months to years.

3) Bacteriological studies are not done at all in the borough offices at the present time.

4) Serological specimens are sent to Manhattan but not preserved in a fitting manner.

The proposal to perform all autopsies in Manhattan is impractical and works an unnecessary hardship on families and funeral directors. At the present time, both parties must wait an overlong time to obtain bodies of Manhattan cases and the situation will surely become worse if the cases from the other boroughs are added to the workload. In addition, there are other factors: the public would be put to great inconvenience and needless expense and effort to make the journey to Manhattan from the other boroughs for the purpose of identifying bodies and to give information of a routine nature. Finally, the District Attorney in each borough outside Manhattan would be put to the needless problem of having to get the Medical Examiner from Manhattan to travel to the site of the Grand Jury or homicide trial to give testimony.

Decentralization, the proponents of this point of view hold, would have the virtue of improving the quality of the work performed in the borough offices. A qualified Deputy Medical Examiner should be assigned to each of the boroughs to serve mainly in an administrative capacity and only to a much lesser extent in professional activities.

It is suggested that the borough offices should seek affiliation with medical schools—two boroughs in addition to Manhattan have schools in their areas. Provision should be made to have hospital laboratories in the respective boroughs perform the Medical Examiner's histology, serology, bacteriology, and routine toxicology; the more difficult procedures may still be done in Manhattan. Rapid tests for alcohol, barbiturates, arsenic, lead, phenothiazines, and salicylates could be done in the hospital laboratories within the boroughs. This arrangement would yield data immediately, or in one to two weeks at the maximum, and the case then could be closed quickly instead of its being delayed, as at present, from 3 to 30 months.

In addition to decentralization there are two other changes that would help to meet the need for skilled manpower not only by augmenting the numbers but also by utilizing them more selectively, appropriately, and therefore efficiently. One category would be assigned mostly to deaths occurring outside the hospital for investigation on the scene. The other would cover deaths occurring in the hospital.

Currently, the Medical Examiner is obliged to go to the scene of every death that is reported. About 50 per cent of these deaths, it has been noted, are clearly the result of natural causes: frequently the case is an elderly person who dies at home and has not been attended by a physician during the week preceding death. The critics of this system argue that it is both unrealistic and wasteful to require that a highly trained forensic pathologist should visit the scene of death in such cases. Indeed, they think it is wasteful to require a physician investigate the case.

In their opinion, the City Charter should be amended to permit the Medical Examiner to engage the services of trained lay investigators—they could be police detectives—who would go to the scene of death and make the preliminary investigation. Then, if the investigation shows no evidence of trauma, crime, etc., the family physician or the physician who pronounced the death should be empowered to issue a death certificate stating the most likely diagnosis from his examination of the body and history from the family.

Such a procedure, it is believed, would correct the present situation in which bodies may remain in the home for many hours—especially if the death occurs between midnight and 7:00 a.m.—till the Medical Examiner arrives to issue a death certificate.

The use of trained lay investigators would eliminate another problem arising from the fact that physicians are very reluctant to work as medical examiners because of the low salaries: $25 per day. This appears to be reflected in the undue turnover of physicians in the system. Also in this connection it is noted that the present staff of investigators, even if they are physicians, are no better qualified for investigative work than trained lay investigators would be.

Under the present law, the assistant medical examiner is required to be "a skilled pathologist and microscopist." But the Office of the Chief Medical Examiner is not complying either with the letter or the spirit of the law. An examination of the qualifications of the current complement of assistant medical examiners reveals that only 20 to 25 per cent of them are qualified pathologists. And this situation, the critics believe, results in part from the fact that the pathologists must visit every scene of death.

If the law were amended as suggested, then a lay investigator who suspects that a death has legal implications would call the forensic pathologist medical examiner on duty for the day, and the latter then would go to the scene of the case himself. This procedure would help to cut down on the work load of the Office of the Medical Examiner, save money for the city, and serve the public better by achieving a more rapid removal of the deceased from homes in cases of natural death.

Given the present scale of salaries, it should be easier to recruit lay investigators who would be trained to a high degree of expertise and would remain in their positions for many years. This system is used in London with maximum effectiveness.

For deaths occurring in a hospital, skilled manpower could also be augmented and used more effectively. The critics of the present system suggest that the Chief Medical Examiner should make use of qualified hospital pathologists. It is proposed that a number of qualified hospital pathologists should be named assistant medical examiners and be authorized to issue death certificates in cases of death in which the hospital is not a potential litigant. Certainly these experienced pathologists would be highly competent to evaluate the cause of death. It would greatly strengthen and elevate the Office of the Medical Examiner to utilize these trained and skilled specialists at any time. At this juncture with prevailing shortage of pathologists their acquisition would be doubly beneficial.

The benefits to be derived from the use of hospital pathologists would become evident to all the parties concerned, proponents of the proposal assert. Deputizing of hospital pathologists would expedite cases in which the hospital is not a potential litigant, the work load of the Office of the Medical Examiner would be cut through the use of a heretofore untapped source of highly qualified professionals.

It should be reiterated that the hospital pathologists serving as assistant medical examiners would perform autopsies on Medical Examiner cases only on order and assignment by the Chief Medical Examiner. In deaths in a hospital in which the institution may be a possible litigant, the hospital pathologist should not serve in the capacity of an assistant medical examiner. Also in deaths that are not medical examiner cases or are released by the Medical Examiner, the hospital pathologist would follow the usual procedure of seeking consent for autopsy from the family.

Another activity of the medical examiner system that involves a waste of time and effort, some observers find, concerns requests for cremation. According to the present procedures, all such requests are forwarded to the Office of the Chief Medical Examiner for clearance by the Department of Health. These requests then are made medical examiner's cases and assigned to the tour assistant medical examiner for investigation.

A more efficient way to handle cremation requests, it is believed, would be to have a lay investigator contact both the doctor who signed the death certificate and the member of the family who authorized the cremation. Then the investigator should decide if there is any reason contraindicating cremation, such as poisoning, abortion, or past accident. If the lay investigator discovers a reason for suspicion, he would be required to notify the forensic assistant medical examiner and have the body sent for autopsy to the appropriate mortuary in the borough.

Mindful of the fact that as many as 50,000 cases, some of them many years old, still remain untyped in stenographers' notebooks, critics of the present system suggest the situation cries out for a remedy. Accordingly, it is proposed that the Medical Examiner should dictate the appropriate material into a machine for recording on a disc. These discs, in turn, would be sent either downtown or to the borough office where a pool of typists would be available to transcribe the material and return it to the assistant medical examiner within one week for checking and signature.

Finally, there is one other matter that demands improvement: certification of death. At the present time certification is dealt with by several deparments of the city government: Health, Hospitals, and the Office of the Chief Medical Examiner. This results in wasteful duplication of paper work. Overlapping and indeterminate jurisdiction causes needless time-consuming effort. A more efficient procedure, the Committee on Public Health suggests, is a central office for the reporting and certification of all deaths.

The Committee has devoted considerable time and attention to its study of the medical examiner system. And while the Committee has high esteem for the professional qualifications of the present Chief Medical Examiner, it believes that the best interest of the people of New York City are more adequately served by an objective examination of both points of view regarding the problem. This, the Committee has attempted to do in the present instance.

## Conclusions

After careful study of the opposing points of view regarding the operation of the medical examiner system, the Committee on Public Health has reached the following conclusions:

1) The Medical Examiner's department should take steps to strengthen the borough offices organizationally and administratively, with provision of necessary facilities and equipment. For special tests, existing facilities outside the department should be utilized. In all boroughs the medical examiner system should be linked more closely with existing medical institutions.

2) The Office of the Medical Examiner should use trained lay investigators to make the on-the-scene examinations in cases of death outside the hospitals and certain deaths inside the hospitals.

3) The Office of the Medical Examiner should utilize heretofore untapped sources of manpower by deputizing qualified hospital pathologists as assistant medical examiners. In that capacity they would perform their functions in all medical examiner cases of deaths occurring in the hospital in which the institution is not a potential litigant.

4) More expeditious methods of record-keeping need to be instituted. To achieve this objective, more extensive use of mechanical and more efficient use of human resources should be made.

5) A central office for the certification of all deaths should be established to facilitate the reporting of deaths and issuance of burial permits.

In the judgment of the Committee on Public Health, these changes give most promise of furthering expedition and of simultaneously raising the level of competence in the operation of the Office of the Medical Examiner. They would minimize delay and inconvenience. But most of all they would bring greater savings to the city, insure a higher level of efficiency in operation, and provide improved quality of services to the people of New York City.

# AVICENNA ON THE LOCATION OF HOUSES

There has just come to hand a new English translation of Avicenna by Lt. Col. Mazhar H. Shah, F. R. C. P. (London), of the Naveed Clinic at Karachi in Pakistan.[1] This volume includes only the first fifth of the famous *Canon*. The translation is based on the original Arabic and on a version in Urdu. It is supplemented by an explanatory introduction, by a summary of the untranslated portions of the *Canon*, and by a biography of Avicenna.

Colonel Shah's devotion to Avicenna proceeds in part from his strong scholarly interest, which was obvious to those who came to know him during his visits to the United States. Apart from this, his work has had an additional motivation that is somewhat exceptional. The creation of the independent state of Pakistan marked the birth of a new country almost totally devoid of modern technical skills. This apparently was true in all or most branches of human activity and was certainly true in medicine. Lacking modern physicians, the Pakistanis turned to their indigenous practitioners of Yunani—i.e. Ionian or Greek—medicine, which had reached them through Arab and Moslem intermediaries. Of those the greatest was Avicenna, whose teachings still live for millions of our contemporaries.

We know that in Western schools of medicine Avicenna's writings were part of the ordinary curriculum at least as late as the 18th century. Morgagni, for example, in a lecture titled *De Via Atque Ordine ab se in Tradenda Publice Medicina et Anatome Servato Epistola* and dated 1761 states that he had regularly used as classroom texts the *Ars Medica* of Galen, the *Aphorisms* of Hippocrates, and the First Fen of the *Canon* of Avicenna.

Colonel Shah's translation includes what Avicenna regarded as fundamentals, i.e., such subjects as the constitutional basis of medicine, the general nature of health and disease, regimen, and principles of therapeutics. With this are included not a few items that are not within the scope of today's textbooks, such as housing.

Since it is likely that some of our readers have problems of housing, either urban or suburban or rural, we append herewith the useful counsel of the renowned Moslem physician.[2]

## The Choice of Site and Construction of Residence

In selecting the site for residence one should consider: (a) the soil; (b) the altitude of the place; (c) whether the site is open or sheltered, (d) whether the water supply is open or covered and low-lying or exposed to breezes; (e) whether the prevailing winds are fresh and cool; (f) whether or not there are seas, lakes, mountains and mines in the vicinity; (g) endemic diseases; (h) general health of the inhabitants, regarding strength, appetite, digestion and dietetic habits; and (i) condition of neighboring houses regarding spaciousness, ventilation and presence of open spaces.

While constructing a house one should be particular in having the doors and windows open toward the east or north. The building should be such that air enters the house from the east or the north and every part of the building is exposed to the sun for the purification of air. Plenty of sweet, pure and clean water should be available nearby and that, too, should be running rather than stagnant in deep and covered wells.

S. J.

*REFERENCES*

1. Shah, M. H. *The General Principles of Avicenna's Canon of Medicine.* Foreword by O. C. Gruner. Karachi, Naveed Clinic, 1966, xl, 459 pp.
2. *Ibid.*, p. 179.

# THE NEW YORK ACADEMY OF MEDICINE

## Eighth Annual Program on

## EMOTIONAL AND PSYCHIATRIC PROBLEMS IN MEDICAL PRACTICE

The spring 1967 session of The New York Academy of Medicine's Eighth Annual Series of Courses on Emotional and Psychiatric Problems in Medical Practice will be held at the Academy beginning on **March 13th.** All physicians in specialty and general practice are eligible.

Each course will consist of seven weekly, small-group, one and one-half hour sessions. Methods of instruction will include didactic and actual case presentations, group discussions and audio-visual aids. In addition to the basic course for beginners, advanced seminars will be offered to registrants who have taken previous courses. The following courses will be offered:

*Problems in Medical Practice*

Special attention will be given to techniques in the diagnosis and practical management of "the difficult patient"; in the observation of anxiety, depression and other emotional conditions; and in the methods and art of the psychiatric interview.

*Problems in Pediatric Practice*

In the basic class typical points of stress in the maturation and development of children will be delineated and considered. In addition there will be emphasis upon the technique of interviewing patients with emotional disorders. In the advanced seminar, instruction will be organized around actual cases according to the preferences of the group.

*Problems in Obstetrics and Gynecology (Seminar)*

This seminar will deal with the psychiatric and emotional problems of women occurring in the practice of obstetrics and gynecology and will include some didactic sessions on sexual problems. Although the course is an extension of the one given in the fall of 1966 newcomers are also welcome.

The program is supported by the United States Public Health Service, is co-sponsored by the New York County Chapter of the American Academy of General Practice, and is acceptable for ten and one-holf hours of Category I credit for its completion.

***Deadline for Registration: Monday, March 6, 1967***

**Fee: $10.00**

*Requests for information should be addressed to:*

Office of Medical Education
THE NEW YORK ACADEMY OF MEDICINE
2 East 103 Street, New York, N. Y. 10029

## The New York Academy of Medicine

## TELEVISED CLINICAL SCIENCE SEMINARS

**Tuesday Evenings, 8:30-9:30 P.M.**

STATION WNYC—TV UHF—CHANNEL 31

**March 7, 1967**

### THE PAINFUL HIP IN THE AGED

J. WILLIAM FIELDING
Director, Department of Orthopedic Surgery
New York Polyclinic Medical School
and Hospital
Orthopedic Surgeon
St. Luke's Hospital

FREDERICK R. THOMPSON
Director, Department of Orthopedic Surgery
St. Luke's Hospital

HUDSON J. WILSON, JR.
Attending Orthopedic Surgeon
St. Luke's Hospital

**March 14, 1967**

### OBESITY

GEORGE F. CAHILL, JR.
Associate Professor of Medicine
Harvard Medical School

### GLAUCOMA FOR ALL PHYSICIANS

EDWIN B. DUNPHY
Henry W. Williams Professor of
Ophthalmology, Emeritus
Harvard Medical School
Ophthalmologist
Harvard University Health Services

*Programs Courtesy of*
*The Bingham Associates Fund, and the*
*Postgraduate Medical Institute, Boston, Massachusetts*

# The New York Academy of Medicine

## TELEVISED CLINICAL SCIENCE SEMINARS

Tuesday Evenings, 8:30-9:30 P.M.

**March 21, 1967**

### CONTROL OF BACTERIAL CROSS CONTAMINATION IN A SURGICAL UNIT

PETER DINEEN
Clinical Associate Professor of Surgery
Cornell University Medical College

DOROTHY ELLISON, R.N.
Head, Department of Operating Room Nursing
The New York Hospital
Associate Professor of Surgical Nursing
Cornell University School of Nursing

CHARLES K. McSHERRY
Clinical Assistant Professor of Surgery
Cornell University Medical College

**March 28, 1967**

### HEADACHE

LAWRENCE E. HINKLE, JR.
Clinical Associate Professor of
Medicine in Psychiatry
Cornell University Medical College

E. CHARLES KUNKLE
Associate Neurologist
Maine Medical Center, Portland, Maine

BRONSON S. RAY
Clinical Professor of Surgery (Neurosurgery)
Cornell University Medical College

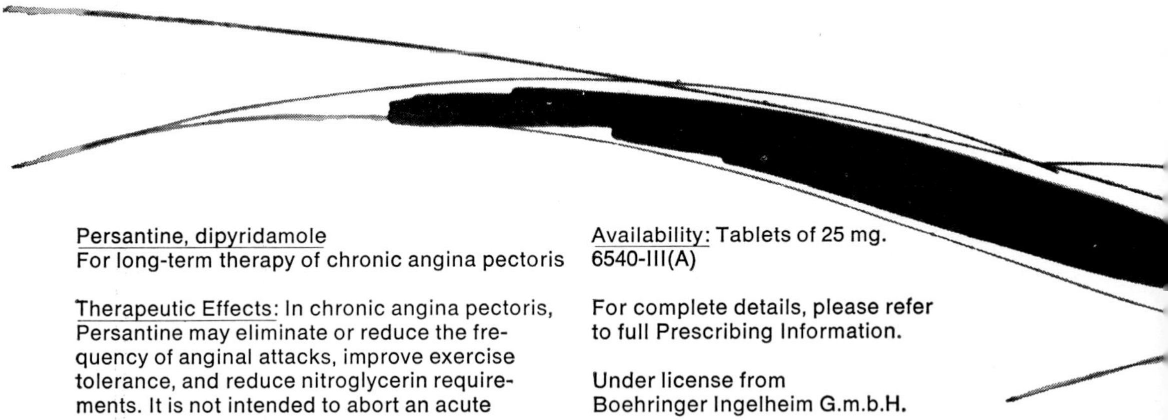

BULLETIN OF
THE NEW YORK ACADEMY
OF MEDICINE

VOL. 43, NO. 4 APRIL 1967

# USE OF RETICULOENDOTHELIAL PHAGOCYTIC FUNCTION AS AN INDEX IN SHOCK THERAPY*

BURTON M. ALTURA**

Assistant Professor, Department of Anesthesiology
New York University Medical Center
New York, N. Y.

S. G. HERSHEY†

Professor, Department of Anesthesiology
New York University Medical Center
New York, N. Y.

A NUMBER of observations from several laboratories, including our own, indicate that tolerance to various types of experimental shock may be associated with the functional capacity of the phagocytic elements of the reticuloendothelial system (RES).[1-8] It has also been reported that the administration of various, apparently unrelated materials such as denatured serum proteins,[6, 8] a variety of biologic agents and suspensions[7, 9-12] as well as certain polysaccharides,[13, 14] lead to an

*Presented at the Scientific Session on Research of the New York Heart Association, held at The New York Academy of Medicine, April 25, 1966. The experiments described in this report were supported in part by Public Health Service Research Grant HE-09042-03 from the National Heart Institute, Bethesda, Md.

**Now in the Departments of Anesthesiology and Physiology, Albert Einstein College of Medicine, New York, N. Y.
†Now in the Department of Anesthesiology, Albert Einstein College of Medicine.

adaptive augmented response in the RES, as manifested by a hyperactivity of the phagocytic behavior of these cells. Typically, stress is promptly followed by depressed reticuloendothelial function, which gradually reverts toward normal in animals that spontaneously recover.[2] Most of these data, however, were derived from studies in which the RES was *deliberately depressed* or *stimulated* by pretreatment with artificial means prior to exposure of animals to *highly lethal stress stimuli;* circumstances that make RES measurements difficult to interpret. Nor were phagocytic indices specifically evaluated as parameters of the course of the syndrome or of the nature of the response to therapy. Studies were initiated, therefore, to determine: 1) whether quantitatively significant sequential changes in reticuloendothelial phagocytic activity develop after relatively mild shock episodes in unpretreated animals and, 2) whether spontaneous or drug-induced recovery from experimental shock is accompanied by and correlates with an adaptive stimulation of the phagocytic cells of the RES. These studies are being done in the hope of deriving data that may serve as diagnostic and therapeutic tissue level indices in the treatment of shock.

## Methods

Rats (female, Wistar strain, 150 ± 15 g. body wt.) anesthetized with pentobarbital, 3.0 mg./100 g. i.m., were subjected to a relatively nonlethal (85 per cent survival) form of intestinal ischemia (SMA) shock by temporary ligation of the superior mesenteric artery for 20 minutes.[15] One hour after release of the ligature therapy with saline (2.0 ml.) or vasopressor* drugs in 2.0 ml. saline was instituted by i.v. infusion via a cannulated femoral vein over a 51-minute period. The vasopressor drugs were given in doses previously determined to raise blood pressure to normotensive levels (100 to 120 mm. Hg); norepinephrine—0.13 μg./min.; angiotensin—0.10 μg./min.; PLV-2 (2-phenylalanine-8-lysine vasopressin)—0.03 μg./min. Control animals were identically prepared but did not receive therapy. A group of sham SMA-shocked rats, similar to controls except that the arterial ligature remained untied, was also prepared. Phagocytic indices were then determined in normal anesthetized rats and in control, treated, and sham SMA-shocked animals at 3 and 24 hours after release of the ligature.

Phagocytic indices (*K* values) were determined by obtaining blood

*Angiotensin (Hypertensin) received through the courtesy of R. Gaunt, Ciba Pharmaceutical Corp. Dr. R. Bircher of Sandoz Pharmaceuticals kindly supplied PLV-2.

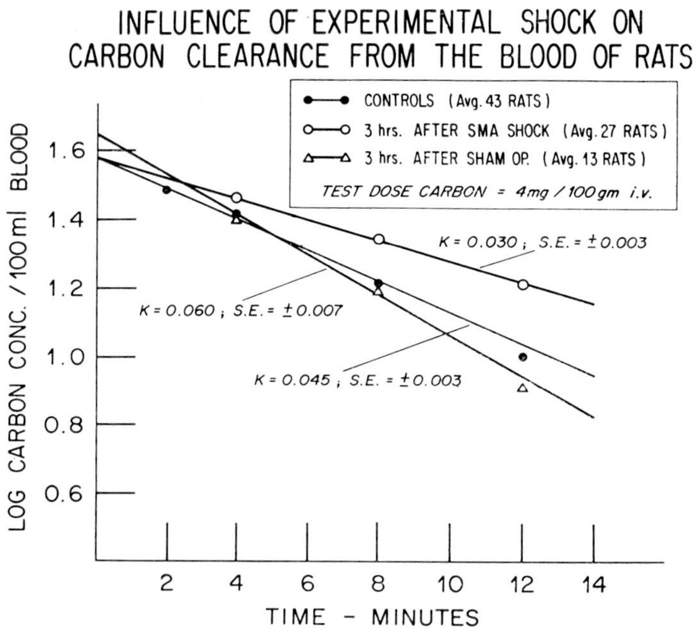


Figure 1.

clearance rates for 4 mg./100 g. of body weight of colloidal carbon (c11/1431*a*, Pelikan-Werke) suspended in calfskin gelatin utilizing a variation of the method of Biozzi *et al.*[16] Precisely timed blood samples of 0.025 ml. were obtained from tail cuts 2, 4, 8, and 12 minutes after carbon injection, hemolyzed in 0.1 per cent $NA_2CO_3$ and carbon concentrations determined photometrically at 675 m$\mu$ (Bausch and Lomb spectronic 20). Differences between mean $K$ values were statistically analyzed by means of Student's $t$ test.

Figure 1 illustrates the carbon clearance rates (slopes of the lines through the plot of log carbon concentration versus time) for normal animals, and for SMA-shocked controls and sham rats 3 hours after release of the ligature. Each point on the upper line represents the average of the values in 27 untreated controls subjected to intestinal ischemia shock while the second line from the top, which shows a steeper slope, represents the average of the values obtained from 43 normal animals. As can be seen, the untreated SMA-shocked rats exhibit a 33 per cent depression in phagocytic capacity after 3 hours ($P < 0.001$ when compared to controls or shams).

Figure 2 compares the phagocytic function at 3 hours in treated and

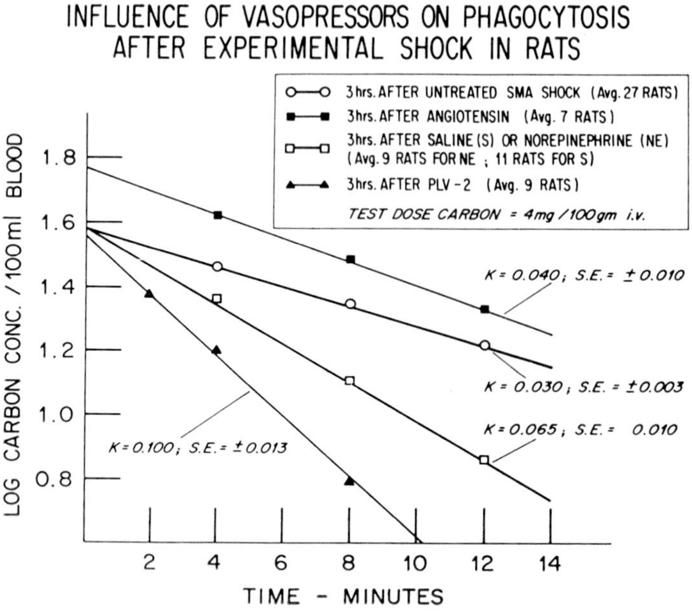


Figure 2.

untreated rats. It is apparent from these data that therapy with saline infusion or norepinephrine, as shown on the third line, results in more than a *100 per cent increase* in over-all phagocytic activity when compared to the untreated intestinal ischemia-shocked animals ($P < 0.01$ and $P < 0.001$, respectively). These data (Figure 2) also show that therapy with PLV-2, as shown by the steepest slope, results in carbon clearance rates that are increased by more than 230 per cent when compared to the untreated intestinal ischemia-shocked rats ($P < 0.001$). PLV-2 treatment results in significantly higher clearance rates even when compared to any of the other therapeutic regimes ($P < 0.01$ in all cases). Therapy with angiotensin results in clearance rates that are not significantly different from the untreated shocked control animals (Figure 2, $P > 0.05$).

Figure 3 compares the phagocytic function of untreated intestinal ischemia-shocked *survivors* (24 hours after release of ligature) to controls and sham-operated animals. It is quite obvious, from the slopes of the clearance curves, that *spontaneously surviving rats* exhibit phagocytic indices that are over *100 per cent increased* when compared to normal unshocked animals ($P < 0.001$).

Figure 4 compares the *K* values of survivors at 24 hours with and without therapy. Analysis of these curves indicates that although ani-

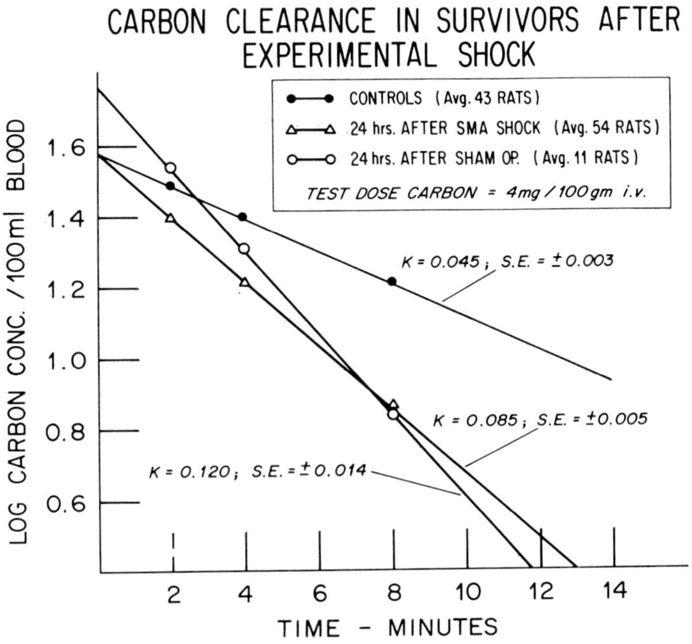


Figure 3.

mals receiving saline or norepinephrine show increased carbon clearances 3 hours after SMA shock (Figure 2), they revert in 24 hours to levels of phagocytic activity that are markedly and significantly decreased when compared with untreated spontaneously surviving rats (P <0.001) or with angiotensin or PLV-2-treated animals (P <0.01). Therapy with PLV-2, a drug that very markedly improves phagocytic function at 3 hours (Figure 2) seems to have predisposed to increased carbon clearance rates even at 24 hours in survivors when compared to spontaneously untreated surviving controls (P <0.01), to normal animals (P <0.001), to saline- (P <0.001) or to norepinephrine (P <0.001)-treated surviving animals. Angiotensin-treated rats, although not exhibiting clearance rates significantly different from untreated spontaneous survivors, are significantly increased when compared to rats treated with either saline or norepinephrine (P <0.01).

## Discussion

Although phagocytic clearance, per se, does not differentiate changes in reticuloendothelial tissue activity from changes in RES blood flow,[17] early changes are most likely due to blood flow, and later changes, in

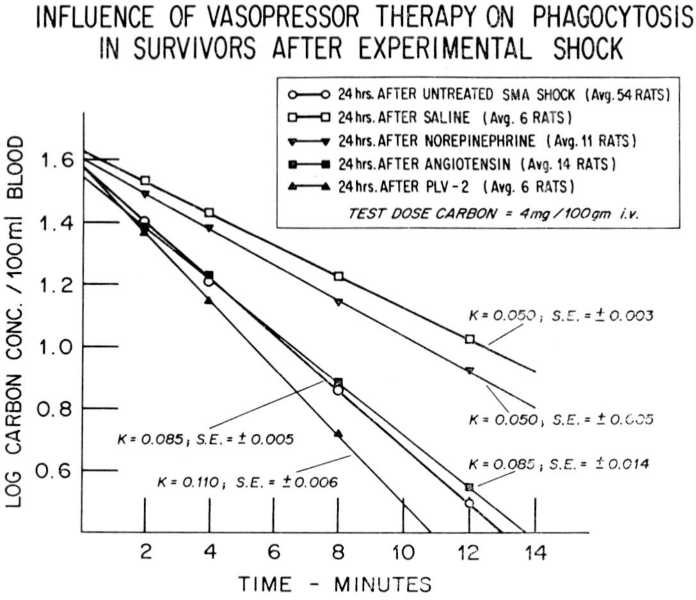


Figure 4.

clinically fully recovered animals not severely stressed, probably reflect adaptive tissue activity. The carbon clearance values found in untreated intestinal ischemia-shocked animals were remarkably consistent with predicted RES adaptive changes; that is, an initial depression followed by a gradual increase, in survivors, to a hyperactive level. PLV-2 (a synthetic analogue of vasopressin), an experimental drug that we have found earlier to induce selective peripheral vascular effects[18-24] not only results in significantly increased survival rates[22-25] when compared with other vasopressor drugs, but also in markedly increased rates of phagocytosis shortly after the onset of shock as well 24 hours later as observed in all survivors.

It is of special interest to note that these data on reticuloendothelial phagocytic function after therapy correlate closely with our previously reported observations on both survival rates and microcirculatory vasomotor behavior in *more severe* intestinal ischemic shock using identical therapy.[21, 24, 25] These reported findings suggest that the normal adaptive responses of the RES can be quantitatively modified by the manner in which therapy directly influences microcirculatory function and integrity. In addition, it is suggested that phagocytic indices or clearances may serve as diagnostic and therapeutic parameters of host responses at a tissue level during and following the course of shock.


## SUMMARY

Studies were undertaken to ascertain whether spontaneous or drug-induced recovery from experimental shock is accompanied by and correlated with a general stimulation of the phagocytic cells of the RES. Rats were subjected to a relatively nonlethal form of intestinal ischemic shock. Therapy with vasopressor drugs (norepinephrine, angiotensin, PLV-2), or saline was instituted by i.v. infusion. Phagocytic indices were determined at 3 and 24 hours in untreated survivors. RES phagocytic activity was depressed 3 hours after shock. However, saline- and norepinephrine-treated animals at 3 hours exhibit over a 100 per cent increase in phagocytic activity while animals treated with PLV-2 showed a 230 per cent increase in phagocytosis. Spontaneously surviving rats (24 hours after shock) exhibited hyperphagocytic indices as did angiotensin- and PLV-2-treated animals, while saline- and norepinephrine-treated rats showed depressed RES activity at 24 hours. These data on RES behavior after shock correlate with previous findings on survival and microcirculatory funtion in more severe intestinal ischemia shock using identical therapy. It is suggested that phagocytic indices may serve as diagnostic and therapeutic indices of the progression of the shock syndrome.


## *REFERENCES*


1. Fine, J., Rutenburg, A. M. and Schweinburg, F. B. Role of the RES in hemorrhagic shock, *J. Exp. Med. 110*:547-70, 1959.
2. Zweifach, B. W. Contribution of the reticuloendothelial system to development of tolerance to experimental shock, *Ann. N. Y. Acad. Sci. 88*:203-12, 1960.
3. Hershey, S. G. and Zweifach, B. W. Adaptation: The key to the problem in shock, *Canad. Anaesth. Soc. J. 8*:529-43, 1961.
4. McKenna, J. M. and Zweifach, B. W. Reticuloendothelial system in relation to drum shock, *Amer. J. Physiol. 187*:263-68, 1956.
5. Smith, J. J. The role of the reticuloendothelial system in shock. In: *Shock and Hypotension,* L. C. Mills and J. H. Moyer, eds. Grune & Stratton, New York, 1965, pp. 327-34.
6. Zweifach, B. W., Benacerraf, B. and Thomas, L. Relationship between the vascular manifestations of shock produced by endotoxin, trauma and hemorrhage. II. The possible role of the reticuloendothelial system in resistance to each type of shock. *J. Exp. Med. 106*:403-14, 1957.
7. Altura, B. M., Hershey, S. G. and Hyman, C. Influence of choline on the reticuloendothelial system and on survival after experimental shock, *J. Reticuloendothel. Soc. 3*:57-64, 1966.
8. Hershey, S. G. and Altura, B. M. Effect of pretreatment with aggregate albumin

on reticuloendothelial system activity and survival after experimental shock, *Proc. Soc. Exp. Biol. Med. 122*:1195-99, 1966.

9. Heller, J. H. Effect of zymosan on the RES. In: *Reticuloendothelial Structure and Function,* J. Heller, ed. Ronald, New York, 1960, pp. 189-94.
10. Cooper, G. N. Functional modification of reticuloendothelial cells by simple triglycerides, *J. Reticuloendothel. Soc. 1*:50-67, 1964.
11. Heller, J. H. Non-toxic RES stimulatory lipids, *Ann. N. Y. Acad. Sci. 88*: 116-21, 1960.
12. Nicol, T. and Bilbey, D. L. J. Effect of various steroids on the phagocytic activity of the reticuloendothelial system. In: *Reticuloendothelial Structure and Function,* J. H. Heller, ed. Ronald, New York, 1960, pp. 301-20.
13. Fitzpatrick, F. W. and DiCarlo, F. J. Zymosan, *Ann. N. Y. Acad. Sci. 118*: 233-62, 1964.
14. Benacerraf, B. and Sebestyen, M. M. Effect of bacterial endotoxins on the reticulo-endothelial system, *Fed. Proc. 16*:860-67, 1957.
15. Rovenstine, E. A., Hershey, S. G., Lanza, S., Baez, A. and Baez, S. Relationship of bowel and liver to drug protection against shock, *Anesthesiology 20*:290-95, 1959.
16. Biozzi, G., Benacerraf, B. and Halpern, B. N. Quantitative study of the granulopectic activity of the reticuloendothelial system. II. A study of the kinetics of the granulopectic activity of the RES in relation to the dose of carbon injected. Relationship between the weight of the organs and their activity, *Brit. J. Exp. Pathol. 34*:441-57, 1953.
17. Benacerraf, B., Biozzi, G., Halpern, B. N. and Stiffel, C. Physiology of phagocytosis of particles by the RES. In: *Physiopathology of the Reticuloendothelial System,* B. N. Halpern, ed. Blackwell, Oxford, 1957, pp. 52-79.
18. Altura, B. M., Hershey, S. G. and Zweifach, B. W. Effects of a synthetic analogue of vasopressin on vascular smooth muscle, *Proc. Soc. Exp. Biol. Med. 119*:258-61, 1965.
19. Altura, B. M. and Hershey, S. G. Pharmacology of neurohypophyseal hormones and their synthetic analogues in the terminal vascular bed: Structure-activity relationships. Proc. 14th Microcirculatory Conference, Atlantic City, April 1966, *Angiology,* 1966. In press.
20. Altura, B. M. Differential actions of polypeptides and other drugs on coronary inflow vessels, *Amer. Heart J. 72*: 709-11, 1966.
21. Altura, B. M. and Hershey, S. G. Effects of vasoactive drug therapy on microvascular injury in shock, *Pharmacologist 7*:144, 1965.
22. Hershey, S. G. and Altura, B. M. Manipulation of the peripheral circulation with vasoactive drugs in the management of shock: A microcirculatory approach, *Schweiz. Med. Wschr. 96*:1467-71, and 1516-22, 1966.
23. Hershey, S. G., Mazzia, V. D. B., Altura, B. M. and Gyure, L. Effects of vasopressors on the microcirculation and on survival in hemorrhagic shock, *Anesthesiology 26*:179-89, 1965.
24. Altura, B. M., Hershey, S. G. and Mazzia, V. D. B. Microcirculatory approach to vasopressor therapy in intestinal ischemia (SMA) shock. *Amer. J. Surgery 11*:186-92, 1966.
25. Altura, B. M., Hsu, R., Mazzia, V. D. B. and Hershey, S. G. Influence of vasopressors on survival after traumatic, intestinal ischemia and endotoxin shock, *Proc. Soc. Exp. Biol. Med. 119*:389-93, 1965.

# TREATMENT OF PULMONARY EMBOLISM WITH FIBRINOLYTIC AGENTS*

EUGENE E. CLIFFTON

Associate Professor of Surgery, Cornell University Medical College
Associate Member, Sloan-Kettering Institute for Cancer Research
New York, N. Y.

PULMONARY embolus remains one of the most common causes of death in postoperative patients and in patients maintained on bed rest for chronic disease or fracture. It is especially high in patients with cardiac disease.[13, 32] Apparently, this incidence has not changed significantly in recent years despite the use of early mobilization and routine anticoagulants,[42] though there has been a decrease in incidence of venous thrombosis with the early prolonged use of anticoagulants.

The incidence of pulmonary embolus or infarct discovered at postmortem varies tremendously, from 10 per cent to 64 per cent depending on the thoroughness of the examination and the type of institution.[12, 18, 21, 32] Clinical diagnosis of pulmonary embolus is even less satisfactory than the poorest postmortem examination. Freiman *et al.* found emboli in 64 per cent of their specially studied postmortem cases; and, in 29 per cent they were obvious. Clinically, only three had been diagnosed, and in two others the diagnosis had been considered a possibility. Coon and Willis[14] reported clinical diagnosis in 7 per cent of their cases, and Uhland and Goldberg[42] in 9 per cent. Donaldson *et al.*[19] found that the diagnosis was made in 50 per cent of the 60 patients who survived more than 2 hours, of a total of 283.

Clinical diagnosis is difficult because of the nonspecific nature of the symptoms and signs, and very few cases will be diagnosed even if suspected. With massive emboli death is frequently so rapid as to make diagnostic studies impossible.[19, 29] Diagnosis by routine plain x-ray films of the chest is equally difficult. The classical diagnostic sign of a triangular shadow based on the pleura is rarely seen; it is due to an infarct and is not a sign of embolus. The most common signs are

*Presented at a meeting of the Section on Surgery, The New York Academy of Medicine, March 15, 1966. This investigation was supported by grants from the National Institutes of Health, Bethesda, Md., and by other institutional funds.

pleural effusion, an elevated diaphragm, a nonspecific infiltrate, or linear densities that usually are seen late.[20, 41]

Electrocardiograph changes are nonspecific and can be considered only confirmatory of a suspected diagnosis. The usual signs are those of rapidly developing cor pulmonale and right heart failure, inversion of S1, Q3, T3, and right bundle branch block.[28, 45, 47, 48] Serum enzyme studies are nonspecific but suggestive.[43]

With suitable equipment, technical ability and facilities, physiological studies may suggest the diagnosis. These include a rise in venous pressure associated with arterial hypotension and tachycardia.[47, 48] More detailed studies will demonstrate respiratory alkalosis, changes in oxygen saturation, and a rise in pulmonary artery pressure.[16, 28, 45]

Angiography will make the diagnosis of a large embolus,[5, 46] and when very expertly performed with the best equipment may demonstrate smaller emboli. The radioactive scanning technique using microaggregates of albumen has been shown to be valuable in patients with large acute emboli causing obstruction of a large pulmonary segment.[44]

It is hoped that with these modern techniques many cases will be diagnosed in the living patient. It must be remembered that all the large series reported to date have been from postmortem studies.[13, 22, 24, 29, 32] Premortem diagnoses have been made in 7 to 10 per cent in these series.[14, 23, 42]

It has been estimated that in a 500-bed hospital about two cases suitable for surgical treatment will be diagnosed each year.[23] In one series of 171 cases collected at postmortem over a 5-year period only 27 survived more than 15 minutes and, of these, 14 were over 70 years of age.[29]

The survival rate following pulmonary embolus is very low.[14, 33, 41] In one series of 136 patients diagnosed premortem 71, or 52 per cent, survived the embolus; 48 per cent died. Of the survivors 10, or 14 per cent, had persistent severe pulmonary disability.[33] Recurrent embolization occurs in a large percentage of untreated cases.[13, 36]

Oral anticoagulants have not been of value in treatment of acute emboli. Heparin has, in general, been thought to be better than oral anticoagulants.[7] Oral anticoagulants have decreased significantly the incidence of recurrence and the mortality with recurrence even more[4, 24, 36] but the failure rate is still high.[31] It has been stated that prophylactic anticoagulant therapy has reduced the incidence of venous thrombus but not of pulmonary embolus.[13, 37]

Vein ligations, either of the superficial or the common femoral, have not been as successful for prevention of recurrence as originally hoped. Failure rates with superficial femoral ligation have been as high as 26.6 per cent.[1, 2, 4, 27] Fatal emboli have occurred after ligation in 5 to 8.2 per cent.[2] Common femoral vein ligation has been more successful, but still with a recurrence rate of about 5 per cent.[2] In one controlled series of two consecutive 5-year periods, one with and one without femoral vein ligation, the hospital mortality from pulmonary embolism was the same in the two periods.[34]

Vena cava ligation or plication has been more successful in preventing subsequent emboli though the percentage recurrence in some series still goes as high as 5 per cent[2, 4] and the mortality is higher than with femoral vein litigation.[1, 2, 4, 17, 36, 49]

The use of fibrinolytic agents might be expected to be useful if given sufficient time to reach adequate levels of treatment. It has been suggested that spontaneous fibrinolytic activity has been responsible when a proved embolus has disappeared without specific treatment.[35] Effectiveness has been demonstrated with experimental emboli.[9, 11, 25] One group also reported four successful clinical cases with acute emboli.[9] Others have also reported satisfactory response in patients.[26]

In recent years surgical extraction of massive emboli using cardiac bypass techniques has been reported more and more frequently.[8, 40] Unfortunately, the total experience from which the cases treated were chosen and the degree of selection used have not been reported.

## Results of Treatment with Fibrinolysin

In this paper I shall report our experience with fibrinolytic therapy for patients with pulmonary emboli, beginning in 1958. Almost all these patients were treated in the Memorial Hospital for Cancer and Allied Diseases, New York, N. Y., and most suffered from cancer (64 per cent); the majority of those treated were postoperative patients (57 per cent). We were asked to see 70 patients who survived more than 30 minutes to 1 hour in the period from 1958 to 1966.

Forty-four patients (Table I) with multiple embolization or massive pulmonary emboli were treated with fibrinolytic agents. Two patients had already had a vena cava ligation. One patient was treated twice for massive embolus, so there were 45 instances of treatment of pul-

TABLE I—CONDITIONS ASSOCIATED WITH PULMONARY EMBOLUS

| | *Total* | | *Postoperative* | |
|---|---|---|---|---|
| Cancer | 29 | (64%) | 14 | (50%) |
| Benign tumor | 1 | | 1 | (100%) |
| Fractures | 2 | | 2 | (100%) |
| Infections | 3 | | 1 | (33%) |
| Other benign disease | 9 | | 8 | (88%) |
| Total | 44 | | 26 | (60%) |

TABLE II—CANCER ASSOCIATED WITH PULMONARY EMBOLUS

| | |
|---|---|
| Renal | 1 |
| Breast | 4 |
| Bladder | 8 |
| Uterus | 5 |
| Stomach | 1 |
| Pancreas | 1 |
| Prostate | 1 |
| Vulva | 1 |
| Undetermined site | 2 |
| Lymphoma or Hodgkin's | 2 |
| Leukemia | 2 |
| Melanoma | 1 |
| | 29 |

monary embolus. Many of those with massive embolus had suffered multiple small emboli before, as has been reported by others.[11] Many of our patients had metastases in the lung or pleura and/or pneumonitis complicating the embolization. It has been demonstrated that the mortality of pulmonary embolus is significantly higher in those with pulmonary disease, or with cardiac disease.

The major failing in this series of cases is the lack of direct demonstration of the embolus by angiography prior to treatment. However, all had the typical clinical picture of embolus and/or EKG and x-ray evidence to support the diagnosis.

The types of cancer associated with pulmonary embolus is shown

Table III—OTHER DISEASES ASSOCIATED WITH PULMONARY EMBOLUS

| | |
|---|---|
| Chronic renal | 1 |
| Fracture femur | 2 |
| Tuberculosis | 1 |
| Prostatic hypertrophy | 1 |
| Endometrial hyperplasia | 1 |
| Pituitary adenoma | 1 |
| Virus infection | 1 |
| Pelvic abscess | 1 |
| Mitral insufficiency | 1 |
| Tbc hip | 1 |
| Ulcerative colitis | 2 |
| Peptic ulcer | 1 |
| None | 1 |
| | 15 |

in Table II. An unsuspected finding in this series was the very high incidence of patients with carcinoma of the bladder. An exact incidence cannot be determined, but it is obvious that the incidence must be very high as compared with breast, cervix, lung, head and neck cancer and lymphoma which are much more common in this institution.

Other diseases associated with pulmonary embolus in this series are shown in Table III. No significance can be attached to these because of the small numbers of cases. It should also be noted that the embolus followed operation in 75 per cent of these patients as compared to 50 per cent of those with cancer (Table I).

## Massive Pulmonary Embolus

There were 14 instances of acute massive emboli in 13 patients[3] (Table IV.) All were in severe shock with absent or minimal blood pressure maintained at adequate levels only by large doses of Levophed or Aramine in all but one case. Nine of the fourteen (65 per cent) survived the acute episode. Five (35 per cent) died during treatment or after failure of treatment without obvious improvement. Three of the five expired 1 to 2 hours after beginning treatment (Nos. 1, 5, and 12). Two of these were treated inadequately (Nos. 1 and 5). One

TABLE IV

| No. pts. | Treatment | Age | Sex | Diagnosis | Treatment | Previous embolus: Yes | Previous embolus: No | Duration in hours | Shock yes | Treatment: Levophed or | Treatment: Aramine | Other | Fibrinolysin: Adequate | Fibrinolysin: Inadequate | Results: Surv. embolus | Results: Died embolus | Results: Died other cause |
|---|---|---|---|---|---|---|---|---|---|---|---|---|---|---|---|---|---|
| 1 | 1 | 62 | M | Ca Bladder | Cystectomy | X | | 3 | X | X | | o2 | | X | | X | |
| | | | | | X-ray ther. | | | | | | | | | | | | |
| 2 | 2 | 64 | F | Ca Breast | Mastectomy | X | | 12 | X | X | | o2 | X | See report | X | | |
| | | | | | | | | | | | | | | | Recurrence | | |
| 2 | 3 | 64 | F | | | X | | 6 | X | X | | o2 | X | | X | | |
| 3 | 4 | 56 | M | Cirrhosis liver | Shunt | ? | | 7 | X | X | | o2 | X | | | | X |
| | | | | Esophageal | | | | | | | | | | | | | |
| | | | | varices | | | | | | | | | | | | | |
| 44 | 5 | 70 | F | Ca kidney | Nephrectomy | | X | 7 | X | X | | o2 | X | | X | | X |
| | | | | | | | | | | | | Heparin | | | | | |
| 5 | 6 | 64 | F | Ca uterus | | | | | | | | | | | X | | X |
| | | | | Pleural effusion | No operation | X | | | X | X | | o2 | | | | | |
| | | | | | | | | | | | | Cortisone | | X | | X | |
| 6 | 7 | 54 | F | Ca bladder | Cystectomy | | X | 24 | X | X | | o2 | | X | X | | X |
| 7 | 8 | 75 | M | Carcinomatosis | Chemotherapy | | X | 3 | X | X | | | X | | X | | |
| 8 | 9 | 64 | F | Fracture hip | Pinned | C.V.A. | | | X | | X | | X | | | X | |
| | | | | Renal failure | Fracture | | | | | | | | | | | | |
| | | | | Thrombosis or | | | | | | | | | | | | | |
| | | | | embolus iliac | | | | | | | | | | | | | |
| | | | | artery | | | | | | | | | | | | | |
| 9 | 10 | 29 | F | Hodgkin's | X-ray ther. | X | | 24 | X | X | | o2 | X | | | X | |
| 10 | 11 | 62 | M | Ca stomach | Irradiation | X | | 24 | X | X | | o2 | X | | X | | X |
| 11 | 12 | 44 | M | Acute pyloneph. | Cystectomy | X | | 12 | X | X | | o2 | X | | X | | |
| | | | | P.O. Ca bladder | Nephrectomy | | | | | | | | | | | | |
| 12 | 13 | 60 | M | Ca prostate | Transurethral | | X | 8 | X | X | | o2 | X | | | X | |
| | | | | | Orchiectomy | | | | | | | Heparin | Excessive | | | | |
| 13 | 14 | 72 | F | Ca uterus | | | | | | | | o2 | | | | | |
| | | | | Thrombo- | Irradiation | X | | 36 | X | X | | | | | | | |
| | | | | phlebitis | | | | | | | | Heparin | X | | X | | X |

TABLE V

| *Total number incidents* | *14* | *Postmortem* | *Embolus Yes* | *Embolus No* | *Infarct Yes* | *Infarct No* |
|---|---|---|---|---|---|---|
| Survived embolus | 9 | | | | | |
| Died embolus | 5 | 3 | 2 | 1 | 1 | 2 |
| Died later of other disease | 5 | 4 | 1 | 3 | 1 | 3 |

was definitely overtreated (no. 12), having received heparin in large doses before fibrinolysin plus excessive treatment with fibrinolysin. I suspect he died of cerebral hemorrhage although a postmortem was not obtained. A postmortem was obtained in three of the five patients who died acutely (Table V). Brief histories of these three patients follow.

The first of these patients, No. 1, Table IV, M. Y., age 58, was treated in 1959. He had a partial cystectomy for cancer of the bladder on July 15, 1959. He had the first of several unrecognized emboli 2 days later. On the 15th postoperative day he had symptoms and signs of a massive embolus with severe shock. He was maintained with large amounts of Levophed for 3 hours and then treatment was started with 75,000 units of Thrombolysin per hour. This dose is now known to be inadequate. He expired 2 hours later, and at postmortem a completely occluding bilateral embolus was found. He also had infarcts in both lower lobes from previous emboli.

The second patient, No. 5, Table IV, had been treated with fibrinolysin for venous thrombophlebitis 1 month before. The treatment was discontinued at the insistence of the controlling service because of ecchymoses and oozing at venipuncture sites and she was inadequately anticoagulated after this. She also had a right pleural effusion and metastases to both lungs. She had phlegmasia cerulea dolens. With the massive pulmonary embolus she was in a state of acute collapse (B.P. of 30/0). She was treated continuously with Aramine and Solu-Cortef for 24 hours and then was seen by us and firinolysin was started. It is doubtful that she was treated adequately because of the previous course of treatment and because she was treated on a weekend, without laboratory control. At postmortem she had a large left pulmonary embolus with some peripheral free area for flow, plus pleural fibrosis and multiple metastases on the right. Note that the good lung was blocked by the embolus.

The third patient, No. 8, Table IV, was treated adequately. This patient, 64 years of age, had severe chronic renal disease. She went into shock suddenly with dyspnea and cyanosis, and the EKG changes were consistent with pulmonary embolus. She also developed signs of impending gangrene of the lower left leg with what was considered a femoral artery thrombosis, or embolus. She was treated for a total of 12½ hours: 2¼ hours with streptokinase, and 10 hours with urokinase. Treatment was adequate. At postmortem there was a residual, partially obstructing thrombus of the iliac artery, but no apparent pulmonary embolus. It is presumed that the pulmonary embolus was lysed in this patient, but that she died of irreversible shock. The fact that the arterial thrombus was not completely lysed is not unexpected since systemic treatment of this duration is not usually adequate for complete lysis of a peripheral arterial thrombus.

Two patients apparently recovered from the embolus after adequate treatment as evidenced by return of normal respiratory and circulatory function without the need for continuation of hypertensive agents, but they died in about 48 hours of other disease (Nos. 3 and 7, Table IV). Neither had an obvious pulmonary embolus at postmortem.

Two patients treated for massive embolus with success are reported in detail.

One patient (S. C.), patient No. 2, Table V, was treated twice for episodes of a massive life-threatening embolus. This 64-year-old woman underwent radical mastectomy on March 1, 1960. In retrospect she had what were, obviously, unrecognized multiple small emboli and, on March 24, 1960, she suddenly went into shock. It was possible to maintain her blood pressure at 100/40 only with very large doses of Levophed. Eight hours after onset, without having shown any improvement, she was started on fibrinolysin treatment. After 6 hours her chest pain and dyspnea cleared and it was possible to discontinue Levophed. She was treated a total of 7 hours. The next day she was treated for 4 hours and had no further treatment. This was obviously inadequate in view of the long duration of the venous thrombosis. She was discharged without anticoagulants on April 6, 1960.

Early the next morning she had a repetition of an acute embolus. She arrived at the hospital by ambulance under oxygen treatment in shock, with blood pressure of 30/0 and again was maintained with large doses of Levophed. She again responded dramatically to fibrinolysin, which was started within an hour. This time she was treated more adequately, for 4 days with Thrombolysin and streptokinase, and then was placed on anticoagulants. She was continued on anticoagulants after discharge and has remained well to the present.

Our most recent case (No. 13, Table IV) was a 72-year-old female with carcinoma of the uterus treated by irradiation. She had been treated previously with fibrinolysin for venous thrombosis of the left leg with success and placed on an oral coagulant, but this was discontinued because of G.I. bleeding. One month later she developed a phlegmasia cerulea dolens of the opposite (right) leg. She also had apparently suffered several small pulmonary emboli. Twenty-four hours after the onset of the phlegmasia she suffered a massive pulmonary embolus and was treated with nasal oxygen and Aramine. When seen 24 hours later she was sitting upright in bed gasping for breath with full nasal oxygen at a flow rate of 6 to 7 l./minute. Fibrinolysin was started immediately. Three hours of treatment were given that night, and 6 hours the next morning. She was then able to lie down and was able to breathe almost normally without oxygen therapy. After 4 days of treatment her phlegmasia cerulea dolens had improved markedly. The fibrinolysin therapy was then discontinued and she was started on intravenous heparin 50 mg. every 4 hours. She remained free of symptoms of the pulmonary embolus, but gangrene of the foot recurred. She was in such poor condition clinically because of uremia and her cancer that the responsible surgical service refused to consider amputation. She expired days later without a recurrence of her pulmonary embolus. At postmortem there were multiple infarcts of the right upper and lower lobes and an old embolus in the right middle lobe artery. She also had an acute myocardial infarct.

During the past year we have seen four other patients with a diagnosis of massive pulmonary embolus using the same criteria who were not treated with fibrinolysin because of lack of sufficient material. All were treated with anticoagulants. All four died, and the three who had a postmortem examination had large emboli.

## Pulmonary Emboli: Not Massive

Thirty patients with multiple emboli or with a single obvious acute embolus, not of the massive type, were treated with fibrinolysin (Table

TABLE VI—MULTIPLE OR SINGLE (NOT MASSIVE) EMBOLI

| | | *Treatment* | | *Results* | | |
|---|---|---|---|---|---|---|
| | *No.* | *Adequate* | *Not adequate* | *Exc.* | *Good* | *Failed* |
| Total | 30 | 25 | 5 | 23 | 5 | 2 |
| Lived | 26 | | | | | |
| Ligated V.C. | 2 | | | | | |
| Recurred late | 2 | | | | | |
| Died | 4 | | | | | |

VI). Three were very close to being massive, and I believe each would have been the type of patient considered a good surgical candidate. Of the 30 patients, 26 (85 per cent) survived. Four (14 per cent) died within 10 days. Postmortem was obtained in all four. One died of a new massive embolus 5 days after completion of treatment that had failed to control her bilateral ileofemoral thrombophlebitis. There were also multiple old infarcts. The second died 9 days after treatment. The cause of death was toxicity from cancer chemotherapy. At postmortem multiple infarcts with small vessel emboli and metastases to the lung were found. The third had small infarcts and emboli and multiple metastases plus lymphagitic spread of cancer. The fourth died 2 days after treatment had been discontinued because of bleeding. This patient also had multiple metastases to the lung and had been treated with chemotherapy. It should be noted that three of the four had extensive pulmonary metastases and two had received chemotherapy.

Of the 25 who survived, embolism recurred early in two, and vena cava ligation was performed in both. One had not been given anticoagulants after the fibrinolysin treatment, though we had recommended it because of the long duration of the primary thrombosis. The second patient was given vitamin K (100 mg. i.v.) and the fibrinolysin therapy, though we demurred, was discontinued because of moderate vaginal bleeding.

Embolism recurred after several months in two patients. One patient, B. F., age 67, was treated at the New York Hospital in April 1960. He had multiple emboli from a severe ileofemoral thrombosis of 2 months' duration. These continued after admission despite adequate treatment with heparin and Coumadin. This patient was seen by us because of progressive cor pulmonale, which was becoming uncontrollable. After 4 days of treatment with fibrinolysin he had complete relief from the embolic manifestations and marked improvement of the cor pulmonale. The thrombophlebitis was improved, but we felt that it was not eradicated; therefore he was sent home on anticoagulant treatment. Nine months later, because of a bleeding ulcer, the anticoagulants were discontinued, and he died 3 weeks later of an acute massive embolus proved by postmortem.

The second patient had an excellent response to treatment with fibrinolysin despite multiple pulmonary metastases of melanoma. He was readmitted 4 months later for chemotherapy of the melanoma. Five months after the original embolus he died and, at postmortem, was found to have a recent right pulmonary embolus plus metastases.

A recurrence of thrombophlebitis without evidence of embolization was observed in three patients treated for pulmonary embolus. None of these was continued on anticoagulant therapy after treatment with fibrinolysin.

It is of some interest that in this group of patients eight (18 per cent) were on anticoagulants at the time of infarction. The adequacy of this therapy cannot be vouched for, but it was under the management of competent internists. This is not a surprising finding, since it has been reported that in general hospitals the incidence of pulmonary embolus in patients under anticoagulant treatment for thrombophlebitis is significant.[7, 13] One of our patients had had a femoral vein ligation and one had had an inferior vena cava ligation. The fibrinolysin treatment was requested in these patients because of recurrent emboli after the ligations.

During this same period only one patient developed a pulmonary embolus while on fibrinolysin therapy for thrombophlebitis. This occurred on the first day of treatment. Fibrinolysin therapy was continued with a complete subsidence of both the pulmonary embolus and the thrombophlebitis. During this period 350 patients were treated for venous thrombosis, giving a very low incidence of pulmonary embolus.

## Discussion

The results reported are not a cause for rejoicing nor are they of a type to warrant a feeling of dismay. The reported mortality rates of diagnosed pulmonary emboli in reported series varies from 23 per cent to 48 per cent.[10, 15, 33, 41] In this series the mortality from the embolus or emboli was less than 21 per cent. The mortality before 30 days from all causes in this group of very sick patients was only 31 per cent. In this same group of patients, in the past year, four patients with massive embolus treated with heparin or Coumadin died from the embolus within 3 days.

Treatment of acute massive embolism is difficult under the best of circumstances. Although interest in surgical extraction is now strong among thoracic surgeons, the probability that this will be a suitable means of treatment for the large number of emboli of this type seems doubtful. As shown by many series, most patients do not survive long enough to reach the operating room;[29] a team must be available at all times, and mortality will certainly be high. Unfortunately, most reports are of a single or a few cases, and none mention the total experience from which the operative cases were chosen. Spencer *et al.*[39] reported two cases, one of which survived (50 per cent survival). Sautter and Emanuel reported two successful cases of five attempted (40 per cent survival).[50] Patou had one survival in three cases (33⅓ per cent). Baker and Wagner[6] reported 13 cases, 9 of whom had embolectomy under bypass with three survivors (33⅓ per cent). No patient with hypotension of less than 100 survived embolectomy.

Treatment with heparin has been successful and may be quite satisfactory in those who will survive a sufficient time to have further thrombosis or if additional embolization becomes a factor. Baker and Wagner[6] mentioned the survival of 2 cases among their 13 treated with heparin and vena cava ligation. Heparin treatment must be carefully controlled and monitored and is just as difficult to manage properly, if not more so, than the fibrinolytic agents. Fibrinolysis has the additional advantage of dissolving the embolus, at least the fresher parts of it, and reopening the channel.

It is conceivable that with the use of partial cardiopulmonary bypass the results of fibrinolysin therapy could be improved markedly; certainly, it would give the agent additional time to dissolve the clot in the patient rapidly progressing to a terminal state.

The fibrinolytic agent to be used is not particularly important so long as it is capable of producing significant fibrinolytic activity *in vivo*, rapidly, and without serious side reactions. Streptokinase, Thrombolysin (SK and plasminogen), and the new agent urokinase all fulfill these requirements. Effective treatment of pulmonary embolus by SK or fibrinolysin have been reported by others.[9, 26, 30]

Treatment with fibrinolytic agents SK, UK, or fibrinolysin (Thrombolysin, Merck Sharp & Dohme) should be instituted as rapidly as possible. A priming dose of 100,000 to 200,000 units should be infused in 10 to 20 minutes and the infusion continued at the same dose hourly until definite improvement occurs. A control sample of blood should be drawn for a dose prediction at the time of starting the treatment, and the dose regulated according to this test and the activity obtained in the course of treatment. Samples should also be obtained for fibrinogen, prothrombin time, and other clotting factors where possible to protect against overtreatment.

Treatment should be continued for several hours until significant improvement is obtained and subsequent courses should be given daily until the primary thrombus has been eradicated. Heparin should be administered between courses to prevent a reaccumulation of clot, and anticoagulation should be maintained after the fibrinolytic treatment is completed, at least until the patient is fully mobilized and returns to normal activities. In patients with diseases subject to rethrombosis, the anticoagulants might be continued indefinitely. Certainly, in two of our reported cases, fatal embolism occurred after discontinuing long-term anticoagulation.

## Summary

Forty-five patients with pulmonary embolus were treated with fibrinolysin. Two had previous vena cava ligations and were treated to prevent exacerbation of the edema and thrombophlebitis.

Fourteen had massive embolism. Nine of these (64 per cent) survived the embolus. Five (36 per cent) died acutely from the embolus or irreversible changes despite apparent dissolution of the clot in three. Five others died of other disease after apparent recovery from the embolism.

Thirty patients were treated for acute single (not massive) or multiple pulmonary emboli. Of these, 25 survived. Of those who survived, two had recurrence of emboli and a vena cava ligation was successful. Two others had late (5 months and 18 months) recurrence of emboli with massive occlusion and death.

[REFERENCES ON FOLLOWING PAGE]

*REFERENCES*


1. Adams, S. T. and DeWeese, J. A. Experimental and clinical evaluation of partial vein interruption in the prevention of pulmonary emboli, *Surgery 57:* 82-102, 1965.
2. Agrifoglio, G. and Edwards, E. A. Venous stasis after ligation of femoral veins on inferior vena cava, *J.A.M.A. 178:*1-7, 1961.
3. Anderson, M. C. and Shields, T. W. Significance of fatal pulmonary embolism in immediate post-operative period, *J.A.M.A. 167:*422-6, 1958.
4. Anlyan, W. G. and Hart, D. Special problems in venous thromboembolism, *Ann. Surg. 146:*499-509, 1957.
5. Baker, R. R. Pulmonary embolism, *Surgery 54:*687, 1953.
6. Baker, R. R. and Wagner, H. N. Pulmonary embolectomy in the treatment of massive pulmonary embolism, *Surg. Gynec. Obstet. 122:*153-16, 1966.
7. Barker, W. F. Management of venous thrombosis and pulmonary embolism, *Surgery 45*(2):198-203, 1959.
8. Beall, A. C., Jr. *et al.* Surgical treatment of pulmonary embolism, *Heart Bull. 13:*41-3, 1964.
9. Browse, N. L. and James, D. C. O. Streptokinase and pulmonary embolism, *Lancet 2:*1039-43, 1964.
10. Byrne, J. J. and O'Neill, E. E. Fatal pulmonary emboli; study of 130 autopsy-proven fatal emboli, *Amer. J. Surg. 83:* 47-49, 1952.
11. Cahill, J. M., Byrne, J. J. and White, R. L. Effect of fibrinolytic agents and anticoagulants on blood clot pulmonary emboli, *Surg. Gynec. Obstet. 116:*486, 1963.
12. Carlo, H. I., Hardy, I. B., Jr., Linton, R. P. and White, P. D. Embolization in cardiac patients, *J.A.M.A. 134:*1447, 1947.
13. Coon, W. W., MacKenzie, J. W. and Hodgson, P. E. Critical evaluation of anticoagulant therapy in peripheral venous thrombosis and pulmonary embolism, *Surg. Gynec. Obstet. 106:*129-36, 1958.
14. Coon, W. E. and Willis, P. W. Deep venous thrombosis and pulmonary embolism: Prediction, prevention and treatment, *Amer. J. Cardiol. 4:*611-21, 1959.
15. Crane, C. Femoral vs. caval interruption for venous thromboembolism, *New Eng. J. Med. 270:*819-22, 1964.
16. Del Guercio, L. R. M., Coomaraswamy, R. P., Feins, N. R. and State, D. The bedside hemodynamic diagnosis of acute pulmonary embolism, *Surg. Forum 15:* 192-194, 1964.
17. DeWeese, M. S. and Hunter, D. C., Jr. Vena cava filter for the prevention of pulmonary embolism, *Arch. Surg. 86:* 852, 1963.
18. Dexter, L., Dock, D., McGuire, L., Hyland, J. and Haynes, F. Pulmonary embolism, *Med. Clin. N. Amer. 44:*1251-68, 1960.
19. Donaldson, G. A., Williams, C., Scannell, J. G. and Shaw, R. S. Reappraisal of the application of the Trendelenburg operation to massive fatal embolism, *New Eng. J. Med. 268:*171-74, 1963.
20. Freiman, D. G., Suyemoto, J. and Wessler, S. Frequency of pulmonary thromboembolism in men, *New Eng. J. Med. 272:*1278-1280, 1965.
21. Gorham, L. W. A study of pulmonary embolism. III. The mechanism of pain; based on a clinicopathological investigation of 100 cases of minor and 100 cases of massive embolism of the pulmonary artery, *Arch. Intern. Med.* (Chicago) *108:*418-26, 1961.
22. Hampson, J., Milne, A. C. and Small, W. P. Surgical treatment of pulmonary embolism, *Lancet 2:*402, 1961.
23. Herman, R. E., Davis, J. H. and Holden, W. D. Pulmonary embolism. A clinical and pathologic study with emphasis on the effect of prophylactic therapy with anticoagulants, *Amer. J. Surg. 102:* 19-28, 1961.
24. Hume, M. Thrombolysis of the experimental radioactive pulmonary embolus, *N. Eng. J. Med. 264:*471, 1961.
25. Israel, H. L., Fisher, G. R., Mueller, O. and Cooper, D. A. Fibrinolysin treatment of thromboembolism, *J.A.M.A. 188:*628-31, 1964.

26. Keisker, H. and Bowers, R. Results obtained by superficial femoral vein ligation, *Surgery 47*:224-9, Feb. 1960.
27. Mackeent, P., Landrigan, P. L. and Dickson, R. C. Early diagnosis of acute pulmonary embolism, *Canad. Med. Ass. J. 85*:233, 1961.
28. Madsen, C. M. and Buhl, J. Fatal pulmonary embolism. Prospects of surgery, *Acta Chir. Scand. 128*:721-8, 1964.
29. McNicol, G. P. and Douglas, A. S. Thrombolytic therapy, *J. Clin. Path. 17*:338-40, 1964.
30. Nusbaum, M. and Blakemore, W. S. Treatment of acute phlebitis, *Surg. Gyn. Obstet. 119*:1107-18, 1964.
31. Parker, B. M. and Smith, J. R. Pulmonary embolism and infarction: Review of the physiologic consequences of pulmonary arterial obstruction, *Amer. J. Med. 24*(3):420-27, 1958.
32. Phear, D. Pulmonary embolism: Study of late prognosis, *Lancet 2*:832-5, 1960.
33. Roe, B. B. and Goldthwaite, J. C. Pulmonary embolism: Statistical study of post-mortem material at Massachusetts General Hospital, *New Eng. J. Med. 241*:679-86, 1949.
34. Sautter, R. D., Fletcher, F. W., Emanuel, D. A., Olsen, T. G. and Lawton, B. R. Complete resolution of massive pulmonary thromboembolism, *J.A.M.A. 189*:948-9, 1964.
35. Schauble, J. F., Anlyan, W. G., Deaton, H. L., Delaughter, G. D., Baylin, G. J. and Lynn, J. A. A study of recurrent pulmonary embolism, *A.M.A. Arch. Surg. 80*:105-11, 1960.
36. Sevitt, S. and Gallagher, N. Venous thrombosis and pulmonary embolism. Clinico-pathological study in injured and burned patients, *Brit. J. Surg. 48*:475-89, 1961.
37. Sevitt, S. and Gallagher, N. Prevention of venous thrombosis and pulmonary embolism in injured patients, *Lancet 2*:981-9, 1959.
38. Sharnoff, J. F., Rosenberg, M. and Mistica, B. A. Seasonal variation in fatal thromboembolism and its high incidence in the surgical patient, *Surg. Gynec. Obstet. 116*:11, 1963.
39. Spencer, F. C., Jude, J., Reinhoff, W. F. III and Stonesifer, G. Plication of the inferior vena cava for pulmonary embolism, *Ann. Surg. 161*:788-801, 1965.
40. Steenburg, R. W., Warren, R., Wilson, R. E. and Rudolf, L. E. New look at pulmonary embolectomy, *Surg. Gynec. Obst. 107*:214, 1958.
41. Stein, G. N., Chen, J. T., Goldstein, F., Israel, H. L. and Finkelstein, A. Importance of chest roentgenography in the diagnosis of pulmonary embolism, *Amer. J. Roentgen 81*:255, 1959.
42. Uhland, H. and Goldberg, L. M. Pulmonary embolism: A commonly missed clinical entity, *Dis. Chest 45*:533-36, 1964.
43. Wacker, W. E., Rosenthal, M., Snodgrass, P. J. and Amador, E. Triad for the diagnosis of pulmonary embolism and infarction, *J.A.M.A. 178*:8-13, 1961.
44. Wagner, H. N., Jr., Sabiston, D. C., Jr., McAfee, J. G., Tow, D. and Stern, H. S. Diagnosis of massive pulmonary embolus in man by radioisotope scanning, *New Eng. J. Med. 271*:377-384, 1964.
45. Wilhelmsen, L., Selander, S. Soederholm, B., Paulin, S., Varnauskas, E. and Verko, L. Recurrent pulmonary embolism, *Medicine* (Balt.) *42*:335-55, 1963.
46. Williams, J. R., Wilcox, W. C., Andrews, G. J. and Burns, R. R. Angiography in pulmonary embolism, *J.A.M.A. 184*:473, 1963.
47. Barritt, D. W. and Jordan, S. C. Clinical features of pulmonary embolism, *Lancet 1*:729-32, 1961.
48. Dexter, L. Thromboemboli as a cause of cor pulmonale, *Bull. N. Y. Acad. Med. 41*:981, 1965.
49. Nabseth, D. C. and Moran, J. M. Reassessment of the role of inferior vena cava ligation in venous thromboembolism, *New Eng. J. Med. 273*:1250-1253, 1965.
50. Sautter, R. D. and Emanuel, D. A. Pulmonary embolectomy utilizing cardiopulmonary bypass. *Amer. J. Surg. 109*:493-95, 1965.

# SIX HUNDRED YEARS OF MEDICINE IN VIENNA*

## A HISTORY OF THE VIENNA SCHOOL OF MEDICINE

ALFRED VOGL

Professor of Clinical Medicine, New York University
President of the Pirquet Society of Clinical Medicine
New York, N. Y.

THE University of Vienna, Austria, which is celebrating the 600th anniversary of its founding, has been the alma mater of many of the members of this audience. In pausing on this occasion to look back over the centuries from the vantage point of 1965, it may be wise not just to reminisce nostalgically about the good old times, but rather to examine critically the kaleidoscopic events of these centuries.

In so doing, we may not only recall the influences to which we were exposed during our formative years, and thus expose the roots of our intellectual development, of our motivations, beliefs, and prejudices, but we may also become aware of some of those related and causal factors in the political, economic, and cultural world of Austria and Europe that shaped the history of the Vienna Medical School.

From such a review we may derive insight, understanding, and a keener appreciation of those factors and forces that over the years have tended either to inhibit or to further the growth of learning in institutions such as the Vienna Medical School. The lessons learned should help us in the search for direction for future goals for ourselves and our younger friends here and abroad.

On March 12, 1365, Duke Rudolf IV of Austria (Figure 1), by-named the Founder (*der Stifter*), obtained permission from Pope Clement VI to establish a university in Vienna. In the words of the papal charter, this act converted the ancient School of St. Stephen's "into a university according to the ordinances and customs observed first at Athens, then at Rome, and after that at Paris."

*Presented at a special meeting of the Pirquet Society of Clinical Medicine, New York, N. Y., on the occasion of 600th anniversary of the founding of the University of Vienna, held at The New York Academy of Medicine, October 13, 1965.

From its inception this new university had a bona fide medical faculty. However, as the historian Josef von Aschbach stated 100 years ago, ". . . it was not much of a medical school during the first 400 years of its existence." In the beginning, the reason was the sorry state of medicine in general in the later middle ages and the paralyzing effect of scholasticism on all learning. Later on, in the 16th and 17th centuries, it was the lack of interest in any scientific endeavors in the war-torn and plague-ridden Vienna of that epoch.

In those early days of the medical school, teaching consisted merely in the reading to the students of some ancient treatises prescribed by the authorities of the university. There were three masters to whom the texts were assigned by drawing lots. The books used were the "*ars parva*" by the Greco-Roman physican Galen, written in the second century A.D., and the "*Canon*" of Avicenna and the "*liber medicinalis*" by Rhazes, both 10th-century Persian-Arabian physician-philosophers. These writings were based essentially on the works of Hippocrates. Criticism or deviations from these doctrines were inadmissible.

The entire study of medicine consisted in memorizing the teachings of Galen and of his commentators (Figure 2). After 2 years of study the successful student would receive his B.A. without ever having seen a patient or the dissection of a body.

The contact of the student with patients began in the third year when he had to accompany a practicing physician on his rounds, watching his master's way of observing the patient, inspecting the ever-present urinal, giving long-winded discourses on the nature of disease and, finally, composing the traditionally very complicated prescriptions. After 2 to 3 years of apprenticeship the bachelor of arts was entitled to obtain a doctor's degree by giving a dissertation on one of the aphorisms of Hippocrates.

The faculty consisted of all the doctors licensed to practice in Vienna and its suburbs. From the early records it becomes apparent that its members were mainly concerned with establishing a professional guild capable of eliminating competition by quacks and foreign graduates and enforcing their more or less important claims, such as that for a privileged spot in the Corpus Christi procession (*Fronleichnams-Prozession*) or exemption from city taxes. They would resolve not to treat any pharmacist who had supplied drugs to a quack, or a patient

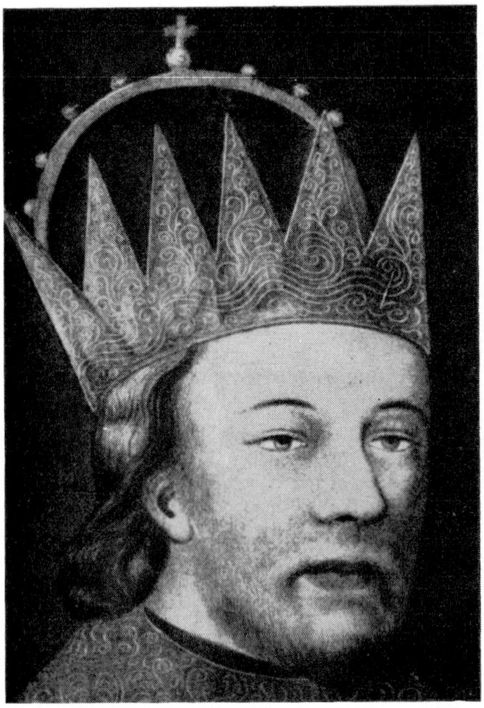

Fig. 1. Duke Rudolf IV, *der Stifter,* 1339-1365.

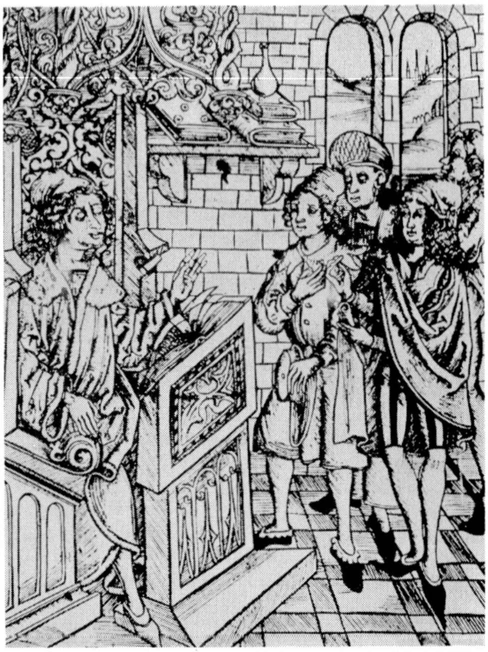

Fig. 2. Teaching of medicine in the 15th century.

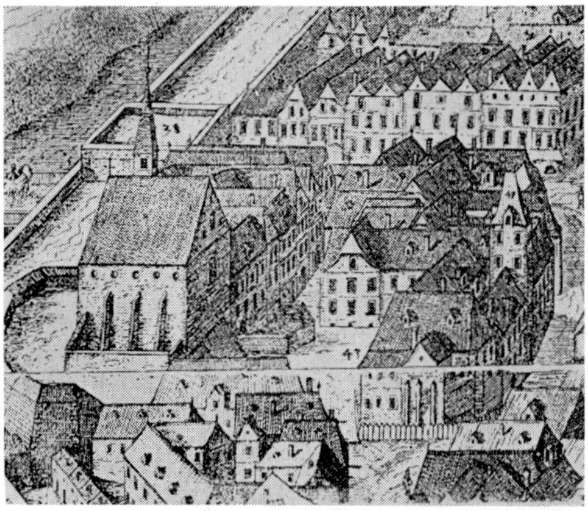

Fig. 3. University Quarter of Vienna in the 14th century.

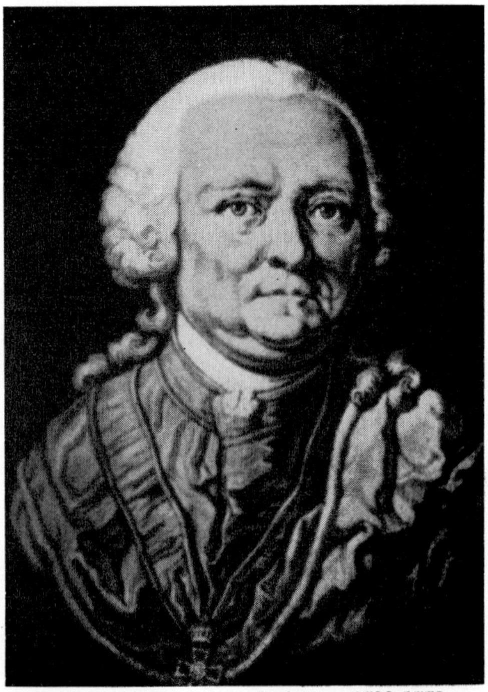

Fig. 4. Gerard van Swieten, 1700-1772.

who had previously been under the care of a nonlicensed healer. Since all other faculties had patron saints, the medical faculty chose two saints, St. Cosmas and St. Damian, as their own protectors and established for them an annual solemn mass at St. Stephen's.

The members of the faculty considered surgical procedures as being below the dignity of a learned doctor and they left cataract, hernia, and stone operations to the migrant healing artists. This attitude prevailed in Vienna at a time when surgery was already developing into a highly respected profession and an important branch of teaching at the faculties of Padua in Italy and Montpellier in France.

The university buildings and the student quarters were located in a cramped area of the city (Figure 3). Later this district had to be walled off in order to prevent the frequent vicious fights between the unruly students and the hostile burghers of Vienna.

Even at the time when the Renaissance and humanism changed the course of Western civilization (around 1500) and produced revolutionary figures on the medical scene, such as Vesalius in Padua, Guy de Chauliac in Montpellier, Lanfranc in Paris, Paracelsus in Basel and Harvey in London, no fresh breeze penetrated the stagnant atmosphere of the medical faculty at Vienna. Here economic and political conditions were at a desperately low level as the result of the religious wars marked by wanton destruction of life, property, and cultural goods.

In 1629, in line with the pious spirit of that time, the university was put under the authority of the College of Jesuits by Emperor Ferdinand II. Under this oppressive regimen the medical faculty remained in its state of lethargy and standstill. Foreign students did not come to Vienna and wealthy Austrians sent their sons abroad to study at the flourishing universities of Italy and France. In 1703 an imperial order suspended the conferral of medical degrees in Vienna because of the poor quality of teaching. The Medical School had reached its lowest status.

During the 17th century only a few members of the faculty are noteworthy for their activities. Among them were Managetta and de Sorbait.

Johann Wilhelm von Managetta, personal physician to three emperors, a man of wide educational background, took vigorous measures to improve the deplorable state of sanitation in Lower Austria and conceived, in an age dominated by the most absurd superstitions, sensible regulations to combat the disastrous epidemics ravaging the country. In Vienna he made himself immortal by inventing the *Wiener Trankel,* a laxative that is still popular there.

Paul de Sorbait, who succeeded Managetta and remained chief of the medical faculty for 25 years, finally managed, against the stubborn resistance of the College of Jesuits, to introduce the teaching of anatomy, which was already well advanced in other medical schools.

The delay in upgrading the medical school in the late 17th and early 18th centuries is difficult to understand. This was an epoch of political and military glory for Austria following the defeat of the Turkish invaders and the victory in the Spanish Wars of Succession. Those were the days of feverish construction of magnificent baroque palaces and churches and of resplendent festivities at the courts of the emperor and the high aristocracy. However, the esteem for university teachers was very low in the same influential circles, and the salaries offered were so inadequate that no man of distinction sought these positions.

It was Empress Maria Theresa who changed this situation radically after her ascendance to the throne in 1740. She must have been painfully aware of the deplorable level of medicine in Vienna and felt the need for vigorous measures to change the conditions. It will be remembered that Maria Theresa's Austria dominated not only a great part of the ancient Holy Roman Empire but also Italy and the Netherlands, two countries in which medical schools were flourishing at that time. They were the regions from which a regeneration of Austrian medicine had to come.

In Italy, around the year 1600, at the University of Padua, Montanus had revived the Hippocratic method of teaching medicine at the bedside. Italian physicians introduced this system to the Netherlands where similar ideas, propagated by the great British clinician Thomas Sydenham, had fallen on fertile ground. In Holland, at the University of Leyden, Hermann Boerhaave was professor of medicine. He was an enthusiastic follower of Montanus' and Sydenham's precepts and had succeeded in making the medical school of Leyden the leading institution of his time by teaching according to the three basic rules of Hippocrates: use common sense instead of unfounded speculations; observe the patient carefully; and rely upon the healing power of nature. The empress turned for advice to Boerhaave who recommended his outstanding disciple, Gerard van Swieten, for the dual position of personal physician to the empress and of protomedicus in charge of medical education in Austria (Figure 4).

Van Swieten's appointment, almost 400 years after the founding of the university, marks the actual beginning of the Vienna Medical School as one of the leading institutions of its kind.

Van Swieten started by removing the obstructive influence of the College of Jesuits, an action that finally made possible systematic instruction in anatomy with regular dissections. The decisive impact of this innovation upon the level of medical education can hardly be realized today. Van Swieten also created the first teaching hospital, even though a modest one, with beds for six males and six females, in the old Burgerspital. He also added to the curriculum the teaching of obstetrics and eye diseases, and appointed another pupil of Boerhaave's, Anton de Haen, as professor of medicine and chief of the new clinic.

De Haen, a devoted teacher, created a clinical school in which new practices were taught, such as attention to all the qualities of the pulse, the taking of a thorough history, and the use of the thermometer. He also laid the very foundation for meaningful clinical investigation by introducing the keeping of detailed case records. De Haen tried to ban the ridiculous polypharmacy customary in the 17th and 18th centuries, and to replace it with diets and hygienic regimes. His teachings had a lasting influence upon the therapeutic orientation of the Vienna medical school, which henceforth required establishment of an exact diagnosis prior to the institution of therapy, and favored a sober and critical approach to any kind of treatment.

It is regrettable that de Haen, although outstanding as a teacher, was too conservative and opinionated to recognize new discoveries; he failed to see the merits of smallpox vaccination or of the most important diagnostic advance of his period: the work of Leopold Auenbrugger (Figure 5). Auenbrugger had invented the method of diagnosing chest disorders by percussion and had described it in a little book *Inventum Novum* in 1761. However, when the influential de Haen belittled this strange new technique of knocking with fingers at the patient's chest and refused to introduce it in his clinic, the whole faculty followed suit and the art of percussion was officially buried. For many years it was practiced only by Auenbrugger and his friends, among them de Haen's successor, Maximilian Stoll. In order to be accepted, percussion had to wait 47 years until Corvisart, Napoleon's

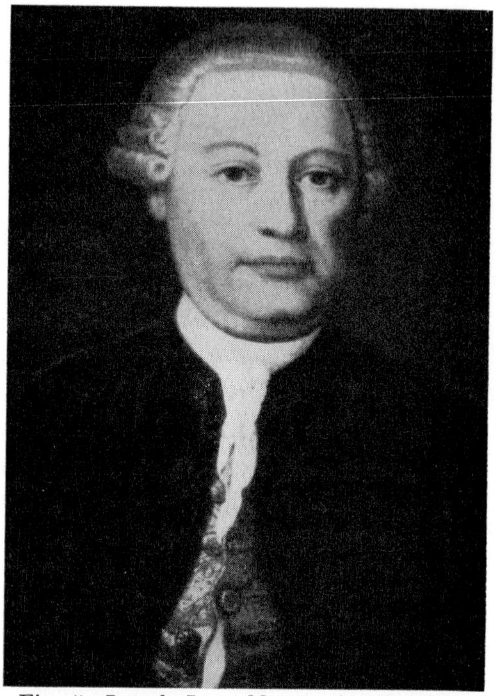

Fig. 5. Joseph Leopold von Auenbrugger, 1722-1809.

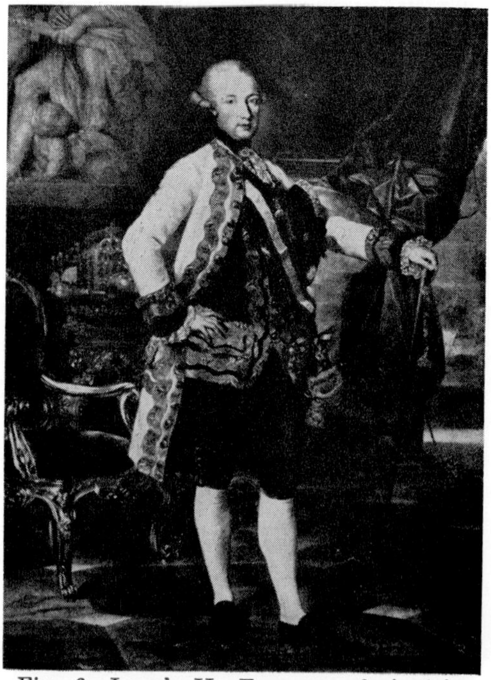

Fig. 6. Joseph II, Emperor of Austria, 1780-1790.

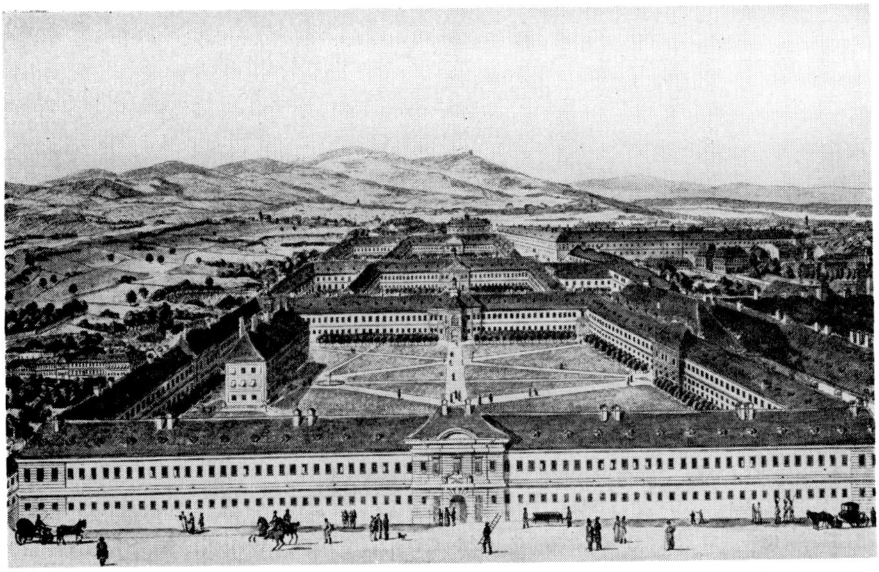

Fig. 7. Allgemeines Krankenhaus in Vienna, about 1800.

personal physician, published a French translation of Auenbrugger's book with favorable comments. Only then was percussion acclaimed as the first real advance in physical diagnosis since the times of Hippocrates. Auenbrugger, incidentally, never received an appointment to the teaching staff of the faculty.

The rise of the Vienna Medical School received a decisive impulse from Emperor Joseph II (Figure 6). He took probably more personal interest in questions of public health and of medical education than any ruler of a large country has ever done before or after him. The creation of the Vienna General Hospital (*das Allgemeine Krankenhaus* shown in Figure 7) was Emperor Joseph's favorite personal project. It was destined to become one of the most famous medical institutions of the civilized world and the home for the Vienna Medical School during its best period. A decision that also had great impact on teaching and studying of medicine in Vienna was Emperor Joseph II's Act of Tolerance, which granted for the first time the admission of Jewish students to the University. This decree not only opened the medical career to a new group of eager and talented students from many parts of Europe, it also changed the composition of the faculty during the following 150 years. During this long period Jewish physicians and investigators made major contributions to medicine and thus enhanced the name of the Vienna Medical School.

The leading physician during Emperor Joseph's regime was Johann Peter Frank. He expounded the then novel idea of the responsibility of the state for maintaining the health of its population. His book, titled *Medizinische Polizey*, was the first comprehensive text on preventive medicine and public hygiene. During his many active years in Vienna he brought about an intimate and fertile relationship with the then eminent Italian medical schools. In the *Allgemeine Krankenhaus*, of which he was director, he founded a pathologic-anatomical museum, and he introduced as an important innovation the isolation of patients with infectious diseases.

The 60-year period between 1745, when van Swieten started his reforms, and 1805, when Johann Peter Frank was forced to resign his position, was an exciting era of progress, which historians later designated the First Vienna Medical School.

This memorable epoch was followed by an abrupt decline, not due to any lack of men of ability but solely because of the oppressive political atmosphere that had settled upon Vienna and Austria. This was the time of all-out reaction against the liberal spirit that had been promoted by Emperor Joseph, it was a period of thought control and mutual distrust, the era of Prince Metternich and of the Biedermeier style with its surface calm and its hated secret police: in short, the era of the Vormärz. The position of head of medical education of Austria fell into the hands of a Baron Stifft, an arch-reactionary who during the 40 years of his dictatorship succeeded in removing virtually all eminent or promising men from their positions and replacing them with servile and politically trustworthy nonentities.

The very few men who survived this purge were able to uphold a certain standard in the faculty despite the discouraging atmosphere permeating it. Among them were two skillful and imaginative surgeons, Vinzenz von Kern and Joseph Wattmann, and the obstetrician Lukas Boer who introduced the teaching of obstetrics as an independent branch of medicine and had the courage to expose the dangers of the then fashionable meddlesome practices of his colleagues.

Shortly after 1840 a miracle happened: out of this political and scientific wilderness, almost suddenly, the Second Vienna Medical School rose like a phoenix from the ashes and brought with it the

Golden Age of medicine in Vienna. This time it was not the doing of a great administrator or reformer, nor had the stifling political atmosphere yet begun to clear. It was solely the result of the fortuitous appearance of the constellation of a few men of genius, endowed also with energy, perseverance, and unlimited devotion to their work. They had converged on the capital of the large Austro-Hungarian Empire from various parts of the multilingual monarchy. Their names were Rokitansky, Skoda, and Hebra.

Carl Rokitansky (Figure 8), born in Koeniggraetz in Bohemia, is one of the great pioneers in medicine and, with Giovanni Battista Morgagni (in Italy) and Rudolf Virchow (in Germany), he became the cofounder of pathologic anatomy as the basis for scientific medicine by correlating autopsy findings with the clinical manifestations of the disease. Rokitansky drew his brilliant descriptions and definitions of morbid entities, many of them previously unknown or misunderstood, from about 100,000 autopsies performed during his career. He recorded his vast knowledge in his *Handbuch der Pathologischen Anatomie*, whose first edition appeared in 1842. This widely read text and his personal teaching for over 40 years had direct influence upon the thinking and practice of medicine of two generations, and the impact of his concepts is still felt in pathology today.

At the same time another Bohemian, Joseph Skoda (Figure 9), born in Pilsen, raised the field of clinical diagnosis to astounding heights by making ingenious use of the newly introduced method of percussion (Auenbrugger) and auscultation (Laennec). He checked his physical findings with the aid of his friend and mentor Rokitansky at the autopsy table and was in this way able to develop a new clinical system of the pathology of the heart and lungs. Skoda's description and interpretation of physical findings in chest diseases were so exact that they are as valid and useful today as they were 150 years ago. This pathfinding work found recognition by his contemporaries only slowly and against the stubborn resistance of the medical authorities in power. They disliked Skoda's fancy and time-consuming methods of physical examination as well as what they called his "therapeutic nihilism," particularly when it became known to have lower mortality than their "active methods of treatment" consisting of blood-letting, purges, and emetics. His opponents succeeded in preventing Skoda from obtaining the chair in medicine until 1846, when he was finally

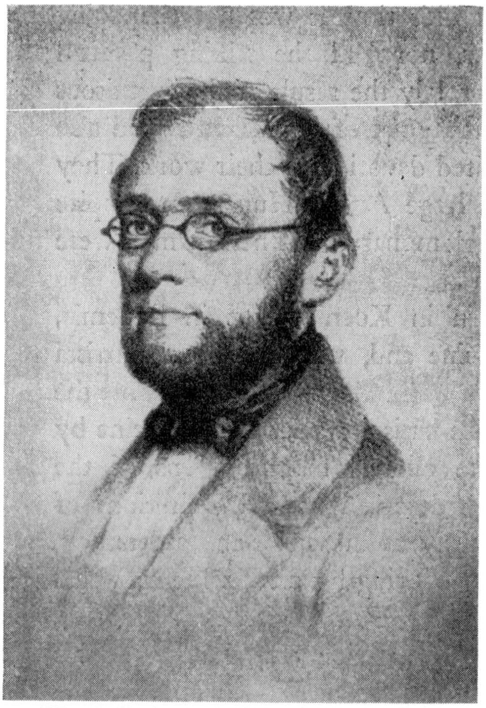

Fig. 8. Carl von Rokitansky, 1804-1878.

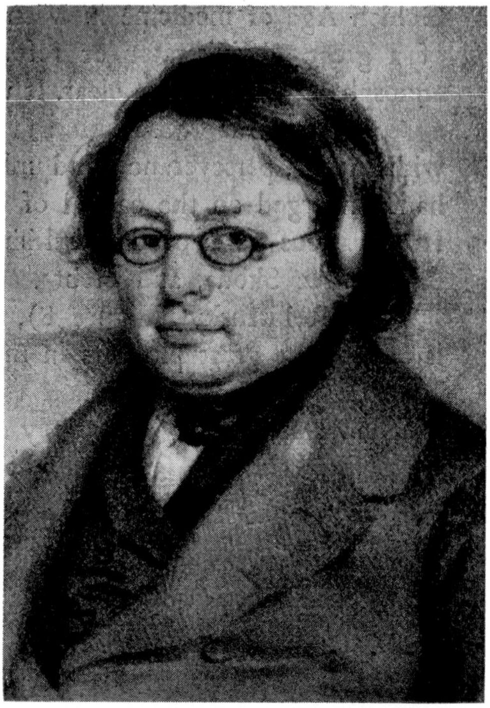

Fig. 9. Joseph L. Skoda, 1805-1881.

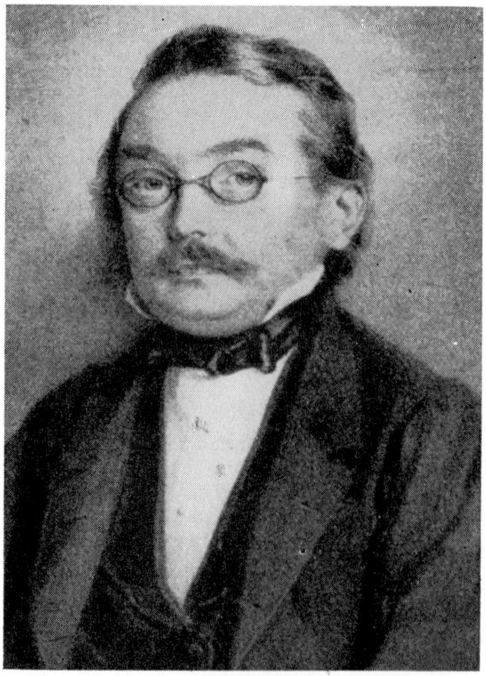

Fig. 10. Ferdinand von Hebra, 1816-1880.

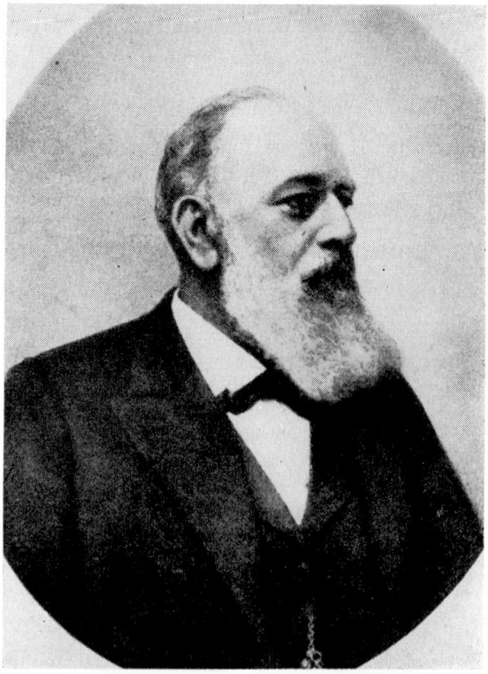

Fig. 11. Theodor Billroth, 1829-1894.

appointed through the energetic intervention of Rokitansky with the help of Archduke Ludwig.

Another great Bohemian of this era was Johannes von Oppolzer who, at Skoda's recommendation, became the chief of the newly created Second Medical Clinic. In contrast to the essentially anatomical concepts of his colleagues Rokitansky and Skoda, Oppolzer emphasized the disturbance of physiologic function in the pathogenesis of disease. This orientation promoted logically a more positive attitude towards active and individualizing therapy, while at Skoda's clinic the guiding principle was still "*primum non nocere*": refrain from any action that might interfere with the natural healing power of the human organism.

Also the development of surgery was decisively influenced by the teachings of Skoda and Rokitansky. Franz Schuh, who was professor of surgery, raised the standard of his specialty when he insisted on pathologic evaluation of operative findings. He evoked the admiration of his colleagues when he performed aspiration of pleural and pericardial exudates, the presence of which had been recognized through physical examination.

A new branch of medicine was born when Skoda entrusted his wards of patients with skin diseases (generally referred to as *Krätzekranke*) to his assistant Ferdinand von Hebra (Figure 10), a Moravian by birth, with the instruction to study the pathology of the skin. Hebra rapidly developed dermatology to a high level. He described, defined, and classified many skin diseases on clinical, pathologic, and parasitologic grounds, and published a monumental atlas of skin diseases. Hebra succeeded in creating in Vienna an internationally renowned school of dermatology. It remained at the same level under his pupil Moritz Kaposi.

The chairs of anatomy and physiology were also occupied by teachers and scientists of outstanding quality: Hyrtl and Brücke. They were colorful characters who were known often to clash violently in their differing estimation of each other's fields and capacities.

Joseph Hyrtl, a Burgenlander, won admiration as one of the great teachers of anatomy, especially of surgical (topographic) anatomy. His text book passed through 22 editions and remained the Bible of anatomy all over the world for two generations.

Under Ernst von Brücke, who had come from Heidelberg, the teaching of physiology developed from virtual nonexistence to an essential part of medical education. During the 40 years of his professorship he trained innumerable students in the fast-expanding field of physiology and in methods of physiologic research. In this way he created the necessary balance against the then prevalent anatomical orientation of the Vienna Medical School.

The attitude of the government towards the leaders in medicine had changed completely during this period. Many professors were honored by the emperor with titles and decorations, and were raised to nobility and appointed members of the Upper House of Parliament.

However, even during this splendid period of progress the voices of reaction were not silenced, and the power of entrenched office holders was still strong. A sad, almost incredible illustration of this fact is the story of Ignaz Philipp Semmelweis. As a young doctor Semmelweis, through keen bedside and autopsy observation, recognized the infectious nature and manner of transmission of childbed fever, the killer of thousands of young women at that time. He reported his findings and recommendations to the Society of Physicians in Vienna in 1847 and again, in a monograph, 14 years later. However, he found himself involved in an unequal battle against a solid front of the obstetricians of the faculty. They were outraged by the effrontery of the young Hungarian who tried to discredit their theories and thus undermine their positions. Despite the active support of Rokitansky and Skoda he was forced out of his position in Vienna, suffered a mental breakdown, and died at the age of 47 in an insane asylum. More thousands of women were to die from childbed fever before Semmelweis' concept gained universal acceptance years after his death.

This cruel interlude is evidence that even during the heroic phase of the School, prejudice, inertia and selfishness were still powerful forces that might easily have led to another decline of the medical faculty at the time when the group of ingenious men who had been in the forefront of progress were getting old. Fortunately, these very same men used the weight of their prestige to have the best possible candidates for any opening at the faculty called to Vienna, no matter what their origin or background. Thus it happened that, through Rokitansky's insistence and against violent opposition, Theodor Billroth (Figure 11), a North German of Swedish ancestry, became professor of surgery in Vienna. With him the school of surgery reached its very

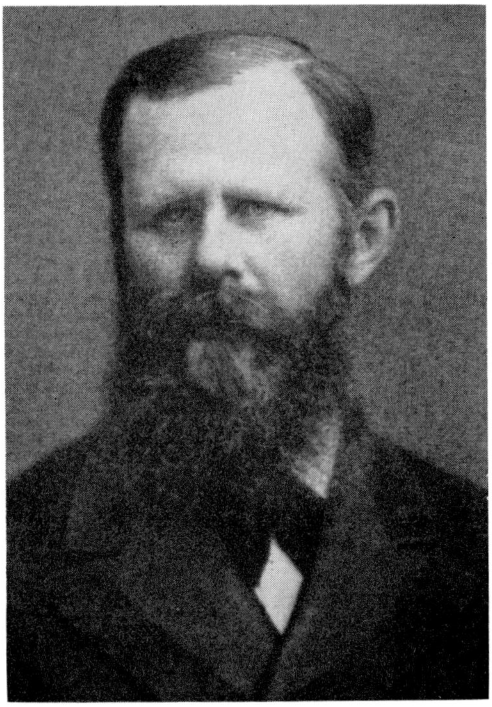

Fig. 12. Hermann Nothnagel, 1841-1905.

culmination. Research and practice advanced brilliantly under his leadership. Elaborate animal experiments were carried out and led to revolutionary progress in operations on the larynx, the esophagus, the stomach, and the bowels. The reputation of Billroth's clinic soon made it an international center for training in surgery, and his assistants were much in demand for leading positions at many universities in Europe.

Billroth, as a teacher, pioneer in surgery, and powerful personality, stood out like a giant within the medical faculty. Fortunately, the other branches of medicine were also represented by eminent men during his time.

To mention only a few:

Hermann Nothnagel (Figure 12), born in Berlin, was one of the last men to master the entire knowledge in internal medicine and neurology of his time. He made significant contributions, especially in the field of gastroenterology and pharmacology, and he had the reputation of being one of the greatest teachers of this period. From Nothnagel's staff came many excellent internists and neurologists who enhanced the reputation of Vienna as a medical mecca around the turn of the century. But outside his scientific achievements, Nothnagel will always be remembered as a fighter for the highest professional standards and as the fearless defender of human rights against the hydra of political anti-Semitism that began to raise its ugly head during his time.

Salomon Stricker, the first professor of experimental pathology, became a legendary figure because of his unorthodox teaching methods and his fascinating lectures during which he demonstrated animal experiments.

Adam Politzer, founder of a prominent school of otologists, developed his field from simple beginnings and wrote a textbook of otology that became a classic.

Hans Horst Meyer, born in East Prussia, was one of the founders of experimental pharmacology and thereby one of the pioneers of rational therapy. His work contributed enormously to the clarification of the action and the value of numerous drugs that had previously been used empirically. Meyer's textbook, *Experimental Pharmacology*, remained the standard text for several decades.

Theodor Meynert, professor of neurology and psychiatry, initiated the study of microscopic changes of the central nervous system, and his successor, Richard von Krafft-Ebing, was the first psychiatrist who ventured to delve into the problems of the psychology of sexual life and its deviations.

The life and work of these men whose activities extended toward or beyond the turn of the century, led into what, for many of us, has been contemporary medicine, the age of increasing specialization. Until World War I, Vienna remained one of the foremost centers of medicine, recognized as a school with a remarkable tradition, staffed with eminent experts, who were highly respected as teachers, investigators, and practitioners. Some of the men whose teachings made a lasting impression upon the older generations of living Vienna graduates were the anatomists Emil Zuckerkandl and Julius Tandler, the pathologists Richard Paltauf and Jakob Erdheim, the surgeons Anton von Eiselsberg and Julius von Hochenegg, the ophthalmologist Ernst Fuchs, the orthopedist Adolf Lorenz, the radiologist Guido Holzknecht, the psychiatrist Julius Wagner-Jauregg, the neuropathologist Constantin von Economo, the gynecologist Ernst Wertheim, and the pediatrician Clemens von Pirquet, the father of the science of allergy.

These men, of a caliber high above average, were able to maintain the reputation of the Vienna Medical School in its increasingly difficult competition with rival schools abroad. All this glory, alas, came to an abrupt end with the outbreak of World War I and the postwar dissolution of the once powerful and wealthy Austro-Hungarian empire.

The small new Austria and its overgrown capital Vienna were too poor to provide the ever-increasing expenses for facilities and salaries of a first-class medical school, and Vienna could no longer attract outstanding scientists from abroad. It was therefore the difficult task of the surviving members of the prewar faculty to maintain its reputation. Perhaps the only prominent newcomer from abroad was the Dutchman Karel Frederick Wenckebach, who promoted the development of cardiology in Vienna. Most of the vacant chairs were filled with pupils of their former occupants, some of them recognized leaders in their field, such as Ernst Peter Pick in pharmacology, Otto Poetzl in neuropsychiatry, and Heinrich von Neumann in otology. Many other appointments made during that period, however, were based more on political expediency than on scientific qualifications. Thus many first-rate candidates for leading positions were not appointed, as for instance the gynecologist and pioneer in endocrinology Josef von Halban, or the innovator of fracture treatment Lorenz Boehler. Many others went abroad and found recognition, among them Carl Landsteiner, the discoverer of the blood groups and Nobel prize laureate, Béla Schick, whose diphtheria skin test had a profound impact on the theory and practice of immunization, Paul Klemperer, the pathologist who originated the concept of connective tissue disease, and Robert Barany, who received the Nobel prize for his work on the physiology and pathology of the organs of equilibrium.

In this period between the two World Wars, in which minor lumina dominated the medical faculty, there lived and worked in Vienna one man whose ideas and teachings had developed outside the official circle of the faculty but were finding a resounding response throughout the civilized world: Sigmund Freud, the revolutionary thinker and creator of psychoanalysis. While the faculty pointedly ignored him and some of its members publicly derided his concepts, Freud stayed on in Vienna and thereby made it the focus of the steadily increasing international attention to the new science. He no doubt attracted personally more disciples, students, and patients to Vienna than any other single clinician in official position at that time.

The continuing deterioration of the level of the medical school in the pre-Nazi era and its disintegration during the Nazi regime and World War II are matters of common knowledge.

After the war little was left but shambles of an old tradition. Out of these and against tremendous odds, a few courageous and devoted men, such as the highly respected internist Ernst von Lauda, tried to rebuild the Vienna Medical School. With total disruption of the continuity of teaching staff and students this was, indeed, a Herculean task. During this relatively short period of reconstruction, no personalities of exceptional rank as teachers or scientists have as yet emerged and no scientific work of outstanding significance has been published. It may take another constellation of the Rokitansky-Skoda-Hebra type to guide the Medical School to new heights.

No one should try to predict the future. The age of "great medical schools" may be over altogether. The leveling influence of easy and rapid communication throughout the scientific world and the free intercourse and exchange of teaching and research staffs of universities will make it increasingly unlikely that any one medical school as such can be greatly superior to others. However, whatever differences there will always be between various schools will depend on the quality of the physical facilities as well as the ability of the teaching staff. The quality of the facilities will necessarily depend on the existing economic conditions, the interest, and the generosity of the community. The quality of the teachers, on the other hand, will depend less on available funds than upon the principles that determine their selection.

With these facts in mind, can we draw any lesson from the history of the Vienna Medical School as to its quality in the future? The rise of the School has in all its phases been associated with times of economic prosperity, with a liberal and progressive atmosphere and with a far-seeing, unprejudiced, and independent policy in the selection of the teaching staff.

Conversely, the School has gone down whenever the country was poor, the atmosphere oppressive, and the choice of men for leading positions dictated by political, nationalistic, or religious motives. The pool of talents from which a small country can draw its leaders naturally is limited. The future can therefore look bright only if every opportunity is given to the most gifted men and if, at the same time, the horizon is searched constantly for new stars. Apathy, jealousy, bias, and the unwillingness to part with the comfortable past have done tremendous harm to the Vienna Medical School again and again, and they would do the same in the future.

In the best tradition of the Vienna Medical School there has been devotion to research by its members and great pride in their discoveries but, at the same time, there has been the firm resolution to remain first and foremost a school in which students are to be educated to become good doctors. These principles must remain the hallmark of the School if it is to regain its position among the best institutions of medical learning of the world.

We salute the Vienna University tonight and wish its Medical School a future true to the ideals of its glorious past.

## Acknowledgments

Figures 1, 3 to 6, and 8 to 12, from Schönberg, L., *Das Medizinische Wien*, 2d. ed. Vienna, Urban & Schwarzenberg, 1947. Reproduced by permission.

Figure 2 is from Castiglioni, A., *A History of Medicine*, 2nd ed. New York, Knopf, 1947. Reproduced by permission.

Figure 7 is reproduced from a colored print by Artaria & Co., Vienna (n.d.). Reproduced by permission.

## *Bibliography*

*Clinical Symposia*, vol. 9. Summit, N. J., Ciba, 1957.

Schrauf, Karl. *Studien zur Geschichte der Wiener Universität im Mittelalter*. Vienna, Selbstverlag, 1904.

Von Aschbach, Josef. *Geschichte der Wiener Universität im ersten Jahrhunderte ihres Bestehens*. Vienna, K. K. Universitätsverlag, 1865.

Wunderlich, Carl R. A. *Ein Beitrag zur Geschichte und Beurtheilung der gegenwärtigen Heilkunde in Deutschland und Frankreich*. Stuttgart, Ebner, Senkert, 1841.

# PSYCHOPATHOLOGY OF AGGRESSION AND VIOLENCE*

GUSTAV BYCHOWSKI

Preceptor, Department of Psychiatry
Mount Sinai School of Medicine
New York, N. Y.
Clinical Professor of Psychiatry
State University of New York Downstate Medical Center
Brooklyn, N. Y.

THE Schilder Society, as you know, is a descendant and a continuation of an analogous society in Vienna, Austria, whose foundation was inspired by Paul Schilder in 1922. I was present at those beginnings, took an active part in the proceedings, and I cherish the memory of intellectual and spiritual stimulation emanating from Paul Schilder.

The historical situation in Vienna of those years created a climate particularly favorable for the study of problems that will occupy us this evening. The disintegration of the Hapsburg monarchy, coming in the wake of World War I, had released powerful social forces and was accompanied by a veritable social and political revolution. Aggression and violence were breaking loose in a country impoverished by the long war and the crushing defeat.

Schilder had a keen eye for all social and political events, and he brought to their study the insights offered by the new psychology being elaborated by Sigmund Freud. Indeed, problems of aggression had occupied him ever since, and he devoted to them many studies, at first alone and then, after moving to the United States, with his co-workers here. He wrote on aggression in children, in man, and in woman; on the impact of cultural factors and ideologies; on aggression in self-defense; and on aggression as related to the openings of the body.

We live in an age of violence, of wars, of the extermination of millions for reasons of perverted racial doctrine and fanatical ideology.

Obviously we are most impressed by events of our own epoch, yet a glance at the past shows that destructive violence was prominent in various periods of history. We may not necessarily agree with all the conclusions of Robert Ardrey, the author of *African Genesis* that

**The Schilder Memorial Lecture,* presented at a meeting of the Schilder Society, New York, N. Y., held at The New York Academy of Medicine, January 27, 1966.

> . . . man had emerged from the anthropoid background for one reason only: because he was a killer. Long ago, perhaps many millions of years ago, a line of killer apes branched off from the non-aggressive primate background. . . . From this branch of apes man emerged with the fashioning of the first true weapons: Far from the truth lay the antique assumption that man had fathered the weapon. The weapon instead had fathered man.[1]

Yet, we must agree that the course of human history seems to be in accord with this thesis, starting from the first chapters of Genesis with the story of Cain and Abel until our own time. In fact, the prohibition of wanton murder in all the moral and religious codes has never prevented homicide from being advocated in the course of history for various reasons, even for the sake of the salvation of the soul. Both facts, the strict prohibition and the breaking through of the homicidal wish, under various disguises and rationalizations, testify to the powerful impact of this repressed drive. We even have reasons to connect it genetically with the primitive cannibalism.

The history of the Holy Inquisition, the persecution of the Cathari, the Albigeois, and all the other religious wars, were worthy predecessors of Stalin's purges and labor camps, and of Hitler's elaborate system of mass extermination.

In an attempt to survey problems of such complexity I shall leave aside the obscure problem of the derivation of the aggressive drive. I shall return to it briefly at the conclusion of this presentation.

By and large, modern psychiatry follows the dualistic doctrine of the founder of psychoanalysis. Eros and Neikos, love and strife, had been postulated as two basic principles already at about 450 B.C. by Empedocles of Akragas.

As a first approach I suggest the division of the phenomena of destructive aggression, according to their origin, into two large groups.

Violent hostility arises in an individual either spontaneously or as a result of an example, indoctrination and, more simply, introjection, that is, absorption of evil, as it were, from the environment.

Obviously, there are situations and configurations in which the child is taught to hate and to use violence as a guiding principle of behavior. This indoctrination may have various origins in familial or social pathology and ideology. We have every reason to believe that in the wake of a protracted war, crimes of violence are on the increase.

The same is true in periods of violent social upheaval.

Claude Brown describes in his autobiography, *Manchild in the Promised Land*, how his father taught him violence as a way of survival in the dark ghetto.[2]

Any fanatical political or ideological indoctrination is usually accompanied by the praise of violence. Here any means is laudable as long as it helps to destroy the adversary. Very often, and we know it only too well from past and recent history, the latter is represented as a deadly enemy so as to make him an object of wrath and destruction.

In the course of individual development we see hostility emerging in the service of the process of individuation.

The ego of the child is at first nonexistent, being undistinguishable from that of the mother: in due time it crystallizes gradually out of this original, so-called dyadic unity. In the course of this process it might be threatened by many factors, yet one of the most important seems to be the symbiotic wish of the mother or, far less frequently, of the father. This symbiotic wish finds its counterpart in the child who, along with his desire for emancipation, does not give up easily the wish to maintain the original unity.[3]

Thus, the increase of hostility at certain turning points of development must be considered as normal.

However, under certain conditions, hostility overwhelms the growing but weak ego and may lead to acts of violence and destruction. This might occur on the basis of such psychopathology as is characteristic of the so-called weak, fluid ego boundaries, for instance, in the clinical group of the schizophrenias.

Here even the individual's own wish to be loved, and the call for love issuing from the other person might be experienced as a threat to the ego which, without being aware, craves just for the very same fusion and complete merging which it consciously abhors.

Some typical erotic constellations may favor such a discharge of hostility. Here belong also various aspects of the oedipal conflict.

Certain acts of violence occur as a defense against the threats of breaking deeply ingrained moral taboos, such as the prohibition of incest or a homosexual gratification.

In attacking the person who, quite unbeknown to himself, mobilizes in him these dangerous and, therefore, repressed ego-alien impulses, the attacker denies and repudiates them vehemently. Periods of biological and, consequently, psychological crisis such as adolesence or menopause might create a particularly favorable background for such reactions.

However, long after the symbiotic relationship has been abandoned, there may exist a psychological situation where the original object of ambivalent love—I call such objects love-hate objects—has become incorporated, as it were, in the unconscious ego of the individual. An emotional situation developing between the latter and a new object of strong emotional involvement may evoke old ambivalence with the consequent desire to get rid of the introject, that is, of the incorporated image of the original love-hate object. Under such dynamic conditions there may occur acts of destructive violence.

Various clinical conditions favor such violent acting out: psychopathy, schizophrenia, epilepsy, and epileptoidy, and, of course, alcoholism, and the addictions. More recently with the advent of the psychomimetic drugs, the use of LSD has been known as an immediate precipitating cause of acts of violence.

Generally speaking, it is important to note at this point that the shifting from destruction in phantasy to violence in action is an event of extreme importance and that it is predicated upon a great number of variables. After all, we must be aware that only a small fraction of destructive phantasies that we know to exist in children and in adolescents and that we observe in our psychoanalytic patients becomes acted out in reality.

Frustrations, oppression, and humiliation in the sensitive period of development contribute to the emergence of reactive hostility. If the original love-hate object is the source of such experiences, then it naturally remains invested with a charge of hostility.

Situations that are directly or symbolically reminiscent of these early deprivations, persons who directly or indirectly evoke the image of the frustrating parent, become a target for destructive hostility. We may say that in such an act the individual attempts to destroy the original love-hate object, as it were, in absentia; or, to use a terminology that I introduced in a former publication, we may describe the aggressive act as an episode in the struggle against the introject.[4]

A great variety of destructive acts may be explained by this mechanism. Their variety is due to the multiplicity of etiological factors and to the richness of unconscious orchestration of the original hostile impulses.

In my doctoral dissertation, *The Psychopathology of Pyromania,* I described a number of individuals of varied clinical classification whose destructive impulses found their outlet in arson.[5]

In the variety of motivations there prevailed a unique combination of a frustrated erotic drive and thwarted primitive aggression. The act of arson appeared, by and large, as a symbolic expression of the destructive wish directed toward a frustrating love object or a generally frustrating life situation. An unrequited erotic wish could be detected under the relatively thin camouflage of symbolism or rationalization.

With my attention directed to these problems, I could demonstrate in the structure of a destructive act by an incipient schizophrenic the combination of symbolism and of a short-circuit compulsive reaction.

This young man was sent for a forensic evaluation to the famous Burghölzli where, at that time, under the direction of Eugen Bleuler, the creator of the concept of schizophrenia, I was serving my psychiatric apprenticeship. The time was the fourth year of World War I. The patient, a quiet and unobtrusive white-collar worker, had posted himself in bright daylight before the window of the Swiss Credit Bank in Zurich, Switzerland, and had smashed it with a stone.

Our explorations revealed that he was opposed to the war, and since, according to him, the war was being promoted by the capitalists, in his act he intended to attack the capitalist system. As you see, this primitive act of protest is reminiscent of contemporary vandalism; yet, it seems more transparent in its meaning and structure.

A more complex orchestration of destructive impulses can be seen in the acts of homicidal cruelty of a sexual delinquent.

As an illustration: many years later and in a different setting, I was able to study a man whom we had to diagnose as a paranoid schizophrenic but who, apart from his crimes, had led a respectable existence as a good family man and as a solid bread winner. As another aspect of his Dr. Jekyll-Mr. Hyde existence, he went prowling at night, assaulted lonely women, stabbed them to death, and raped them.

It appeared that in his hapless victims he was symbolically destroying his mother who had frustrated him in many ways in his childhood. She drank heavily and apparently went through psychotic episodes, abandoning the little boy to the care of a cruel, sadistic father. It was from him that the little boy absorbed the wrath which he then directed at his victims as the innocent maternal substitutes. In this, too, he was following the pattern of his father, who had mistreated the mother, trying to "reform" her and punishing her by measures of sadistic cruelty. Obviously, the boy was not exempt from these ministrations.

The characteristic split in the personality of this man, which allowed him to lead his double existence, with his crime remaining undetected for a long time, points to schizophrenia, a term introduced by Bleuler and derived from the Greek word for splitting. The lack of emotional reaction to his crime, complete absence of feelings of regret or guilt, points to another important trend, namely to the dynamic weakness of the superego.

This latter characteristic is shared by some schizophrenics with a large group of psychopaths who provide us with numerous examples of crimes of violence.

In classic psychiatry these psychopaths were said to have moral insanity, a term introduced by William B. Pritchard. Today this illness is described under various names, among them moral agnosia or moral imbecility. It is related on the one hand to psychopathy, on the other to the group of schizophrenias.

What all individuals thus affected have in common is the lack of empathy with other human beings: they lack the basic ability for identification that is the foundation of the social and human bond. In a progressing schizophrenic process this defect may precede by a long range the emergence of any other symptoms. Hence a particularly brutal crime of violence, committed against a close friend or relative, strikes even the closest environment like lightning.

It seems that in a time of general unrest, with its weakening of religious and moral norms in the group climate of alienation, such crimes are on the increase. This appalling phenomenon would require a much deeper and broader sociological and psychopathological analysis than we can offer in this place and at this moment. Suffice it to say that in our contemporary social climate certain psychopaths find encouragement and stimulation that trigger their reactions and even provide certain rationalizations.

I must mention here that in the epileptoid group and in the so-called driven psychopath the charge of primitive violence is particularly heavy, while the dynamic weakness of inhibitions and the low threshold of stimulation provide for an easy discharge of violence. Unfortunately, the very same individuals are inclined to use narcotics and stimulants which, in addition to alcohol, help the dynamic shift toward uncontrolled instinctual discharge.

Absorption of violence from a hostile, often psychopathic parent who, by his harsh and cruel handling of the child, has exposed him to endless frustrations and humiliations, may lead to the development of an individual imbued with wrath and emanating hatred. Given some personal magnetism and a favorable historical and sociopolitical situation, such an individual may grow to become a political leader who will satisfy his sadistic impulses and his lust for power under the guise of fanatic ideology. I have given a detailed analysis of such leaders in my studies of some past and recent dictators. The sinister figures of the latter have cast a dark shadow over the last decades of our history.[6]

Analysis of dictators has demonstrated in their personality makeup one element of great importance that they share with many other persons inclined to the use and promotion of violence: intense narcissism. Overemphasis on one's own ego leads to great vulnerability, with exaggerated reactions to real or imaginary frustrations, humiliations, or slights. On the primitive level of functioning these reactions manifest themselves above all in anger, culminating at times in rage and violence.

Many other factors may contribute to such aggressive hyperreactivity. As an example of the complexity involved let me mention the importance of the impairment of the physical or psychological functioning. An ego whose "effectance" is seriously impaired is naturally limited in its opportunities for gratification and discharge of socially acceptable aggression.[7]

If, as an example, we take a boy handicapped by infantile or spastic paralysis, or by limited intellectual abilities, it is easy to see that his occasions for frustration are much more numerous than for his contemporaries not having such handicaps.

It is also evident that severe economic deprivations that affect the essential human needs contribute substantially to the increase and violent discharge of destructive aggression. John B. Watson, creator of the behavioristic system of psychology, said that "hampering of bodily movement brings out the series of responses we call rage." It is clear that this statement should be taken in more than a literary sense.[8]

All these data gathered from observations of individual pathology, especially from the study of aggressive delinquents, can be easily applied to the flare-up of group violence among the underprivileged and oppressed minority groups.

Since we are a group of physicians gathered here to pay tribute to the memory of an illustrious colleague, we should consider the problem of aggression in a biological and evolutionary perspective. Such a point of view may offer an outlook for the future.

In the animal world, aggression serves above all the instinct for self-preservation. In Spinoza's words "every creature wants to persevere in its existence." Thus, aggression secures the acquisition of food and the defense of the territory, yet this aggression has nothing in common with the sadistic cruelty that we encounter in man. Cruelty does not belong to the essence of the predator, as poignantly illustrated in an Indian tale about a tiger cub brought up by goats. After a happy childhood as a goat he is reminded by an adult tiger of his true essence. As Konrad Lorenz, one of the leading ethologists of our time, puts it: "The lion in the dramatic moment before the leap on his prey is by nc means angry."

The aggressive drive plays also a most significant part in the preservation of the species. Animal studies show in a most impressive way the intricate interweaving of "love" and "strife" in an infinite variety of ingenious ritualized patterns of courtship, friendship, and fighting ceremonies. Lorenz, who has devoted a recent book to the study of aggression in the animal world, has shown that the social bond and the bond of friendship are based on evolutionary overcoming of original hostility. Aggression, which originally served to achieve the mastery of the female and to frighten away rivals, when inhibited becomes transmuted into protective domination of the female and of the offspring. According to Lorenz: "We find a personal bond, an individual friendship only in animals with highly developed intraspecific aggression; this bond is the stronger the more aggressive the respective animal species."

In summing up his phylogenetic considerations Lorenz says: "The intraspecific aggression is millions of years older than personal friendship and love. There exists, to be sure, intraspecific aggression without its counterpart (love) but, conversely, there is no love without aggression."[9]

While this evolutionary point of view offers some perspectives and hopes for the overcoming of intraspecific aggression in man, ethological studies offer eloquent analogies for the understanding of the psychopathology of individual and social aggression.

The changes in homeostasis, that is, in the emotional balance of relationships within an animal group can trigger the increased release of intraspecific aggression. This is especially conspicuous when natural (or experimental) conditions interfere with the normal outlets of the aggressive instinct. In such a case the aggression can easily turn against the members of one's own group or even nearest family.

A most suggestive analogy with human groups is provided by the intense hostility of some animal groups towards the outsider of the same species. A member of a rat colony, for instance, may become an object of hostility and rapid destruction after he has been put for a few days in a different rat colony or simply been rubbed with the soil of another group. The implications for human sociology or, rather, pathology are too obvious to be emphasized.

In man the process of socialization implies the curbing and domestication of instincts. These inevitable frustrations lead, in the last analysis, to what Freud described as discontent of civilization.[10] They are a source of psychic tension both within the individual as well as within the social group.

In the course of evolution the orchestration of basic instinctual impulses became infinitely complex as a result of symbolic implications and the creation of codes and powerful systems of values.

The eruption of violence is predicated upon changes in the intensity of all the variables responsible for the control and the socialization of the aggressive drive.

Here belongs love as the most powerful antidote against hate; the gratification of basic vital needs; economic security and political balance; ability to form and to maintain the social bond based on sympathy and empathy with fellow men; and, finally, in a general sense of the meaning and value of human existence.

In conclusion we must ask: Would it be really too optimistic to hope that with our increased insight into the mainsprings of human behavior and with the technological advances that should make secure all the basic needs of man, we might learn to control and discipline the urge for destruction and violence? Obviously prevention and education should be our primary goals here. This brief survey of the complex problems involved seems to offer clear if not easy guidelines. After all we belong to a profession whose essence is always to hope and never to give up. In this we are truly human.

## REFERENCES


1. Ardrey, R. *African Genesis.* New York, Atheneum, 1961.
2. Brown, C. *Manchild in the Promised Land.* New York, Macmillan, 1965.
3. Mahler, M. S. Thoughts about development and individuation, *Psychoanal. Stud. Child 18*:307-24, 1963.
4. Bychowski, G. Struggle against the introjects, *Int. J. Psychoanal. 39*:182, 1958.
5. Bychowski, G. Psychopathology of Pyromania (Zur Psychopathologie der Brandstiftung), *Schweiz. Arch. Psychiat. Neurol. 5*:29, 1919.
6. Bychowski, G. *Dictators and Disciples from Caesar to Stalin.* New York, Intern. Univ. Press, 1948. (German edition with new chapters on Hitler and Stalin, Munich, Szezesny, 1965.)
7. Term "effectance" introduced by Robert White in: Ego and reality in psychoanalytic theory, *Psychol. Issues 3*:33, 1963.
8. Watson, J. B. *Behaviorism.* New York, Norton, 1930, p. 154.
9. Lorenz, K. *Das Sogenannte Böse: zur Naturgeschichte der Aggression,* Vienna, Borotha-Schoelder, 1963. Quotations translated by the author. (English edition, *On Aggression,* New York, Harcourt, Brace, World, 1966.)
10. Freud, S. *Civilization and its Discontent.* Standard Edition, vol. 21.

# ANNUAL MEETING OF THE NEW YORK ACADEMY OF MEDICINE

## ADDRESS OF THE RETIRING PRESIDENT*

John L. Madden

President
The New York Academy of Medicine

I should first like to present to you the highlights of the activities of the major sections of The New York Academy of Medicine during the past year and then pause for a few moments to look into the Academy's immediate future.

The Committee on Medical Education, chaired by Dr. M. Ralph Kaufman and with Dr. Aims C. McGuinness as its Executive Secretary, has continued its expressed interest in the televised clinical seminars presented every Tuesday evening over station WNYC-TV, Channel 31. The videotapes of these various seminars are circulated on loan to institutions throughout the country.

The Committee works in close harmony with the officers of the 16 sections of the Academy, which include the most recently founded Section on Plastic and Reconstructive Surgery. This new section held its inaugural meeting on November 11, 1966; more than 400 persons were in attendance.

The Committee on Medical Education is now in the process of reviewing its goals for the future, and it plans many departures from its present program.

I am truly sorry to relate that Dr. McGuinness, who has been a stalwart of the Academy since 1959, has left our ranks. He has become Associate Executive Director of the Educational Council for Foreign Medical Graduates, effective January 2 of this year. He leaves us with

*Presented at the Annual Meeting of The New York Academy of Medicine, January 5, 1967.

a void to fill and has our heartiest best wishes for continued success in this new and most important educational endeavor.

The Committee on Public Health, chaired by Dr. Arthur Fischl, and headed by Dr. Harry Kruse as its Executive Secretary, has continued its constant pursuit of excellence in all matters affecting community health. Foremost and of general current community interest has been its report on air pollution. It should be of interest to note that in 1926, 41 years ago, the Committee published the findings of a 6-year study relative to this problem. Subsequent reports on the pollution of water and air were presented in 1931, 1957 and, most recently, in 1965.

Chronic bronchitis and pulmonary emphysema are the most rapidly growing causes of death in people over 50 years of age, and air pollution is believed to be a responsible cause. Accordingly, the importance of an early solution to this health menace is self-evident. It is heartening to everyone here, I am sure, that you, Mayor Lindsay, have already initiated the proper corrective measures against this menace. The Committee is also actively engaged in an effort to improve the psychiatric services in New York City. The manifold activities of this Committee and the many constructive tasks that it is undertaking should be a true comfort to the medical profession and the citizenry at large.

The Committee on Special Studies, which is chaired by Dr. Norton S. Brown and has Mr. Harry Becker for its Executive Secretary, is a pioneering leader in the socioeconomic aspects of health care. The activities of this Committee have gained widespread national recognition. The Committee has sponsored special seminars for health and public interest groups in New York City. One of these was held with the State Commission of Health and Welfare on policies and procedures for the administration of Medicaid.

The annual spring Health Conferences sponsored by this committee have become increasingly popular and, during the past 3 years, they have been oversubscribed. The 1966 Health Conference was entitled "New Directions in Public Policy for Health Care." More than 500 professional persons from all parts of the nation participated in this forum.

The national interest in the work of this Committee is exemplified by the fact that 5,000 additional copies of the special issue of the *Bulletin* of the Academy devoted to the papers presented at this conference are almost sold out. The Academy is indebted to this Committee for its splendid leadership and devoted labor in matters pertaining to health care.

The Committee on Library is chaired by Dr. Bronson S. Ray, and the Library itself is under the capable guidance of Miss Gertrude Annan. When one speaks of The New York Academy of Medicine, one speaks reciprocally of the Academy Library. They are truly inseparable. Through the years there has been a progressive parallel between the growth of the Academy and that of the Library. Annually the budget of the Library has amounted to approximately 45 per cent of the total budget for the Academy. In 1967 this sum represents in round figures $500,000.

In the future, expenses must of necessity increase if the established reputation of the Library, which is both national and international, is to be maintained. No library in New York City or in the whole of the nation gives so much for so little as does our own, and its ever pressing needs should be supported to the utmost.

The great increase in the cost of scientific libraries and the increasing demands for service have resulted in mounting expenses that are a true source of concern. We hope that federal aid may be forthcoming in support of these expenses. New equipment has already been added to increase the types of service available. This includes a Polaroid camera to make prints and transparencies, a microfilm reader, and an IBM system for cataloging. Support of the Library is in truth support of the Academy itself.

The last but not the least important item for consideration is finance. The Academy's finances are the province of our business manager, Mr. Robert Brereton. The problems in the financial management of the Academy are the same as those that affect the country at large, and they include primarily the sharp increase in inflation. This has particularly affected salary costs, which represent 70 per cent of our total annual expenditure.

The Academy expenses have increased at a more rapid rate than income, yet Mr. Brereton has done the noble job of balancing the budget without allowing this task to impair the progress of the Academy. To him we are indeed most grateful for a job well done.

What is the future of The New York Academy of Medicine? There is an old saying that you either move forward or backward; there is no standing still. The New York Academy of Medicine, since its founding in 1847, 120 years ago, always has moved forward and has always been a perpetual leader in its field. It may be stated with understandable and justifiable pride that the medical profession and the citizens of New York and, yes, the nation at large, owe much to the exemplary qualities of leadership that the Academy has provided through the years.

The immediate future, with its rapidly changing concepts that affect the entirety of medical care, would appear offhand to pose a challenging problem. The Academy not only has met this problem head-on but has anticipated it well in advance. This forward outlook has resulted in the formulation of recommendations that happily have proved acceptable to the proper authorities in both city and state government. In fact, The New York Academy of Medicine, by its recognized preeminence in the whole field of health care, is constantly being asked for advice, guidance, and recommendations relative to the vexing problems that confront both the medical profession and various governmental authorities. This is an acceptable and proper function of the Academy, and the fellowship have every reason to be proud of its accomplishments.

The immediate problem that the Academy must solve, and solve quickly, is that of physical expansion. Geographic circumstances, fortuitous and unplanned, have projected the Academy into a position between two rapidly developing medical centers, namely, the New York Medical College and The Mount Sinai School of Medicine. The Academy must of necessity participate as an equal partner in this development so that it may serve with continued excellence the professional needs of the community.

The Council of the Academy is most cognizant of its responsibility in this regard and has duly authorized its Building and Planning Committee, under the aegis of Dr. Robert Levy, and in close alliance with Dr. Howard Craig, to proceed forthwith as it sees fit to complete this most necessary and essential task. I sincerely request that the fellowship of the Academy, its friends and admirers, give their wholehearted support to this undertaking, the largest assumed by the Academy since it moved to its present location in 1927, 40 years ago. I have the utmost confidence that this project will come to complete fruition within the foreseeable future.

In closing, I wish to express my sincere appreciation to the members of the Council and of the Board of Trustees, to the Committees and membership of the 16 different sections that represent the Academy, and to the fellowship at large for their unwavering support during the past 2 years. Due public homage must also be paid to Dr. Anthony Cipollaro, our retiring and most efficient Recording Secretary.

I have been truly fortunate in that my term of office has coincided with the last 2 years of Dr. Howard Craig's 20 years of devoted service to the Academy. These 2 years have proved the most informative and enjoyable that I have ever experienced. To you, Howard, I shall be ever grateful.

The Academy is indeed fortunate in having Dr. James E. McCormack as a most worthy successor to Dr. Craig, and we all wish him well for his inevitable success as the new director of The New York Academy of Medicine. Dr. McCormack is joined by Dr. Preston Wade, a renowned surgeon, as the new president of the Academy, and I can assure you that this union augurs well for the continued preeminence of The New York Academy of Medicine.

# ADDRESS OF THE INCOMING PRESIDENT*

PRESTON A. WADE

President
The New York Academy of Medicine

In electing me president of The New York Academy of Medicine for the next 2 years, you have given me a flattering and challenging assignment. The history of the Academy is a long record of many remarkable achievements, and the officers of the past have been physicians of great distinction who have left an enviable record. It is now my duty to take up where they have left off, and I do so with great sincerity and with a realization of the great responsibility I have assumed.

I am embarrassed to have to admit that the frailties of the flesh have made it necessary for me to default in my very first official duty as president: namely, to act as presiding officer on this occasion. I trust I shall not fail you again, and I shall do my best to carry out my duties henceforth.

It is just 120 years ago this month that The New York Academy of Medicine was formally founded. The description of the meeting at which it was founded, as related by Philip Van Ingen in *The First Hundred Years*, his history of the Academy, is most amusing. The official description of the dinner of the Society for the Relief of Widows and Orphans of Medical Men indicates that "every delicacy of the season abounded upon the festive board—and the sparkling wine circulated freely about the table." It continues: "After eight formal toasts had been offered and responded to, many volunteer toasts were given and throughout the evening many excellent songs and stories were given. Later, the meeting was organized to discuss the propriety of establishing a local medical voluntary association having for its objects the purification of the professional body." Thus was conceived The New York Academy of Medicine.

The objectives of the Academy, as written at its founding, do not

*Presented for Dr. Wade by Dr. Frank Glenn at the Annual Meeting of The New York Academy of Medicine, January 5, 1967.

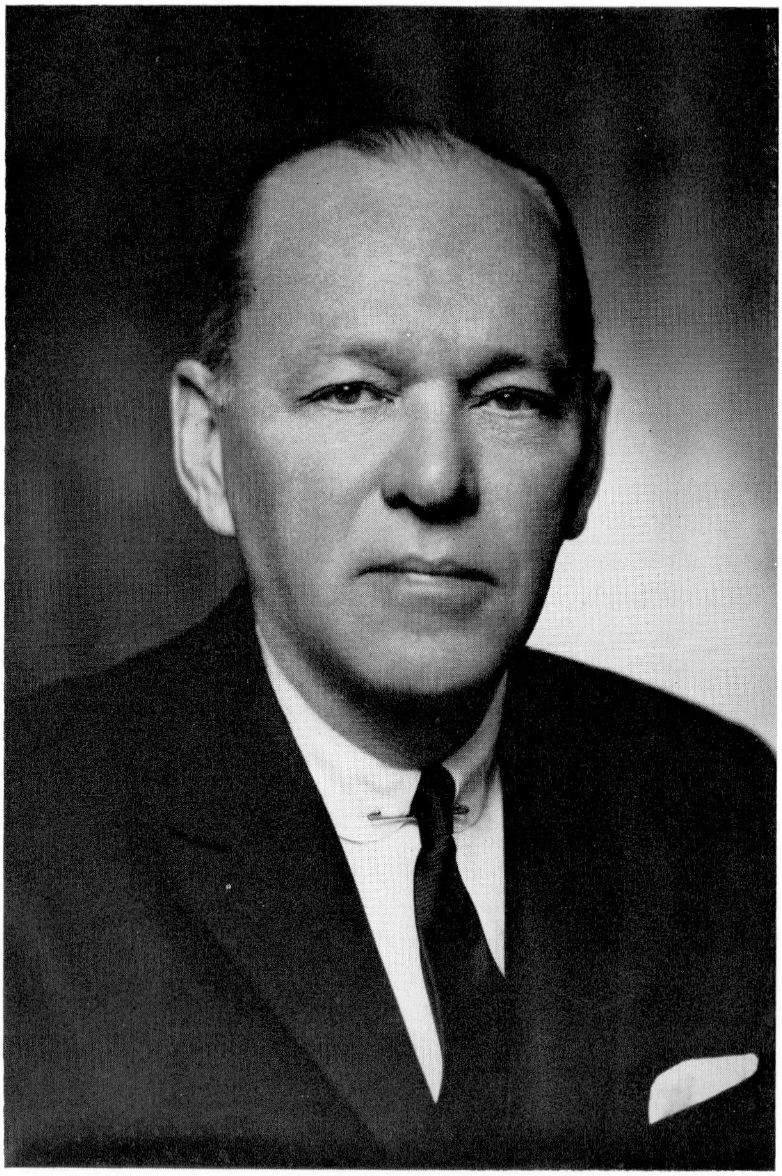

PRESTON A. WADE

differ greatly from the objectives now current in our constitution. After reading the story of the dinner at which the organization was founded a cynic might smugly say the Academy seemed to have been conceived in ribaldry, but he would be forced to admit that the original objectives and ideals were sound, and that they have surely proved to be so over the past century and more.

Modern science has advanced in explosive fashion of late years, and medicine has developed so rapidly and has included in its development such marvelous technological advances that the entire medical field has changed. We sometimes worry that these advances will so change the doctor-patient relationship that the physician will be pictured as a scientific observer of facts compiled by computers fed by technicians who alone will have contact with the patient. Other problems worry us in medicine today, and many of these problems are said by some to be capable of wrecking medicine as we know it. Others feel that modern sociological changes will lower the quality of medical care. A glance at our history over the past 120 years will show us that medicine in the New York area in particular has weathered crises and troublesome times on many occasions, and we have still advanced. Each crisis has been considered the most serious ever affecting the profession at the time it has occurred. So, now, we shall surely weather the present threats to our profession, and The New York Academy of Medicine will, I am sure, take its place, as always, in the center of the scene and will contribute to the solution of the problems affecting the health of our community and of the nation.

I am sorry that I shall not be present at the presentation of the Academy Medal to our distinguished scientist, Dr. Donald D. Van Slyke, and I shall miss not being able to take part in the well-deserved tribute to Dr. Howard Reid Craig, who has meant so much to the Academy over so many years.

I should like to hear Mayor John V. Lindsay's address, for I know he has a great understanding and concern for the health problems of the city. We are most fortunate that the mayor is willing to devote his time on this occasion to give us his ideas about the improvement of medical facilities.

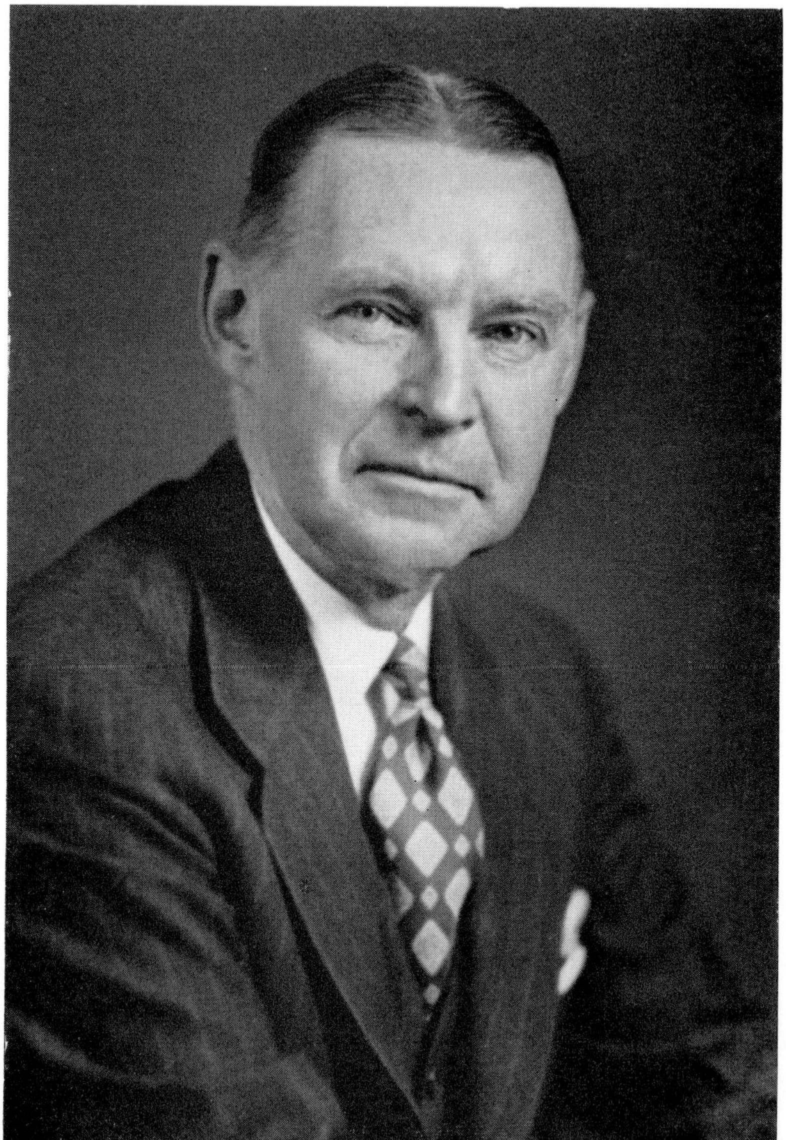

Howard Reid Craig, M.D.

# CITATION AND PRESENTATION* OF THE ACADEMY PLAQUE TO HOWARD REID CRAIG, M.D.

GEORGE BAEHR

Emeritus Director of Medicine
The Mount Sinai Hospital
New York, N.Y.

THIS YEAR the Academy will celebrate its 120th birthday. It reached its pinnacle of maturity during the last two decades under the leadership of our retiring director, Howard Reid Craig. I hesitate to think what could have happened at the Academy during this critical period in American medicine if the officers of the Academy had acted unwisely in the year 1946 and had chosen as our director someone less attuned to the rapidly changing world of public health, medical practice, and social welfare—someone less tactful and wise in handling the multifarious activities of the Academy's fellowship and its working committees. I hope I may be forgiven for harboring the thought that perhaps the Committee on Awards was guilty of an oversight in not awarding two plaques this year—one to Howard and another, in absentia, to the wise trustees of the Academy who selected him to be its director 20 years ago.

I can report that the Committee on Awards was unanimous and enthusiastic.

Presidents of the Academy come and go—usually after a term of 2 years. Occasionally one may be reelected for another term under some exceptional circumstances. Thereafter we politely vanish into academic obscurity, unless it is discovered that we can add, subtract, and multiply. In recognition of such talent we may be elected to a seat on the Board of Trustees—the guardian of the Academy's endowment fund and its budgetary expenditures. But policy decisions, as you know, are the responsibility of the Council of the Academy whose membership is composed of the chairmen of the standing committees

*Given at the Annual Meeting of The New York Academy of Medicine, January 5, 1967.

in addition to the officers elected by the general fellowship.

I tell you this so that all may realize that the role of the director is not merely administrative. Equally, or more important, is his role in the transmission and maintenance of policies and programs from one presidential administration to another.

The first full-time director of the Academy was Linsly R. Williams. He took office in January 1924 when we were still housed in the old building on West 43 Street, 3 years before we moved to our present site. Williams had formerly served as Deputy Commissioner of Health of New York State under the great Hermann M. Biggs, the first state health commissioner appointed by the governor under the public health laws of 1913, which he and Homer Folks wrote for the State Legislature in that year. As the Academy's first director, Linsly Williams expanded its public health activities through a newly established Committee on Public Health Relations. This committee was created by the Academy to take over the work of the health section of the Municipal Research Bureau, a voluntary agency for the improvement of public affairs on which Linsly Williams, Charles A. Dana, and James Alexander Miller had represented the Academy. After the Academy Committee on Public Health Relations was established, Dana and Miller served successively for many years as its chairmen and, later, Dana and Miller served as presidents of the Academy. During the past 40 years the important work of the Public Health Relations Committee has greatly enhanced the public image of the Academy as an institution
greatly enhanced the public image of the Academy as an institution
especially to our first director for these accomplishments.

Williams was succeeded as director in 1934 by John A. Hartwell, formerly professor of surgery at Cornell. He served as a most dynamic director of the Academy during the critical years after the Great Depression. He was drafted by the governor to be chairman of the medical section of the State's Emergency Relief Bureau. Under his influence a system of medical care for the indigent was adopted which was the forerunner of social legislation inaugurated since that time by federal, state, and local governments.

"Josh" Hartwell was followed in 1939 by Herbert B. Wilcox, formerly professor of pediatrics at the Babies' Hospital. He enlarged the Academy's interest in maternity and infant care and in medical education, and he promoted the growth of the library.

But in my experience of more than 50 years at the Academy, the most effective director of all was Howard Craig. He came to us in 1946 following a miraculous recovery from an illness which had incapacitated him temporarily for pediatric teaching at Babies' Hospital and for private practice. I believe it was "Bert" Wilcox who first called our attention to his availability and to his personal qualities, for which we shall be ever indebted to him.

Having had the privilege of serving as president of the Academy during the transition period (1945 to 1948), I recall the Howard Craig of that time as a modest, soft-spoken, and diffident young man (or so he seemed to me), who grew daily thereafter in stature and influence. We soon learned to recognize that his gentle demeanor was misleading, for behind it lies the strength, the wisdom, and the quiet determination of a statesman. Every department of the Academy has felt his ever watchful influence. The business management of the Academy was completely reorganized on a sound managerial basis under his direction. Our library has developed at a more rapid rate. New ventures in public service have had their roots in the Academy, such as the creation of a Community Blood Bank and the establishment of a Central Deposit Library to serve medical schools and research institutions throughout this part of the country. A Committee on Special Studies was established to reexamine objectively the relations of medicine to society in the tradition of the monumental studies conducted by the Academy in the years 1944 to 1947, which culminated in the publication of *Monograph Studies* by a special Committee on Medicine and the Changing Order. We are now face to face with the problems of medical education predicted by that Academy committee.

Behind these and many other developments in public affairs in which the Academy has participated during the last 20 years we can discern the unobtrusive guidance and the expertise of a skillful and diplomatic leader. As time moves on, even directorships must change. But we can take comfort in the assurance that Howard has agreed to be available hereafter as a consultant.

On behalf of the Academy fellowship, I have the honor to present this plaque to you, Howard Craig, in commemoration of your distinguished services to the Academy and, may I add, also as a symbol of our deep personal affection for you and for your wife Agnes, whom we all love and admire.

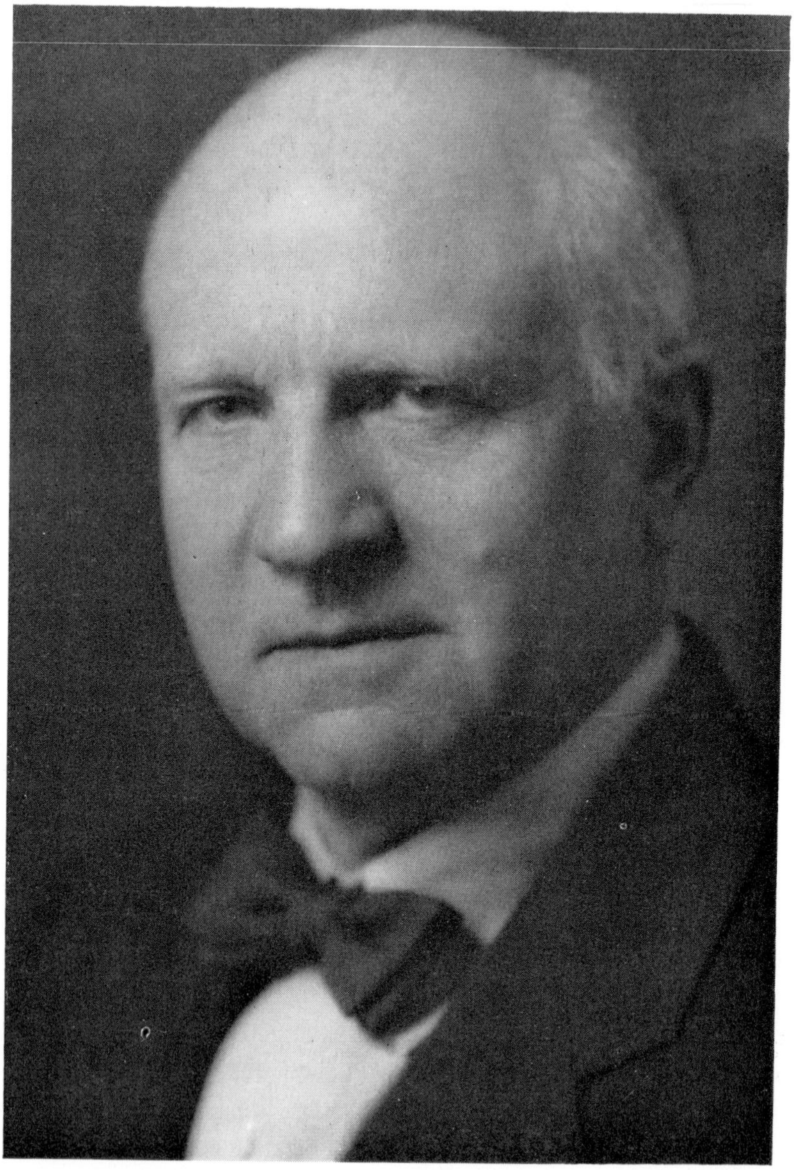

DONALD D. VAN SLYKE

# CITATION AND PRESENTATION* OF THE ACADEMY MEDAL TO DONALD D. VAN SLYKE

MICHAEL HEIDELBERGER

Emeritus Professor of Immunochemistry
Columbia University College of Physicians and Surgeons
Adjunct Professor of Pathology
New York University School of Medicine
New York, N.Y.

It is a great joy for me to give the citation in connection with the award of the Academy's medal for outstanding contributions to medical science to Dr. Donald D. Van Slyke. In the early 1920's, as a young, comparatively unknown organic chemist, I was sent by Dr. Simon Flexner, who was the organizer and Director of the Rockefeller Institute (now the Rockefeller University), from its laboratories to its hospital to learn enough biochemistry from Dr. Van Slyke to qualify for a position elsewhere. Learn biochemistry I did, first as a member of the Van Slyke-Hastings-Stadie-Neill team that studied the oxygen-binding and other properties of hemoglobin, then by absorption as I watched the Van Slyke blood-gas apparatus develop from a hand-shaken glass contraption into the beautiful precision machine it soon became, not only for the accurate measurement of the blood-gases, but also for amino nitrogen and many other vitally important determinations urgently needed in clinical medicine and in general chemical science. During those latter four years, in which I was really working with Dr. Oswald T. Avery, not once did Van, as we all affectionately called him, hint that he might have other and perhaps better uses for the considerable fraction of his none-too-large laboratory footage that I occupied. During this period Van also developed his quantitative theory of buffer action, and I shall never forget my consternation, tempered with flattered pleasure, when he brought around copies of the finished paper to us junior co-workers for constructive critical comment. It took me weeks to recover enough of my long-unused

*Given at the Annual Meeting of The New York Academy of Medicine, January 5, 1967.

calculus to follow through intelligently to the end.

Donald Dexter Van Slyke was born in Pike, N. Y., in 1883. Christening with double letters seems to have been a family habit, for Van's father was Lucius L. Van Slyke, an amiable, bewhiskered gentleman who was head of the Experiment Station at Geneva, N. Y., and who obviously took great pride in his son on his visits to the Rockefeller Institute, where Van had become chemist to the Hospital in 1913. Although trained as an organic chemist, with finishing touches on amino acids under Emil Fischer in Berlin, Van soon became an excellent clinician. For this I have the word of Dr. Edgar Stillman, who was for many years on another of Van's teams studying kidney function, metabolic diseases, and connective tissues. Since 1948, when he became an emeritus member of the Rockefeller Institute, Van has been senior scientist and guest investigator at the Brookhaven Laboratories and has been in charge of clinical chemistry in its large hospital as well. In his spare time from these duties he is writing a book on the manometric methods he did so much to develop.

Van, of course, has been the recipient of numerous awards, honorary degrees, presidencies of scientific societies, and honorary memberships in foreign academies and societies. I shall not bore you with the long list, which you will find in *Who's Who* and in *American Men of Science*, but shall single out only two which, I hope, gave Van as much joy and pleasure and stimulation as they did those of us who also had the privilege of participating in these events:

One example was the Honorary Presidency of the International Congress of Clinical Chemistry in Stockholm in 1957, at which biochemists from all over the world did honor to him, and the other was the *Symposium on Chemistry in Medicine* held at Brookhaven, N. Y., in 1963 on the occasion of Van's 80th birthday, at which his patience and endurance put to shame many of his younger colleagues.

And now we happily and affectionately add one more honor to the long list: namely, the Academy's medal, with the hope that your "outstanding contributions to medical" and biological science will continue well into the next decade of your rich and busy life.

# GOVERNMENT AND COMMUNITY HEALTH

*The Anniversary Discourse**

THE HONORABLE JOHN V. LINDSAY

Mayor of the City of New York

I AM deeply conscious of the honor that you do me on this occasion. I am a layman in your eyes—a lawyer and a government official. Yet you have invited me to address a meeting that for you is one of the great occasions of the year, and you constitute one of the most distinguished medical assemblages in our city. I approach my task with a mixture of humility and pride—pride that you have asked me to be here; humility before the vast problems you have asked me to discuss.

When Dr. Howard Reid Craig took time from his many duties at the end of last year to brief me on the nature of this gathering, he asked me to talk, not primarily about the immediate issues facing us in City Health Services, but on a wider theme. I shall try to comply.

First, however, I wish to say a few words about three people, two institutions, and a single issue that is, for all of us in New York City, an immediate one.

As a postscript to the tributes already paid here to Dr. Craig I wish to pay my respects, on behalf of the people of the city of New York—as you, Dr. George Baehr, already have done on behalf of The New York Academy of Medicine—to a great human being who has served us all so well for so long, whose theoretical "retirement" begins today.

Dr. Craig, I am grateful, as so many of my predecessors have been, for your wise guidance. I know that the many services you have rendered to the city over the years will not terminate with your official retirement. Indeed, I made sure of their continuation by asking you to serve as chairman of the Medical Advisory Committee to my Commission on the Delivery of Personal Health Services.

We in the city are grateful for the willingness and enthusiasm with which you took on this vital and challenging job. None of us envies

*Presented at the Annual Meeting of The New York Academy of Medicine, January 5, 1967.

Dr. James E. McCormack as he succeeds you—but to him we all extend good wishes as he does so.

The honor conferred on this occasion on Dr. Donald D. Van Slyke, one of the finest of medical scientists, increases the sense of humility I feel in appearing before you. At the same time it enables me to join you in doing honor to the important facet of medicine he represents.

Although I am here tonight to discuss with you aspects of the application of medical knowledge to the community at large, I am deeply cognizant of the vital contributions of both basic and clinical research. Without the scientific work of men such as yourself, Dr. Van Slyke, there would be no health services to administer, for governments to finance or plan, or for us patients to come to for treatment.

The third individual whom I wish to single out lacks the lifetime of clinical experience that you, Dr. Craig, had before you became executive head of this great institution. The man I have in mind does not pretend to the scientific bent or stature of yourself, Dr. Van Slyke.

He is, however, a Fellow of this Academy, where he has spent rewarding hours at your meetings, in the exemplary library you maintain, and in service on your working committees. He is a relatively young man of courage, imagination, and vision, and he has a humane determination to bring the best in health services to the people of this city.

He is Dr. Howard J. Brown, Health Services Administrator of the City of New York, and I appreciate the sense of public service that moved him to accept the great challenge I asked him to face last June. I am grateful for the decisiveness and tenacity with which he has moved forward, with innovation and yet with respect for the retention of all that is worthwhile, in tackling the almost superhuman problems that have confronted him.

The two institutions I want to talk about are, of course, the Health Services Administration of the City of New York and The New York Academy of Medicine. Although one is new and the other is established, they have much in common.

The Academy, as I see it, tries to encompass the whole of medicine and health. You have a great library, one of the greatest in the world. You have committees on public health and on special studies. You concern yourselves with the latest advances in methods of delivering health services, as evidenced by the great work of your Committee on Medicine in the Changing Order in the 1940's and the Committee on Social Policy for Health Care in the 1960's.

You are as active in the clinical as in the scientific and social aspects of medicine. You have groups at work in mental health and in public health. Your staff has medical men and lay administrators working in close collaboration with private practitioners, with organized medicine, with voluntary hospitals–with government departments, with medical schools, and with health insurance plans.

You view medicine as a comprehensive social activity directed to the benefit of man, independent of party faction and above public controversy.

The city's goals in moving toward the creation of a Health Services Administration are not entirely dissimilar. Our hope has been, and I believe that it can be realized, to achieve functional coordination of the several separate agencies responsible for the over-all health and medical problems of the city. We must build a capability in the public sector with which to attack those problems in a unified and effective manner.

In doing so, we can learn much from this Academy, which–as Dr. Craig has so often said–has a clear wish to help all those who have common health plans. I ask you on behalf of this young administration to help us–and I thank you for the help already given for so long a time to programs formulated to improve the health of the people of this city.

At the outset of my talk, I said that I should mention three individuals, two institutions, and one immediate issue. That issue, familiar to all of you, is the implementation of the Medicaid Program in New York City.

Medicaid and its predecessor, Medicare, may represent to later generations the most significant, progressive, conscientious social legislation enacted by Congress during the mid-part of this century. Medicaid offers enormous opportunities to the private and public sectors of our city's health structure. Unfortunately, the Act also presents enormous administrative headaches–not in New York alone, but in every city in the country. The cause of the trouble has been that Congress failed to recognize the consequences of the varying and complex eligibility requirements it wrote into the law. The result of that failure in New York City is that registrations for the Medicaid program have fallen well behind our original expectations.

As many as 4 million New Yorkers are eligible to participate eventually in Medicaid. But only about 720,000 persons have been registered here since the legislation was signed last May 1, and 600,000 of them are welfare recipients whose enrollment was virtually automatic.

We are processing additional applications covering about 60,000 persons, and we expect to have enrolled a total of between 1.5 and 2 million persons by October 1, the end of our year-long preregistration campaign.

The figures, nonetheless, are somewhat disappointing, for we had counted heavily on Medicaid to relieve the city of many of the financial strains placed upon us by our continuing responsibility to provide health care to the needy. Until Medicaid, the city bore most of the burden of providing medical care to New York's indigent. The Medicaid program, however, grants us an average reimbursement of about 75 cents in state and federal funds for every dollar we spend in providing care for Medicaid registrants. We have expected to receive about $200 million in state and federal funds.

Our disappointment has several sources, most of them, as I have said, the result of unforeseen administrative problems. One difficulty is that many persons, chiefly in the lower income groups, ordinarily do not plan for their future health. As a result, they do not explore their eligibility for Medicaid assistance until they, or a member of the family, are taken ill.

Second, many New Yorkers have misconceptions about the program; they often do not understand that they can retain their resources and assets and still be eligible for Medicaid. For example, a family of four with an income of $6,000 a year can qualify even if it has $3,000 in savings. Also, ownership of a home and personal property does not disqualify an applicant for Medicaid if he meets the customary financial limitations.

Third, the application forms for Medicaid cards are entirely too complicated. A trained registrar needs almost an hour to make one out, and the applicant who is unfamiliar with government paperwork is likely to give up after an hour's effort. Since registrations began, about 123,000 applications have been distributed throughout the community and only 33,000 have been returned for processing—a clear indication of the complexity of the forms.

The Department of Welfare, which has a superlative administrator in Commissioner Mitchell I. Ginsberg, is charged with registering applicants for Medicaid. It has petitioned the New York State Board of Social Welfare for a simplification of the enrollment forms. We hope state authorities will agree that applications less demanding of the applicant will help us greatly in placing more eligibles on the Medicaid rolls, thus reducing the drain on the city's scarce reserves.

The department, in an enterprise conducted jointly with the new Human Resources Administration, is launching a community education campaign called a "Medicaid Alert." Its purpose is to reach into the neighborhoods for eligible families, rather than wait for them to come to us. During the alert, hundreds of antipoverty and welfare workers will call on families to explain Medicaid to them, to inform them how benefits can be obtained, and to help them register.

In summary, we are moving as rapidly as we can to establish enlightened Medicaid procedures as efficient, or more efficient, than those in any city. I am optimistic about our ability to create a model for other cities chiefly because the reorganization of city government begun last year equips us with the administrative framework to do so. Medicaid cuts across many social welfare services, including health, hospitals, welfare, and the antipoverty program. All, however, are now under the direction of two administrations—Human Resources and Health Services. I think we were very fortunate and—if I may say so—farsighted in laying the groundwork for a streamlined city administration at the same time that Medicaid became law.

In 1882 the English statesman, Lord Lytton, said: "Government is neither more nor less than the trustee and guardian of the collective interests of the state."

If one element of that collective interest surpasses all others in importance, it undoubtedly is the public health. It should be the very cornerstone of all government concern.

But it is increasingly difficult to disentangle the problems and responsibilities of health from the other facets of community need. Health is an all-pervading matter of concern reaching into every department of life. In so doing, it touches on every facet of government.

Government health departments have been, historically, the gatherers of unconsidered trifles, their growth being determined less by logic than by convenience. They have accumulated a variety of functions that were performed—often inadequately—by other medical services. But in recent years our society has invested its government, its trustee and guardian, with new responsibilities for health and with new financial powers to implement those responsibilities. At the same time that it has invested its government with these new powers, it has created, by thoughtless "internal combustion," vast new problems, problems unimaginable to preceding centuries, problems that our evolving medical structure and hierarchy has failed to solve. We in government must create a new vision of our role as guardian and trustee, so that we can cope with these demands and difficulties.

We also must find a new basis for cooperation with the medical profession so that the staggering battles that must be faced can be fought in unity and partnership.

This Academy already is on record with a series of trenchant statements on current issues that provide a framework within which I can discuss the topic of "Government and Community Health."

I believe your policy statement of July 1965 on the role of government tax funds in problems of health care is as cogent a summation as I have seen on the subject. I hope you will forgive me if I borrow rather freely from it tonight.

Your statement began by stating the belief of the Trustees and Council that:

> In the United States today a serious gap exists between the state of health of significant numbers of people and that state of health which would be attainable if the best of present-day medical knowledge were more universally available and more fully utilized by the people of this country.

The Academy went on to say:

> A major goal of our democratic society must be that all people have the assurance of an equal opportunity to obtain a high quality of comprehensive health care . . . the availability of health services, as a matter of human right, should be based on health need alone, not on a test of ability to pay.

The statements express a heritage of the people of the United States: that health, like education, must be accessible to all; that medical and hospital services, like schools and universities, must be matters of public concern. How is that concern to be expressed? Again, this

Academy has anticipated us. "The attainment of the goal of equal access to a high quality of comprehensive health care," it has said, "requires that governmental and voluntary agencies must work together."

Here, I believe, is the essence of our mutual responsibility: How can we best create and sustain a partnership between public and private effort, between government and voluntary services?

Both are concerned with identifying the reasons health services are not more universally available to people, and with taking whatever actions are necessary to make them available.

Government is well placed, perhaps better placed than the private sector to obtain the data on which to build objectives and goals from which needs and demands can be deduced. Its resources and its records, its ability to demand that standards of record-keeping be adhered to, its access to whole populations—all these make government the logical location of the over-all planning functions.

We must not forget that the public has placed its welfare, its health, its education, and its safety in the hands of its elected representatives. If health in this day and age is a right, no longer a charity, then the government, as the public's trustee and guardian, must always exercise vigilance and vision to see that that right is fully realized. Cooperation with the voluntary sector is the historic duty of government, but in the last analysis goverment exists to ensure that the health assets available shall be available to all, to ensure that priorities are fixed, and that gaps are filled.

In the words of Disraeli: "Power has only one duty, to secure the welfare of the people."

Government must set priorities on public expenditure. It must set standards for the health care services supplied throughout its own and other agencies, for here it fulfills its perpetual duty to protect the people. And government should provide most—but by no means all—of the financing. In this context, it seems to me that it is the federal government's financial resources, rather than the city's or the state's, on which we must rely. As the Academy's policy statement puts it:

> The varying fiscal capacities and efforts of the several states have resulted in an uneven and inadequate level of many of those health services that are required in the national interest. When the nation as a whole suffers from such varying levels of essential health

services, the resources of the federal government must be utilized for establishing and maintaining standards of service, as well as for an equitable basis of financing throughout the nation.

It seems clear to me that only official health agencies should be assigned responsibility for the administration of tax funds allotted to health purposes. Only such agencies can combine public responsibility and accountability and the other functions of public administration with the professional skills, concern, and consultation required for setting standards and for continuous evaluation of program quality and over-all effectiveness.

This rather heavy assignment of the various roles of government and of tax funds implies tremendously important planning, coordinating, and so-called "watch dog" roles for government. But it implies neither total government control of all health services, nor actual government operation of them. There is, in fact, only one "health system"; but there are different ways of operating different branches of it.

The great contribution of the United States to constitutional theory is that of "checks and balances." In many spheres of life, outside of the governing process itself, that approach has proved eminently workable. The Securities Exchange Commission works well, but it does not operate the Stock Exchange. The antitrust laws have not placed business in the United States in the hands of Washington, D.C. All children of certain ages must go to school, but not all schools are government-operated.

The successful provision of health care calls for systematization of health services—but not for governmentalization. Acceptable health care for all the people demands that patients have a say—directly and through their representative governments—in the services that they receive.

The charter of the World Health Organization, to which the United States is a signatory, stipulates that "Governments have a responsibility for the health of their peoples which can be fulfilled only by the provision of adequate health and social measures." The charter also says that "informed opinion and active cooperation on the part of the public are of the utmost importance in the improvement of the health of the people."

There is, too, a difference between what Wendell Berge called "the organization of medicine" and "the technology of medicine." The technology of medicine means "all those arts of diagnosis, therapeutics, surgery, radiology, dentistry and the like, which constitute the profession of medicine." The organization of medicine means "all the arrangements, social and economic, by which medical service is made available."

"It is idle," Berge says, "to dispute as to which is the more important; for there must be a medicine to practice, and there must be arrangements for bringing physician and patient together. It is no veiled mystery as to which is the more backward.

"In the advance of the art of medicine, the medical profession has done a brilliant job. In the face of this advance it is all the more tragic that progress in the organization of medicine has lagged, and because of this lag the nation has not had the full benefit of medicine's superlative performance."

I do not presume to advise you on the technology of medicine. But as a sometime patient, and as one who is responsible for one arm of government, I believe I am qualified to discuss the organization of medicine.

It is a measure of the stature of this Academy that many times it has invited a layman into its midst to comment on such matters. It is apparent that you have realized—ahead of many others—that in medical care, as in other fields, the practitioner is not necessarily the best organizer.

In industry there are, on the one hand, engineers of many kinds and, on the other, men concerned with administration, management, and distribution.

In medical care there are, on the one hand, practitioners, generalists, and specialists of all the healing arts and, on the other, those concerned with organization. The latter have studied it and have applied to it the same objective measures of scientific inquiry that the practitioner applies to his study of the patient. While those who are concerned with organization may be medically qualified, they may also be nonprofessional people.

This, of course, is a distinction that holds good in many fields of human endeavor. It is a distinction that is perhaps hardest for the practitioner to accept in those spheres in which the practitioner has functioned for a very long time as an isolated student of his craft. It appears that only within the last 100 years has science come of age in the technology of medicine. The practice of medicine depended so much on the individual for countless centuries that the advent of laboratory science was accepted only after acute dislocations.

The technology of medicine has outstripped not only its organization, but also the sciences that are basic to the technology of medicine: the physical and natural sciences; and these, in turn, have outstripped the sciences that are basic to organization: the social and behavioral sciences. Nevertheless, in the field of behavioral science great strides have been made in recent years.

Last May, at the centennial meeting of our city's Board of Health—the retention of which we have been so careful to ensure under recent reorganization plans—I said:

> This Administration recognizes its responsibility to join with its health officials in setting and meeting increasingly higher levels of standards in public health. The responsibility of Administration lies, I believe, in making possible more effective use of an always-limited resource, in providing improved relationships with related agencies, in encouraging the recruitment of outstanding persons, in improving the administrative process, and in providing the funds which make possible the vital work of public health.

But to meet all these duties requires today, and will require increasingly in the future, a new vision of what the challenges are.

Dr. Cecil Sheps has quoted Dr. John B. Grant as saying: "When setting up a program, set it up so that 20 years hence it will still be progressive."

We must face the fact that the next 25 years may produce developments in social health that will outstrip in radical change the developments of the last 100. Thus for a program conceived today to be progressive in 25 years, it must verge on the revolutionary. Any planning that we do must be broadly based and as capable of growth as possible.

This involves, of necessity, a rationalization of our present structure and a realignment of the apparatus we have inherited: one that has grown over the years more by the stress of necessity than the compulsion of logic.

It has been a privilege to have had your attention for so long, just as it has been for me an education and an inspiration to find in the work and in the words of The New York Academy of Medicine a striving for that same partnership between the professional and the public servant, between the public and private agencies, that I believe is a necessity. It is essential if we are to achieve the conquest of the gap between available knowledge and its effective application to the needs of men, if we are to achieve the goal of equal opportunity to obtain a high quality of health care, and if we are to approach the goal of health as a right for all the people.

# AMBULANCE SERVICE IN NEW YORK CITY*

REPORT BY THE
COMMITTEE ON PUBLIC HEALTH
THE NEW YORK ACADEMY OF MEDICINE

AMBULANCE service in New York City, which is said to be the forerunner of civil ambulance services throughout the world, was initiated in the decade following the Civil War. In 1869, Dr. Edward B. Dalton, in his capacity as Sanitary Superintendent, presented to the Metropolitan Board of Health a plan for ambulance service to be operated from Bellevue Hospital in the north, and from its Center Street branch in the south.

It was a novel idea for a city, according to Dr. E. H. L. Corwin, former Executive Secretary of the Committee on Public Health of The New York Academy of Medicine, who reviewed New York City's ambulance service for the United Hospital Fund in 1937.

The new plan went into operation in 1870. Five ambulances, built to Dr. Dalton's specifications and assigned to the two hospital units, answered 1,812 calls during the first year of operation. The example set by Bellevue Hospital and its branch was soon followed by other institutions in New York City and gradually the ambulance became a recognized part of the armamentarium of many hospitals. In 1873, ambulance service was established for the first time in Brooklyn.

With the multiplication of ambulances, the need for some kind of regulation became apparent in order to prevent unnecessary and sometimes competitive runs. The Police Department, acting without any special warrant of law, but simply because its officers were nearest the problem of handling street accidents, assumed authority. Districts were assigned to individual institutions but these could not be laid out in a satisfactory manner because of the clustering of hospitals in certain areas and the limited radius of horse-drawn vehicles. In Brooklyn and Queens, the authority was centered partly in the Police Department and partly in the Department of Health.

However, as the city grew and new institutions were founded, there were considerable shifts in the boundaries of the districts. In 1926 the Committee on Public Health became aware of the need to organize ambulance service in New York City on a more efficient basis. In the following year, the Committee issued a report which suggested that all the ambulance service in the city should be carried on by the Police Department.

From 1909 till 1929, when the Department of Hospitals was established, the operation of ambulances in the city was under the supervision of a Board of Ambulance Service. The president of the Board was the Commissioner of Police. With the creation of the Department of Hospitals—a development in which the Committee played an important part—the ambulance service in muni-

*Approved by the Committee on Public Health, January 23, 1967.

cipal hospitals was brought under the control of the Commissioner of Hospitals. The new Commissioner of Hospitals soon advanced a proposal to improve the ambulance service in the city. According to the Commissioner's plan, the Police Department would have charge of the city's ambulance service. This plan received the endorsement of The New York Academy of Medicine.

Under the plan, responsibility for the operation of emergency ambulance service was divided between the Police Department and the Division of Ambulance Service of the Department of Hospitals. The latter agency was to serve in a supervisory capacity while the dispatching of ambulances was to be handled through the lines of communication maintained by the Police Department in each borough.

In 1934 the Committee on Public Health made a special study of ambulance service at the request of the New York State Department of Social Welfare. The Committee found that the rules and regulations governing the ambulance service of all hospitals in New York City, as formulated by the Division of Ambulance Service of the Department of Hospitals, "are quite satisfactory and the enforcement of these rules should be supervised in a more systematic way than perhaps has been the practice in the past."

As regards the use of interns on the ambulance service, the Committee stated that "interns should be allowed to practice under the regulations of the hospitals in which they are serving."

But while the ambulance service in New York City was believed to be superior to that of other large cities in the country, it still left much to be desired.

The United Hospital Fund conducted a survey of the operation of the ambulance service in New York City in 1937. In the report of the survey were listed nine recommendations aimed at improving the situation.

By 1947 the Hospital Council of Greater New York had published its Master Plan for Hospitals and Related Facilities. As a supplement it issued in 1950 a lengthy report entitled *Emergency Ambulance Service in New York City.* For, it explained in its preface, "Emergency ambulance service is an integral part of any over-all plan for medical and hospital facilities and services."

Actual operation of the ambulances in the emergency ambulance service was the responsibility of the individual hospitals that buy the vehicles, maintain them, and hire the personnel to staff them, the Hospital Council report stated. It pointed out that ultimate control of the emergency ambulance service rests with the Commissioner of Hospitals, as represented by the Division of Ambulance Service. The division exercised general supervision, consisting largely of the issuance of minimum regulations, preparation and negotiation of contracts in the case of voluntary hospitals, development of reporting forms and compilation and publication of statistics.

The dispatching of ambulances rested with a single agency, the report continued. All calls from citizens, physicians, or policemen were routed to the telephone switchboards of the Police Department in each borough. In turn, the Police Department's Communications Division maintained direct lines of communication with the hospitals operating ambulance service.

It used to be customary for a hospital to notify the Police Department whenever an ambulance was under repair, the report said. Notification also was required when an ambulance was "taken off service for repairs, lack of chauffeur or attendant, or for any duty not a part of the emergency service." But in 1950 a new regulation was instituted to provide that the Police Department be informed of every departure from and return to the ambulance station. The purpose of the new provision was to reduce the number of calls that the hospitals were unable to answer.

In reply to the question: "Who should operate the emergency ambulance service?" the Hospital Council compared the advantages and disadvantages of three municipal agencies: the Department of Hospitals, the Fire Department, and the Police Department. It observed that the Police Department is uniquely qualified for the task of operating the emergency ambulance service.

The Police Department, the Hospital Council noted, is always the first authority to receive information, whether from citizens or policemen, about accidents or other emergencies. Moreover, the citizen is used to seeing the policeman on his beat or the police patrol car cruising about. In addition, members of the Police Department are experienced in making responsible judgments in the matter of eliciting information as to the nature of the illness or injury and the need for a physician to proceed to the scene of the call.

Concluding its report, the Hospital Council suggested that the following elements would add up to a good system of emergency ambulance service for New York City:

1) Centralized operation by a single municipal agency; this agency to buy, equip, maintain and repair vehicles, hire and direct staffs for all ambulances, and dispatch the vehicles as required.

2) A larger number of ambulance stations; there is no reason why hospitals should serve as ambulance stations.

3) Just as it is desirable to relieve hospitals of their emergency ambulance functions, it is equally desirable to interest them in rendering emergency medical care within hospital walls. Transportation service is not properly the mission of a hospital while medical care is.

4) Physicians to respond to emergency ambulance calls only when needed. It is possible to move a patient quickly to a place where he may receive medical care. Rapid communication gives the hospital advance notice of the patient's impending arrival, enabling it to prepare for prompt diagnosis and treatment. On the other hand, the medical care that can be given by ambulance physicians is of inferior caliber.

5) Adoption of a two-way radio hook-up. Such radio communication permits flexibility in the deployment of vehicles, contributes to the efficiency of operation, and facilitates action on requests for medical assistance at the same time that it reduces the number of such requests. However, the benefits of a two-way radio system cannot be fully realized under an emergency ambulance system that falls short of unitary administration.

Following consideration of the recommendations proposed by the Hospital Council in its publication *Emergency Ambulance Service in New York City,* the Committee on Public Health issued a report which was generally in agreement with the position of the Hospital Council. Furthermore, it expressed its willingness to cooperate in bringing about an improvement in the operation of the existing ambulance service. But an editorial appearing in the *New York Times* on November 1, 1952 indicated that little progress had been made in the two years subsequent to the report.

> Outrageous delays in getting ambulances to the scene of illness or accident, which occur from time to time in New York, can only be matched or surpassed by the length of time it has taken the city administration to come to grips with the question and make up its mind about remedies of jurisdiction. The problem was studied in 1950 by the Hospital Council of Greater New York. Then it was studied by the Hospital Department phase of the Mayor's Management Survey. Then it was studied by the Police Department phase of the Mayor's Management Survey.
>
> First we get a bill in City Council to coordinate the whole ambulance service for city and voluntary hospitals within the Police Department. Then we get another bill to coordinate within the Hospital Department. . . .

This state of delay was further confirmed by an article appearing in the same paper on December 14, 1952:

> A plan to centralize emergency ambulance service in New York under one municipal agency appears no closer to adoption today than when it was proposed two years ago by the Hospital Council of Greater New York.
>
> Emergency ambulances are operated by municipal and voluntary hospitals, are dispatched by the Police Department and are under the general supervision of the Department of Hospitals.
>
> Under the Hospital Council plan one department, Police or Fire or Hospitals, would undertake complete operation, including dispatching, maintenance and supervision.
>
> The principal obstacles to centralized operation are the large outlay involved and the unwillingness of city departments to assume responsibility for the service. . . .
>
> Authorities indicated that ambulance service was "adequate" at present, but the latest annual report of the Department of Hospitals noted a disturbing "trend." . . .

Despite the general tone of discouragement in the news item, there was one encouraging note:

> One suggestion of the Hospital Council has been adopted and is working well. Installation of two-way radio for emergency re-routing of ambulances while in transit, has been completed in Brooklyn, Richmond and the Bronx. . . .

In 1950, there were 45 hospitals—12 municipal and 33 voluntary—operating ambulances in the emergency service in New York City. Among them, the ambulances made 343,000 emergency calls during the year, with 53 per cent of the total handled by voluntary hospitals. By 1963, the annual total of emergency calls increased to 373,000 while the number of hospitals participating dropped to 39—15 municipal and 24 voluntary—by spring 1964.

A study of the situation by the Hospital Review and Planning Council, issued in 1964, showed that municipal hospitals were caring for more than 61 per cent of the total load—a reversal of the picture seen 14 years before.

This report outlined uniform minimal standards for the emergency rooms in hospitals as an important part of an emergency ambulance program.

On the heels of the report by the Hospital Review and Planning Council there appeared a series of articles about the local ambulance service in the now-defunct *New York Hearld Tribune.* The writer of the articles pointed out that among the most serious defects in the New York City system are the lack of trained attendants and the shortage of available vehicles.

An effort to improve the training of ambulance personnel was begun in September 1965. All personnel was scheduled to have American Red Cross Advanced First Aid certificates by December 31, 1966. But the training program is considered far from satisfactory by several observers, including Dr. Robert H. Kennedy, Director, Field Program of the Committee on Trauma of the American College of Surgeons. Dr. Kennedy has been studying emergency care throughout the country for the past six years. In his opinion, the training program in New York City does not go far enough inasmuch as it fails to include the employees of voluntary hospitals who answer 40 per cent of the city's emergency calls.

"In fact," the writer of the *New York Herald Tribune* series states, "the voluntary hospitals are not under the direct control of any city official. The hospitals are paid $35,000 to $40,000 a year for each ambulance they place on emergency duty."

A further complication surrounding the problem of coverage stems from the fact that some voluntary hospitals in strategic locations refuse to run ambulances or even to take emergency cases carried by city ambulances. Some of the 83 voluntary hospitals would like to accept ambulance cases but their emergency facilities are considered inadequate.

Then there is the matter of the number of ambulance stations—six fewer in 1965 than in 1950, when a study commission recommended doubling the number. This forces some hospitals to cover huge districts. For example, Kings County, the city's largest hospital, runs ambulances eight miles through one of the city's most crowded areas.

Another problem is the "sick" calls. Every day and all day, New Yorkers with minor or imaginary illnesses call police to get an ambulance. The service is free and it ties up ambulances that might serve a more important use somewhere else in the city.

Many of the shortcomings of the system are counterbalanced by the work of the Police Department, it has been shown. All city policemen are required to have at least 16 hours of first-aid training and members of the Emergency Service Division receive intensive training every year.

The 26 emergency service station wagons patrolling the city 24 hours a day often can reach emergency victims within a few minutes with the equipment and trained men that could mean the difference between life and death.

In the concluding article of the three-part series, the *Herald Tribune* writer suggests that the basic elements of an improved ambulance system are already in use in other cities or have been recommended for New York by city officials and medical experts.

"Under the proposed system, the city would have thousands of ambulances instead of the present 110." The new ambulances would be specially designed police cars, manned by policemen. "Each patrol ambulance would carry equipment that could save as many as 8,000 lives a year in New York City."

However, the new system would eliminate one service that New York City, unlike almost all other cities, provides at the present time. They could no longer transport "sick" cases; they would be used only for emergencies. Transport of patients between hospitals would continue to be the responsibility of the hospitals.

The final article ventures the prediction: ". . . abolishing the traditional New York system would almost certainly meet with vehement opposition, despite its multitude of faults." Listed among the probable objectors were the voluntary hospitals that now run ambulances, and unions representing the present drivers and attendants.

Some reforms have been made in the ambulance system since Mr. David C. Dimendberg became director of the service for the Department of Hospitals. But, he concedes, the reforms are only a "patch-up" job. The major weaknesses are built in. There are not enough ambulance stations to provide reasonably quick service and authority is divided so that no official can order mandatory training for all attendants.

Additionally, the service has failed to keep pace with advances in medical science. An official of the National Resuscitation Association has estimated that approximately 8,000 new victims of heart attacks, choking, windpipe obstructions, drownings, and poisoning might be saved if they received oxygen within 4 minutes.

In 1964, according to a spokesman for the Department of Hospitals, the ambulance service answered 394,719 calls but 176,936 were clearly not emergencies. There were 89,430 transfers, 42,187 unnecessary calls, 16,722 dead when the ambulance was called, 19,668 not removed and 9,029 return home trips for patients who had walked into hospitals.

The remaining 217,783 calls, which might have been emergencies, included all sick calls. The drivers of ambulances say that sick calls make up the majority of their calls. Only 80,954 cases were serious enough to require admitting anyone to a hospital.

## Summary of Situation

To sum up the existing situation, the principal complaint is over inordinate delays in the emergency service. In addition, in the opinion of experts in ambulance service, the level of skill and competence of the attendants should be raised in order to become adequate and satisfactory.

The reasons for the shortcomings in the ambulance service are not difficult to fathom:

1) The ambulance service is too frequently diverted from its primary emergency function by unrelated calls. At the present time every call for an ambulance is answered without question. Too often the ambulance service is abused as free transportation for the most trivial reason: to rush an actress to a theater, to answer a call for toothache, or to spare a citizen from losing his parking space in front of his house. While the ambulance is on this capricious errand, it cannot respond to a true emergency. Unjustifiable and unnecessary calls are costly and time-consuming and thereby waste the time and funds of the ambulance service.

2) Another source of diversion of ambulances from their primary emergency function is the use of transfer of patients between hospitals. While the ambulances are engaged in transfer, they are not available for emergencies. These two uses of ambulances—emergency and transfer—are separate and unrelated. But use in transfer may interfere with answering emergency calls. The use of ambulances for transfer of patients as well as for emergency calls tends to create confusion and delay and leads to impairment of the system.

3) Lack of a means of intercommunication between dispatcher, ambulance,

and hospitals allows no flexibility that might overcome some delays, expedite movement, and generally shorten the time in transit. Police cars and taxicabs have demonstrated the effectiveness of intercommunication for quick deployment.

4) Geographically the ambulance stations are not now well distributed for coverage of emergencies. The hospital-based ambulance service is not well adapted for city-wide coverage. Hospitals are not located in relation to the need for ambulances. As might be expected, those using the most ambulance service are most removed from hospitals. Long running time increases the delay.

5) Hospitals are not equally equipped for emergency service. Some are not prepared to handle all types of emergencies.

Not unrelated to this inadequacy are those occasions when hospitals refuse to accept an ambulance delivery. In some instances refusal may arise from lack of a proper emergency service.

6) The central authority now in the Department of Hospitals does not in reality have the complete and firm force and power necessary for meeting its responsibility. The 28 hospitals operating ambulances each have a voice in the management of the ambulance service along with the Department of Hospitals and the Police Department. Under the contracts presently in force, the city does not pay to the voluntary hospitals the full cost of their operating ambulances. Under the existing arrangement and circumstances, it is difficult for the administrator to exercise full control, apply necessary pressures, and bring about desirable changes.

7) Ambulance drivers and attendants generally are poorly trained. Even before that, the low salaries offered do not attract a high caliber personnel. In city hospitals drivers are paid from $99 to $125 per week. Attendants receive from $79 to $100 per week. Improvement of salaries is complicated by differences between civil service and non-civil service status as well as by wage schedules for comparable positions in other departments of the city government.

Despite efforts to improve the situation by training programs, these are neither systematic nor extensive enough to be complete in their effect.

Finally, there is the question: Who should run the ambulance service? There are obvious reasons for placing ambulance service under hospital administration. The hospital is the ultimate destination of the patient. And the ambulances also are used for transfer of patients from hospital to hospital or hospital to home.

But just as obviously there are reasons for not placing administration of the ambulance service in the Department of Hospitals. Some of the reasons have just been enumerated in considering existing shortcomings. The location of hospitals is ill-adapted for ambulance stations. The divided use of ambulances for emergency and transfer presents problems. Under the present arrangement the Department of Hospitals has difficulty in operating full and complete authority. All these disadvantages must be weighed against the advantages.

Then too, there are strong arguments in favor of putting complete control of the emergency ambulance system under the Police Department. Police precincts provide better geographical districting for the service. The police already are doing everything except moving the patient to the hospital. The police are the first on the scene. They are equipped, in many instances, to handle emergencies. Furthermore, the nature of their organization requires them to use the hospital to obtain data for the full report regarding the patient. Finally, the policemen are highly intelligent, are already trained in first aid, and have the organization for providing additional training as needed systematically and completely.

It has been asserted that the Police Department is at present experiencing a shortage of manpower. If the Police Department was to assume authority and direction of the emergency ambulance service it might seem that manpower woud have to be taken into consideration. Yet in fact there need be little or no increase in the existing manpower to operate the emergency service since the drivers of the present patrol cars would assume the new functions in new vehicles. The only time taken out of their usual duties would be that necessary for retraining or continued training.

## Recommendations

Regardless of where the administration of ambulance service is placed, there are several changes that should be made. The Committee on Public Health makes these recommendations:

1) Emergency ambulance service should be restricted to true medical emergencies. There should be guidelines defining a true emergency call and the responsibility for decision should be on the citizen and not on the dispatcher. Where a person is not able to move or only with difficulty, is in severe pain or injured, cannot use his private car or taxicab, and cannot reach his doctor, the situation would be a true medical emergency. Cases of doubt should be resolved by answering the call.

If the citizen is just seeking medical attention he should direct his call to the County Medical Society Emergency Service. Furthermore, when Medicare and Medicaid are in full operation they should be of assistance in providing medical care. Finally, if the Bronx Medical Care Project to provide family physicians and storefront clinics proves practicable, it might be applied throughout the city.

2) An intercommunication system should be established between the dispatcher, ambulances and hospitals.

3) Hospitals should upgrade their emergency service.

For six years the Field Program of the Committee on Trauma of the American College of Surgeons has been trying to improve the care given in hospital emergency departments. For the last 4 years the U. S. Public Health Service has been making similar efforts. In 1966 the American Medical Association directed its attention to the movement.

The American College of Surgeons has formulated a set of standards for emergency departments in hospitals which has been reprinted by the Joint Commission on Accreditation of Hospitals. This trend of events indicates the need for improvement in emergency departments in hospitals.

Furthermore, there should be a central directory listing the status and capabilities of the emergency department of every hospital in New York City.

Every hospital should be required to accept all ambulance deliveries that it is qualified to handle. Upon refusal of acceptance a full explanation in writing should be filed.

4) It is the Committee's belief that the division of authority and separation of duties between the Hospital and the Police Departments is at the wrong

point. At present the police are responsible for dispatching and the Department of Hospitals for the rest of the operation. The Committee would point out that there is a natural division in the ambulance service according to the uses to which it is put: emergency or transfer. In the opinion of the Committee, these two operations should be kept separate.

5) As for location of ambulance stations and the use of trained personnel, these two conditions are linked closely with the selection of the department for the administration of the ambulance service. Solution of these two problems would depend largely on that decision.

6) The Committee has carefully considered all the arguments about who should be in charge of the ambulance service. After much deliberation it has concluded that the emergency service should be placed entirely under the Police Department while the transfer of patients should remain under the administration of the hospitals. On balance, there are real advantages in placing the Police Department in full control over the emergency service.

The department already has 26 emergency vehicles. Many of the existing ambulances in the city are of ancient vintage and should be modernized. If the police were in charge of the emergency service it would be possible for the patrol cars to be modified station wagons that would serve as ambulances. Hence, the change of vehicles to the modified patrol cars for purposes of ambulances, rather than replacement of the standard ambulances, would come at an appropriate time. Furthermore, it could be brought about in an orderly way since patrol cars are replaced at regular intervals.

The police could make the emergency ambulance service a special division of its department. Training of police for this division could be incorporated into the Police Academy.

The operation of the emergency ambulance service under the police would be on the basis of precinct which would enhance its effectiveness. There are areas of the city that are far removed from ambulance stations but are patrolled by the police. Therefore, the response would be more prompt and the running time much shorter under a system operated entirely by the police than under the present system of hospital-based stations even with outposts.

It is estimated that the additional time required by police for operating the emergency service would be offset to a large extent by the saving of time now wasted unavoidably by them. For example, recently three squad cars were kept 30 minutes handling traffic at the scene of an accident while awaiting the arrival of an ambulance. The police are usually first to arrive on the scene. If one of the police cars had had the responsibility and authority to remove the patient to an appropriate reception facility in this instance much of their time and effort would have been saved. Patrolling police cars equipped as ambulances with intercommunication could quickly respond to an emergency and carry out the entire mission.

By placing the emergency ambulance service completely under the Police Department, it is quite possible that the improvement in operation might be achieved without too high an additional cost. That improvement would come by ending delays in answering calls and by having more highly trained personnel in attendance. Not to be overlooked is the good will that would accrue for the Police Department as it was observed in the performance of its errand of aid and assistance.

Emergency ambulance service is already being successfully operated by the police in two cities: Cleveland, Ohio, and Louisville, Ky.

Quite a different function for the ambulance is the transfer of a patient from one hospital to another or, in case of discharge, to his home. These movements on order are part of the business of the hospital and naturally its responsibility. Hence, the Committee on Public Health would recommend that a hospital authority retain control and operation of an ambulance service for transfer and discharge.

It would probably be an unnecessarily expensive service for each hospital to maintain its own ambulances just for transfer. But the hospitals could join in operating a transfer ambulance service of suitable size.

For 30 years there have been complaints about the ambulance service in New York City and it has long been regarded as far from satisfactory. Over that period several surveys have not brought improvement. Action to better the service is long overdue. The Committee on Public Health strongly advocates that the city administration move without delay to remedy the situation. It is to be hoped that the points raised in this report will be carefully considered by the administration.

## SCURVY DURING MAGELLAN'S VOYAGE

THE story of Magellan's great deed is well known to inhabitants of the oblate spheroid that he circumnavigated. Born about 1480, Ferdinand Magellan participated in voyages to India, Africa, and the Indonesian archipelago between 1505 and 1510. The voyage for which he is chiefly remembered began at Seville, Spain, in August 1519. Included among his companions was Antonio Pigafetta, an Italian of Vicenza. The flotilla of five ships crossed the Atlantic, traversed the Straits of Magellan, and passed into the Pacific. In the Philippine Islands, in April 1521, Magellan was killed. In the summer of 1522 the one ship remaining of the original five reached Spain.

For the best extant record of the voyage we are indebted to Pigafetta, who is thought to have prepared his account at the request of Pope Clement VII. The original manuscript is believed to have been written in the Venetian variant of Italian, and a manuscript in that language is preserved at the famous Ambrosian Library in Milan.

The following excerpt has been translated from "*Il Primo Viaggio Intorno Al Mondo di Antonio Pigafetta*," edited by Camillo Manfroni, and published at Milan in 1928 (pp. 110-11).

> We had been three months and twenty days without taking refreshment of any kind. We ate biscuit which was no longer biscuit but powder with handfuls of maggots because these creatures had eaten the good part. It smelled strongly of rat urine. We drank water that was yellow and putrefied for many days, and we ate certain cowhides which were placed over the main yard so that the yard should not break the shrouds, hardened by sun, rain, and wind. We left the hides in the sea for four or five days. . . . Many times we ate sawdust. Rats were sold for half a ducat each, when we could get them.
>
> But above all other calamities this was the worst: in some men the gums grew over the teeth, both lowers and uppers, so that they could not eat in any way and thus they died of this sickness. Nineteen men died and also the [Patagonian] giant and an Indian from the land of Brazil. Twenty-five or thirty men became sick, some in the arms, in the legs or other places, so that few remained healthy. By the grace of God I had no sickness.

S. J.

## WILLIAM CLOWES CHIRURGIAN, to his louyng frend Iohn Banister.

THY noble skill in Surgerie (for so we call it heer,)
Thyne honest lyfe, and faythfull hart vnto thy countrey deer,
Well knowen to me (good Banister) thy poore and loyall frend,
I would I could in skilfull Verse so cunnyngly commend,
As well I know it well deserues both prayse and prayse agayne.
And sure I am that this thy toyle, and heere employed payne
For paynting out the frame of man, in this our mother toung,
Culd out of learned Latine workes, heerehence hath onely sprong
That thou thereby thy countrey men mighst further much in skill:
And geue them light that earst they lackt, as sure (I hope) it will.
Thou wrightst not for the learned sort (I know) that were but vayne,
But hopest to helpe the meaner folke. And so, I trust thy payne
Shall wynne such prayse of skillfull men, as paynfull toyle may craue,
And as a mynde that meaneth well of duety ought to haue.
If errour ought hath scapte thy penne, or paynter hapt to hault,
Let that no whit dismay thy mynde. None scapes deuoyd of fault.
Where skillfull men geue iust reproofe, with carefull payne amend it.
Regarde not much the rascall sort that blyndly reprehend it.
For as we know that men be men, and easely apt to stray:
So Enuyes Imps do bend them selues to sclander euery way.
My selfe of late haue tryed in that so small a worke of myne,
Wherein I sought no prayse to winne, nor get a name deuine,
But onely to content my frendes, whose earnest suyte to craue it,
I could in no wise satisfie, but so, as they might haue it.
Yet some I found with readyer tounges forthwith to reprehend it,
Then fraught with skill to frame the like, or ought perhaps to mend it.
But who so ready to controll, or fit to carpe, and clatter,
As he that hath the dymmest sight, and iudgement in the matter?
What if I did somewhat omit? What if the Print was lame?
What if I meant at leasure more to haue enlargd the same?
How euer it be, I neuer meant to please eche curious hed,
Syth who so toyles him selfe in that may bryng a foole to bed.
Wherfore my good and honest frend referre the whole successe
Of this, and all thy toyles to hym that will thy trauailes blesse.
And as thou hast by labours great, obteined a grounded skill,

(*Continued*)

And settled sight in Surgery, so I exhort thee still
By skillfull workes the fame of such a facultie to rayse,
Wherein we know most famous Clerkes haue, often, spent their dayes,
And trauailes great: in hope thereby immortall fame to winne,
Whose worthy workes do well bewray their paynfull toyle therein.
I speake not of the famous Greekes, and fathers of the Artes:
Nor Guidoes workes, nor Vigoes workes that write of other partes:
But of the whole Anathomie Vesalius passyng well.
Collumbus and Fallopius workes, how much they here excell.
Whose skilfull pennes haue paynted so ech part and peece of Man,
As none lookes now to better it, (I thinke) nor euer can.
Whose lastyng fame no age shall once be able to deface.
Among the which (good Banister) I wish to thee a place.
And so Adeiwe. And thou (good Reader) pardon I thee pray
My penne that in this homely ryme hath raungd to farre astray.
But three fold wayes enforst thereto. For zeale vnto my frend.
For wronges of myne. For my professed Art. And so I end.

———

From: Banester, John. *The Historie of Man*, London, 1578.

---

***Advance Announcement***

The May 1967 issue of the *Bulletin* will contain papers that were presented at the Fifth Annual Meeting of the

***CAREER SCIENTISTS OF THE HEALTH RESEARCH COUNCIL OF THE CITY OF NEW YORK***

held at the Academy December 5, 1966.

Dr. Howard J. Brown, Health Services Administrator, gave a talk on *The Impact of the New Legislation on Health Services,* and Mayor John V. Lindsay gave the closing address.

Also included in the issue will be abstracts of the scientific papers submitted to the meeting by the career scientists and their colleagues.

Reprints of the entire proceedings available from:

Health Research Council
125 Worth Street
New York, N. Y. 10013

Reprints of individual papers or abstracts may be obtained by writing to the respective authors.

*Advance Announcement*

## NEW YORK HEART ASSOCIATION

The June 1967 issue of the *Bulletin* will contain papers that were presented at the Association's Conference on

## POSSIBILITIES AND ACTUALITIES IN THE DELIVERY OF MEDICAL CARE

which was held November 21, 1966, at the Hotel Waldorf-Astoria.

Dr. Alfred P. Fishman, President of the New York Heart Association, was chairman of the conference.

### IMPACT OF MEDICARE AND MEDICAID

THE MUNICIPAL HOSPITALS
Howard J. Brown, M.D.
Health Services Administrator of the City of New York

THE VOLUNTARY HOSPITALS
Martin Cherkasky, M.D., Director, Montefiore Hospital and Medical Center

IMPACT OF MEDICARE ON MEDICAL EDUCATION
John H. Knowles, M.D., General Director, Massachusetts General Hospital

PROSPECTS OF FEDERAL PROGRAMS
John W. Cashman, M.D.
Chief, Division of Medical Care Administration, USPHS, Arlington, Va.

### OVERVIEW OF INTERNATIONAL TRENDS IN MEDICAL CARE

Stanley W. Olson, M.D., Baylor University College of Medicine, Houston, Texas

### ROLE OF REGIONAL MEDICAL PROGRAMS IN IMPROVING THE DELIVERY OF MEDICAL CARE

George James, M.D., Dean
Mount Sinai School of Medicine, New York, N. Y.

FEDERAL PROGRAMS
Robert Q. Marston, M.D., Associate Director
National Institutes of Health, Bethesda, Md.

THE NORTHWEST PROGRAM
John R. Hogness, M.D., Dean
University of Washington School of Medicine, Seattle, Wash.

THE CONNECTICUT PROGRAM
E. Richard Weinerman, M.D.
Yale University School of Medicine, New Haven, Conn.

THE NEW YORK CITY STORY
James E. McCormack, M.D., Director
The New York Academy of Medicine

Reprints of the entire group of the conference papers, as published in the Bulletin, will be available from: New York Heart Association, 10 Columbus Circle, New York, N. Y. 10019.

Reprints of individual papers presented may be obtained by writing to the respective authors.

**The 1967 Health Conference of The New York Academy of Medicine**

**Thursday and Friday, April 20 and 21**

# Planning for Community Health Services—Perspectives for Action

**APRIL 20 — 9:00 A.M.**

***Keynote Speech***

**THE COMPLEXITY OF THE TASK**

THOMAS MCKEOWN, M.D., Professor, Department of Social Medicine
The Medical School, Univ. of Birmingham, Edgbaston, Birmingham, England

*Commentary:*

RAY E. BROWN, Director, Graduate Program in Hospital Administration
Duke University, Durham, N. C.
LEWIS THOMAS, M.D., Dean, School of Medicine
New York University, New York, N. Y.

***First Panel***

**THE POTENTIAL OF PLANNING**

WILLIAM H. STEWART, M.D., Surgeon General, Public Health Service
U.S. Department of Health, Education, and Welfare, Washington, D.C.

**1:30 P.M. *Second Panel***

**THE PLANNING PROCESS: GOAL SETTING AND EVALUATION**

*Panel Chairman:* PAUL DENSEN, Deputy Administrator
Health Services Administration, New York, N. Y.

*Panel Participants*

AVEDIS DONABEDIAN, M.D., Professor of Public Health Economics
School of Public Health, University of Michigan, Ann Arbor, Mich.
WILLIAM GORHAM, Assistant Secretary for Program Coordination
U.S. Department of Health, Education, and Welfare, Washington, D.C.
BERNARD G. GREENBERG, Professor of Biostatistics
School of Public Health, University of North Carolina, Chapel Hill, N.C.
HERMAN HILLEBOE, M.D., Professor of Public Health and Administrative Medicine, School of Public Health and Administrative Medicine, Columbia University, New York, N. Y.

**6:00 P.M. *Banquet Address***

**THE URBAN CRISIS AND FEDERAL-STATE-LOCAL RELATIONS**

*Banquet Chairman:* BYARD WILLIAMS, M.D.

*(Continued)*

## The 1967 Health Conference of The New York Academy of Medicine

*(Continued)*

### APRIL 21 — 9:00 A.M.

***Third Panel***

**PLANNING FOR HEALTH CARE: PROBLEMS AND SOLUTIONS**

*Panel Chairman:* DONALD ELLIET, Chairman
City Planning Commission, New York, N. Y.

*Speaker:* LEONARD S. ROSENFELD, M.D., Director, Division of Medical Services
Hospital Review and Planning Council of Southern New York, Inc., New York, N. Y.

***Panel Participants***

JAMES CAVANAUGH, M.D., Director
Office of Comprehensive Health Planning and Development
Public Health Service
U.S. Department of Health, Education, and Welfare, Bethesda, Md.
JOHN J. HANLON, M.D., Public Health Director
Detroit and Wayne County, Detroit, Mich.
JERRY OSTERWEIL, Chief, Technical Programs Assistance Branch
National Institute of Mental Health, Chevy Chase, Md.
EDMUND PELLEGRINO, M.D., Director, Medical Center
Professor and Chairman, Department of Medicine
State University of New York, Stony Brook, N. Y.
HANS B. C. SPIEGEL, Assistant Professor, Department of Urban Planning
Columbia University, New York, N. Y.

**1:30 P.M.** ***Fourth Panel***

**NEW CONCEPTS IN PLANNING FOR MORE EFFECTIVE USE OF RESOURCES, MANPOWER AND FACILITIES: ALLOCATION OF CURRENT RESOURCES AND PLANNING FOR FUTURE REQUIREMENTS**

*Panel Chairman:* CECIL SHEPS, M.D., General Director
Beth Israel Medical Center, New York, N. Y.

*Speaker:* EUGENE A. STEAD, JR., M.D., Chairman, Department of Medicine
Duke University, Durham, N. C.

***Discussants:***

H. JACK GEIGER, M.D., Professor of Preventive Medicine
Tufts-New England Medical Center, Boston, Mass.
FRANK REISSMAN, Professor of Educational Sociology
New York University, New York, N. Y.

**3:00 P.M.** ***Conference Summary***

**NEW DIMENSIONS IN PLANNING FOR THE HEALTH SERVICES**

*Chairman:* MILTON TERRIS, M.D.
THOMAS MCKEOWN, M.D.

BULLETIN OF
THE NEW YORK ACADEMY
OF MEDICINE

VOL. 43, NO. 5 MAY 1967

# MANAGEMENT OF URETEROPELVIC OBSTRUCTION*

ORMOND S. CULP

Chief, Section of Urology
Mayo Clinic and Mayo Foundation
Rochester, Minn.

PROLIFIC literature on ureteropelvic obstruction, replete with platitudes, admonitions, innovations, and technical minutiae, has pointed up two irrefutable facts: 1) not all obstructions are amenable to the same type of operation, and 2) the ideal, foolproof technique for any type remains elusive.

From August 1950 to January 1966 my colleagues (Drs. J. H. DeWeerd, D. C. Utz, and P. P. Kelalis) and I performed 708 operations on 652 patients because of ureteropelvic obstruction. Our combined experiences have raised several pertinent questions regarding this clinical entity. These constitute the nucleus of this presentation. It is quite improbable that the same answers ever will be elicited from all urologists. Consequently it is hoped that our concepts and convictions will be provocative as well as informative.

Diagnosis of ureteropelvic obstruction usually is obvious during excretory or retrograde pyelographic studies, but *are urographic impressions dependable?* Some kidneys are able to cope with the reduced

*Presented at a combined meeting of the Section on Urology, The New York Academy of Medicine, with the New York Section of the American Urological Association, Inc., New York, N. Y., held at the Academy, March 30, 1966.

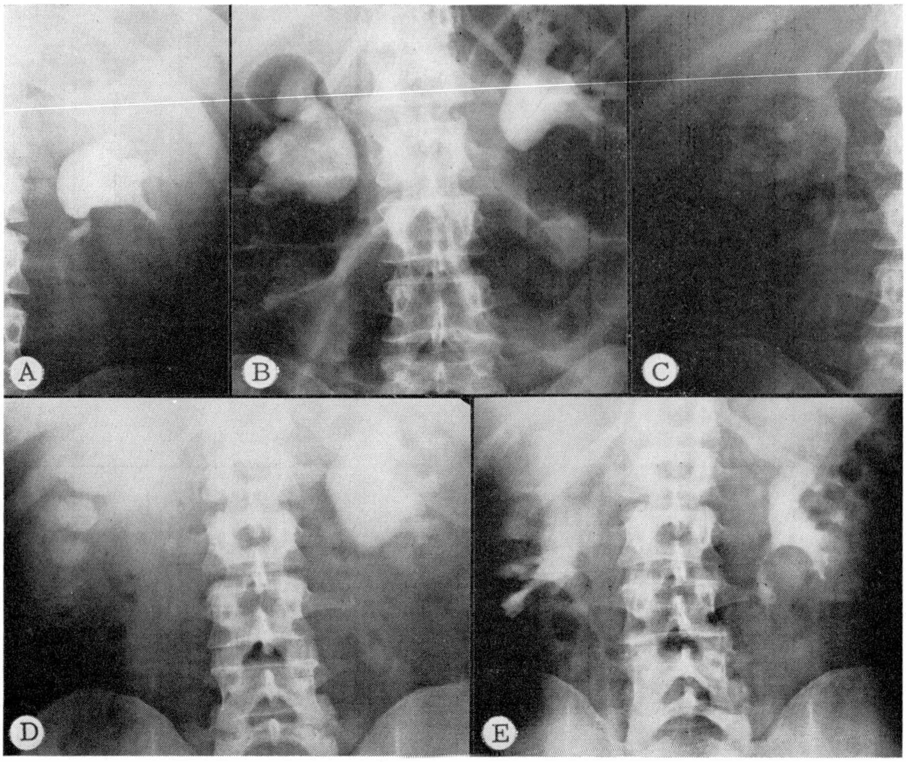


Fig. 1. Excretory urograms showing ureteropelvic obstruction. *A*) Solitary left kidney with pyelectasis only, which has not changed in 25 years. *B*) Bilateral pyelectasis but only right kidney symptomatic. *C*) Same patient as in *B* after successful repair of right ureteropelvic obstruction; left pyelectasis has not changed during 15 years. *D*) Both kidneys obstructed and symptomatic. *E*) Same patient as in *D*), showing postoperative changes. Left kidney was operated on 3 months after right pyeloplasty.

urinary volume that ensues during dehydration preparation for excretory urography and, therefore, appear relatively normal roentgenographically. The same kidneys may exhibit spectacular differences during diuresis. Both types of excretory urograms will be advisable when the nature of the patient's discomfort suggests renal origin.

Children with presumptive ureteropelvic obstruction warrant studies to exclude ureteral reflux. Frequently they have simulated stasis in the renal pelvis due to the decompensating column of regurgitated urine. Elimination of the reflux can result in dramatic reversion to a normal ureteropelvic transition.

It is best to have thorough knowledge regarding the *entire* ureter before formulating definitive therapy. The calculated risk of iatrogenic infections in these cases can be minimized if retrograde pyelographic studies are deferred until the patient is hospitalized and ready for operation during the same anesthetic period.

## When is Surgical Intervention Indicated?

When renal function is excellent and calyces are well preserved, and when the patient has no pain, pyuria, or calculi, it is foolhardy to tamper with the ureteropelvic region (Figure 1*A*). Yet, patients continue to be subjected to unpredictable operations solely because of pyelectasis and bizarre complaints.

Admittedly, renal pain can simulate a great variety of disorders, notably gastrointestinal disease. Evaluation of the discomfort can be extremely difficult. Relief by temporary indwelling-ureteral-catheter drainage is much more pathognomic than reproduction of the pain by retrograde pyelography. Too frequently the unstable victim is a fertile field for suggestion.

When in doubt, it will be prudent to "watch" the kidney with periodic urographic and urinary studies. Some obviously obstructed ones without cortical damage will never change.

An especially tempting situation is the case of bilateral obstruction in which the more advanced symptomatic side has been repaired successfully (Figures 1*B* and *C*). Despite an overwhelming desire to correct the quiet, incipient, contralateral ureteropelvic obstruction, it will be wise to wait and be sure that such measures are justified.

But this admonition to be cautious must not be misconstrued as endorsement of needless procrastination. When both kidneys are obstructed and symptomatic, both sources of obstruction must be eliminated (Figures 1*D* and *E*). Hopefully the delay between operations will not exceed 3 to 6 months.

## When Patient has Bilateral Obstruction, Should the More Advanced Side Always be Corrected First?

Table I summarizes treatment to date in 152 patients with bilateral ureteropelvic obstruction. More than half the nephrectomies in the group with unilateral pyeloplasty were performed elsewhere. Many of the 67 untreated contralateral kidneys will require some type of operation eventually, including selected nephrectomies. Of the 31 patients

TABLE I.—BILATERAL URETEROPELVIC OBSTRUCTION

| *Treatment* | | *Patients* |
|---|---|---|
| Bilateral pyeloplasty | | 17 |
| Both sides at Mayo Clinic | 13 | |
| One side done elsewhere | 4 | |
| Unilateral pyeloplasty | | 104 |
| Opposite side: Nephrectomy | 34 | |
| Nephrostomy | 3 | |
| Untreated | 67 | |
| Nephrectomy: other side untreated | | 31 |
| Total | | 152 (23%) |

with only nephrectomy to date, minimal pyelectasis predominates in the untreated kidneys. But it is imperative to follow these kidneys carefully because the degree of dilatation often progresses with the increased postoperative functional load.

Some obviously useless kidneys must be removed initially because of sepsis or pain. Others must be sacrificed because of trauma, neoplasm, debilitating symptoms, and a variety of diseases.

One must digress from comprehensive considerations to make a special plea for those patients who are operated on primarily to remove calculi. Too frequently the responsible ureteropelvic obstruction continues to be ignored. Secondary pyeloplasties can be disgustingly difficult, if not impossible.

## How Can One be Certain that the Ureteropelvic Juncture is Truly Competent?

Careful dissection may reveal high insertion of the ureter, localized constriction, a narrow ureter that tapers over a variable distance, or a long diminutive segment. But less than one third of the ureteropelvic obstructions in this series had demonstrable mechanical barriers. Calibration was deceiving and virtually useless. Many junctures accommodated large instruments but the pelves failed to empty promptly. Physiologic obstructions were more common than anatomic ones.

Some very sophisticated measures are being utilized for evaluation of the ureteropelvic juncture. Pressure gradients between the pelvis and the ureter have been especially illuminating. For practical purposes, any abrupt transition between pelvis and ureter indicates obstruction.

Table II.—PREVIOUS OPERATION(S) ON SAME KIDNEY

| Initial procedure | Total | Subsequent treatment Pyeloplasty | Nephrectomy |
|---|---|---|---|
| Pyeloplasty | 26 | 13 | 13 |
| Removal of calculi | 18 | 14 | 4 |
| Nephrostomy | 11 | 9 | 2 |
| Nephropexy | 5 | 3 | 2 |
| Division of vessels | 4 | 2 | 2 |
| Partial nephrectomy | 1 | 1 | 0 |
| Total | 65 | 42 (65%) | 23 (35%) |

When in doubt, simple distention of the pelvis with saline and observation of peristalsis and emptying ability usually will be diagnostic. Indeed, any time the ureteropelvic juncture can be identified, a pathologic state exists. Transition between the normal pelvis and ureter always is funnel-shaped.

The risk of unnecessary revision of the ureteropelvic juncture seems to be significantly less than the risk of difficulties inherent in secondary operations.

Table II summarizes experiences with 65 kidneys that had been operated on previously. Although 65 per cent were salvaged eventually, far too many earlier procedures were devoted solely to removal of calculi, nephropexy, or division of aberrant vessels. One patient with only two thirds of one kidney remaining still had untreated ureteropelvic obstruction.

## Does any Particular Type of Patient Predominate in a Large Series of Ureteropelvic Obstructions?

Ages of the patients varied from 10 days to 79 years (Table III). It is noteworthy that 50 per cent of the individuals were 40 years old or older when they were first seen. Twice as many males as females were operated on under the age of 20 years. Yet there was no significant difference in total sex distribution. Right and left kidneys were affected about equally.

When the 652 patients included in this study were first seen, their renal status varied tremendously. Some were azotemic; others had uncontrollable infection; some had mild symptoms but severe hydronephrosis; others had severe symptoms and mild hydronephrosis.

TABLE III.—AGE AND SEX

| *Years* | *Males* | *Females* | *Total* | % |
|---|---|---|---|---|
| <1 | 6 | 0 | 6 | 1 |
| 1-9 | 30 | 17 | 47 | 7 |
| 10-19 | 47 | 27 | 74 | 11 |
| 20-29 | 49 | 38 | 87 | 13 |
| 30-39 | 53 | 58 | 111 | 17 |
| 40-49 | 66 | 64 | 130 | 20 |
| 50-59 | 50 | 68 | 118 | 18 |
| 60-69 | 33 | 30 | 63 | 10 |
| 70-79 | 8 | 8 | 16 | 2 |
| Total | 342 | 310 | 652 | |

## How Does One Choose Between Nephrectomy, Nephrostomy, and Some Type of Pyeloplasty as the Initial Treatment of Choice?

Such decisions can be difficult. Many obvious factors and other less tangible ones must be weighed differently in comparable clinical situations. It is unlikely that the choice of operations can ever be based on arbitrary rules, rigid prerequisites, or didactic formulas.

Of all patients treated by pyeloplasty, 74 (19 per cent) had only one kidney capable of sustaining life, because the contralateral one had been removed in 23 cases, was functionless in 23, was diminutive in 11, and was congenitally absent in the remaining 17.

Extenuating circumstances left little or no therapeutic latitude in 30 per cent of the entire series. Many kidneys undoubtedly would have been sacrificed if there had been a reasonably normal-appearing one on the other side.

## What are Acceptable Indications for Primary Nephrectomy?

When one kidney is useless (Figure 2*A*) and the other appears normal, choosing nephrectomy entails no mental gymnastics. Hydronephrotic sacs in this series contained as much as 8,000 ml. of urine. When an unexpected neoplasm is encountered, as was true in five patients, the wisdom of nephrectomy is obvious if the other kidney is capable of sustaining life. If the kidney is studded with cortical abscesses, as in 10 instances in this series, nephrectomy is highly desirable. If unanticipated leukoplakia threatens to compromise the result and the

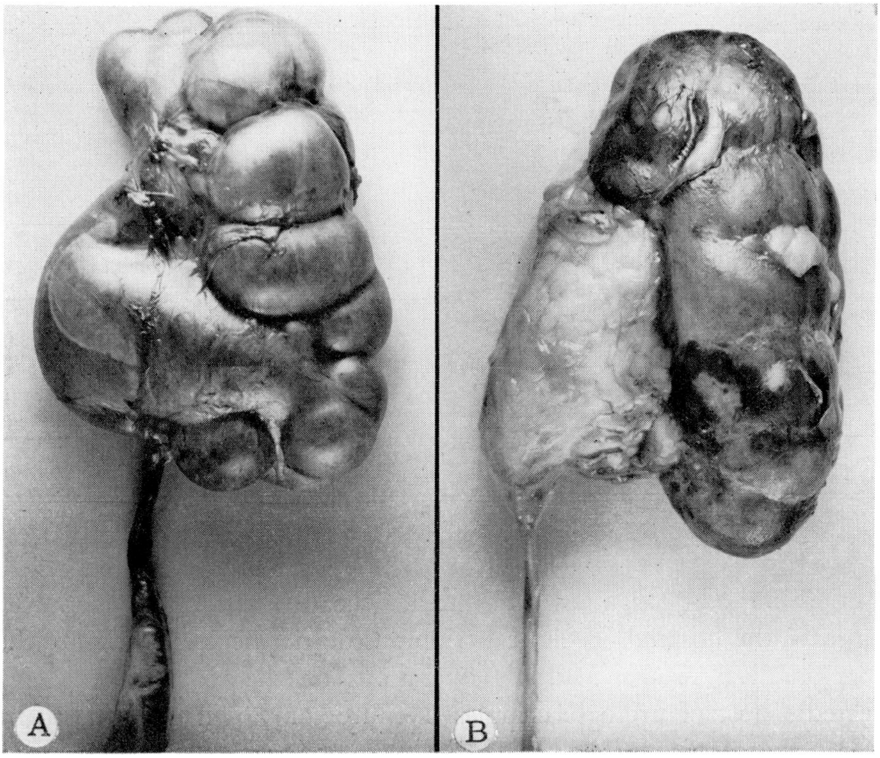


Fig. 2. Kidneys with ureteropelvic obstruction. *A*) Useless because of complete cortical destruction. *B*) Equivocal degree of hydronephrosis.

kidney is expendable, as in four cases, it should be removed. Other unique situations, including some bizarre anomalies, may point up nephrectomy as the procedure of choice despite reasonably good renal function.

When the benign hydronephrotic kidney seems to have equivocal value (Fig. 2*B*), therapeutic decisions can be truly soul-searching. There are no infallible indices of salvageability of kidneys. Saving patients will continue to be more important than saving a few extra nephrons. Two seldom-mentioned factors warrant serious consideration when there is a good contralateral kidney.

1) *Rehabilitation.* Too frequently surgeons forget that the patient should again be able to be a useful citizen. Executives do not have to face the same physical demands that confront laborers. The poor man's urinary tract should not be sold short because of his social or economic

TABLE IV.—PATIENTS WITH NORMAL OTHER KIDNEY

| *Age, years* | *Total* | *Treatment* *Pyeloplasty* *Patients* | *%* | *Nephrectomy* *Patients* | *%* |
|---|---|---|---|---|---|
| <1 | 1 | 0 | | 1 | |
| 1-9 | 28 | 16 | 79 | 12 | 58 |
| 10-29 | 113 | 63 | | 50 | |
| 30-49 | 175 | 93 | | 82 | |
| Total | 317 | 172 (54%) | | 145 (46%) | |
| 50-59 | 89 | 37 | | 52 | |
| 60-69 | 49 | 7 | 21 | 42 | 41 |
| 70-79 | 10 | 1 | | 9 | |
| Total | 148 | 45 (30%) | | 103 (70%) | |
| Grand Total | 465 | 217 (47%) | | 248 (53%) | |

position, but surgeons must look farther ahead than the day John Doe can leave the hospital. Technical triumphs do not necessarily assure the most practical results. Multiple operations on the same kidney have created a host of urologic cripples. Nephrectomy will continue to be prudent in many instances.

2) *Age.* Although chronologic age can be most deceiving, one should be reluctant to perform any type of pyeloplasty if the patient is more than 60 years of age. Indeed, doubts exist about the virtues of such procedures after the age of 50 if the other kidney has good function. Infections can be deep-seated and refractory, vascular lesions are common, results are unpredictable, and risks of secondary nephrectomy in the older age groups cannot be ignored.

Influence of age in this series is summarized in Table IV. Not all the 465 patients with grossly normal contralateral kidneys had the same functional potential in the obstructed one. Although pyeloplasties outnumbered nephrectomies in the entire series, more kidneys were removed than were saved in the unilateral group. In patients of 50 or more years there were more than twice as many nephrectomies as pyeloplasties. Seventy-nine per cent of the plastic procedures were on patients less than 50 years of age.

In the entire series, 313 kidneys were removed, including the secondary nephrectomies.

## What is the Legitimate Role of Preliminary Nephrostomy?

Attitudes regarding simple drainage of an obstructed kidney have changed. Unless the patient's general condition is truly precarious, it is wise to correct the obstruction during the primary operation. Usually this requires astonishingly little more operating time and it is unlikely that the surgeon will ever have a better opportunity to foster a good result.

There is one notable exception. Occasionally a kidney that cannot be sacrificed is so large that anatomic relationships are widely distorted. A plastic operation is not feasible until the entire renal mass shrinks and appropriate deployment of tissues can be made precisely. Even extensive resection of the dilated renal pelvis will not suffice in these situations.

Preliminary nephrostomy alone was employed for 14 kidneys in 10 patients. None of these seemed to be expendable at that time. Several pelves contained more than 1,000 ml. A few calculi were removed simultaneously. Blood-urea values ran as high as 339 mg./100 ml. In that particular case the value dropped to 48 within 8 months.

Plastic needles, customarily employed for parenteral administration of fluids, have been especially useful as nephrostomy tubes in infants, children, and young adults. They can be inserted under local anesthesia.

Of the 14 kidneys with preliminary nephrostomy drainage in this series, 10 have been salvaged by pyeloplasties that were performed from 1 week to 4 years later. Three patients with bilateral nephrostomies had such good results after pyeloplasty on the better kidney that the other one was removed. One patient awaits further treatment.

## What Type of Pyeloplasty Offers Best Results?

It is generally agreed that any acceptable pyeloplasty must provide: 1) dependent drainage, 2) good funneling, and 3) adequate caliber. Failure to fulfill all these prerequisites permits continued urinary stasis and compromises the result.

Furthermore, he who elects to treat ureteropelvic obstructions must be prepared to cope with five basic situations that pose dissimilar technical problems: 1) high insertion of the ureter on an extrarenal pelvis, 2) an obstructed juncture that already occupies a dependent position, 3) aberrant vessels or fibrous bands, 4) postoperative stenoses, and 5) "microureter." The last entails variable segments of diminutive ureter that may taper just below the ureteropelvic juncture or extend through-

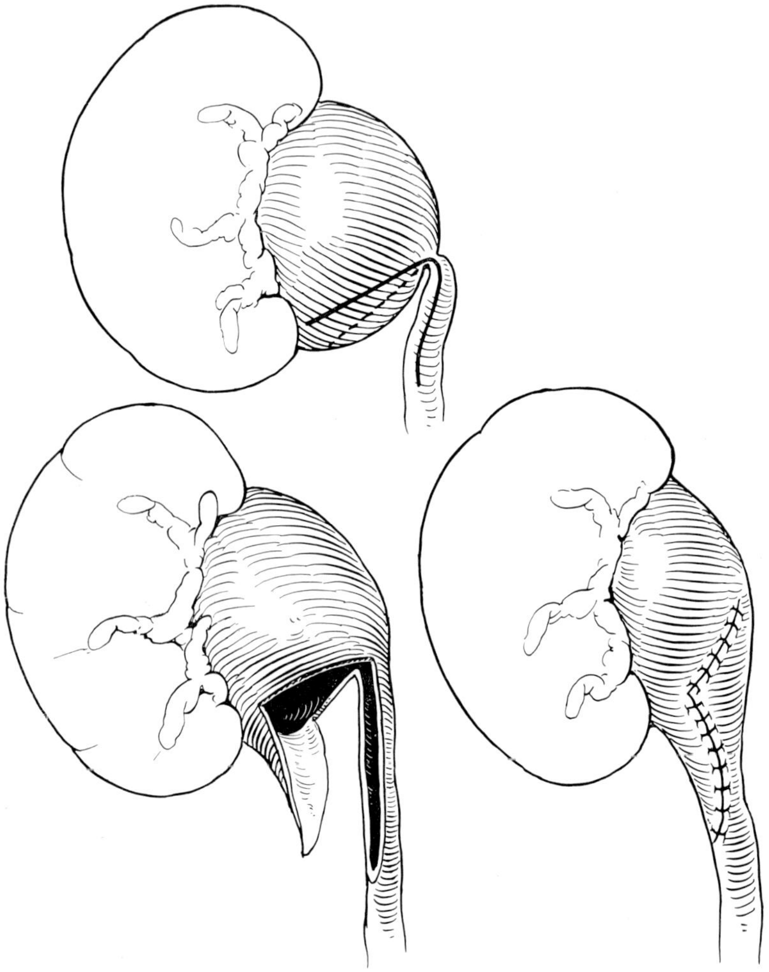

Fig. 3. Foley Y-plasty for high insertion of ureter. (Figures 3, 4, 5, 7, 9, and 10 are reproduced by permission of the Canadian Medical Association from Culp, O. S., "Choice of Operations for Ureteropelvic Obstruction: Review of 385 Cases," *Canad. J. Surg.* 4:157-65, 1961.)

out the lumbar region. To date, "microureters" seem to be normal structurally and are best described as "sending a boy to do a man's job." Additional anatomic and physiologic studies of these oddities are under way and will be reported later.

Choice of operations for these five categories offers as much individuality as the selection of a club for a particular shot on a favorite golf course. The wood or iron best suited to one man's ability may be

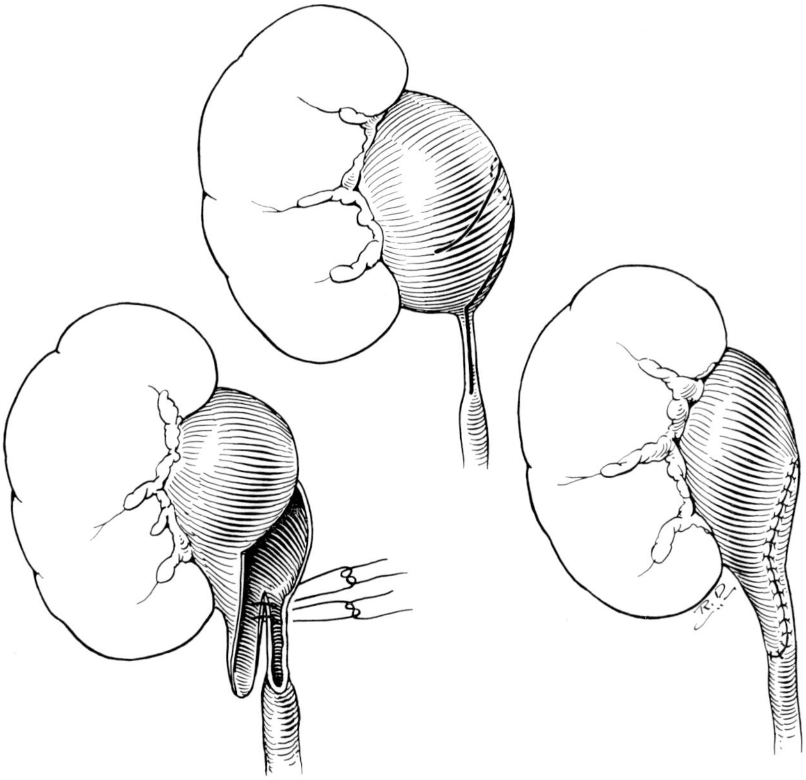

Fig. 4. Spiral-flap technique for dependent ureteropelvic obstruction.

inadequate for his partner. But even so, there are limits to this flexibility if one ever hopes to shoot par. Furthermore, the sharpest distinction between the amateurs and the professionals is the ability to "pitch from the rough to the green." It is axiomatic that any surgeon should utilize those techniques that serve him best, provided his results are comparable to those of others.

When the ureter has a high insertion on an enlarged extrarenal pelvis, the well-known Y-plasty has been preferred (Figure 3). The conversion of a Y-shaped incision to a V-type closure was not new, but Foley was the first to project this concept into a three-dimensional operation.

When performed properly the Y-plasty creates a V-flap that literally falls into its new position. Unfortunately, the Foley Y-plasty has been abused. Many surgeons have failed to appreciate its fundamental

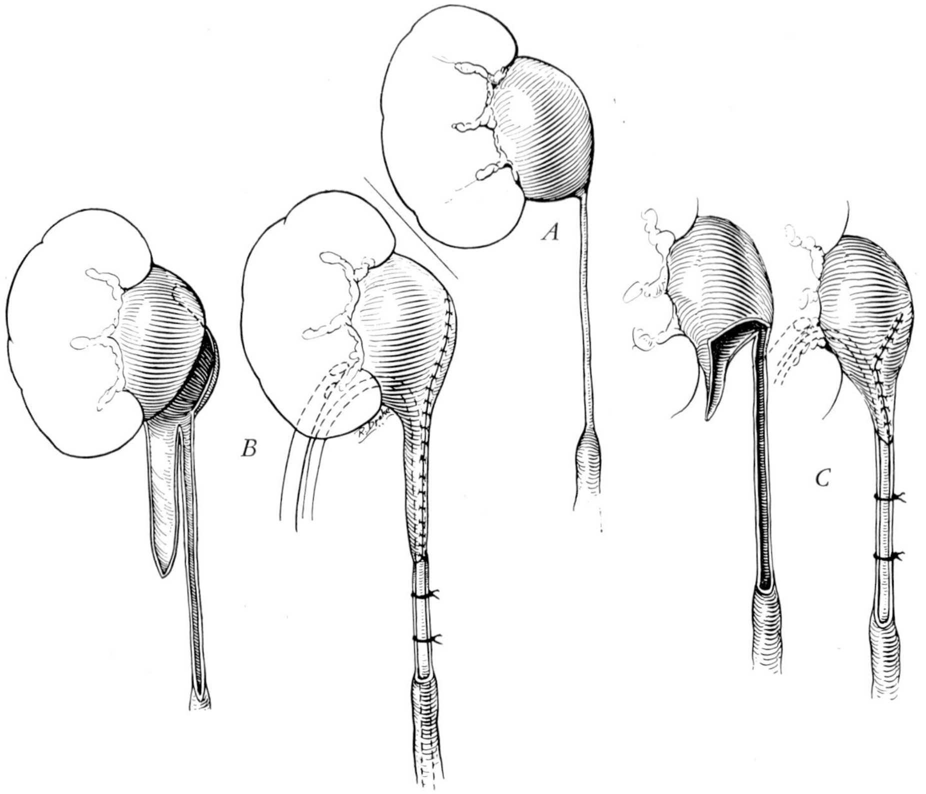


Fig. 5. *A*) Typical long stricture or "microureter." *B*) Intubation ureterotomy combined with spiral-flap procedure. *C*) Davis's operation combined with Y-plasty.

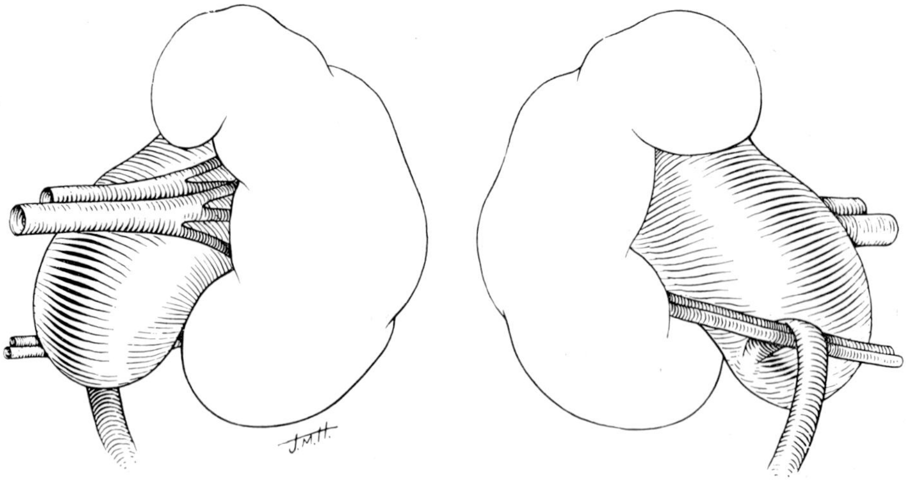


Fig. 6. Hydronephrosis aggravated by aberrant renal vessels.

mechanical principles. One limb of the Y must be on the *anterior* surface of the pelvis and the other on the *posterior* surface. Both limbs must be generous to create a truly dependent V-shaped flap. Dainty localized revision of the high insertion per se does not suffice. The tail or stem of the Y must be on the *lateral* aspect of the ureter and carried on to a point well below the lower limit of the extrarenal pelvis, regardless of the adequate caliber of the upper portion of the ureter.

Some enterprising surgeons have attempted to use the Y-plasty in situations that were not suitable for this type of repair. It must be remembered that the Y-plasty was designed for and should be confined to kidneys with high insertion of the ureter.

Many constricted ureteropelvic junctures already occupy a dependent position, as shown in Figure 4. The Y-plasty would create angulation or tension. Dissatisfaction with other plastic procedures in cases of this type prompted the evolution of the "spiral flap" that incorporates commendable features of the three-dimensional Foley operation.

The converging incisions have a broad base, are slightly longer than the ureteral constriction, and follow the spherical contour of the pelvis to avoid undesirable angulation at the base.

Scardino was thinking along the same lines when he proposed his vertical-flap operation. But the spiral method affords opportunities for longer flaps to bridge longer narrowings.

When performed properly the "spiral flap" operation likewise creates a new, dependent, funnel-shaped juncture free of tension. Many questions and even more doubts have been raised regarding the practical ratio between length and width of such flaps. Intensive studies were made of the blood supply of the renal pelvis and upper end of the ureter in both normal and hydronephrotic kidneys. A consistently rich anastomotic pattern of vessels was found in all cases. It is doubtful whether any exacting proportions are necessary when creating flaps of pelvic wall. I have employed some that were 10 to 15 cm. long with only 2-cm. bases and had no problems. Nevertheless, it is wise to avoid sharply pointed tips. Even an overlapping rounded end is preferable.

Some constrictions are far too long to be amenable to any type of revision of existing tissues (Figure 5*A*). The temptation to stretch a short flap must be avoided. Problems of this type have been managed best with Davis's intubated ureterotomy.

Intubation alone sometimes still leaves an abrupt transition from the

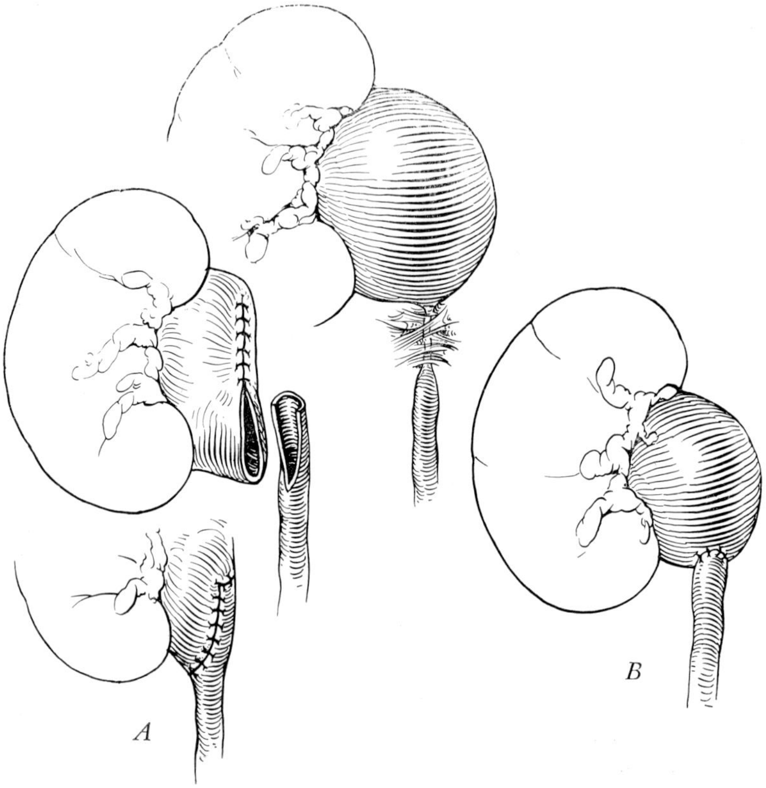


Fig. 7. *Inset,* Postoperative or inflammatory ureteropelvic obstruction. *A*) Reimplantation with spatulation of ureter. *B*) Simple approximation of ureter to dependent portion of pelvis.

pelvis to the ureter. To ensure adequate funneling, it is preferable to combine intubated ureterotomy with the spiral-flap procedure (Figure 5*B*) or with the Y-plasty (Figure 5*C*).

Admittedly, there are a few well-documented examples of ureteropelvic obstruction due entirely to aberrant vessels. But more commonly they aggravate rather than produce obstruction (Figure 6). The policy in this series has been to preserve anomalous blood supply. Two patients had only division of aberrant vessels. Both patients were relieved of pain but their renal pelves remained unchanged. In general, revision of the ureteropelvic juncture also will be advisable.

Frequently the ureteropelvic region is encased in scar tissue (Figure 7). If the pelvis and ureter can be freed sufficiently, one of the previously described techniques is preferred. But too often the entire fibrotic

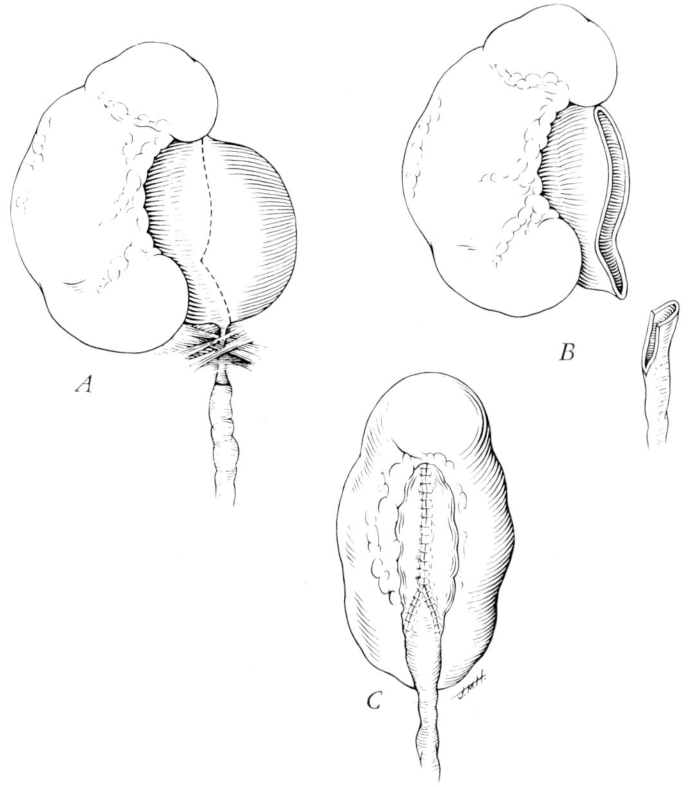


Fig. 8. Dismembered Y-plasty. *A*) Outline of portion to be excised. *B*) Configuration of remaining pelvis and spatulated end of ureter. *C*) Inverted Y-type of anastomosis.

mass must be excised. Reimplantation becomes imperative. The manner in which this is accomplished depends upon the amount of ureter that can be freed. Every effort should be made to create a funnel between pelvis and ureter. Simple approximation (Figure 7*B*) must be deplored because results have been atrociously poor. If pelvis and ureter can be freed for only short distances, simple spatulation (Fig. 7*A*) can create a satisfactory new transition.

There has been considerable championing of the dismembered Y-plasty (Figure 8), not only for cases of this type but also for *primary* revision of the ureteropelvic region. This technique requires a substantial amount of mobile pelvic and ureteral tissue.

Further cineradiographic studies should resolve conflicting views regarding the virtues of preserving ureteropelvic continuity.

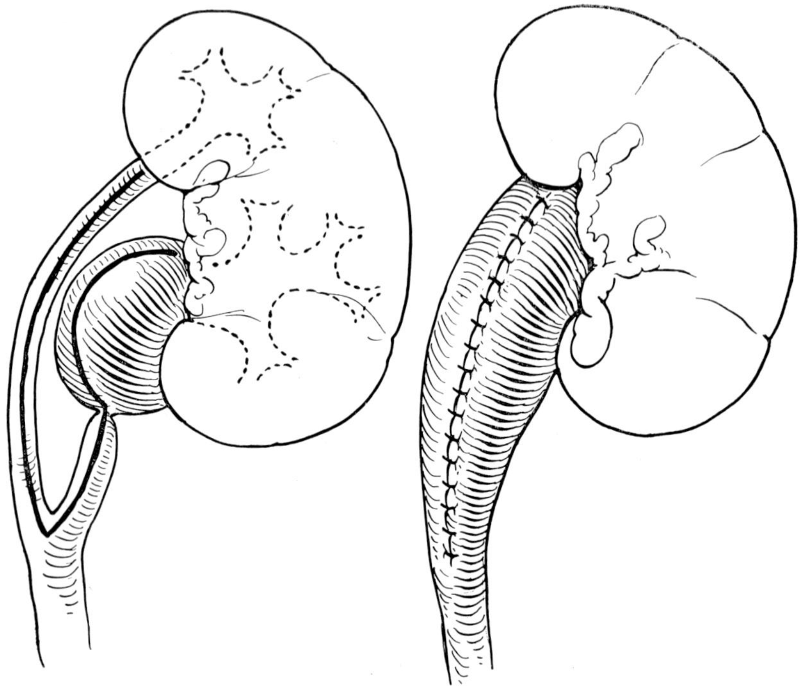

Fig. 9. Elimination of ureteropelvic obstruction in lower segment of duplicated renal pelvis by anastomosis of pelves and ureters.

Y-plasties, spiral flaps, intubated ureterotomy, and reimplantation accounted for 97 per cent of the pyeloplasties in this study. In 10 cases, unique situations were treated by unorthodox measures.

Obstruction confined to the lower segment of a duplicated pelvis was remedied by joining the two segments of pelvis and partially duplicated ureters (Figure 9).

A solitary, grotesque, cake kidney had obstruction high in the renal sinus. Some of the medial cortex was resected so that the side-to-side anastomosis could be extended into the dependent portion of the pelvis. This failed and nephrostomy drainage was continued. Similar principles were employed with good results in four horseshoe kidneys after each isthmus had been divided.

A simple Heinecke-Mikulicz operation was tried in two early cases. Only one was successful. The failure was rectified later by a spiral-flap procedure. It is regrettable that this was not employed initially. The Heinecke-Mikulicz is a treacherous maneuver because it tends to replace one type of obstruction with an equally dangerous one.

As mentioned previously, two patients had only division of aberrant vessels with questionable results.

None of the last four procedures could truly be considered an operation of choice.

## How can Postoperative Results be Evaluated?

All formulas for gradation of postoperative results have been inadequate. None is flexible enough to compensate for the original renal status of the individual or for the indeterminate recuperative power of the affected kidney. Isotope renograms have been promising but disappointing.

Although 35 per cent of the patients subjected to plastic procedures now have normal pyelograms and no pain, infection, or calculi (Table V), the most spectacular results were in individuals with kidneys incapable of resuming normal size or configuration because of permanent cortical damage. For example, a man aged 37 had advanced hydronephrosis and a blood-urea value of 146. The latter dropped to 34 after pyeloplasty. The solitary kidney drains promptly but the pelvis is not normal and remains infected. The operation obviously was successful but the patient can hardly be considered well.

Probably the most significant confirmation of success has been the fact that 107 patients with calculi in their obstructed kidneys have had no recurrences to date following simultaneous pelviolithotomy and pyeloplasty.

Failures usually are evident soon after operation. Additional elapsed time generally reveals further improvement rather than belated deterioration. For example, a 21-year-old Brazilian consistently had 500 ml. of residual urine in her solitary kidney after a Y-plasty and was assumed to have a poor result. After 1 year of continued nephrostomy drainage the renal pelvis emptied promptly and completely when the tube was clamped. She now is free of tube, symptoms, and infection.

There were two late failures. These kidneys were removed 3 and 7 years after pyeloplasties because of persistent infections and increasing drug allergies despite less hydronephrosis. Perhaps nephrectomy was the initial operation of choice in both cases.

Results of 381 pyeloplasties are shown in Table V. The four hospital deaths were due to rupture of an aneurysm of the circle of Willis

TABLE V.—RESULTS OF 381 PYELOPLASTIES

| Basic type | Total | Died | Failures Patients | % | Now normal Patients | % | Others Patients | % |
|---|---|---|---|---|---|---|---|---|
| Spiral flap | 171 | 2 | 10 | 6 | 64 | 37 | 95 | 56 |
| Y-plasty | 139 | 0 | 6 | 4 | 53 | 38 | 80 | 58 |
| Intubation ureterotomy | 37 | 1 | 5 | 14 | 9 | 24 | 22 | 59 |
| Reimplantation | 24 | 0 | 3 | 13 | 6 | 25 | 15 | 63 |
| Others | 10 | 1 | 2 | 20 | 2 | 20 | 5 | 50 |
| Total | 381 | 4 | 26 | 7 | 134 | 35 | 217 | 57 |

(one case), coronary occlusion (one case) and renal insufficiency (two cases). Both of the last two patients were azotemic on admission and had multiple calculi. One had been operated on previously elsewhere. Their operations on the ureteropelvic juncture did not prolong the procedures unduly. They probably were doomed from the beginning.

Two late failures due to uncontrollable infection were mentioned previously. Of the other 24 that were evident early, one is in a patient who has a functionless kidney and has refused further treatment because of lack of symptoms. Five kidneys were salvaged by repeat pyeloplasties. These were performed from 3 weeks to 6 months after initial efforts. Secondary plastic procedures seem to be most promising when a substantial time interval can be interposed between operations.

Thirteen kidneys were removed. Many of these probably should have been extirpated initially. Perhaps some could have been salvaged; but the effort did not seem to be justified under the circumstances.

Nephrostomy drainage was continued in the remaining five cases because the kidneys were not expendable. This proved to be a poor solution to a bad problem. Three patients died of renal insufficiency in 2, 3, and 5½ years respectively. One patient was converted to an ileal ureteral substitute 7 years later and is still alive 14 years after the initial procedure. The fifth patient in this small group removed his nephrostomy tube at home soon after dismissal from the hospital and is alive but not well 12 years later. Nevertheless he may have added to his own longevity.

Despite all extenuating circumstances, seven failures occurred under seemingly ideal conditions.

## Why do Failures Occur after Pyeloplasty?

All failures, especially the inexplicable ones, have been studied in detail in hope of finding a responsible and controllable common denominator. Ureteritis and periureteritis produced ureteral stenosis in each patient who underwent subsequent exploration. But the cause of this fibrosis remains obscure. Failures occurred with and without splints, infection, and calculi, and with all degrees of postoperative drainage from the incision. None of the strictures occurred at the end of the splint. Theories have been advanced regarding possible allergies to absorbable sutures, composition of tubes, and so forth. None is tenable.

It is especially noteworthy that 111 consecutive pyeloplasties were performed without a failure. Then there were two failures in rapid succession. Inexperience is not the explanation.

Histologic study was made of 50 normal ureteropelvic regions in kidneys that were removed because of hypernephroma and of 50 obstructed junctures obtained by nephrectomy or autopsy. Many types of special tissue stains were used. All degrees of hydronephrosis were included.

The obstructed juncture invariably was accompanied by hypertrophy of the muscularis of the pelvis, but occasionally the pelvic musculature was replaced by diffuse fibroelastic tissue. It was concluded that perhaps intrinsic alterations of the pelvic wall might preclude normal healing and function. But so far this theory has not accounted for all subsequent failures, despite routine biopsy of the renal pelvis. To date, one can merely conclude that the healing properties of some ureters and pelves are unpredictable.

## Should Ureteral Splints (or Stents) be Employed and Should Urine be Diverted?

In recent years there has been increasing enthusiasm for abandoning ureteral splints and diversion of urine. The wisdom of abruptly discarding *all* tubes in *all* cases is viewed with skepticism. Of late, about 50 per cent of patients have been treated by tubeless methods.

These patients were selected on the basis of the caliber of ureter with which the flap of pelvis was to be anastomosed. Some had infection. A few had calculi. Most had bulbous dilatation just below the obstruction (Figure 10*A*). This permitted accurate approximation of tissues in contrast to the difficulties encountered when only a thin rib-

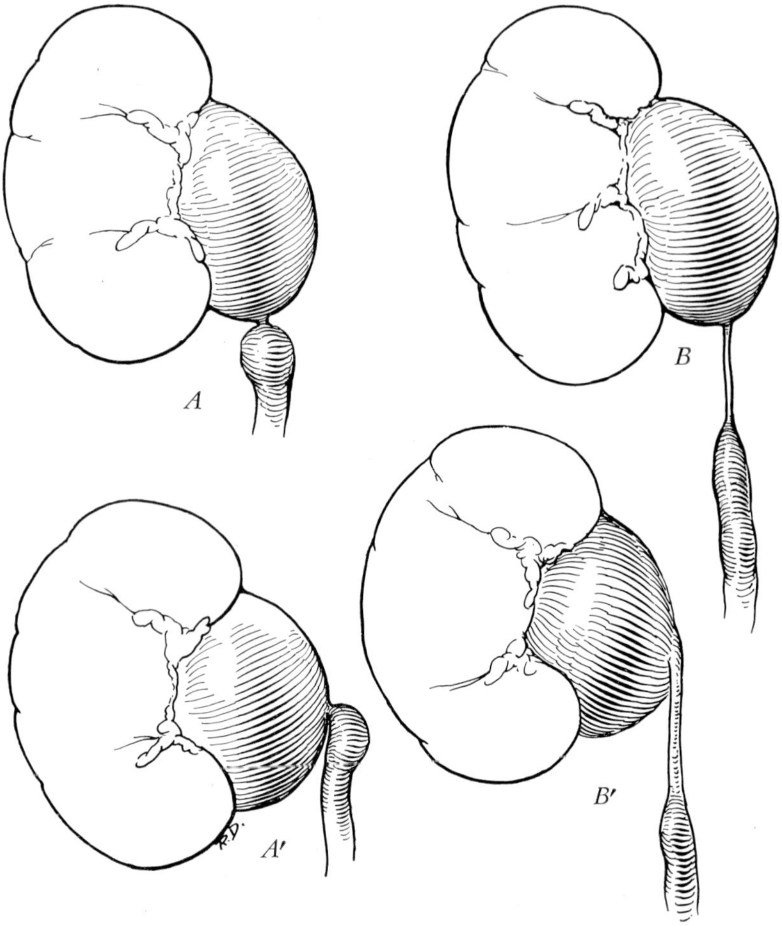


Fig. 10. Types of upper end of ureter. Bulbous dilatation associated with dependent juncture and A′) high insertion of ureter. Narrow ureteral segment with B) dependent juncture and B′) high insertion.

bon of ureteral tissue was available for a significant distance (Figure 10*B*). In the latter situation the two parallel rows of sutures can be so close to each other that viability of the intervening tissue may be jeopardized. Splinting still seems to be prudent in these cases.

Despite careful selection of candidates for the tubeless techniques, four failures occurred. Two of these followed spiral-flap operations and two were the aftermath of Y-plasties. One of the latter kidneys was saved later by *intubation ureterostomy combined with Y-plasty*.

A few other pertinent facts became self-evident in this group. When all goes well there is no question about the reduction in postoperative morbidity, despite the slower return of pelvis and calyces to normal. A few patients never leaked urine, had no infection, and were out of the hospital within 1 week. Others were less fortunate.

Urinary drainage persisted for as long as 28 days, with an average of 12 days, despite meticulous suturing. A constant urinary poultice is annoying, uneconomical, and demands continued hospitalization. Indwelling ureteral catheters reduce this morbidity but they usually must be kept in place for several days and they preclude customary ambulation. Ureteral catheters were inserted because of copious flank leakage in 12 cases. They usually were dramatically effective, but they defeated the basic therapeutic concept.

In recent years, constant seepage of urine from the incision has been avoided by inserting a Hemovac tube with multiple openings through a stab wound below the incision and attaching it to suction. The patients have been dry and more comfortable but the duration of drainage has not been reduced even though the gradual decrease could be measured accurately.

With nephrostomy, ureteral splinting, and a leg receptacle for urine, most patients have been ambulatory the next day and out of the hospital on or about the seventh postoperative day, but their urine has been infected.

Delayed intrarenal bleeding can be especially harassing. One patient was ready to leave the hospital on the eighth postoperative day when excretory urography failed to visualize the operated kidney. Retrograde pyelography revealed a pelvis filled with blood clot. A nephrostomy tube would have been welcomed at this point. Indeed, it might have prevented this predicament. After 10 days of lavage with streptokinase-streptodornase (Varidase) through indwelling ureteral catheters, the pelvis became free of clot. Fortunately, the kidney appeared normal a year later. Another such experience was encountered; but that kidney eventually had to be removed.

## If One Decides to Splint Ureter and Divert Urine, What Method is Preferred and for How Long?

Soft rubber splints (10 to 16 F) have been much more satisfactory than plastic ones. It is imperative to avoid excessively large splints because they can produce ischemia. An extra aperture is made in the intrapelvic portion. This has been a welcome auxiliary outlet for urine when the nephrostomy tube has become dislodged or obstructed.

With Y-plasties and spiral-flap operations a whistle-tip urethral catheter of appropriate size is passed down the ureter a reasonable distance and left in place for 2 weeks. One must remember that a Robinson or solid-end catheter will serve as a cork instead of a conduit!

With intubated ureterotomy and reimplantation, a Levin tube of proper size is used to splint the *entire* ureter for 4 to 8 weeks. In recent months, Silastic-coated tubes have been employed and much less edema has seemed to develop at the operative site.

It is wise to pass Braasch bulbs and calibrate the *entire* ureter from above to be sure that other segments of relative narrowing do not exist. Any that are detected should be incised as advocated by D. R. Smith, W. R. Smart, and others.

All splints are brought out through a lower calyx adjacent to a nephrostomy tube. The latter usually is a 22 F urethral catheter that is removed 24 hours after removal of the splint, provided clamping of the nephrostomy tube is not followed by pain, fever, leakage, or residual urine in the pelvis. It is noteworthy that delayed pyelograms made after injection of contrast medium through the nephrostomy tube do not always reflect the true result because of edema at the operative site and the viscosity of the contrast medium.

During the period of splinting and diversion, the nephrostomy tube is attached to a plastic receptacle on the leg during the day and to a bedside bottle at night. The splint is occluded with heavy silk and is incorporated in the dressing. It is thereby less likely to be dislodged than if it is connected to the drainage system.

Interrupted 000 or 0000 chromic sutures are used throughout the closure of the urinary tract. Mannitol is administered as soon as closure has been completed. Some type of sulfonamide or antibiotic is given during convalescence, especially after removal of all tubes, in hope of sterilizing the urine.

## Should One Anticipate any Special Complications?

Except for the flagrant failures after plastic procedures and the varying degrees of urinary infection that accompanied splinting and diverting catheters, these operations were followed by the same major complications that can be anticipated in any large surgical series. There was nothing unique in the successful management of sequelae. For example, patients with presumptive or obvious phlebothrombosis in a lower extremity did not develop hematuria during controlled anticoagulation therapy.

## What Type of Follow-up Study is Indicated?

An excretory urogram usually is made before the patient is dismissed from the hospital. Another at home 6 months later is advised and a request is made to have the films forwarded for comparison. The patient is urged to return for thorough study 1 year later—sooner if symptoms referable to the urinary tract develop.

Every effort should be made to sterilize the urine. This invariably entails cooperation with the home-town physician. It may necessitate early return of the patient if the response to antibacterial drugs is disappointing.

Cine and retrograde radiographic studies usually are deferred until the patient returns and are governed by clinical indications.

## Conclusion

No one harbors any illusions that the therapeutic plan outlined in this presentation is the best. Nevertheless, my associates and I have found that the Y-plasty and the spiral-flap operation seem to have comparable value, and intubation ureterotomy is so effective, even in adverse situations, that splints cannot be condemned.

Reimplantation was employed mostly in disheartening predicaments but served a most useful purpose. Less orthodox methods are justifiable infrequently.

The ureteropelvic juncture always has been and no doubt always will be treacherous ground that should command everyone's respect. It is not the realm of the faddist. In the parlance of the horsey set, injudicious selection of patients and poor choice of operations constitute a daily double that will pay off only with grief and disappointment.

*Proceedings of the Fifth Meeting of the*

# CAREER SCIENTISTS OF THE HEALTH RESEARCH COUNCIL OF THE CITY OF NEW YORK

*held at*

THE NEW YORK ACADEMY OF MEDICINE

December 5, 1966

Officers and Members of the
Health Research Council . . . . . . . . . . 379

Program of the Meeting . . . . . . . . . . . 380

Health Services: The Impact of New Legislation
*Howard J. Brown* . . . . . . . . . . . 381

Closing Address
*John V. Lindsay* . . . . . . . . . . . 388

Abstracts of Presentations by Career Scientists . . . 392

Roster of Career Scientists . . . . . . . . . 429

# THE HEALTH RESEARCH COUNCIL OF THE CITY OF NEW YORK

JOHN V. LINDSAY, *Mayor of the City of New York*
HOWARD J. BROWN, *Health Services Administrator*

*Officers*

COLIN M. MACLEOD,* *Chairman*
FRANK L. HORSFALL, JR.,* *Vice Chairman*
GEORGE S. MIRICK,* *Scientific Director*
MARION C. MORRIS, *Assistant Scientific Director*

*Members*

LEONA BAUMGARTNER*
DETLEV W. BRONK
HOWARD J. BROWN*
TIMOTHY W. COSTELLO
HOWARD REID CRAIG
JOHN E. DEITRICK
PAUL M. DENSEN*
LUDWIG W. EICHNA*
SAUL J. FARBER*
EDWARD FISCHEL
MITCHELL I. GINSBERG
LEO GOTTLIEB
FREDERICK O'R. HAYES
AUSTIN N. HELLER
MILTON HELPERN
DAVID M. HEYMAN
GEORGE K. HIRST
JANE H. HOEY
FRANK L. HORSFALL, JR.*
GEORGE JAMES*
MARCUS D. KOGEL*
MRS. ALBERT D. LASKER
JOHN S. LAUGHLIN
RACHMIEL LEVINE*
COLIN M. MACLEOD*
MACLYN MCCARTY*
WALSH MCDERMOTT*
AIMS C. MCGUINNESS
H. HOUSTON MERRITT
GEORGE S. MIRICK*
ROBERT S. MORISON
JOHN H. MULHOLLAND
QUIGG NEWTON
FAIRFIELD OSBORN
MARVIN E. PERKINS
GERARD PIEL*
EMANUEL R. PIORE
HANS POPPER
CHARLES F. PREUSSE
MARIO A. PROCACCINO
ALEXANDER ROBERTSON*
BERTON ROUECHÉ
ROY C. SWAN, JR.
JOHN V. TAGGART*
JOSEPH V. TERENZIO
LEWIS THOMAS
HARVEY J. TOMPKINS
BETHUEL M. WEBSTER
ABRAHAM WHITE
S. BERNARD WORTIS

*Member of the Executive Committee.

# PROGRAM

*Opening Address*, Colin M. MacLeod, *Chairman*
The Health Research Council

Saul J. Farber, *Chairman*
The Association of Career Scientists

1. INFECTIOUS HEPATITIS: EVIDENCE FOR TWO DISTINCTIVE PATTERNS OF THE DISEASE
   Joan P. Giles, New York University School of Medicine

2. REPLICATION OF GROSS LEUKEMIA VIRUS IN THYMIC CULTURES WITH INDUCTION OF CELLULAR NEOPLASTIC TRANSFORMATION
   Harry L. Ioachim, Columbia University College of Physicians and Surgeons

3. A MECHANISM FOR THE ANTITUMOR, ANTIVIRAL AND AMEBICIDAL ACTIVITIES OF EMETIN
   Arthur P. Grollman, Albert Einstein College of Medicine

4. RNA VIRUSES: MECHANISM AND INHIBITION OF VIRAL RNA SYNTHESIS
   Joseph T. August, Albert Einstein College of Medicine

5. INCREASED NET SYNTHESIS OF LECITHIN BY PHAGOCYTIC CELLS ENGULFING PARTICLES
   Peter Elsbach, New York University School of Medicine

6. STUDIES ON SICKLE-CELL ANEMIA: IRREVERSIBLY SICKLED CELLS
   John F. Bertles, St. Luke's Hospital Center

7. PLASMA DIAMINE OXIDASE AS AN INDEX OF "HIGH RISK" PREGNANCY
   A. Louis Southren, New York Medical College

8. A NEW FORM OF CONGENITAL ADRENAL HYPERPLASIA
   Maria I. New, Cornell University Medical College

9. AUTOMATED HEMODIALYSIS IN A MUNICIPAL HOSPITAL
   Eli A. Friedman, State University of New York Downstate Medical Center

CLOSING ADDRESS

The Hon. John V. Lindsay, *Mayor of the City of New York*

# HEALTH SERVICES: THE IMPACT OF NEW LEGISLATION

Howard J. Brown

Health Services Administrator of the City of New York

I should like to amplify the statement made by Dr. Colin M. MacLeod, your chairman, about the support of the mayor for the Health Research Council. Mayor John V. Lindsay was here on this occasion, as was Donald Elliott, the new chairman of the Planning Commission, and we are here because we feel very strongly about our research scientists. There is no question that the support of the Career Scientists will be continued. If there is any question it is only that of how rapidly we can afford to expand additional programs.

I am happy to discuss the problems of the new health legislation with this group for this reason: it is through your approach, your knowledge, and your leadership, and only through them, that many of the answers and the implementation of the new legislation will be provided. I know that some of you are laboratory scientists, only peripherally concerned with the practice of medicine. But only when the scientific approach that you use in your research is applied to the delivery of medical care shall we find solutions of the problems that we face now. We lack any scientifically based notion of how to deliver personal health services. This, to me, is the basic problem of properly implementing Medicaid and Medicare.

As you well know, because you work in our hospitals, the administration of health services by city governments to date has been largely a matter of providing services for the poor. The mandate given to us by new legislation is clear: we must now move to carry out the legislative decree to eliminate the gap in health services between the poor and the rich.

It is quite clear that the economically segregated part of our city hospital is no longer acceptable. Indeed, in an administrative sense, I can tell you that it will not work and that it must go. We must head toward

*Presented at the Fifth Annual Meeting of the Career Scientists of the Health Research Council of the City of New York, held at The New York Academy of Medicine, December 5, 1966.

a goal in New York City of a series of community hospitals that will treat patients in "one-level" facilities irrespective of their income. This is at the heart of our reform of the city hospital system. It is also clear that we are going to have only one class of patients, each of whom may be involved in the teaching and research program. Since teaching and research improve the quality of care, we wish to extend their benefits to all levels of income. It is the academic people and research scientists who have kept our city hospitals functioning and have made our teaching hospitals the places from which most informed people seek their major care.

The motive of service in our city hospitals has been a major factor in attracting the first-rate doctors who now staff them. But of equal importance has been their desire to do research and to teach. These motives have served to maintain our city hospitals as valuable institutions, and the Health Research Council has played a central role in keeping this resource viable.

The two areas in which there is now substantially more money for care are ambulatory services and chronic care in nursing homes. This is the first time in the history of our government that there has been adequate money to support important programs in these areas. Also, the new legislation includes money for the development of comprehensive programs for children. And this year the antipoverty bill included $60 million for health demonstrations on a community basis.

We now need to develop—and we need your help in developing it—a scientific model for the delivery of personal health services, with emphasis on ambulatory and chronic care. We must look at this in a hard-headed scientific way, using real data as the basis for recommendations. We are told that young physicians want to specialize and are not interested in delivering personal care in clinics and nursing homes. I submit that the reason physicians feel this way is that a scientific role has been worked out for inpatient care, particularly in the treatment of highly specialized problems. However, once outside the inpatient service we find that many of our present methods of delivering care are so irrational and so foreign to the scientific approach that a doctor must function as an entirely different type of person.

Let us say the frontline physician—either in community practice or on outpatient service—takes care of 2,000 people if he does his proper share. Even when the doctor works 10 hours a day, each patient will receive less than a half hour of his time—far too little for a good work-up. The physician sees many people but has little to do with pathology—too little to maintain his competence.

The problem is intensified when one distinguishes between organic disease, which the physician treats, and psychiatric and social problems that he scarcely has time to diagnose, much less treat. This is clarified by comparing studies of general and pediatric practice in England with studies in this country—such as the Baltimore Study of Chronic Illness. The Baltimore study shows a much higher incidence of organic disease than is found in studies of general practice. This reflects to some extent the greater time spent in the Baltimore scientific study and the greater skill of the specialized diagnosticians. Indeed, looking at the diagnoses reported in this study, one finds that they are diagnoses that a practicing physician *would make* if he could leisurely contemplate his patients; an impossibility in caring for 2,000 of them.

When one comes to psychiatric care there is a great difference between the incidence of psychiatric disease reported by frontline doctors and that revealed by such studies as the Midtown Manhattan Study* or George A. Silver's demonstration studies of family health.** This again suggests that the more time one spends with a patient the more psychiatric diagnoses one encounters. The same thing is true of social problems.

Anyone who has dealt with the problems of the poor knows that medical problems cannot be treated apart from social problems; separate treatment is almost impossible. Several studies have shown that the physician deals with more social problems than any other professional in the community. There are more problems in his field of activity than he can handle, and the more time he spends with people the more problems he finds. It is quite clear that no physician treating his sample of the population can deal with the full extent of the problems that are present. A physician may not even proceed rationally in deciding upon what problems he should concentrate.

Studies of frontline physicians show that many in practice deteriorate scientifically. This is simply because there is not enough of the

*Thomas A. C. Rennie Series in Social Philosophy, vols. 1 and 2. Vol. 1: Srole, L. *et al., Mental Health in the Metropolis,* New York, McGraw-Hill, 1962; vol. 2: Langer, T. S. and Michael, S. T., *Life Stress and Mental Health,* New York, Macmillan, 1963.

**Silver, G. A. *Family Medical Care.* Cambridge, Mass., Harvard Univ. Press, 1963.

kind of disease that is taught in medical school to keep a physician competent if he practices frontline medicine. A physician will probably see one neoplasm a year, perhaps several anemias, and may have infrequent opportunity to work up his cases of hypertension for etiology. His problems are such that scientific research is required to work out rational solutions of them. As an administrator I say that if we do not provide the required assistance, doctors with the greatest scientific knowledge will not retain interest in delivering frontline care.

So now federal funds have become available to deliver personal health services. But in New York City we lack any accepted scientific model as to how to proceed. As we plan medical care programs, we ask for some hard data on what we are and should be doing. I hope some of you will get tired of the laboratory and turn to the community and develop a research model for answering some of these questions. This includes the scientific knowledge that many of you have developed for inpatient services. Hopefully, scientific approaches can be developed for other medical and social problems.

It seems to me critically important that in each portion of this city we have a strong hospital with resources for scientifically based care at the core of our program. We are attempting to draw lines on the map that will assure this, but it will require some understanding. For example, there have been questions about the withdrawal of Columbia University from Bellevue, but very few people have applauded the notion of increased participation of Columbia at Harlem and Delafield hospitals, which can be of immense value to those communities. We must support, for example, the Catholic hospitals in southern Queens and northern Brooklyn and Staten Island, and help them develop programs that will convert them into medical centers. We must support them because low-income areas need this kind of resource. There are some areas where smaller hospitals must be merged to create such scientific resources. In addition to general-care beds, we are also speaking of psychiatric facilities; the Community Mental Health Board is planning a series of community mental health centers throughout the city. Also, we need nursing homes and chronic-care beds.

Anyone who has worked in a city hospital knows that the central problem is the congestion of patients who have no choice but to remain in bed there. The only way in which the services can be unclogged is to develop social facilities in the community and a program of ambulatory care that will induce the right kind of doctor to practice in the community. A major thrust of the Health Services Administration is to develop community programs that will tie together the general-care hospital, the chronic-care hospital, and the psychiatric facility. We are proposing to do this with grant funds from the Children's Bureau and the Poverty Program, and with financial help from Title 19. We are proposing to use the 25 Health Department Centers as facilities in which we can develop these community programs. They can provide the interrelation between nursing homes or chronic-care facilities, general-care facilities, and psychiatric facilities. Only when we develop a rational program shall we make these institutions workable and make them human in terms of service to people.

One of the reasons that community services have not developed is the absence of a manageable science of ambulatory care and social service. The basic problem in dealing with low-income people is poverty rather than health or other problems. We have not yet developed the social techniques required, but we should not allow this lack of knowledge to isolate the ambulatory services from the scientific standards of our teaching or university centers. Therefore I see in our community centers a partnership between the health scientists and the social scientists. I do not agree with those who suggest that the frontline doctor of the future should be a combination of practitioner, social scientist, and social worker. It is not that I do not dream of 50,000 Renaissance men; it's that each of these areas requires a degree of scientific knowledge that no one group of professionals can encompass. I think the doctor of the future should be even more specialized and more scientifically based and probably increasingly restricted in his area of expertise, so that as we develop our programs we can unite the kind of scientific medicine he exemplifies with new social insights and new ways of dealing with the problems of society. We are working on this, and we are thinking in terms of a plan by which physicians may continue to deal with those problems in which they are competent and thus retain their competence. At the same time new disciplines must be developed that will enable individuals to deal with the broader social welfare problems of patients. We are working closely with the City University of New York and the Human Resources Administration to develop courses that will teach these disciplines for the social welfare programs of the neighborhood. But we need young scientists who will keep up with the new group of social scientists and document the hard facts that will make these rational programs.

We are now organizing a system for Medicaid or Title 19 of the new legislation, using data-processing equipment to provide data about neighborhoods or health districts as census tracts. This will provide knowledge that will enable us to measure and apply standards of medical care services and their relationship to the needs of patients. For example, the problem of high-risk pregnancies described at this conference by Drs. A. L. Southren and A. B. Weingold highlights one way in which data might be used to deploy professionals in a given neighborhood. We need to develop in our low-income neighborhoods organized programs for the frontline care of patients; we shall start with the Health Centers in New York City's Health Department. Doctors in these health centers must participate in the intellectual excitement that is created in institutions where scientists such as you work.

We have not used modern machinery to the extent that we could. There is the prosaic matter of allowing doctors to dictate all information. We could automate many diagnostic and screening procedures, as is being done by the Kaiser Foundation Hospital in Oakland, Calif. We are going to have to automate most preventive and early diagnostic services. Of still greater importance is the training of additional health professionals to deal with minor ailments and social problems and to make the role of the physician more efficient in terms of his competence as well as in terms of his time.

Research such as many of you are doing will do more to shape the pattern of health services in this country than economic changes or changes in patterns of service that the administration works out. Imagine the changes in frontline practice if we had a vaccine for all virus infections, or if we had a breakthrough in neoplasms. For example, the advent of the Salk vaccine enabled us to let poliomyelitis be handled by nurses rather than by doctors, and we can now proceed to do the same with measles. On the other hand, this would not necessarily produce simplification of practice. Many of you can tell me what might happen if hemodialysis became an accepted part of community practice. If Methadone maintenance works out as the solution for most of the narcotic addicts in the city, imagine the deployment of resources to carry that out.

To sum up: the biggest opportunity presented by the new legislation is financial support for good community programs of medical care. How well these are developed will depend a great deal on whether scientists will apply factual data rather than platitudes in planning and developing frontline medical care. We shall have patterns that, because of the work of scientists, will require change. This may well be a change that will shift tasks from the doctor to other professionals, and back again, if it complicates the management of these problems. But if we can conceive and work out a rational program it can now be supported. I hope that each of the research institutions of the city, which you represent, will join the Health Services Administration in trying to develop community research laboratories to supply the hard data that will make these years productive for the citizens of New York.

# CLOSING ADDRESS*

THE HONORABLE JOHN V. LINDSAY

Mayor of the City of New York

It is a pleasure to be addressing for the second time this distinguished group of our city's scientists. One of the things that makes this city unique is the Health Research Council. No other city in this country that I know of has a tax-supported granting agency to fund the cost of research into urban sociomedical problems. As you know, the state contributes approximately one half of the Health Research Council's budget.

I am aware of our colossal burden of delivering health services not just to our 8 million people but to all the people of the region who use this city's facilities but do not reside in it. Yet I suspect that we are ahead of most communities in this country in developing solutions. More than one third of this city's population receives its medical care at public expense, which gives some idea of the nature of our burden. City, state, and federal governments contribute more than a half billion dollars annually to finance that care, but the overwhelming bulk of these funds comes from the city itself.

In New York City we have 21 municipal hospitals, more than are maintained in any other city in this country. We operate and staff the hospitals and carry their cost by arrangements with other levels of government for partial funding. It is clear, of course, that capital improvements are needed to strengthen this structure. We also need trained personnel at professional and nonprofessional levels. But many of these problems can be solved by research, and this government is committed to the need for research in the delivery of health services. Its role is critical. I wish that it were possible for us to fund more greatly than we have in the past the work of the Health Research Council. What the Council does in the field of medical research unquestionably has an impact on the Department of Health, Education, and Welfare in Washington, D.C., and its constituent agencies. Un-

*Presented at the Fifth Annual Meeting of the Career Scientists of the Health Research Council of the City of New York, held at The New York Academy of Medicine, December 5, 1966.

doubtedly, the Council leads the country in this regard.

The Council's Career Scientist program, which gives institutions employing these scientists 5-year grants as their salary, has brought top talent to New York City. The Council has been able to attract many of the best scientists in the country. I understand that 183 Career Scientists are now being supported through the Health Research Council. The city's annual contribution to their support is about $13,500 each, which is supplemented by their respective institutions.

Project grants made by the Council to support basic or applied research in specific phases of health complement these individual grants. They lead to a greater concern on the part of the health community at large in such problems as the delivery of medical care services and environmental questions such as air pollution and narcotics addiction.

In the latter areas the Health Research Council has set an example for the nation. The Council finances the renovation of facilities for research not only in city-owned buildings but also in medical schools and voluntary hospitals. In the past 5 years your Council has created over 100 laboratories for research on city health problems, one example being the conversion into laboratories of the open porches at Kings County Hospital.

I am also conscious of the fact that for every dollar invested in the Health Research Council we bring into the city through public and private resources approximately 5 to 6 dollars in additional research funds. This means that during the past years an estimated 100 million dollars annually has been brought here from outside the city.

I want to tell you something about the stress and strains under which the city government operates in providing more money for research, and for other needs of the people. We have the biggest expense budget in this country: 4.5 billion dollars, with projections of over 5 billion dollars for the next fiscal year. Only the federal government exceeds this figure. The budgetary pressures in the oncoming fiscal year rise almost 100 per cent from inescapable mandated costs over which neither I nor any other official of the city government has any control whatsoever.

We face the constant addition of pupils in primary, secondary, and higher education. We are at this moment going through collective bargaining with police, fire, sanitation, welfare, and other workers: our welfare case load is still increasing.

Here in New York City we have stretched ourselves almost as far as possible in doing our share of providing operating budget funds. We can get greater performance out of the governmental apparatus. We shall do so by reshaping and restructuring, by attracting better men at all levels, by shaking out and weeding out, attracting professionals and urbanists to top posts, by instituting modern budget practices. This will take time, but it can be done.

This city has probably taxed itself to the point where it cannot go much further. When a city gets to a certain tax level, citizens say, "Okay, we'll move." That's why the apportionment of the resources and revenues increasingly is a national problem.

I have never seen reorganization occur in any level of government—federal, state, or local—without the development of growing pains in the process. Let us hope that the Health Research Council will not only give us recommendations and suggestions but will work with us in implementing this administration reform.

The last thing in my mind, or Dr. Howard Brown's, is to neglect research or basic public health. We shall never neglect these, since we recognize their vital importance in the delivery of health services. What we have before us is a monstrous administrative job. The problem of putting together the revolution known as Medicare in this country is one that has thrown many communities of the nation into chaos. Some of them have literally thrown up their hands, and are saying they cannot cope with it. Here in New York City we think we are emerging with a structure that will enable us—after many headaches—to have a system that can administer both Medicare and Medicaid.

I am grateful to the medical community for its support of Dr. Howard J. Brown, our able and distinguished Health Services Administrator. I cannot tell you how much of his energies and his resources Dr. Brown has poured into his task. Fortunately, he is a young man and can stand the pressures of giving leadership of this kind.

I am grateful also to the health community for supporting my selection of Joseph Terenzio as Commissioner of Hospitals. Dr. Terenzio is not a medical man but a lawyer by profession. After being graduated from the Yale School of Law he immediately took his doctorate in Hospital Administration. For the past decade and a half he has been a hospital administrator of great distinction in the Brooklyn-Cumberland Medical Center. That great medical facility was unhappy at losing him, but it supported Dr. Terenzio's move here because it was for the larger good.

It is our commitment to see that in all this reorganization there emerges an administration in which public health and health research play primary roles. We also want to administer these services efficiently, even though many communities consider them unadministrable.

The Health Services Administration and its component parts are being designed to deliver the best possible health services to the people. These parts include the research in which you are engaged, without which it is impossible to deliver the best health services. I appreciate your support.

Where there are growing pains and differences of opinion on reorganization, let us know about them. Perhaps we can clarify, perhaps we can change, perhaps we can adjust as we go. The important thing is to keep open the channels of communication.

## Abstracts

*An asterisk indicates that the author is a Career Scientist of the Health Research Council of the City of New York

### *RNA Viruses: Mechanism and Inhibition of Viral RNA Synthesis*

J. T. August*

Department of Molecular Biology
Albert Einstein College of Medicine
New York, N. Y.

Enzymic studies of viral RNA synthesis provide an insight into the mechanism of RNA virus reproduction and indicate an approach to the control of these organisms. This investigation has been performed with an extensively purified (500-fold) RNA-dependent RNA polymerase found in *Escherichia coli* infected with the RNA bacteriophage $Q\beta$. With this enzyme, synthesis of RNA with properties similar to those of the template RNA is achieved. The reaction has certain unique characteristics. The requirement for template is satisfied only by $Q\beta$ RNA and certain synthetic polynucleotides. This template specificity is found to involve the initiation of RNA synthesis as measured by the formation of a 5′-nucleoside triphosphate terminus. Chain initiation occurs only with GTP, and polynucleotide synthesis takes place only when there is transcription of cytidine. The association of enzyme and nucleic acid has also been characterized by studies of the inhibition of the reaction. In contrast to the specificity of initiation, inhibition occurs with a variety of polynucleotides. These observations suggest the possible use of chemotherapeutic agents to block the action of viral RNA polymerase and, thereby, virus reproduction.

### *Elimination of Agranular Endoplasmic Reticulum in Regenerating Liver*

F. F. Becker* and B. P. Lane

Department of Pathology
New York University School of Medicine
New York, N. Y.

Following 70% hepatectomy of the rat, augmentation of ribonucleic acid synthesis occurs in the residual hepatocytes and, concurrently, their cytoplasmic organelles undergo lysosomal degradation. This study attempts to evaluate the relationship between nuclear preparations for mitosis and cytoplasmic alterations. Hyperplasia of the agranular endoplasmic reticulum (AER) was produced by the administration of 100 mg. phenobarbital/100 g. body weight for 3 days. Seventy per cent hepatectomy or sham operation was performed 24 hours after the last injection and liver biopsies were studied by electron microscopy and histochemically. Phenobarbital treatment induced hyperplasia of the AER and an increase in associated TPNH-cytochrome c reductase, which was unaffected by sham operation. In contrast, 70% hepatectomy eliminated some of this hyperplastic membrane system by lysosomal phagocytosis. The presence of hyperplastic membranes did not inhibit completely the mitotic response that followed 70% hepatectomy when phenobarbital-treated and -untreated rats were compared. Therefore, the stimulus imparted to the hepatocytes by 70% hepatectomy results in cytoplasmic dedifferentiation and eventual cell division despite intense stimulation of cytoplasmic organelle formation and function.

## *Studies on Sickle-Cell Anemia: Irreversibly Sickled Cells*

J. F. Bertles,* E. Roth, and V. Anku

Department of Medicine
St. Luke's Hospital Center
New York, N. Y.

The presence of severely deformed erythrocytes (irreversibly sickled cells, or ISC's) in peripheral blood led to the original description of sickle-cell anemia (Hb SS disease); their role in pathogenesis has remained obscure. Current explanations of their existence assert that ISC's are relatively old erythrocytes that have suffered prior sequestration in areas of low $O_2$ tension. Old erythrocytes in Hb SS disease should, through processes of selective destruction, contain more Hb F than young erythrocytes, whereas low Hb F content presumably facilitates ISC formation during sequestration. Experiments were conducted to resolve these conflicting predictions.

Thin films of blood from Hb SS patients were stained for Hb F by the Kleihauer-Betke technique, and optical densities of the projected images of individual cells were measured with a gun-type photometer: mean values for ISC's were consistently less than half those for non-ISC's. Following ultracentrifugation of Hb SS erythrocytes, fractions taken along the packed cell columns were analyzed for proportions of alkali-resistant hemoglobin. This value increased in parallel with increasing specific gravity, then fell sharply as the proportion of ISC's rose to over 90% in the heaviest fraction. Cell content of total hemoglobin (MCH) was constant in all fractions: thus absolute amounts of Hb's F and S per cell varied reciprocally. In contrast, Hb A/cell in thalassemic erythrocytes is constant, but Hb F/cell varies markedly (D. Loukopoulos and P. Fessas).

These data, providing information on a morphologically curious cell, support the concept that cell content of total hemoglobin limits synthesis when a predetermined MCH is achieved. Syntheses of $\beta^s$ and $\gamma$ chains in Hb SS disease continue in individual cells until an MCH of normal magnitude is reached, regardless of relative amounts of Hb's F and S formed. Synthesis of $\beta^s$ chains predominates in cells destined to become ISC's.

## *Quantitative Assay and Properties of Adenyl Cyclase*

M. W. Bitensky,* E. A. Gamache, and J. W. Clancy

Department of Medicine
New York University School of Medicine
New York, N. Y.

Adenyl cyclase is a membrane receptor site for several hormones. These molecules regulate the synthesis and degradation of glycogen through the intermediacy of organ specific adenyl cyclases that transform hormonal messages into appropriate intracellular enzymic responses.

Previous adenyl cyclase assays have suffered from insensitivity, nonlinearity, and dependence upon coupled enzyme systems. The present method, which uses the heavy particulate fraction of rat brain, is also applicable to muscle and kidney. Six $\times$ $10^{-4}$ $M$ $C^{14}$ ATP was used as substrate. Labeled

3′5′-AMP (CAMP) was cleanly separated from the reaction mixture. Descending thin layer chromatography was used with two successive solvent systems on ion exchange cellulose. Cold marker facilitated retrieval of product for scintillation counting. Concomitant phosphodiesterase activity was measured using tritiated CAMP.

The assay detected levels of CAMP below $8 \times 10^{-8}$ *M*. The reaction was linear for at least 4 minutes; during this time between $10^{-6}$ and $5 \times 10^{-6}$ *M* CAMP was produced by 2 to 7 mg./ml. of brain protein. Brain adenyl cyclase was inhibited 50 per cent by $5 \times 10^{-5}$ *M* methyl mercuric ion. Cysteine, however, did not improve enzymic activity when present during preparation or assay. Linearity was affected by the buoyancy of enzyme particles. Salt concentrations greater than 0.01 *M* caused flocculation with resulting activity loss. Phosphodiesterase activity was present in the heavy particle preparations and was not removed by washing. Even in the presence of aminophylline, between 15 and 30% of product was destroyed.

The described assay provides direct *in vitro* quantitative measurement of adenyl cyclase. The rat brain enzyme contains one or more sulfhydryl groups that are available for reaction with organic mercurials. Buoyancy of the enzyme particles is dependent on ionic strength. Accurate estimation of adenyl cyclase activity requires correction for contaminating phosphodiesterase activity.

## *Experimental Fetal Growth Retardation*

W. A. Blanc* and Joseph Cuneo

Department of Pathology
Columbia University College of Physicians and Surgeons
New York, N. Y.

Reduction of uteroplacental blood flow in one uterine horn of pregnant rats was achieved by Wigglesworth's technique (ligation of uterine vessels at lower end of one horn on the 17th day of pregnancy). Cesarian section was performed on the 21st day. Fetal death or stunting occurred in fetuses located near the ligation. The most stunted fetus was compared with the corresponding fetus in the normal horn and a statistical analysis of 35 such pairs was carried for fetal weight and organ/fetal weight ratio of all organs. Stunted newborns had a mean weight of 2.77 g. vs. 4.76 g. for controls. The liver, lungs, and kidneys were the most stunted, and were affected more than the fetus as a whole, whereas the brain, placenta, and heart were least affected. The ratios for thymus, spleen, pancreas, and submaxillary gland were not statistically different from those of controls. These observations are, in part, comparable with those made in human newborns in maternal hypertension and "placental insufficiency." Histologically the organs differed little from those of control fetuses, except for lack of glycogen in livers of stunted fetuses. Even very stunted organs appeared to have matured normally. These experiments extend and confirm Wigglesworth's data on the weight of liver, brain, and placenta. They support the suggested relationship between uterine blood flow and fetal growth. They show an interesting discrepancy in the effect on growth and on maturation. *(Supported by Public Health Research Grant HED 00.743 from the National Institutes of Health, Bethesda, Md.)*

# *Clinical, Structural, and Functional Studies of Hemoglobin$_{Gun\ Hill}$, a β Chain Abnormality*

T. B. BRADLEY, JR.,* AND R. F. RIEDER

Albert Einstein College of Medicine and Montefiore Hospital and Medical Center
New York, N. Y.

A Caucasian man and one of three daughters had compensated hemolysis and an abnormal hemoglobin. Hemoglobin$_{Gun\ Hill}$ ($Hb_{GH}$), 20% of the total hemoglobin, migrated like Hb C during starch gel electrophoresis at 8.6. An additional minor (2.5%) component was present anodal to the major abnormal band. The $Hb_{GH}$ components were separated from Hb $A_2$ by carboxymethyl cellulose chromatography. An accelerated turnover of $Hb_{GH}$ relative to Hb A *in vivo* was indicated by the specific activities of the hemoglobins both after i.v. administration of $Fe^{59}$ and after *in vitro* incubation of reticulocytes with leucine-$C^{14}$. Although the α and β chains of $Hb_{GH}$ were indistinguishable from those of Hb A after urea/starch gel electrophoresis, the abnormality was localized to the β chains by hybridization with Hb H. Peptide maps of aminoethylated β chains showed an abnormality in the region of peptides βTpX-XI. An alteration in the molecular size or configuration of the major component of $Hb_{GH}$ was suggested by a low sedimentation velocity and by relative retardation during gel filtration. Oxygen equilibrium studies of the major component revealed an abnormally high $O_2$ affinity, absence of heme-heme interaction, and presence of a Bohr effect. The extinction coefficient at 430 mμ of the deoxy form of both abnormal components was lower than that of deoxyhemoglobin A, resembling the hemoglobins that do not undergo conformational changes during reactions with oxygen.

# *The Critical Site and Residues for Hemoglobin Function*

R. W. BRIEHL*

Department of Physiology
Albert Einstein College of Medicine
New York, N. Y.

Structure-function relations in hemoglobin (Hb) may be a prototype for such relations in a whole class of (allosteric) enzymes. Much is known about all levels of structure of Hb and about the critical properties of function (heme-heme interaction, Bohr effect, low oxygen affinity) but local molecular mechanisms of function are unclear.

Human HbA shows two classes of ultraviolet difference spectra reflecting interactions of aromatic amino acids: 1) pH-dependent spectra. Carbon monoxide (CO) HbA shows peaks at 288½ and 281 mμ (therefore chromophore is tyrosine) with m*M* difference extinction coefficient (δ) 1.0. $pK' = 7.38$ (3°); $\Delta H = 6$ kcal/mole (therefore the perturbing group is histidine). Oxy-, met-, and cyanmetHb have the same spectrum. In deoxyHb the spectrum is much smaller ($\delta = 0.2$). 2) Form-dependent spectra. Among CO-, oxy-, met-, cyanmetHb there is no protein-dependent difference spectrum. Compared to deoxyHb these forms show peaks at 291½ and 284 mμ (therefore chromophore in tryptophan) with $\delta = 1.0$. Isolated HbA subunits ($\alpha^A$, HbH, $\alpha^A$ and $\beta$APCMB) lack the spectra of HbA, which therefore depend on interchain interactions. Dimeric ($\alpha\beta$) Hb (in 3 *M* KCl) retains the spectra; therefore they depend on contact between unlike chains.

There are 3 Tyr residues per $\alpha$ chain (B5, C7, H23*, nomenclature of Perutz) and 3 per $\beta$ chain (Cl, H8*, H23*). Tryp is present at A12$\alpha$ and $\beta$ and C3$\beta$. On the basis of the known 3-dimensional structure the *p*H-spectra are due to Tyr C7$\alpha$ perturbed by His FG4$\beta$ and the form-spectra to Tryp C3$\beta$. In tetrameric Hb with dyad symmetry there are 2 types of $\alpha$-$\beta$ contact, $\alpha_1\beta_1$ and $\alpha_1\beta_2$ (Perutz). C7$\alpha$ and C3$\beta$ both lie in $\alpha_1\beta_2$. Since the spectra persist in dimeric Hb, $\alpha_1\beta_2$ is retained and $\alpha_1\beta_1$ is broken. Since functional properties remain in the dimer and are known to depend on an interchain contact, the contact critical for function is $\alpha_1\beta_2$.

C3$\beta$ can form a bridge between vinyl groups of $\alpha$ and $\beta$ hemes thus forming a large interchain $\pi$-electron system; the $\beta$-chain (allosteric) shift (Perutz) which occurs with deoxygenation and on which function depends is parallel to the C-helices and changes the environment of C3$\beta$. Accordingly the C-helices (and neighboring FG corners) of the $\alpha_1\beta_2$ contact, and in particular residue Tryp C3$\beta$, are of critical importance in the functional properties of hemoglobin.

## *Perfusion of the Liver After Portacaval Shunt*

R. C. BRITTON,* A. B. VOORHEES, JR., AND J. B. PRICE, JR.

Department of Surgery
Columbia University College of Physicians and Surgeons
New York, N. Y.

Critics of the side-to-side portal vein to vena cava anastomosis for relief of portal hypertension argue that loss of hepatic perfusion may result from drainage of arterial inflow into intrahepatic portal radicles and then retrograde out through the shunt without effective perfusion of hepatocytes. Catheterization studies have demonstrated that retrograde flow does occur and have permitted sampling of hepatic vein, retrograde portal, and arterial blood for comparative extraction studies. Cineangiography has provided a gross estimate of the volume of retrograde portal flow. This value multiplied by the arterial-portal difference of bromsulfthalein (BSP), yields the portal removal rate that may be subtracted from the total removal rate to yield a corrected hepatic vein removal rate. A corrected hepatic vein flow may then be estimated from the Fick formula (see formula below).

The removal rates (flow × arteriovenous difference) of oxygen, BSP, glucose, and ammonium were then compared in nine patients after operation. All patients had retrograde flow ranging from 440 to 1750 cc./min. Although the extraction per cent of the test substances averaged greater by the hepatic vein than by the portal route, the average removal rates were larger by the retrograde portal route. There were individual variations in the proportion of flow by both routes and their respective removal rates. In two patients the venous-arterial glucose difference was larger in retrograde portal blood. It was concluded that retrograde portal flow after side-to-side shunt provides quantitatively significant hepatic perfusion.

$$\text{Estimated hepatic vein flow} = \frac{\text{Total BSP removal rate—portal removal rate}}{(0.01) \times \text{arterial—HV difference}} \times \frac{1}{1 - \text{Hct}}$$

## *Electrolyte Concentrations, Potassium Flux Kinetics, and the Metabolic Dependence of Potassium Transport in Human Platelets*

H. J. CARROLL*

Department of Medicine
State University of New York Downstate Medical Center
Brooklyn, N. Y.

F. GORSTEIN* and E. PUSZKIN

Department of Pathology
New York University School of Medicine
New York, N. Y.

Blood from normal human donors was collected in siliconized glass or in plastic vessels using acid citrated dextrose as the anticoagulant. The intracellular concentrations of sodium (39 mEq./l. platelet water), potassium (114 mEq./l. platelet water) and water (74.6% by weight) were determined by centrifugation of platelet-rich plasma and direct analysis of the packed platelets, with corrections for plasma trapped in the platelet buttons. The rate of flux of potassium across the platelet membrane was determined with radioisotopic potassium (K42) using standard kinetic technics. The flux rate was determined to be 112 mEq./l. platelet water per hour. In about one third of the preparations intracellular potassium appeared to be distributed in two compartments with different rates of exchange with K42. All intracellular potassium appeared to be exchangeable.

The metabolic dependence of potassium flux was studied by metabolic inhibition achieved by the use of cyanide, iodoacetate, ouabain, and anoxia. It was concluded that an active transport mechanism is present in the platelet membrane that transports potassium inward against a concentration gradient using ATP derived equally well from either glycolysis or respiration.

Ethylenediaminetetra-acetic acid (EDTA) was shown to inhibit glycolysis in platelets, probably through chelation of Mg. The production of lactate in the presence of EDTA virtually ceased but recommenced with the addition of Mg.

Clumping of platelets with ADP appeared not to alter their ability to pump potassium.

## *Further Characterization of the Pulmonary Blood-Gas Barrier*

F. P. CHINARD,* W. PERL, AND A. C. DELEA

Cardiorespiratory Research Unit
New York University Medical Division
Goldwater Memorial Hospital
New York, N. Y.

An earlier report** presented a hypothesis on the role of water as a major determinant of the permeability characteristics of this barrier. On the basis of indicator dilution experiments, it was proposed that water in the barrier was structured as in normal pure water in hydrogen-bonded tetracoordinated clusters. Solutes such as ions, which disrupt normal water structure, are excluded from the barrier while solutes such as inert and

*******Advances in Respiratory Physiology*, C. G. Caro, ed. London, Arnold, 1966.

respiratory gases, hydrocarbons, and short-chain alcohols enter the barrier either because they do not disrupt the clusters or because they enhance their formation. The hypothesis is supported by the results of subsequent studies with a number of other solutes of different types. In keeping with predictions based on viscosity effects, formamide and acetamide do not enter the barrier freely; propionamide and benzamide do. The monohydric alcohols from C-1 through C-4 also enter the barrier freely and have outflow patterns and distribution volumes almost identical to those of water. However, the alcohols from C-5 through C-8 have apparent extravascular volumes of distribution increasingly larger than the volumes of water as the chain length increases. The complete recovery of these alcohols in arterial blood (in contrast to the losses of the inert gases and $CO_2$) does not support a distribution into the gas phase but rather concentration in a nonaqueous barrier compartment. These experiments provide supporting *in vivo* evidence for the existence in the barrier of a significant lipid phase that has the important potential of rapid exchange with the vascular compartment.

## *Concepts and Patterns of Assistance to Failing Circulation*

R. H. CLAUSS*

Department of Surgery
New York University School of Medicine
New York, N. Y.

The incidence of circulatory failure may be decreased and survival following cardiac resuscitation increased through the use of new concepts of function and interrelationships of lungs and heart and vasoactivity. The prevalence of arterial hypoxia suggests that altered gas transport in the lung may aggravate existing heart disease, inciting failure of the circulation. Observations will be reported that confirm the work of West, demonstrating that nondependent portions of lung may have near-optimal gas exchange, and alveolar-arterial gradients may be used to quantify abnormal ventilation-perfusion relationships. Analysis of gas tensions in blood of pulmonary veins and peripheral arteries demonstrates that changing body position can yield far greater increase in blood oxygen content than ventilation with high concentrations of oxygen.

Vasoconstriction is as common in hypoxic states, congestive failure, and pulmonary edema as it is in hypovolemia and shock, and may be overcome. The virtues of the concept of flow through capillaries has been documented by visualization of changes in microcirculation and determination of oxygen tension in lymph. The per cent saturation of oxygen in central venous blood, a reliable index of cardiac function, may be maintained or restored to normal through early and continued treatment with precise doses of adrenergic stimulating or blocking drugs and fluid and electrolyte adjustment.

## *Kinetics of Antibody Formation in Multiple Myeloma*

L. A. CONE* AND C. CHIN

Department of Medicine
New York Medical College, New York, N. Y.

The relative rate of antibody synthesis as well as its molecular class have been studied in normal humans and in patients with various acquired immunologic deficiency disorders. Both groups of patients were immunized with 5 × $10^9$ plaque-forming particles of $T_2$ coliphage and serial bleedings were assayed for neutralizing antibody. The 19 and 7S antibodies were distinguished by sensitivity to 2-mercaptoethanol (2ME). Most normal individuals demonstrated an exponential rise in 2ME sensitive antibody by 3 days following immunization. This increase terminated within the next 4 days, by which time the 7S antibody was detectable. The doubling time of the early 19S response was approximately 10 hours, while the early 7S response averaged 20 hours. In patients with multiple myeloma the latent period was prolonged by 24 to 48 hours and the doubling time for 19 and 7S production rates were also increased. Those patients with lower levels of IgG globulin produced quantitatively less antibody at a slower rate. The patients with normal levels of nonmyeloma IgG globulin or with IgA myeloma globulin were found to have normal kinetics of antibody synthesis.

## *Translational Control of Gene Expression Regulated by a Hormone*

R. P. COX* AND M. J. GRIFFIN†

Department of Medicine
New York University School of Medicine, New York, N. Y.

The alkaline phosphatase activity of certain HeLa cell lines is markedly increased (5- to 20-fold) during growth in medium containing a glucocorticoid hormone such as prednisolone (Δ' hydrocortisone). The kinetics of enzyme induction and studies using inhibitors of protein synthesis show that *de novo* protein synthesis is required for prednisolone induction of alkaline phosphatase in HeLa $S_3$ cell cultures. However, there is neither an increased rate of alkaline phosphatase synthesis nor a hormone-mediated decrease in the catabolism of the enzyme since both chemical and immunological method show that despite a 5- to 10-fold increase of enzyme activity in induced cells the number of alkaline phosphatase molecules is about the same in induced as in uninduced cultures. Moreover, the physical and chemical properties of the induced enzyme differ from the base level alkaline phosphatase with regard to heat inactivation at 64.5°C., speed of elution from Sephadex G-200 and enzyme activity at all substrate concentrations tested. The base level and the induced enzyme, however, are similar with respect to certain other properties such as their Michaelis constants, electrophoretic mobility, and the degree of inhibition produced by various inhibitors of the enzyme. These findings suggest that prednisolone mediates a conformational change in alkaline phosphatase during its synthesis. Such alterations might lead to an increase in the number of catalytic sites or lowering of the energy level of the enzyme-substrate transition state. The induction by a glucocorticoid hormone of increased alkaline phophatase activity in HeLa cell cultures therefore may occur at the level of protein synthesis (translation) as a result of a steroid mediated alteration in the conformational state of the enzyme. Maximal enzyme induction is not attained until the base level enzyme has been replaced by enzyme synthesized in the presence of the hormone. *(Supported by Research Contract U-1296 from the Health Research Council of the City of New York.)*

†Present address: Oklahoma Medical Research Foundation, Oklahoma City, Okla.

## *Lipid Metabolism in Aortas of Hypertensive Rats*

M. M. DALY*

Departments of Biochemistry and Medicine
Albert Einstein College of Medicine
New York, N. Y.

The composition of aortic lipids is altered in rats with renal hypertension. The concentrations of phospholipid and of free and esterified cholesterol are above normal while the concentration of triglyceride is essentially unchanged. The possibility that these changes may be related to synthetic activity in the vessel was investigated by studying the incorporation of acetate-1-$^{14}$C into aortic lipids *in vitro*. A relative increase in the fraction of acetate incorporated into phospholipid and cholesterol would suggest that aortic synthesis is a major factor contributing to the changes in composition. Whole thoracic aortas from hypertensive rats and from normotensive controls were incubated in the presence of acetate and then divided into a preparation of media plus intima and another of adventitia plus residual media. Lipids were extracted and fractionated into classes by thin-layer chromatography, and the radioactivity in the fractions measured. The difference between the amounts of acetate incorporated into lipid by tissues from the two groups of animals was greater in media-intima than in adventitia-media. Significant amounts of acetate were incorporated into all classes of lipids, but media-intima preparations from hypertensive rats incorporated three to eight times as much acetate into all classes of lipids as controls. The results reveal no significant shift in the pattern of incorporation of acetate into lipids by aortas of hypertensive rats, and may reflect a general increase in the metabolic activity of the tissue.

## *Electron Microscopy of Human Leukemia Cells in Tissue Culture*

E. P. DE HARVEN*

Cytology Division
Sloan-Kettering Institute for Cancer Research
New York, N. Y.

Cell cultures originating from human acute leukemias and lymphomas were studied to find out if these cells are associated with virus particles recognizable under the electron microscope. The examined material consisted of two groups of cultures: the first originating from cases of acute leukemia in American patients, and the second from biopsies of African Burkitt's lymphoma. From the cytological point of view, most of these cultured cells resemble large undifferentiated blasts or stem cells. After several months in continuous culture, it becomes difficult to differentiate between cultures of myelocytic or lymphocytic origin. The prominence of cytoplasmic polyribosomes and the large size and striking electron density of the nucleoli were frequently considered as indicating the blast character of most of these cells. In all the observed cultured cells mitochondrial alterations were noticed consisting of mitochondrial gigantism frequently associated with the presence of conspicuous 30Å filaments, probably DNA. As far as the presence of virus particles is concerned, a clear difference seems to exist between cell cultures of American and African origin. In cultures of Burkitt's lymphoma cells and confirming the observations of Epstein (M. A. Epstein *et al., J. Exp. Med.* *121*:761, 1965) characteristic herpeslike particles have been observed at various phases of their maturation. These particles resemble viruses of the herpes group and were observed almost exclusively in degenerating cells in intentionally "aged" cultures (1 week without refeeding). The significance of these particles remains obscure since: 1) their infective properties have not yet been demonstrated, 2) they were never observed in biopsy material from Burkitt's lymphoma, 3) their presence in degenerating cells is not a classical feature for that type of virus, and 4) their presence seems, in our series, restricted to cell cultures of African lymphoma origin. Similar particles were not so far observed in any of the cell lines of American origin, even when these were submitted to the same aging procedure. (*Supported in part by Health Research Council of the City of New York, Contract I-325, and Public Health Service Research Grant CA 08748 from the National Cancer Institute, Bethesda, Md.*)

# *Glucuronic Acid Conjugation of Steroids in Crigler-Najjar Syndrome*

W. D. DRUCKER,* T. ENGEL, A. MEISLIN, H. JIRKU, M. LEVITZ, AND R. DAVID

Department of Medicine
New York University School of Medicine
New York, N. Y.

The possibility that there are many hepatic glucuronyl transferase systems, each specific for a limited number of substrates, was examined in this study. Radioactively labeled steroid hormones of varied structure were infused intravenously into a 3-month-old female, MG, with congenital absence of bilirubin glucuronyl tranferase (Crigler-Najjar syndrome). For comparison, studies were also made in a 3-month-old female, JP, who had trisomy-21 but was otherwise normal. Complete urine collections were made following steroid infusions and the distribution of radioactivity among various urinary metabolites was determined. Following tetrahydrocortisone (THE) infusion, 27% of counts recovered in the urine of MG were extractable with $CH_2Cl_2$ after $\beta$-glucuronidase hydrolysis *vs.* 49% in JP. After cortisol, 21% of recovered counts were extractable after hydrolysis in MG *vs.* 42% in JP. Thus, there was a 50% reduction in the excretion of metabolites conjugated at the 3 position (3-glucs.) of C-21 steroids bearing a $17\alpha$-hydroxyl group. After a loading dose of unlabeled THE, the findings were similar as with tracer doses. The excretion of etiocholanolone and androsterone glucuronosides (3-glucs., C-19 steroids) and testosterone-gluc. (17-gluc., C-19 steroid) was comparable in both infants. The excretion of tetrahydroaldosterone-gluc. (3-gluc., C-21 steroid lacking a $17\alpha$-hydroxyl group but bearing an 18 oxygen function), acid hydrolyzable aldosterone (18-gluc., C-21 steroid) and estriol-gluc. ($16\alpha$-gluc., C-18 steroid) was normal in MG. The results indicate that in this patient with congenital absence of bilirubin glucuronyl transferase, glucuronic acid conjugation is not uniformly impaired at all sites of the steroid molecule or even at the 3 position of all C-21 steroids. The existence of multiple glucuronyl transferase systems with different substrate specificities is suggested.

## *Increased Net Synthesis of Lecithin by Phagocytic Cells Engulfing Particles*

P. ELSBACH*

Department of Medicine
New York University School of Medicine
New York, N. Y.

Phagocytosis is associated with striking morphologic alterations involving membrane structures. Earlier studies of formation of macromolecules during phagocytosis have revealed only a small increase in *de novo* synthesis of membrane constituents such as phospholipids. Thus, no convincing biochemical counterpart for the morphologic changes has yet been found. The present *in vitro* study is aimed at exploring recently discovered alternative pathways of phopholipid (lecithin) synthesis as a possible source of membrane material during phagocytosis. Homogenates of rabbit leukocytes and alveolar macrophages contain enzymes that directly convert lysolecithin to lecithin. Resting intact cells, incubated in a medium containing $^{32}P$ lysolecithin, also incorporate $^{32}P$ radioactivity into cellular lecithin. Accumulation of $^{32}P$ lecithin proceeds linearly for at least 30 minutes. At equivalent substrate concentrations whole granulocytes incorporate considerably more lysolecithin into lecithin per mg. protein than do intact macrophages while homogenates of both cell types are more active than whole cells. However, the quantity of labeled lecithin associated with intact granulocytes after 30 minutes amounts to as much as 5% of total leukocyte lecithin. In macrophages this percentage does not exceed one. In the presence of polystyrene particles, incorporation of exogenous lysolecithin into lecithin is stimulated by 50% or more. Almost all of the newly formed lecithin remains associated with the cells; apparently little is released or exchanged with medium lipid. Since lysolecithin is a normal constituent of plasma, direct conversion of medium lysolecithin to cellular lecithin can therefore account for considerable addition of membrane phospholipid, especially by granulocytes. It is proposed that this mechanism of net lecithin synthesis provides building blocks for the increased membrane formation that accompanies phagocytosis.

## *Divergent Effects of Divalent Ions on Acetylcholine Release*

D. S. FELDMAN*

Division of Neurology, Department of Medicine
State University of New York Downstate Medical Center
Brooklyn, N. Y.

Acetylcholine (ACh) release at the motor nerve terminals of the rat hemidiaphragm was estimated in an *in vitro* system as the rate of appearance of miniature end-plate potentials (m.e.p.p.). Spontaneous m.e.p.p. frequency (2/sec.) is augmented by exposure of preparation to 20 m$M$ K to about 120/sec. This high rate continues for more than eight hours and reflects continuing synthesis of quantal packets of ACh. When Ca ion concentration is increased above normal (2 m$M$) in the presence of 20 m$M$ K a decline in m.e.p.p. frequency is observed proportional to the logarithm of the concentration. The low m.e.p.p. rate continues for the duration of exposure to high Ca and is reversible. When Ba is substituted for Ca at the high concentration a slow return in m.e.p.p. frequency to its previous augmented level occurs. No change in m.e.p.p. rate occurs with interchange of bathing solutions between 2 and 16 m*M* Ba concentrations unless the preparation has been previously exposed to Ca-containing solutions. After Ca depletion of a preparation by prolonged (3 to 6 hr.) exposure to a chelating agent, m.e.p.p.s. are no longer observed; 2 m*M* Sr in the calcium-depleted preparation (K normal — 5 m*M*) gave a m.e.p.p. rate of 0.69 $\pm$ 0.10; and 2 m*M* Ba under similar circumstances gave a rate of 4.1 $\pm$ 1.4. In the presence of an augmenting concentration of K (20 m*M*) Ba (2 m*M*) gave a rate of 138 $\pm$ 41, and Sr of 107 $\pm$ 16 in the previously Ca-depleted preparation. The results suggest: 1) Ba and Sr can substitute for Ca in the ACh release process; 2) Ba can displace residual bound Ca; 3) these ions bind with different coefficients to unknown intermediates involved in release of ACh; and 4) Ba and Sr lack the stabilizing capacity of Ca on the membrane. They support the hypothesis that free Ca ions interact with an intermediate in the process of ACh release at the mammalian neuromuscular junction. *(Supported in part by Grant NB 07004, National Institute of Neurological Disease and Blindness, and I-502, Health Research Council of the City of New York.)*

# *Renal and Metabolic Response to Various Sodium Salts in Experimental Burns*

C. L. Fox, Jr.,* and J. Stanford

Departments of Microbiology and Surgery
Columbia University College of Physicians and Surgeons
and
First Surgical Division, Bellevue Hospital
New York, N. Y.

Despite recent emphasis on the use of isotonic saline in the early therapy of burns, the effect of various Na salts on renal function has not been delineated although therapy is guided by urine output. The rapid onset of metabolic acidosis and NaCl retention after injury, and the known diuretic action of alkaline Na salts suggested a comparison of 0.15 molar solutions of Na acetate, bicarbonate, chloride, lactate, phosphate, succinate, etc. and mixtures such as Ringer's lactate. After i.p. administration of 150 ml./kg. body wt. in two doses, urine was collected for 24 hours from groups of 5 to 10 mice and analyzed for Na, K, Cl, urea, osmolarity, and *p*H. *Normal* mice yielded maximal output of urine, Na and Cl after NaCl but one tenth or less of these outputs was excreted by burned mice. In contrast, *burned* mice excreted maximal amounts of urine, Na, K, and urea following Na acetate or $HCO_3$, and these outputs were several-fold greater than after NaCl. In *normal* mice, alkaline Na salts yielded outputs similar but slightly less than NaCl. Ringer's lactate or similar Cl solutions alone or containing dextran or THAM yielded outputs only slightly greater than NaCl. Potassium and urea excretion were maximal in *burned* mice after alkaline salt therapy and minimal after NaCl in *normal* mice. Acute survival was approximately equal with these Na salt solutions but the relatively smaller excretion after NaCl was reflected in analyses of skin and muscle 24 hours postburn; these gained up to one third more water, Na, and Cl than tissues of mice treated with alkaline Na salts. Insensible water loss in the first 24 hours postburn was greater in normal than in burned mice. The earlier excretion and greater output of urine and solutes after alkaline Na salts suggest their preferential use *initially* in therapy. Clinical trials have been in accord with these findings. *(Supported by Grant GM 08582 from the National Institutes of Health, Bethesda, Md.)*

## *Automated Hemodialysis in a Municipal Hospital*

E. A. Friedman*

Department of Medicine
State University of New York Downstate Medical Center
Brooklyn, N. Y.

In September 1965, a 14-bed hemodialysis center, supplied by an automated dialysate delivery system, commenced operation. Concentrated, acetate-buffered dialysate is diluted 34:1 with filtered, heated tap water by matched proportioning pumps. Prior to delivery through polypropylene tubing to individual patient stations, dialysate electrical conductivity, temperature, and flow rate are monitored. Each patient's station is equipped with a dialysate hemoglobin detector, flow meter, temperature sensor, negative pressure monitor, and venous return pressure sensor. Activation of any of the central or patient station high-low alarms causes audible and visible signals and interrupts dialysate flow. Sterilization of the central diluting unit, patient stations, and connecting tubing is effected by flushing hot water through the entire system. Fifteen men and five women, aged 17 to 57 years, with terminal renal failure, have been maintained as active outpatients while undergoing twice-weekly overnight hemodialysis. Renal function inadequate for life preservation was documented by endogenous creatinine clearance values of less than 2 ml. per minute, 24-hour urine outputs of less than 400 ml., and the failure of conservative medical management. Dialyses are conducted by specially instructed nurses under the supervision of on-call physicians. Seventeen patients have returned to full-time work or home responsibilities and three are partially rehabilitated. Complications of the therapeutic regimen include infection and clotting of arteriovenous cannulae, secondary and tertiary hyperparathyroidism, subclinical peripheral motor neuropathy, and abnormal carbohydrate tolerance. Persistent anemia has necessitated transfusion of 0.5 to 4.0 units of packed erythrocytes per patient per month to maintain a venous hematocrit of 25 per cent. Posttransfusion hepatitis has occurred four times. Serious psychiatric problems have not been encountered. Long-continued intermittent hemodialysis is an effective method of life prolongation and rehabilitation for selected patients with renal failure.

## *An Unusual Effect of Aspirin and Other Nonsteroid Anti-Inflammatory Drugs on Serum Albumin*

D. A. Gerber*

Department of Medicine
State University of New York Downstate Medical Center
Brooklyn, N. Y.

Almost all work on the mechanism of action of aspirin and clinically similar nonsteroid anti-inflammatory compounds has concerned mediators of inflammation, mitochondrial enzymes, and oxidative phosphorylation. The present report concerns evidence that almost all nonsteroid anti-inflammatory drugs (e.g., aspirin) interact with serum albumin in a unique manner. Thus it was found that the nonsteroid anti-inflammatory drugs had the ability to alter the tertiary configuration of serum albumin molecules so that they reacted more rapidly with 65 $\mu M$ dithiobisnitrobenzoic acid at 30° C. (*p*H

7.4). A total of 180 compounds were studied, each at a concentration of 0.67 m*M*. These compounds were chosen at random to include commonly used drugs and commonly occurring biologicals and drugs with anti-inflammatory activity. Thirteen compounds accelerated the reaction between serum albumin and dithiobisnitrobenzoic acid. They were, in order of decreasing effect: indomethacin, oxyphenbutazone, phenylbutazone, flufenamic acid, ibufenac, salicylic acid, dichlorotolylanthranilic acid, hydroxydione, lauryl sulfuric acid, gentisic acid, mefenamic acid, aminophylline, and acetylsalicylic acid. Except for hydroxydione, these compounds are all known to be anti-inflammatory. No measurable effect was associated with the other 167 compounds tested, a group that included only one nonsteroid anti-inflammatory compound, aminopyrine. The administration of 3 g. of aspirin per day to human subjects produced a 33% increase in the reactivity of the subjects' serum albumin and provided direct evidence that the concentration of salicylate present in the serum of patients receiving therapeutic doses of aspirin is adequate to produce profound effects on this reaction. Salicylate did not reduce protein disulfide bonds, and the SH group was a necessary part of the reaction. These studies demonstrate an effect of therapeutic concentrations of nonsteroid anti-inflammatory compounds on a simple chemical reaction involving a serum protein and an aromatic disulfide, and may provide assistance in screening compounds for anti-inflammatory activity.

## *Infectious Hepatitis: Evidence for Two Distinctive Clinical, Epidemiological, and Immunological Patterns of the Disease*

J. P. Giles* and S. Krugman

Department of Pediatrics
New York University School of Medicine
New York, N. Y.

As a result of the endemic environment, 1153 cases of infectious hepatitis with jaundice have been observed at the Willowbrook State School, Willowbrook, N.Y., during the past 12 years. Second attacks of hepatitis have occurred in 63 or 5.5% of this group. Recent studies have indicated that two immunologically distinct types of infectious hepatitis virus may be responsible for second attacks of the disease in certain patients. The two types of virus have been designated MS-1 (derived from the serum of a patient during the first attack) and MS-2 (derived from the serum of the same patient 6 months later during the second attack of hepatitis).

The distinctive characteristics of the two types of infectious hepatitis are as follows: 1) incubation period—ranges from 31 to 53 days for MS-1 as compared with 41 to 108 rays for MS-2; 2) abnormal serum transaminase activity—relatively short for MS-1 (3 to 15 days), relatively long for MS-2 (35 to 200 days); 3) thymol turbidity—significantly elevated for MS-1, frequently normal for MS-2; 4) contagion—MS-1 was highly contagious for all 6 intimate presumably susceptible contacts, MS-2 spread to only 2 of 5 presumably susceptible contacts; 5) immunity—patients who had an MS-1 infection were resistant to subsequent exposure to MS-1, patients with an MS-2 infection were later exposed to MS-1; their response was compatible with an MS-1 type of reaction.

These studies provide evidence for the presence of at least two types of infectious hepatitis.

## *Pacing on Demand in Atrioventricular Conduction Disturbances of the Heart*

R. H. Goetz*

Department of Surgery
Albert Einstein College of Medicine
New York, N. Y.

In pacing on demand, ventricular stimulation is coupled to the preceding QRS complex and takes place only after a preset time interval following ventricular depolarization has been exceeded. Pacing on demand eliminates many of the dangers inherent in other pacemakers—arising from a competition between the intrinsic and electrical rhythm for capture of ventricular contraction—such as competitive or summated beats, repetitive ventricular contractions, and ventricular fibrillation caused by stimuli falling into the vulnerable period of the cardiac cycle. Pacing on demand has been found particularly valuable in patients who may revert to normal 1:1 conduction.

Therefore, pacing on demand was found to be the ideal mode of pacing in the coronary care unit, i.e., in patients who may come back to a normal sinus rhythm or in patients with a partial dissociation and unstable rhythm. External and implanted units have been tested. A method of checking the units out prior to implantation has been developed and is working satisfactorily.

In pacing on demand the electrode that delivers the electric impulse also monitors the electrocardiogram for the purpose of programming the pacemaker. It is, therefore, important to protect it from stray currents and leaking electric appliances. This has been achieved by special electronic circuitry. Conventional epicardial wire and uni- or bipolar catheter electrodes presently used with conventional pacemakers may be employed.

## *Chemical Mechanisms of Metabolic Inhibition*

I. Goodman,* J. W. Scherrer, and A. P. Olenczak

Departments of Biochemistry and Surgery
Columbia University College of Physicians and Surgeons
New York, N. Y.

The present study was initiated to explore by means of model systems the alternate chemical reactions possible between metabolic inhibitors and the functional groups normally present in enzymes. Representative metabolite analogs of amino acids, corticosteroids, carbohydrates, purines, and pyrimidines were treated at near physiological conditions in dilute solution ($10^{-3}$ to $10^{-5}$ $M$) with compounds bearing the main functional groups normally present in proteins. These included the amino acids serine, tryosine, cysteine, and histidine. Rates of reaction between inhibitor and amino acid in the absence of enzymes were determined by organic functional group analysis, or by spectrophotometry. Some members of every group of analogs examined were found to react with the sulfhydryl group of cysteine to form stable products. Present results support the view that many inhibitors generally classed as isosteric antimetabolites may function by a mechanism of sulfhydryl-group linkage.

# *Metabolic Interactions Between Intracellular Compartments of Intact Cells*

E. E. GORDON*

Department of Medicine
Albert Einstein College of Medicine
New York, N. Y.

L. ERNSTER

Wenner-Gren Institute
Stockholm, Sweden

Fractionation of tissue cells has led to a characterization of the metabolic profiles of each of the cell components, i.e., mitochondria, microsomes, nuclei, and cell sap. Information concerning the metabolic interactions between cell components has accumulated less rapidly. The present studies were undertaken to explore characteristics of intracellular transport systems in intact Ehrlich ascites tumor cells. Two transport systems were studied: 1) transfer of reducing equivalents from the extramitochondrial space to the mitochondrial compartment, and 2) a $K^+$-proton exchange between these two compartments. The experimental approach involved the use of inhibiting and stimulating agents with well localized and defined sites of action. The contribution of extramitochondrial-reduced pyridine nucleotides for mitochondrial oxidation was assessed after inhibiting Krebs cycle activity with arsenite, fluorocitrate, or fluoroacetate. The results of these studies indicate that these cells are unable to transport hydrogen from extramitochondrial-reduced pyridine nucleotides to the mitochondrial DPNH oxidase system. Thus, in the absence of an effective mitochondrial mechanism, the major pathway for oxidation of extramitochondrial-reduced pyridine nucleotides is pyruvate reduction to lactate. Other experiments provide evidence for an energy-dependent $K^+$-proton exchange across the mitochondrial membrane of intact $K^+$-depleted Ehrlich ascites tumor cells. In the presence of valinomycin, one observes a $K^+$-dependent $O_2$ uptake and proton release that is independent of the active transport of $K^+$ across the plasma membrane. As much as 50% of the high energy intermediates synthesized in the mitochondria can be utilized for the mitochondrial transport system. Studies of these two transport systems demonstrate the feasibility of this approach for the investigation of complex intracellular metabolic pathways in the intact cell.

## *Lipid Composition of Normal and Leukemic Human Leukocytes*

E. L. GOTTFRIED*

Department of Medicine
Albert Einstein College of Medicine, New York, N. Y.

The lipids of human leukocytes vary with cell type and source. Earlier studies in this laboratory indicated that differences in phospholipid content between preparations of normal and abnormal leukocytes were due primarily to the predominance of a particular morphologic cell type. Significant differences in lipid composition have now been found between normal lymphocytes and polymorphonuclear leukocytes (isolated from blood with glass-bead columns), abnormal leukocytes from cases of acute and chronic leukemia, and polymorphonuclear leukocytes from human peritoneal exudates.

Lipids were extracted from suspensions of isolated leukocytes and analyzed for total lipid, phosphorus, cholesterol, and plasmalogens. Neutral lipids and phospholipids were studied by thin-layer chromatography. In general, the major phospholipids were (in order of descending concentration) lecithin, ethanolamine phosphatide, phosphatidyl serine plus phosphatidyl inositol, and sphingomyelin. The neutral lipid fraction contained primarily free cholesterol, with some triglyceride but little esterified cholesterol. Normal lymphocytes contained about half as much total lipid per cell as normal polymorphonuclear leukocytes, a similar cholesterol:phospholipid ratio, a somewhat lower proportion of ethanolamine phosphatide, and a higher proportion of lecithin. Normal mature leukocytes, when compared with immature cells of the same series, had a higher total lipid content per cell, with much more cholesterol and a higher cholesterol:phospholipid ratio. There was little difference in total lipid phosphorus per cell, but relatively less lecithin and more sphingomyelin.

These findings may reflect differences in the relative content of various intracellular organelles, as well as possible differences in the quantity and composition of the plasma membrane.

## *A Mechanism for the Antitumor, Antiviral, and Amebicidal Activities of Emetine*

A. P. GROLLMAN*

Department of Medicine
Albert Einstein College of Medicine, New York, N. Y.

A recent report that the amebicidal alkaloid, emetine, showed a dramatic therapeutic effect against granulomatous conditions in man stimulated this investigation of its mode of action. It will be shown in the present report that emetine is a potent, specific and selective inhibitor of protein synthesis. In emetine-treated mammalian cells, certain effects are observed that are secondary to the inhibition of protein syntheis. Host cell DNA synthesis is markedly reduced, and the replication of polio virus and vaccinia virus is prevented. Comparison of the inhibitory activity of related alkaloids allows a structural model to be formulated for the observed biological activity. The amebicidal properties of emetine, the known toxic effects of the alkaloid in man, and the effects of the drug on granulomas and mammalian cell viruses are readily explicable on the basis of the presently reported effects of emetine on protein synthesis. The present findings offer a molecular basis for the pharmacologic and therapeutic action of emetine. *(Supported by grants from the National Institutes of Health, Bethesda, Md., and The National Science Foundation, Washington, D.C.)*

## *Solubilization and Activation of Bilirubin Glucuronyl Transferase*

E. Halac* and A. Reff

Department of Pediatrics
New York University School of Medicine
New York, N. Y.

Bilirubin is eliminated by the liver after being conjugated through an acyl bond with glucuronic acid (GA). Other compounds are conjugated through an ethereal or an N-C kind of linkage. The glucuronidation of these compounds is catalyzed by glucuronyl transferase. Studies have been reported where results obtained with phenolic type of acceptors have been extrapolated to the conjugation of bilirubin. This extrapolation would be valid only if a single enzyme would be responsible for the transfer of GA to different acceptors.

In agreement with data obtained by others from *in vivo* experiments we have obtained *in vitro* evidence in favor of the plurality of this enzyme system. This information has been obtained after defining the optimum conditions for the *in vitro* assay of bilirubin glucuronidation and after solubilizing the enzyme. This has been accomplished by the treatment of liver microsomes with EDTA and deoxycholate. EDTA dialysis induces a tenfold activation of bilirubin glucuronide synthesis by liver homogenates. The *in vitro* activity thus obtained equals the hepatic capacity for clearance of bilirubin measured *in vivo* by B. Billing *et al.*

---

## *A New Pyrazinamide Diuretic: Reduction of the Kaliuretic Action of Ethacrynic Acid in Man*

J. G. Hilton,* S. Alter, and P. Cushman

Department of Medicine
St. Luke's Hospital Center
New York, N. Y.

An undesirable feature of ethacrynic acid (E.A.) as a diuretic is its accompanying kaliuresis. MK870 is a pyrazinamide with limited natruretic potency but capable of significantly diminishing $K^+$ secretion at the distal tubular exchange site in dogs. Accordingly, the two drugs were studied singly and in combination in patients with edema refractory to conventional diuretics. Modified balance studies were performed on the metabolic unit with daily weights, 24-hour urine electrolyte excretion, and plasma electrolyte measurements. Given alone, MK870 had minor effects on Na, K, and water excretion. E.A. alone exhibited natruresis and weight loss together with hyperkaliuria and consequent hypokalemic alkalosis. E. A. plus MK870 produced augmented natruresis and weight loss and, in addition, a blunted kaliuresis and prevention of or, in some cases, reduction in severity of hypokalemic alkalosis. In conclusion, it is suggested that E. A. (100 mg. o.d.) plus MK870 (20 mg.) is a useful combination in patients with refractory edema resulting in augmented Na excretion and reduction in the hypokalemia seen with E. A. alone.

## *Replication of Gross Leukemia Virus in Thymic Cultures with Induction of Cellular Neoplastic Transformation*

H. L. Ioachim*

Department of Pathology
Columbia University College of Physicians and Surgeons
New York, N. Y.

Gross leukemia virus (GLV) is the inducive agent of spontaneous leukemia in AkR mice. To develop a system for the study of its replication *in vitro,* cultures of embryonal rat thymus were infected with GLV grown for long intervals and periodically explored for infectious virus particles. Bioassays in susceptible animals were positive up to 100%, and electron micrographs of cultures (L. Berwick) confirmed the presence of abundant virus particles. Examination of stained coverslips, periodically removed, indicated morphological transformation of the thymic cells. Isotransplantation of these cultures resulted in tumors at the site of injection with the histological pattern of reticulum cell sarcomas. These tumors are serially transplantable and continue to carry the initial GLV as demonstrated by electron microscopy. Long-term replication of GLV in thymic cultures is important for establishing a constant source of virus, as well as for the study of virus-cell interrelationship. Neoplastic transformation of cells *in vitro* with GLV reveals a previously unknown potential of this virus and provides the system to study these events. *(Supported by Grant CA-06215-06 from the National Cancer Institute, Bethesda, Md.)*

## *Association of Altered Phospholipid Composition of Erythrocytes with Hereditary Nonsperocytic Hemolytic Disease*

E. R. Jaffé, E. L. Gottfried,* and T. B. Bradley, Jr.*

Department of Medicine
Albert Einstein College of Medicine
New York, N. Y.

This investigation was concerned with a family in which a fairly well compensated hemolytic disorder (mild jaundice, splenomegaly, reticulocytosis 6 to 15%) was documented in six members and was presumed to be present in eight others. Consistent changes in the lipids of RBC in hemolytic disorders have not been reported, except in acanthocytosis, in which mild hemolysis may occur. The individual phospholipids of RBC were determined by quantitative thin-layer chromatography. The proportion of lecithin in the RBC of affected members of this family was increased (34.1 to 38.4%) and was normal (29.7 ± 1.6%) in the cells of unaffected relatives. The alteration appeared to be an absolute elevation in lecithin content, rather than a decrease in other phospholipids. The difference between the proportion of lecithin in RBC of affected family members and of normal subjects was highly significant, $p < 0.001$. RBC from other patients with hereditary hemolytic disorders and comparable levels of reticulocytosis had normal phospholipid compositions. Stained peripheral blood smears revealed occasional target cells and slight anisocytosis, poikilocytosis, and polychromatophilia. Osmotic fragility was reduced and the increase in fragility after 24 hours of incubation was less than that observed with normal cells. Autohemolysis after 48 hours was increased slightly and was corrected to nearly normal by addition of glucose. Utilization of glucose and production of lactate by the RBC were increased, the activities of 15 enzymes of the RBC were normal or elevated, and the ATP content was normal. Heinz bodies were not seen, even after prolonged incubation, and an abnormal hemoglobin could not be demonstrated. RBC life-span in the propositus was reduced ($Cr^{51}$T1/2 = 10.6 days), but compatible normal cells survived normally (T1/2 = 28 day). A causal relationship between the altered phospholipid composition and the hemolytic disorder has not been established, but both appeared to be inherited as autosomal dominant characteristics.

## *Growth-Related Modulation*

R. I. JAHIEL*

Department of Public Health
Cornell University Medical College
New York, N. Y.

Clones of human heteroploid cells differing in colonial morphology provide simple systems to study factors regulating the shape and orientation of and contact between cells growing *in vitro*. The sequence of morphological changes during colonial growth, in uniform environmental conditions, of five clones derived from a HeLa-S3 strain, was studied with quantitative morphologic methods. The nature of the changes and the time at which they occur are characteristic, heritable features of each clone. A detailed analysis of the change from diffuse to compact colonies during colonial growth of one of the clones will be presented. The term growth-related modulation is introduced to describe heritable, reversible changes in cell morphology that are associated with definite stages of colonial growth. Growth-related modulation will be analyzed in terms of: 1) recovery from trauma incident to plating, 2) changes secondary to cell-cell interactions, 3) modification of medium induced by cells, 4) modification of substratum induced by cells, and 5) random events. The relevance of the concept of growth-related modulation as an analytical tool in the study of cell differentiation *in vitro* will be discussed.

## *Sodium Taurolithocholate: Effect on Bile Acid Excretion and Liver Function*

N. B. JAVITT* AND S. EMERMAN
Department of Medicine
New York University School of Medicine
New York, N. Y.

Since lithocholic acid is a normal fecal bile acid, is occasionally detectable in conjugated forms in bile, and causes a local inflammatory reaction, the effects of parenteral admission of the taurine conjugate on bile acid excretion and liver function were determined in hamsters and rats. Sodium taurocholate, taurochenodeoxycholate and/or taurolithocholate were given by intravenous infusion (0.1 to 1.6 $\mu$mole/min.) or injection (13 $\mu$moles) to animals and bile collected quantitatively from a polyethylene cannula inserted in the common duct during pentobarbital anesthesia. Total bile acid excretion was estimated enzymatically (steroid dehydrogenase) and taurolithocholate-$C^{14}$ by radioisotopic and chromatographic techniques. Bilirubin, glutamic-pyruvic transaminase, and 5′-nucleotidase were estimated in serum obtained from cannulated and noncannulated animals at appropriate intervals. Administration of sodium taurolithocholate alone caused a rapid fall in bile acid excretion followed by elevated serum enzyme levels, hyperbilirubinemia, and bilirubinuria. These effects could be prevented by simultaneous administration of either sodium taurocholate or taurochenodeoxycholate. These bile acid salts were found to enhance the rate of excretion and recovery of sodium taurolithocholate in bile. Prevention of the deleterious effects of sodium taurolithocholate is attributable to the solubilizing properties of micellar solutions of the other bile acids.

## *The Reaction of the Conjugated Nitro-Olefins with Protein*

A. S. JOSEPHSON*
Department of Medicine
State University of New York Downstate Medical Center
Brooklyn, N. Y.

The conjugated nitro-olefins may be found in exhaust products of the internal combustion engine. These compounds can provoke delayed hypersensitivity responses in the guinea pig. This immunologic activity has been correlated with the ability of the nitro-olefins to form addition products such as thio-ethers with 1-cystein.

Studies of the interaction of the conjugated nitro-olefins were carried out by incubation at *p*H 7.2 of a representative nitro-olefin, 2-nitro-2-butene, with solutions of human serum albumin, human gamma globulin (Cohn FII), and egg-white lysozyme. Some denaturation of the gamma globulin was noted. Both the lysozyme and albumin, when obtained free of the unreacted nitro-olefin, had a yellow color. Increases in the optical density at 260 to 265 mμ of solutions of both these proteins were noted. This is the region of maximal absorption of 2-nitro-2-butene. In addition, olefinated serum albumin solutions exhibited a new absorption peak at 305 mμ. The electrophoretic mobilities of the olefinated and native albumins were compared on starch gel and cellulose acetate supporting media. The olefinated albumin showed a more anodal migration. Similar studies of olefinated egg-white lysozyme indicated the presence of two bands, compared with the single band of native lysozyme. Assays for enzymatic activity of the olefinated and native egg-white lysozyme indicated a loss of ability of this enzyme to lyse the microorganism *Micrococcus leisodeikticus* after reaction with the olefin. Similar enzymatic loss was noted when human tear lysozyme was olefinated.

These studies, indicating a reaction of the nitro-olefin with protein, are consistent with their immunologic activity. They also indicate that this reactivity may cause inactivation of an enzyme involved in resistance to infection.

## *Fibroblast Renewal Associated with Epithelial Renewal in the Rabbit Gallbladder and Colon*

G. I. Kaye,* N. Lane, R. M. Maenza, and R. R. Pascal

F. Higginson Cabot Laboratory, Division of Surgical Pathology
Departments of Pathology and Surgery
Columbia University College of Physicians and Surgeons
New York, N. Y.

As a result of combined physiological and electron microscopic studies of fluid transport in the gallbladder and colon, it has been shown that maximal absorptive activity occurs at the crests of the mucosal folds in the gallbladder and at the free surface of the colonic mucosa (*J. Cell Biol.*, *27*:50A, 1965; *30*:237, 1966).

Related *in vivo* and *in vitro* studies of gallbladder mucosa labelled with $^{3}$H-thymidine followed by autoradiography have demonstrated that epithelial cell replication is localized in particular sites even though the gallbladder epithelium consists of a single cell type. These sites, the valleys between mucosal folds, can now be considered analogous to the bottoms of the crypts of the intestinal mucosa, and they are, therefore, complementary to the sites of maximal absorptive function.

Electron microscopic studies have shown an adepithelial fibroblast sheath that is multilayered in the germinative zones but that forms an incomplete sheath subtending the absorptive zones of the epithelium.

The autoradiographic studies show that division of the cells of this fibroblast layer occurs during the same experimental period during which epithelial cell division is seen following a pulse of $^{3}$H-thymidine. There is also incomplete evidence that these fibroblasts migrate in association with the epithelial cells. This suggests that a specialized fibroblast population may play a vital role in the differentiation and migration of the epithelial cells and basement membrane.

## *Ventricular Diastolic Compliance in Human Subjects*

N. KRASNOW,* D. N. SUMMERS, S. AHMED, R. LEVINE, B. WECHSLER, M. FOX, AND R. RABINOWITZ

Department of Medicine
State University of New York Downstate Medical Center
Brooklyn, N. Y.

The distensibility and elasticity of the left ventricle in diastole is of significance for physiologic studies, especially where pressure is used as an estimate of ventricular volume and when various hemodynamic interventions are imposed. Previous studies have been performed only in animals. In subjects with mitral stenosis whose natural disease acts as an indwelling orifice flowmeter, it is possible by measuring simultaneously cardiac output, ventricular volume (thermodilution method) and left atrial and ventricular pressures, to determine at 0.04-second intervals of diastole the ventricular inflow, volume (V), and radius (r), and to construct curves of $\Delta P/\Delta V$, total pressure/volume (P/V), tension-length (T/r) and elasticity (T vs. $\Delta r/r$). These curves in the resting condition were compared with changes after isoproterenol (0.8-4.0 $\mu$g./min. i.v.), l-norepinephrine (12-22 $\mu$g./min. i.v.), supine leg exercise, lanatoside C (0.6-1.0 mg. i.v.), and electrically induced tachycardia (rates 60 to 158/min.) in 33 subjects. One subject was studied during coupled extrasystolic potentiation.

The curves of distensibility, P/V, were similar to those of T/r, and were generally linear or slightly curvilinear, without evidence of plasticity. There was no significant change in shape of these curves, or of the slope of $\Delta P/\Delta V$, indicating unchanged distensibility or stiffness ($\Delta T/\Delta r$), regardless of left- or rightward shifts of the absolute P/V curve. Elasticity was linear until after onset of ventricular systole, at extensions up to 16% of initial length. There was no effect on the slope of T vs. $\Delta r/r$ (elastic modulus). The data indicate that catecholamines, digitalis, exercise, induced tachycardia, and coupled pacing shift P/V and T/r curves primarily by their effects on systolic functions and end-systolic volume "set," without affecting diastolic mechanical properties.

---

## *Monoamine Oxidase Activity of Brain Tissue in Experimental Puppies*

M. LENDING* AND A. L. SOUTHERN*

Department of Pediatrics
New York Medical College, Flower and Fifth Avenue Hospitals
New York, N. Y.

Monoamine oxidase (MAO) content of specific areas of brain tissue was determined in a series of control puppies and those subjected to 3 hours of hypoxia and hypercapnia. Our modification of the radioisotopic assay procedure of Otsuka and Kobayashi (*Biochem. Pharmacol. 13*:995, 1964) was used. Similar results were obtained in the control and hypercapnic puppies. However, in the hypoxic animals the combined pituitary and hypothalamic areas showed a definite elevation of MAO titers and the cerebellum a definite diminution of enzyme activity. Other areas studied, i.e., pons, stem, thalamus, and cerebral cortex showed no changes. See accompanying table.

MEAN MAO UNITS/G. BRAIN TISSUE

| | | | | | | *Cortex* | | |
|---|---|---|---|---|---|---|---|---|
| | *P and H** | *Thalamus* | *Stem* | *Pons* | *Cerebellum* | *Anterior* | *Central* | *Posterior* |
| Control | 95,485 | 96,382 | 83,831 | 88,166 | 77,715 | 86,281 | 93,727 | 97,046 |
| Hypercapnia | 95,300 | 90,904 | 89,625 | 92,597 | 81,226 | 92,203 | 91,884 | 100,282 |
| Hypoxia | 121,445 | 93,980 | 79,305 | 88,168 | 56,034 | 87,501 | 85,894 | 85,702 |

*Pituitary and hypothalamus.

## *An Immunochemical Study of the $Le^a$ and $Le^b$ Blood Group Antigens*

D. M. MARCUS,* A. P. GROLLMAN,* AND R. E. ROSENFIELD

Albert Einstein College of Medicine and The Mount Sinai Hospital
New York, N. Y.

Anti-$Le^a$ and anti-$Le^b$ isoagglutinins are weak nonprecipitating antisera that usually require fresh, enzyme-treated cells to yield reproducible results. The poor and variable reactivity of anti-$Le^b$ sera with $A_1$ and B cells has precluded general agreement on the specificity of these sera, and the inhibition of many anti-$Le^b$ sera by H substances has led some investigators to question the existence of an anti-$Le^b$ specificity distinct from anti-H. Antisera to $Le^a$ and $Le^b$ substances isolated from ovarian cysts were prepared in goats. The precipitation of $Le^a$ substance by its antiserum was inhibited by oligosaccharides of known $Le^a$ specificity, but not by oligosaccharides possessing A, B, H, or $Le^b$ specificity. The anti-$Le^b$ precipitin reaction was inhibited by an oligosaccharide possessing $Le^b$ activity, but not by oligosaccharides with A, B, H, or $Le^a$ activity. After absorption with Le(a–b–) cells the anti-$Le^a$ serum agglutinated Le(a+b–) cells strongly, and Le(a–b+) cells weakly. The absorbed anti-$Le^b$ serum reacted strongly with Le(a–b+) cells and to a lesser degree with Le(a+b–) cells. A sample of 312 bloods obtained from Negro, Puerto Rican, and Caucasian donors were typed with the goat antisera. Nineteen per cent were Le(a+b–), 72% were Le(a–b+), and 9% were Le (a–b–). These results were independent of ABO type. The production of precipitating Lewis antisera of defined specificity by immunization of goats with purified ovarian cyst mucopolysaccharides has made available strong reagents for blood typing. Moreover, it affords an opportunity to detect and measure these antigens in mucous secretions, and on the surface of erythrocytes and other cells.

## *Purification and Properties of the 5′-Nucleotidase of* Escherichia coli

H. C. NEU*

Department of Medicine
Columbia University College of Physicians and Surgeons
New York, N. Y.

A cobalt-stimulated 5′-nucleotidase has been purified some 2,000-fold from *Escherichia coli* by means of the osmotic shock treatment of Neu and Heppel followed by DEAE and hydroxylapatite column chromatography. The enzyme is highly pure as indicated by disc gel electrophoresis, molecular sieve chromatography and sedimentation properties. The molecular weight calculated from sucrose-density gradient centrifugation and sephadex chromatography is about 53,000. The enzyme is stimulated about 100-fold by $5 \times 10^{-3}$ *M* Co++ at *p*H 6 and about 200-fold when Co++ and Ca++ are present. The cobalt requirement can be partially replaced by Mn++. The enzyme in dilute solution is unstable in the absence of albumin. The *p*H optimum is 6.0 with essentially no activity at *p*H 4 and 8. The enzyme is inhibited by 0.1 *M* Zn++, but it is not inhibted by up to 0.3 *M* phosphate. It is active against all 5′ ribo- and deoxyribonucleotides with optimal activity against 5′ AMP. The enzyme is inactive against 2′, 3′, or cyclic phosphates. It will cleave the 5′ phosphate of di- and triphosphates only in the presence of cobalt because of the metal chelate formed by the nucleotide and cobalt. It has not been possible to separate the 5′-nucleotidase and UDPG-pyrophosphatase activity of the enzyme, and ratios of specific activity remain constant through purification. The enzyme is shown to be located between the cell wall and the periplasmic membrane. Within the cell a protein inhibitor has been found that inhibits the activity against AMP, ATP, and UDPG. The role of the 5′ nucleotidase and its inhibitor remain unclarified. Both are constitutive. A similar 5′-nucleotidase activity and inhibitor activity has been found in *Salmonella typhimurium, Proteus mirabilis,* and *Klebsiella aerobacter.*

---

## *A New Form of Congenital Adrenal Hyperplasia*

M. I. NEW* AND R. E. PETERSON

Departments of Pediatrics and Medicine
Cornell University Medical College
New York, N. Y.

A new form of adrenal hyperplasia in a 12-year-old boy is described. The unique features of this syndrome are: 1) classical signs of hyperaldosteronism, i.e., benign hypertension, hypokalemic alkalosis, low plasma renin, expanded plasma volume, and hyperaldosteronism unresponsive to sodium restriction or sodium administration; 2) low normal plasma levels of cortisol, corticosterone but elevated plasma aldosterone levels; 3) elevated plasma ACTH levels; 4) sluggish response to ACTH administration of the baseline low normal urinary free cortisols, 17-hydroxycorticoids, and 17-ketosteroids, pregnanetriols and pregnanediols; 5) normal response of plasma testosterone to chorionic gondatrophin administration; 6) decrease of aldosterone production to low levels and marked fall in elevated blood pressure following treatment with glucocorticoids; 7) after 4 months of continuous therapy with prednisone, blood pressure has remained normal and the aldosterone response to sodium restriction and sodium administration returned to normal. Extensive metabolic studies and steroidal determinations utilizing the double isotope dilution derivative technique indicate that an overproduction of an ACTH-dependent adrenal steroid (or steroids) was responsible for the syndrome. On the basis of steroidal data obtained, a partial 17-hydroxylase defect in the adrenal and not the gonad appears to explain the syndrome best. This form of hypertension is noteworthy because it is alleviated by medical treatment and may be misdiagnosed as primary hyperaldosteronism. See accompanying table.

BASELINE VALUES

| *Urine aldosterone* | *Plasma aldosterone* | *Plasma ACTH* |
|---|---|---|
| 17-26 μg./d | 24 mμg. % | 1.5 mUnit % |
| (normal 14) | (normal 3-15) | (normal 0.3-0.7) |

## *Measurement of Exchangeable Intracellular Thyroxine in Man*

J. H. Oppenheimer*
G. Bernstein and J. Hasen

Division of Medicine
Montefiore Hospital and Medical Center
and
Department of Medicine
Albert Einstein College of Medicine
New York, N. Y.

The differential exit of exchangeable intracellular thyroxine (T4) and I-125 albumin from plasma during the first 4 hours following their simultaneous administration can be used to calculate the size and kinetic characteristics of the total intracellular (= extra-albumin) compartment of exchangeable T4. The analysis is based on the demonstration that the kinetics of I-125 albumin distribution are representative of those of the other T4-binding plasma proteins and that I-131 T4 does not mix more rapidly in the total plasma protein compartment than does I-125 albumin itself. A closed two-compartmental model is used to calculate the appropriate fractional transfer contestants and the permeability characteristics of the hypothetical membrane separating the two compartments. In normal subjects, approximately 37% of tracer thyroxine is ultimately distributed to the intracellular compartment. The unidirectional cellular clearance is approximately 43 ml./min., far in excess of the normal metabolic clearance. Partition of T4 between cellular and extracellular compartments depends on the relative strength of binding by plasma proteins and by as yet unspecified intracellular factors. In patients with thyrotoxicosis, congenital decrease of thyroxine-binding globulin, and subjects receiving infusions of dipenylhydantoin, an increased fraction of administered I-131 T4 is distributed to the cellular compartment. Conversely, in patients with hepatic cirrhosis there is diminished cellular uptake of I-131 T4. Direct external hepatic measurements and liver biopsies indicate that the liver is an important component of the intracellular space. Radioautographic and chromatographic studies in experimental animals confirm the intracellular localization of I-125 T-4 shortly after injection and indicate that the rapid reversible interchange of T4 between cellular and extracellular compartments is not accompanied by a net metabolic transformation of the tracer. These findings emphasize the importance of intracellular factors in the regulation of the circulating thyroxine concentration.

## *Infrared Spectroscopic Examination of Cornea and Lens of the Human Eye by the Attenuated Total Reflectance Technique*

F. S. Parker* and M. D'Agostino

Department of Biochemistry
New York Medical College
New York, N. Y.

Recent studies on aorta and other tissues (*Bull. N. Y. Acad. Med. 42*:415, 1966) have shown the value of the attenuated total reflectance technique (ATR) in demonstrating biochemical lesions. The methodology has been extended to the study of cornea and lens autopsy specimens of wet, normal and diseased tissues. A thallium bromide-iodide trapezoidal plate 50 × 20 × 1 mm. with ends beveled at 45° was used in contact with tissue on one side only in a Wilks ATR unit in a Perkin-Elmer model 521 with a 621 Nernst glower. A wire screen was used in the reference beam. Many absorption bands are common to most types of biological tissue, although direct *transmission* IR methods on wet cornea do not even allow these bands to appear. In a comparison of normal lens nucleus with cataractous lens the following differences are found: band shoulder around 3100 $cm.^{-1}$ compared to shoulder missing; band around 1740 $cm.^{-1}$ compared to band missing; in normal lens 1450 intensity is greater than that of 1385, whereas in cataractous 1450 intensity is less than that of 1385. Intensities of bands of 3000 to 2800 range are quite different for normal and cataractous. Band shapes differ from 1550 to 1500. In normal cornea 2950 intensity is greater than 2850; in opaque cornea 2850 has the greater intensity. The 1630 and 1545 bands are much deeper in the normal than in the opaque specimen. Around 1400 and 1100 to 1000 band shapes are different. At 960 no band appears in normal cornea, but a weak band is present in the opaque specimen. The ATR method obviously demonstrates gross chemical changes, and should be helpful in elucidating pathological eye biochemistry.

## *Metabolic Alteration in the Aging Erythrocyte*

S. Piomelli* and J. Miraglia

Department of Pediatrics
New York University School of Medicine
New York, N. Y.

Metabolic alterations occur in the red cells that ultimately lead to disapperance from the circulation. In order to evaluate the mechanism of red cell aging, rabbit erythrocytes (free of leukocytes and platelets) were fractionated in groups of progressively mean age by ultracentrifugation in high density discontinuous gradient of bovine serum albumin. The efficiency of fractionation was evaluated by dating the cells with $Fe^{59}$ and glycine-2-$C^{14}$ pulse labeling.

When the red cells were nitrited and incubated with glucose, with and without methylene blue, a sharp decrease was observed in the capacity to reduce methemoglobin (mthgb.) in the older cells. The NADH pathway in the older cells was intact, both in the level of NADH-generating enzymes (3-phosphoglyceraldehyde dehydrogenase and lactic dehydrogenase) and of the transporting enzyme ("diaphorase"). In fact, the capacity to reduce mthgb. was not altered when lactic acid or glyceraldehyde were used as a substrate instead of glucose. The NADPH-dependent pathway showed a marked decrease in the older red cells. This was found due to a reduction in one of the NADPH-generating enzymes (glucose-6-phosphate dehydrogenase); neither 6-phosphogluconate dehydrogenase nor mthgb. reductase activity were found decreased in the older red cells. As the defect in mthgb. reduction is observed even in absence of methylene blue and thus of stimulus to NADPH production through the pentose pathway, the primary defect must lie in glucose utilization. The activity of hexokinase in the older red cells was found to be one third of the youngest red cells. Hexokinase, the lowest activity enzyme in the red cells, is probably a rate limiting step in glucose utilization. A decrease in hexokinase in the aging erythrocyte explains the diminished utilization of glucose through glycolysis as well as the pentose shunt and it might be one of the important factors in red cell senescence and death.

---

## *Autoimmune Response to Thermal Injury*

F. T. Rapaport*

New York University Medical Center
New York, N. Y.

K. Kano and F. Milgrom

State University of New York
Buffalo, N. Y.

The inability of the severely burned mammalian host to resist invasion by frequent pathogens (*Pseudomonas pyocyanea,* e.g.) and suggestions of the release of altered tissue constituents from the site of injury, raise the possibility that severe burns may induce alterations in host immunological function. This possibility has been explored by a study of serum and thoracic duct lymph obtained from burned Fisher rats at various times after injury. Rats received 15% body surface area full-thickness skin burns by timed contact with a metal plate (250° C.). Serial thoracic duct lymph samples were studied for: 1) total lymphocyte output, and 2) presence of autoantibodies directed against normal Fisher rat erythrocytes. Sera obtained during the same periods from burned animals, as well as sera and thoracic duct lymph samples obtained from normal animals were studied in similar fashion. Results of studies in 60 consecutively burned rats and in 12 normal controls indicate that: 1) there is a sharp decline in the total lymphocyte output in burned animals within the first 24 hours after injury; this effect is still in evidence as late as 56 days after injury; 2) burn lymph contains a 7S antibody capable of specifically agglutinating normal Fisher erythrocytes; 3) this autoantibody is absent in burn sera or in normal lymph. The results indicate that severe burns may induce in Fisher rats a state of autosensitization to their own erythrocytes and a fall in the total circulating lymphocyte count. These observations may have a possible bearing upon the course and prognosis of severe thermal injury. *(Supported by Contract NONR-4503, Office of Naval Research, Washington, D.C.; by Public Health Research Grant GM 12748-01 from the National Institutes of Health, Bethesda, Md.; and in part by a grant from the John A. Hartford Foundation, Inc., New York, N. Y.)*

## *Biological Alterations in Human Recipient Reactivity to Skin Allografts*

F. T. RAPAPORT* AND H. S. LAWRENCE

New York University Medical Center
New York, N. Y.

J. DAUSSET AND J. M. CONVERSE

University of Paris
France

Leukocyte surface antigens detected by hyperimmune sera obtained from multiparous women and polytransfused patients have been shown to be active as transplantation antigens. In addition, mechanical disruption and differential centrifugation of blood leucocytes has yielded cell-free cytoplasmic particulate components capable of inducing allograft sensitivity in man.

In an attempt to facilitate the survival of human skin allografts, 31 healthy subjects selected by leukocyte grouping techniques were pretreated with cytoplasmic leukocyte extracts obtained from the prospective graft donors. The preparations were injected by the intradermal, subcutaneous, and intramuscular routes, in doses varying from 4 to 500 times the concentration capable of inducing graft sensitivity. Two weeks later, the recipients were tested with skin allografts obtained from the same donors. The mean survival time of skin allografts in this group of individuals was 15.6 days. The longest graft survival (graft still intact at 68 days) was noted in a donor-recipient combination in whom no major leukocyte group incompatibilities were detectable. These data are in contrast with the mean survival time of 10.1 days previously observed in 71 normal, untreated, randomly selected subjects.

The combined use of leukocyte grouping techniques and pretreatment with cytoplasmic extracts of leukocytes may offer an approach to the conditioning of human recipients to skin allografts. Further progress in this direction awaits the availability of a soluble, biologically active preparation of transplantation antigens suitable for intravenous use. *(Supported by a grant from the John A. Hartford Foundation, Inc., New York, N. Y.)*

## *Single Neurone Activity in Hippocampus and Amygdala of Man*

M. RAYPORT*

Department of Neurological Surgery
Albert Einstein College of Medicine
New York, N. Y.

P. BUSER

Laboratoire de Neurophysiologie Comparée
Faculté des Sciences, Université de Paris
Paris, France

J. BANCAUD AND J. TALAIRACH

Service de Neurochirurgie Fonctionelle
Hôpital Sainte Anne
Paris, France

Previous exploration of cortical epileptiform spike foci of man with one and two microelectrodes have revealed that more than one pattern of intracortical slow potential distribution and of single neurone discharge underlie the generation of the epileptiform spike recorded at the pial surface, these intracortical activities resembling those observed in cortical evoked potentials in the experimental animal. Neuronal activity patterns implied by Jackson's classic hypothesis of "excessively discharging gray matter" were not observed (M. Rayport and H. J. Waller, 1961-66). These findings being consistent with the possibility that a preponderance of spike foci in cortex exposed at craniotomy are the result of projected activity from deep gray matter, single neurone recording was undertaken in the hippocampal formation and amygdala in patients with intractable epilepsy.

During stereotaxic-EEG exploration, tungsten microelectrodes with tip diameters of 1-3 micra have been oriented according to the anatomical criteria of the Talairach school and advanced with a micromanipulator mounted on the stereotaxic instrument. Single neurone recordings have been made during spontaneous electrical activity with the subject awake or in light sleep; during attention and higher mental performance (naming, reading); during olfactory and electrical neocortical and rhinencephalic stimulation and electrical after-discharge; during interictal epileptiform EEG phenomena; during spontaneous and bemegride-induced seizures.

## *Abnormal Composition of the Lipophilic Components of the Brain Gangliosides in Infantile Amaurotic Idiocy (Tay-Sachs Disease)*

A. ROSENBERG*

Departments of Biochemistry and Medicine
Columbia University College of Physicians and Surgeons
New York, N. Y.

Monosialoganglioside lacking a galactose residue accumulates in the degenerating brain of children with Tay-Sachs disease. This study provides new clues to the chemical aberration leading to the degenerative process. Fatty acids of gangliosides were identified by gas liquid chromatography, sphingosine by examination of permanganate-periodate oxidation products. Fatty acids and sphingosine of gangliosides from diseased brain were compared with those of the various brains of normal humans and rates of varius ages. Tay-Sachs gangliosides had an unusually high content of stearic acid and sphingosine almost exclusively of the 18-carbon variety. Gangliosides from the brain of normal children had a lower content of stearic acid and almost equal quantities of 18- and 20-carbon sphingosine. The pattern found in the gangliosides of the diseased brain was that found in the gangliosides of the brain of the normal human and normal rat immediately after birth. These results indicate that a failure of chemical development may underlie the massive accumulation of monosialoganglioside that accompanies degeneration of the brain in Tay-Sachs disease.

## *Evidence for Evolutionary Changes in Fat Cell Physiology*

D. Rudman,* M. Di Girolamo, and L. A. Garcia

Department of Medicine, Columbia University Division
Goldwater Memorial Hospital
New York, N. Y.

The rat's fat cell performs four functions, each of which is hormonally regulated: conversion of glucose to fatty acids (FA) (lipogenesis); uptake of extracellular triglyceride-FA; storage of FA as intracellular triglyceride (TG); and mobilization of stored TG. This laboratory has now examined *in vitro* patterns of glucose metabolism and hormonal responsiveness of adipose tissue (AT) of 6 mammalian species, and other laboratories AT of 3 additional mammalian, 4 avian, and 3 insect species. Results of all these studies show: 1) vertebrate fat cells utilize glucose as the major extracellular carbohydrate, but insect fat cells use trehalose instead; 2) among vertebrate AT, conversion of glucose to FA is a major pathway in rodents of Muridae and Caviidae families but not in rodents of Cricetidae family, in the lagomorph order, or in the bird class; 3) insulin stimulates glucose transport into fat cells of Muridae and Caviidae but not of Cricetidae or lagomorph mammals, or of birds; 4) stored TG is mobilized by insect AT as diglyceride but by vertebrate AT as FFA; and 5) in rodent and lagomorph mammals, pituitary peptides stimulate FFA mobilization; in all other mammal and bird species tested, catechol amines are the principal stimuli of this process. These data indicate major alterations in the lipogenic and mobilization functions of the fat cell during invertebrate and vertebrate evolution.

## *Metabolism of Hyaluronateprotein in the Wrist Joint of Calves*

J. I. Sandson*

Department of Medicine
Albert Einstein College of Medicine
New York, N. Y.

Hyaluronateprotein (HP) is a large polymer that is responsible for the viscosity of synovial fluid (SF). Since the protein moiety of HP can be labeled with $I^{131}$, the metabolism of HP in SF can be approached experimentally. HP, isolated from bovine SF by ultrafiltration on 0.1 $\mu$ millipore filters, contained 3% protein. Bovine HP was labeled with $I^{131}$; free $I^{131}$ was removed by sequential dialysis, zone electrophoresis, and ultrafiltration of HP-$I^{131}$. One ml. HP-$I^{131}$ (100 $\gamma$ HP, 1 to 10 microcuries $I^{131}$) was injected into the wrist joint of a calf. The rate of removal of HP-$I^{131}$ was determined in two ways: 1) by daily aspiration of SF and serial determination of specific activity $\frac{I^{131}\ (\text{CPM/ml.})}{\text{HP}\ (\gamma/\text{ml.})}$ of HP isolated from each sample of SF, and 2) by daily external counting of $I^{131}$ over the joint. For 7 to 14 days determinations of $I^{131}$ were performed on the blood, urine, and stool. When the values for specific activity of HP-$I^{131}$ were plotted on semilog paper, a straight line was obtained. The half-life of HP-$I^{131}$ varied from 15 to 24 hours in 6 experiments performed in 4 different calves. Two straight lines could be extrapolated from the curve obtained when the data from external counting were plotted. During the first 4 to 6 days of the experiment the rate of removal of HP-$I^{131}$ from the joint was similar to the half-life of HP-$I^{131}$ in the SF. After the sixth day the rate of removal of $I^{131}$ from the joint slowed markedly. Within 1 hour after injection of HP-$I^{131}$ into the joint, $I^{131}$ appeared in the blood. Within 24 hours a significant amount of $I^{131}$ was found in the urine. Very little $I^{131}$ appeared in the stool. Throughout the experiment the HP-$I^{131}$ in SF remained nondialyzable; the $I^{131}$ that appeared in the urine was dialyzable. Thus far the data obtained in the studies indicate that: 1) HP is rapidly removed from SF; 2) HP does not appear to be degraded in the SF; 3) HP is not removed from the joint as rapidly as from the SF; 4) HP is degraded either in the joint or elsewhere in the body after it is removed from the joint, and 5) some of the degradation products of HP are excreted in the urine.

## *Adaptive Regulation of the Biosynthesis of a Specific Cell Protein: Apoferritin*

D. SCHACHTER,* Y. YOSHINO, AND J. MANIS

Department of Medicine
Columbia University College of Physicians and Surgeons
New York, N. Y.

The biosynthesis of apoferritin *in vitro* is a useful probe for studying cell differentiation, i.e., regulation of the synthesis of specific proteins. Apoferritin binds and stores iron to yield ferritin, and both forms of the protein can be crystallized or readily quantified and isolated as immune precipitates. For *in vitro* studies slices of rat liver (or spleen, duodenum, or kidney) are incubated with $C^{14}$-leucine, subsequently apoferritin and ferritin are isolated by precipitation with specific antiserum, and both net synthesis and incorporation of $C^{14}$ are estimated. Doses of 1 to 9 mg. Fe/100 g. rat given 2 to 24 hours prior to sacrifice enhance incorporation of $C^{14}$-leucine into apoferritin by liver slices *in vitro* up to tenfold, and net synthesis is observed. Actinomycin D, an inhibitor of DNA-dependent RNA synthesis, markedly inhibits this adaptive response to Fe. Moreover, Fe administration increases the subsequent incorporation of $C^{14}$-orotic acid, given as a 10-minute pulse to intact rats, into the rapidly labeled fraction of liver nuclear RNA. Thus iron appears to act on a genetic locus to increase apoferritin synthesis. Following actinomycin D the capacity to synthesize apoferritin decreases with a half-life of about 4 to 5 hours, and this may reflect the half-life of the corresponding messenger RNA. *(Supported by Public Health Service Research Grant 04407 from the National Institute of Arthritis and Metabolic Diseases, Bethesda, Md.)*

## *Enzyme Induction in Regenerating Rat Liver*

I. SEIDMAN,* G. W. TEEBOR, AND F. F. BECKER*

Department of Pathology, New York University School of Medicine, New York, N. Y.

It is well known that changes in the physiologic status of an animal (administration of hormones, starvation, etc.) results in predictable alterations in the activities of many enzymes in the liver and other tissues. Hepatomas, however, have been shown to be largely unable to respond to these stimuli with the expected changes in enzyme activity. Some workers feel that this absence of normal enzymatic regulatory mechanisms may represent a fundamental biochemical lesion in malignant neoplasms. The activity of the hepatic enzyme tryptophan pyrrolase (TP) is increased several times within a few hours after cortisone administration. This effect of cortisone is absent or markedly reduced in hepatomas.

The induction of TP by cortisone was studied in regenerating rat liver in an attempt to determine whether a dividing but nonneoplastic population of cells would respond normally to steroid administration. At various times after 70% hepatectomy, adrenalectomized rats were given cortisone i.p. They were sacrificed 4 hours after steroid administration, and TP activity was assayed. Sham-operated adrenalectomized rats were used as controls.

The results show a marked decrease in the degree of TP induction in the regenerating liver, beginning at a time coinciding with DNA synthesis. This suggests that the findings observed in hepatomas may not be specific for neoplasms.

## *The Diagnosis and Therapy of Shock, Using Physiologic Correlates Quantified with a Bedside Computer*

J. H. SIEGEL* AND L. R. M. DEL GUERCIO*

Department of Surgery, Albert Einstein College of Medicine, New York, N. Y.

Cardiovascular dynamics and oxygen consumption were measured in patients in shock from sepsis, hypovolemia, or pulmonary embolus, and five physiologic correlates immediately derived using an Olivetti Programma 101 bedside computer: 1) net vascular tone; 2) effective oxygen transport; 3) relative peripheral shunting; 4) pulmonary venoarterial admixture; and 5) ventricular function. Each of these was graphed as the patient's condition indicated on a nomogram for that particular function previously derived from analysis of 84 patients. This analysis showed that, compared both to normal and nonseptic shock patients, patients in septic shock have a net vascular tone that is decreased to a degree comparable to that found in severe liver disease. Determination of the effective oxygen transport and relative peripheral shunting functions has enabled discrimination of a hyperdynamic and hypodynamic group amongst the patients in septic shock. Both relative peripheral shunting and pulmonary venoarterial admixture were greater in the patients in hyperdynamic septic shock than in any other group, and correlated well with the severity of the shock. Evaluation of the ventricular function relationships showed that decreased cardiac function is a factor relatively early in the clinical course of nearly all patients in septic shock, and that a worsening ventricular function relationship is associated with a deteriorating clinical course. This myocardial failure can often be reversed by administration of an inotropic agent. Using computer determinations of these physiologic correlates and the appropriate nomograms, it is possible to follow an individual patient's clinical course and make therapeutic decisions at the bedside based on the nature and extent of the individual deviation from normal.

## *Oxandrolone in the Treatment of Short Stature*

E. H. SOBEL* AND H. K. BETTMANN
Department of Pediatrics
JACK GELLER
Department of Medicine
Albert Einstein College of Medicine
New York, N. Y.

Six boys and two girls, aged 4 to 18 years, were treated with oxandrolone, 0.2 mg./kg. daily during the second 6 months of an 18- to 24-month period. Measurements of height and of skeletal age were made at the beginning and at 6-month intervals, and results were evaluated in terms of increments in height age and in skeletal age. The rate of increase in height age was significantly increased in the 6 months of treatment. This analysis was made by applying the one-tailed ranking test to the difference between height age advance during treatment and that before treatment for each child individually. Similar analysis of increments in skeletal age showed no difference attributable to treatment. The average 6-monthly increment in skeletal age minus height age was calculated for each child for the 12 to 18-month period that included treatment and post-treatment follow-up. This number was subtracted from the increment in skeletal age minus height age during the 6 months preceding treatment. Analysis of these figures showed no significant effect, by either T test or ranking test. However, 2 of the 8 children showed an excess increase in skeletal maturation: one of 6 months and one of 12 months. This observation indicates that caution should be exercised when this drug is used in an effort to improve rate of growth.

## *Plasma Diamine Oxidase as an Index of "High Risk" Pregnancy*

A. L. SOUTHREN*
Department of Medicine
A. B. WEINGOLD
Department of Obstetrics and Gynecology
New York Medical College, New York, N. Y.

The definition of "high risk" pregnancy is currently based upon clinical parameters, many of which have been shown to be inadequate guides to the outcome of a particular pregnancy. In the present study, serial plasma diamine oxidase (DAO) titers (radioassay procedure) were determined in a series of subjects with 1st and 2d trimester complications of pregnancy in an attempt to delineate further the "high risk" group. DAO titers within the normal range consistently indicated the maintenance of pregnancy into the 3d trimester. For this reason the plasma DAO assay is uniquely applicable to problems of the first trimester unlike estriol determinations, which assume prognostic significance toward the latter half of pregnancy. A falling or persistently low level of plasma DAO in early pregnancy was associated with significant fetal wastage. There were, however, some pregnancies with abnormal enzyme titers that continued to successful term deliveries. Despite these live births there is evidence to suggest that infants born of these pregnancies have an increased incidence of neurological impairment. Thus, serial plasma DAO titers appear to be of value both in the identification of the "high risk" group of pregnancies and in the selection of the infant who will require long-term comprehensive observation.

## *DNA, RNA, and Protein Synthesis in Human Lymphocytes Stimulated with Phytohemagglutinin (PHA)*

J. E. Ultmann,* R. A. Arthur, and A. N. Zeitlin

Department of Medicine
Columbia University College of Physicians and Surgeons
Medical Service, Francis Delafield Hospital, New York, N. Y.

When PHA is added to suspensions of blood lymphocytes there occurs a prompt increase in the rate of desoxyribonucleic acid (DNA), ribonucleic acid (RNA), and protein synthesis. A period of growth commences and, during the succeeding 72 hours, a majority of the cells undergo enlargement (transformation) and some enter mitosis. In the present study, the effect of actinomycin D (5 $\gamma$/ml.) and of puromycin (10 $\gamma$/ml.) on DNA, RNA, and protein synthesis *in vitro* of PHA-stimulated normal lymphocytes was measured employing $^3$H-thymidine, $^3$H-uridine, and $^3$H-leucine. Cultures were set up in triplicate employing the technique of Bach and Hirschhorn (*Science 143:* 813, 1964). Inhibitors were added at the same time as the tracers and isotope incorporation was studied over a 4-hour period. DNA synthesis in PHA cultures is minimal on day 1; however, it increases 20- and 42-fold compared to controls on days 2 and 3 respectively. On days 1, 2, and 3, PHA stimulates RNA synthesis 5-, 13-, and 15-fold, respectively, compared to controls; protein synthesis is increased 3-, 6-, and 14-fold. Actinomycin D inhibits the synthesis of RNA 100%, DNA 80%, and protein 50%, compared to untreated PHA cultures. The results are consistent with the view that actinomycin D, by completely blocking DNA-template function in RNA synthesis, inhibits formation of new RNA(s) and thus inhibits formation of new protein. This decrease of protein synthesis or the direct inhibition by puromycin leads to a decrease of enzyme(s) essential for DNA synthesis. Continuation of protein synthesis at a reduced rate following actinomycin D supports the hypothesis that a portion of the messenger templates is stable.

---

## *Effects of Infusion of Recirculated Pump-Oxygenator Blood*

F. J. Veith,* J. W. C. Hagstrom, S. L. Nehlsen, and M. Deysine

Departments of Surgery and Pathology
Cornell University Medical College

Second Surgical Division, Bellevue Hospital, New York, N. Y.

Pulmonary damage of obscure etiology occurs after pump-oxygenator procedures. To study its pathogenesis, dog blood was recirculated through a sterile system containing heat and gas exchangers. Aliquots of this blood or its derived plasma or washed cells were infused intra-arterially into 10 dogs, or intravenously into 5. Portal, systemic and pulmonary, hemodynamics and pulmonary function and morphology were monitored before, during, and after infusion. Recirculated blood or plasma infusion by either route regularly produced elevation of pulmonary vascular resistance, compliance and impaired gas exchange. Morphologically, recipients showed varying degrees of pulmonary damage characterized by hemorrhage and edema. Distinctive periarterial hemorrhage was an early or minimal finding that preceded all other changes, and was identical to that in lungs of patients dying after cardiopulmonary bypass and in dog lungs after venovenous bypass. Unrecirculated blood and washed cells failed to produce these changes. These results exclude many proposed causes of postperfusion damage and indicate that it results primarily from injury to small arteries or their vasa vasorum, mediated by a plasma alteration or factor that exerts specific effects on noncapillary pulmonary vasculature and is unaffected by passage through a capillary bed.

## *Biochemical Investigation of the Inherited Variation in Drug (INH) Acetylation*

W. W. WEBER* AND S. N. COHEN

Department of Pharmacology
New York University School of Medicine
New York, N. Y.

Many drugs are metabolized in the body by reaction with endogenous compounds to form inactive derivatives (e. g., by acetylation or glucuronidation). We are investigating the biochemical basis for the genetically determined variation in the rate of enzymatic transfer of the acetyl group from acetyl coenzyme A to isoniazid (INH) and sulfonamides in man and the rabbit. Our investigations involve the comparison of the acetyltransferase obtained from various INH inactivator genotypes and rely upon knowledge of both the relationship between enzyme concentration and activity and the characteristic kinetic constants of the enzyme.

We have studied the kinetics of the inactivation of INH by acetyltransferase partially purified from rabbit liver (300-fold from the $10^5 \times g$ supernatant). Our initial rate data show that the reaction obeys "ping-pong" kinetics, i.e., the enzyme oscillates between free enzyme and another stable form. The latter is probably acetylated enzyme, since our product inhibition studies show that coenzyme A is a competitive inhibitor with respect to INH and a noncompetitive inhibitor with respect to acetyl coenzyme A.

An enzyme that obeys "ping-pong" kinetics cannot be saturated readily with both substrates, so that the rate of drug acetylation *in vitro* may not be proportional to enzyme concentration. Moreover, the $K_m$ determined with one substrate, in such a system, varies with the concentration of the other substrate, and therefore any single, experimentally determined $K_m$ is not necessarily characteristic of the enzyme. Thus, a more complete kinetic evaluation is necessary to determine the characteristics of each INH acetyltransferase before comparisons of the enzyme derived from the various inactivator genotypes can be made. Such an evaluation of our kinetic data will be presented.

The significance of these findings for studies of other reactions that proceed by complex mechanisms will be discussed with special reference to specific human pharmacological and genetic studies.

# *Effect of Polyene Antibiotics on Lysosomes and Artificial Lipid Structures*

G. WEISSMANN*

Department of Medicine
New York University School of Medicine
New York, N. Y.

Polyene antibiotics such as amphotericin B and filipin kill susceptible cells by reacting with their limiting membranes. Since fever and renal lesions are the toxic effects of polyene antibiotics, their effect on lysosomes and mitochondria was studied. Whereas filipin and etruscomycin (low molecular weight polyenes too toxic for clinical use) disrupted lysosomes from liver, spleen, and leukocytes at both acid and neutral *p*H, amphotericin B and nystatin were only disruptive for *kidney* lysosomes at acid *p*H. Polyenes were effective at concentrations above $10^{-5}M$, and none of the antibiotics proved injurious to mitochondria. Since such differences might result from differences in lipid composition of the target membranes, artificial lipid structures were prepared that resemble natural membranes in response to lytic agents (*J. Molec. Biol. 13*:253, 1965). Filipin and etruscomycin induced leak of marker molecules from phospholipid/long-chain anion spherules prepared in the absence of cholesterol. Amphotericin B and nystatin, in contrast, preferentially disrupted spherules prepared with cholesterol; the leaks induced by these varied directly with the molar ratio of cholesterol. Neither variations in sign or amount of charged components of the spherules affected polyene action, as shown by varying the molar percentages of cationic stearyl amine and anionic dietylphosphate from 5 to 20% of the total spherule lipid. It was concluded that polyene antibiotics can rupture synthetic membranes by interactions with membrane phospholipids alone; however, some polyenes (amphotericin B) require an optimum phospholipid/cholesterol ratio. The toxicity of the polyene antibiotics may be due to their interaction with membrane components common to both microorganism and host.

# Career Scientists of The Health Research Council of the City of New York*

THE COUNCIL OF THE ASSOCIATION OF CAREER SCIENTISTS
OF THE HEALTH RESEARCH COUNCIL OF THE CITY OF NEW YORK

Saul J. Farber
C. Andrew L. Bassett
Matthew J. Freund
Jerome P. Parnell

A

Alexander, Hattie E.
Dept. of Pediatrics
Columbia Univ. Coll. of Phys. & Surg.

Al-Askari, Salah
Dept. of Urology
New York University Medical Center

August, Joseph T.
Dept. of Molecular Biology
Albert Einstein College of Medicine

Auld, P. A. McF.
Dept. of Pediatrics
Cornell University Medical College

B

Bank, Norman
Dept. of Medicine
New York University Medical Center

Bassett, C. Andrew L.
Dept. of Orthopaedic Surgery
Columbia Univ. Coll. of Phys. & Surg.

Becker, Frederick F.
Dept. of Pathology
New York University Medical Center

Beller, Fritz K.
Dept. of Obstetrics and Gynecology
New York University Medical Center

Benacerraf, Baruj
Dept. of Pathology
New York University Medical Center

Benjamin, William
Dept. of Medicine
Columbia Univ. Coll. of Phys. & Surg.

Bennett, Dorothea
Dept. of Anatomy
Cornell University Medical College

Berkovich, Sumner
Dept. of Pediatrics
S.U.N.Y. Downstate Medical Center

Bernheimer, Harriet P.
Dept. of Medicine
S.U.N.Y. Downstate Medical Center

Bertles, John F.
Dept. of Medicine
Columbia Univ. Coll. of Phys. & Surg.

Bitensky, Mark W.
Dept. of Medicine
New York University Medical Center

Blanc, William A.
Dept. of Pathology
Columbia Univ. Coll. of Phys. & Surg.

Brachfeld, Norman
Dept. of Medicine
Cornell University Medical College

Bradley, Thomas B., Jr.
Dept. of Medicine
Albert Einstein College of Medicine

Briehl, Robin W.
Dept. of Physiology
Albert Einstein College of Medicine

Britton, Richard C.
Dept. of Surgery
Columbia Univ. Coll. of Phys. & Surg.

Brooks, Dana C.
Dept. of Anatomy
Cornell University Medical College

Burman, Sheldon O.
Dept. of Surgery
New York Medical College

C

Camerini-Davalos, R. A.
Dept. of Medicine
New York Medical College

Canfield, Robert E.
Dept. of Medicine
Columbia Univ. Coll. of Phys. & Surg.

Carroll, Hugh J.
Dept. of Medicine
S.U.N.Y. Downtown Medical Center

* As of October 15, 1966.

Chambers, Robert W.
Dept. of Biochemistry
New York University Medical Center
Chinard, Francis P.
Dept. of Medicine
New York University Medical Center
Christian, Charles L.
Dept. of Medicine
Columbia Univ. Coll. of Phys. & Surg.
Clauss, Roy H.
Dept. of Surgery
New York University Medical Center
Cohen, Burton D.
Metabolism Laboratory
Bronx-Lebanon Hospital Center
Cohen, Morton I.
Dept. of Physiology
Albert Einstein College of Medicine
Cone, Lawrence A.
Dept. of Medicine
New York Medical College
Corcos, Josue M.
Dept. of Medicine
New York Medical College
Cox, Rody P.
Dept. of Medicine
New York University Medical Center

D

Daly, Marie M.
Dept. of Biochemistry
Albert Einstein College of Medicine
Darnell, James E., Jr.
Dept. of Biochemistry
Albert Einstein College of Medicine
Davis, Robert P.
Dept. of Medicine
Albert Einstein College of Medicine
de Harven, Etienne P.
Dept. of Cytology
Sloan-Kettering Institute
Del Guercio, Louis R. M.
Dept. of Surgery
Albert Einstein College of Medicine
Dorn, Gordon L.
Dept. of Genetics
Albert Einstein College of Medicine
Dreizen, Paul
Dept. of Medicine
S.U.N.Y. Downstate Medical Center
Drucker, William D.
Dept. of Medicine
New York University Medical Center
Dunham, Edward T.
Dept. of Physiology
Albert Einstein College of Medicine

E

Elsbach, Peter
Dept. of Medicine
New York University Medical Center
Enson, Yale
Dept. of Medicine
Columbia Univ. Coll. of Phys. & Surg.

F

Feigelson, Philip
Dept. of Biochemistry
Columbia Univ. Coll. of Phys. & Surg.
Feldman, Daniel S.
Dept. of Neurology
S.U.N.Y. Downstate Medical Center
Fikrig, Senih M.
Dept. of Pediatrics
New York University Medical Center
Fox, Charles L., Jr.
Dept. of Surgery
Columbia Univ. Coll. of Phys. & Surg.
Franklin, Edward C.
Dept. of Medicine
New York University Medical Center
Freund, Matthew J.
Dept. of Pharmacology
New York Medical College
Friedman, Eli A.
Dept. of Medicine
S.U.N.Y. Downstate Medical Center

G

Gerber, Donald A.
Dept. of Medicine
S.U.N.Y. Downstate Medical Center
Gesner, Bertram M.
Dept. of Medicine
New York University Medical Center
Gidez, Lewis I.
Dept. of Biochemistry
Albert Einstein College of Medicine
Gilder, Helena
Dept. of Surgery
Cornell University Medical College
Giles, Joan P.
Dept. of Pediatrics
New York University Medical Center

Goetz, Robert H.
Dept. of Surgery
Albert Einstein College of Medicine
Goodman, DeWitt S.
Dept. of Medicine
Columbia Univ. Coll. of Phys. & Surg.
Goodman, Irving
Dept. of Biochemistry
Columbia Univ. Coll. of Phys. & Surg.
Gordon, Edwin E.
Dept. of Medicine
Albert Einstein College of Medicine
Gordon, Harry H.
Dept. of Pediatrics
Albert Einstein College of Medicine
Gorstein, Fred
Dept. of Pathology
New York University Medical Center
Gottfried, Eugene L.
Dept. of Medicine
Albert Einstein College of Medicine
Grant, Lester H.
Dept. of Medicine
New York University Medical Center
Grayzel, Arthur I.
Dept. of Medicine
Albert Einstein College of Medicine
Greenbaum, Lowell M.
Dept. of Pharmacology
Columbia Univ. Coll. of Phys. & Surg.
Griffiths, Sylvia P.
Dept. of Pediatrics
Columbia Univ. Coll. of Phys. & Surg.
Grollman, Arthur P.
Dept. of Medicine
Albert Einstein College of Medicine
Gurpide, Erlio
Dept. of Biochemistry
Columbia Univ. Coll. of Phys. & Surg.

H

Haft, David E.
Dept. of Medicine
New York Medical College
Halac, Elias
Dept. of Pediatrics
New York University Medical Center
Hays, Richard M.
Dept. of Medicine
Albert Einstein College of Medicine
Heinemann, Henry O.
Dept. of Medicine
Columbia Univ. Coll. of Phys. & Surg.
Herbert, Victor D.
Dept. of Hematology
The Mount Sinai Hospital
Hilton, James G.
Renal-Endocrine Laboratory
St. Luke's Hospital
Hirschhorn, Kurt
Dept. of Medicine
New York University Medical Center
Hollenberg, Milton
Dept. of Medicine
Cornell University Medical College
Holt, L. Emmett, Jr.
Dept. of Pediatrics
New York University Medical Center

I

Ioachim, Harry L.
Dept. of Pathology
Columbia Univ. Coll. of Phys. & Surg.

J

Jaffé, Ernst R.
Dept. of Medicine
Albert Einstein College of Medicine
Jahiel, Rene I.
Dept. of Public Health
Cornell University Medical College
James, Leonard S.
Dept. of Pediatrics
Columbia Univ. Coll. of Phys. & Surg.
Javitt, Norman B.
Dept. of Medicine
New York University Medical Center
John, Erwin R.
Dept. of Psychiatry
New York Medical College
Josephson, Alan S.
Dept. of Medicine
S.U.N.Y. Downstate Medical Center

K

Kao, Frederick F.
Dept. of Physiology
S.U.N.Y. Downstate Medical Center
Karpatkin, Simon
Dept. of Medicine
New York University Medical Center
Kavaler, Frederic
Dept. of Physiology
S.U.N.Y. Downstate Medical Center

Kaye, Donald
Dept. of Medicine
Cornell University Medical College

Kaye, Gordon I.
Dept. of Surgical Pathology
Columbia Univ. Coll. of Phys. & Surg.

Kelly, William G.
Dept. of Pharmacology
Columbia Univ. Coll. of Phys. & Surg.

Kinney, John M.
Dept. of Surgery
Columbia Univ. Coll. of Phys. & Surg.

Korein, Julius
Dept. of Neurology
New York University Medical Center

Krasnow, Norman
Dept. of Medicine
S.U.N.Y. Downstate Medical Center

L

Lamm, Michael E.
Dept. of Pathology
New York University Medical Center

Langner, Thomas S.
Dept. of Psychiatry
New York University Medical Center

Lee, Kwang S.
Dept. of Pharmacology
S.U.N.Y. Downstate Medical Center

Lending, Miriam
Dept. of Pediatrics
New York Medical College

Lesser, Gerson T.
Dept. of Medicine
New York University Medical Center

Levine, Bernard B.
Dept. of Medicine
New York University Medical Center

Levine, O. Robert
Dept. of Pediatrics
Columbia Univ. Coll. of Phys. & Surg.

Lieberman, Marvin
Committee on Special Studies
The New York Academy of Medicine

Louria, Donald B.
Dept. of Medicine
Cornell University Medical College

M

MacLeod, John
Dept. of Anatomy
Cornell University Medical College

Marcus, Donald M.
Dept. of Medicine
Albert Einstein College of Medicine

Marmur, Julius
Dept. of Biochemistry
Albert Einstein College of Medicine

Marsh, Donald J.
Dept. of Physiology
New York University Medical Center

May, Charles D.
Dept. of Pediatrics
New York University Medical Center

Miescher, Peter A.
Dept. of Medicine
New York University Medical Center

Miller, Orlando J.
Dept. of Obstetrics and Gynecology
Columbia Univ. Coll. of Phys. & Surg.

Moreno, Augusto H.
Dept. of Surgery
New York University Medical Center

Morse, Jane H.
Dept. of Medicine
Columbia Univ. Coll. of Phys. & Surg.

Moser, Hermann A.
Dept. of Biochemistry
Columbia Univ. Coll. of Phys. & Surg.

N

Neu, Harold C.
Dept. of Medicine
Columbia Univ. Coll. of Phys. & Surg.

New, Maria I.
Dept. of Pediatrics
Cornell University Medical College

O

Oppenheimer, Jack H.
Endocrine Research Laboratory
Montefiore Hospital

Orti, Eduardo
Dept. of Pediatrics
S.U.N.Y. Downstate Medical Center

Ovary, Zoltan
Dept. of Pathology
New York University Medical Center

P

Parker, Frank S.
Dept. of Biochemistry
New York Medical College

Parnell, Jerome P.
Dept. of Anatomy
S.U.N.Y. Downstate Medical Center
Paulsen, Elsa P.
Dept. of Pediatrics
Albert Einstein College of Medicine
Phillips, Louise L.
Dept. of Obstetrics and Gynecology
Columbia Univ. Coll. of Phys. & Surg.
Piomelli, Sergio
Dept. of Pediatrics
New York University Medical Center
Piore, Nora K.
Dept. of Economics
Hunter College
Plentl, Albert A.
Dept. of Obstetrics and Gynecology
Columbia Univ. Coll. of Phys. & Surg.
Potter, Jacobus L.
Dept. of Medicine
New York University Medical Center

R

Ranney, Helen M.
Dept. of Medicine
Albert Einstein College of Medicine
Rapaport, Felix T.
Dept. of Surgery
New York University Medical Center
Rayport, Mark
Dept. of Neurological Surgery
Albert Einstein College of Medicine
Ribble, John C.
Dept. of Medicine
Cornell University Medical College
Richter, Goetz W.
Dept. of Pathology
Cornell University Medical College
Rifkind, Richard A.
Dept. of Medicine
Columbia Univ. Coll. of Phys. & Surg.
Rosenberg, Abraham
Dept. of Biochemistry
Columbia Univ. Coll. of Phys. & Surg.
Rothenberg, Sheldon P.
Dept. of Medicine
New York Medical College
Rothfield, Lawrence I.
Dept. of Molecular Biology
Albert Einstein College of Medicine
Ruben, Robert J.
Dept. of Otolaryngology
New York University Medical Center
Rudman, Daniel
Dept. of Medicine
Columbia Univ. Coll. of Phys. & Surg.

S

Sandson, John I.
Dept. of Medicine
Albert Einstein College of Medicine
Schachter, David
Dept. of Medicine
Columbia Univ. Coll. of Phys. & Surg.
Scheinberg, Labe C.
Dept. of Neurology
Albert Einstein College of Medicine
Seidman, Irving
Dept. of Pathology
New York University Medical Center
Shapira, Daniel
Dept. of Surgery
Albert Einstein College of Medicine
Shinowara, George Y.
Dept. of Pathology
New York University Medical Center
Siegel, John H.
Dept. of Surgery
Albert Einstein College of Medicine
Silber, Robert
Dept. of Medicine
New York University Medical Center
Silverman, William A.
Dept. of Pediatrics
Columbia Univ. Coll. of Phys. & Surg.
Simon, Eric J.
Dept. of Medicine
New York University Medical Center
Siskind, Gregory W.
Dept. of Medicine
New York University Medical Center
Snyderman, Selma E.
Dept. of Pediatrics
New York University Medical Center
Sobel, Edna H.
Dept. of Pediatrics
Albert Einstein College of Medicine
Solish, George I.
Dept. of Obstetrics and Gynecology
S.U.N.Y. Downstate Medical Center
Soskind, Leo
Dept. of Neurological Surgery
New York University Medical Center
Southren, Aaron L.
Dept. of Medicine
New York Medical College

Speirs, Robert S.
Dept. of Anatomy
S.U.N.Y. Downstate Medical Center

Spritz, Norton
Dept. of Medicine
Cornell University Medical College

Steinberg, Israel
Depts. of Radiology and Medicine
Cornell University Medical College

Stracher, Alfred
Dept. of Biochemistry
S.U.N.Y. Downstate Medical Center

Stuckey, Jackson H.
Dept. of Surgery
S.U.N.Y. Downstate Medical Center

Summers, Donald F.
Dept. of Microbiology
Albert Einstein College of Medicine

Switzer, Sam
Dept. of Medicine
Albert Einstein College of Medicine

T

Taketomo, Yasuhiko
Dept. of Neurology and Neurosurgery
St. Vincent's Hospital

Tobin, Mark S.
Dept. of Medicine
Brookdale Hospital Center

Turino, Gerard M.
Dept. of Medicine
Columbia Univ. Coll. of Phys. & Surg.

U

Ultmann, John E.
Dept. of Medicine
Columbia Univ. Coll. of Phys. & Surg.

V

Vande Wiele, Raymond L.
Dept. of Obstetrics and Gynecology
Columbia Univ. Coll. of Phys. & Surg.

Veith, Frank J.
Dept. of Surgery
Cornell University Medical College

W

Wallach, Stanley
Dept. of Medicine
S.U.N.Y. Downstate Medical Center

Warner, Jonathan R.
Dept. of Biochemistry
Albert Einstein College of Medicine

Weber, Wendell W.
Dept. of Pharmacology
New York University Medical Center

Weinstein, I. Bernard
Dept. of Medicine
Columbia Univ. Coll. of Phys. & Surg.

Weissman, Gerald
Dept. of Medicine
New York University Medical Center

Weitzman, Elliot D.
Dept. of Neurology
Albert Einstein College of Medicine

Weser, Elliott
Dept. of Medicine
Cornell University Medical College

Windhager, Erich E.
Dept. of Physiology
Cornell University Medical Center

Winkelman, James W.
Dept. of Pathology
New York University School of Medicine

Winters, Robert W.
Dept. of Pediatrics
Columbia Univ. Coll. of Phys. & Surg.

Wittner, Murray
Dept. of Pathology
Albert Einstein College of Medicine

# THE MUNICIPAL HOSPITALS OF NEW YORK CITY*

REPORT BY THE
COMMITTEE ON PUBLIC HEALTH
THE NEW YORK ACADEMY OF MEDICINE

A CONTEMPORARY observer may see more than a hint of irony in the fact that the New York City hospital system had its faint beginnings in a "Publick Workhouse and House of Correction" built in 1736 on the present site of City Hall. One room in the House of Correction was set apart as a hospital ward with six beds.

Early in the second decade of the 19th century, the institution was moved to Bellevue Farm fronting on the East River. Two hospital pavilions were established near a pesthouse which had been erected some years earlier. As a result of various changes—the removal of children, prisoners, the mentally ill—the buildings on the Farm became devoted exclusively to the care of the sick. This is how the present Bellevue Hospital evolved. In 1837, the pesthouse was moved to Blackwell's Island and was named the Smallpox Hospital of the City of New York.

Five years before the American colonies declared their independence from the British, a charter was secured by a corporation known as The Society of the Hospital of the City of New York in America. Because of the war, the hospital was not opened till 1791. In 1810, the name of the corporation was changed to The Society of the New York Hospital.

The first organized outpatient program was begun in 1791 when the New York Dispensary was opened as a result of the combined efforts of the Reverend John Rogers and the City Medical Society. The Dispensary gave aid to "persons who, when deprived by disease of the earnings of their daily labor are also deprived of the means of procuring the medical assistance necessary for their relief."

In the wake of an epidemic of yellow fever that struck New York City in 1798, many pregnant women were left destitute in consequence of the death of their husbands. A group of sympathetic persons, including Dr. David Hosack, organized the Society of the Lying-In Hospital. But the Society was unable to raise sufficient funds to establish a separate institution and, in 1801, its leaders entered into an arrangement with New York Hospital to provide a special lying-in ward. The Society contributed funds toward the maintenance of the ward. The arrangement lasted for 26 years and was terminated by the action of the governors of New York Hospital. But by then there was in operation a New York Asylum for Lying-in Women.

The annals of the city reveal that from the earliest days there was great concern about the mentally ill. The almshouse was their first refuge. In 1826, separate wards were opened at Bellevue for the care of these patients. Even earlier, the Society of the New York Hospital tried to accommodate mental patients.

*Approved by the Committee on Public Health, February 6, 1967.

A special building to house the mentally ill was erected in 1808. But this facility soon proved to be inadequate, and a new building was opened in 1821. Called the Bloomingdale Asylum, it was located not far from the present site of St. Luke's Hospital.

Work on the so-called Municipal Lunatic Asylum on Blackwell's Island was begun in 1835 but was not completed till 13 years later. And although the hospital had been planned for 200 patients it immediately had a population of 400 mentally ill. Thus it is clear that overcrowding in institutions for the care of the mentally ill is an old story in New York City.

Specialization—except for the treatment of contagious and mental diseases—was not a significant factor in the hospitals during the early days of the 19th century. The first specialized hospital was the Eye Infirmary, established in 1818. Three years later, the institution was incorporated as the New York Eye Infirmary and shortly afterwards a department for the treatment of diseases of the ear was added. In 1856, the New York Eye and Ear Infirmary settled at its present location and a new building was erected to accommodate inpatients as well.

The development of hospitals in Brooklyn followed a similar pattern. In 1832, the first hospital provision was made in connection with the poorhouse at Flatbush. Later, a lunatic asylum was erected within the boundaries of the poorhouse property. This hospital quickly became overcrowded and, in 1845, a new building for the care of the mentally ill was opened.

A new institution known as the Brooklyn City Hospital was incorporated in 1845 and began to operate under the auspices of the Brooklyn Association for Improving the Condition of the Poor. Before the hospital building was erected, patients were treated at the Brooklyn City Dispensary.

In the 10 years between 1850 and 1860, 12 hospitals and 5 or 6 independent dispensaries came into existence, and the hospitals already functioning were developed further. The impetus for this development derived chiefly from two sources: the growth of the city; and the great advancement of medical knowledge that took place at that time. Within this period, Bellevue Hospital became an important teaching institution. The City Hospital on Blackwell's Island, known later as the Charity Hospital, was placed under the direction of the Medical Board of Bellevue Hospital.

Prior to 1848 responsibility for medical work at Bellevue was vested in a so-called Resident Physician who was appointed by the Common Council. In that year, a reform was instituted whereby the hospital was governed by a board of eminent medical men, and regular instruction in clinical practice was begun. Conditions improved very rapidly and, in 1861, a medical school was opened in conjunction with the hospital.

Another important development became apparent at that time. Hospitals no longer were regarded as institutions for the poor exclusively. They began to be patronized by patients who were able to pay for service. St. Vincent's Hospital, built in 1850, was the first to provide comfortable private rooms for paying patients. It also was the first denominational hospital in the city.

The opening of St. Vincent's Hospital was followed quickly by the establishment of St. Luke's Hospital and of the Jews' Hospital of the City of New York—the forerunner of The Mount Sinai Hospital. The first hospital to be built by an immigrant group was the German Hospital now known as Lenox Hill Hospital. Also during this period there came into existence the Home and Hospital for

Colored People, now known as Lincoln Hospital.

Grants by New York City and the state led to the establishment of the Woman's Hospital, which is closely associated with the name of Dr. J. Marion Sims. In 1853, the Infirmary for Women and Children was established in order to give indigent women the opportunity to consult physicians of their own sex, to assist educated women in the study of medicine, and to form a school of instruction in nursing and public health.

One year before the German Dispensary was organized in 1856, a number of German physicians and surgeons in Brooklyn combined to institute a charitable medical service in their community. This was merged shortly thereafter with the newly founded St. John's Hospital. In the following year, the Long Island College Hospital was incorporated for the dual purpose of "maintaining a public hospital" and "for promoting medical science and instruction in the department of learning connected therewith."

The first hospital in Queens was St. John's, founded in 1861, the same year in which the Samuel R. Smith Infirmary was started on Staten Island.

A school for professional nurses was begun in 1873 at Bellevue Hospital. This was in response to the keenly felt need to replace almshouse and penitentiary inmates who worked as hospital helpers. The school at Bellevue was directed by a nurse who had organized a nursing school at St. Thomas Hospital in London; she was chosen by Florence Nightingale.

In rapid succession, hospitals of one kind or another were established in various sections of what came to be the five boroughs of the City of New York. Scientific development, individual initiative, philanthropy, the burgeoning population, and the rapid extension of the city boundaries combined to produce a considerable number and variety of medical institutions. But the situation was far from satisfactory, according to some observers. An examination of the trend of hospital development showed a lack of a conscious directing agency.

In 1875 the hospitals treating contagious diseases were placed under the jurisdiction of the city's Department of Health, which had been established a short time earlier. In general, it was noted that the hospital situation and the responsibility for the sick poor was in a confused condition. Inasmuch as municipal hospitals had developed in connection with relief of the poor, most of the city hospitals had evolved under the aegis of the overseers of the poor. In 1902 Bellevue and several other municipal hospitals in Manhattan and the Bronx were removed from the Department of Charities and placed under the jurisdiction of a Board of Trustees appointed by the mayor. This action was taken with a view to freeing the hospital system from political interference.

By 1911 there existed three groups of hospitals maintained by the city: one under the direction of the Department of Health; a second group supervised by the Department of Welfare; and a third group consisting of a number of hospitals located in various parts of the city. The lack of one central authority was reflected in the considerable variation in the medical standards of the respective institutions. Waste and corruption also were factors that diminished the effectiveness of the municipal hospital system.

Early in 1911 the Committee on Public Health of The New York Academy of Medicine was called into being at the request of the Bureau of Municipal Research, a voluntary agency engaged in studying the problems of the New York City government. One of the charges to the new Committee was the responsibility for scrutinizing the budget of the hospital system. In fact, for a long time thereafter, an annual scrutiny of the budgets of the city's hospitals was a regular activity of the Committee.

Very soon after it was established, the Committee recognized the need for a single Department of Hospitals administered by a commissioner. The Committee made efforts in 1911, 1921, and again in 1925 to win acceptance for its recommendation to establish a Department of Hospitals. In 1927, the Committee joined with a group appointed by the mayor to work out a plan for consolidation of the municipal hospitals. Most of the recommendations advanced by the Committee on Public Health were accepted, and the Department of Hospitals came into being in 1929.

The Hospital Council of Greater New York was established in 1938 to coordinate and improve the hospital and health services of New York City through planning the development of these services in relation to measured community needs and the available resources. Its Master Plan, issued in April 1947, was intended to serve as a flexible guide to the development of hospital and health services for the people of New York City. This plan recommended the establishment of three types of general care hospital: community; regional; and central. In addition to providing the general services of a community hospital, the latter two types of institutions were to have a larger scope in their range of specialties and would serve a wider area. The need for general care beds in each area in each borough was estimated.

In 1961 the Hospital Council of Greater New York was converted by law into the Hospital Review and Planning Council of Southern New York, Inc., and its domain was expanded from the five boroughs of New York City to include the 14 counties comprising the southern tier of New York State.

In 1966 the number of general hospitals in New York City had reached 129, of which 77 were voluntary, 17 municipal, and 35 proprietary. These figures attest to the remarkable growth of hospitals in New York City over 2 centuries.

This sketch, depicting the development of hospitals and, particularly, of the municipal hospital system, provides background and perspective on the present situation. It also shows that the very beginning and early work of the Committee on Public Health was closely linked with the city hospitals.

## Mounting Troubles

For many years the municipal hospital system has been showing signs of rigidity and deterioration traceable to the mode of operation imposed by the city government. Controls and restraints instituted in the name of good government under the professed intent to keep things honest and fair had been proliferating over the years. Narrow budgetary policies and Civil Service restrictions combined to put the administration of the Department of Hospitals in a straitjacket. Red tape and bureaucracy ruled supreme as the hospital system, and the individual units were all the while weakening. Unionization of personnel was one more drain. To compound the difficulties, the city pursued a policy of providing capital funds for construction of hospitals but of being miserly in their maintenance. It is impossible to overestimate the shackling and paralyzing effect of these policies and practices; they alone would have dragged down a healthy system. But upon this rapidly declining system already beset, overburdened, and strangled, came demands from another quarter.

In 1919 the American Medical Association had emphasized that the primary purpose of a hospital internship was the training of a physician. The full impact of this pronouncement was not felt until much later. An intern and residency program was developed, and hospitals had to have an acceptable program before they could receive approval. The medical schools of the United States did not graduate enough physicians to fill all the openings for interns in hospitals. The growth of specialization, the method of distributing interns, and the conditions for approval of an educational program had the effect of favoring hospitals affiliated with medical schools. Many nonaffiliated hospitals resorted to interns trained abroad; other hospitals were not able to obtain any interns.

Because of the decline of many of the municipal hospitals and the shortage of interns created by a demand that exceeded supply, the municipal hospitals were among those that were less successful in obtaining medical manpower. A shortage of nurses became equally critical.

In this desperate situation, the city turned to the expedient of affiliation. An extensive program of contracts was entered into by the city in 1961 whereby medical schools and well-staffed voluntary hospitals acted in essence as employment agencies for medical manpower in the municipal institutions. It should be said at once that the effects of the affiliation program were not uniform. Undoubtedly some affiliations improved the situation; others were less successful.

In retrospect it is possible to recognize mistakes made in the rush of arrangements. For one thing, not all hospitals should have been affiliated. Second, a weak municipal hospital should not have been affiliated with a weak voluntary. Third, disruption of some experienced attending services that were already functioning had serious effects. Finally, in some instances there was dual authority with all its complications.

Under the pressure of meeting educational demands superimposed upon a system under administrative restrictions set by the city government, the total weight of the handicaps was so severe that the stresses and strains began to show. Beginning in the mayoralty campaign in 1965 and continuing until the present time, there have been almost continuous headlines about the unsatisfactory operation of municipal hospitals in New York City. There has been no lack of surveys and recommendations. One survey after another has revealed shortcomings; many of these defects are neither recent nor secret. It would be difficult to add any new discoveries of faults in the hospital system. The list of inadequacies is fairly long, and it would serve little purpose to reiterate them as well as the spectacular and dramatic charges that have appeared almost daily.

## Deliberations and Conclusions

The Committee's approach to the present situation in the municipal hospital was strictly positive and constructive. Its primary concern was that the people of New York City should receive excellent hospital care in these municipal institutions. Its objective was therefore that these hospitals be lifted to such a level that they can perform their service and responsibilities in an exemplary manner.

The Committee first reviewed the various shortcomings of the municipal hospitals and system as currently reported. In this way it catalogued and appraised the nature of the defects and impairments. Then came the search for the causes and reasons for these unsatisfactory conditions in order to find a way to overcome or obviate them.

It came to the conclusion that the primary and ultimate cause of the present difficulties was a combination of three restrictive and self-defeating circumstances that have prevailed for years: 1) inappropriate administrative procedure and practice; 2) budgetary restrictions; and 3) limitations in the personnel system.

Red tape and bureaucracy explain much of the difficulty, which has become further complicated by shortage of medical manpower.

It became clear that the most effective remedy would come from reviewing the role of the hospitals and finding a suitable and proper scheme of organization, management, and administration.

At first thought the primary question would seem to be how to improve the municipal hospitals by removing these barriers and impediments. On further reflection it was realized that other recent events had changed the order of questions to be answered. What had been the first question had been superseded. The primary question had become: Are municipal hospitals needed and, if so, what is their purpose? The answer to that question was prerequisite to posing the problem of their improvement.

The original purpose of the municipal hospitals was to care for the indigent. But it may be presumed that the need they have served will soon disappear, now that Medicare and Medicaid have been enacted. Under these laws it is expected that there will be no more indigent patients. Hence the need for the municipal hospitals on that basis will no longer exist.

It is the opinion of the Committee on Public Health that the beds in the municipal hospitals are needed; therefore, the hospitals are needed, but not all the municipal hospitals are worth saving. The buildings are in various stages of obsolescence. It may cost as much to modernize as to build in some instances; hence the most obsolete should be discontinued and new buildings constructed as needed. The condition of the building, location, and the number of beds needed would have to be considered in reaching a decision about the future of each hospital. Those hospitals that are to be retained should no longer be municipal institutions. They should be converted into autonomous community hospitals.

These autonomous community hospitals should be open institutions capable of providing progressive care, including long-term care. Great emphasis should be placed on avoiding duplication of services and equipment as well as authority and location.

With the conversion of the municipal hospitals to autonomous community hospitals, the need for a municipal Department of Hospitals and a Board of Hospitals would no longer exist and they should therefore be abolished. By removing the city from the management of hospitals the difficulties of administrative, budgetary, and personnel practices could be obviated, and a hospital system that would meet the demands of the future could be developed. For it is the opinion of the Committee that the hospitals must have a new organization and administration as well as a new role.

The transition of the municipal to the autonomous community hospitals should be stepwise in orderly progression. The Hospital Review and Planning Council of Southern New York surveyed the physical plants of the city in 1965. These data could be used in conjunction with a Master Plan. As a pattern, the Master Plan of 1947 would be helpful. Its concept is still timely. On the basis of age, condition, capacity, and location of a hospital, as well as avoidance of duplication, the Council could determine which hospitals should be retained and which should be dropped. It could advise on new construction or improvement of an existing plant. All the recommended changes could be effectuated in an orderly way.

Each municipal hospital that is converted to an open autonomous community hospital should be controlled and operated by a trusteeship. The trustees should be public-spirited, knowledgeable citizens drawn from the immediate community. For selection of them, various methods are possible.

The board of each community hospital would be responsible for its total operation. This latter term includes finance, maintenance, and all the nonprofessional and housekeeping activities, as well as the professional services. Management and administration would be responsible to the board.

It is the Committee's further recommendation that a Hospital Authority should be created over all these newly-established community hospitals upon their conversion from municipal status. This Authority should be a quasi-official body. Existing voluntary hospitals and all new establishments in the future should also come under the Hospital Authority.

One of the Authority's functions would be to serve as a central clearing house on finances for the new hospital system. It is amply clear that the hospital of the future will derive most of its income from government funds. Indeed, that point has already been reached by many institutions. Funds for this source are available for both capital construction and maintenance.

The Authority's functions in finance should be of adequate latitude. If the Hospital Review and Planning Council recommended that hospitals be located in specific areas at present without convenient and ample facilities, funds for construction become an immediate consideration. If necessary, the Hospital Authority could float bonds for construction in these areas.

Another function of the Hospital Authority would be to make policy. For example, the present budgetary practices of hospitals do not include provision for depreciation and amortization of future replacements. If this prudent policy were practiced, funds for replacement would be available when the plant becomes obsolete.

The Authority would also provide information and advice to the individual hospitals under its jurisdiction.

The functions of all bodies at present primarily concerned with hospitals should be reexamined in the light of the proposed system. Duplication and functions no longer necessary should be eliminated. New and additional functions should be explored. Perhaps some groups upon reconstitution could be suitably incorporated into the newly created Hospital Authority.

The Committee recommends that the present state of affiliation should be reviewed. It is recognized that it would be difficult and, in instances, ill-advised, to disturb existing relations. Nevertheless, there should be a reexamination of all the present arrangements. As a temporary measure those that are desirable and justifiable should be retained. Any abuses should be abolished; any mistakes rectified.

For the future, in the new setting, any contemplated affiliation should be highly selective. The type of affiliation as well as of the institutions should be carefully considered. Mistakes of the past should be avoided.

These points should be particularly borne in mind:

1) Affiliation should not be construed as necessarily a permanent arrangement.
2) Not all hospitals should be affiliated. Some will not need to be.

3) Two weak hospitals should not be affiliated with each other.

4) There should be no dual authority.

Medical schools could play an important role in the new hospital system. Where feasible, the Central and Regional hospitals under the Master Plan could be associated with them.

Under the proposed system the present new unit of health services in the city government created by executive order in the mayor's reorganization plan would be unnecessary. Hospitals are a large part of the health services. With removal of the hospitals from municipal management those departments performing health services that remain would not justify a superstructure and additional executive level either on grounds of interrelation or longitudinal administration. These functions could be performed effectively by the individual departments. Any benefits claimed for the superstructure of health services could be achieved in a simpler and less expensive way.

## Recommendations

The Committee on Public Health recommends that:

1) The status of each municipal hospital should be reviewed on the basis of its age, condition, capacity, and location to determine whether it should be retained in operation, renovated, or discontinued when feasible, according to a Master Plan.

2) Those hospitals that are to be retained should no longer be municipal institutions but should be converted into autonomous community hospitals. These autonomous community hospitals should be open institutions capable of providing progressive care, including long-term care.

3) With the conversion of the municipal hospitals to autonomous community hospitals, the need for a municipal Department of Hospitals and a Board of Hospitals would no longer exist, and they should therefore be abolished.

4) The transition of the municipal to autonomous community hospitals should be accomplished in orderly progression.

5) Each municipal hospital that is converted to an open autonomous community hospital should be controlled and operated by a Trusteeship. The Trustees should be public-spirited, knowledgeable citizens drawn from the immediate community.

6) A Hospital Authority should be created over all these newly-established community hospitals upon their conversion from a municipal status.

7) The present state of affiliation should be reviewed. For the future, any contemplated affiliation should be highly selective and not necessarily permanent.

8) Under the proposed system the present new unit of health services in the city government created by executive order in the mayor's reorganization plan would be unnecessary.

# WEAVERS AND COMPUTERS

It is a well-known fact—indeed, almost an axiom—that the *New York Times* compensates the New Yorker for the thousand inconveniences, the myriad annoyances, and the *n*-fold exasperations of daily life in the metropolis. This feat the *Times* accomplishes by simple delivery of the news. Encyclopedic in scope, variegated in content, and correct in expression although imperfect in proofreading, the *Times* daily deposits on one's doorstep a conspectus of all that happens in the world and on the nearest planets. This alone makes it worth one's while to live in New York.

Pouring forth its news in abundance, the *Times* must relegate to inner or posterior pages much material that would deserve greater prominence. Therefore the reader is well advised to read each issue through to the end.

On November 17, 1966, those who followed this salutary principle found on the 60th page of the newspaper an article by Bernadette Carey titled "Quick, Compute Me a Nice Tapestry." This surprising contribution explained a new system called "textile graphics" introduced by Janice Lourie of the International Business Machines Corporation.

Mrs. Lourie is engaged in developing new applications for computers. She is said also to have the hobby of weaving textiles. It was natural for her to combine her work with her hobby. This marriage of interests has resulted in "textile graphics," a system for designing textiles by means of an electronic pencil that writes on an oscilloscopic screen connected to a computer. The system has much in common with computerized devices that are beginning to be used for the editing of manuscripts at the University of Pittsburgh and other centers of culture.

To the physicians who read about Mrs. Lourie in the *Times* her work must have seemed utterly remote from medical interests. But a connection is readily demonstrated.

The modern computer is descended from the Hollerith punch-card machine, which was created by Herman Hollerith at the suggestion of Dr. John Shaw Billings (1838-1913), a foremost authority on public health, creator of the *Index-Catalogue*, and architect of the Johns Hopkins Hospital, the New York Public Library and the Peter Bent Brigham Hospital. The Hollerith machine was first used for the eleventh census of the United States, in 1890.[1]

The Hollerith punch-card device is descended from the perforated cards used to guide the work of the famous Jacquard tapestry looms. The system of Jacquard (1752-1834) is considered the culmination of advances made by Bouchon (1725), Falcon (1728) and Vaucanson (1745). The recent application of computers to medical diagnosis can be regarded as a remote descendant of these devices, just as it is also a descendant of the Morgagnian clinicopathological correlation and of the elaborate indices in the *De Sedibus*.[2] The lines of descent are long and they have not ended.

S. J.

*REFERENCES*

1. Billings, J. S. Mechanical methods used in compiling data of the 11th United States Census. *Proc. Amer. Ass. Adv. Sci. 40*:407-409, 1892. See also Rogers, F. B. *Collected Papers of John Shaw Billings*. Chicago, Med. Libr. Ass., 1965, pp. 7 and 207.
2. See also *Bull. Hist. Med. 35*:489-496, 1961 (esp. p. 492 and n. 13).

# The New York Academy of Medicine

## TELEVISED CLINICAL SCIENCE SEMINARS

Tuesday Evenings, 8:30-9:30 P.M.

STATION WNYC—TV UHF—CHANNEL 31

---

**May 2, 1967**

### TROPICAL DISEASES IN AMERICAN TRAVELERS

B. H. KEAN
Professor of Medicine (Tropical Medicine)
Cornell University Medical College

DONALD W. HOSKINS
Assistant Professor of Medicine
Cornell University Medical College

**May 9, 1967**

### IMMEDIATE MANAGEMENT OF THE ACUTELY INJURED

CHARLES F. SCHETLIN
Assistant Professor of Clinical Surgery
New York University School of Medicine
Associate Attending Surgeon
St. Luke's Hospital

RICHARD B. STARK
Associate Professor of Surgery
Columbia University College of
Physicians and Surgeons
Attending Surgeon in Charge of
Plastic Surgery
St. Luke's Hospital

(Continued on following page)

(*Continued*)

**May 16, 1967**

## INFECTIONS OF THE URINARY TRACT

EDWARD H. KASS
Director, Channing Laboratory
Boston City Hospital
Associate Professor of Bacteriology
and Immunology
Harvard Medical School

EDWARD W. HOOK, JR.
Professor of Medicine
Cornell University Medical College

**May 23, 1967**

## SEIZURE DISORDERS

SIDNEY CARTER
Professor of Neurology
Columbia University College of
Physicians and Surgeons

ARNOLD P. GOLD
Assistant Professor of Clinical Neurology
Columbia University College of
Physicians and Surgeons

JAMES F. HAMMILL
Assistant Professor of Clinical Neurology
Columbia University College of
Physicians and Surgeons

**May 30, 1967**

## COMPLICATIONS OF ANTIMICROBIAL THERAPY

EDWARD W. HOOK, JR.
Professor of Medicine
Cornell University Medical College

DONALD KAYE
Assistant Professor of Medicine
Cornell University Medical College

JOHN C. RIBBLE
Assistant Professor of Medicine
Cornell University Medical College

BULLETIN OF
THE NEW YORK ACADEMY
OF MEDICINE

VOL. 43, NO. 6 JUNE 1967

*New York Heart Association*

# CONFERENCE ON POSSIBILITIES AND ACTUALITIES IN THE DELIVERY OF MEDICAL CARE

*Held at the Hotel Waldorf-Astoria, New York, November 21, 1966*

## *Foreword*

The rapid and profound changes in the means for financing and delivering medical care led the New York Heart Association to devote its annual conference on problems in public health to this topic.

Medicare, Medicaid, and the federal program of grants for Regional Medical Programs in heart disease, cancer, and stroke are the major factors in the new developments, and the conference accordingly centered on them. Under the stimulus of these programs, the major medical centers in the country, where high-quality medical care has been concentrated, are attempting to find ways in which to extend quality care more widely, while maintaining high standards. The public, through the formation of local committees of responsible community groups, is indicating in a more effective way than ever before what its needs are and what is expected in medical services.

As a result, a new partnership is emerging among the federal and state governments, the medical centers, and the public in developing flexible, dynamic, high-quality medical care programs for everyone. This can come about only through a continuing exchange to which the New York Heart Association hoped to contribute by convening this conference. The speakers, invited from near and far corners of the United States, were selected because of their direct involvement with the various expanding medical care programs made possible by recent legislation. It is our hope that the presentations will be found informative and will bring about increased understanding of the portent of these programs for the future.

ALFRED P. FISHMAN, *President*
NEW YORK HEART ASSOCIATION

# MUNICIPAL HOSPITALS*

HOWARD J. BROWN

Health Services Administrator of the City of New York

It is a pleasure to be here and to discuss the effect of the new Medicare legislation on the city hospitals. The New York Heart Association has an historic role in upgrading hospital care through its setting of standards. I know this because I used to be an attending physician in one of the Association's approved clinics at the Beth Israel Medical Center and have had an opportunity to sit on one of its committees in which strengthening and broadening its role were considered.

I am taking the basic theme of this conference, *Possibilities and Actualities in the Delivery of Medical Care,* and I am going to dwell more on the possibilities than on the actualities. For we are in a year in which there is a ferment of increasing dissatisfaction with our municipal health services. And for the Health Services Administration I wish to say that only important innovations can bring about solutions for our problems. Or, to put it in another way, simply putting more money into our present programs may improve them, but will not produce the solutions desired.

We are at the end of a period in the administration of city hospitals and shall enter a new one, if not this year, then next. The legislation of this year reflects the desire for new programs. Medicare in essence will finance the present state of affairs. Medicaid, however, allows and suggests comprehensive programs. Children's Bureau grants are available for introducing comprehensive services for children. Last year the Office of Economic Opportunity made grants to develop totally new community programs of care, and this year it increased the money available to about $60,000,000. This act suggests that while the actuality can be simply more of what we have had, the possibility exists for new programs of care for our city hospitals.

The city hospitals and health clinics do more than care for the acutely ill in hospital beds; their clinics and emergency rooms provide

*Presented at the *Conference on Possibilities and Actualities in the Delivery of Medical Care,* held by the New York Heart Association at the Hotel Waldorf-Astoria, New York, N.Y., November 21, 1966.

over 6,000,000 ambulatory visits a year. While the number of beds in city hospitals has been declining, the number of ambulatory visits has been increasing over the last decade. Both in our public home infirmaries and in our general-care hospitals we provide nursing home and custodial care, and in our clinics and mental wards, almost all the psychiatric care for the poor. Solo private practice is passing in low-income neighborhoods because doctors are abandoning them. Our city hospitals are the family doctors for the poor and their low-income neighborhoods. For the first time adequate financing is now available to develop good community health programs. And a basic task for the Health Services Administration is to put together personal health services now scattered in the departments of Health, Hospitals, Mental Health, and Welfare into neighborhood programs of comprehensive personal health care: preventative, diagnostic, therapeutic, and rehabilitative.

The model for this combination has been worked out at the Gouverneur Ambulatory Care Unit on the Lower East Side in New York City and is being reproduced in Watts, in Los Angeles, by the University of Southern California, and in Chicago by the University of Illinois. In this model a patient may have a personal physician and is treated with kindness, but he also has access to all levels of care. High scientific standards are incorporated.

As a keystone of these new programs we shall renovate and update all our district health centers and relate these to hospitals. Medicaid can finance programs that can relieve congestion in our clinics and emergency rooms but, more important, it can bring a neighborhood orientation, the services of a personal physician, and attention to health needs in a social context. While our nursing homes should be attached to general-care hospitals, it is of equal or greater importance that these be related to organized community-care programs so that the aged ill can participate in various levels of care, of which bed care is only one level. The architectural model for our chronic care facilities can be seen in Zurich or in other communities of Switzerland.

The model for emergency rooms may be seen here in the New York Hospital and at the Cincinnati General Hospital. We have developed architectural plans for the type of neighborhood ambulatory care units we want. And so this better programming is the major possibility of the new legislation and of the new coordination of services envisioned in the Health Services Administration.

And now as to actualities. The city hospitals suffer from the "syndrome of the poor law hospital": a syndrome well known to the medical schools in all large cities, for it is common to such hospitals as the Detroit General and the Chicago-Cook County, as well as to municipal hospitals in New York City. There may be an excellent medical staff, and emergencies and critical matters may be well handled. However, there are also antiquated and poorly maintained plants, shortages of supplies and supporting staff, and the personnel is too busy to be always thoughtful. And the day-by-day problems are not well handled.

Medicaid and Medicare can act to lead to reform of these conditions. The major force leading to this reform will be greater public involvement, more patients' rights, and a demand for greater public accountability.

The public accountability must be developed for both the city and the voluntary hospitals. It will of course include public financial reports with careful audits, and it will include assurance of scientific standards, but it must provide accounting of social responsibility. Important to this is the concept of equal access and the provision of a community program.

As long as the city hospital system serves as the residual system for the voluntary hospitals it will always be inferior, for it will be forced to accept the patients not wanted by the professionals and by the administrators of the voluntary hospitals.

Development of this public accountability is essential for reform of the administrative problems of the city hospital; for only when equal access is assured to the voluntary hospital can there be the necessary freedom to use different administrative mechanisms in the city hospitals.

As I have repeatedly announced, we are proposing that our city hospitals become community hospitals that treat persons of all income levels. This is important for several reasons. For one thing, treating only the many-faceted and complicated social and health problems of the poor is wearing to the staff. Of equal importance is it that other income groups are better complainers and will effectively insist on better amenities. Such groups will demand better facilities, more courtesy, and more attention to their demand for personal relationships.

Teaching can be carried out on all income levels. This is being done in Chicago and Detroit. Teaching upgrades quality of care, and other income groups deserve this higher quality as well as the poor. Social problems of other income groups are more manageable to the medical student, and I suspect that learning from all segments of society will result in a better balanced and more human physician. Whatever the truth, patients will have equal rights, and teaching will necessarily be organized to reflect this goal.

The money is at hand to rebuild our city system. Health services have the top priority in the capital budget, and funds are and will be available to renovate our hospitals and to replace obsolete plants. Medicare and Medicaid provide reimbursement of costs and, as we increase our expenditures, these will be reimbursed. Ninety-five per cent of inpatients and about 90 per cent of outpatients are now eligible for Medicare and Medicaid.

There has been much discussion of where new money will go. Since this represents cost reimbursement, it will all go into health services.

Now there is the possibility this year of extra money, in a sense. However the amount of this is as yet uncertain, and is probably overestimated. The Charitable Institution Budget, which pays voluntary hospitals, and payments to private physicians and voluntary clinics will increase, both because of higher payment rates and greater utilization. Since 25 per cent of this is city money it must be balanced against the greater reimbursement in the Department of Hospitals. The result will be a constant expenditure of local tax levy funds, with the increasing state and federal aid providing the money for improvement of the system. Other unknowns at this time are the final rates of reimbursement to be set by the state, and the extent to which patients will leave the city system. To enroll perhaps 3 million people is a vast job and it will take some time to complete. But the important matter is the fact that there will be cost reimbursement.

In meeting our goals for the hospitals and to use the new financing it is necessary to deal more positively with administrative problems of operation:

1) There are certain restrictions in the state and local laws caused by overcentralization and the excessive size of government operation; these result in perpetuation of outmoded traditions of public service. New construction and renovation of facilities are considerably delayed by a provision in the state law that requires multiple contracts for

projects. Without a change in this law, we shall always have difficulty in obtaining speedy renovation and construction. City charter provisions surrounding purchasing make it a long procedure, and they often prevent individualization of choice: a need that is important in the health services. Classification and description of personnel legally required by Civil Service prevent the individualization and change in personnel required for the health industry. These are problems that could be overcome to a large extent by appropriate changes in the law.

2) Decision-making is overly centralized not only in the departments of hospitals and health but in the extent to which decisions for change must also be made in other city agencies, often only by the highest official. To relieve the tremendous pressure on a budget director, a mayor, or a deputy mayor, crude instruments of control such as line budgeting and required accruals have been set up. This means that often important decisions about details of operation can be made only at the level of the mayor, or by the budget director. The job of steering even the creation of a single new post through this maze can be very time-consuming. Securing an increase in salary can be a major task unless one talks to the mayor about it.

3) There is a traditional reluctance on the part of local government to pay competitive salaries to professional and managerial people. In the health field, with its extensive educational requirements and competitive pressures, this causes shortages that constitute a serious handicap. Local governments across the country have not solved this problem, nor have past administrations in New York City. Both this and the difficulty of working with the other requirements of local government have too often deterred both professionals and effective administrators from accepting positions in government. Those who do accept them often experience over the years a loss of initiative because of the complexity of this system. Another tradition of government has been its inability to withstand local community pressures for health facilities that do not represent the most valid use of community resources. Again, this must seem unimportant, but it is essential that the public have an understanding of the problems faced in New York City in improving the health care services: both to obtain public support and to allow the time necessary to effectuate the basic changes required.

In summary: I have discussed some of the possibilities and actualities. The possibilities include broadly comprehensive programs of a human, personal, and neighborhood quality. The possibilities include hospitals, psychiatric programs, and nursing homes of which we as a city can be proud. The extent to which possibilities become actualities will depend on the involvement of what has been missing today—the informed patient and public.

# VOLUNTARY HOSPITALS*

MARTIN CHERKASKY

Director
Montefiore Hospital and Medical Center
New York, N. Y.

THERE is still considerable confusion about the Medicaid Law (Title 19) over how the voluntary hospitals will be paid; how private physicians will be paid, and so forth. There are also significant areas of unresolved problems with regard to Medicare, particularly under Part B, and payments for the services of hospital-based doctors. Despite this, however, this extraordinary social legislation has already had a major effect on this country's voluntary hospitals and will in due course produce a major revolution in the voluntary hospitals: in the areas of finance, patient population, doctors' services, education, public accountability, and control. I should like to touch on each of these points.

In the past, voluntary hospitals have managed to survive by piecing together income from third parties such as Blue Cross and commercial insurance companies; by income from city, state and federal government programs; by self-paying patients; and by the uncertain and fluctuating support of philantrophy. As the country became affluent and third-party insurance grew, the role of philanthropy in maintenance changed significantly. While our situation at Montefiore Hospital may not be typical in all respects, the trend is quite clear. In 1950, with an operating budget of less than 4 million dollars, somewhat more than 1 million dollars was available from philanthropic sources. In 1966, with an operating budget of 18 million dollars, there was approximately $900,000 available from philanthropy. Income from philanthropy decreased from almost one third of the budget to less than 5 per cent of our operating budget.

Each of these sources of payment was governed by different criteria: Blue Cross and other third parties theoretically paid close to cost; the private patient paid what the traffic would bear to subsidize the inadequate payments of the municipality or of welfare departments; while philanthropy tried to fill the gap. In most instances, the inability of

*Presented at the *Conference on Possibilities and Actualities in the Delivery of Medical Care,* held by the New York Heart Association at the Hotel Waldorf-Astoria, New York, N. Y., November 21, 1966.

philanthropy to shoulder ever increasing operating commitments resulted in the necessity for great economies in operation. With the hospitals forced into such fiscal straightjackets, only a few—with easier access to funds or associated with medical schools—were able to take full advantage of the explosion in medical science. These institutions are truly magnificent medical care institutions of high quality and have great opportunity for communal service.

Other voluntary institutions have not fared so well. Indeed, some of the difficulties gleefully pointed out in the municipal and proprietary hospitals are *not* unknown to many of our voluntary hospitals. Another result of this underfinancing has been the obsolescence of voluntary hospitals, a situation that in New York City alone would require more than $400 million to correct. At one fell swoop many of these fiscal inequities and instabilities will be substantially corrected by this new Medicare-Medicaid legislation with many immediate and long-range results.

First, a practice that has long been undesirable will become unnecessary: that of overcharging patients who pay their own way to cover costs for those who do not. Second, all patients who come into the institution virtually without exception will be able to pay the full, legitimate cost of their hospital expense either through their third parties or through Medicaid and Medicare, for the Medicare payment formula was designed to pay full cost and, presumably, Medicaid will follow suit. Third, it will be possible to redirect philanthropic contributions. Instead of attempting to provide large amounts of money—which proved to be inadequate—in an effort to defray the enormous operational costs of modern hospitals, philanthropies, it is hoped, will reexamine their roles and earmark their monies for some of the risk undertakings, such as new program developments and the breaching of new frontiers. With such flexibility in the use of these funds as "seed monies," these new programs and undertakings, when proved feasible, can then be incorporated into hospital operations to be financed by more stable and continuing fund sources.

The control of money is of course closely related to the control of enterprises, and hospitals are no exception. Philanthropic funds, at one time very significant, and at all times visible, were the base for the lay control of hospitals by a small segment of the population. The changing sources of fundamental fiscal support will increasingly sensitize our

**CHANGING SOURCES OF FISCAL SUPPORT:**

*Montefiore Hospital, 1965 and 1967*

| 1965 (%) | 1965 | | 1967 (est.) | 1967 (est.) (%) |
|---|---|---|---|---|
| 48.0% | $7,700,000 | Blue Cross | $5,100,000 | 25.5% |
| 10.6 | 1,700,000 | Municipality | 2,300,000 | 11.5 |
| 23.9 | 3,800,000 | Direct Pay | 3,300,000 | 16.5 |
| 6.9 | 1,100,000 | Philanthropy | 800,000 | 4.0 |
| 10.6 | 1,700,000 | Other | 1,400,000 | 7.0 |
| 0 | 0 | Medicare | 7,100,000 | 35.5 |
| 100.0% | $16,000,000 | TOTAL OPERATING BUDGET | $20,000,000 | 100.0% |

**Nearly 50 per cent of hospitals' 1967 budget will come from tax funds, with precipitous drop in share from Blue Cross.**

voluntary institutions to new forces and new voices. To get an idea of the magnitude of the change in financing, a quick look at the fiscal activity of Montefiore Hospital is enlightening.

Excluding all related enterprises and examining the operation of the hospital alone, a comparison between 1965 and our projection for 1967 is shown in the accompanying table. You will note that income from tax funds was about 10.5 per cent in 1965 and that in 1967 it will be at least 47 per cent. Blue Cross' share of income has dropped precipitously from about 48 per cent to about 25 per cent. In my view, when Medicaid is fully taken into account, the income from tax sources will rise even more, with a concomitant decrease in Blue Cross payments.

I noted previously the disastrous obsolescence that has enveloped the voluntary hospitals because of general omission of monies for depreciation and capital allowances. The Medicare payments and presumably the Medicaid payments and the present Blue Cross formula now provide percentages for capital replacement. This means that if we can once get the voluntary hospital system into a state of good repair, there will be a constant flow of monies to keep them up-to-date.

I have devoted so much of my time to money rather than program, about which I am more concerned, because the finances largely determine the nature of the program and also its possibility. For the first time this industry, considered the third or fourth largest in the country, will move into a period of sound and stable financing, and the hand-to-mouth existence that debilitated this vital resource should be behind us.

While again it is too early to draw definitive conclusions, there is already evidence that the character of the patient population in the hospital has changed, and this will probably continue. When we enfranchised almost 20 million elderly people in the United States who have a high degree of medical risk and a disproportionate per cent of long-term disease problems, we anticipated that the number of older people in the hospitals would rise, and that hospital stays would lengthen. From July 1 through October 31, 1966, Montefiore hospitalized 7 per cent more people over 65 than in the previous year. That patients will stay longer is proved by the fact that despite maximal demands on our beds (over 95 per cent occupancy) we discharged 80 fewer patients in October 1966 than in October 1965. This reduction was achieved despite the fact that our Utilization Committee has been functioning aggressively. This demand for inpatient beds under Medicare and the expected demand under Medicaid make it clear that Utilization Committees, which were set up in response to the law, are going to have to operate in an extremely effective manner if we are not going to be faced with an enormous demand for beds—a demand that we can ill afford to meet, that we should find difficult to maintain and impossible to staff.

Voluntary hospitals in other ways have begun to feel the impact of Medicare and to anticipate the effect of Medicaid. We realize that if we are to make the best use of the precious, costly inpatient bed, if we are to serve all the community and not just the old, we must use every device that serves patients well and that spares the hospital bed for its narrow and specific purpose. To do this, the hospitals have begun to look at their "outpatient departments" in a new way. Until now these departments have been a drain on resources. They were avoided by the better doctors, were hardly used in teaching, and were considered fit for the poor only. The outpatient department now, however, looms large as a means of providing good-quality care and avoiding or shortening inpatient stay. This has been possible before, but only now is the money available to run costly ambulatory services, through Medicare and Medicaid.

Home care has long been talked about as a superb means of providing care to patients within their own homes with great benefit to the patient at a cost markedly less than that of hospital care. Yet this superb device for the care of patients has shown almost no growth in 20 years. More recently, new interest in home care has increased with home-care programs in various stages of development in many communities.

The reason is clear: the pressure for beds—due to the large numbers of long-term illnesses the hospitals must now deal with—plus the monies available under both Part A and B of Medicare have provided the proper combination of need and money to galvanize institutions into action.

The nursing home now takes on special significance to the hospital, for if it is *not* available, the ability to discharge hospital patients will be seriously compromised. Many hospitals are planning nursing home units as a part of their institutions to insure the ready discharge of patients and to make their hospital beds more useful. Further, the requirement of the Medicare Law that nursing homes must have a transfer agreement with hospitals has awakened the interest of the hospitals in the conditions in the nursing homes to which they will discharge their patients. We can look forward to the day when the term "general hospital" will cover not only the services and facilities we know now but will also include a nursing home, a group practice unit, and a home care program.

The key professional figure in hospitals and in all our health services is the doctor. Doctor-hospital relations are already undergoing significant change, which will accelerate because of Medicare-Medicaid legislation. First, the contribution by the doctors of free services to the indigent is finished. Doctors in and out of hospitals will be paid for virtually all medical services. The reluctance of the doctor to work in the outpatient departments has already been lessened in these last few months, for adequate payment for such service is now available. Many more doctors will go on full or part-time salary as Medicare and Medicaid people provide the funds to make this possible. Many doctors who fought the concept of the employment by hospitals of people on a full-time plan will have a change of heart as they are offered attractive paid hospital positions. There are, of course, negatives. Most serious is the elimination of hospital-based specialists such as radiologists and pathologists from inclusion in the hospital reimbursement formula—with the provision that these doctors will be paid by Part B and have separate billing. This prospect has already produced great bitterness in some instances between hospitals and their radiologists—between whom mutually satisfactory relations had been hitherto enjoyed. Separate billing produces a costly administrative problem. It threatens the full-time system, and it will soon increase the cost of medical care significantly, without increasing the quality.

The great expenditure through public funds for physicians' services will bring these physicians under greater and, in my view, appropriate examination with regard to the quality of their services. This matter of the quality of medical care is of importance not only to hospitals but also to the entire society. Medicare provides for virtually no standards of quality for doctors' practice. While the fate of Medicaid will be governed by state and local standards, the reluctance of official agencies to face the wrath of organized medicine has resulted, so far as I can tell, in virtual abandonment of any attempt to set adequate standards for the quality of medical care to be purchased by these public funds. I quote from a resolution passed by the policy-making committee of one of our local medical societies:

> *Certification of Physician's Competency*
>
> RESOLVED: That the Society is unalterably opposed to any system of self-imposed certification of a physician's competency by any governmental agency other than that which is currently the practice.
>
> *Supervision of Quality of Medical Care*
>
> RESOLVED: That the Society is unalterably opposed to any governmental agency evaluating the quality of medical care; and be it further
>
> RESOLVED: That the Society formally approved the continuation of the evaluation of quality care under the criteria that now exist.

Someone must assume the leadership in linking Medicaid money to *quality*. We in the voluntary hospitals must seize the opportunity offered by the Medicaid legislation to develop organized programs of ambulatory care of high quality to serve the public, and to establish the standards that all ambulatory care should achieve.

One of the immediate problems that has faced those voluntary institutions that have a large commitment to graduate teaching at the intern and resident level has been the virtual disappearance of that group of patients upon whom this entire generation and previous generations of physicians were educated—that is, the service or ward population. Every patient will in due course be a private patient and not someone who, under the old arrangement, could be managed primarily by the resident. I am certain that John Knowles will cover this situation in some detail—I should merely like to note that, particularly in surgery, the entire independent nature of the surgeon and his practice will necessarily give way to the "team" approach if we are to continue our educational activities as, of course, the public interest requires.

I should now like to touch upon public accountability and control. Voluntary hospitals have had great freedom to decide what they will do and what they will not do. They have been able, within limits, to decide whom they would care for and what their patient population would be. They have had the freedom to decide what programs they would undertake and those they would decline. This freedom to move and decide has often been related to notions of excellence and creativity; and this, in some measure, is true. Some of our institutions are marvels indeed; but it has become increasingly clear that with greater complexity, rapidly rising costs, greater expectation on the part of the public, these private institutions have not been in fact as responsive to community need and concern as might seem desirable. Even before Medicare and Medicaid, public controls beyond licensing were introduced in our state by the Metcalf-McClusky bill and the Folsom legislation, which strengthened and put teeth in community planning. Hospital construction, whether in existing institutions or in the building of new ones, is now allowed only where it will serve community needs. It is a virtual certainty that with a major part of the financing from tax sources, our voluntary hospitals will become, in effect, public utilities; our governing boards will necessarily take on the complexion of the community we serve; our every move will necessarily answer the question of community interest before it satisfies self-interest. I am not concerned about autonomy, some of which will be lost. My own view is that a blending of voluntary effort with governmental support will free our institutions to realize their full promise in serving our society.

# IMPACT OF MEDICARE ON MEDICAL EDUCATION*

John H. Knowles

General Director
Massachusetts General Hospital
Boston, Mass.

What is good for medical education is good for the care of the patient, and what is good care of patients is good medical education. Teaching and the care of patients are inseparable elements, and the inferior quality of one is reflected ultimately in the other. One cannot attain the highest quality of care without the best teaching and, just as importantly, one cannot enjoy excellence in teaching without demonstrating that the medical wants and needs of the patient-community are being served in optimal fashion. I believe that the first function of any hospital worthy of the name—regardless of the adjective used to describe it—is to care for the sick, and that the attitudes, values, and allocation of resources must reflect this primary concern. Once this is established, teaching and research are added to improve the quality of existing service and to provide for the long-range interests of the community and nation. Woe be unto the hospital that says its first function is teaching and research, and therefore "we need some selected patients to carry out our teaching and research programs"! This, I might add, is the only kind of hospital that should fear the effects of Medicare. I wish to establish these values as those of the hospital I represent.

Medicare has had *no* impact on medical education, if one is referring to visible and established change in undergraduate or graduate educational programs in medical schools and teaching hospitals, or even to alteration of premedical requirements for admission to medical school.

If, however, one is referring to the emotional, intellectual, and financial impact on medical faculties and teaching hospital administrators, there has been considerable turbulence, although there is still no change as yet, of course. All of us have indulged in recurrent debates, which have centered around two questions: 1) What will happen to the teach-

*Presented at the *Conference on Possibilities and Actualities in the Delivery of Medical Care,* held by the New York Heart Association at the Hotel Waldorf-Astoria, New York, N. Y., November 21, 1966.

ing function when everyone is entitled to a private physician and a semiprivate bed? 2) How can we collect fees for professional service under Part B of Title 19, thereby getting our collective hands on what could be enormous sums of money?

Let me say immediately that, first and foremost, I believe these are the wrong questions, as they concern themselves with means and not *ends*. Believing with a passion that excellence in teaching and excellence in patient care are inseparable and interdependent, I should rather see us concern ourselves with the following question, in place of the two just cited.

How can we improve the quality of our care and the quality of our teaching so that the public and our community will be assured of what they want and need: personal care, continuing and comprehensive care, and technically excellent care?

This question asks us to review and improve our goals—for if we accomplish this, we need not be concerned with such questions as what will happen to our teaching patients, or how we can collect the money available for professional care. Simple enough, but problematic and perhaps a reflection of the distorted importance of means such as teaching and research, rather than the ends of teaching and research—the care of the sick and injured and the prevention of disease, all to improve and enhance the quality of life.

Specifically I wish to make certain suggestions for changes at various levels of medical education, changes that must occur if the medical world is to have a hand in shaping legislation in the years to come and, indeed, if it is to adapt successfully and meaningfully and supply solutions to the socioeconomic problems of medical care—problems that have been pushed to the forefront by Medicare.

## Undergraduate, Premedical Education

Undergraduate education in the university becomes differentiated into the special interests of natural and physical science and of mathematics once the individual has declared himself a premedical student. There are at present no social science requirements for admission to medical school. (Of 96 medical schools, 2 require "political science," 3 require "other," and 12 require "unspecified."[1]) There are two opposing views of this, expressed by well-intentioned educators, looking for the best balance between depth and breadth in college education. One view is that breadth is especially necessary for the future doctor and that the humanities and social sciences must receive their full measure of attention along with the biological and physical sciences. Sir Robert Platt has noted in this regard: ". . . the paradox that medicine has won its place in the university not through its humanism, but through becoming a science, and the influence of the university has been to put it further from and not nearer the humanities."[2]

The other view is that the steadily increasing period of medical education must be shortened, and that this can be accomplished by more intensive instruction in the "medical" sciences in college, which therefore will not be repeated in the first year or two of medical school.[3] There is merit here but the intellectual acceleration and constriction of the student's interests may not be desirable. In this view, the humanities and social sciences become embroidery to the physical and biological sciences and mathematics.

The fact is that the undergraduate has little choice today if he wishes to leave little to chance on applying for admission to the medical school. As the Assistant Dean for Admissions of the Faculty of Medicine of the Harvard Medical School stated in answer to the question of how best to gain entry: ". . . the humanist dedicated to working with people but fearing mathematics, who hopes that science will be a minor part of his medical education, stands little chance of being accepted to medical school."[4]

There are two problems here. One is concerned with the prematurely acquired specialism and expertise, the other with the almost universally accepted notion that knowledge of the physical and biological sciences and mathematics (to the inevitable exclusion or competitive underemphasis of the humanities and the social sciences) represents the best preparation for medical school and hence for one's life in medicine.

The hazards of specialism have been discussed by Harlow Shapley, himself a noted scientist, in a general criticism of the undergraduate curriculum:

> Must we climb steeples? In other words, how far should we permit ourselves to go in specialism? Intellectual isolation may be an attempt to escape responsibility.
>
> The habit of steeple-climbing has, alas, helped to divert us from our civic duties. The intellectual, in spite of his specialization, should he not be a soldier in the army that makes democracy and Christian

ethics work?[5]

Shapley admits, however, that some steeple-climbing is necessary for the premedical student "unless the specialized professional training in medicine be prolonged still further toward middle life."

Granted at least some necessary premedical steeple-climbing in the curriculum, is it necessarily true that the steeple to be climbed is the one built with the materials of physical and biological science? Can the medical intellect function only or best on a foundation of natural science? Certainly it is true for those who plan a career in medical research, but is mathematics necessary to the successful practice of medicine? Can intellectual development suitable for a doctor be developed otherwise than through the study of the physical and biological sciences? Why did Virchow say that medicine is a social science and politics was nothing but medicine on a large scale? Why did L. J. Henderson refer to the practice of medicine as "applied sociology"? Could it be that man is, indeed, a social as well as biological animal? Is there *social,* as well as biological ease and disease? And can dis-ease in one system give rise to dis-ease in the other? The answers are obvious. The methods and content of scientific thought are vital disciplines for all educated men, but where does that leave the remainder of the liberal and general education? Is there anything in the humanities and social sciences that relates to medicine or, more importantly, to the well-educated man that we want our doctor to be? Does the following statement by President Nathan M. Pusey of Harvard relate in any way to our physician or, let us say, his collective self, the American Medical Association?

> The humanities have a very special place in a university, especially perhaps because of the pleasure they give, but also because of the heightened effects which experience of them can produce in individuals in terms of enlivened imagination, increased responsiveness, broadened interest, clarified purpose and in the end also, quickened ethical sense.[6]

My view is very simple; premedical education should be horizontal without steeples, for I believe that medicine is a social as well as a physical and biological science, and that it needs the humanities and social sciences and the effects of their study as never before in the history of man. Let the differentiation occur in medical school and beyond, but let us *educate* the man in college.

## Graduate, Medical School Education

Science pervades all for the first 2 years in medical school that is biological and physical science. The last chance to treat at least some of the aspects of medicine with the disciplines of the social sciences* is taken only in several of the present medical schools of this country. Why this exclusion? Not enough time in an already overcrowded curriculum? The "nonscientific" nature of their results? Perhaps all these reasons must be taken into account, but just as important has been the complete segregation of schools of public health from the mainstream of medicine. Such schools do utilize the social sciences when considering the subjects of medical administration and the formulation, organization, and implementation of public health programs. Quite clearly, human attitudes, beliefs, and values play a determining role in the utilization of health services by the recipient public as well as in the implementation of programs by the purveying members of the health profession. Sociological research in medical care has given us invaluable information in many spheres. A brief list of such studies would include the analysis of health wants and needs of communities; the influence of prepaid insurance programs on the utilization of health services; the dynamics of solo versus group practice of medicine; role expectations among the various categories of health workers, including doctors, nurses, social workers, dietitians, and medical scientists; the influence of social and economic class on the receipt and utilization of services; the evaluation of types of organizations designed to give comprehensive, continuing medical care in ambulatory clinics, extended care facilities and homes; the internal organization of the hospital with its paradoxical arrangements of authority and responsibility; the public's attitude toward the general hospital, the mental institution, the public health unit, and so on; the assessment of medical care programs for special population groups such as the medically indigent, dependents of military personnel, the chronic physically and mentally ill; the effect of cultural determinants on the utilization of health services; and the recruitment, development, organization, and retention of health personnel.

Clearly, the results of such studies have tremendous implications for all of us interested in the health of our communities, whether we be the professional purveyors or the inexpert recipients of medical care. The

*The social sciences include sociology, political science, economics, and cultural anthropology. History is usually included but used to be considered a part of the humanities. Psychology in all its forms is included and is "behavioral science."

rational organization, distribution, and utilization of limited and costly health resources are of central importance. The rationalization of the behavior of doctors, nurses, administrators, patients, and so on should facilitate the provision of high-quality medical care for all our people.

I believe that the social science of medicine must be available to the student and its thread should be woven through the 4 years of medical school. To name one subject, the social history, economics, political science, and social psychology of third-party payment for medical services, culminating in Public Law 89-97 in 1965, would be interesting to some of our students. Then, in addition to producing biologists and practicing physicians, we might produce sociologists (and medical administrators) *and* practicing physicians. Or, why not settle for a complete product: a well-educated physician! I have written of this extensively elsewhere and shall not repeat it here.[7-11]

## Postgraduate, Teaching Hospital Education

Here, certain aspects of our current practices must be challenged and changed.

1) Is it true that the best teaching and the best care of patients (remember, they are inseparable and interdependent) are carried out with the *least* supervision of and the most responsibility for the patient by the house staff? Are we adequately grading and individualizing the degree of responsibility for our doctor-in-training in this regard?

2) Do we not persist with certain aspects of the old indentured apprentice system in our teaching hospitals, and should we not develop a corporate responsibility, with a visible organizational (over-all hospital) structure to review, scrutinize, and improve our programs in graduate education? The Millis Commission suggests this. I heartily agree, while disagreeing with its suggestion that the American Medical Association control the evolution of such programs on a national basis. I believe that medical schools and teaching hospitals should carry it out as their corporate responsibility locally *and* nationally in the public interest.

3) Should not the conceptual attitudes of those dedicated to ambulatory services, social service departments, and social psychiatry interests become an integral part of graduate education for *all* in teaching hospitals? Shouldn't we extend our intellectual gaze to the community and bring extended care facilities onto our main educational realm?

Should we not have discovered the great educational opportunities in utilization committees a long time ago and how can we exploit their educational values for the resident staff as well as the visiting physician?

I could ask many more questions. Quite clearly, I cannot answer them all, but I believe I am asking some of the right questions. Let me summarize by reviewing our experience with Medicare at the Massachusetts General Hospital since July 1966.

1) There has been a marked increase in utilization of the hospital by those over 65 years of age, both inpatients (by roughly 10 per cent) and outpatients (70 per cent increase). At the moment, our facilities are overstrained and our short supply of manpower overworked.

2) The patients have not left our teaching (i.e., ward) services, nor have they demanded semiprivate rooms with gray-haired private doctors (except in rare instances). Tradition and the habit of our community will give us ample time to improve our *ends* so that there will never be a mass exodus of patients from teaching hospitals, save for those hospitals that put the care of the patient second and not first. (Coincidentally we have an equally pressing problem in how to extend the full benefits of teaching to *all* our patients, private or teaching service!) Personal, continuing, comprehensive, technically competent, appropriately utilized care, all in a dignified social and physical environment of one class (not two or three classes!) will assure us all the patients in the world.

3) The lack of quality and quantity in extended care facilities has reached critical proportions and is adversely affecting us and our community. Our institution could be transformed into a chronic hospital and nursing home, which would not be the best way of providing acute, curative care for the community or for our doctors in training. In a very subtle fashion, social problems will change our functions of care and teaching—for the best, we hope. Shall we be able to shape the changes or merely remain the passive or even the negativistic recipients of social change? Again, in order to shape and cause change, our educational system must change.

4) We are *not* collecting fees under Part B for our teaching services. We do not believe, at this moment, that any special or privileged group in the hospital should collect these fees, be they house staff or visiting surgeons or hospital administrators. Teaching and supervision of house staff and patients can be carried out and any expense reimbursed the

hospital under Part A, if necessary. What we are doing is reviewing our *ends* of excellence in patient care, which therefore requires excellence in teaching. If improvements are needed, and I believe firmly that they are, and if money is required, we shall find the necessary money to improve our functions. We shall not undergo the self-deceptive subterfuge of collecting money under Part B for functions that haven't changed over the years and for which charges have never been made. The vacuous argument is voiced that if we collect money from Medicare patients under Part B, the patient will somehow think he is getting "private care," or the doctor-patient relation will be improved. I do not believe this thought justifies the dignification of debate.

Medicare has had a large impact on all of us in just the first 5 months of its operation. Yes, over the long run, its effect will be to change medical education for the better, force hospitals to provide one intellectual atmosphere—technically and socially—for the sick, force medical schools and teaching hospitals to extend their influence and standards to extended care facilities, foster increased use of ambulatory facilities and domestic services, and encourage regional planning and coordination with other regional care facilities. Finally, it will force medical educators to change medical curricula and premedical requirements so that the intellectual tools of the social sciences can be brought to bear on the social problems of medicine, just as the natural and physical sciences have been so fruitful in the advance of medicine as a biological science. At the graduate, house-staff level in the teaching hospital, we shall establish corporate and organizational responsibility with the medical school for graduate education while we focus on ways to improve our ends—first, the best care of the sick, which implies, second, the best teaching in their care. One social and physical environment, one teaching environment, and one standard for *all* our patients, whether they are private or "ward" patients. It will not be easy to attain this end but, once it is attained, we need not fear any adverse effects of Medicare nor be concerned with means and administrative gimmicks. We hope that we can look to Medicare for improvement in our care of the sick and in our teaching.

*REFERENCES*

1. Nourse, E. S., ed. *Medical School Admission Requirements: U.S.A. and Canada, 1966-67*, 17th ed. Evanston, Ill., Ass. Amer. Med. Colleges, 1966, p. 3.
2. Platt, R. Progress report to Thomas Linacre: Reflections on medicine and humanism. Linacre Lecture, 1963. *Univ. Quart. 17*:327-40, 1963.
3. Cope, O. and Zacharias, J. *Medical Education Reconsidered.* Philadelphia, Lippincott, 1966.
4. Culver, P. J. What shall I tell my son or daughter? *Harvard Med. Alum. Bull. 38*:19, 1964.
5. Shapley, H. *The View from a Distant Star.* New York, Basic Books, 1963, p. 143.
6. Harvard University. *Annual Report of the President, 1961-1962.* Cambridge, Mass., Harvard Univ. Press, 1962, p. 21.
7. Knowles, J. H. Medical education and the rationalization of Health services. In: *Views of Medical Education and Medical Care.* J. H. Knowles, ed. Cambridge, Harvard Univ. Press. To be published.
8. Knowles, J. H. Medical center and the community health center, *Bull. N.Y. Acad. Med. 40*:713-43, 1964.
9. Knowles, J. H. Experts, enclaves and the public interest, *Conn. Med. 30*:743-48, 1966.
10. Knowles, J. H., ed. *Hospitals, Doctors and the Public Interest.* Cambridge, Mass., Harvard Univ. Press, 1965, p. 333.
11. Knowles, J. H., ed. *The Teaching Hospital: Evolution and Contemporary Issues.* Cambridge, Mass., Harvard Univ. Press, 1966, p. 152.

# PROSPECTS OF FEDERAL PROGRAMS*

JOHN W. CASHMAN

Director, Division of Medical Care Administration
Public Health Service
U.S. Department of Health, Education, and Welfare

A TECHNIQUE of high school debaters is to open a speech by retreating to the dictionary, and my being assigned the title "Prospects of Federal Programs" almost justifies this technique. The dictionary, in a burst of optimism, defines "prospects" as meaning both "that which is hoped for" and "probable result."

While I may be qualified to discuss the *hopes* we hold for federal programs in the health care field, it may well be that the *probable results* will relate more closely to the remarks of the distinguished speakers who have preceded me this morning than to my own prophetic observations.

Nor is this false modesty on my part. In this country health care is a partnership that involves every public and private agency and resource. The areas we are covering today–municipal hospitals, voluntary hospitals, medical education, and private practice–collectively comprise the major portion of the machinery and manpower that the nation applies to the care of health.

Federal programs are designed to implement federal legislation. In the health field federal legislation is the end product of a long process of consultation and discussion to which every group in the country that participates in the health care partnership is invited to make its contribution. In a democracy the *legislative* branch of government authorizes action to meet the expressed needs of the people, and the *executive* branch of the government establishes programs responsive to those needs.

Medicare and Medicaid (and sometime, some*how* we must find better words than these!) do not represent federal inventions, put forward as patented panaceas for national health care problems. As carried out they will represent the majority judgment of informed opinion in

*Presented at the *Conference on Possibilities and Actualities in the Delivery of Medical Care,* held by the New York Heart Association at the Hotel Waldorf-Astoria, New York, N. Y., November 21, 1966.

this country—both expert opinion and lay opinion—concerning feasible methods for expanding the quantity and improving the quality of health care.

It might be well to stress that the animated discussion that continues to surround Medicare and Medicaid should not blind us to the far broader picture of the full range of federal health programs. In recent years federal legislation has created many new health programs. All these must be taken into account in understanding the basic philosophy and evaluating the potential impact of the massive effort now being made on a national scale to raise standards of health care. Merely to list a few major pieces of recent legislation in this area is sufficient to suggest the scope of current activity: the Heart Disease, Cancer and Stroke Act; the Health Research Facilities Act; the Community Health Services Extension Act; the Mental Retardation Facilities and Community Mental Health Centers Construction Act; the Health Professions Educational Assistance Act; the Manpower Development and Training Act; the Medical Library Assistance Act.

In any brief presentation of the "prospects of federal programs" it is manifestly impossible to explore the full range of these national health undertakings, but we must bear in mind, as we consider Medicare and Medicaid, that these challenging activities must always be viewed against a background of the *total* federal health program. They were by no means designed to stand alone. Their effectiveness will be conditioned by progress achieved through many other major federal programs and through related private programs.

Nor should we think of Medicare and Medicaid as Siamese twins. Coupled they certainly were in Public Law 89-97, the Social Security Amendments of 1965. And, in application to individual cases, one program will frequently supplement the other. Each program emphasizes comprehensive health care and quality health care. Despite similarities, however, Medicare and Medicaid represent two quite different philosophies, two quite different approaches to solution of the problem of financing health care. Medicare embodies the health insurance approach; Medicaid illustrates the medical assistance or welfare approach.

In this country the principle of health insurance has been accepted as sound for many years. Medicare applies this principle to all United States citizens 65 years of age or older in a program carried out under federal auspices. Medical assistance for the needy has been a part of welfare programs in this country ever since such programs have existed. Medicaid introduces a coherent pattern into this situation by making federal grants to states contingent upon the development of state plans that meet uniform quantitative and qualitative requirements for health care.

Medicaid differs from Medicare in containing a built-in feature that provides for gradual extension of coverage. Starting with specified groups of individuals initially eligible for health services, the law requires that states broaden the scope of care and services by liberalizing the eligibility requirements for medical assistance "with a view toward furnishing by July 1, 1975, comprehensive care and services to substantially all individuals who meet the plan's eligibility standards with respect to income and resources, including services to enable such individuals to attain or retain independence or self-care."

As of July 1, 1967, state plans will be required to provide at least the following array of health services: hospital inpatient and outpatient services, laboratory and x-ray services, skilled nursing home services, and physicians' services. This is roughly equivalent to the basic services available under Medicare, although home health services are also specified under Medicare and skilled nursing home services are identified as "extended care services" following hospitalization.

It is evident that both programs are designed to foster comprehensive health services.

"Comprehensive" is the key word in health care. It is also, I suggest, the key word in federal health programs. Medicare and Medicaid are, essentially, financing mechanisms—broadened applications of traditional methods for paying health care costs. In themselves they do not create health care facilities, resources, or personnel.

They pay bills.

In the health area, as in every other aspect of our society, effective "demand" is a financial fact. The health professions do not operate independently of the economic laws that regulate the life of this country. Thus the availability of payment—from some source, public or private—activates the delivery of every health service.

When the demand for material goods exceeds the supply, we call the result "inflation." If health resources and personnel do not increase in proportion to increased demand the same phenomenon occurs. If you will recall the major federal health programs which I mentioned a few moments ago you will note that each was designed to expand our national physical health plant, our national professional or trained health manpower pool, or our national health research capacity.

That is why I stressed that progress under these other federal programs, and private programs of a similar nature, will greatly affect progress achieved under Medicare and Medicaid.

Through the Hill-Burton program the federal government has been active for almost 20 years in the field of hospital construction and, more recently, in the construction of long-term care facilities. The Federal Housing Administration and the Small Business Administration have likewise made contributions in the private sector of the latter field.

Also on the physical plant side of the health picture there have been significant advances in recent years in our national supply of specialized facilities—research, diagnostic, and treatment centers designed to satisfy a diverse group of medical needs.

Health services are delivered *in* facilities but *by* individuals. Without adequate manpower all plans for health care are meaningless. That is why the federal government is investing more heavily in programs of education and training, not only for physicians and nurses and other individuals dedicated to professional disciplines but also for those thousands of essential adjuvant workers without whom the health professions cannot function effectively.

We have been listening this morning to perceptive analyses of the problems and opportunities and challenges experienced by our two greatest health resources, our hospitals and our physicians. Clustered around these basic resources are the other health facilities and health personnel. The fusion of all these into a national endowment for the delivery of health services is the instrumentality of planning, and the united complex is energized by our methods of national financing for the care of health.

Very generally indeed I have tried to convey some impression of the federal involvement in every segment of this vast and intricate national enterprise. Only against such a background can specific mechanisms such as Medicare and Medicaid be usefully appraised.

In this perspective, the two goals I wish to emphasize today stand forth in a sharper light. I have pointed out that comprehensive health care is built into both the Medicare and the Medicaid programs. We can accept nothing less. Modern health care *is* comprehensive health care.

Quality health care is the other inevitable, self-defined goal of any modern health program, and both Medicare and Medicaid were planned to provide nothing less than a high quality of health services.

The review of utilization, a proved technique for supporting efficient care in our leading hospitals, has been made a statutory requirement for all hospitals and extended care facilities that participate in the Medicare program. When the Medicaid program is fully developed throughout the country, skilled nursing home services will be made available under standards comparable to those of Medicare, and the advantages of utilization review will be still further extended.

The review of utilization is also a vital component of continuing medical education as well as an invaluable contribution to the achievement of that *continuity of care* that modern medical practice requires. Continuity of care is the link between our two major goals—comprehensive health care and high quality of health care. It is likewise a connecting link between medical education and medical practice.

Here we see the impossibility of divorcing the financial component of health care from the other elements in the health care universe—construction, research, education, planning, and the rest. The need for continuity of care for any individual patient can be recognized, analyzed, and demonstrated; plans can be made for meeting that need through coordination of health services. But these plans cannot be carried out without adequate financial support.

By the same token, the most far-reaching and generous arrangements for financing health care in this country will prove only ironic disappointments for the people of the United States unless the physical and manpower resources of this country are equal to the task of delivering comprehensive, high-quality health services in the volume required. Not only must the total national volume of available health services be adequate, but the distribution of services must be accurately geared to the needs of every geographical area and every group within the population. In the context of health service the terms "rich" and "poor" cannot be permitted to apply to any state or county or city or precinct, or to any minority group in the country.

Senate Bill 3008, enacted into law by the last session of Congress, was designed to coordinate our national system of public health services by comprehensive planning and by channeling funds into areas of greatest need.

When this legislation is implemented by the 50 states through the development of comprehensive plans for the expenditure of funds for public health services, we shall have created a system for combining the values of federal financial support and thorough sensitivity to local health needs.

Planning is a traditionally and incessantly abused word. But the state plans I speak of will not be paper plans. They will not be made by one group of people to be carried out by another group in the interests of a third group. State planning councils under S. 3008 will have both lay and professional members; they will represent both the consumers and the providers of health services. They will include the agencies that must carry out the plans.

And, as the years go on, it is anticipated that these state plans will have an increasingly strong impact on the delivery of all health services within each state, through their influence on coordination of services, both public and private, on manpower utilization, and on education and training.

Have we strayed too far from Medicare and Medicaid?

I do not believe so. I think that focusing our discussion on the mechanics of these two programs, or defending the purposes of these programs, or stressing the potential accomplishments of these programs, would have been a myopic contribution to today's forum.

Medicare and Medicaid are not to be considered as sacred cows. They are to be judged on the basis of the extent to which they speed up or slow down our progress toward reaching our national health goals.

These programs were created by Congress to give wider application to the advances of medical science in our generation. They are aids for harvesting the fruits of progress in the health fields. Other programs were designed to assist in the sowing and cultivating of the crops.

If today one is optimistic concerning the "prospects of federal programs" in the field of health care, then Medicare and Medicaid contribute to that optimism. But any mood of informed optimism must be based on a complete survey of the entire range of health programs.

Clearly, I should not be here today if I were not optimistic about the future of health care in the United States. My optimism, however, is not derived exclusively from observation of federal programs. It is also derived from recognition of the unprecedented advances in medical research in this generation, from the inspiring new developments in medical education, and from the dedication to duty of the health professions.

Achievement of national goals in the delivery of health services is a gigantic task. But the United States today is a nation committed to revolutionary advances in the quality of living.

# OVERVIEW OF INTERNATIONAL TRENDS IN MEDICAL CARE*

STANLEY W. OLSON

Professor of Medicine
Baylor University College of Medicine
Houston, Tex.

In the past year I visited Australia, New Zealand, Great Britain, Sweden, and Canada, and spent considerable time looking at their medical schools and examining their medical care arrangements. I found the health needs and expectations of the people of these countries to be remarkably alike but, despite this similarity, the structural forms of their health services were quite different. The principal value in taking a firsthand look at these diverse arrangements is the improved perspective and clearer focus it gives to what one sees when examining the health care system in our own country.

The purpose of my visit was to observe the relationships between the organization of medical care and medical education, especially at the graduate level. I had two primary reasons for making such an inquiry. The first reason had to do with the major changes now taking place in our health care system—changes resulting from strong social forces not peculiar to this country alone—changes that will surely influence the clinical setting in which medicine will be taught. The second reason was the concern I felt over the growing imbalance between specialism and general practice in this country. The medical schools, including my own, are contributing to this imbalance, but we have not found an effective way to change the situation. Our graduates at Baylor University College of Medicine are not unique in seeking specialty training—85 per cent of all United States medical graduates do so. Contributing strongly to the trend toward specialization are the rapid advances in medical knowledge, the nature of the clinical experience students acquire in our teaching hospitals, and the more secure position enjoyed by the specialist in obtaining hospital practice privileges.

The time available to me in each of the countries I visited varied

*Presented at the *Conference on Possibilities and Actualities in the Delivery of Medical Care,* held by the New York Heart Association at the Hotel Waldorf-Astoria, New York, N. Y., November 21, 1966.

from 1 to 4 weeks, scarcely enough to become conversant with the many diverse aspects of health care organization. However, with the kind assistance of knowledgeable persons I was able to identify some of the more prominent elements influencing the development of specific programs and to appreciate the interplay of economic, cultural, professional, and educational factors.

I was struck by the fact that none of these countries any longer has charity hospitals. The institutions that had formerly served this purpose had become general hospitals with the introduction of a universal health insurance or comprehensive social security schemes. The hospitals, for the most part, still have large open wards built on the Florence Nightingale pattern, but are neat and well lighted and serve the general public very well. Funds for construction of new hospitals are becoming available and new hospital designs are being adopted.

Australia, alone, has a voluntary system of health insurance but, like the others, it requires direct government subsidy. The insurance schemes are quite similar in that they all offer hospitalization without charge. They vary greatly, however, in administrative arrangements for meeting hospital costs. In great Britain and New Zealand almost all hospital funds come from the central government; local boards of trustees manage the hospitals, but their authority over finances is limited. Canada and Australia are alike in that funds allocated to the states or provinces from the federal government are distributed through state agencies to the local hospitals. Sweden follows a very different pattern. The local district, corresponding to our county, devotes about 80 per cent to 90 per cent of the taxes it collects to the support of health care. The federal government provides advice and guidance, but decisions are made locally as to where hospitals shall be built, what they shall contain, and how they shall be operated. The hospitals are well managed, and the people are highly satisfied. Teaching hospital costs there are largely borne by the federal government, which supports all higher education.

One finds that medical benefits for patients while in *hospital* are almost wholly covered by the health care scheme. Ambulatory medical benefits vary, however, in that medical services are free in some countries as, for example, Great Britain, while others require additional payments by the patient to the physician. Ordinarily if the patient is a pensioner—i.e., receiving assistance from the government for basic living expenses—he is not required to make additional payments.

In New Zealand the medical benefit is designed to favor the general practitioner; in Australia the insurance benefit cannot be more than 90 per cent of the physician's charge. Canada is in transition, for the government has announced a nationwide system of medical benefits but has postponed implementation until 1967 or 1968. Saskatchewan has already adopted a provincial plan of compulsory medical insurance over the severe objection of the medical profession—peace, however, reigns for the moment.

Pharmaceutical benefits are free in Great Britain and New Zealand. In Australia patients pay the first 50 cents of the cost of a prescription.

Understandably, the average person reacts favorably to measures such as these, as they relieve him of worry and concern about the payment of hospital and medical bills. This reaction of the public was epitomized in a conversation I had with the cabdriver who took me to the Waikeri Hospital in Dunedin, New Zealand. He judged from my accent that I was an American and by my destination that I was a physician. I tried to get more than full value for my fare by questioning him about his reaction to the medical care he received under social security. He said this: "We get *good* care. If I go to a doctor I may have to pay him 3 or 4 bob in addition to what he gets from the government, but if I get sick and go to the hospital it won't cost me a farthing. I'll lose my wages but I won't have either a doctor bill or a hospital bill to worry about." Then he looked slyly over his shoulder and said, "I hear this really is a worry in the United States! I've got six kiddies and if they get sick it would set me back a pretty penny to pay for their care if we didn't have socialized medicine. I hear your people are worried about socialized medicine. All I can say is they have nothing to fear." This worthy hackman may not know whether his medical care is good or bad. He has no way of judging whether the long-range health policies adopted by his country will lead to improved medical standards or poorer ones. But he will support with his vote the politician who pledges to maintain or increase his health benefits and will oppose anyone who tries to take them away.

Imposition of governmental restrictions, especially on hospital budgets, can be frustrating to administrators, board members, and physicians. Decisions are always made by people but the basis for restrictive decisions may be either political expediency or the operation of the principle of administrative uniformity. Professor John Beck is physician-in-chief to the Royal Victoria Hospital in Montreal. In a recent paper delivered to physicians from the United States he made these comments about the "dangers inherent in the medico-socio-economic changes taking place in Canada . . . as seen through the eyes of a departmental head."

> Perhaps first and foremost is the increasing governmental control of medical education and clinical care. . . .
>
> Failure of government to recognize special financial needs of teaching hospitals above and beyond those of community hospitals.
>
> Failure of government to supply and of the public to understand the need for funds for construction and equipment of new facilities and the improvement of existing areas, including those for training of paramedical personnel. . . .
>
> An inadequate supply of patients for teaching at all levels. This entails, in the most gloomy outlook, the complete disappearance of out-patient clinics. . . .
>
> Continued pressure for an increased output of physicians, with over-all reduction in quality, emanating not only from government but also from the medical profession at large, the latter because of an increased work load. . . .
>
> Failure to provide realistic house officer salaries. . . .
>
> Failure of the government to support adequate numbers of full-time teachers. . . .
>
> Failure by government to insist on maintenance of a differential fee structure for specialist and general practitioner services. . . .
>
> An ever widening gap between supply and demand for health personnel. . . .
>
> The greatest danger . . . concerns the expense of such programs to the public purse and the inevitable competition for the tax dollar. The expensive investment required to supply facilities for education and research proffers little political advantage whereas diversion of funds for personal health services is a major political weapon.[1]

Professor Beck may betray excessive concern in his comment, but he is a thoughtful person, and his observations confirm many remarks made to me by academic persons around the world.

The main difficulty with governmentally supported health services, however, is a much graver problem than administrative inadequacy or even political expediency. When a new health care system is put into effect there is little time or opportunity to change the existing mechanism for the delivery of health services, and it must be imposed upon an arrangement likely to have grave defects. Dr. Gordon McLachlan, of the Nuffield Provincial Hospitals Trust, London,[2] puts it this way: "In the health *service* field, accurate relevant information, scientifically compiled, about the quality and scale of medical care needed, regrettably, is still wanting. It would, of course, be idle to suggest that policies should wait on the results of empirical research; but it is important to get into focus the perspective of needs and priorities for change. Thus even if the structural panaceas which are from time to time dreamt up, were accepted, and brought into being immediately, the fact by itself would contribute little to answering the universal and perplexing questions relating to the reality of the times—i.e., the deployment of skills and money available, and the establishment of policies concerned with the rate and direction of the development of health services in totally different kinds of areas."

My inquiry into the relationship of general to specialty practice yielded some interesting but not very helpful information. The problem of general practice is a universal one. Everyone wishes that more interest would be shown in the field by young medical graduates, but little is offered in the way of definitive training or prestige and status for those who do enter it. What happens, therefore, to bring new medical graduates into general practice is more the result of economic and administrative forces than of educational, scientific, or social influences.

Great Britain has a roughly equal division between general practitioners and specialists. The salaried positions in the hospital system are restricted in number and are open only to specialists. A little less than half the graduates of the medical schools can be accommodated in such positions. Intensive training for a period of 7 to 8 years is required to secure full specialty status and appointment to a consultantship. A young physician may spend 3 to 4 of these years taking additional training and passing the examination of one of the Royal Colleges before he knows for sure that he will obtain a senior registrarship, which is the door leading to consultantship. Unsuccessful candidates have virtually no alternative but to go into general practice or to emigrate. General practitioners are paid on a capitation basis and, with panels of 2,500 to 3,500 patients, earn an average of $7,000 to $9,000 per year. Consultants start at a salary of about $12,000 and may earn, through confidential merit ratings, up to twice that amount. The discrepancy in financial incentives offered to physicians is a stimulus to secure specialty training. For those who do enter general practice there are few inducements, other than the physician's own sense of personal obligation, to improve his knowledge or to raise his standard of practice.

In Australia and New Zealand, on the other hand, the economic arrangements clearly favor the general practitioner. Surgical specialists make a reasonably good living, but specialists in medicine and pediatrics have a most difficult time and may end up by practicing general medicine; some emigrate to Great Britain or to the United States.

Seventy per cent of Sweden's physicians practice in hospitals. This includes house officers and full-time salaried specialists. Young physicians spend an average of 4 years in hospitals after graduation, and most of them hope for a permanent salaried appointment. Of those who go into private practice, most practice as specialists, many in 12- to 15-man clinics. Relatively few become general practitioners but of those who do many serve also as salaried district health officers performing both public health functions and caring for patients at the rates established by the compulsory health insurance system.

Sweden is the one country where I found the proportion of general practitioners to be less than in the United States. In response to a recent governmental decision the faculties of the six universities have set about the task of doubling medical graduates by 1975. The sharp increase in physicians will undoubtedly increase the ratio of general practitioners to specialists.

The situation in Canada is much the same as in the United States. About 60 per cent of physicians are specialists and about 75 per cent to 80 per cent of graduates seek training for a special field.

One may say, therefore, with some confidence that, in the absence of external controls, medical graduates today will pursue specialty practice in preference to general practice. Those who do go into general practice have an uncertain medical future. Most, except in Australia and Canada, will have no hospital privileges and will be handicapped in keeping abreast of medical advances. Hanging over the general practitioners of Commonwealth countries is the shadow of the capitation system that Great Britain has adopted. The fear is that labor governments, which are in general opposed to fee-for-service medical practice, will put pressure on the medical profession. It is anticipated that the specialists in such a circumstance will "cave in" and will accept full-time salaried hospital positions, leaving the general practitioner vulnerable to imposition of the despised capitation system. This underlying fear may well account for the subtle resistance on the part of organized medicine in Australia and New Zealand to changes that would ameliorate the less than satisfactory arrangement under which the specialist works.

Having looked at the broad aspects of the financial and professional elements in the organization of medical care in these several countries, we might now find it useful to get some judgment of the quality of what has been accomplished. Sir Douglas Robb, a thoracic surgeon and now chancellor of the University of Auckland, reviewed several years ago the development of health services in New Zealand, the first of these countries to adopt a universal health scheme. He says in his general evaluation, "The whole thing, in every particular, has been an exercise in supplying services [in novel ways] to the people. [We have seen] why the emphasis was on service and why those planning it were unable or unwilling to include in their view any serious consideration for quality. Medical, hospital, other services were going on—let us make them free or more generally available. No question was asked whether they were worth having as they were or whether they could be made better. The politician had to get into office and stay there, and official medicine had to secure the best bargain it could. It was not, as might be ideally hoped, an opportunity for an all-around review and improvement. The old wine was to be distributed in new bottles—let the purveyors of the product take care of its quality at their own expense.

"Whether any country as it bends itself to the seemingly inescapable task of providing smaller or larger doses of state medicine will ever be able to look at it more constructively is doubtful. Certainly New Zealand did not and has not yet done so 20 years later. Any important reform or betterment must still come up the hard way through enlightened and tenacious individuals or institutions which are most unlikely to be paid to think it out or provide it."[3]

Sir Douglas' judgment of state medicine may be factually correct but the picture is not quite so universally depressing as he makes it out to be. The quality of hospital medicine in both Great Britain and Sweden is high. The main difficulty is the waiting period for elective procedures. Unfortunately the quality of general practice is not of the same standard.

Investigators in many countries, aware of the lack of quality controls, are now actively engaged in health care research. They are acquiring a body of factual information about the distribution of medical services, including the incidence of medical conditions encountered in practice and in hospitals—the extent of both recognized and unrecognized health needs—how physicians work or fail to work with associated health personnel—and information about many other related aspects of the total health care environment. Ultimately information of this kind, when verified and refined, will form a basis for making sound plans and for making equitable adminstrative decisions. One might compare this recent exploration of the relatively new field of medical care research with our early scientific studies, which later came to have such a profound effect on the practice of medicine. The lag in application to ongoing problems is regrettable but inevitable.

Is there any consistent pattern discernible in the varied responses made by these several countries to the health needs of their people that would be of value in our own planning? I doubt that we in this country would wish to adopt any of these schemes, but perhaps we can heed some of the warnings based on the experience they have acquired over the past quarter century—McLachlan has advised us not to rely on "structural panaceas"; Beck has indicated the dangers to medical education of governmental influences that fail to respond to the needs of quality education and research; and Sir Douglas Robb has told us to beware of dispensing the old health care wine in new bottles.

In our response to demands for change we should make intelligent efforts to avoid the dangers to which we have been alerted. Valid reasons exist for expecting that we in this country shall chart our own course, avoiding known rocks and shoals but perhaps encountering new ones:

1) Our economic resources are substantial and we are prepared to use them to establish the highest standard of health care.

2) As a people we have prided ourselves on voluntarism as opposed to compulsion. Both private education and private hospitals have achieved high standards in this country.

3) Our hospital system is strong. It has grown strong through the support of voluntary health insurance, private philanthropy, and a creative, governmentally supported hospital construction act.

4) Our medical schools have developed strong programs of research

and research training, accomplished initially through the effort of private philanthropy but maintained and expanded chiefly by the National Institutes of Health.

Health legislation recently adopted by Congress, rather than portending the imposition of governmentally determined patterns of health care, as feared by some, can instead become the vehicle for modifying the delivery of health services in keeping with the most authentic tradition in the United States. The enactment of Medicare legislation together with Title 19 will relieve voluntary health insurance organizations of a heavy burden of responsibility that they found they could not in any case meet through premiums from subscribers. These organizations are now in a favorable position to experiment with the provision of wider coverage of medical benefits, and with greater standardization of premiums and benefits for both medical and hospital insurance.

The time is now favorable also for the medical profession to cooperate in making prepaid medical care (including x-ray and laboratory examinations) for ambulatory patients more readily available. This step will go a long way toward reducing those hospital costs created by unnecessary hospitalization of patients for diagnostic purposes. Our Blue Shield plans for payment of medical costs have not worked as well as they should because they have not had the full support of the medical profession. In contrast, the Manitoba Medical Service in Canada has shown what can be accomplished voluntarily by a united profession. One hundred per cent of the physicians in that province have signed contracts agreeing, first, that they will limit their charges to subscribers to the schedule of fees adopted and published by the Manitoba Medical Service and, second, that they will accept that share of their total charges, which income from premiums will support. The physicians currently receive an 80 per cent proration of their fees from regularly enrolled subscribers and a 70 per cent proration of fees from pensioners whose premiums are paid by the province. Manitoba Medical Services has enrolled 55 per cent of the entire population in the province.

The full exploration of the possibilities of voluntary health insurance can challenge the best efforts of consumer groups, employers, insurance carriers, hospitals, clinics, and the medical profession. Failure to develop a satisfactory basis for a broadly based and adequate voluntary system will surely result in the adoption of a compulsory one: first for hospitalization, including medical care in hospital, and then for ambulatory medical benefits.

We can make good the time we have left for experimentation in still another way. In enacting the Regional Medical Program for Heart Disease, Cancer and Stroke and Related Diseases, Congress has put into the hands of the people a means for examining closely the basic health requirements of each region. It has even left to institutions and public and professional representatives the determination of what should constitute a medical region. The opportunity exists to conduct the planning that Sir Douglas Robb doubted would ever be accomplished. We can now identify our current assets in personnel and facilities, and we can establish experimental programs to explore ways of uniting the resources of each region for greater effectiveness. It is significant, I believe, that this program has been made a division of the National Institutes of Health. The tradition of that organization for making awards on the basis of merit will assure that the funds expended will be for projects of scientific value.

Given sufficient hard information about our health needs and resources and given flexibility in determining which programs are effective and which are not, we shall be in a sound position to ascertain whether we can obtain high-quality care for all our people under an expanded system of voluntary health insurance. If it appears that further direct government aid is in fact necessary, we can hope to establish a basis for directing this support in constructive ways that will advance health standards rather than retard them.

We face twin evils: on the one side, a laissez-faire attitude toward health care; on the other, a desire for the imposition of politically sponsored "structural panaceas" to meet the clamor for public support of health costs. We must protect ourselves from both.

We can avoid the dangers to the right and the left only by establishing a rational basis for meeting health needs—a task of no mean proportions. Such a basis will be established, if at all, only by intelligence, persistence, and hard work. A health care system that will serve us well should be consistent with our traditional preference for voluntarism, should stimulate and attract superior people to join the health field, should encourage the advancement of knowledge and, in the end, should result in the highest standard of health attainable.

*REFERENCES*

1. Beck, J. C. Impact of paid hospitalization and total medical care on the university hospital. Presented at the Annual Meeting of the Association of Professors of Medicine, Atlantic City, April 30, 1966. Unpublished.
2. McLachlan, G., ed. *Problems and Progress in Medical Care.* London, Oxford Univ. Press, 1964, p. 8 of introduction.
3. Robb, D. New Zealand medical services: An appraisal, *Canad. Med. Ass. J. 82:* 490-97, 1960.

# REGIONAL MEDICAL PROGRAMS: A REVIEW*

ROBERT Q. MARSTON

Associate Director, National Institutes of Health
Director, Division of Regional Medical Programs
Bethesda, Md.

My interest in Regional Medical Programs developed primarily from what was said in the Coggeshall report.** Published shortly after the *Report of the President's Commission on Heart Disease, Cancer and Stroke*, that report addressed itself to the problems of the medical schools of this country and came to grips with some of the very same problems that came to light during the legislative process that led to passage of Public Law 89-239.

At about that same time I also had conversations with Dr. Carleton B. Chapman and others that reflected the interest of the American Heart Association in Regional Medical Programs, its role in the legislative process, and the potentialities of the law if passed.

The immediate impetus for the law was the *Report of the President's Commission on Heart Disease, Cancer and Stroke*. The emphasis of the recommendations of that group lay in the relationship of science and service in medicine. Following publication of the report, Dr. Edward W. Dempsey, the special assistant for Health and Scientific Affairs to the secretary of the U.S. Department of Health, Education, and Welfare, and Surgeon General of the U.S. Public Health Service William H. Stewart, previously Dr. Dempsey's assistant, became the key persons to draft the legislative proposals introduced by the administration. There were several fundamental elements in that original draft. These included proposals for the development of workable cooperative arrangements among the health resources of the nation and for the use of competitive grants rather than formula grants.

The administration's proposal went through the Senate hearings virtually intact but after extensive hearings by the House Committee on

*Presented at the *Conference on Possibilities and Actualities in the Delivery of Medical Care*, held by the New York Heart Association at the Hotel Waldorf-Astoria, New York, N.Y., November 21, 1966.

**Coggeshall, L. T. Planning for Medical Progress Through Education. Evanston, Ill., Assn. Amer. Med. Colleges, 1965.

Interstate and Foreign Commerce, held under the chairmanship of Representative Oren Harris of Arkansas, a number of changes were made. These emphasized the need to develop cooperative arrangements among existing institutions and reflected the conviction that local initiative should play a determining role in the development of regional programs. The belief was expressed that the advisory groups should be broadly representative of all the health interests of the region and should include practicing physicians and members of the public.

Congress was also concerned with the manpower problem. During the hearings it was stressed that there was a need for careful planning to meet manpower needs throughout the nation. As a result, Congress emphasized that training and continuing education be a major part of the programs and included the opportunity for use of funds under the program to encourage such plans to meet these manpower problems.

Shortly before passage of the bill, the decision was made that the administrative implementation of the program should take place within the organizational framework of the National Institutes of Health. This decision emphasized the fact that the concept of the Regional Medical Programs was focused on the interaction between the development of new knowledge and the improvement in medical care achieved by the application of that knowledge.

The purposes of the programs are contained in the law and provide for:

> ". . . grants to encourage and assist in the establishment of regional cooperative arrangements among medical schools, research institutions, and hospitals for research and training (including continuing education) and for related demonstrations of patient care in the fields of heart disease, cancer, stroke and related diseases . . . affording to the medical profession and the medical institutions of the Nation, through such cooperative arrangements, the opportunity of making available to their patients the latest advances in the diagnosis and treatment of these diseases, and . . . improving generally the health manpower and facilities available to the Nation. . . ."

The law requires that these purposes should be achieved without "interfering with the patterns or the methods of financing of patient care or professional practice, or with the administration of hospitals, and in cooperation with practicing physicians, medical center officials, hospital administrators, and representatives from appropriate voluntary health agencies."

During the spring of 1966, the staff of the Division of Regional Medical Programs proposed regulations and guidelines for the implementation of P.L. 89-239. It is important to recognize that there are no provisions for construction. Congress specifically eliminated such authority with the statement this would not hamper the program during the first three years. However, Congress also indicated that such funds might be requested appropriately on the basis of demonstrated need. Most of us have come to share the feeling that the availability of construction funds in the initial phases of the program might have complicated the task of defining and implementing the program to date.

Applications for planning grants started to arrive in April 1966. We were surprised at the number. During the three months of April, May, and June, a total of 39 applications were received. These were for areas that varied in size from a part of one state with a population of a few hundred thousand, to multiple state regions with a population of many millions.

The review of these applications began in April. From the beginning, certain areas of emphasis became apparent together with certain problems. On the one hand was a major focus relating continuing education to patient care; on the other was the need for evaluation. In saying that we did not have a national plan, the question arose as to whether we were going to set up a mechanism for project-by-project evaluation along the lines that many others experienced in the field of grant awards had come to expect. We found that we were facing the possibility of receiving long lists of meritorious projects that might have no relation to the development of comprehensive Regional Medical Programs.

Increasingly this has been viewed as a program to allow additional opportunities for those responsible for regional health resources to establish meaningful priorities in terms of developing ways for dealing with advances in the diagnosis and treatment of heart disease, cancer, and stroke. It has also become apparent that funds are available not only to support high priority items once chosen, but also to develop a process for determining those priorities.

The legislative authority came about because there was a concern, which eventually became a conviction in Congress, that scientific advance will increasingly affect the quality of service. It was the feeling that the problems in the relationship between the development of new knowledge and its application had received too little attention in the past.

It has been over a year since the legislation establishing the Regional Medical Programs was passed. During that time, I believe we have reached a stage in the implementation of the program in which we have the support and commitment of many institutions and organizations throughout the United States for the development of plans. We shall soon be faced with the implementation of the second phase of the program, the development of operational applications as they will be proposed individually by the regions.

The actual definition of the programs will be determined to a great extent by the persons who will be conducting them. This is true not only on the regional level, but also on the national level. About 65 persons outside of government have already been involved as consultants to the division. They have given many days to discussions and have played a major role in the implementation of the initial stages of the program. In addition to these, there are individuals and groups all over the nation who have taken part in discussions and made commitments of time and effort in advisory capacities. There have been organizations, such as the American Heart Association, that have held meetings throughout the country to discuss ways in which they can help implement the program.

After initial experience with the first planning grants, certain facts were brought more clearly into focus and, as a result, the job of the division staff became easier in terms of defining the program to others. In groups with which we met we found an increasing number of persons involved in Regional Medical Programs on the local level. Many of these people, in turn, are now describing the programs through speeches and publications.

How do we see the progress of the program at this time?

From an analysis of the applications that we have received, it is certain that an unusual degree of cooperation is being achieved. The composition of Regional Advisory Groups shows that practicing physicians and medical school and medical center officials each make up about 20 per cent of the advisory groups. Hospital administrators, representatives of the voluntary health agencies and other health professions and public health officials, each account for about 13 per cent of the total.

Public members, including lawyers, industrialists, labor leaders, and housewives account for about 8 per cent.

There are others who have been involved. We see in about half of the applications that representatives of state governments have been included. State health officers, and appropriate members of state Boards of Health, members of regional and areawide planning groups, and representatives of voluntary health organizations, particularly the heart associations and cancer societies, have been included in all of the applications reviewed.

The review groups have developed competence in reviewing applications for planning grants. They are now facing new problems in defining adequate review processes for operational grants. But the important part of the review process is that it has identified and communicated the fact that the evaluation of the programs is also a responsibility of the regions themselves, and not of representatives of the federal government.

Another consideration is that of continuing education. It received attention in Congress, and it has continued to receive attention throughout the country. We have seen a type of enthusiasm in this area of the program that will lead to rapid and effective action. However, experts in the field of continuing education have emphasized the need to utilize the cooperative arrangements possible under this program to introduce a new level of effective relations between patient care and continuing education. This is one of the areas on which we are focusing, in terms both of recruitment and of working with other national voluntary and governmental groups.

A third area of concern at present is the fact that we do have a report to make to Congress in June of 1967. We are planning a national conference in mid-January of several hundred people from all areas of medicine and health and all sections of the country to obtain additional material for this report.

A final area concerns the mechanisms by which in the future we may evaluate the program—not simply as to its over-all effectiveness in terms of impact on quality, but as to which activities implemented by Regional Medical Programs were most effective in terms of providing the highest quality of service to the largest number of people, which is the sum of all the goals.

# THE NORTHWEST PROGRAM*

JOHN R. HOGNESS

Dean, School of Medicine
University of Washington
Seattle, Wash.

DURING the past 2 years, a staggering array of new health legislation has been passed by Congress and introduced into our society, all of it aimed at improving the quality of medical care available to all of the people in the United States. Most of these measures, such as Medicare, introduced to meet specific needs, have therefore had specific purposes. The social impact of most of these specific programs will be apparent in a very short time. This is not true of the Regional Medical Programs legislation. This legislation has very broad purposes indeed, and its impact will not easily be measurable for several years. Legislation defining the Regional Medical Programs emphasizes principles and concepts rather than specific programs or procedures. Perhaps more than any other federal health legislation, it assures local control over local programs. In addition it is apparent that the administrative guidelines developed subsequent to the passage of this legislation indicate that all programs shall be locally conceived, locally developed, and locally administered.

There is very little question in my mind that the Regional Medical Programs Bill is the most important single piece of legislation in the health field to have passed Congress in several decades. I believe that it is far more significant and potentially more far-reaching in its implications than is Medicare. Furthermore, even though the current legislation requires that Regional Medical Programs be related to heart, cancer, stroke and other related diseases, I fully expect that if they are successful these programs will be broadened to include the entire field of medicine within a very short time.

This legislation, then, offers a challenge, a challenge to all health professions, to the universities and their medical schools, to hospital administrators, to voluntary health agencies, and to health departments.

*Presented at the *Conference on Possibilities and Actualities in the Delivery of Medical Care,* held by the New York Heart Association at the Hotel Waldorf-Astoria, New York, N. Y., November 21, 1966.

Above all, a challenge to work together, for it seems apparent that there is one word that more than any other describes the purpose, spirit, and value of the Regional Medical Programs, and that is cooperation. We have all been offered a challenge and an opportunity to develop a new pattern of medical care in the United States, a pattern which, if well developed, can bring us to a new position of leadership in world medicine and in the provision of health care to the people of the United States.

The Regional Medical Programs must be viewed in the broadest possible context. We must recognize the many changes that are occurring in our society today that make it appropriate for us to be considering such concepts as are embodied in Regional Medical Programs. First, many dramatic changes have occurred in the understanding of health matters by the general public and in popular expectations. At the same time, there has been an increasing awareness on the part of many representatives of the public that there are wide disparities between the quality of medical care offered to different groups and individuals throughout this country.

On the other hand, we must recognize that the nature and orientation of the universities of this country are changing rapidly and that their medical schools are changing even faster. Universities are becoming more concerned with and involved in the affairs of the community. Some schools are changing more rapidly than others, but the changing role of the university is inevitable. The medical schools, even more conspicuously than their other counterparts within the university system, are becoming increasingly involved with the community in the solution of common problems. Classical examples of this are the increasing involvement of medical schools in programs for research and training in mental retardation, in environmental and other aspects of public health, in continuing education and, of course, most classically, the involvement of medical schools in the Regional Medical Programs. The Regional Medical Programs are a major step, and the most significant step so far, in the development of "the new medical center." In fact, in this context we should really speak of the "new university" since so many of the aspects of the Regional Medical Programs are interdisciplinary and involve faculties from nonmedical parts of the university. The Regional Medical Programs legislation, therefore, is very timely indeed.

As this change occurs it will have a profound effect on the delivery of health care in the United States. It is a change for the better, and I believe it can make the private practice of medicine much more stimulating and much more attractive. For the setting in which a man practices is the most important single factor determining the quality of medical care he provides.

I should like now to review with you the status of the Regional Medical Program for the states of Washington and Alaska. I shall review the development of this program and its present condition, not because it is the best program or the first program but because, to date at least, it illustrates how a cooperative program can be developed. At the outset it must be recognized that problems to be encountered in the many diverse areas of this country will differ from region to region, and that no one pattern can be successful in another region. For example, we in the Northwest are in some ways fortunate in establishing the Washington and Alaska plan, that there is only one large university medical center in the region. On the other hand, we have special problems of distance different from those encountered in New York, since the state of Alaska is larger than the states of Texas, California, and Montana put together, and logistical problems are enormous.

With the knowledge that legislation relating to Regional Medical Programs for heart, cancer, and stroke was contemplated by Congress, a number of preparatory steps were taken within the Northwest region. During the early phases of the development of the proposed legislation, long before any legislation had passed Congress, the dean of the School of Medicine held a number of discussions with an advisory group consisting of the president and president-elect of the Washington State Medical Association, the president and president-elect of the King County Medical Society, a group that had been created about 2 years previously to discuss matters of common interest. This group discussed, frankly and openly, the impending legislation and its implications. About the same time, the dean initiated a number of discussions with the president of the University of Washington, attempting to define the over-all university position on this legislation and the possible role that the university might play should the legislation pass.

Then, about one and one-half years ago a meeting of representatives of the State Medical Association, the King County Medical Society, directors of Washington State and King County Health Departments, and representatives of the Washington State Hospital Association was called. This group again discussed the possible implications of the impending legislation and began to explore means by which it might be implemented. Concomitantly, three committees of physicians, one in the area of heart disease, one for cancer, and one for stroke, were constituted and were asked to survey extant facilities and resources.

Shortly after this, the dean entered into a series of protracted discussions with Dr. Carl Schlicke, president of the Washington State Medical Association, regarding the implications of the bill then before Congress. When the bill was passed by the House, these discussions were intensified, and they resulted in the firm conviction that whatever action was to be taken to implement the legislation in the region should be taken jointly, with full cooperation between the School of Medicine, the Washington State Medical Association, county medical societies, the Washington State Hospital Association, the Washington State Dental Association, the Washington State Nursing Association, voluntary health agencies, and health departments within the state. As soon as the legislation had passed Congress, Dr. Schlicke and I jointly requested an interview with Governor Daniel J. Evans of the State of Washington to review with him the implications of the bill and our desire to proceed in a cooperative fashion in implementing its provisions. We found the governor well informed of the provisions of the bill, and he encouraged us to develop specific plans for application for a planning grant. Governor Evans indicated approval of the general approach suggested, gave approval of the suggestion that the School of Medicine act as the agent for the region, and agreed to appoint the lay members of the Regional Advisory Group that was to be constituted.

At about the same time, there was a growing realization among the group involved in discussions that our large neighbor to the north, Alaska, had very definite and specific problems in the matter of delivery of health care. There was also a realization that Alaska did not have direct access to its own large medical center. It was therefore increasingly apparent that Alaska should be invited to participate with us in the development of a Regional Program. With this in mind, we entered into a number of discussions with the Commissioner of Health and Welfare for the state of Alaska, the president of the Alaska State Medical Association, and other representatives of health organizations in the state. Through Governor William A. Egan of Alaska we formally invited Alaska to participate in the program with us as two co-equal states. Governor Egan accepted this invitation with enthusiasm, as did members of the professions and hospitals in the state of Alaska. Governor Egan designated the lay members of the Regional Advisory Group who represent Alaska and approved the participation of other health care professionals in the advisory group. Since Alaska is naturally related to the state of Washington by transportation, communication, and economic and social ties, and since the pattern of referral and consultation of patients from Alaska has traditionally been to the state of Washington, the union of these two states in our region for programs in heart, cancer, and stroke seemed quite logical.

In October 1965, over a year ago, the dean of the School of Medicine, after consultation with representatives of the Washington State Medical Association, the King County Medical Society, and other representatives of interested agents and groups, entered into negotiations with Dr. Donal R. Sparkman, a physician in the state of Washington who has had extensive experience in the practice of internal medicine and cardiology, has been on the clinical faculty of the School of Medicine for many years, and is highly regarded by that faculty as a teacher and by the practicing profession as a physician. Dr. Sparkman in recent years had held a full-time position with the Washington State Department of Vocational Rehabilitation; therefore, in addition to his participation in many national organizations, he has had extensive experience with practicing physicians, with the academic community, and with state agencies. Dr. Sparkman was given a full-time faculty appointment at the University of Washington and was appointed coordinator of Regional Medical Programs on March 1, 1966. This appointment was made long before the planning application for the Washington-Alaska Region was approved. In fact, it was made before the application was formulated.

Now began the task of explaining the program and developing support among the various component medical and other health care groups. Dr. Schlicke, president of the State Association, and I made visits to every county society in the state of Washington to discuss the implications of this program. In October 1965 a meeting of the faculty of the School of Medicine was called by the dean. The legislation was again reviewed, item by item, and in general discussions the implications of the legislation for the School of Medicine, the university and the community as a whole were brought out. In early November 1965, a conference on Regional Medical Programs was held at the University's experimental forest site, Pack Forest, which is in a beautiful setting approximately 2 hours south of Seattle. Approximately 60 members of the practicing profession from throughout the states involved and 35 members of the full-time faculty of the School of Medicine as well as representatives of the State Hospital Association, the state and county Departments of Health, and representatives of the Idaho State Medical Association attended this 2-day conference. The entire conference was devoted to discussion of the implications and potentials of recent legislation in heart, cancer, and stroke. A representative of the secretary of Health, Education, and Welfare and a representative of the American Medical Association attended the conference and discussed some of the pros and cons of the legislation. During the conference, the participants, particularly the representatives of the faculty of the School of Medicine and of the practicing profession, had an opportunity to discuss the program together. It was a lively and cordial discussion, and one that was received enthusiastically by all present.

After this conference, plans for an application to develop a Regional Medical Program in Washington and Alaska proceeded in earnest, with the support of all groups involved. The dental and nursing associations in both states, the hospital association, the voluntary health agencies, the health departments, were all asked to nominate representatives who might serve on the Regional Advisory Group. In addition, as mentioned before, lay members of the group from the states of Washington and Alaska were appointed by Governors Evans and Egan. As the application progressed, it was reviewed by the advisory group and was approved by this group before it was submitted.

The Washington-Alaska planning application has now been approved and funds have been made available to develop planning and to implement the program. We have been able to proceed so rapidly that we hope to enter an operational phase and implement many of the programs that are being developed within the coming year. Time does not permit me to review all the projects that may be initiated in the early phases of this program. However, I should like to mention a few. First, a health manpower data bank is being established; it will be maintained by the Washington State Medical Association. This data bank will provide information on health care statistics, manpower, etc., for the regions of Alaska and Washington for any interested party. The task of accumulating these large quantities of information about manpower has already begun. Second, we are proceeding with the appointment of a great number of persons with different and varying backgrounds to the staff of the Regional Medical Programs. These will include economists, sociologists, hospital administrators, additional physicians, and other health-care personnel concerned with the large field of continuing education, as well as biostatisticians and systems analysts, to name a few. Cooperative efforts between participants in this program based in the medical school and members of the faculty in other departments in the rest of the university have already developed. It is anticipated that joint appointments will be made, and the many talents of the faculty of the university outside of the medical school will be called upon with increasing frequency.

A study of physicians' use of medical libraries throughout the region is being undertaken. It is essential in the provision of improved facilities for physicians and other health personnel that all be made aware of existing library services, and some of the problems associated with the use of such services must be studied more carefully. Such a study is essential in the development of a Regional Medical Library now being planned for the region.

It has become apparent in recent months that there is a very serious shortage of x-ray therapy technicians, particularly in the smaller communities throughout the region. In addition there is a great shortage of health physicists to provide consultation service to radiation therapy units throughout the region. It is therefore our intention to proceed rapidly with the development and sponsorship of training programs for additional x-ray technicians and with the development of a physics consultation service that will be available for all hospitals that provide radiation therapy in the region.

Since communications are paramount in the development of improved medical care, and in the provision of better and more up-to-date information to physicians and other health care personnel within the area, a pilot television network that links the Seattle area and the Yakima area* has been proposed. It is anticipated that regularly scheduled conferences—medical, surgical, pediatrics grand rounds, tumor conferences, and so forth—that were held at the university and at other large medical

*Yakima lies about 150 miles southeast of Seattle.

facilities in the Seattle area will be transmitted on a two-way basis through closed-channel television to the Yakima area. In addition, the availability of this television circuit will provide ready consultation for physicians and others in the area. Should this venture prove to be successful, it will be extended throughout the states of Washington and Alaska until the entire area is equipped. It is possible that because of the size of the area involved, it will be necessary for us to develop our own Tel-star unit for communication. Furthermore, it is recognized that this system is only the beginning of a rather massive communication system that must be introduced into the area to provide better service for practitioners in outlying areas. It is anticipated that immediate two-way television consultation, assistance in interpreting electrocardiograms, and other increasingly complex tests, medical library service, including immediate reference service, will ultimately be available to every physician throughout the region by means of an elaborate communication system.

Needless to say, continuing education is one very important aspect of the Regional Medical Programs. We are intensifying our continuing education projects, in part by increasing the number of circuit courses in which members of the faculty participate. In presenting these courses a group of faculty members will travel throughout the region, discussing problems with practitioners and bringing them up to date on most current aspects of medicine in a very informal way. All of us, faculty and practitioners alike, realize that continuing education programs are still unsatisfactory, and we are seeking better methods of providing such education.

Other programs that are contemplated are:

1) An increasing emphasis on the early detection of cancer, particularly by financing and sponsoring universal use of Papanicolaou smears and wide-spread breast examination.

2) The introduction of intensive coronary care units, where appropriate, in smaller institutions throughout the two states.

3) The development of cardiac rehabilitation clinics and stroke rehabilitation clinics throughout the region.

I am certain that, in terms of the ultimate potential of this program, we have merely begun to scratch the surface. As I have emphasized repeatedly, the program is and must be built on cooperation among existing institutions and organizations and the people in them. It is geared to provide a maximum of local initiative, local option, and flexibility. These options and this flexibility have been developed as deliberate public policy. We have here a great opportunity for creativity, an opportunity to develop new and improved methods and systems of health care, an opportunity to utilize these systems in research and teaching programs, and most particularly an opportunity to make the private practice of medicine and the practice of the other health professions throughout any area more exciting, more attractive, more productive, and intellectually more rewarding.

# PLANNING AND ORGANIZATION OF THE CONNECTICUT REGIONAL MEDICAL PROGRAM*

E. RICHARD WEINERMAN

Professor of Medicine and Public Health
Yale University School of Medicine
Director of Ambulatory Services
Yale-New Haven Medical Center
Member, Planning Committee
Connecticut Regional Medical Program

New Haven, Conn.

## INTRODUCTION

A significant change has occurred in United States social policy on medical care. The development of federal support for the planning of regional medical programs throughout the country marks a new level of acceptance of public concern for the organization as well as the financing of personal health services. Assignment of central responsibility for such regional planning to medical teaching centers represents a new kind of partnership among government, university, and community.

Shortly after Public Law 89-239 was enacted, studies of its possible implementation in Connecticut were under way. An application for a regional planning grant was approved in June 1966 in the first group of such awards announced by the new Division of Regional Medical Programs of the National Institutes of Health. This report will attempt to summarize the guiding concepts and the initial steps taken in the planning and organization of the Connecticut program.

Dr. George James has alluded here and elsewhere[1] to the challenging new potentials for improvement in the standards of medical care inherent in this legislation. Dr. Robert Q. Marston has clearly delineated the desired features of regional planning efforts from the viewpoint of the administrative federal agency, emphasizing the guidelines recently promulgated by his office.[2] Dean John R. Hogness has summarized the underlying principles and the long-range objectives of such rationalization in medical education and medical care in one large area. It is our

*Presented at the *Conference on Possibilities and Actualities in the Delivery of Medical Care,* held by the New York Heart Association at the Hotel Waldorf-Astoria, New York, N. Y., November 21, 1966.

hope that the project now under way in Connecticut can emerge as a model directly reflecting these principles.

## Guiding Principles in the Connecticut Program

A rich literature of concept and experience is available as background for these new efforts in regional planning.[3-10] In addition, the Connecticut planners have been guided by more recent analyses of the implications of the new legislation.[1, 2, 11-13] The initial policy decisions of the Connecticut plan can be briefly summarized as a basis for description of the project itself:

1) A single planning body, representative of all regional interests, is authorized to undertake the development of the regional program.

2) A noncategorical approach is emphasized, with the objective of an integrated regional plan for general health service, training, and research—*not* segregated into the specific areas of heart disease, cancer, and stroke. This decision was fortified by the recent statement in the published *Guidelines for Regional Medical Programs* prepared in Dr. Marston's office[2]: "Because of the broad scope of heart disease, cancer and stroke, it would be difficult and perhaps detrimental to some types of medical services and educational activities if a rigidly categorized approach were adopted for all relevant program elements."

3) Decentralized patient care services are stressed, with maximum effort devoted to the improved delivery of care at the community level. The regional centers are envisaged as supporting resources rather than magnets for the centralization of services.

4) The echelon model is accepted—essentially that of local service arrangements relating to community general hospitals which, in turn, affiliate with regional medical centers—as the framework for the coordination of all aspects of personal health service within a delineated area.

5) An academic partnership is established, linking the two university medical centers in the region: the independent and well-established Yale-New Haven Medical Center and the newly developing state-owned University of Connecticut Medical-Dental Center near Hartford. Thus, the basis is provided both for the unified planning activity now under way and, ultimately, for the specialized central resources of the regional network.

6) A threefold objective is envisaged in the regional medical program: *a*) to achieve greater operational efficiency on the part of the

cooperating institutions and agencies, *b*) to make available more productive and effective training opportunities for all classes of health personnel, and *c*) to enhance the quality and the accessibility of medical care within the area.

7) The concept of "action-research" is favored as the basis for the preparatory planning efforts—combining the techniques of field survey, epidemiological and operational research, experimental demonstration, and continuous program evaluation. Pilot feasibility projects are scheduled early in the planning phase, concurrent with the base-line inventory studies.

8) Interregional cooperation is recognized as an essential component of both planning and operation. The most carefully delineated regional program cannot stand in splendid isolation. In the Connecticut situation, close liaison is maintained with both a New England-wide coordinating body and the planning activities in neighboring New York State.

9) The maintenance of close academic interrelationships is considered to be of significant value, both to the regional planning effort and to the teaching and research activities of the participating universities. Thus, the individuals recruited to the planning staff of the Regional Medical Program hold academic appointments at Yale or the University of Connecticut, take active part in the academic goings-on, and—in turn—make the regional planning activity itself available as both classroom and laboratory.

10) Maximum use is made of previous experience with regional programming within the area as the starting point for the new projections. A particularly rich experience is available in Connecticut, since state public health and district planning agencies, hospital associations, mental health authorities, and university researchers have all been involved in such efforts.[14] Since the suggested subdivisions for the area by no means coincide in any two of the previous studies, the planning staff starts out with a challenging problem in synthesis as well as with a rich store of available data.

Two recent congressional enactments further complicate this problem of duplication of planning efforts. One is the recently passed Senate Bill 3008, now Public Law 89-749, the *Comprehensive Health Planning and Public Health Service Amendments of 1966*, which provides authority and funds to state (rather than regional) planning agencies. The other is the little-noted program for *Community Health Planning Grants for*

*Heart Disease, Cancer and Stroke,* administered by a unit of the Public Health Service quite distinct from Dr. Marston's Division of Regional Medical Programs, and apparently seeking to encourage local community (rather than state *or* regional) efforts in "the planning and coordination of health activities."[15] Unless some resolution of these seemingly contradictory jurisdictions is achieved, both in and out of Washington, grants will become necessary for planning among the planners. It is our hope in Connecticut—where, fortunately for us, state and region essentially coincide—to coordinate the activities of all these planning grant programs.

## Organization of the Project

*Delineation of the region.* On the basis of the previous regional studies and the current assessment of communication and medical care flow lines, it has been tentatively decided that the unit of regional planning should be the State of Connecticut. Recent studies by a team from the Yale Medical School have indicated that medical care for state residents is essentially contained within the state boundaries—except for the eastern border areas—and that the existing Yale-New Haven Medical Center already serves as a statewide referral resource.[14]

This is by no means a distortion of the general definition of a health service region—that is, a logical and functionally integrated area that contains a self-sufficient network of health and medical resources. While these criteria are closely met by the conditions within our state boundaries, in many other sections of the country the most natural regions will be either divisions of large and populous states or combinations of portions of various states. The State of Connecticut—with its 2,850,000 population, its compact area of 5,000 square miles, its interlaced transportation and communications systems, its closely associated and fully accredited group of 35 community hospitals, its university medical centers in the two major urban locations, and its cooperative professional groupings—constitutes an almost ideal regional unit. This cooperative spirit is exemplified by a recent statement from the president of the State Medical Society, who is himself a member of the Advisory Board of the Regional Medical Program:[16]

> The State of Connecticut is fortunate to be one of the first four regions in the Nation to receive planning grants under P.L. 89-239. It is not without responsibility. The accomplishments of this pioneer

project will receive wide scrutiny. We enter this exploratory phase of the program with confidence in the wisdom of those who will direct and supervise. . . .

This may well be the heralding of a new era in town-gown and government-professional relationships—*if* the planning responsibilities are carried out wisely.

*Planning authority*. One month after the enactment of the Regional Medical Program legislation, the governor of Connecticut assembled a broadly representative statewide committee to recommend means of implementing the new law. Meanwhile, officers and faculty members of the Yale-New Haven Medical Center and the newly planned University of Connecticut Medical-Dental Center had been meeting jointly to consider the response of the two academic institutions to the challenge posed by Congress. The university group, recognizing both the new social responsibility and the opportunity to enrich the teaching and research activities, submitted a proposal to the Governor's Committee that called for a single state-planning agency under the aegis of the two medical teaching centers acting conjointly, with careful provision for representative advisory bodies and with authorization to apply for a single regional planning grant. After careful discussion and with important modifications of the original recommendations, the advisory committee—which included representatives of state health agencies, medical society, hospital association, voluntary agencies, and the public—adopted these recommendations, which were promptly implemented by the governor.[17]

*Joint University Planning Committee*. Accordingly, a Planning Committee was established by the two university medical centers, consisting of the two deans, hospital administrators, and faculty members experienced in various aspects of medical care organization and research. Four months later, a completed grant application was ready to be submitted to the National Institutes of Health (N.I.H.), describing the rationale for a Connecticut regional delineation, the capacities of the two universities as planning agents, the anticipated planning program, and the organization of advisory bodies and project staff. Consultation had been sought from the Division of Regional Medical Programs at the N.I.H., the assistance of the newly constituted Advisory Board was solicited, and frequent meetings were held with planning authorities in neighboring states. After careful consideration of the possibility of participating in a New England-wide planning activity, the decision was made to cooperate fully with other regional planning groups but to submit an application for a single Connecticut program. With the announcement of the Connecticut grant as one of the first in the country, the current preparatory effort was under way.

*Project organization.* The new entity, established by the two university medical centers for the purposes described in the grant application, is called the Connectitcut Regional Medical Program. It operates by virtue of the delegated responsibilities of the two medical school deans. Its essential elements are a Regional Advisory Board, four affiliated Health Service Conferences as described below, the project staff, and the continuing joint university Planning Committee.*

Consistent with the provision of the new law and with the objective of maintaining an advisory body small enough to be efficient and influential, the Advisory Board is composed of 14 members widely representative of interests and areas within the region, but selected as individuals rather than as formal organizational delegates. Among the seven physicians are the state health officer, leaders of professional associations, and community practitioners. Other members bring backgrounds in industry, labor, nursing, hospital management and public welfare. The elected chairmen of the four affiliated conferences are regular voting members. The two deans and university hospital administrators have ex officio status without vote.

The Advisory Board from its inception has been intimately involved with the design of the original grant application and the initial organization of the program.

In the effort to involve all the important health resources in the region, yet still to maintain the effective small size of the Board, a unique plan has been devised for establishing four specialized Health Service Conferences to assist the Advisory Board, with voting representation as indicated above. These conferences are comprised as follows: 1) presidents of the governing bodies of Connecticut hospitals, 2) chiefs of medical staffs of these hospitals, 3) administrators of the hospitals, and 4) representatives of a wide variety of public and voluntary health agencies in the State. The various conferences have met, have studied the planning materials so far assembled, and have elected their officers

*Since this writing, a series of task forces have been appointed, representative of a variety of statewide interests, charged with the responsibility for developing information and recommendations in 9 or 10 specific areas (i.e., manpower, long-term care, continuing education, etc.).

and Advisory Board representatives.

In preparing the original grant application, it was envisioned that the project would involve planning in relation to the three aspects of research, training, and patient care. Accordingly, the proposed planning staff includes, in addition to the over-all director, an associate director for each of these broad areas, with appropriate assistants. The staff roster also includes positions for a communications specialist, for various technical consultants and for supporting clerical personnel. In all, the staff components represent about 70 per cent of the total two-year planning grant of $400,000.

Connecticut has been fortunate in having been able to attract as director of the regional planning program Dr. Henry Clark, former Administrator for Health Affairs at the University of North Carolina—a man with rich experience in regional-university affiliations and in health service organization.[12] Since the detailed content of the planning program is only slowly emerging from the discussions of the advisory groups, it has been decided to conduct the initial phase of exploratory study and pilot activities by taking advantage of the specialized skills and interests of selected present members of the two university faculties. In this way the basic explorations can be started while the director gains time for the careful recruitment of the full-time staff members. The first such appointment to the full-time planning staff has involved a specialist in community organization with long experience in the Connecticut setting.

*The planning process.* The goal of the project is to develop a detailed plan for a system of cooperation among health services and facilities within the region for purposes of obtaining more efficient administration, conjoint training of health manpower, and elevated standards of patient care. To be involved are relationships among general and special hospitals, long-term care facilities, community health agencies, and private and group medical practitioners. Emphasis in the administrative component is to be on such matters as common record and procedural systems, joint purchasing and use of major capital resources, and new methods of communication. Educational goals involve region-wide residency training programs, continuing education arrangements for practitioners, technician training with temporary stand-in replacements, and the like. Provision for a two-way flow of patients, specimens, consultants, information and supportive personnel is the goal of the medical care planning component.

The informational support for the development of the ultimate regional plan is to be derived from both research and pilot demonstration. The research aspect includes analysis of available data on health problems and resources, conduct of new studies of need and use of health services in the region, and evaluation of special pilot efforts. From these studies, from the deliberations of staff and advisory bodies, and from the active involvement of a wide variety of professional and consumer groups in specially designated "task forces" will emerge the building blocks with which the plan for the on-going regional medical program will be constructed.

*Research components.* While the final design of the research phase of the project is not complete, the major components can be outlined:

1) Delineation of the borders and subdivisions of the region, through studies of population characteristics, geographic factors, lines of communication and transportation, trade and market movements, distribution of services and facilities, etc. Much of this material has already been compiled.

2) Inventory of health services and educational resources within the region, using both available sources of information and fresh surveys of location, characteristics, and adequacy of existing personnel and facilities.

3) Assessment of assets and deficiencies in meeting needs for personal health care, based upon sample surveys of health-related attitudes, knowledge and behavior in the regional communities, analysis of available indices of health status, medical examination of population subsets, analysis of patterns of utilization of existing services, and measurement of quality medical care services.

*Pilot demonstration projects.* With the dual objectives of exploring new patterns of regional cooperation and of early involvement of maximum numbers of local community participants, plans are now being developed for the conduct of small pilot projects during the survey and research phase of the 2-year program. This will provide information on the feasibility of various approaches for possible inclusion in the long-range program. It is hoped that such "action-research" will give impetus to the concept that regional medical planning and organization is a continuous process of interplay between theory and practice.

A number of specific projects are now in the design stage:

1) Regional relationships in laboratory services, with special attention to possibilities of wider use of automated central procedures and rapid electronic communication with local service activities.

2) Cooperative medical library arrangements, again with exploration of modern processing techniques.

3) Testing of new designs for special intensive and extended care units in community hospitals.

4) Trial programs for training of new kinds of technical aides and patient care assistants.

5) Exploration of methods of uniform systems of medical records throughout the region, with possibilities of central computer storage and rapid recall and transmission procedures.

6) Development of affiliation agreements between university medical centers and community hospitals on the one hand, and between general hospitals and long-term facilities on the other.

*Time sequences in the planning process.* At the end of the 2-year planning period, a general program for a regional system of health service and training should be described—with provision for continuing research into improved methods of organization, for continuing experimentation with new methods of delivery of patient services, and for continuous evaluation of experience with the various components of the regional system. In order to accomplish these goals within the time allotment, an interlocking sequence of activities has been projected:

1) The survey-research activities begin at once and continue through the full planning period. The basic data required for the delineation of a tentative regional plan should be compiled during the first project year.

2) Feasibility studies of various service and training components begin after six months or so of basic preparation, and continue throughout the planning period.

3) Outlines for a preliminary "master plan" are prepared after the first year of planning activities, and serve as the basis for field trials, demonstration projects, and further feasibility studies during the second year.

4) A final regional medical program is completed at the end of the two-year grant period and is the template for the operation of the over-all service and training network.

It is to be hoped that key members of the planning staff will be available for supervision of the operating program itself, as will the members of the various advisory and community groups. At this point also, the sponsoring universities will begin to utilize the regional program for student participation and for its own research efforts.

## Problems and Potentials

Quite aside from the many obvious problems of organization, research, and public relations in such a planning effort, the success of both the preparatory and the operational phases will depend to a very large measure on the resolution of difficulties which are common to all efforts to rationalize the provision of medical care in the United States. The enabling legislation itself is restrictive with respect to disease categorization, injunctions concerning change in the system of financing of medical care, conflict between political jurisdictions, and the like. Other federal programs, particularly PL 89-749, threaten possible administrative complications. Time and money allotments are tight. Talent in the field of regional medical organization is sparse, and now the recruitment efforts are highly competitive. General and professional political conflicts come into sharp focus when region-wide collaboration is on the agenda. The independence of autonomous institutions, such as voluntary hospitals, is hard to reconcile with cooperative regionalism. Economic barriers to patients hoping to make full use of the echelons of service are often prohibitive. The solidarity of the long-term interest of the universities is yet to be tested.

Nonetheless, the prospects for the introduction of order into the patchwork array of United States medical care services have never been brighter. The key concepts—those of region, of social planning, of academic involvement, of experimentation, of self-evaluation, of standards—these are the long-awaited ingredients of quality needed for effective social progress in the organization of personal health services in the United States. Public Law 89-239 sets the stage for the drama to come. We in Connecticut are excited to be part of Act I.

*(REFERENCES ON FOLLOWING PAGE)*

*REFERENCES*


1. James, G. Implications of the Heart Disease, Cancer and Stroke program: an interpretation, *Med. Opinion Rev. 2:* 112-23, 1966.
2. Division of Regional Medical Programs, National Institutes of Health. *Guidelines—Regional Medical Programs.* Washington, D.C., Govt. Print. Off., 1966.
3. Consultative Council on Medical and Allied Services. *Interim Report on the Future Provisions of Medical and Allied Services.* Dawson Report. London, Ministry of Health, 1920.
4. Mountin, J. W., Pennell, E. H. and Hoge, V. M. *Health Service Areas—Requirements for General Hospitals and Health Centers.* Public Health Bulletin No. 292. Washington, D.C., Govt. Print. Off., 1945.
5. Anon. *The Bingham Associates Fund.* Boston, the Fund, 1945.
6. Weinerman, E. R. Medical schools and the quality of medical care, *New Eng. J. Med. 239:*810-17, 1948.
7. Lembcke, P. A. Regional organization of hospitals, *Ann. Amer. Acad. Polit. and Soc. Sci. 273:*55-61, 1951.
8. Pellegrino, E. D. Role of the community hospital . . . in continuing education—the Hunterdon experiment, *J.A.M.A. 164:*361-65, 1957.
9. Roemer, M. I. and Morris, R. C. Hospital regionalization in perspective, *Public Health Rep. 74:*916-22, 1959.
10. Joint Committee of the American Hospital Association and Public Health Service. *Areawide Planning for Hospitals and Related Health Facilities,* Public Health Service Publication No. 855, Washington, D.C., Govt. Print. Off., 1961.
11. Report of the Committee on Interstate and Foreign Commerce. *Heart Disease, Cancer, and Stroke Amendments of 1965,* H. R. 3140, 89th Congress, House Report No. 963. Washington, D.C., Govt. Print. Off., 1965.
12. Clark, H. T. Challenge of the regional medical programs legislation, *J. Med. Educ. 41:*344-61, 1966.
13. Russell, J. M. New federal regional medical programs, *New Eng. J. Med. 275:*309-12, 1966.
14. Thompson, J. D. *et al. Study of Hospital Service Areas in Service Regions for the State of Connecticut.* New Haven, Conn. Hosp. Plan. Commission, 1966.
15. Goodman, G. E., Gainey, C. D. and Graber, J. B. Community health planning grants for heart disease, cancer, and stroke. *Health, Education, and Welfare Indicators,* Sept., 1966, pp. 13-24.
16. President's page, *Conn. Med. 30:*663, 1966.
17. Ebbert, A., Jr. A look at Public Law 89-239: the Heart Disease, Cancer and Stroke Program, *Conn. Med. 30:*664-69, 1966.

# THE NEW YORK CITY STORY*

James E. McCormack

Director
The New York Academy of Medicine
New York, N.Y.

The Regional Medical Programs authorized just over a year ago are sometimes referred to under the label of Regional Medical Complexes. In New York City "complex" is an especially good word since the complexity and the complications of the local situation are so great.

For simplicity, I should like to tell the story in three parts: first, what has happened thus far in relation to the regional concept; second, what are some of the assets available to a regional program here; and, third, what are some of the things that could be done under the program.

Before proceeding, however, permit me to reemphasize two obvious points: a) a planning grant normally precedes an operational grant, and b) when the stage of the operational grant is reached it is not intended that the money be used for hospitalization costs unless the care of the particular patient relates to teaching and research.

I make these rather obvious observations because those who are impatient in the desire to get on with an operational grant should acknowledge that Congress was very wise in recognizing that a program of this dimension—a program based on new concepts of social and public health policy—had to be staged, with assessment and planning as one stage and implementation or operation as the second—even though the two stages may overlap.

## What Has Been Happening in New York City?

To my knowledge at least four local institutions have prepared planning grant applications. In some only one disease was considered; in others only a limited part of the metropolitan region was to be covered. As the situation has evolved there has developed a conviction that a planning grant should be sought for a region that includes all the

*Presented at the *Conference on Possibilities and Actualities in the Delivery of Medical Care,* held by the New York Heart Association at the Hotel Waldorf-Astoria, New York, N.Y., November 21, 1966.

five counties within the city limits and, probably, also Westchester, Nassau, and Suffolk counties. To be sure, the U.S. Surgeon General could designate as a region any geographic division such as, for example, the area from 14th Street south to the Battery; these sites once constituted the city limits. However, it would seem that the entire city and the adjacent counties constitute a more appropriate region for the purposes of this program.

In the spring of this year representatives of several local medical organizations, as well as the deans of all the local medical schools, requested The New York Academy of Medicine to participate in forging a program for New York City that would represent all the various interests that must be represented in a community effort such as the authors of the Regional Medical Programs concept had in mind. Several meetings were held with representatives of appropriate and interested agencies, including the deans of all the medical schools in the city, members of the Upstate Planning Group concerned with the regional health program and, on a few occasions, representatives of the National Institutes of Health.

After serious review of the implications for future operational grants, especially in relation to the many ways in which activities and interests of the local medical schools overlap, it was decided that the most feasible way to approach the matter would be for the medical schools to form a corporation, including in this corporation The New York Academy of Medicine.

Request for a charter for this new corporation is now before the Regents in Albany, and a draft is being prepared of an application for a planning grant to be made by "The Associated Medical Schools of Greater New York"; this application should be submitted in the near future. This approach to forming a new corporation was predicated on two principal facts: one, a growing belief that as more and more of these large-scale programs develop, the medical schools must cooperate in realistic fashion in joint efforts within the community; the other is the success of a joint venture started a few years ago by the Academy of Medicine and the local medical schools with a few related institutions. I refer to the Medical Library Center, sometimes described as a repository library. This library has helped to alleviate the inexorable pressure for space in the member libraries by its willingness to accept and house old and infrequently used material, thereby minimizing unnecessary duplication. The Medical Library Center operates an interlibrary loan service whereby, on a daily basis, material is transported by truck between participating libraries.

In addition, the Medical Library Center maintains a Union Catalogue of all the periodical holdings, not only of the member libraries, but of other valuable collections in the metropolitan area, such as those in museums, botanical gardens, and at Brookhaven: a total of 68 libraries. A catalogue on magnetic tape for computer searching makes it possible to explore the assets of all the significant libraries in the area.

Obviously, this cooperative enterprise makes scientific information available to researchers as quickly and conveniently as possible, at the same time relieving pressure upon the participating libraries.

Located physically adjacent to the Academy of Medicine Library, the Medical Library Center bulwarks the huge collection in the Library of the Academy, which has been serving de facto as a regional medical library because of its size and tradition and because the medical school library resources cannot be dissipated or diverted from their primary purpose of serving a specific faculty and student body.

## What Are Some of the Assets upon which a Program Might Be Planned?

Indeed, the wealth of assets contributes to the complexity of the planning. There are seven medical schools within the city limits and two more are planned in the region as defined. There are 156 hospitals in the city limits and at least 68 more in Nassau, Suffolk, and Westchester. There are about 18,600 registered physicians in New York City and an additional 4,000 or more in the adjacent three counties. Within the city limits of New York City there are 10 per cent of all the internships and 12.8 per cent of all the residencies in the country.

All these data, impressive as they are, are purely quantitative, and someone has suggested that it might be appropriate to enumerate some relevant contributions to the advance of medical science made in New York City. Certainly in recent days the profession and at least some of our hospitals have had a pretty bad press image, and it may not be inappropriate to remind even this audience that the first cardiac catheterization in this country was done in New York City, a development which catalyzed advances in cardiology from all points of view: research, diagnosis, and therapy. The now widely used functional classification of heart disease was introduced in New York City. The first clinic specifically for ambulatory care of cardiac patients was started in New York City, the technique of visualization of heart chambers and great vessels by injection of radiopaque substance was also developed in New York City. Similarly, the transaminase test useful in management of acute myocardial infarction was introduced here. The first use of synthetic textiles as blood-vessel replacements took place in New York City.

Perhaps it is appropriate to point out that the Papanicolaou technique of exfoliative cytology, so important in the cancer field, was developed in New York City, as also was the first chemical test for cancer (acid phosphatase).

Finally, Ralph Chester Williams' *The U.S. Public Health Service: 1798-1950* reminds us that a tiny laboratory established in Staten Island's Marine Hospital for sick and disabled sailors was the beginning of medical laboratory research in the Public Health Service and was designated the Laboratory of Hygiene. "It was the embryo of the largest medical research organization in the world—The National Institutes of Health." The chain is a direct one: Dr. Joseph Kinyoun's laboratory grew into the Laboratory of Hygiene of the United States Public Health Service; the name of the Laboratory of Hygiene was changed about 25 years ago to the National Institutes of Health.

These various contributions of which we boast in our shameless effort to bask in reflected glory were made in a variety of hospitals, government and private, and in various medical schools; many of them involve more than one institution. Increasingly, progress is made today by joint effort, and there will be more of this joint effort in the future, not less.

## What Do We Visualize as the Areas that Can Be Explored and Exploited When and If a Grant is Made to the New York City Region?

Obviously, we do not have a precise protocol since we do not yet have a grant or a staff, but the people involved in discussions to date have already found enough areas worthy of study to make us confident that progress can be made if support is forthcoming.

We cited earlier some fairly impressive statistics—now let us cite a few facts suggesting that the situation could be improved.

The ratio of physicians to population is higher in New York City than in any other community except, perhaps, the District of Columbia with its large population of federally employed physicians.

Similarly, the ratio of hospital beds for the United States is 3.7 beds/1,000 population, whereas in New York City the ratio is about 8.1/1,000.

But what has not been emphasized is that a large number of physicians in New York City have no hospital connection. A study done 15 years ago indicated that over 5,000 of the physicians then licensed in New York City had no hospital appointment and that, of these 5,000, about 2,500 were considered in practice. How many physicians today lack any hospital appointment and how does one best bring to these physicians the newest advances in "heart disease, cancer and stroke?"

We seem to have enough physicians in this region, but what about the shortage of personnel in other health professions about which we read almost every day? Since so many of the newer techniques require a team of trained persons rather than a heroic solo effort, a recent statement made by Secretary John W. Gardner of the Department of Health, Education, and Welfare is especially significant. Mr. Gardner said: ". . . shortages in nursing and subprofessional fields are the most serious barriers to the achievement of the health goal of the American people."

How can a planning grant be used to stimulate programs for training more laboratory technicians and nursing and allied personnel? Certainly with the great hospital and educational resources we have boasted of, more people ought to be trained in the allied health professions in the New York region.

In an area that contains only one medical school and one large medical center and a relatively homogeneous population, planning a program must be relatively easy. None of these conditions prevails in New York City. It is a simple matter to superimpose on a map of the metropolitan area the location, the capacity, and the average census of each of the hospitals in the region, but to suggest that this tells all we should know about unmet needs in specific areas is somewhat of an oversimplification. A person who is relatively close to hospital X as the crow flies may prefer to use hospital Y, which is in another neighborhood altogether, because of convenient and rapid transportation, or because his doctor is not connected with hospital X, or for various other reasons.

A series of television commercials has drawn attention to the well-known fact that New York City is the largest, or certainly one of the largest cities in the world of this or that ethnic group—Negro, Puerto Rican, Hebrew, Italian, Irish, Polish, German, etc. Various groups, quite naturally, tend to colonize the city in neighborhood arrangements, and recently these neighborhoods have been changing much more rapidly than in an earlier day. The earlier neighborhoods are recalled by the continued existence of the French Hospital, the Swedish Hospital, and the Caledonian Hospital. The German Hospital has long since changed its name to Lenox Hill Hospital. The Mount Sinai Hospital of New York was started under the name of The Jews' Hospital in New York.

One of the problems that besets the provision of medical care in New York—the great cultural and ethnic diversity of its population—also presents a great opportunity. Perhaps no other city in the world today contains communities of such diverse origin and ways of life. New York contains within its city limits meaningful social units of persons from such groups as: Mohawk Indians, Sephardic Jews, Hassidic Jews, Lebanese, Armenians, Maltese, Finns, Chinese, Japanese, West Indians, Moslems, and many more.

To a remarkable degree, many of these groups still preserve their old ways and customs of living, their old dietary patterns, and their original languages. There are over 100 foreign-language newspapers published in New York City on a monthly, weekly, or daily basis. Indeed, there are 26 dailies in 14 foreign languages.

The identification of these groups and a study of their way of life in this great city could provide a rich opportunity for epidemiological studies of many kinds in relation to heart disease, cancer, and stroke, and it could also provide a rich opportunity for the study of the medical practices and response to medical care programs of these ethnically and culturally diverse groups.

One goal of the new program is to increase the *number* of patients brought to treatment for heart disease, cancer, stroke, and related diseases. Thus it is desirable to go beyond hospital and other official records and gather morbidity data by means of a population health survey to obtain estimates of *untreated* ailments in various parts of the metropolitan area. This would make it possible to select institutions for participation in this program on the basis of the *need* rather than merely the *demand* for treatment. Such a survey could estimate, for example, the number of apparent stroke victims who have not received rehabilitation, the number with recent histories of coronary disease who are not now under medical supervision, etc. Some of these data may, of course, already have been gathered by the New York City Department of Health's periodic household survey. However, as with other kinds of demographic data, it will be a major task of the planning staff to canvas various agencies and determine which data can be retrieved from their files and which must be obtained through a new research study.

One thing, I trust, is clear from this recital. There is no intention of cutting up the city under the regional program and parceling out blocks of territory to the various medical schools. The intention rather is to use all the agencies that can contribute to a concerted effort to bring better health care to more people.

If the regional concept is designed to make the high level of excellence that presumably prevails in the teaching centers available to every patient, this must be done without jeopardy to the teaching and research programs of these centers. It must be done by strengthening the outposts of health services in thc neighborhoods where people seek health services.

The Congress has said in effect that quality of medical care is the people's business; this means it is the business of the community: that is why this conference was convened.

# SUMMATION*

GEORGE JAMES

Dean, Mount Sinai School of Medicine
New York, N. Y.

It is a difficult task that has been wished upon me: to attempt to summarize this afternoon's discussion, with a few nods toward what happened this morning.

Some of us like to divide people and programs into two major categories, those that primarily consider long-term plans, and those that accentuate short-term planning.

This morning we heard a great deal about short-term plans, the immediate provision of resources to make possible the distribution of medical care without reference to financial barriers. But even this morning we noticed a few angry young men who were rebelling against past traditions that have impeded progress. We noted that the legislation considered this morning was not necessarily conducive to improvement of quality of medical care, and these angry young men were reacting as people who like to look at long-range goals. They like to ask these questions: "Where is all this heading? Where shall we be 30 years from now? Where should we be?"

It is amazing that in this country so little attention has been paid to long-range goals. Our Canadian brethren have instituted a remarkable 2½-year study, recently published as *The Canadian Royal Commission Report on Health,* in which they establish health goals for a generation. I look for the day when we shall attain the intellectual, emotional, and political maturity in this country to engage in such a project.

To a great degree, people look on medicine as a political science. It is a matter of meeting the demands of people. Of course, as political creatures, we must meet these demands.

Short-range goals are being attained. But we must constantly look ahead to the long-range goals, to demands for services that people should have but do not have. Remember Dr. Ray E. Trussell's study in New York City, in which he showed by medical audit that 40 per cent

*Presented at the *Conference on Possibilities and Actualities in the Delivery of Medical Care,* held by the New York Heart Association at the Hotel Waldorf-Astoria, New York, N. Y., November 21, 1966.

of the medical care being received by one part of the population was inadequate, even though 95 per cent of the people who were receiving this care thought it was of high quality.

We must make sure that the needs of people are met, and take steps to see that they are met, even though there is not at the moment an awareness of this need.

The theme that I believe ran through this afternoon's program was the dynamism of public health, and the fact that there is a need for change, and that change is in the air.

The very pluralism of the nation's approach is a safety factor.

We may argue about aspects of Medicare. We may be a little concerned over the long-range implications of Senate Bill 3008's comprehensive planning measure that gives planning grants to states and to agencies within states. But all in all, we do have these programs, and we have a Regional Medical Program, too, which accentuates high quality.

In regard to the Regional Medical Programs: we are here dealing with a project very loosely defined in federal legislation, one in which the true pattern that will develop will again depend far more upon how it is implemented through the review process. This review, as Dr. Robert Q. Marston has mentioned, has a great responsibility, and he has wisely involved many people in these deliberations. For these people will determine the pattern of the first few grants, and after that the pattern of the next few grants, and eventually that of the entire program.

Essentially, all the medical schools in this nation are now becoming involved. Their ivory towers are crumbling. They are looking at their communities. They are being asked, and they are asking themselves the question, "What can we do to spread this high quality of medical care more widely in our area?"

John Millis, president of Western Reserve University, has a statement he likes to make. He says, "Let us be careful when we institute change that we do not replace the old orthodoxy with the new."

When we become enamored of this or that principle, such as the continuous, patient-centered, family-centered, all-stage-of-disease approaches to medical care—it is easy to try to replace the old orthodoxies with the new.

It is far more important that we always remain flexible, that though orthodoxy be established, new approaches must always be tried. We must approach a host of short-range goals, realizing always that they are fleeting in essence, and that we are capable and wish to be capable constantly of reevaluating and changing them.

It is obvious that a state with one medical school has an easier time of rationalizing a great deal of individual points of view within its boundaries.

We in New York City, with seven medical schools, have a tremendous task. The fact that under the stimulation of the Regional Medical Programs seven deans are meeting once a month, and are planning not only to institute Regional Medical Programs but several other joint programs also, is itself an amazing contribution of this legislation.

I believe that the realistic programs, the tailor-made, evolutionary programs based upon local centers of excellence, with constant opportunity to return to Washington for supplemental grants, will give us the opportunity to make of the Regional Medical Programs a vital force for the future.

Local initiative is a key, and local cooperation is another. Cooperation between schools has not been an element for which our medical schools have been famous in the past. When it comes to emphasizing full community service, these schools are indeed at the start of a new era.

All the programs you have heard discussed will have an amazing impact upon what comes ahead. None of us knows where this will lead, but all of us, I believe, have faith that we are out for high-quality, comprehensive health and medical care for our population as an inalienable right, and we are here to do everything we can to attain this goal.

# MEDICAL AND BIOLOGICAL RESEARCH ON HUMAN BEINGS*

A STATEMENT BY THE
COMMITTEE ON PUBLIC HEALTH
THE NEW YORK ACADEMY OF MEDICINE

CLINICAL research on human beings is a topic that is being discussed with increasing frequency in the press, periodicals, and medical journals. Indeed, it is a topic of the times. Perhaps attention was first directed to limited and specific aspects of it. But subsequent consideration has gone far beyond the initial issue.

As it has been explored in both breadth and depth it has been found to be somewhat more complex than had at first appeared. This subject has its moral, ethical, and legal as well as medical aspects. Furthermore, although it is not difficult to give voice to beliefs in the abstract, it is less easy to transmute them into concrete terms for application.

Despite the profusion of utterances about research on man there is still some confusion and misconception. To clarify the subject, the Committee on Public Health has been led to make a positive statement.

At the outset one important basic fact should be realized. Research on humans is absolutely essential if there is to be progress in the knowledge of diseases and their prevention, treatment, and cure. This dictum is inescapable. If a procedure or project shows merit and promise as well as safety after preliminary work on animals, there comes a time sooner or later when it must be tested on man.

It should be distinctly understood that clinical research may carry an element of risk, which is variable. Fortunately, in most research harm does not eventuate. But where there is risk, it must always be weighed against the benefits. Research on man therefore necessitates a medical decision in which risk has been calculated. Unless the benefits are in proportion to the risk, the latter is not likely to be taken.

At this point, lest generalizations about clinical research become misleading, it should be stated that study on humans is a broad generic term that comprises three different categories:

1) Clinical research with professional care in which a new therapeutic measure is used in the hope that it will save the patient's life, reestablish his health, or alleviate his suffering.

2) Clinical research combined with professional care with the objective of acquisition of new medical knowledge. Here the patient may not directly benefit, but the hope is for more enlightened management in the future for patients with the same disease.

3) Clinical research that is neither therapeutic nor directed toward acquiring knowledge of a specific disease. The purpose of the research is not necessarily to benefit the patient or to provide information on the disease he may have. Rather, it may be to obtain chemical, physiological, or pharmacological information. It may be conducted on normal subjects with a view to gaining further understanding

*Approved by the Committee on Public Health, March 6, 1967.

about the functioning of bodily systems.

Between as well as within each category there are differences in risk, and even more in risk:benefit ratio. Unless these differences are observed, they can be the source of misconception, misstatement, and misapplication.

Lack of discrimination can occur in attempts to protect the patient through control of research by law. It is exceedingly difficult to draft a bill that will protect the patient in any contingency but is not unduly and unwarrantedly restrictive of research. It is not easy to frame a bill that is flexible and suitable for all kinds of research. Efforts to minimize risk and maximize benefits by law can lead to an indiscriminate and rigid statute. The most damaging effect of such a law is that it may distort, impede, even halt, research. The usual provision in law is the requirement of an informed consent from the patient. This requirement on the one hand may lead to difficulties over interpretation of the amount of disclosure and whether it should be of an oral or written nature. On the other hand, if it is not appropriately applied it may impair or distort research.

Actually it is important to note that further statutes are unnecessary. Amid all the hubbub about the safety of clinical research, it may not be generally known that the public already has a large measure of protection.

As one source, the role of the physician should not be forgotten. His motivation and interest are identical with the patient's: that nothing untoward happen to the latter. Basic is the physician's desire to heal. If something goes amiss in research it is not likely to be fruitful for the patient, for humanity, for the physician, or for the science of medicine. Then too, the physician's reputation is always at stake.

As another source of protection to the patient, there are reminders, guidelines and restraints, many self-imposed by the profession, to reenforce the proper procedure. Among the safeguards for the public are the many codes: the Nuremberg Code, with its 10 points; the World Medical Association's Declaration of Helsinki; the stand of the American Medical Association; statements by the United States Public Health Service, Académie Nationale de Médecine (France), The French Academy of Moral and Political Sciences; and the pronouncements of the Roman Catholic Church as expressed by Pius XII. In all of them, safety of the patient is paramount. Certainly there is no lack of guidelines for clinical investigations on human subjects.

Besides this guidance, there are mandatory requirements controlling much of clinical research in the United States. By far the greatest part of it is conducted under federal grants-in-aid or contracts in which suitable precautions are invariably a requirement in the agreement that must be met. Clinical research is usually conducted under the auspices of a responsible medical institution such as a medical school or hospital with a review committee passing upon the procedures. Linking a stipulation for protection of the patient with the provision of research funds is a highly effective means of fostering observance of safeguards.

There is also a statutory provision for the protection of the public in one type of clinical research, the clinical testing of investigational drugs. Under the Federal Food, Drug, and Cosmetic Act the investigator must obtain informed consent of the subject.

Finally, surveillance that all precautionary requirements are completely observed is an important provision for the protection of the patient or subject. The few difficulties of record have arisen largely from remissness in surveillance.

It should be reiterated that this system of protection covers in general all clinical research. If vigilance in surveillance were extended and emphasized by existing research committees no further legislation would be needed.

In summary, this is the situation. For the future, medical research is the only hope for the prevention or conquest of disease. In any medical research, studies on man are the ultimate and necessary step. But along with the chance of benefit from saving life, routing disease, bringing comfort, or acquiring knowledge, there may be some risk. Whether to try some procedure or product on man should be a physician's and patient's decision, in which the readiness for application, the need, the relative safety, and the chance of benefit or success, enter into calculation. For the protection of man against overzealous investigators, clinical research is already subject to enough guiding principles, contractual stipulations, and regulations. In the rare instance of nonobservance, the final responsibility is with the institutional administration for failure in its surveillance. Further legislation could add nothing to existing protection. Indeed, it could distort, hamper, impede, even destroy research. If any further action needs to be taken, it would be to extend the already widely prevalent requirements of institutional auspices to all clinical research and to emphasize the serious responsibility for maintaining surveillance.

# POLYBIUS ON MEDICINE AND HISTORY

So far as we can judge by fragmentary evidence, it would seem that medicine has always interested the layman, although the character and intensity of that interest may well have varied in the course of the centuries. Even in antiquity medicine was often mentioned or used as an example or an analogy. This is noticeable especially in the Platonic dialogues. At least one ancient medical writer, Aulus Cornelius Celsus, is supposed to have been not a physician but a lay encyclopedist.

Apart from this, medicine and historiography show one interrelation of a special and specific kind. This consists of the fact that the physician who writes the clinical history of a patient employs methods which are strikingly similar to those employed by the historiographer. Both men work by collecting evidence, evaluating it, and placing it in meaningful chronological sequence. This similarity deserves more elaborate consideration than can be given here, but we may extend the resemblance by observing that histories are often written in order to explain how a certain condition of affairs came into existence. This is altogether identical with the clinician's attempt to explain how his patient came to be sick: i.e., a present state is explained by reference to antecedent conditions.

It has already been mentioned that ancient writers sometimes used medicine as an analogy to illustrate or prove a point. In this category belongs the curious statement of Polybius that is reproduced herewith.

Polybius, one of the greatest although not necessarily the most captivating of the ancient historians, was born at Megalopolis in Arcadia about 208 B.C. and lived till about 126 B.C. He was a close friend of the younger Scipio and witnessed the destruction of Carthage in 146 B.C. Well qualified by political and military experience, he wrote a history in 40 books, of which only the first 5 have come down to us complete. He laid great stress on personal experience and first-hand evidence. In the passage quoted herewith* he attacks a contemporary historian named Timaeus for ignoring these essentials:

*Polybius XII. 25*d*-25*e*, translated by W. R. Paton. Loeb Classical Library. London, Heinemann, 1925. Reprinted by permission of Harvard University Press.

"Besides the above-mentioned faults another thing remains to be noticed about Timaeus. Having lived for nearly fifty years in Athens with access to the works of previous writers, he considered himself peculiarly qualified to write history, making herein, I think, a great mistake. For as medicine and history have this point of resemblance, that each of them may be roughly said to consist of three parts, so there is the same difference in the dispositions of those who enter on these callings. To begin with, as there are three parts of medicine, first the theory of disease, next dietetics and thirdly surgery and pharmaceutics [*a sentence only partly legible in the MS.*], the study of the theory of disease, which is derived chiefly from the schools of Herophilus and Callimachus at Alexandria, is indeed an integral part of medicine, but as regards the ostentation and pretensions of its professors they give themselves such an air of superiority that one would think no one else was master of the subject. Yet when you make them confront reality by entrusting a patient to them you find them just as incapable of being of any service as those who have never read a single medical treatise. Not a few invalids indeed who had nothing serious the matter with them have before now come very near losing their lives by entrusting themselves to these physicians, impressed by their rhetorical powers. For really they are just like pilots who steer by book. But nevertheless these men visit different towns with great parade, and when they manage to collect a crowd, throw into the greatest confusion and expose to the contempt of their audience men who in actual practice have given real proof of their skill, the persuasiveness of their eloquence often prevailing against the testimony of practical experience. The third quality, which in every profession gives the true habit of mind, is not only rare but is often cast into the shade by gabble and audacity owing to people's general lack of judgement. In the same fashion systematic history too consists of three parts, the first being the industrious study of memoirs and other documents and a comparison of their contents, the second the survey of cities, places, rivers, lakes, and in general all the peculiar features of land and sea and the distances of one place from another, and the third being the review of political events; and just as in the case of medicine, many aspire to write history owing to the high opinion in which the science is held, but most of them bring to the task absolutely no proper qualification except recklessness, audacity, and roguery, courting popularity like apothecaries, and always saying whatever they regard as opportune in order to curry favour for the sake of getting a living by this means. Some of those again who appear to be justified in undertaking the composition of history, just like the theoretical doctors, after spending a long time in libraries and becoming deeply learned in memoirs and records, persuade themselves that they are adequately qualified for the task, seeming indeed to outsiders to contribute sufficient for the requirements of systematic history, but, in my own opinion contributing only a part. For it is true that looking through old memoirs is of service for knowledge of the views of the ancients and the notions people formerly had about conditions, places, nations, states, and events, and also for understanding the circumstances and chances which beset each nation in former times. For past events make us pay particular attention to the future, that is to say if we really make thorough inquiry in each case into the past. But to believe, as Timaeus did, that relying upon the mastery of material alone one can write well the history of subsequent events is absolutely foolish, and is much as if a man who had seen the works of ancient painters fancied himself to be a capable painter and a master of that art."

S. J.

***Advance Announcement***

The August issue of the Bulletin will be devoted to the publication of papers presented at the

*CONFERENCE ON BURNS AND*
*FLAME-RETARDANT FABRICS*

that was held at the Academy last December, under the auspices of the American College of Surgeons, the National Fire Protection Association, the Academy's Section on Plastic and Reconstructive Surgery, the Division of Accident Prevention of the U.S. Public Health Service, in cooperation with the American Academy of Pediatrics, the American Public Health Association, and the National Safety Council.

The nature and extent of the burn problem, its medical and surgical aspects, the present technology and efforts to develop and apply flame-retardant fabrics, and the roles of government, industry and other agencies in controlling the problem of fires in clothing will be discussed in 22 papers by physicians and surgeons, by technicians and managers of the textile industry, and by executives in various government departments.

Advance orders for copies of this issue may be sent to:

Editor, Bulletin of The New York Academy of Medicine
2 East 103 Street, New York, N.Y. 10029

## BATHING IN VIENNA

The system established for private bathing in Vienna, from its convenience, deserves particular notice; for, besides accommodations at the baths, called the Diana and Emperor's baths, you may, at any time, by sending an order a few hours previously, be furnished from them with a warm bath in your own lodging. This is done by putting the hot water into small casks, formed of staves at least two inches in thickness, which are conveyed to any part of the city or suburbs upon carriages resembling our brewers' drays. A bathing vessel is brought at the same time, and placed in your chamber, and is filled from these casks, of which a sufficient number are left to be added to the rest, to keep up the temperature. When confined in these thick casks, the water will retain considerable heat for twenty-four hours. The apparatus is removed by the same persons who brought it; and the whole charge does not amount to more than eighteenpence or two shillings, according to the distance of your abode from the public baths.

From: Richard Bright, *Travels from Vienna through Lower Hungary.* Edinburgh, Constable, 1818, p. 88.

### *Bowen-Brooks Scholarship For Advanced Study Abroad*

In the current year the Committee on Medical Education of The New York Academy of Medicine will award *one* Bowen-Brooks Scholarship in the amount of $5,200 for the *academic year 1968-69*.

This scholarship was established by the donor to provide aid for advanced study abroad in a clinical subject in preparation for the practice of medicine or surgery in any of their branches.

As stipulated by the donor of the fund, candidates must be *male* interns or residents in voluntary, municipal or Veterans Administration hospitals in New York City.

The course of study, the auspices under which it is to be taken, and the place or places where the study is to be pursued must receive the approval of the Committee. Applicants are favored who, from their records, show themselves capable of advanced work in clinical medicine. The Committee stipulates that the study be pursued abroad, preferably in Great Britain or in continental Europe.

The deadline for receipt of applications is *November 1, 1967*. Applicants will be required to appear before the Awards Committee for a personal interview at a meeting to be held in December. Announcement of the award will be made in late December.

Requests for application forms should be addressed to:

Office of Medical Education
The New York Academy of Medicine
2 East 103 St., New York, N.Y. 10029

## *The Glorney-Raisbeck Fellowship in the Medical Sciences*

The Glorney-Raisbeck Fellowship in the Medical Sciences for the academic year beginning July 1, 1968 will be awarded by the Committee on Medical Education of The New York Academy of Medicine for one year of research or study, in the United States or abroad, in any field of medicine or its allied sciences.

The fellowship, which carries a stipend of $7,500, is open only to citizens of the United States who are holders of the M.D. degree and who are located in the New York metropolitan area. Applicants must have demonstrated potential for productivity in research and teaching.

An applicant should be prepared to give assurance that he will have an institutional appointment which will enable him to carry out the purposes of his program of research or study. Such institutions will be encouraged to supplement the fellowship stipend. The fellowship *is not available* for supplementation of residency salaries.

The deadline for receipt of applications is *November 1, 1967*. Applicants will be required to appear before the Awards Committee for a personal interview at a meeting to be held in December. Announcement of the award will be made in late December.

Requests for application forms should be addressed to:

Office of Medical Education
The New York Academy of Medicine
2 East 103 Street, New York, N.Y. 10029

# TELEVISED CLINICAL SCIENCE SEMINARS

**Tuesday Evenings, 8:30-9:30 P.M.**

STATION WNYC—TV UHF—CHANNEL 31

**June 6, 1967**

## ELECTROLYTE DISTURBANCES IN INFANTS AND CHILDREN

CHESTER M. EDELMANN, JR.
Assistant Professor of Pediatrics
Albert Einstein College of Medicine

LAURENCE FINBERG
Chief, Division of Pediatrics
Montefiore Hospital and Medical Center
Professor of Pediatrics
Albert Einstein College of Medicine

LEONARD S. TAITZ
Assistant Professor of Pediatrics
Albert Einstein College of Medicine

**June 13, 1967**

## REDUCING THE CLEFT PALATE HANDICAP

WILLIAM H. CANFIELD, Ed.D.
Associate Professor of Speech Pathology
Adelphi University
Consultant, Speech Pathology
St. Luke's Hospital

RICHARD B. STARK
Attending Surgeon in Charge of Plastic Surgery
Director of Cleft Palate Clinic
St. Luke's Hospital

EDWARD STROH, JR., D.D.S.
Director, Department of Dentistry
St. Luke's Hospital
Director, Department of Oral Surgery
Metropolitan Hospital

**June 20, 1967**

## HEADACHE

LAWRENCE E. HINKLE, JR.
Clinical Associate Professor of
Medicine in Psychiatry
Cornell University Medical College

E. CHARLES KUNKLE
Associate Neurologist
Maine Medical Center

BRONSON S. RAY
Clinical Professor of Surgery (Neurosurgery)
Cornell University Medical College

**June 27, 1967**

## PANCREATITIS AND ITS MANAGEMENT

DAVID A. DREILING
Chief of Surgery, City Hospital Center at Elmhurst
Director of Animal Research, The Mount Sinai Hospital

HENRY D. JANOWITZ
Head, Department of Gastroenterology
The Mount Sinai Hospital
Clinical Professor of Medicine
The Mount Sinai School of Medicine

O. D. KOWLESSAR
Associate Professor of Medicine
and Director, Division of Gastroenterology
New Jersey College of Medicine
and Dentistry

BULLETIN OF
THE NEW YORK ACADEMY
OF MEDICINE

VOL. 43, NO. 7 JULY 1967

# SOME CONSIDERATIONS IN THE THERAPY OF PINEAL TUMORS

*Rudolf Virchow Lecture**

LEO M. DAVIDOFF

Professor Emeritus
Department of Neurological Surgery
Albert Einstein College of Medicine
New York, N. Y.

THE 100 years of the 19th century are, medically speaking, in many ways like the legendary days of old. Not because of their remoteness in point of time—I was born in the 19th century myself—but because giants such as Pasteur, Koch, Lister, and Rudolf Virchow walked the earth. To state that Virchow is, even today, a three-dimensional figure would be to neglect at least half a dozen other dimensions of his richly endowed personality. He was physician, pathologist, epidemiologist, anthropologist, archeologist, sociologist, historian, linguist, political scientist, and practicing politician. And he stood in the top rank of each of these disciplines.

As a very young man he set his goal as "an all-around knowledge of nature from the deity down to the stone." What is more, his great mind, coupled with his small but rugged physique, unbounded energy, and a

*Based on a lecture given before the Rudolph Virchow Medical Society in the Ctiy of New York at a meeting held at The New York Academy of Medicine, October 3, 1966. By special arrangement this paper will also appear in the *Proceedings of the Rudolf Virchow Medical Society in the City of New York.*

long life, permitted him to come very close to achieving his aim.

His productivity is not only astonishing, it is almost unbelievable. Ackerknecht[1] states:

> Besides his research, crystallized in more than two-thousand papers and books, besides his academic and popular teaching, his traveling, his political and administrative work, besides his editorial and organizational activities, he still found time to arrange and label with his own hands more than twenty-thousand preparations and four-thousand skulls for his Institute collection.

Politically he was always on the side of liberalism, and he even helped man the barricades in the unsuccessful German revolution of 1848. After a period of quiescence, he reentered the political arena as a member of Parliament and was such a goad in the side of Bismarck that the chancellor actually challenged him to a duel. One cannot help thinking, when visualizing such an encounter between the spunky little *Geheimrat* and the "Iron" Chancellor, of David and Goliath. Only this time no miracle from heaven could have saved the miniature defendant, for Virchow—David—was an atheist or at least an agnostic and certainly did not believe in heaven. However, he averted the disaster in his own forthright way. He simply refused to fight—with swords, that is.

While Virchow is best known to us as the discoverer of cellular pathology, he was responsible for so many discoveries in morphological as well as physiological pathology that it is not at all surprising to find that he was also the first to describe the appearance of tumors in the region of the pineal body, which is the subject of this lecture. His report on these lesions largely reflects the doubts and uncertainties still existing concerning them today.

In his famous book, *Die krankhaften Geschwülste*,[30] he states (the translation is mine):

> I add here a type of tumor, namely the hyperplasia of the pineal; I cannot decide whether it is to be considered, in the narrowest sense, a glioma. In view of our lack of knowledge of the function of this organ and its parts, I cannot draw any firm conclusion as to whether the increase in these elements should not rather be classed with the neuromas. I can state nevertheless that some gliomas of the brain highly resemble the hyperplastic tumors of the pineal grossly and in their individual elements. No one, to my knowledge, has ever estimated the neuronal nature of the pineal cells.

Indeed, no firm concept of the function of the pineal body exists to this day.

In a recent review entitled "The Pineal Gland," Richard Relkin[23] pointed out that in fishes, amphibians, and lacertilian reptiles the pineal gland is primarily a photoreceptor organ in which distinct sensory cells resembling retinal cone cells are found. In mammals there are no sensory cells, the pinealocyte being a secretory cell.

As for proof concerning its secretory activity, neither extirpatory experiments nor experiments in which there were injections of pineal extracts or implants of pineal tissue have given clear-cut answers.

The consensus is that the pineal secretes an inhibitory hormone causing retardation of sexual maturation until puberty, when the gland atrophies and the maturing secretions of the pituitary, adrenal, and gonadal glands go into high gear. These impressions are derived from the rare clinical cases in prepubertal male children with tumors in the pineal region who develop macrogenitosomia praecox, whereas occasional cases also having tumors in this location are associated with delayed puberty. Correlations of such clinical manifestations with this type of tumor tend to show that parenchymatous pineal tumors display a high degree of association with depressed gonadal function, whereas nonparenchymatous lesions such as gliomas, or those teratomas that destroy the normal pineal and contain no neoplastic pineal tissue may be associated with pubertas praecox. Thus, according to this theory, pineal hyperfunction is associated with delayed pubescence, and hypofunction with advanced puberty. However, this is still a highly theoretical concept.

Moreover, Virchow's confusion derived not only from a lack of knowledge concerning the function of the pineal, but also from the considerable variation in the microscopic appearance of these tumors.

When Bailey and Cushing[4] presented their work on the *Classification of the Tumors of the Glioma Group on a Histogenetic Basis* in their classical monograph in 1926, they included eight cases of pineal tumor, three of which they named pineoblastoma, and five pinealoma. As time passed, this proved to be an oversimplification, and it failed to cover a number of tumors in this region clearly not eligible for such classification. Thus Bochner and Scarff[5] described a teratomatous lesion of the pineal containing elements from all three embryonal layers, including fully developed teeth, as well as pineal tissue. This tumor was primary in the pineal region, and they theorized that there is "inherent multipotentiality in the primitive cells of the pineal body similar to that found in the cells of the testes and ovary." However, as late as 1941, Globus[10] still clung to the histogenetic origin of these tumors and felt that he was able to match each of the 12 cases he reported with some stage in the histogenesis of the pineal. It is important to note, by the way, that Globus found the majority of the tumors on which he reported to be invasive lesions.

It remained for Dorothy Russell[25] to point out in 1944 that the resemblance of the so-called pinealomas to embryonic pineal tissue is only superficial and is suggested by their mosaiclike appearance. The large spheroidal cells so conspicuous in this tumor, unlike similar cells in the embryonic pineal body, lack the blepharoblasts and the silver-staining qualities of these cells, while the smaller cells of the tumor are really only smaller examples of the spheroidal cells, and not lymphocites. Moreover, in two of Dr. Russell's cases, which were studied in serial sections, she found teratoid elements, and she felt that those neoplasms making up the majority of pineal tumors that Bailey, and also Globus, had called pinealomas, are really atypical teratomas resembling the spheroid-cell carcinomas of the testes. As further proof of the independence of these tumors from the pineal, she called attention to the occurrence of these very tumors in other sites along the midline structures of the brain, such as the hypothalamus, the so-called "ectopic pinealomas." In such cases a perfectly normal pineal body is usually found in the normal anatomic position. This is not to say that true pinealomas do not occur but, in her opinion, they are very rare.

Horrax and Wyatt,[16] however, reported in 1947 three cases of "ectopic pinealoma," in one of which they demonstrated (and in a second one they presumed) a continuity of the tumor with that in the original site in the region of the pineal, with extension to the hypothalamus by way of the lateral walls of the third ventricle. The third case, however, was definitely primary in the neighborhood of the optic chiasm.

In 1949, Walton[31] reported two cases of teratomas in the hypothalamic region that contained pineal tissue. This he felt was due to the polypotentiality of these tumors. He argued, then, that they should thus be called teratomas in the hypothalamus, rather than ectopic pinealomas; with this opinion I am inclined to agree.

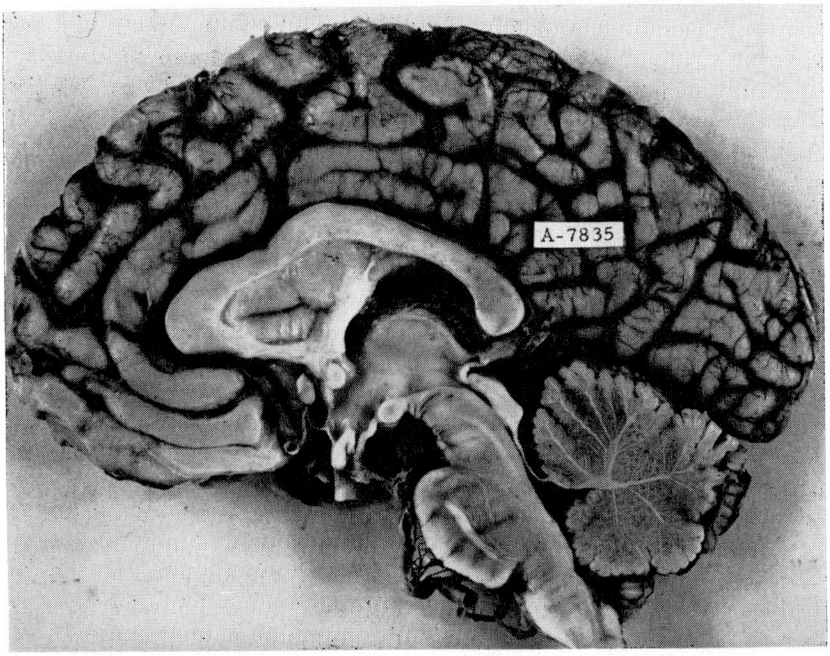


Fig. 1. Midsagittal section of a normal brain, showing the relation of the pineal body to the quadrigeminal plate and the latter's relation to the aqueduct of Sylvius.

In 1957 Løken[19] described three cases of tumor in the hypothalamic region, all of them histologically resembling Russell's atypical teratomas.

Russell's thesis was strongly supported by N. B. Friedman[9] in 1947, when he reported on his study of 23 cases of pineal tumor found in the collection of the Armed Forces Institute of Pathology, Washington, D.C. Ten of these, identical in appearance with the spheroid cell carcinoma of the testes—thus the atypical teratoma of Russell, Friedman felt, could as well be called "seminoma" or "germinoma." Five others were true teratomas, or teratomatous carcinomas, and eight were gliomas. Friedman's observation that the germinoma is extraordinarily sensitive to radiation will find support when we come to a discussion of the treatment of these neoplasms.

This brief discussion by no means covers all the possible types of tumors in the pineal region, nor the extensive literature on this aspect of the problem, since it is my purpose on this occasion to concentrate primarily on the *treatment* of these rare but interesting neoplasms.

For the same reason we need not tarry very long on the diagnosis.

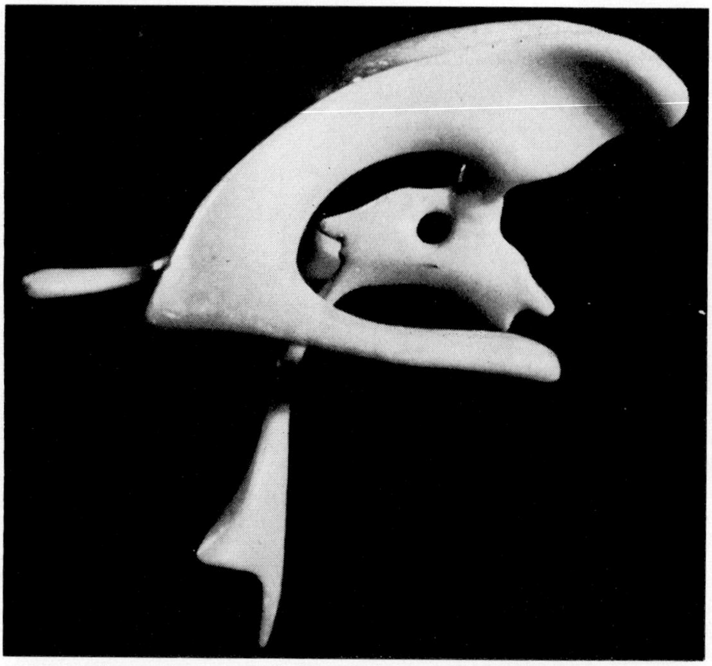

Fig. 2. A mold of the cerebral ventricular system, graphically presenting the possibility of a "bottleneck" in the aqueductal region.

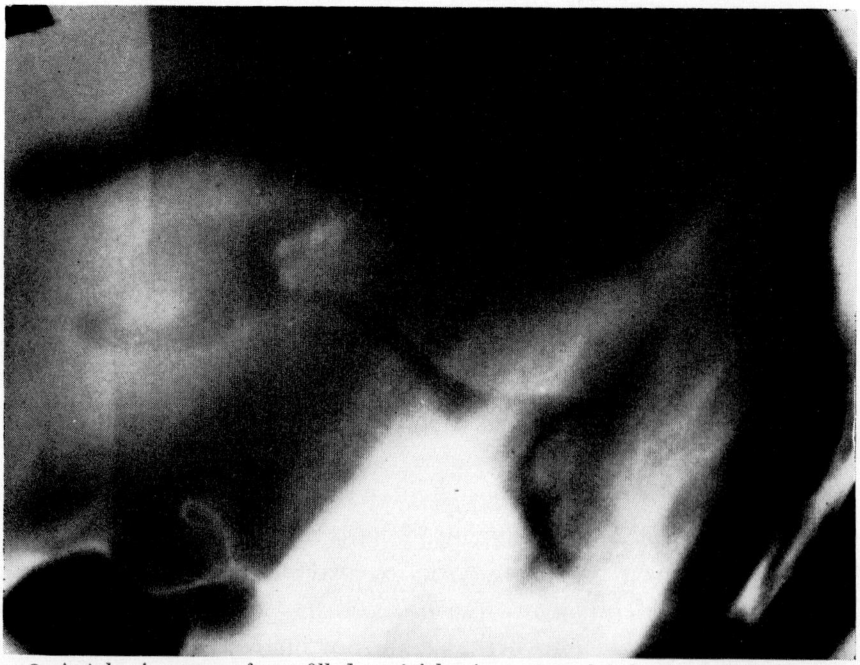

Fig. 3. Autolaminagram of gas-filled ventricles in a normal individual. This shows the unobstructed aqueduct of Sylvius in its normal relation to the third and fourth cerebral ventricles.

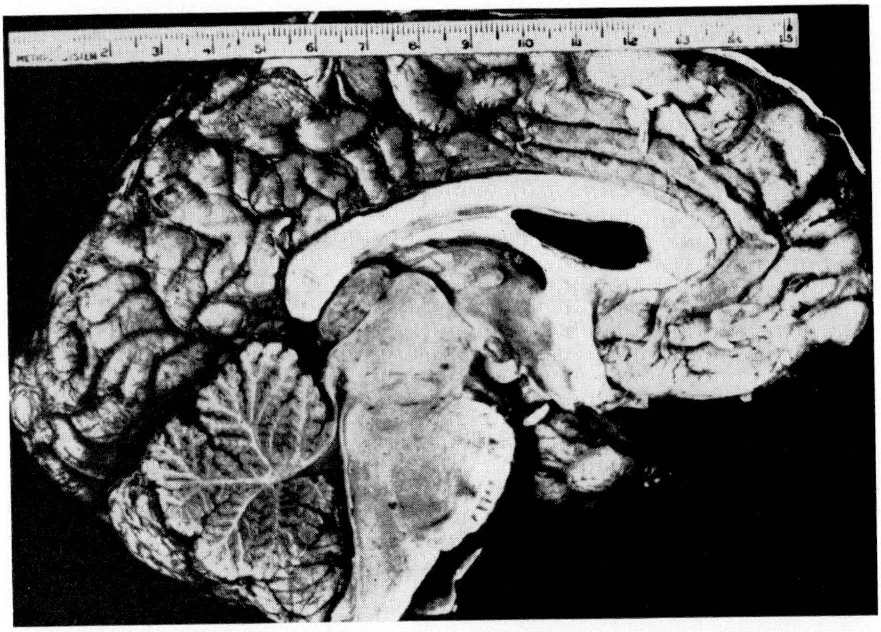

Fig. 4. Sagittal section of brain in a case with a small tumor in the pineal region, showing already the obliteration of the aqueduct and the dilatation of the third ventricle. Reproduced by permission from Horrax, G., and Bailey, P. Pineal pathology: Further studies, *Arch. Neurol. Psychiat.* *19*:394-415, 1928.

The major point about the clinical aspect of the problem is to remember that the pineal body is located just above the quadrigeminal plate, and that the quadrigeminal plate forms the roof of the aqueduct of Sylvius. Figure 1 shows a sagittal section of a normal brain. Here one sees that the cavity of the lateral ventricle is hidden by the septum pellucidum, but its outlet into the anterior part of the third ventricle by way of the foramen of Monro is clearly visible. The cerebral fluid then passes backward and leaves the third ventricle via the aqueduct of Sylvius. The quadrigeminal plate is well seen here, and also the pineal above it. After passing into the fourth ventricle by way of an unobstructed aqueduct, the fluid leaves the fourth chamber by way of the foramina of Magendie and Luschka and passes into the subarachnoid spaces, to bathe the base and the convexities of the cerebral hemispheres and then to be reabsorbed into the general blood circulation through the arachnoidal villi. Figure 2 shows the lateral view of a mold of the cerebral ventricular system, which graphically presents the relatively narrow aqueduct. Figure 3 shows a lateral laminagraphic ventriculogram of this area as it appears in a normal individual. Since the lumen

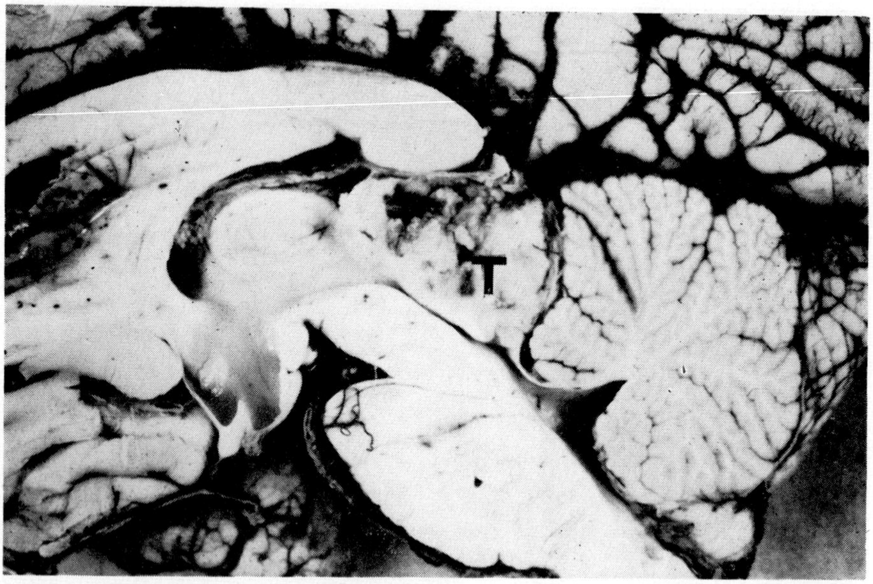


Fig. 5. Midsagittal section of the brain in a case of a large pineal tumor (T). The third ventricle is ballooned out, and the lamina terminalis is almost paper-thin.

of this narrow aqueductal passageway varies in the diameter of its cross-section from only 1 mm. to 3 mm., it is easy to see how any—even a minor—degree of pressure on the roof would obstruct the passageway and produce obstructive hydrocephalus. Now see, in Figure 4, what happens when even a small tumor occupies the region of the pineal. The fluid meets a block at the aqueduct, and the ventricular system ahead of the block dilates like an artificial lake behind a dam. Note particularly the stretching of the anterior wall of the third ventricle. Figure 5 shows a sagittal section through a brain specimen harboring a larger pineal tumor. I call your attention to the even greater thinning-out of the lamina terminalis. And Figure 6 shows how it looks when the brain specimen is x-rayed. Note how the tumor, which is denser than the surrounding brain because of calcium deposited in it, bulges into the posterior border of the third ventricle. The next, Figure 7, represents the lateral ventriculogram made during life in this patient, in which the characteristic deformity may again be noted.

Anyone would deduce from all this that the symptoms and signs of tumors in the region of the pineal would necessarily fall into four broad categories: 1) those of increased intracranial pressure due to obstructive hydrocephalus; 2) those of interference with the function

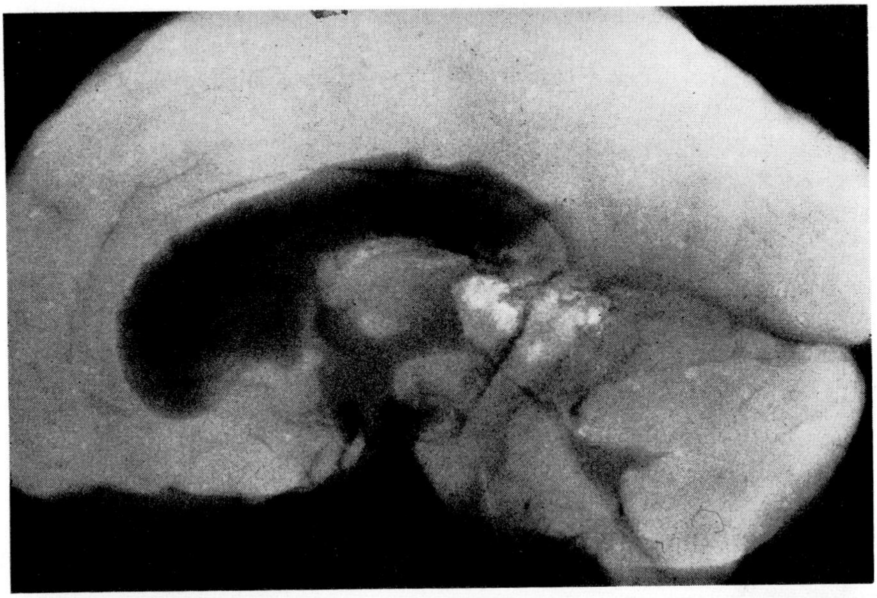

Fig. 6. Same case as in Figure 5. A roentgenogram of the brain, postmortem, showing the ballooned-out third ventricle, and the thin, elongated aqueduct of Sylvius.

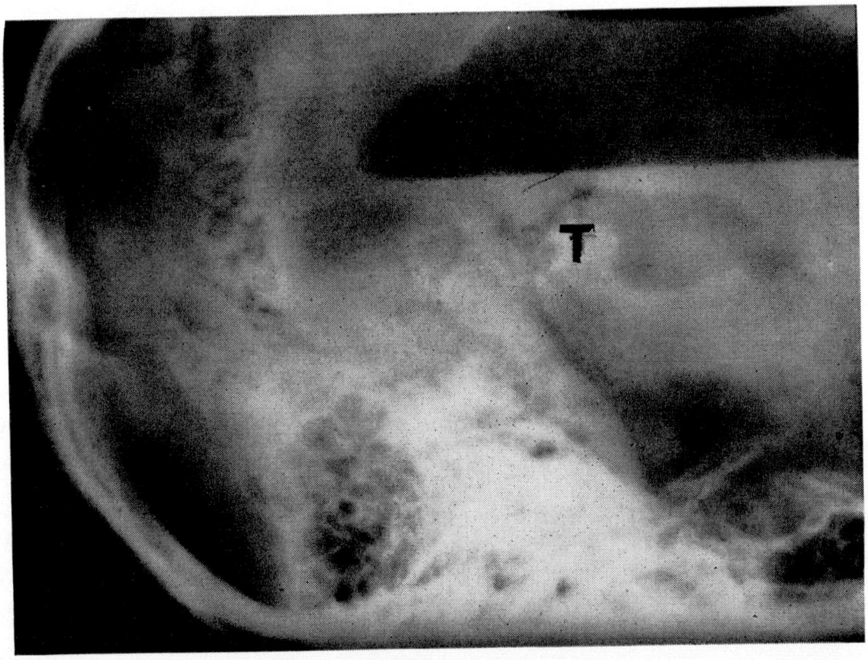


Fig. 7. Same case as in Figures 5 and 6. This shows the indentation by the tumor (T) into the posterior border of the third ventricle.

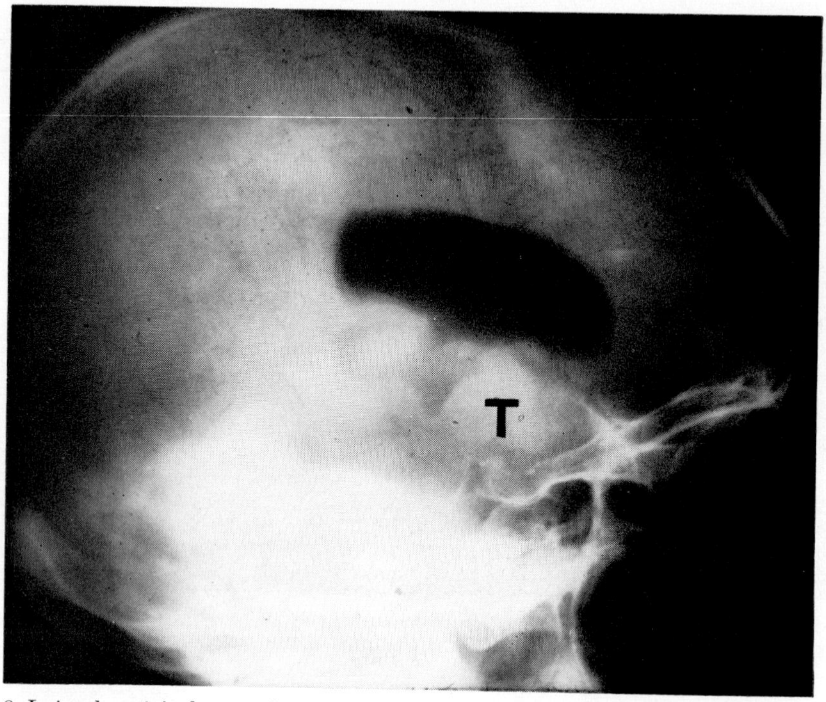


Fig. 8. Lateral ventriculogram, brow-up position, showing the indentation of the anterior border of the third ventricle by a tumor (T) at the foramen of Monro.

of the quadrigeminal plate and the midbrain generally; 3) those of interference with the function of distant parts of the brain, such as the hypothalamic-pituitary region; and 4) those less-well-understood endocrine manifestations due to depression or hyperactivity of pineal secretion, if any.

Since it has also been observed that the majority of patients with this disease are young males, a theoretical classical case—which, by the way, almost never happens—therefore would be that of a boy, let us say 8 years of age, complaining of severe headache and vomiting. He may also be suffering from double vision, and may have been observed to be partially deaf, unsteady of gait, and spastic. If, on examination, he proves to have a cracked-pot sound on percussion of his head (Macewen sign), due to spreading of the cranial sutures; papilledema; extraocular muscle disturbances, particularly limitation of upward gaze; pupils that respond poorly to light; partial or complete deafness; cerebellar ataxia and bilateral Babinski signs; and if, in addition to all this, he shows signs of advanced gonadal maturation, the presumptive diag-

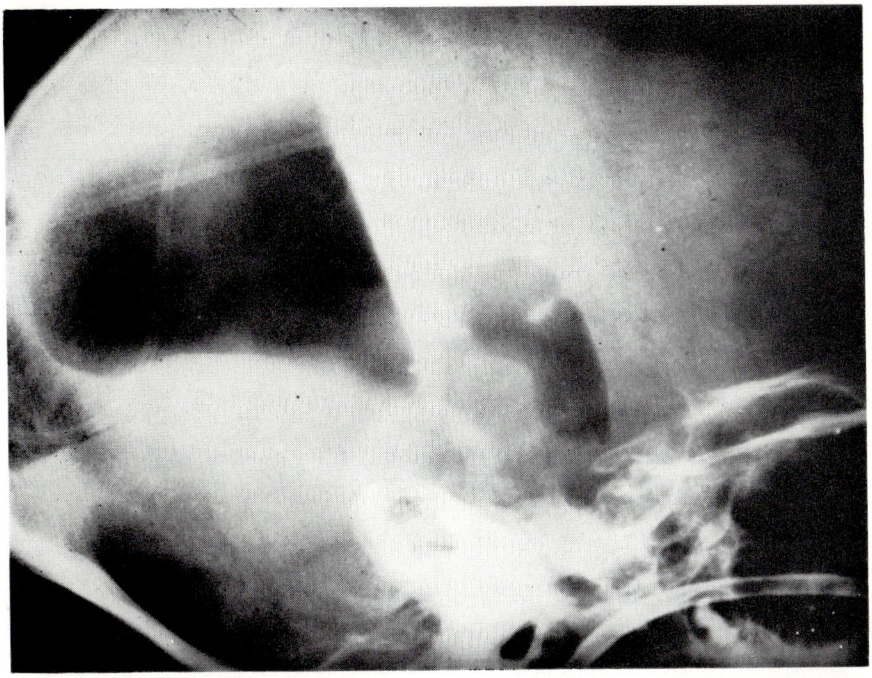

Fig. 9. Lateral ventriculogram, brow-down position, outlining dilatation and anterior angulation of the aqueduct of Sylvius resulting from a tumor of the cerebellum.

nosis of tumor in the pineal region will almost certainly prove to be correct. Unfortunately for the clinician, it almost never happens that way. Clinically, pubertas praecox is a rare accompaniment of pineal tumor, and signs of increased intracranial pressure plus cerebellar dysfunction are most prominent. Thus, especially in preventriculography days, these cases were frequently mistaken for tumors in the cerebellum. What is more, exploration of the posterior fossa not only failed to reveal the lesion, but was often followed by death.

Ventriculography has largely eliminated this uncertainty. And this diagnostic procedure, with due precautions into which I need not go, should be carried out in almost any case in which increased intracranial pressure due to obstructive hydrocephalus is encountered. This would include cases with tumors of the anterior third ventricle obstructing the foramen of Monro, tumors in the region of the pineal that we are chiefly concerned with here, and tumors in the posterior fossa obstructing the inlet of, or the outlet from, the fourth ventricle.

Figure 8 is from a lateral ventriculogram in a case of tumor of the anterior part of the third ventricle. Note that the foramen of Monro is

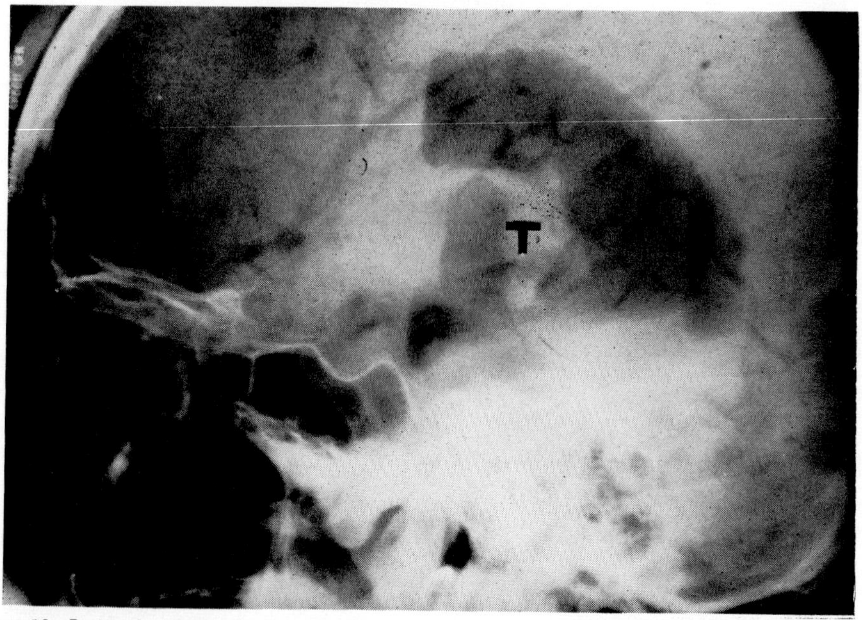

Fig. 10. Lateral ventriculogram, brow-down position, from another case of tumor of the pineal. The third ventricle is dilated and indented posteriorly by the tumor (T), and the aqueduct is not visualized.

dilated, and that the gas in the dilated third ventricle shows a projection of tumor into it on its anterior border. The next view, Figure 9 in this group, is from a patient with a cerebellar tumor. Here the whole of the dilated third ventricle is visualized, but the aqueduct is also dilated, and its caudal end is kinked forward by the forward thrust of the tumor in the posterior fossa.

Contrast this with the next illustration, Figure 10, from another patient with a tumor of the pineal, to which I again call your attention. The lateral ventricles, the foramen of Monro, and the *anterior* portion of the third ventricle are all dilated, and the outline of the tumor is seen projecting into its posterior border.

In any case in which a midline tumor obstructing the free passage of cerebrospinal fluid is suspected, and the ventriculograms show the protrusion of a mass into the posterior border of the third ventricle such as this, a diagnosis of tumor of the pineal region is justified and is most likely to be correct.

So much for the diagnosis.

We come now to the question of treatment, which is my point of emphasis on this occasion. Before doing so, however, let us stop for a moment to gain perspective. Brain tumors in general are relatively rare lesions, making up only 0.06 to 0.15 per cent of all the causes of death. Moreover, pineal tumors are rare tumors among the already rare intracranial tumors, making up only 0.4 to 1.0 per cent of intracranial neoplasms.

Why, then, have I chosen to present, before a general medical audience, a discussion involving technical neurosurgical problems, matters of neurosurgical judgment, and related radiotherapeutic considerations in so rare, limited, and highly specialized an area of medical interest? Indeed, I do so with apologies to all of you. However, certain principles and philosophical concepts of therapy are involved here that are equally valid in many other situations in the treatment of human ills, and they make this discussion—so, at least, I hope—worthy of your time and attention.

I can still remember many a doctor's consulting room, a few generations ago, conspicuously displaying the framed motto: "*Primum Non Nocere.*" While Latin is no longer the common language of scholars and physicians, the principle—First of all, do no harm—should still be our guide, in whatever language we communicate.

*And the direct surgical attack upon these tumors was in the past—and still is, by and large—a harmful procedure.* This is due, for the most part, to two factors: first, the dangerous location of these tumors and, second, their infiltrating character, which makes it impossible to eradicate them surgically in toto, even after Scylla and Charybdis are successfully circumvented.

Since the early decades of this century, various approaches have been made to reach the lesion surgically. Thus, in 1907 Theodor Krause suggested trying to approach them through the posterior fossa, transtentorially; and Brunner, as reported by Rorschach in 1913, attempted but failed in removing a pineal tumor by this route. Puusepp in 1914 ligated the lateral sinus, divided the tentorium, and thus reached the tumor site, but the patient died in this attempt.

In 1921 Dandy,[6] who was a bold, resourceful, and skillful surgeon, exposed the parieto-occipital region of the brain on the right (that is, the nondominant) side, divided the large draining veins that passed from the cerebral cortex to empty into the superior longitudinal sinus, then retracted the hemisphere away from the falx cerebri. Upon reaching the splenium of the corpus callosum he divided this structure, and in this way visualized the tumor through a tangle of the great vein of Galen and its tributaries. The first case, after all this, proved on exposure to be a widely infiltrating glioma which he could not even *attempt* to remove. The second case was a patient from whom he succeeded in removing a well-demarcated mass, which proved to be a tuberculoma. The patient died 8 months later, presumably from a spread of her disease to other parts of the brain. The third patient reported upon in his paper survived the operation but died 48 hours postoperatively. No wonder that 4 years later, in 1925, when Horrax and Bailey[14] reported 12 verified cases from Harvey Cushing's clinic, they had all been verified postmortem. All had ended fatally *without* operation because they had been considered inoperable.

Harvey Cushing himself, in 1926,[4] was extremely pessimistic about the future treatment of these lesions. He felt that it was improbable that we should ever be able successfully to extirpate them in view of their inaccessible position. He believed, from all points of view, that they are most unfavorable lesions.

In 1931 Van Wagenen,[29] faced with a case of pineal tumor, tried a new approach. He exposed the posterior half of the right cerebral hemisphere; entered the dilated lateral ventricle by a temporo-occipital cortical incision; then, locating the bulge produced by the tumor on the medial side of the ventricle, he transected the medial side of the brain, thus reaching the tumor. Even then he had to leave some of the tumor behind because it was so intimately involved with the great vein of Galen. Postoperatively the patient was incontinent, sluggish, and had impaired memory. These symptoms largely cleared up, and the patient received x radiation. She was followed for 15 months, when she was lost to follow-up. As a result of this experience, Van Wagenen concluded that perhaps a better way to treat these patients is to do a subtemporal decompression first, followed by roentgen irradiation; then, when recurrence of symptoms occurs, as he believed it usually would, the radical approach should be tried.

In 1932 Harris and Cairns[11] wrote up an extensive study of the diagnosis and treatment of pineal tumors, and included a report of one case operated upon by Cairns. This male patient, 20 years of age, was first mistakenly explored for a cerebellar tumor, and actually improved for 6 months. The second operation was by Dandy's method, but the right internal occipital vein had to be cut in order to get the tumor out.

The patient was conscious following removal of the tumor. However, he had a left hemiplegia, left homonymous hemianopsia, and was noisy and incontinent. These signs cleared up in about 4 weeks, but he was left with poor memory. In spite of this heroic effort, he began to show signs of a recurrence of tumor about 9 months after the operation. He was then given some radiation therapy, which was admittedly inadequate because, among other things, the patient could not be made to lie still during the treatments. Nevertheless, he showed some improvement until some months later when he fell, struck his head, and again showed progressive signs. Radiation was resumed, with the patient sedated with Nembutal for each treatment. He improved steadily and seemed to be in good condition 13 months after the operation, when the report was made.

In 1935 McLean[20] reported another fatality following radical removal of a pineal teratoma.

In 1936 Dandy[7] published another report. Since the 1921 paper, he had had seven fatalities postoperatively, then three patients that survived. Of these, one died 3 months postoperatively, cause unknown; the second survived 2 years and 6 months, and then died of a recurrence of his tumor; and the third was living 4 months postoperatively when the paper was written. In 1936 also, another paper by Horrax[12] included a report on two more cases. One patient, a middle-aged woman, survived a partial extirpation of her tumor, was given irradiation, and was doing well 18 months later. The other patient was a boy of 10 years, with pubertas praecox and a tumor located but not verified in the pineal region; he was finally doing well after having had a subtemporal decompression as well as several courses of radiation therapy.

The next year, in 1937, Kahn[17] contributed his experience with two cases of pineal tumor. One was a patient operated upon by Max Peet in 1929; the patient was still living then and had received postoperative irradiation. The second was a patient upon whom Kahn himself had operated. This patient was alive one year later, but was somewhat below par in his intellectual functions and seemed to have a permanent left homonymous hemianopsia. The year 1937 also saw another report by Horrax[13] upon a case of a patient with a huge tumor (70 g.), in which he had to resect the right occipital lobe of the brain in order to deliver the mass. The postoperative course was agonizing, and ended fatally in 3 months.

Baggenstoss and Love[3] in 1939 wrote a general report on the experience of the Mayo Clinic with pinealomas; 10 cases had been seen there in 23 years. They did not report upon early or late results of treatment, but their attitude was distinctly gloomy since they stated: "The treatment of pineal tumors carries a high mortality, and the results of therapy at present are unsatisfactory."

More than 20 years after the description by Dandy of his radical operation for pineal tumors, Horrax, who had made many studies on these lesions, reported together with Daniels[15] upon four patients with such tumors, three of whom had had only subtemporal decompression and radiation therapy, and the fourth, radiation therapy alone; all four patients had recovered and were leading useful lives 18 to 30 months after treatment.

In 1943 W. O. Russell and Ernest Sachs[26] had collected from the literature 32 cases of patients with tumors of the pineal who had been treated by direct attack upon the tumor; only three of these patients had survived the immediate postoperative period.

Toward the end of the 1940's the impact of this holocaust began to trouble even the most intrepid surgeons. Torkildsen, who in 1939 had invented a method of circumventing an obstruction to the cerebrospinal fluid by leading the stream by way of a permanent tube from a lateral ventricle into the subarachnoid space, suggested the use of this method in tumors of the pineal region. He wrote an article[28] in 1948 entitled, "Should extirpation be attempted in cases of neoplasm in or near the third ventricle of the brain?" He answered his own question in the negative, and reported on eight cases of pineal tumors treated by his shunting method. Three of these patients were living and well 7 years and 6 months, 4 years and 6 months, and 2 years respectively after operation. In the same volume of the *Journal of Neurosurgery*, Ward and Spurling[32] presented their experience with "The conservative treatment of third ventricle tumors." They had collected the cases of 14 patients with appropriate symptoms and typical ventriculograms, sufficient to make the diagnosis of a tumor in the pineal region. Each was treated with subtemporal decompression and "intensive radiation." Two of these patients failed to respond to treatment, and proved to have cysts obstructing the aqueduct. Six patients had malignant gliomas, in whom conservative treatment failed. They were then operated upon by direct approach, and were all dead within 3 years. Six patients were alive and well approximately 6 to 16 years after subtemporal decompression and radiation therapy.

The largest experience with the surgical treatment of pineal tumors from a single institution was reported by Ringertz, Nordenstam, and Flyger[24] in 1954 from the Serafimerlasarettet in Stockholm. In a period of 25 years, from 1926 through 1951, 65 such cases had been seen, and 51 had grossly total or partial extirpation of the tumor by the Dandy technique. In addition to an immediate operative mortality of 58.8 per cent, six of the *survivors* died in less than 10 months postoperatively. Only seven patients were living 5 to 20 years postoperatively, and two of these had had only cysts instead of solid tumors.

However, as late as 1960 this radical operation was still being reported for the treatment of pineal tumors. Thus Kunicki[18] presented eight cases that year in which the Dandy procedure was used. Actually six of them survived the operation, but all showed poor memory and masklike immobility. Three had left hemiplegia, and one had left homonymous hemianopsia. The average stay in the hospital following operation was 4 months. The follow-up of the six survivors also showed many disturbing aspects. One patient, after 30 months, was attending school, but was aggressive, quarrelsome, and lacked perseverance. A second patient was blind, but was seemingly well otherwise; but he had received postoperative radiation therapy. The third patient was normal and attending school, but he too had had postoperative radiation. The fourth patient died after 6 months, cause unknown. The fifth patient was working as a farm hand 70 months postoperatively, but had also been given postoperative radiation. After 2 years of relative good health, the sixth patient died in a psychiatric hospital.

Thus we see that only in the three cases in which Kunicki was led to use postoperative irradiation did the patients do reasonably well.

At the present time so many mechanical, chemical, and electronic devices are available for our use that what was impossible only 20 years ago has become a matter of daily achievement. However, modern methods utilizing stereotactic instruments thus far have not shown any great promise, although experience is still limited. Thus, Radanowicz-Harttmann[22] reported two cases, in one of which a preliminary Torkildsen procedure was done, followed by Yttrium 90 implantation into the tumor by stereotactic means. The patient died a few days later, and the postmortem examination revealed a very large and very hemorrhagic tumor. The second patient in whom a similar procedure was planned got only as far as the Torkildsen, and then died of a pulmonary embolus. At postmortem an ependymoma was found, with infiltration of neighboring structures.

Incidentally, both of these patients showed reactive meningitis to the tube used for the Torkildsen shunt. With the selection of minimally reactive tubing for the shunt, this complication usually can be avoided, but not always. It is one of the prices one sometimes must pay for leaving foreign material implanted in patients' bodies for an indefinite period of time.

The present official neurological attitude toward these lesions was summarized by Zülch[33] in the 1965 English edition of his book, *Brain Tumors: Their Biology and Pathology*. In this work he stated: "Operation, even 'total extirpation,' seldom insures freedom from recurrence. Besides, total removal is difficult due to the pinealomas' close relationship to nervous centers and important blood vessels, and their growth by infiltration in the marginal zone."

## My Own Material

One day, about 6 months ago, while thinking about an appropriate subject for this lecture, I had a follow-up visit from a vigorous, healthy-looking, youngish man of 36 whom I had treated for a pineal tumor in 1943—that is, 23 years previously. This man had by now attended high school and college, was a successful teacher and had a family consisting of a wife and three children. It occurred to me, then, to check up on my own experience with these lesions and report to you on them on this occasion.

I found 14 cases of tumors in the pineal region in my own series that fit the diagnostic criteria already mentioned. The only exception was one patient in whom the ventriculographic studies were unsuccessful, so that the posterior border of the third ventricle was not visualized. However, he had clinical signs of increased intracranial pressure, obstructive hydrocephalus, and paralysis of upward gaze, and most likely had a pineal tumor.

Three of the 14 cases had been treated by direct approach to the tumor, and all three had died postoperatively. One of these was a 27-year-old woman upon whom I did a subtemporal decompression, which was followed by radiation. She failed to get relief, was taken to Baltimore, Md., where Dandy removed a tumor from her pineal region, but she died in the immediate postoperative period. The second patient was a boy of 9 with macrogenitosomia praecox. I succeeded in partially removing a tumor diagnosed as "pinealoma" at the time—that was in 1936. The boy was confused and right hemiparetic after the operation, but was beginning to do well, when he managed to get his fingers under the dressing and rip his wound wide open. It was immediately resutured, but he developed fulminating meningitis and died two months after the operation. The third patient in this group was a 22-year-old girl who died 4 days after a radical removal of the tumor by the Dandy technique.

Nine of the other 11 patients were treated by perforating the thinned-out anterior wall of the third ventricle to bypass the dammed-up fluid; one had a Torkildsen procedure, and one only a subtemporal decompression. In all these patients, operation was followed by radiation therapy. One of them died 3 years and 6 months after treatment, with uncontrollable recurrence of the lesion and, eventually, multiple spinal cord implantations of tumor. Another died 16 years after treatment. The remaining 9 patients are alive, respectively 9, 10, 12, 14, 16, 18, 19, 23, and 24 years following treatment. One patient, during 9 years of follow-up, has had two recurrences of focal symptoms without recurrence of papilledema, suggesting that the shunt is working while the tumor is periodically becoming reactivated. Each time, so far, she has responded to further radiation therapy. The other eight patients are not only alive, but are functioning normally in a variety of life situations.

The history of events in one of these cases may perhaps be made a little more vivid for you by describing its progress, and I have accordingly chosen to give you the details in the case of the young man who sparked my interest in the choice of subject for this paper.

*S. B.; Jewish Hospital of Brooklyn, N. Y., No. 268735.*

This boy was first seen by me on September 27, 1943, when he was 13 years of age. He had been healthy until a few months previously, when he began to have severe headaches associated with vomiting. Four or five weeks before the above date, his left eye became crossed, and he complained of double vision. These symptoms were progressive, but no other neurologic symptoms could be elicited.

On examination the child was extremely uncomfortable, holding his head and moaning. He was lethargic and uncooperative until he vomited, and then seemed a little more responsive. The right pupil was slightly larger than the left. Both reacted sluggishly to light. There was bilateral external rectus weakness. Upward gaze could not be tested because of lack of cooperation. Bilateral papilledema was noted. A suggestive left Babinski sign was recorded. The general physical examination revealed no abnormalities.

Routine blood and urine tests were all normal.

Plain x rays showed the skull to be within normal limits.

Cerebral gas ventriculograms were reported as showing: "Symmetrically dilated lateral ventricles and a dilated anterior portion of the third ventricle. There is a deformity of the posterior portion of the third ventricle characteristic of a tumor in the region of the midbrain, such as a pineal tumor."

On October 1, 1943, a right frontal craniotomy was performed, and the very thinned-out lamina terminalis was punctured. An incidental small subtemporal decompression was added for good measure.

He did extremely well postoperatively. His headaches subsided, the papilledema disappeared, and he became alert, bright, and cooperative in a matter of days.

Eleven days after the operation he was discharged from the hospital, to be treated with radiation to the tumor site on an ambulatory basis.

Between October 18, 1943, and January 21, 1944, he received three courses of x radiation, each consisting of about 1,000 r, to the tumor site.

Meanwhile he had remained symptom-free and, on examination on November 17, 1943, he looked well, had no diplopia or headaches. The decompression area was level and soft. The pupils still did not react well to light, and some limitation of upward gaze was present. The optic discs appeared to be within normal limits.

In November 1945 he again complained of mild headaches, and his optic discs showed some venous congestion. Because of this he was given an additional, similar, course of radiation therapy.

From then on to the present, I either saw him personally, or heard from him by letter, at approximately yearly intervals. In his last letter he wrote: "In answer to your letter, I am in excellent health. I have had absolutely no trouble in regard to my head. As you may know from my previous letters, I am married and the father of two boys, with a third on the way. I am in my eleventh year of teaching. I thank you for your continued interest. . . .

Seven other patients in this group present essentially similar pictures, and the young woman previously mentioned with the 9-year follow-up after treatment, who was again having trouble, is once more responding to radiation therapy.*

## Discussion

The radical surgical treatment of tumors originating in the pineal region, after 50 years more or less of bold, aggressive efforts on the part of several generations of neurosurgeons to extirpate them, is even to this day dismally unsuccessful. What the future may hold, when stereotactic methods are more skillfully used than they are today, is uncertain. I have grave doubts as to their applicability to these or, for that matter, to any other intracranial lesions that infiltrate neighboring brain structures. This would be particularly true in the region of the midbrain, where so many vital brain mechanisms are located. The reason for my skepticism is that the destructive agents that can be delivered through a probe, whether it be supercold, superheat, or a radioisotope implant, are totally necrotizing. The margin between the zone of necrosis and the neighboring brain would have to be so exquisitely placed as to destroy all the tumor and yet spare all the surrounding brain. This, I submit, would be extremely difficult if not impossible to do. However, assuming even that it could be accomplished, it would be necessary either to carry the effect of the destructive agent deliberately into the neighboring brain tissues in cases of infiltrating tumors and thus destroy vital brain elements, or leave the infiltrating portions of the tumor behind, thus guaranteeing recurrence.

The advantage of roentgen irradiation therapy over these methods is the relatively selective destructive effect on the tumor cells, and the resistance of normal neuronal elements to the same dose of radiation. Ideally, of course, one should have an agent that would destroy the tumor completely and leave normal tissue completely unharmed. If such an agent existed, our search for the cure of cancer would have come to an end. Unfortunately, this is seldom true. However, in some cases of highly radiosensitive tumors, such cures are occasionally

*Following this treatment she had another remission lasting about 8 months. Tumor symptoms then again recurred, and she died after an attempted radical operation by another surgeon.

achieved; and some, among the tumors under discussion, belong to this group.

I believe, therefore, that now and for the foreseeable future the most promising treatment for tumors in the pineal region is radiation therapy. I am purposely not going into a discussion of the type of radiation used, since this has changed over the years both in the efficiency of the source of radiation and the accuracy of focus on the lesion. Suffice it to say that the cases with the longest follow-up obviously received the least sophisticated forms of therapy. This would indicate that some of these tumors are remarkably sensitive to radiation. As my old grandmother used to say, "If God wills it, even a broomstick can shoot."

Prior to the application of radiation therapy to the tumor itself, these patients are in urgent need of relief from increased intracranial pressure produced by the obstruction of the aqueduct. This, in my estimation, cannot be achieved adequately in the majority of cases by just a simple subtemporal decompression, and some form of shunting procedure is preferable to bring about this result.

It may be of some interest to you to review, briefly, the history of the diversion of the cerebrospinal fluid stream past an obstruction. As early as 1908 it was suggested by Anton,[2] and done by Von Bramann, that a hole be punctured in the corpus callosum, which forms the roof of the lateral ventricles (Balkenstich). This is theoretically logical and technically not difficult to perform, but due to the thickness of the corpus callosum and the relatively small and collapsible subarachnoid spaces into which the fluid escaping through this hole would have to enter in order to be reabsorbed, this method does not work.

In 1923 Mixter[21] inserted an urethroscope into the dilated lateral ventricle of a hydrocephalic child, and then, under direct vision, passed the instrument through the dilated foramen of Monro and punctured the thinned-out floor of the third ventricle with a probe inserted through the urethroscope. The communication was still functioning a few weeks afterward, when the report was published, but no follow-up appeared later.

Stookey and Scarff[27] in 1936 advocated the puncture of the thinned-out lamina terminalis by way of a right transfrontal craniotomy, to permit the cerebral fluid to pass into the roomy cisterns of the base of the brain and thus rejoin the cerebral fluid stream on its way to absorption. They took the additional precaution of puncturing the posterior wall of the third ventricle to place this cavity in communication with the pontine cistern as well. This addition can be, I believe, theoretically dangerous and, in my experience, is not necessary. However, their approach to the lamina terminalis is direct and simple to carry out, and I am convinced that the opening produced in the floor of the ventricle in most cases remains open and continues to function.

Dandy[8] in 1945 advocated the puncture of the lamina terminalis through a temporal approach, but this was a personal preference and, insofar as I could see, had no advantages over the anterior approach.

In 1939 Torkildsen described a new method for shunting cerebral fluid around an obstruction by the insertion of a tube into a dilated lateral ventricle through a burr hole in the skull, and then leading it out over the skull but under the scalp into the subarachnoid space in the cisterna magna and upper cervical spinal canal—a method referred to previously.

Since I have a personal revulsion against leaving foreign substances of any kind permanently in the human body, and since the Stookey-Scarff procedure has worked well in my hands, I have seldom made use of the ingenious procedure of Torkildsen.

One proof of the efficacy of the third ventriculostomy, in the immediate postoperative phase at least, is the prompt relief the patient feels from the headaches and vomiting, and the relatively early subsidence of the papilledema. If a patient has only a subtemporal decompression, without a third ventriculostomy, these symptoms disappear much more slowly under the favorable effect of radiation therapy, and the decompression site bulges and is tense for a long time. Whereas, when the ventriculostomy is done and a deliberate decompression is also made, or a small defect in the skull is left perforce, the intracranial contents do not bulge through the defect, and the skin that covers the defect is soft and relaxed almost immediately, even before radiation therapy is instituted.

One might raise the question of whether a permanent communication is necessary, since it may be expected that in favorable cases the disappearance of the tumor under radiation therapy will relieve the obstruction and make the shunt superfluous. It would be difficult to answer this question categorically. It may well be that in some cases the radiation retards or arrests the growth of the tumor rather than destroys it. In this situation the shunt would be a permanently necessary ingredient in the satisfactory circulation of the cerebrospinal fluid. On the other hand, if the normal diameter of the lumen of the aqueduct of Sylvius becomes reestablished, it is possible that the reduction in size of the ventricles may thicken the anterior wall of the third ventricle sufficiently to close off the artificial opening. If, on the other hand, it remains permanently open, and the circulation of the cerebral fluid utilizes both passages, I can see no harm in it. It would seem to me much less desirable, if a patient no longer needed the bypass, to have one by the way of an implanted plastic tube. This is another reason for not using the Torkildsen procedure, unless an initial puncture of the lamina terminalis should fail to do the job.

One other weakness in the course of treatment previously outlined in these cases, other than its failure to cure *all* the patients, is the use of radiation therapy on lesions that are unverified histologically. Radiotherapists are unhappy about treating unverified lesions, particularly when they are asked to apply their rays to tumors in the pineal region that could be anything from teratomas, germinomas, gliomas, and pinealomas to tuberculomas, metastatic carcinomas, or benign cysts. However, in view of the tremendous risk to the patient from attempts to obtain a biopsy, I have found all the radiotherapists with whom I have worked to be understanding and cooperative. After all, it is better to have a living patient, restored to good health, whose diagnosis lacks the stamp of certainty that the microscope provides, than it is to have beautiful microphotographs from postmortem specimens.

ACKNOWLEDGMENT

I am indebted to Dr. Mannie M. Schechter for all illustrations used in this paper, except Figure 4.

*REFERENCES*

1. Ackerknecht, E. H. *Rudolf Virchow, Doctor, Statesman, Anthropologist.* Madison, Wisconsin Univ. Press, 1953, 304 pp.
2. Anton, G. and von Bramann, F. G. Balkenstich bei Hydrozephalien, Tumoren und bei Epilepsie, *Münch. Med. Wschr. 55*:1673-77, 1908.
3. Baggenstoss, A. H. and Love, J. G. Pinealomas, *Arch. Neurol. Psychiat. 41*: 1187-1206, 1939.
4. Bailey, P. and Cushing, H. *Classification of the Tumors of the Glioma Group on a Histogenetic Basis with Correlated Study of Prognosis.* Philadelphia, Lippincott, 1926, 175 pp.
5. Bochner, S. J. and Scarff, J. E. Teratoma of the pineal body: classification of the embryonal tumors of the pineal body: Report of a case of teratoma of the pineal body presenting formed teeth, *Arch. Surg. 36*:303-29, 1938.

6. Dandy, W. E. Operation for the removal of pineal tumors, *Surg. Gynec. Obstet. 33*:113-19, 1921.
7. Dandy, W. E. Operative experiences in cases of pineal tumor, *Arch. Surg. 33*:19-46, 1936.
8. Dandy, W. E. Diagnosis and treatment of strictures of the aqueduct of Sylvius (causing hydrocephalus), *Arch. Surg. 51*:1-14, 1945.
9. Friedman, N. B. Germinoma of the pineal: Its identity with germinoma ("seminoma") of the testis, *Cancer Res. 7*:363-68, 1947.
10. Globus, J. H. Pinealoma, *Arch. Path. 31*:533-68, 1941.
11. Harris, W. and Cairns, H. Diagnosis and treatment of pineal tumors, with report of a case, *Lancet 222*:3-9, 1932.
12. Horrax, G. Further observations on tumor of the pineal body, *Arch. Neurol. Psychiat. 35*:215-28, 1936.
13. Horrax, G. Extirpation of a huge pinealoma from a patient with pubertas praecox: A new operative approach, *Arch. Neurol. Psychiat. 37*:385-97, 1937.
14. Horrax, G. and Bailey, P. Tumors of the pineal body, *Arch. Neurol. Psychiat. 13*:423-70, 1925.
15. Horrax, G. and Daniels, J. T. Conservative treatment of pineal tumors, *Surg. Clin. N. America 22*:649-59, 1942.
16. Horrax, G. and Wyatt, J. P. Ectopic pinealomas in the chiasmal region; report of three cases, *J. Neurosurg. 4*:309-26, 1947.
17. Kahn, E. A. Surgical treatment of pineal tumor, *Arch. Neurol. Psychiat. 38*:833-42, 1937.
18. Kunicki, A. Operative experiences in eight cases of pineal tumor, *J. Neurosurg. 17*:815-23, 1960.
19. Løken, A. On the relation of atypical pinealomas to teratoid tumours, *Acta Path. Microbiol. Scand. 40*:417-24, 1957.
20. McLean, A. J. Pineal teratomas, with report of a case of operative removal, *Surg. Gynec. Obstet. 61*:523-33, 1935.
21. Mixter, W. J. Ventriculoscopy and puncture of the floor of the third ventricle, *Boston Med. Surg. J. 188*:277-78, 1923.
22. Radanowicz-Harttmann, B. von. Pinealome: Pathologisch-anatomische Untersuchung von zwei Beobachtungen, *Conf. Neurol. 26*:104-18, 1965.
23. Relkin, R. The pineal gland, *N. Eng. J. Med. 274*:944-50, 1966.
24. Ringertz, N., Nordenstam, H., and Flyger, G. Tumors of the pineal region, *J. Neuropath. Exp. Neurol. 13*:540-61, 1954.
25. Russell, D. S. The pinealoma: Its relationship to teratoma, *J. Path. Bact. 56*:145-50, 1944.
26. Russell, W. O. and Sachs, E. Pinealoma. Clinicopathologic study of seven cases with a review of the literature, *Arch. Path. 35*:869-88, 1943.
27. Stookey, B. and Scarff, J. Occlusion of the aqueduct of Sylvius by neoplastic and non-neoplastic processes with a rational surgical treatment for relief of the resultant obstructive hydrocephalus, *Bull. Neurol. Inst. N. Y. 5*:348-77, 1936.
28. Torkildsen, A. Should extirpation be attempted in cases of neoplasm in or near the third ventricle of the brain? Experiences with a palliative method, *J. Neurosurg. 5*:249-75, 1948.
29. Van Wagenen, W. P. Surgical approach for the removal of certain pineal tumors: Report of a case, *Surg. Gynec. Obstet. 53*:216-20, 1931.
30. Virchow, R. *Vorlesungen über Pathologie. Die krankhaften Geschwülste,* vol. 2. Berlin, Hirschwald, 1864-1865, p. 148.
31. Walton, K. Teratomas of the pineal region and their relationship to pinealomas, *J. Path. Bact. 61*:11-21, 1949.
32. Ward, A. and Spurling, R. G. Conservative treatment of third ventricle tumors, *J. Neurosurg. 5*:124-30, 1948.
33. Zülch, K. J. *Brain Tumors: Their Biology and Pathology,* 2d. Amer. ed. New York, Springer, 1965, 326 pp.

# THE HOUSE OF MEDICINE*

H. D. KRUSE

Executive Secretary, Committee on Public Health
The New York Academy of Medicine

THE Mad Woman of Chaillot confined her daily reading to one day's newspaper of a number of years past. Her explanation was simple: the news was especially good that day. Her rationale is so tempting that I toyed with the idea of redelivering a message of some vintage year. But discretion has tempered my impulse; instead, like a bride, I have selected something old and something new.

The old is that inevitable process: change. In the abstract, change per se as a process is not new. There is nothing more constant, more unchanging than change. Concretely, change may bring novelty, difference and, we hope, freshness. The time, the place, the characters, the circumstances and results in change are usually different. It is the working of a very old process that brings the new look.

For the new, I shall trace the high points of change in the environment, in the list of more prevalent diseases, and, in the main, in systems and institutions dedicated to combatting and overcoming disease and maintaining health. In the course of examining this latter sector, four main lines must be traveled: medical education; medical practice-medical care; hospitalization; and public health. It is little short of impossible to discuss one of these topics without bringing in the others. Playing a variety of roles, the physician is a prominent performer on all four stages.

In a previous message I went in some detail into the profound changes in the environment. Here it is sufficient only to touch upon the imposing list. Almost nothing in life is like what it was. The frontier days with virgin lands beckoning for settlement in ever-onward expansion and venting restless urge have given way to an era of a different kind of pressure: population pressure. More and more people are scrambling to share in the available remaining resources. What immigration started, prolongation of life has continued. With that longer survival

*Presented at the Annual Meeting of the Committee on Public Health of The New York Academy of Medicine, January 9, 1967.

came not only a swell in population but a change in its age distribution. There is a larger proportion of elderly people. Diplomatically speaking, survival was highly selective by sex. There are of coure no old ladies; only old men. Yet biologically woman points to an actual selectivity as evidence of the superiority of the female of the species.

As the population swelled there was a series of changes in transportation and communication. The swaying stagecoach and prairie schooner gave way to the hissing, panting iron horse roaring over ribbons of steel. And then came the motorized carriage, the automobile that now zooms over thousands of miles of concrete. Finally, the graceful flight of planes in the sky became a familiar sight. Now more and more planes winging their way through the skies and whisking at ever-increasing speed have shrunk time in traversing long distances.

This ease of travel encouraged frequency of movement with resulting increased mobility and migration. This is a nation on the move. With this enhanced movement the population has undergone a geographic shuffling. Urbanization, suburbanization, megalopolis attest to the new centers of attraction in this pattern of flocking and clustering.

No less wondrous is the acceleration of communication. From the pony express to telegraph, telephone, radio, television, and telstar, the succession of triumphs has brought instant pushbutton communication. We have not learned how to avoid or stop crime and war, but we can watch them from afar while they are happening.

Mechanization has advanced to an amazing degree. More recently in this electronic age, computers and automation have brought a new system of performance and control and have already altered the modes of many tasks. Not touched by human hands is a statement that more and more is literally true.

In this wonderful world of technology—with its synthetic fibers, contraceptives, jet engines, atomic submarines, space capsules, trips to the moon, and open heart surgery—nuclear, electronic, chemical, and mechanical marvels vie for the national accolade.

In this whirling kaleidoscopic world man might expect to find one spot intact: his home, that shelter in which he seeks surcease and to which he repairs to nurse and restore his battered and wounded ego. He returns only to find that his castle is open under new management. The princes and princesses have usurped his power, leaving him only an empty title. There are men who still insist that they run things at home. Some men do: the lawn mower, the washing machine, the vacuum cleaner, and errands. On the totem pole the positions have shifted. The small fry, once exploited, oppressed and lowest in rank, have climbed to the top. Much else is different in the domestic haven. Home and family life are not the same.

Life has changed so rapidly in so many ways that modern man has not had time to adjust, to adapt completely to the new order. He is searching for the pattern, the way of living in the new world.

Science has brought about many of these changes in the world around us. Even science in medicine has played a part in the transformation. Developments in these areas have had their effect on health and disease, some good, some problematic. On the bright side, the national death rate has been halved in the past 60 years. Life expectancy at birth has been extended by 40 per cent. Survival of infants and prolongation of life are largely attributable to medical advances.

Balancing these highlights are the somber points. We have not moved entirely out of our unsanitary past. We still pollute streams but we do it in part in a new way with new pollutants. Dirty air, principally a problem of concentrated people, has accompanied urbanization. Even this pollution has its new elements.

The picture of the sociomedical ills of mankind has been retouched with magnification here, minimization there, and substitution at several points. Many current juvenile problems—surging venereal disease, illegitimacy, drug addiction, glue sniffing, pep pills, goof balls, pot—are ultimately traceable to the family. Originally these irregularities in behavior were regarded as sins and crimes. Only recently has their medical component been recognized.

In addition to these communal disruptions of adolescent behavior, there is a new order of diseases according to their frequency in producing death and morbidity. During the past 60 years the ranking of diseases as causes of death has shifted. At the turn of the century five infectious diseases were among the 10 principal causes of death in the United States. Pneumonia and tuberculosis occupied the undesirable first and second places. By 1964 only one infection was among the top 10 killers and it was in fifth position. Now in the table of fatality, communicable diseases have been replaced by degenerative processes among the elderly. Diseases of the heart, cancer, stroke and trauma are the most prominent in applying the coup de grâce. Likewise the ranking producers of morbidity and disability have undergone alteration.

This change in the nature of the nation's health problems fell upon the medical profession with such suddenness that it was not entirely prepared to combat the new forces of disease. Saving of life in infancy and old age had created problems of disease in old age. There were effective arms against communicable disease; but new weapons were needed, many yet to be discovered, to combat degenerative disease.

While these changes in environment and man's ills and afflictions were occurring, the structure, system, and organization of medicine and public health were also changing. As all these wonders, some incredible, were transforming this planet into a new and different world, and while the cavalcade of diseases paraded by, medicine with its mission to combat and rout or control disease was being recast and reshaped. Medical practice, public health, medical education, and hospitals underwent change.

In their beginnings, clinical medicine and public health were quite different from each other in means and mode. Indeed, they developed separately. Medicine was on a one-to-one basis: physician vis-à-vis patient in the provision and receipt of care. Management of the patient and treatment of disease were the principal functions of medical practice and, for a long time, they were largely empirical. Public health, on the other hand, was concerned with diseases in the mass, mostly epidemic. Its social element was therefore of a larger scope than that in medicine, yet it was less personal. This approach in public health was the answer to the problem of combatting transmissible and communicable diseases on a large scale. Its aim was to control the situation by preventing spread. For then, as now, it was easier to prevent than to overcome, especially when specific remedies were lacking. Measures taken by public health were largely social and environmental, particularly those that required no effort from the populace. Sanitation, safeguarding the water supply, sewage disposal, quarantine, and isolation were the main courses of action.

Then came the era when both medicine and public health were placed on a scientific basis. Discoveries in bacteriology, immunology, chemotherapy, and nutrition provided new and effective weapons. Vaccines, diagnostic and therapeutic sera, antibiotics and proper diets brought a favorable change in the odds in the battle with disease and death. This scientific age led to profound changes in the training, equipment, and deployment of the medical forces and in their theater of action. Medical education underwent a change in character that was reflected in the content, method of instruction, and even the teachers. The rapid and evergrowing accumulation of new knowledge necessitated division of subjects and specialization. Full-time teaching staffs, at first preclinical and then clinical, came into being. Even postgraduate education was affected. With the expanded body of knowledge to be covered, the resulting division and specialization, together with the demand for ever-higher standards of performance, a longer period of training was deemed essential. Intern and residency programs were introduced.

These developments occurred pari passu with the drastic change in medical practice and were in preparation for its new form. Specialty boards had been created and specialization was to grow by leaps and bounds.

Meanwhile, hospitals had been transformed from dens of despair and death to havens of life, confidence, and hope. No longer were they the end of the line; rather, they had become the repair and restoration stations on the speedway called the marathon of life. Three events gave hospitals a new function in addition to their new performance in life saving and restoration: the declaration that the primary purpose of a hospital internship was the training of a physician; the system of accreditation of hospitals leading to improvement of their physical facilities; and the provision for approval of hospitals for intern and residency programs that moved them toward assuming an educational function. In passing it should be noted that these nonofficial and voluntary developments raised standards far above any imposed by law.

As these developments gained full force, they had their effects, four of which may be mentioned.

1) Instruction was conducted more and more by hospital-based full-time clinicians and less and less by attending physicians.

2) The increase in specialists reached the point where they were in the majority; concomitantly, general practitioners became a smaller and smaller minority.

3) Hospitals were increasingly the site where medicine was practiced; this arrangement supplanted home and office visits.

4) Medical schools in the United States did not produce graduates in sufficient numbers to meet the needs of hospitals for interns. Demand

exceeded supply. A shortage of interns occurred most acutely in those hospitals not affiliated with medical schools. Into this breach came the immigration of foreign interns.

While medicine was in ferment, public health was not exactly quiescent. Science, waving its wand over the domain of public health, had brought it a new outlook and broadened its approach to its responsibilities. Programs were introduced that required personal, individual, one-to-one application. Case-finding for tuberculosis required x-ray screening. Prenatal and well-baby clinics necessitated personal examination, serological tests, and vaccinations. It was a new and different age in public health.

In this review of developments it is helpful to examine the record of how health services and personnel have been deployed according to the natural history of disease.

It is obvious that prevention is preferable to treatment, whether judged by time, expense, or results. Indeed, it is most desirable when no successful treatment is available. Failing prevention, early detection becomes the second line of defense. The earlier a disease is recognized and combatted, the less time it has had to progress and the easier it is to arrest and reverse. Consequently, there is less damage in the early than in the late stage.

When disease has reached its manifest stage, it is then more firmly entrenched and requires commensurately active counter measures. And finally, when disease has run its course or has been brought under control, there is the aftercare period.

Preventive services largely take two forms: prophylactic sera and vaccines, and health education. Much of the prophylaxis by serology is conducted by pediatricians. Health education is carried on in the private practice of both obstetrics and pediatrics, as well as prenatal and well-baby clinics. It is more formally the program of health departments. Thus, preventive services are performed by both clinical medicine and health departments.

Likewise, the responsibility of early detection is shared by both clinical medicine and public health. Part of the value of prenatal and well-baby clinics lay in the opportunity for early detection. Furthermore, Papanicolaou smear, breast examination, and chest x ray are measures designed for early detection.

But the management of active disease is largely the function of clinical medicine aided and assisted by public health. As for aftercare, it is still mostly social, shouldered by social agencies.

In sum, clinical medicine is concerned mainly with the management of sick persons and their diseases, with some activity in prevention and early detection. In contrast, health departments are concerned mainly with maintaining health, prevention, and early detection and, to a lesser extent, with playing an accessory role in clinical medicine.

Under some circumstances in the normal course of medical practice the physician can advance or may arrest the normal course of public health practice. This has been expressed more broadly yet concisely by the assertion that the physician has become a part of the public health team. In its turn, almost as if to reciprocate, public health has increasingly included the individual approach. At the same time, to meet a growing demand, public health has also become increasingly occupied with the administrative practice of medicine. On this basis a closer association between clinical medicine and public health is said to be discerned.

It would be a mistake to overestimate and exaggerate the degree and magnitude of approximation of the two disciplines and thereby convey the misleading impression of their association and integration. The fact is that by their very nature, aims, and functions they are different. That they have points of contact is undeniable. But disease and health are different; just as curative medicine is not the same as maintenance of health and preventive medicine. In his provocative topical page in the *British Medical Journal*, Pertinax has asserted that the term "National Health Service" is a misnomer. It should be, he maintains, "National Medical Service."

Still another development should be especially noted because of its tremendous impact on medical science, medical education, medical practice, hospitals, and public health. It was the growing participation of government in promotion of health and medical care. It materialized in a number of forms, each a story in itself. Stimulus, guidance, and money were powerful prods, persuaders, and providers. The creation and expansion of the U. S. Public Health Service from its small beginnings, and later the establishment of the National Institutes of Health, were tremendous developments. Specialization occurred during the period of expansion in the Public Health Service and the state and local health departments. In recent years there have been vast federal funds, first for research, then for buildings and teaching. These funds were administered by the Public Health Service. The Hill-Burton Act breathed new life into hospitals across the nation.

For several reasons, the cost of medical care had been rising. The elderly especially, with their reduced income, higher sickness rate, and longer periods of hospitalization, felt the pinch acutely and distressfully. Over the past decade there has been gradually emerging a new social policy that would have the government take broader responsibility for the health of its citizenry. After 10 years of public outcry and exhaustive, at times sharp, debate, what is popularly called Medicare and Medicaid finally became law. It was designed to ensure medical care and hospitalization for the elderly as well as to bring benefits for the young. No longer was heard the plea of some years ago:

Oh, to be in England
Now that health is free!
Not a farthing needed
For an appendectomy.
Dentures for the asking,
For husband, child, or spouse;
Oh, to be in England
Now that health is "on the house."

Less heralded, less discussed, and perhaps less fully recognized was the legislation for regional centers for cancer, heart, and stroke. In some quarters it was the clarion call for medical schools to become more community-minded.

On history's clock this revolution in biology and medicine has occurred in a relatively short period of time. Since time slips by unnoted and reshaping in numerous respects may occur unobtrusively by steps, the extent and rapidity of the shifting scene may not be readily grasped. We may be taken aback by the sudden realization that it has been only a little over 50 years since the death of Robert Koch, and some of the pioneers of nutrition are still amongst us. This extensive renovation of medicine has happened within a half century.

It would have been unusual if these sweeping changes in the medical scene had occurred without flaw or fuss. Then too, life provides a seemingly inexhaustible supply of problems. As soon as one is overcome another is ready to take its place. At this juncture three problems emerged into prominence. First, even after federal legislation to soften the financial blow, the cost of medical care is still a pressing concern, and the likelihood of even greater trouble in the future overhangs it.

Second, the deafening clamor for a decade over Medicare drowned out the voices of those who were convinced that even under the circumstances existing then, there was a shortage of medical manpower. If Medicare became a reality, the short-handed situation might become critical. Passage of Medicare and Medicaid and the regional medical system was viewed by some as accentuating the manpower gap.

A third concern, less spectacular and less seldom heard among public complaints but always in the forefront of part of the profession's consciousness, especially since 1910, was the quality of medical care. In the discussions over provision of public medical care programs it was sometimes mentioned. As government ensured greater quantity of medical programs, concern about their quality became increasingly voiced.

Today, in the midst of expanding medical programs, these three concerns loom large: the cost of medical care; sufficient manpower and facilities; and the quality of medical care. As the first receives some relief, the latter two gain more attention. With changes in society, the character of disease, medicine, and public health moving concurrently, it is indeed still a time of *Sturm und Drang*. Concern over the cost of medical care, adequacy of manpower, and the quality of medical care lead directly to a look at medical education, medical practice, and hospitalization.

The official professional pronouncement, almost a vaunt, is that this nation has the best medical care ever provided anywhere. But even the best, so long as it has not reached perfection, is improvable and can benefit by amendment. Even the smoothest system can stand occasional adjusting. Without denying the merit of the medical system, some friendly critics believe that its blemishes and flaws amount to problems, and that if these were corrected, it would be still better.

There has accrued a veritable catalog of critical questions and comments, both spoken and written from time to time, that indicate sensitive points in the cost of medical care, manpower, and quality of medical care. Although each item could certainly start almost unlimited debate, they can be given here only barest mention.

In federal legislation providing the means for hospital and medical care, realization may fall short of expectation. Coverage may not be as complete as many envision. Catastrophic illness still remains a problem. The overhead on official programs of medical care and hospitalization bears watching. Instances of administrative costs consuming too much, even most of the substance, and of "chiseling" are not entirely unknown. Ways must be found to lower the cost of hospitalization or to shift the schedule of values. Unless a solution is found, hospitalization may create poverty faster than antipoverty programs can abolish it.

In the area of manpower, specialists have been increasing, general practitioners declining, until the former now outnumber the latter. Much time and a vast amount of money are invested in the education and training of specialists. When they practice below their qualifications, both time and money are wasted. Under the present system and trend the medical education production line becomes slowed and clogged. So far as possible it would appear that the training of doctors in number and type should match the nature and amount of illness prevalent.

There is need to differentiate training, education, and practice. If there was reason 30 years ago to proclaim that the primary purpose of the hospital internship is training and that the secondary purpose is patient care, is it useful or judicious to continue the refrain? Patients in a hospital need medical care and young physicians need training.

The system of approving hospitals for intern and residency training was created in full knowledge that medical schools in the United States did not graduate enough physicians to fill openings. The flat assertion that not all hospitals need interns is open to question. Under the present definition, category, and function, it may in one sense be true. But it is more difficult to argue that hospitals do not need to have 24-hour qualified medical coverage and performance of duties regardless of what the personnel are called. The need for coverage and the belief that a certificate of approval will attract graduates accentuate the imbalance between the openings in hospitals and the output of medical graduates.

Several questions have been raised about the intern and residency program. Was the length of the residency determined arbitrarily or on justifiable grounds that would stand reexamination on a realistic basis with consideration of all factors? It has been intimated from time to time that there is a discrepancy between the training programs on paper and in actuality. One of the arguments advanced for the training program was that the young physicians in training were supposed to work under experienced men. But it is readily admitted that most of the instruction is conducted by residents. It has been asserted that soon there will be a generation of medical graduates who will have been taught by instructors who have never practiced outside the hospital.

There has been criticism over the allotment of interns and the lack of realistic rules governing the number requested. In the past the dual appointment as professor of a department and physician-in-chief in an affiliated hospital was regarded as a superhuman responsibility. Now the same person has been asked to take on a third role: that of scientific investigator. Does conducting research necessarily make a better teacher or clinician? Should department heads be chosen on the total amount of their research grants? Should interns and residents be used in research? What is the cost of the intern-residency training to a hospital?

World powers have usually had medical graduates in such profusion that they could be sent abroad. By what reasoning are foreign graduates of foreign medical schools accepted as interns when it is almost certain that they would not have been accepted as students in American medical schools?

Eli Ginzberg has advanced a novel argument on the value of keeping medical manpower in tight supply. In any event, there is lack of precise data on the number and kinds of physicians needed to care for all the prevailing illness now or in the immediate future. Yet plans for constructing many more medical schools are under way without benefit of that information. Is it in the public interest when medical schools are built, not in fulfillment of an over-all national or local plan, but just to ensure an institution's supply of interns?

Despite the boast that the United States has medical care of the highest quality, it is criticized from two sources: one, the public, the other within the ranks. There have been four or five publications on the shortcomings of the modern-day physician, who has been described as having a slipping halo, more recently a sickly image. Sometimes reflecting a sense of loss, the longing for the old-time physician is said more in bereavement for departure of the old than in reproach of the new. But in actuality, says William R. Carson, the nostalgic complainers and detractors are engaging in shadow boxing. "The brutal truth is that this imaginary figure of humanitarian perfection, this all-knowing and sympathetic expert in human relations, has no more substance in reality than Peter Pan or the Loch Ness monster." It is myth more than legend. Carson points out that physicians themselves have joined in the "ritualistic adulation of an illusory figure that never was, to accord it respect it never experienced, endowing it with a nobility it never possessed, and prestige it never knew." He points out that "every generation has tried its healers and found them wanting." However, he agrees that there was "one period when the medical profession seemed to come closest to fulfilling the public concept of what a doctor should be." It was during the 1920's and 1930's that the profession was made up of a "product of the new medical system which combined the scientific knowledge of the new with the humanitarian devotion of the old." At that time the image of the hospital changed from a den of death to a house of hope. Carson accords no little importance to the adoption of the color white in both the hospital setting and the garb of the medical personnel. In fact, he traces the decline of the doctor's image to the date that the interior decorator was allowed to invade the operating room and apply his pastel shades.

Specifically, the public complains most about unavailability, inattention, distraction, lack of compassion, lack of humanitarianism, impersonal attitude, and a hurried manner with sharply curtailed time. Not to be overlooked are the public's great expectations, indeed unrealistic expectations in medical care. To quote Carson again, "the most the doctor can do is to bring postponement in the duel with death whereas the patient expects the repeal of natural laws." Certainly it is true that the public has higher standards of health along with its expectations. These expectations have been heightened by more research, more money spent on research, and more publicity on discoveries in research. Also to be mentioned is the vast amount of money spent by the public on health as manifestation of its interest.

Modern-day practice of medicine has also drawn comment from those within its ranks, usually the veterans. Briefly, they charge that scientific medicine neglects the heart of medicine. They object to both manner and procedure. They deplore the impersonal, hurried, even inattentive manner and argue for a return to the personal and humanitarian touch. Second, they object to the use of too many tests, many of which they regard as unnecessary. Relatedly, they criticize the lack of inspection and observation of the patient. In short, they believe that the technic of examining a patient has been lost with more and more dependence on what tests will show.

Medicine in the United States is not alone in realizing that everything is not completely rosy and in indulging in self-examination and soul-searching. Recently Professor Henry Miller in an article entitled "Fifty Years After Flexner" described the plight of medicine in Britain even more somberly. He was devastating in his critique. Here and abroad medical care is a lively and timely topic.

At home the murmurs and mutters have not gone unheard. There is evidence of awareness of pressing problems and concerns. Deliberations have yielded a number of reports with recommendations designed to alleviate the difficulties. In medical education there has been the Blain report, followed by the Bayne-Jones report, followed most recently by the Millis report. The so-called Coggeshall report set forth the position of the Association of American Medical Colleges, and recently the Academy of General Practice has released its report. Harvard Medical School has added to the pronouncements. In medical practice there is the so-called DeBakey report on heart, cancer, and stroke. Perhaps the latest report on hospitals came from the Folsom Committee in New York State.

To meet these criticisms there is little evidence of a desire or need to turn back the clock. Admittedly the advances for the most part have been fundamentally sound and good. But as in all periods of rapid transition there are troublesome spots. It may prove more difficult to improve something generally good than to rectify a bad situation.

What is the role of the Committee on Public Health in this era of dizzying whirl in medicine and health? It occupies a unique place in that it stretches across the full expanse of health care. Over the 55 years of its history it has worked on hospitals, clinics, medical practice, community ills, and public health. It was either magnificent foresight or happy circumstance that when the By-Laws of the Academy were being written many years ago, this Committee was specifically charged to concern itself with the provision for the sick, and with the practice of medicine, hospitals, and public health. Besides its experience and ability in fulfilling the responsibility, this Committee wears a shining badge of honor: the reputation of working in the public interest. Today it is as needed, ready, willing, and able as at any point in its long history. Now is another high moment of challenge and opportunity.

To take just one sector of medicine and health, there is much talk today about the quality of medical care. If the Committee on Public Health did not coin the phrase, it surely gave meaning to it long ago. It did not just talk about it, it showed how it could be done. In its pioneer fashion it led the way. Its hospital study in 1924, its obstetrical study in 1933, its infant and maternal care study in 1952, its perinatal study in 1955, its study of blood in 1958, are evidence that the quality of medical care can be investigated and improved. Those who have gone before on this Committee have left a remarkable record as a rich heritage.

The poet has caught the true spirit of this Committee and put it in words:

> There are two kinds of people on earth today;
> Just two kinds of people, no more, I say.
> The two kinds of people on earth that I mean
> Are the people who lift and the people who lean.
>
> WILCOX

The Committee's character and influence displayed in its lifting has a timeless quality.

> Its echoes will "roll from soul to soul,
> And grow forever and for ever."
>
> TENNYSON

# NICHOLAS ROMAYNE: FIRST PRESIDENT OF THE COLLEGE OF PHYSICIANS AND SURGEONS, NEW YORK CITY

BYRON STOOKEY*

THE last half of the 18th century and the first quarter of the 19th were a time of great progress in the United States both in the practice of medicine and in the development of medical education. No one was more qualified by talent and training, or more dedicated and fruitful in his efforts to advance these aspects of medicine than Nicholas Romayne. Yet upon his death in New York on July 21, 1817, at the age of 61, no cognizance of the fact was taken by the faculty of the College of Physicians and Surgeons, which he had founded and, at its inception, had largely financed out of his own funds. Romayne had been the first president of the college and also the first president of the newly-formed Medical Society of the County of New York. A formal notice of his death was placed in the New York newspapers by the county and the state medical societies. Members were urged to attend the funeral of their former president at his late residence, 49 Chambers Street at 5 o'clock on July 25th, and were requested to wear the usual badge of mourning for 30 days. That the faculty of his own school did not even record his death in its minutes is the more amazing since a short time later David Hosack delivered a eulogium at the College of Physicians and Surgeons in memory of Dr. Caspar Wistar of Philadelphia, Pa., who had never had a faculty appointment in New York City.

However, at the first quarterly meeting of the Medical Society of the County of New York after Romayne's death, held at Washington Hall on October 5, 1817, it was moved by Dr. William Hammersly, seconded by Dr. William Moore, and unanimously agreed upon that: "The public papers of this city having announced since the last meeting of this Society the death of Nicholas Romayne, M.D., the first President

*Dr. Byron Stookey died October 20, 1966. This is the last of a series of studies on medical education in early New York that Dr. Stookey prepared in anticipation of the 200th anniversary of the medical school of Columbia University (King's College) being celebrated this year. For other publications in the series see *Bull. N.Y. Acad. Med. 41*:1037, 1965 (footnote).

of this Incorporation, which occurred in this city on the 21st of July of the present year, therefore Resolved that in testimony of the respect which the Society bears to the memory of the deceased member and in consideration of the services which he has rendered to it, this mark of their respect be recorded in their minutes and registered in their archives."

A recent article[19] refers to Nicholas Romayne* as the ". . . stormy petrel of American medical education." Even a superficial review of the early years of New York medicine makes it obvious that this designation might more appropriately have been applied to David Hosack.

Nicholas Romayne,[11] born in September 1756, was the eldest of five children of John Romeyn,** of New York City, and Juliana McCarty, both parents being of ". . . great moral and Christian worth." Following Nicholas were three sisters, Rachel, Jane, and Susan, and a brother, Jeremiah, the youngest of the family. Nicholas and Jeremiah attended the Hackensack Academy, Hackensack, N.J., where they received scholarly training in the classics from Peter Wilson, educated in Aberdeen, Scotland, who subsequently, having been considered for the presidency of Queen's College, New Brunswick, N.J., accepted the chair of Greek and Latin languages at Columbia College. Jeremiah, like several of the family's close relatives, became a Dutch Reformed clergyman.

Nicholas Romayne began his medical studies in King's College Medical School in 1774, at the age of 18; however, shortly after the outbreak of the Revolution in 1775 he went abroad to study at Edinburgh, where he received his medical degree in 1780. Thanks to the thorough classical training given him by Peter Wilson he was able to read without difficulty the *Aphorisms of Hippocrates* in Greek and to write in Latin the thesis for his medical degree, *De Puris Generatione*, without the aid of the commonly employed translator. In addition to his knowledge of the classical languages he spoke both Low Dutch and French fluently.

Romayne's Edinburgh thesis was dedicated to Peter Middleton, Samuel Clossy, John Jones, and Samuel Bard, professors in King's College Medical School under whom he had begun his medical education, and to Anthony Van Dam, a distinguished New York citizen whose niece, Susannah Van Dam, he married. That Romayne was highly

*The portrait in that article is not an authentic one of Nicholas Romayne. The same portrait in Claude Heaton's articles was put in by the editors and not by Dr. Heaton, who recognized that the painting was mislabeled.

**Nicholas Romayne changed the spelling of his family name to facilitate pronunciation.

DISSERTATIO INAUGURALIS,

DE

PURIS GENERATIONE:

QUAM,

ANNUENTE SUMMO NUMINE,

Ex Auctoritate Reverendi admodum Viri,

D. GULIELMI ROBERTSON, S. S. T. P.

ACADEMIÆ EDINBURGENÆ PRÆFECTI;

NEC NON

Ampliſſimi SENATUS ACADEMICI conſenſu,

Et nobiliſſimae FACULTATIS MEDICÆ decreto;

PRO GRADU DOCTORATUS,

SUMMISQUE IN MEDICINA HONORIBUS ET PRIVILEGIIS RITE ET LEGITIME CONSEQUENDIS;

Eruditorum examini ſubjicit

NICOLAUS ROMAYNE,

AMERICANUS,

Societatis Regiae Medicae Edinburgenae Socius.

Nec non

Societatis Phyſicae Socius Honorarius.

Ὁ βίος βραχύς, ἡ δὲ τέχνη μακρή, ὁ δὲ καιρὸς ὀξύς, ἡ δὲ πεῖρα σφαλερή, ἡ δὲ κρίσις χαλεπή. *Hippocrat. Aph.* I. *Sect.* I.

Octavo kalendas Julii, hora locoque ſolitis.

EDINBURGI:

Apud BALFOUR et SMELLIE,

Academiae Typographos.

M,DCC,LXXX.

Fig. 1. Title page of Nicholas Romayne's thesis on *The Formation of Pus*, Edinburgh, 1780. Reproduced by courtesy of The New York Academy of Medicine.

considered by the Van Dams is shown by the will of Sarah Van Dam, Anthony's sister, dated March 4, 1791 and proved December 1, 1792, in which she not only gave one sixth of her estate to her niece Susannah Romayne, but also left to her great-niece, Susan Romayne ". . . in consideration of the many services paid me by her parents, Nicholas and Susannah, my household furniture and plate."[17]

Before returning to the United States in 1782, Romayne had spent several years in travel and study at Leyden, Paris, and London. No physician in America had had as extensive and thorough a foreign education as Nicholas Romayne when, on his return, he landed in Philadelphia, where he remained until after the British evacuated New York in November of 1783.

Had it not been for Romayne's New York ties he might well have

Celeberrimis Viris,

PETRO MIDDLETON,
SAMUELI CLOSSY,
JOANNI JONES,
SAMUELI BARD,

Dignissimis in Academia Novi Eboraci Medicinae
PROFESSORIBUS;

Nec non,
Ornatissimo Viro,

ANTONIO VAN DAM,

De Civitate eadem,

NICOLAUS ROMAYNE

Felicitatem.

*Cum nulli sint, amplissimi Viri, quibus plus debeam, quos cariores habeam, aut qui meam observantiam magis quam vos mereantur; ob vestra enim beneficia in me collata, quae alta manent mente reposta, vobis, Praeceptores, omnem aetatem colendi, quorum sub auspiciis animum ad Artem Apollinarem primum appuli; necnon, tibi, optime Virorum, cui maxime devinctus sum, Dissertationem hancce, exiguum grati animi testimonium, consecrare volo.*

Dabam ex Collegio Edincensi
Idibus [illegible] Junii [illegible]

Fig. 2. Dedication of Nicholas Romayne's thesis. Reproduced by courtesy of The New York Academy of Medicine.

remained in Philadelphia, where he was welcomed both by the medical profession and society. It was during his stay there that he met William Blount, a member of the Continental Congress, then in session in that city, to whom reference will subsequently be made. Blount found Dr. and Mrs. Romayne's parties appealing, was attracted by their friends, and realized the potential value to himself of Romayne's foreign connections.

The New York to which Nicholas Romayne returned was a far different city than he had known—barricades and breastworks still stood at street intersections, trees had been cut down for firewood, King's College had been used as a barracks and later as a hospital, and its "philosophical" paraphernalia destroyed and scattered. The disastrous effects of the extensive fires of 1776 and 1778 were still apparent, and even several of the churches had been used as riding academies. Most of the loyalists had fled, taking with them as much of their belongings as they could. Funds available for the college and the medical faculty were extremely limited.

In May 1784 King's College, having become Columbia College by act of the legislature, came under the control of a Board of Regents of the University of the State of New York, of which Nicholas Romayne was an original member. This board reserved the authority to confer degrees beyond the Master's, including the M.D. degree. The Columbia medical faculty was reorganized at this time with Romayne as "professor of the practice of physic." And when, in April 1781, the Legislature restored to Columbia a self-perpetuating board of trustees consisting of 24 members, Romayne was an original member. He held the position until 1793.

As a trustee of Columbia, Romayne was precluded from becoming a member of the faculty and was thus prevented from using his great talent as a teacher. He consequently followed the system commonly used in Edinburgh, where outstanding physicians and the professors in the medical school often conducted private classes. These private lectures, in which he was assisted by Dr. Benjamin Kissam and Dr. William Moore, were carried on at the Alms House and at the Bridewell, attracting a number of students. Romayne was an energetic and fluent teacher, capable of lecturing on any medical subject, and he drew students from Canada as well as from many parts of the United States. In January 1791 he submitted a memorial to his fellow regents informing them that since 1787 he and his associates had conducted a private medical school in which all of the major branches of medicine were taught. He urged the regents to grant a charter. The memorial stated that during the winter sessions, beginning the first Monday in November and ending the third Saturday in April, lectures were delivered, two a day for 5 days a week, on the practice of physic, anatomy, the Institutes of Medicine, midwifery, and surgery. During the summer sessions, from the first Monday in May to the third Friday in August, the lectures were on chemistry, botany, and materia medica. Throughout the year clinical lectures were given on Saturdays at the Alms House and at the Bridewell. A second memorial, presented February 1791, was signed by Drs. Sir James Jay, Knt. (elder brother of John Jay), Benjamin Kissam, Richard S. Kissam, Samuel L. Mitchell, William Moore, Samuel Nicoll, and Nicholas Romayne.

Before action could be taken by the regents, however, a remonstrance was presented signed by John Bard, as president, and James Tillary, secretary of the local medical society, opposing the grant of the charter. The legislature, nevertheless, on March 24, 1791,[15] passed *An Act to Enable the Regents of the University to Establish a College of Physicians and Surgeons within this State*. Because of this action, Columbia College appointed a committee to study the problem of medical education in the college. This committee resolved: "That it will be proper at present to have lectures in chemistry, anatomy and the practice of physic read in Columbia College and that Dr. Romayne (who already has a considerable number of pupils (56) under his tuition and has been in the habit of teaching) be nominated Lecturer."

With the imminent threat of the formation of another medical school in New York City, John Bard, ever solicitous for the future of his son Samuel, joined with the local medical society in urging the trustees of Columbia to greater action. The trustees thereupon formed a committee in January 1792 which, on February 1, requested the regents to suspend action on the establishment of a second school, and promised that the principal medical subjects would be faithfully taught at Columbia. With this assurance the regents informed the Senate that they had postponed action on the founding of the College of Physicians and Surgeons with the expectation that the efforts of the Columbia medical school would be efficient and permanent.

Dr. Romayne had notified the trustees some weeks earlier that he had planned to resign all his connections with Columbia College as of May 10, 1792. With the announcement of the action of the regents, Romayne sent the following letter to the Trustees of Columbia:[20]

> . . . It gives me, however, much satisfaction to reflect, that under very disadvantageous circumstances, in direct opposition to the unwearied efforts of some of my fellow Trustees, without the smiles of many of them, against the steady exertions of some of the Regents of the University, and the combined Faculty of New York, who have seldom been confined within the limits of Decency or Truth in

their sentiments with respect to me, I have greatly contributed to draw the public attention to the present state of Literature in Columbia College, and which is likely to be of some immediate advantage, and must contribute to her future prosperity. My pupils, at my request, are mostly matriculated in the Album of the College, of which for the present year according to Academic Rules they are alumni. Many of them are gentlemen of Genius and worth. I have evidenced their studious attention, the progress they have made in the acquisition of knowledge; and I have a due sense of the eminent abilities which some of them possess. It may be of some service to Columbia College, that some of them be admitted to medical honours before the period fixed for my resignation—some of them would do no dishonour to the first Universities in Europe—some benefit may also be derived from this, by such persons as the Trustees may think proper to employ as teachers in future in the different branches of Medicine. I have only to request that the Trustees will be pleased to come to some early determination on this subject.

I have the honour to be,

Gentlemen

Your Obedient Servant

N. Romayne

To the Trustees of Columbia College, New York

Romayne's previously submitted resignation was now accepted, effective May 10, and immediately the students receiving their medical instruction from him at Columbia resigned in a body, though two of them subsequently withdrew their resignations. With characteristic resourcefulness Romayne at once secured temporary lecture facilities in the City Hall.[7]

It will be recalled that Nicholas Romayne belonged to an old Dutch family and that therefore, quite naturally, he sought to place his school under the aegis of Queen's College at New Brunswick, N.J., whose charter had been granted by the Dutch Reformed Church in 1766. He petitioned the trustees on April 10, 1792,[9] informing them that he had for some years been teaching the various branches of medicine and had 56 students in attendance at his school. He also pointed out that by patronizing medical education the influence of Queen's College would be extended and its resources increased.

Romayne's petition was referred to a committee of the trustees consisting of Col. Frederick Frelinghuysen, the Rev. Peter Studiford, and Dr. Lewis Dunham. After some investigation of his students Romayne was appointed professor of physic and authorized to form a medical faculty, in which he was joined by Dr. Richard S. Kissam and Dr. William Moore. Queen's College agreed to confer the degrees of Bachelor of Medicine and Doctor of Medicine on recommendation of the professors. The college would receive £5 for the bachelor's degree and £10 for the doctor's. In 1792 three Bachelor of Medicine and four Honorary Doctor of Medicine degrees were granted, and in 1793 six Doctor of Medicine and three Doctor of Medicine ad eundum—a total of 16 degrees. Shortly after 1793 Queen's College, because of lack of funds, was forced to suspend both its collegiate and medical activities.

Dr. Romayne wrote to the trustees of Columbia College on June 20, 1793:[21]

> As I propose to sail for Europe as soon as the arrangement of my domestic concerns will permit, and my return to my native Country being among the more uncertain Events of my life, I beg leave to resign the appointment, which I have the honour to hold by the Act of the Legislature of the State, as one of the Trustees of Columbia College.
>
> Wherever in the order of things, I may hereafter reside, I shall always be happy in promoting the general interests of literature; and the Trustees of Columbia College may be assured, I will take much pleasure in rendering them any services, if ever they be pleased to favour me with their commands.
>
> I shall make such arrangements with Col. Livingston before my departure for the liquidation and payment of the Debt due the Trustees from the late Company of underwriters, for the payment of which I have made myself responsible as I am persuaded will be satisfactory.

Stimulated by Romayne, a committee of the faculty of the Columbia Medical School, headed by Samuel Bard, made an announcement assuring the public ". . . of their most faithful and strenuous exertions to render the important Branch of Education committed to their care as complete and extensive as possible . . . and of increasing the Fame and extending the usefulness of the College."

Romayne did not leave New York for two years, maintaining his residence at 23 John Street until he sailed for Europe in June 1795. In

December of that year he became a licentiate of the Royal College of Physicians (London), which gave him the right to practice in England.

Romayne may have been influenced to go abroad at this time by William Blount, who had interested Romayne in his extensive land scheme in the territory over which he had been in charge. Blount had been appointed by George Washington governor of the territory south of the Ohio river and was in charge of Indian affairs from 1790 to 1796; in both posts he had aquitted himself efficiently. In the Tennessee constitutional convention of 1796 he was made one of that state's first United States senators.

Blount[16] became interested in extensive land investments on his own behalf in the territory over which he had presided; however, he overextended himself in these commitments and repeatedly found himself in serious financial straits. In an attempt to secure his holdings he grew involved in a direct scheme to unite the frontiersmen and the Creek and Choctaw Indians with England to take over West Florida and Louisiana, fearing that if this land and the Mississippi river were to pass under French control, as had been rumored, the entire territory would be in jeopardy and his own large holdings lost, as well as the returns he had promised to Romayne.

Jay's treaty with England in 1795 caused French animosity, which resulted in the commandeering and seizure of United States ships as French prizes. The Directory had recalled the French minister to the United States and had refused to receive Charles Pinckney, our minister, when he arrived to relieve James Monroe.

The Thomas Pinckney Treaty of 1795 with Spain granted free navigation on the Mississippi and set up the boundaries of East and West Florida and Louisiana; however, by subsequent *secret* treaty with Spain the territory was to be returned to France. Blount's financial difficulties became most serious early in 1797, causing him to go to New York in an attempt to bolster his position and to delay action on a protested note. At this time Blount urged Nicholas Romayne to persuade his friends to become purchasers of some of his extensive lands, for he feared the loss of the glittering financial gain that he had persuaded Romayne might accrue. Romayne refused at this time to enlist further support by his friends.

Shortly thereafter President John Adams was informed of Senator Blount's secret activities in international affairs and of his enlistment of

Romayne's assistance. On July 3, 1797, after returning to Washington, Blount walked into the Senate to find it in a noisy and tumultuous session; the clerk was reading some of his correspondence that had been intercepted. By a vote of 25-1, Blount was expelled from the Senate.[27] He fled from the city on horseback, taking backroads to Tennessee where, in 1798, despite the action against him in Washington, he was elected to the state senate. His impeachment trial began in December 1798; however, the United States Senate ruled that its senators were not impeachable and the affair was dropped. Meanwhile, on orders of the president, Dr. Nicholas Romayne was arrested at his house in New York early on the morning of July 12, 1797, a week after Blount's episode in the Senate, and was taken to Philadelphia to testify before a committee of the House of Representatives.

The Blount-Romayne affair must be considered in its historical background of Franco-American diplomatic relations, commonly known as the XYZ Affair. When the French Directory refused to receive our minister in 1797, President Adams sent a three-man commission to France, but Talleyrand, the foreign minister, refused to receive them and it was said that he had demanded £50,000 before he would permit the Directory to deal with them. A letter of October 31, 1797,[13] from Rufus King, minister to Great Britain, to U.S. Secretary of State Timothy Pickering, raises the probability, to judge by the reputed financial machinations in ranks as high as Talleyrand's, that the scheme involving Blount and Romayne may well have included Count de Moustier, former French minister to Washington, and Marquis Las Casas, Spanish minister to London, who presumably, according to Rufus King's letter to our secretary of state, ". . . was to support the Scheme at Madrid, and by his influence procure the King's sanction. De Yrujo who, as I am informed was privy to these conferences, and who was soon going to America, was to act as Las Casas' Agent in that Country." It would appear probable that these men, having established intimate relations with Romayne, may have used him to further their own ends with the expectation of tremendous financial returns.

Robert Troup, distinguished New York lawyer, in writing on June 24, 1800,[14] to his friend Rufus King, a letter which he gave to Nicholas Romayne to deliver in person, said, ". . . I cannot charge the Doctor [Romayne] with intending to do his country the least degree of injury. His imagination was heated with an idea that the French were negotiating with the Spaniards for those countries, and that the possession of them by the French would prove a source of the greatest mischiefs to us. Hence he thought it not amiss, provided he could make a great man of himself, to form a combination with the British government to defeat the plan of the French, and thereby give us friendly neighbours.'

Nicholas Romayne is listed in the New York City directory from 1797 to 1800 as living first at 23 John Street and then at Corlaers Hook. Always interested in his native city, he presented to the Common Council in July 1799 a street plan, which was adopted, for the improvement of Corlaers Hook.[8] (This area is now, under the same name, an extensive park and housing development along the lower East River Drive.) Somewhat earlier he had dealt in real estate, including the purchase of Fraunces Tavern from George Powers, warden of St. Ann's church in Brooklyn. This property he subsequently sold at considerable profit.

When Romayne went abroad in 1800, he left for England with the expectation of possibly remaining there. A few months after his arrival he became a Fellow of the Royal College of Physicians of Edinburgh—the first United States citizen to attain this honor. His stay abroad was short, however, for we find him listed in the New York City directory of 1804-1805 as living on Orchard Street, and the following year at Corlaers Hook.

On April 4, 1806, the New York State Legislature passed a bill that created the Medical Society of the State of New York and authorized the formation of societies in each county.* Nicholas Romayne, as already mentioned, had in 1791 petitioned the regents of the University of the State of New York to establish a College of Physicians and Surgeons and had obtained enabling legislation to effect this. Since he was one of the most able, versatile, and highly trained physicians in the state, it was quite natural that the newly formed Medical Society of the County of New York should turn to him for leadership. At the society's first meeting on July 1, 1806, with 102 physicians present, he was first elected chairman of the meeting, then president of the society, and a delegate to the meeting of the Medical Society of the State of New York to be held in Albany in February 1807.

*When Dr. Asa Fitch of Washington County, Dr. John Stearns[26] of Saratoga County, and Dr. Alexander Sheldon of Montgomery County, the last-named, fortuitously for the cause, being the newly elected speaker of the House, presented a memorial on February 25, 1806, requesting the state legislature to sanction the formation of a medical society they intended it for their three counties. Instead, thanks to the foresight and backing of the Honorable William W. Van Ness, when the matter came to a vote on April 4, 1806, a bill was passed to include the whole state, creating the Medical Society of the State of New York with each county authorized to form its own society, to be represented by delegates to the state society, and to appoint 3 to 5 censors to examine and license applicants for the practice of medicine.

Upon his arrival at the Albany meeting, Romayne found that certain practitioners of physic residing in New York, had signed a memorial to the legislature against establishing a College of Physicians and Surgeons in the City of New York, since the Columbia Medical School had existed for a number of years and had diligently taught the branches of medicine; the formation of another medical school was therefore opposed. Romayne[22] considered it unwise to air professional disputes before the legislature; instead, it seemed expedient to present the plan for the institution of a College of Physicians and Surgeons to the chancellor and Board of Regents. Accordingly, he was invited to meet with them on March 2, 1807, when he laid before them the many advantages to be gained for the public, as well as for the profession, by the formation of another medical school, especially since the population of the city had nearly trebled since 1790. His plan was referred to a committee that weighed both Romayne's appeal and the remonstrance from some members of the county society. The committee and the Regents nevertheless ". . . *agreed without one dissenting voice* to grant a charter for establishing a College of Physicians and Surgeons in this city" (italics the author's). And the regents ". . . by virtue of the act entitled, 'An act to enable the Regents of the University, to establish a College of Physicians and Surgeons within the state,' passed the 24th day of March, 1791, and we do by these presents, Ordain, Grant, and Declare, That a *College of Physicians and Surgeons, for the promoting of medical science, and diffusing the knowledge of the healing art*, shall be, and is hereby established in the city of New-York, in this state. . . ." The charter granted March 12, 1807,[23] was signed by Morgan Lewis as chancellor and Francis Bloodgood as secretary.

At a special meeting of the county society called on Monday, March 23, 1807, for the purpose of considering the action of the regents and Romayne's report, the members voted overwhelming approval. The charter of the new college was then read and adopted, and 500 copies were ordered printed. Surely this culmination of his hope and effort must have given great satisfaction to Romayne, as must also his election as president of the Medical Society of the State of New York for the years 1809 and 1810, and as first president of the new College of Physicians and Surgeons, a post he held from 1807 through 1810.

Though the charter had been granted, *no funds were made available.* Stepping into the breach, Dr. Romayne gave his personal note for $4,000,

Report AND Address,

DELIVERED BY THE

PRESIDENT,

TO THE MEDICAL SOCIETY OF THE COUNTY

OF NEW-YORK;

TOGETHER WITH THE

Charter

OF THE

COLLEGE OF PHYSICIANS & SURGEONS

IN THE

CITY OF NEW-YORK.

PUBLISHED BY ORDER OF THE SOCIETY.

NEW-YORK:

PRINTED BY JAMES CHEETHAM.

1807.

Fig. 3. Report and address delivered by Nicholas Romayne, President of the Medical Society of the County of New York, March 23, 1807. Reproduced by courtesy of the New York-Historical Society.

followed by another for $1,000 and a third for $700 (not a trivial sum in those days) to enable the medical school to begin. Thanks to his help, it did begin in rented quarters at 18 Robinson Street in November 1807. Romayne concluded his opening address by saying:[25] "Confiding in the constituted authorities of the state, and in their fellow-citizens for protection and support, the trustees, professors, and teachers of this College, will exert their humble efforts to fulfill their respective duties to the public with assiduity, zeal and attention." At the end of its second year the school moved into its own quarters in Magazine Street, now Pearl Street; the building had been purchased and largely financed by Dr. Romayne.

Dr. David Hosack, a graduate of the Medical College of Philadelphia in 1791,* was appointed professor of botany in the Columbia Medical School in 1795 and of materia medica a year later. Both of these appointments he continued to hold while he *simultaneously* sought a professor-

*In the catalogues of Columbia College for *both* 1815 and 1826 Hosack listed, following his name, "M.D. Edinburgh"—a wholly unfounded claim.

AN

ADDRESS,

DELIVERED AT THE

COMMENCEMENT OF THE LECTURES,

IN THE

COLLEGE OF PHYSICIANS AND SURGEONS

IN THE

CITY OF NEW-YORK.

*By NICHOLAS ROMAYNE, M. D.*

*PRESIDENT OF THE COLLEGE, FELLOW OF THE ROYAL COLLEGE OF PHYSICIANS OF EDINBURGH, LICENTIATE OF THE ROYAL COLLEGE OF PHYSICIANS OF LONDON, &c.*

*PUBLISHED BY ORDER OF THE COLLEGE.*

NEW-YORK:
PRINTED BY COLLINS AND PERKINS,
Printers to the College of Physicians and Surgeons.
1808.

Fig. 4. Title page of Nicholas Romayne's address at the opening of the College of Physicians and Surgeons, delivered November 10, 1807. Reproduced by courtesy of the New York-Historical Society.

ship in the newly formed College of Physicians and Surgeons. Since botany had been his major interest and since he had been teaching materia medica he was, quite naturally, given the chair in these subjects.

Inasmuch as the professors' remuneration depended upon the number of students taking their courses, and fewer took botany than the more important clinical subjects of surgery and midwifery, Hosack demanded during the first session to be made professor not only of surgery but also of midwifery. He wrote the following letter to Romayne, president of the Medical School and newly designated president of the Medical Society of the State of New York.[1]

New-York, Feb. 10th, 1808

My Dear Sir,

I have good reason to believe that it is not your intention to procure the appointment of the Professorship of Surgery and Midwifery for me. I need not relate the circumstances which have led to this opinion, nor the direct information I have received. If so, I have only to remark, that I abandon the Institution in toto. *I do not choose to be Botanist*, or *Midwife* to it, if unaccompanied with a more respectable appointment.

I cheerfully give up Materia Medica and Botany when you please, which afterwards can be arranged for Gillespie, MacNeven, etc. But if Dr. Smith is appointed Professor of Anatomy and Surgery, DeWitt to Chemistry, and I not made Professor of Surgery and Midwifery, I now request you, as President of the College, to communicate to the Regents my resignation of the appointment which they have bestowed upon me.

I can spend my time more profitably, than by teaching unproductive branches to the College of Physicians. I am very candid with you Doctor, as I have ever been; but I must not be neglected.

I am, Sir, yours,

D. Hosack

Dr. Nicholas Romayne
President of the Medical Society, Albany.

Hosack had up to this time shown great interest in botany, as evidenced by the botanical garden that he had established and that he had been trying by various means to sell at great profit. Being denied the chair of surgery and of midwifery, he began to do what he could, as a trustee and through DeWitt Clinton, mayor of New York, Elisha Jenkins, secretary of state of New York, Daniel Tompkins, governor of New York, and other influential friends, to disrupt the newly formed College of Physicians and Surgeons, which closed, finally, in 1811.

Interference in the affairs of the medical school began during its second session when, on February 13, 1809, the regents demanded that the faculty examine and report to them on the qualifications of all candidates for the degree of Doctor of Medicine.[2] Up to that time, however, the faculty, because of the as-yet-brief existence of the school, had not considered *any* candidate worthy of the degree. Nevertheless DeWitt Clinton and Elisha Jenkins in their report, March 5, 1810,[3] stated that the committee had been informed that "... several candidates were examined in 1809 and that some of them were adjudged qualified to receive the said degree of Doctor of Medicine." The report further held that ". . . the advancement of the highest Seminaries of learning depends not on the reduced price of education, but on the talents, the industry and the reputation of the Professors: and without sufficient encouragement to ensure these qualifications, no medical school can become great and respectable. But as the Regents are not provided with means to compensate the Professors . . . *it is fit they should receive a liberal sum from such Students as attend their Lectures*" (italics the author's).

At the same time, without the concurrence of the faculty, the regents stated over the signature of F. Bloodgood,[4] secretary, that ". . . the professor of Anatomy and Surgery and the professor of Chemistry shall each be entitled to receive a sum not exceeding twenty dollars, from each Student, for every course of Lectures, and all other professors shall each receive a sum not exceeding fifteen dollars for their courses of Lectures respectively delivered in said College." These were higher charges than the students could afford. Regrettably, this arrangement also did away with *free tuition for a student from each county* so essential for the development of medicine throughout the state. Romayne insisted that a total of $60 a year was as much as medical students could afford and would provide adequate remuneration to "respectable" professors. He appropriatedly stated, "But a College of Placement cannot be supported by Students–It would require national resources." Ten years later the student fees had risen to approximately $180. Hosack required his students to take both the practice of physic and midwifery, for which he charged $30 a course.

In March 1810 the diploma agreed upon and registered by the faculty was discarded; a new diploma was made, to be dispensed by the regents without the faculty's consent.[5]

The new regulations by the regents authorized the chancellor of the University *in his discretion* to authenticate and fix the seal of the University to diplomas during the recess of the regents, and specified that after *each* professor had examined a candidate for the degree of Doctor of Medicine the approval of *only three* was required for the granting of the degree. This violated the provision in the charter requiring the approval of *all* the professors before a degree could be granted.

On April 1, 1811, the regents finally having abrogated the charter, Hosack, again with the influence of his good friend DeWitt Clinton, sought to have the faculty of the Columbia Medical School unite with the College of Physicians and Surgeons, which would have destroyed the Columbia school—and this while he was still a member of the Columbia faculty where he had for many years been honored with a professorship! A public announcement of the appointment to professorships in the College of Physicians and Surgeons included the names of some of the professors in the Columbia Medical School. To the embarrassment of Hosack, three of these, Wright Post, William Hammersley, and James S. Stringham, appointed without their approval or consent, in an open letter in the *New York Evening Post,* April 8, 1811, repudiated the announcement, saying that they felt ". . . it a duty which they owe to themselves, as well as to the honourable the Board of Trustees of Columbia College, and the public, to say that the arrangement had been entered into without their knowledge, approval, or consent." In consequence of this refusal the long-standing annual allowance for the support of Dr. Wright Post's anatomical museum in Columbia Medical School was withheld.

About a week later, Dr. Archibald Bruce,[6] already on the faculty of the College of Physicians and Surgeons, who had been nominated by Hosack to continue as professor of mineralogy and pharmacy in the latter's proposed reorganization, wrote to Daniel D. Tompkins, chancellor of the University, "I take the earliest opportunity of informing you, that I cannot, under present circumstances, consistent with the respect I owe the profession and my own character, accept the same."

The following letter from Hosack to Samuel Bard,[12] then living at Hyde Park, 75 miles from New York and retired from practice, clearly reveals the former's scheme in relation to both medical schools:

To Dr. Samuel Bard

New York, April 9th, 1811

So important a change as is contemplated in our medical school can not take place without creating some disorder—The Regents have manifested a very liberal disposition by giving to each gentleman in the two medical schools a place in which he can be useful to the community and at the same time be profitably employed as it regards interest—We have however some men among us who will be blowing coals let the consequences be what it may that does not place them at the head—Romayne has accordingly been at work to prevent Bruce and Miller from partaking in the new college and another had had so much influence as to make Post, Hammersley, and Stringham decline—But the new institution will still be preserved and excepting Post all the other resignations will be of no moment. If Anatomy, Surgery, Practice of Physic, Midwifery, and Chemistry are well taught they constitute the most essential part of every medical school and will insure it success.—Smith, MacNeven, DeWitt, Rodgers and myself are determined to do our duty [sic] and we are convinced we shall receive the most liberal support from the Regents and the Legislature—we have funds—we have the Botanic Garden and Anatomical Museum—Chemical apparatus and we have the determination of the students to support us—neither shall these men prevent our success: in a short time Post will be brought in—I am convinced we shall make it honourable to all concerned—it is our intention to continue to educate one pupil from each county gratis—*this will assure us the support and approbation of the community and the Legislature*—I hope therefore you will not be discouraged but *will retain at least your nominal place—activity on your part will not be necessary*—The Regents having looked to you and elected you unanimously. I am sure you will be disposed to use your own influence to calm any irritation which may be at first created—you appear to anticipate very properly a little ferment from the change—and with you I think it well to let it subside—you will receive immediately your official notice from the Regents—they will all be sent out at the same time. [Italics the author's.] DR. HOSACK

DR. S. BARD

The ructions that arose at this time have been blandly dismissed as springing from ". . . feuds, animosities and recriminations," whereas they were engendered by Hosack's ambition and intrigue.*

The College of Physicians and Surgeons which, as has been said, Nicholas Romayne founded and largely supported out of his own funds, and of which he had been the first president, was now con-

*In 1817, Hosack, hard pressed financially, reduced the requirements for the degree of Doctor of Medicine—the student being at liberty to attend any course or courses he thought expedient, his attainments, and not the number of courses or years of study, being the sole criterion for an M.D. degree, provided he had attained the age of 21. This abuse of the qualifications for a degree and the consequent debasement of the licence to practice led, in 1819, to a series of charges preferred by the County Medical Society concerning the government of the College of Physicians and Surgeons and the excessive student fees. These and other charges culminated on April 11, 1826, in the resignation of the faculty, led by Hosack. Hosack was now, however, financially independent, having on February 26, 1825, 10 months after the death of his second wife, married the rich widow of Henry C. Coster through whom, according to Pintard,[18] he came into $300,000—a tidy sum indeed, even for that time.

trolled by Hosack and his influential friends. Never willing to accept defeat, Romayne immediately organized a rival medical school, the Medical Institution of New York, housed in a new three-story building especially erected for it on Duane Street, in time for the opening of the winter session on November 4, 1811. The following constituted the faculty:

Archibald Bruce, M.D., Professor of Materia Medica and Mineralogy;
Nicholas Romayne, M.D., Professor of the Institutes of Medicine and Forensic Medicine;*
Valentine Seaman, M.D., Professor of Anatomy, Physiology and Surgery;
Thomas Cock, M.D., also Professor of Anatomy, Physiology and Surgery;
Mr. John Griscom, Professor of Chemistry and Natural Philosophy;
Robert Bayard, M.D., Professor of Midwifery and Diseases of Women and Children;
John Watts, Jr., M.D., Professor of the Practice of Physic.

Romayne and the faculty deemed it essential to have a collegiate connection, and again they turned to Queen's College and to its new president, John H. Livingston, to whom Romayne wrote on October 8, 1811, informing him that a faculty had been formed, a building procured, and a large number of students enrolled—100 in the first-year class, 51 in the second, and 37 in the third. Ever solicitous for the advancement of students from the more distant parts of the state, Romayne accepted, as he had at the College of Physicians, one student from each county without charge on the recommendation of the president of the County Medical Society.

Discussions were held with the trustees of Queen's College on December 14, 1811, relative to the school's becoming the Medical Faculty of Queens College, and a memorial to this effect was drawn up and signed by Archibald Bruce, Nicholas Romayne, John Watts, Jr., Robert Bayard, John Griscom, Valentine Seaman, and Thomas Cock. The last three ". . . as members of the Society of Friends except only to the forms of address, but agree in substance."

Dr. John Watts, Jr., was designated to represent the faculty and

*Dr. Romayne's course on forensic medicine was the first to be given in America in any collegiate institution. This was followed by Dr. Stringham's lecture on this subject in 1814.

to meet with President Livingston on January 21, 1812, when agreement was immediately reached, and on the same day the Trustees resolved to establish the connection with the medical school and created[10] ". . . the professors of the Medical Institution in form and in fact the Medical Faculty of Queen's College." The professors were to assume entire responsibility for both the finances and the success or failure of the medical school. A candidate for the degree of doctor of medicine was required: to have studied medicine for three years, to present a thesis, to be of good moral character, and to be considered competent, before his degree could be signed by the president of the college, a number of trustees and *at least five* of his professors. The only fee paid to the college by the candidate was for his diploma, in an amount determined by the faculty. Tuition fees were paid to the professors.

The Medical Institution of New York presented a memorial to the New York Legislature in 1815, and again in 1816, requesting incorporation of the school. In an attempt to block such action by the legislature a counterremonstrance was presented by Dr. John W. Francis, a protégé of Hosack's, in 1815; and, in 1816, Hosack himself led a delegation to Albany which, through a successful appeal to DeWitt Clinton and Simeon DeWitt, surveyor-general of the State of New York, was able to block the request of the Medical Institution.

Unfortunately Queen's College was shortly thereafter again in financial difficulties, involving not only the undergraduate but also the graduate departments; and, in 1816, it was once more forced to close all but part of its theological training. During the 4 years of the existence of the Queen's College Medical School as The Medical Institution of the State of New York only 21 students were considered by the faculty to have qualified for the medical degree—evidence of the high standards maintained.

The closing of the school and the consequent end of his teaching career were a severe blow to Romayne, and preceded his death by only a year.* Throughout his career his innate talents and the un-

*As Romayne's wife and daughter had died a number of years earlier, he left no direct descendants. His will, probated August 11, 1817, named as his heirs his sisters Jane, Rachel, and Susan; his brother Jermiah and Jeremiah's eldest son; a kinsman, John, son of Casparus Romayne; a cousin, Benjamin, son of Thomas Romayne; the eldest son of a cousin, John Romeyn; and the son of Dirck Romeyn. As executors the will listed Romayne's sister Rachel; his brother, the Rev. Jeremiah Romeyn; a cousin, John, son of Dirck Romeyn; and a friend, Hon. John Rutherford of Sussex County, N.J.

Romayne's constant concern for others is evidenced in the conclusion of his will, which reads,[28] ". . . having in my early life felt and experienced want and difficulties and while I had to attend to Literary persuits to provide for the day which was pressing over me. I leave a competency to some and an ample fortune to others who by care and attention prudence and economy and confining and moderating their views and desires may enjoy and possess many earthly comforts themselves and leave the same to their successors."

equaled advantages of his European training had been unfailingly focused on his paramount aim of establishing high standards of medical education in his city and state, with particular concern for medical students in the more remote parts of the state. To this end his resources, both mental and material, were lavishly and unstintingly given. Such conflicts as he had were, in the main, with those less able and less highly trained, whose vision was less far-reaching, and whose purposes were less disinterested.

The high-mindedness of Romayne's life-long ambition and effort can be summed up by his own concluding remarks in his report to the Medical Society of the County of New York on March 23, 1807, when he obtained overwhelming approval for the establishment of the College of Physicians and Surgeons,[24] ". . . I pray Almighty God that this Institution may in its operation be useful to this Nation and be handed down with honour to the latest posterity."

## *REFERENCES*


1. College of Physicians and Surgeons in the City of New York, *Exposition of the Transactions Relative to the College of Physicians and Surgeons in the City of New York, from Its Establishment until the Assumption of the Charter, by the Regents of the University.* Report by a committee of the members of the college comprehended in the charter. New York, Collins, 1812, p. 12.
2. *Ibid.,* p. 10.
3. *Ibid.,* p. 12.
4. *Ibid.,* p. 14.
5. *Ibid.,* p. 10.
6. *Ibid.,* p. 41.
7. Common Council of the City of New York. *Minutes (1784-1831).* New York, City of New York, 1792, vol. 1, p. 709.
8. Common Council of the City of New York. *Minutes (1784-1831).* New York, City of New York, 1817, vol. 2, p. 559.
9. Demarest, D. D. *Rutgers (Queen's) College and Medical Degrees.* Trenton, New Brunswick Historical Club, 1894, vol. 2, p. 54.
10. Demarest, W. H. S. *A History of Rutgers College, 1766-1924.* New Brunswick, Rutgers College, 1924, 570 pp.
11. *Dictionary of American Biography,* D. Malone, ed. New York, Amer. Council of Learned Societies, 1943, vol. 16, pp. 127-128.
12. Hosack, D. *Letter to Samuel Bard, April 9, 1811.* MS., New York Academy of Medicine.
13. King, C. R. *Life and Correspondence of Rufus King, 1787-1801.* New York, Putnam, 1894, vol. 3, pp. 236-237.
14. *Ibid.,* pp. 258-259.
15. *Laws of the State of New York,* 14th session. An Act to enable the Regents of the University to establish a College of Physicians and Surgeons within this state. Albany, Child, Swaine, 1791, chap. 45, p. 34.
16. Masterson, W. H. *William Blount.* Baton Rouge, Louisiana State Univ. Press, 1954, 378 pp.
17. N.Y. (City) Surrogate's Court. Abstracts of Wills on File, vol. 14 . . . 1786-1796. In: *Collections of the New York Historical Society for 1905,* vol. 38, pp. 223-24.
18. Pintard, J. *Letters from John Pintard to His Daughter Eliza Noel Pintard*

*Davidson, 1816-1833.* New York, N. Y. Hist. Soc., 1941, vol. 4, p. 39.

19. Rogers, F. B. Nicholas Romayne, 1756-1817: Stormy petrel of American Education, *J. Med. Educ. 35*:258-63, 1960.
20. Romayne, N. *Letter of resignation, Feb. 1, 1792.* MS., Columbia University.
21. Romayne, N. *Letter, June 20, 1793.* MS., Columbia University.
22. Romayne, N. *Report and Address Delivered by the President, to the Medical Society of the County of New York; Together with the Charter of the College of Physicians and Surgeons in the City of New York.* New York, Cheatham, 1808, p. 6.
23. *Ibid.*, p. 14.
24. *Ibid.*, p. 10.
25. Romayne, N. *An address Delivered at the Commencement of the Lectures in the College of Physicians and Surgeons in the City of New York.* New York, Collins, Perkins, 1808, p. 39.
26. Stearns, J. An account of the origin of the law "to incorporate Medical Societies for the purpose of regulating the practice of Physic and Surgery in this State"; passed April 4, 1806, *N. Y. Med. Phys. J. 7*:380-384, 1828.
27. United States Congress. House of Representatives. *A report of the committee . . . appointed to prepare and report articles of impeachment against William Blount, a Senator of the United States, impeached of high crimes and misdemeanors. . . .* [Containing letters to and from Nicholas Romayne.] Washington, D.C., John Fenno, 1798, 160. pp.
28. N.Y. (County) Surrogate's Court. Original will on file. In: *Liber 54*:240-43.

# THE MICHAEL M. DAVIS COLLECTION OF SOCIAL AND ECONOMIC ASPECTS OF MEDICINE

LEE ASH

Library Consultant
New Haven, Conn.

THE Library of The New York Academy of Medicine is the fortunate and grateful recipient of one of the most outstanding gifts offered to any medical library in many years in the form of personal files and memorabilia. The records of Dr. Michael Marks Davis, one of the fathers of public medical care (now in the 88th year of his life), have given the Academy 52 vertical file drawers of correspondence, confidential reports, special surveys, scarce pamphlet and document publications, clippings, and ephemera relating to the legislation, organization, and economics of government-sponsored public medical care in the United States and foreign countries.

The active life and many public services of Michael Davis need not be described here since they are a matter of record in the usual biographical sources, such as *Who's Who in America*. Suffice that, in entrusting these files to The New York Academy of Medicine, Dr. Davis has made a lasting memorial to himself and to the devoted medical men, social workers, and political movers who followed his leadership by demonstrating their belief in public and governmental health security measures.

Dr. Davis' tremendous file—well over 400,000 pieces—which is certain to attract other similar gifts to the Academy, covers the period of his most valiant efforts, from the late 1920's to 1966, the year that witnessed the consummation of Medicare, a great step forward in government health services. Thus the files are in themselves unique source material for studying some of the most important legislative advances in the history of our country. All sides of every aspect of the problem are covered, and drawer after drawer contains material—most of it unpublished—on the arguments against "socialized medicine" as well as far-seeing statements by legislators and physicians who have acknowledged government and community responsibility to support protective health care and medical insurance programs. Of course there will be other advances, new changes, and radical improvements in public medical care but, reaching to the year of 1966 (the terminal year of his major efforts), Dr. Davis' records form a treasure of resources for study of the increasingly important problems of medical economics and social security.

The files are divided into six major groupings that form the basis of a singularly effective classification of the materials they contain, a classification that will enable future students to approach the mass without the usual confusion found in so many collections of personal papers deposited in libraries.

To enhance the usefulness of the classification there is a descriptive master index of 61 pages, listing the various file folders within each major grouping, drawer by drawer. This index alone will save thousands of dollars and hundreds of hours of professional and clerical time that would otherwise have to be spent sorting, calendaring, and describing the contents of the files in order that researchers might make use of the material.

The six major groupings determined by Dr. Davis are as follows: I. Medical Economics and Sociology (8 file drawers); II. Medical Care (21 drawers); III. Legislation (5 drawers); IV. Organizations (10 drawers); V. Medical Care in Foreign Countries (4 drawers); and VI. Personalities (4 drawers). In the following paragraphs I shall attempt to describe some of the most important items contained in each group and try to suggest the quality and flavor of this invaluable resource.

## I. Medical Economics and Sociology

These eight file drawers contain material that is concerned, essentially, with the cost of medical care and with special studies by, for, and about the Committee on the Costs of Medical Care, including confidential reports in typescript carbon copies by such eminent authorities of the 1930's as Haven Emerson, Louis I. Reed, and C. Rufus Rorem. A great deal of the material concerns Michael M. Davis' evaluations of the work of this important committee and its implications for the development of its recommendations, made during the period of Davis' term as director of Medical Services of the Julius Rosenwald Fund during the depths of the depression, when the health needs of the population were in great flow and public resources at their lowest ebb. The files, at this point, are filled with publications, special studies, reports, drafts of minutes of committee meetings, and special groups concerned with public income data, taxes, and similar material (with much of a contemporary and ephemeral nature) concerning President Franklin D. Roosevelt's Committee on Economic Security and the Advisory Council on Economic Security, from the time of its establishment by executive order on June 29, 1934. This is supplemented by special studies (some undertaken by Dr. Davis or his associates) on the program of grants-in-aid for rural hospital services, and of Social Security programs. Many special studies, both published and unpublished, are in this group of files, such as those on the attitudes of Roman Catholics toward Social Security, the report of the Michigan *Governor's Study Commission on Prepaid Hospital and Medical Care Plans* (1962), etc.

Original questionnaires returned by certain labor unions, requesting information on their attitudes toward and experience with medical care and hospital insurance, are in one of these drawers, along with manuscript reports, typescripts of articles, addresses, etc., concerned with Blue Cross (including its early history)—much of it separately classified by subject or by states of the Union.

Material on state, industrial, and cooperative medical plans, comprehensive group medical plans, and union health programs fills the next few drawers, providing a mine of information on social trends in the past three decades. This is material that cannot be duplicated and does not appear in any other library collection as a unit standing ready for the analyses of scholars of the future who will build on the experience detailed in the records of the Davis Collection.

This running descriptive record of appraisal can only suggest the contents of the collection, but the excitement that is generated by examining such a trove of unusual material carries the examiner breathlessly from drawer to drawer. Appraisals—whether for monetary or quantitative evaluation—must be objective and, in line with this purpose, I have considered the whole of the collection and its parts in relation to similar source records in other places. In a word, there is no comparison that can be made, even in special libraries devoted to the main subjects of these files.

## II. Medical Care in the United States

Here again, confidential reports made for foundations in the United States on the subject of medical care abound, and the files are replete with correspondence, publications, clippings, and other documentation on the distribution of medical care, medical care for dependents of military personnel, home care, and social medicine.

Material contained in the file drawer on various diseases is somewhat less interesting and less valuable, probably because these seem not to have been of primary interest to Dr. Davis and his colleagues in their broad approach to the problems of universal health. Most of the material here is in the nature of secondary sources and, although there are some scarce or unusual reports (e.g., *The Middle Atlantic Educational Congress on Vision in Defense Industry*, April 1942—a 218-page transcript), the bulk of this one drawer is probably duplicated by the Academy's holdings. Apparently Dr. Davis used this file merely for background information.

When we go on to national affairs and social planning, however, we return to a principal interest of Dr. Davis', and again we come onto a number of unusual documents—published and unpublished—such as the interesting literate study that Benjamin C. Gruenberg made for the Committee on American Museum of Hygiene of the American Public Health Association in 1937, *A Museum of Health* (72 pp.). And so it goes, on and on, covering early antipoverty programs, population problems, regional and medical programs for heart disease, cancer, and stroke, urban renewal and urban planning, health conditions in the United States, etc., with a great deal of material on the problems of youth in urban communities. The administration of medical research comes into its own throughout the records of these files, and there is a great deal of valuable material, much of it wholly ephemeral and not retained elsewhere, on various special, typical, and particular public or private health surveys. The file on Health in Wartime provides a special source on health problems in defense migration, the effect of war (usually referring to World War II) on the medical profession, the war and medical manpower, hospital and health center requirements in defense areas, etc.

This section of the files also contains much stimulating material of an historical nature on rural economic conditions from the 1930's through the 1950's, and on rural health problems and programs, especially with regard to national and state government interest in health security measures for farm and migrating laborers. The section continues with extensive material in the nature of private reports, correspondence, surveys, and publications on group practice of medicine, including files on specific organizations, and on prepayment plans made by specific labor unions, much of it not available elsewhere.

Major divisions of Section II of the files also include subdivided groups of folders on medical education (federal aid, intern training, regional cooperation, etc.), medical personnel, and physicians (choice and change of doctors, discrimination in medicine, the involvement of druggists, ethics, fee-splitting, etc.), specialists, dentists and dentistry, medical social workers, nurses and nursing, etc.

Several drawers are filled with reports, correspondence, and publications on hospitals, including some complete and some broken files of newsletters and reports of hospital councils and organizations, as well as privately conducted surveys and studies of hospitals, their services, administration, and financing. Obviously, Dr. Davis' view of public medicine was over-all and complete, and his files include an accumulation of years concerning the American Hospital Association and its various subsidiary parts, much of which is supplemented in the extensive separate correspondence files that make up a part of this gigantic collection.

The bulk of the files (21 drawers) of the collection are in this Second Section, "Medical Care in the United States," and this brief description continues now to give a summary review of the further inclusiveness of Dr. Davis' working papers. There is a large file on public medical care programs, particularly as they concern the aged and aging, public welfare projects, public health, and workmen's compensation (with detailed studies of variations, laws, etc.).

Of special interest is a drawer devoted to some of the restricted records of the 1952 hearings of The President's Commission on the Health Needs of the Nation and other related confidential transcripts, correspondence, etc. There is a very complete file on the Salk Vaccine debate of 1955 which, besides containing hearings and releases from the U.S. Department of Health, Education, and Welfare and from the Committee for the Nation's Health, has Dr. Davis' comments (manuscript lecture notes, correspondence, etc.), on all aspects of the argument. Also included is a valuable collection of different organizations' official and unofficial statements on the subject.

Problems of Veterans Administration medical care programs and a small file on the War Stabilization Board Report on Health, Welfare, and Pension programs are housed in a large file drawer, three quarters of which is taken up by an extensive record related to Medicare, which bridges a break in Dr. Davis' collection between Section II, Medical Care, and Section III, covering federal and state legislation for public health care under the Social Security program and other forms of state-administered medical care.

## III. Legislation

The National Health Insurance Legislation file contains original texts of bills, committee hearings, and basic data in the form of official publications and statements of organizations and individuals (clippings, correspondence, published releases, etc.). There are also folders of correspondence and other expressions of different and differing attitudes as evidenced by labor, "organized medicine," commercial, and political organizations. The whole picture of a nation concerned is here —and there are files of statements by personalities in all fields, newspaper and columnist's comments, articles from all kinds of magazines, along with radio and television publicity, and cartoons. What a mass of primary source records for study of the history of one of the greatest social actions of the United States! This record is, in fact, the very substance of history itself.

Not only the early health insurance bills and actions sponsored by Flanders and Herter in 1949, the Humphrey Cooperative Health Act of 1949, and the Taft-Smith-Donnell action of 1946, 1947, and 1949 are here, but these records are accompanied by Dr. Davis' complete files of correspondence, clippings, confidential reports, and annotated copies of published items referring to these legislative movements. Most inclusive are the files on the Wagner-Murray-Dingell bills and their evolution from previous legislative proposals dating back more than 30 years.

In addition to these specific files there are two whole file drawers crammed with material on legislation since 1950, and two more stuffed with pertinent publications, reports, correspondence, and ephemera relevant to legislation prior to 1950, public assistance and child welfare, mental health, and state legislation, including sickness and disability insurance programs to be paid for by the state.

There are, further, materials on the legal aspects of hospitals, their medical staff relations, and licensing laws regarding hospitals and convalescent institutions. The file on legal suits and medical societies is especially fascinating, including as it does a unique scrapbook of newspaper clippings on "The A.M.A. Trial" of 1941, when the American Medical Association was indicted for alleged violation of the antitrust act. This, along with trial records of other legal actions affecting medical organizations, optical rebates, and so forth, give us a substantial corps of reference materials not easy to come by and, in most cases—particularly where Dr. Davis' correspondence or ephemera are added—not to be duplicated in any other collection.

## IV. Professional Organizations

Samples of special reports, annual reports, and letters to and from Dr. Davis concerning the work of various organizations are included in this part of the collection, which is grouped into the following sections: *a*) Professional Organizations; *b*) General Organizations; *c*) International Organizations; *d*) Political Organizations.

Much of the material here would be difficult to find, but some of it may already be in the Academy's Library. A large part of Dr. Davis' intrinsic interest in the dozens of organizations represented in this portion of the collection is more substantially supported by correspondence located by subject designation elsewhere in the files and, also, in the large part of the collection devoted to "Personalities," which will be described later. There is considerable material on rural or farm organizations and on a number of temporary groups.

One of the chief values of the section devoted to organizations, however, is the inclusion of a good deal of material on groups now defunct or inactive, along with publications derived from them; also, many publications that are now unobtainable from organizations that are still existent are in the file drawers at the Academy. This section of the collection is not a stable one, however, in terms of completeness, and it will be necessary to check it against the Academy's present holdings.

In addition to the miscellaneous organizations just commented upon, there are two drawers devoted to Dr. Davis' complete file of records, correspondence, interviews, confidential reports, etc., concerning the Committee for the Nation's Health, with articles promoted or arranged for by the committee in various publications, 1948 to 1956; there are also memoranda, minutes, and financial statements. Dr. Davis was, of course, chairman of the Executive Committee of the Committee for the

Nation's Health. This is an absolutely unique and basic record of the work and administration of one of the most effective instruments for public education with regard to medical security ever to be active in this country. The work of the Committee for the Nation's Health, its internal administration and public programs, will serve as a model for many other social drives in the future. Likewise, the similar files of the Committee on Research in Medical Economics (CRME), also in two more drawers, gives the Academy a corner on research in the field of medical economics. The unique, priceless archives of these two organizations will undoubtedly be the cornerstone of a research collection that will be of growing importance to all branches of the medical profession. Acquisition by the Academy of this material is a gift that merits solemn and continuing thanks to the donor.

The American Medical Association was, naturally, of prime interest to Dr. Davis and his colleagues in the various committees and groups with which he worked toward the goal of government-sponsored or government-supported health plans. Four file drawers contain basic studies of the A.M.A. and its organization, with detailed publications, reports, correspondence, clippings, and private studies gathered from many sources. There are folders of correspondence with several individuals and officers of the A.M.A., with a good deal of supplementary material such as reports of the association's meetings, speeches made to them, etc. The A.M.A. files continue with a drawer on medical societies (state and county) filled with correspondence as well as with clippings and other secondary source records of "position statements" made by auxiliary groups across the country during the years of the great debate on "socialized medicine."

Not less interesting are the files on the A.M.A.'s public relations programs, with confidential internal documents of policy and procedures (some conducted by outside surveyors), and documentation of the high-gear efforts of the association to publicize its views about publicly supported health programs. The file contains fascinating documentation on the crisis in the mid-1940's when a noted public relations counseling firm withdrew from its association with the A.M.A. in a dispute over purpose and intention. Such historic items are of the record and would not be found in any other collection. The bitter battles of the A.M.A. against the programs of the Committee on the Costs of Medical Care, the Committee on the Nation's Health, and findings or recommendations of these and similar bodies are all exposed in Dr. Davis' collection—a picture of social turmoil in professional-societal relations in flux over many, many years.

One drawer contains "The A.M.A.-Record," with extensive coverage—in confidential correspondence, secret reports, brochures, clippings, and other published or unpublished formats—of documentation that is beyond value for historical consideration of the battle of the A.M.A. Campaigns and samples of advertising literature are described (with numerous actual examples), the 1948 assessment of $25 and reactions to it, attitudes toward health insurance, folders on medical ethics and economics, tax exemption, etc. Position papers and studies on various legislation such as compulsory health insurance, disability insurance, family doctors, federal aid, health care for the aged, public school systems, Social Security, and veterans care are only a part of this exciting story of social change. The files will surely be required by many scholars, legislators, and administrators who will build publicly supported health plans in the future.

This "record" is further extended by files describing the "A.M.A. in Politics," the National Professional Committee for Eisenhower (1952), action in political campaigns, "Doctors for Nixon-Lodge," and similar efforts that were made over the years to bring the proper forces into line for political action. It is all rather a desperate story, and Dr. Davis' files enhance a view of political battles that is not otherwise available in such completely documented form. Take, for example, the folders on the famous Whitaker and Baxter activities of 1952 to 1954 and the campaign to fight for voluntary medicine described as "one of the choicest plums and hottest potatoes in U.S. public relations," or the file on the National Physicians Committee, and the lobbying activities of the various medical organizations other than the A.M.A. What a tremendous source for a study of the record of power politics in the milieu and annals of professional medicine a hundred years from now! Dr. Davis was in the center of it all, and his letters, special studies, and clippings documenting the course of events is remarkably complete and disturbingly revealing.

## V. Medical Care in Foreign Countries

This section of the collection contains much public documentation and correspondence with leaders and private physicians concerned with social medicine and public health abroad. Most of these folders are devoted to the era in Great Britain that preceded and followed the Beveridge Plan, and are abundantly supplemented by comments (in print and letter form) made by practitioners, consultants, and specialists referring to the National Health Service Act and all aspects of its administration. There is a long correspondence with Sidney Lamb, one-time secretary of the International Hospital Association and secretary of the Merseyside Hospitals Council (Liverpool) who devoted so many years to the cause of improved hospital care in Great Britain and elsewhere, a correspondence containing warm and sensitive expressions of hopefulness for "the health help needed by the people of all countries."

Much of the foreign material from Great Britain, the Continent, Asia, Africa, Canada, Australia, and New Zealand appears in the form of published and unpublished reports, most of it probably not duplicated in other collections on the social and economic aspects of medicine, health insurance, etc. One especially interesting part of the files at this point is correspondence and other material originating in the United States and commenting on the National Health Service in Great Britain —a remarkable display of varieties of opinion both favorable and hostile.

## VI. Personalities

If my description of the Davis Collection has stimulated some enthusiasm or curiosity on the part of readers up to this point, let me say that perusal of the four closely packed drawers on personalities shows them to be an even more valuable and exciting part of the files. Here we have Dr. Davis' correspondence, notes, comments, clippings, personality evaluations, and memorabilia to, from, and about all of the leaders associated with him in his multifarious activities. I cannot take space to write in detail about these file drawers but there are remarkably full folders about such dynamic personalities as, for example, Elin Anderson whose grass-roots pioneering efforts brought more adequate medical service to thousands of people in the United States; other names follow in a list of movers and shakers on the social scene there, such as: Dr. George Baehr, Harry Becker, Dr. George Berry, George Bugbee, Morris L. Cooke, Thomas E. Dewey, Oscar Ewing, Dr. I. S. Falk (an exceptionally long file dating from 1933 to 1954), Dr. Channing Frothingham, Sir William Jameson, Mr. and Mrs. Albert D. Lasker, Dean

Leonard Mayo, Dr. James C. McCann, Dr. Frederick D. Mott, Anna M. Rosenberg, Adlai Stevenson, Senator Robert Taft, President Harry S. Truman, Albert W. Whitney, and hundreds of others. Most of the files contain correspondence of greater or lesser significance; many are reflections of Dr. Davis' numerous activities and include his terse comments—sometimes kindly, sometimes stringent and critical.

## VII. The Book Collection

In addition to the 52 file drawers described above, Dr. Davis has given the Academy about 250 monograph publications relative to his fields of interest, and sets of bound volumes of ephemeral reports of such organizations as the Committee for the Nation's Health (which do not appear in the files).

This remarkable collection is a unique record of a great period in the health services of the United States. It is surely among the most important acquisitions the Library of The New York Academy of Medicine has received in its entire history. Over the years it will prove to be a jewel box of resources in a field of medicine that is continuously growing in importance, for until this time the story has been inadequately documented by materials of such a personal nature as Dr. Davis' collection.

# THE PSYCHOTIC SON OF BENJAMIN RUSH

The versatile and impetuous Benjamin Rush (1745-1813) was one of this country's first great physicians. In combining a medical career with an active career in politics he did what few of our professional colleagues have done. Indeed the combination is rare with us although common among Latin Americans.

Rush's medical reputation was large during and immediately after his lifetime. It rested partly on his numerous writings, partly on his great experience as a teacher, and partly on his contributions to psychiatry. As the terrible story of yellow fever recedes into the background of time, it carries with it Rush's sanguinary therapeusis, and we begin to feel that the lasting eminence of Rush is based on his work in mental disease, which is symbolized by the psychiatric division of the Pennsylvania Hospital. But to this a pathetic story is attached. The following narrative has been taken from the *Autobiography* of Samuel D. Gross, Philadelphia, G. Barrie, 1887, vol. 1, pp. 377-379.

* * *

I became acquainted with Mr. Forrest under peculiar circumstances. In the summer of 1828 Professor George McClellan called at my office at Library and Fifth Streets, in this city, to ask me if on the morrow I would accompany Mr. Edwin Forrest to the Pennsylvania Hospital, adding that the young actor was studying the character of Lear and was anxious to see a Mr. Rush, who had long been confined in that institution on account of insanity. My answer was, "Certainly; it will afford me much pleasure to be of service, in any manner possible, to you or to your friend." Punctually at twelve o'clock, the hour appointed for our meeting at McClellan's house, we were presented to each other; and Forrest and I strolled off, talking pretty briskly as we passed along, to the office of the steward, to whom I introduced my companion. In a trice we were at the desired spot. Mr. John Rush was a son of Dr. Benjamin Rush, and had been educated for the Philadelphia bar, then perhaps the most famous bar in the United States, adorned as it was by many of the leading minds of the country. The case of Rush was a singularly melancholy one. In an evil hour the young lawyer quarrelled with his bosom friend, a Mr. Bingham, who occupied a high position in the social circle. A meeting took place soon after—in Canada, I believe—and Rush killed his adversary. Remorse seized him, and in a short time he became a victim of incurable insanity. At the time of our visit the insane were confined in the basement story of the building; and Rush was in the habit of pacing to and fro in the corridor, with his hands behind his back, engaged in incoherent mutterings, in which the word "Bingham" was conspicuously noticeable. He was then an old man, although he was still erect, with a handsome, open, manly countenance. Through the grating in the heavy iron door of the corridor Forrest stealthily studied the conduct of the demented duellist. He visited the hospital a number of times, and finally came away perfectly convinced of the madness of Lear, as graphically portrayed by Shakespeare. Forrest thenceforth made a special study of the character, and how faithfully he delineated it is too well known to require comment.

In 1837, at an advanced age, Rush died in his cell, the light never having reëntered his soul. His illustrious father, who was the author of a work on the Mind, which is still frequently quoted with approbation, was not able to discover among his remedies any balm for his unfortunate son.

Except at an occasional visit to the theatre at Louisville, New York, and Philadelphia, in which I saw Forrest in some of his great characters, such as Hamlet, Lear, Othello, Brutus, Virginius, and Richard III, I did not meet him again until June 1870 when he came to my office with his sister, Miss Eleanora Forrest, who had a cancer of the mammary gland, for which my advice was sought. We shook hands cordially, I said, "Mr. Forrest, do you remember the summer of 1828, in which, in the company of a young man who had been introduced to you by Dr. George McClellan, you visited the Pennsylvania Hospital to see Mr. Rush, an insane inmate?" "I recollect the circumstance," he replied, "but have forgotten the name of the gentleman." "I am that man," I said, when he again grasped my hands. "Well, I am very glad to see you after so long a separation, during which we have both grown older, and, I hope, a good deal wiser."

S. J.

## *Bowen-Brooks Scholarship For Advanced Study Abroad*

In the current year the Committee on Medical Education of The New York Academy of Medicine will award *one* Bowen-Brooks Scholarship in the amount of $5,200 for the *academic year 1968-69.*

This scholarship was established by the donor to provide aid for advanced study abroad in a clinical subject in preparation for the practice of medicine or surgery in any of their branches.

As stipulated by the donor of the fund, candidates must be *male* interns or residents in voluntary, municipal, or Veterans Administration hospitals in New York City.

The course of study, the auspices under which it is to be taken, and the place or places where the study is to be pursued must receive the approval of the Committee. Applicants are favored who, from their records, show themselves capable of advanced work in clinical medicine. The Committee stipulates that the study be pursued abroad, preferably in Great Britain or in continental Europe.

The deadline for receipt of applications is *November 1, 1967.* Applicants will be required to appear before the Awards Committee for a personal interview at a meeting to be held in December. Announcement of the award will be made in late December.

Requests for application forms should be addressed to:

Office of Medical Education
The New York Academy of Medicine
2 East 103 St., New York, N.Y. 10029

***Advance Announcement***

The August issue of the Bulletin will be devoted to the publication of papers presented at the

*CONFERENCE ON BURNS AND FLAME-RETARDANT FABRICS*

that was held at the Academy last December, under the auspices of the American College of Surgeons, the National Fire Protection Association, the Academy's Section on Plastic and Reconstructive Surgery, the Division of Accident Prevention of the U.S. Public Health Service, in cooperation with the American Academy of Pediatrics, the American Public Health Association, and the National Safety Council.

The nature and extent of the burn problem, its medical and surgical aspects, the present technology and efforts to develop and apply flame-retardant fabrics, and the roles of government, industry, and other agencies in controlling the problem of fires in clothing will be discussed in 22 papers by physicians and surgeons, by technicians and managers of the textile industry, and by executives in various government departments.

Advance orders for copies of this issue may be sent to:

Editor, Bulletin of The New York Academy of Medicine
2 East 103 Street, New York, N.Y. 10029

BULLETIN OF
THE NEW YORK ACADEMY
OF MEDICINE

VOL. 43, No. 8 AUGUST 1967

# CONFERENCE ON BURNS AND FLAME-RETARDANT FABRICS

## *Opening Remarks**

PAUL V. JOLIET

Chief, Division of Accident Prevention
U.S. Public Health Service
Arlington, Va.

As your general chairman, I shall start by emphasizing what I consider the great importance of the subject matter under discussion.

There is much to cover on our agenda. Each topic has been carefully selected in the hope that each presentation will contribute to the objective of the conference—namely, the reduction of burns from clothing and other fabric fires.

Those of us in the U.S. Public Health Service who work full time in the field of injury prevention are concerned over the serious, complex problem of injuries and deaths due to fire. We must be concerned—

*Presented at the *Conference on Burns and Flame-Retardant Fabrics,* held at The New York Academy of Medicine, December 2 and 3, 1966. The conference was sponsored by: the New York and Brooklyn Trauma Committee of the American College of Surgeons, Chicago, Ill.; The National Fire Protection Association, Boston, Mass.; the Section on Plastic and Reconstructive Surgery of The New York Academy of Medicine; and the Division of Accident Prevention of the U.S. Public Health Service, Washington, D.C. The conference was held in cooperation with the American Academy of Pediatrics, Evanston, Ill.; the American Public Health Association, New York, N. Y.; and the National Safety Council, Chicago, Ill.; and was supported by a grant from the U.S. Public Health Service.

Since this conference was held the Division of Accident Prevention has become the Injury Control Program, National Center for Urban and Industrial Health.

fire and explosion are the second leading cause of all nontransportation accidental deaths in the United States. Eighty per cent of these deaths occur in the home. Nonfatal injuries from fire and explosion, as estimated by the National Health Survey, are suffered by more than 250,000 persons each year.

One important segment of this problem is burn and asphyxia associated with clothing and fabric fires. If we consider the sequence of events that precedes the injury, we can identify 1) a source of ignition coming in contact with 2) combustible clothing or fabric worn by 3) children, elderly persons, and other high-risk groups.

This conference is being held to find a way to interrupt this sequence. We are here to consider practical approaches to the modification of the fabric to render it flame-retardant and to make it available in the market place. We sincerely solicit the full cooperation of the textile industry, retail merchants, professional groups, and the volunteer organizations in this country in this effort. We want to create a demand for flame-retardant clothing for children, elderly persons, handicapped people, people in high-risk occupations, sportsmen who must protect themselves from serious and disabling burns.

I think that our meetings here will prove to be unique as well as constructive. They should be unique because of the subject matter designated for a formal conference. They should be constructive because of the excellent agenda and the unusually high caliber of our speakers.

They are all leaders in government, industry, the health professions, and the consumer public.

I know that our program was carefully prepared. Those who appear on it as principals were chosen, not at random to fill a spot, but because of their individual qualifications and because of their abilities to express themselves lucidly.

# CONFERENCE ON BURNS AND FLAME-RETARDANT FABRICS

## *Welcoming Remarks**

JOHN L. MADDEN

President
The New York Academy of Medicine

IN the name of The New York Academy of Medicine and its Director, Howard R. Craig, I welcome you. Dr. Craig, after 20 years of devoted service, will be succeeded next month by Dr. James E. McCormack, who is present on this occasion.

When I received a call from my good friend, Robert H. Kennedy, asking me to make a few welcoming remarks, I was glad, of course, to do so. However, when he sent me a copy of the program, I noticed that 30 minutes had been alloted to my welcoming remarks. However, I wish immediately to allay your fears and promise you that I shall speak but a few minutes. Despite Dr. Kennedy's most kind comments about delaying my departure for Spain, I wish to assure you that in coming here to welcome you I have suffered no inconvenience and certainly no imposition.

I have had the pleasant occasion of reviewing in depth your program for the *Conference on Burns and Flame-Retardant Fabrics* and I believe it the most impressive and the most comprehensive coverage of the many and varied aspects of burns that I have seen. The Program Committee is to be congratulated on a job exceedingly well done. I am confident that your deliberations in the ensuing 2 days will prove most informative and beneficial to each and every one who has the privilege to be in attendance. I wish you well and I thank you.

*Presented at the *Conference on Burns and Flame-Retardant Fabrics,* held at The New York Academy of Medicine, December 2 and 3, 1966. The conference was sponsored by: the New York and Brooklyn Trauma Committee of the American College of Surgeons, Chicago, Ill.; The National Fire Protection Association, Boston, Mass.; the Section on Plastic and Reconstructive Surgery of The New York Academy of Medicine; and the Division of Accident Prevention of the U.S. Public Health Service, Washington, D.C. The conference was held in cooperation with the American Academy of Pediatrics, Evanston, Ill.; the American Public Health Association, New York, N. Y.; and the National Safety Council, Chicago, Ill.; and was supported by a grant from the U.S. Public Health Service.

# WHY ARE WE HERE?*

RICHARD A. PRINDLE

Assistant Surgeon General
Director, Bureau of Disease Prevention and Environmental Control
U.S. Public Health Service, Wash.ngton, D.C.

SINCE I am on the program to deliver what is known as a keynote address, I shall attempt to state where I think we are and where I hope we are going.

This *Conference on Burns and Flame-Retardant Fabrics* follows by about four years the *Textile Flammability Conference* held in Boston, October 2 and 3, 1962, and attended by many of you here today.

The Boston conference, to the best of my knowledge, was the first attempt by qualified representatives of industry, government, and the medical and public health professions to hold a frank and open discussion of this subject. The purpose of that conference was to define an extremely serious national health problem—namely, the problem of burns resulting from the ignition of clothing, or other material such as bedding, draperies, upholstery fabrics, and household furnishings.

The purpose of *this* conference is to develop a plan of action, using all present knowledge and resources to make flame-retardant fabrics more readily available to the public in the United States.

Simply stated, flame-retardant fabrics may be defined as materials that are so slow to burn that, if they are ignited, serious injury from burning will not result.

To begin with, we know that much of the everyday clothing worn in this country burns readily when ignited. I need not elaborate on the tremendous loss of life, the human suffering, the emotional shock, and the cost that result from such burns.

And even as we recognize the Boston conference as our first unified assault on this problem, we acknowledge, too, with appropriate appreciation, the incentive of the National Fire Protection Association in generating that meeting in collaboration with the U.S. Public Health

*Keynote address presented at the *Conference on Burns and Flame-Retardant Fabrics,* held at The New York Academy of Medicine, December 2 and 3, 1966. The conference was sponsored by: the New York and Brooklyn Trauma Committee of the American College of Surgeons, Chicago, Ill.; The National Fire Protection Association, Boston, Mass.; the Section on Plastic and Reconstructive Surgery of The New York Academy of Medicine; and the Division of Accident Prevention of the U.S. Public Health Service, Washington, D.C. The conference was held in cooperation with the American Academy of Pediatrics, Evanston, Ill.; the American Public Health Association, New York, N. Y.; and the National Safety Council, Chicago, Ill.; and supported by a grant from the U.S. Public Health Service.

Service. This was a bold and daring step to try to bring together in one joint meeting all the people and interests that needed to be unified, for it well might have resulted in complete fragmentation of the effort, since there was bound to be divergence of method and opinion. However, the need for unification was paramount.

Today the sponsors of the previous meeting acknowledge with gratitude the additional formal support given to the second conference by the New York and Brooklyn Trauma Committee, the American College of Surgeons, and The New York Academy of Medicine's Section on Plastic and Reconstructive Surgery.

In considering our mission here, let me discuss first the extent of the problem of burns from ignited clothing. Exact statistics are difficult to obtain, but our Division of Accident Prevention has made some determinations that clearly demonstrate the need for action.

Each year, many scores of thousands of persons in this country are burned in fabric fires. Add to this the tragic fact that most burns from ignited clothing occur among children and the elderly—the members of our society least able to defend themselves in such emergencies.

Little girls' dresses and nightwear, for example, can go up quickly in flames, and the amount of heat generated is sufficient to produce the most serious form of deep burning. A deep burn over a large area is the explanation for the severity of such cases. Here is an illustration of such a case from U.S. Public Health Service files:

A 2-year-old girl opened the oven door of a gas stove and used it to climb to the top of the stove in order to reach her pet bird, which was perched on top of the refrigerator. It is believed that she hit a burner knob while climbing up and ignited her quilted cotton housecoat and cotton flannel pajamas. Her mother was outdoors at the time.

Over 51 per cent of the child's body surface was burned. The burned area covered her back, a small section on the back of the head, the right front of the body, the front of the right leg, a small section of the left thigh, and most of the right arm and hand. Eleven skin grafts were necessary.

The child's mother blamed herself for the accident and developed a serious emotional problem. The child was hospitalized 97 days. The cost of her treatment—$12,460—was partially covered by private insurance but primarily by the state's Crippled Children's Services.

The proper treatment and care of a severely burned patient consumes an inordinate amount of professional attention. The patient needs surgeons, nurses, physiotherapists, dietitians, and laboratory specialists. He may require 30 to 50 pints of blood and many times as much nursing attention as most other patients.

To sum up: of all accident victims, those suffering from severe injuries from burns usually present the most difficult medical problems, and require the greatest amount of nursing and supportive care. There is, once again, the terrible emotional experience of the patients and their families, and the staggering expense. And a large number of these severe burns are associated with fires in clothing and other fabrics.

At this point, let me set forth some of the divergent opinions that, I am sure, are represented here and that doubtless will come into some sort of confrontation before we adjourn.

In the first place, we in the U.S. Public Health Service think that progress in the flame-retardant fabric field should be more effective and should move much more swiftly. In short, we submit that not enough of these fabrics are being made available to the consumer in the United States; and yet a manufacturer in this country now produces the fiber used to make garments that are sold for the protection of English children. For example, one child's night robe in England is made of a flame retardant, man-made fabric that has originated in the United States, and yet no such garment is sold in the United States for the protection of children here.

Is this situation circumstantial, or is it deliberate, or is it due to lethargy or, if you will pardon me for being so direct, is it simply a laissez-faire attitude carried to the highest degree?

Even the industrial interests involved in the various approaches to flame-retardant fabrics seem to be somewhat at variance on the question of why the United States consumer has only limited access, or is completely denied access, to the end product.

As to the individual fabrics, I am sure we can all agree that wool can be eliminated as a subject of contention. Wool fibers are comparatively flame-resistant in their natural state. Wool will ignite, but it will burn very slowly and the fire will usually go out by itself. Therefore, wool is not often found among the fibers worn by individuals severely burned by ignited clothing. Wool, however, is not the only fabric used today in the manufacture of clothing.

As to other fabrics with which we are familiar in the U.S. Public

Health Service: let me cite a number of conclusions based on evidence in our files.

Natural fibers of plant origin—that is to say, cotton and viscose rayon—tend to burn fairly quickly, but they can be treated with chemicals that make them flame-retardant. An exception here is a very sheer garment that does not possess enough body for the chemical additive without adversely affecting the feel or texture, or if you prefer, the "hand," as it is called in the industry.

Modacrylic fibers possess a quality not normally provided by other synthetics in that they are inherently flame-retardant. They do not support combustion when exposed to flame or heat. Other affirmative qualities of the modacrylic fibers must be known to most of you.

A new member of the nylon family does not support combustion. It was used in the space suits of the Mercury and Gemini astronauts and is part of the apparel of military flyers and fire fighters. All but one of the drivers in the Indianapolis 500 Race this past Memorial Day wore flame-retardant uniforms made from this material. We hope it will be available to the general public before too long, for it has potential uses as underwear, play clothing, children's sleepers, bathrobes, bedding, and other articles.

Glass textiles are fire-resistant for the life of the fabric and, although washable, need no special treatment or handling to maintain this characteristic.

Synthetic fibers cannot be treated to make them flame-retardant. However, it is possible to weave inherently flame-retardant modacrylic fibers with other synthetic or natural fibers, thus producing a fabric that will not easily support combustion. Our records indicate that the minimum amount of modacrylic fiber necessary in a blend with some other fibers to produce a satisfactory degree of flame retardancy is about 40 per cent.

All of these fibers and fabrics I have reviewed can be produced, are being produced, and are available in limited quantity for use in home furnishings and clothing.

To summarize: flame-retardant material in one form or another is available for almost all our fabric needs, not only for use by the military, by fire fighters, or by race drivers, but also for use by the private citizen. Even so, our technology can and should develop better and cheaper processes for producing flame-retardant clothing.

As a physician, as a public health officer, and as a citizen, I ask why all these materials are in such short supply—especially clothing and furnishings for the very young and very old people, who suffer the highest incidence of clothing burns?

The usual reasons given are these: flame-retardant fabric is naturally unattractive because it automatically identifies with tragedy. It must be sold like insurance—a thing that is good to have but that, it is hoped, one will never need. Fire resistance is said *not* to be a good selling point.

The argument also is made that flame-retardant items are too costly for acceptance by the consumer and that, in addition, the public does not like the feel of the product. It is said further that some chemically treated fabrics lose their fire-resistant qualities when laundered, and that their tear and rip strength is also adversely affected.

Some of these arguments, which once may have been valid, now may be without substance. Technology in the field is progressing. The ability of the consumer to be more discriminating in the market place is becoming more apparent.

For example: assume that bedsheets treated for fire resistance are 50 per cent more expensive than untreated sheets. If they contribute to the saving of a life, or to the prevention of accidental burn due to ignited bedding, and if this fact is properly advertised, would not large numbers of housewives buy them? And what about aggressively sales-minded hotel managers?

In spite of all our warnings, tens of thousands of people are going to smoke in bed or in an easy chair, and they are going to fall asleep and, with considerable frequency, they are going to start fires.

Let us look briefly at the case of a careless smoker—again, from a report from our files at the U.S. Public Health Service. A 59-year-old man burned himself while lighting a cigar. He dropped the match and ignited the top of his long cotton underwear. He died on the 66th day of hospitalization. As he was on social security, the County Welfare Department defrayed the cost of $14,348.

Even if the cost still is a deterrent, even if the texture seems overly stiff to some people for some uses, life-saving material should be made available to the general public. Let the housewife determine for herself what she wants for herself, for her family, or for her home and, *above all,* allow her the privilege of deciding whether she can afford to buy assured safety.

While I cannot pose as an economist or as a marketing analyst, am I naïve to ask about volume production, volume sales, and the corresponding lowering of retail prices? We paid $75 for one 10-cc. vial of penicillin in 1943. Today, through improved technology and volume production, 10 cc. of a vastly improved penicillin can be purchased for 17 cents.

Surely United States business imagination, ingenuity and, above all, sales ability can do better than merely say that "we cannot develop the volume because we do not have the product, and we can't distribute the product because we can't be sure of the volume."

It is my feeling that this conference will have to come to grips with some of these basic issues. Can the same society, the same combination of government, profession, and industry now preparing itself for a flight to the moon, retreat timidly from so heavy a responsibility? Can we continue to deny to the little girl playing near an open flame the same protection that is available to, and in some instances required of, race drivers, airmen, firemen, spacemen, and steelmen?

But let me go into the problem of accidental injury from fire as we have found it in the U.S. Public Health Service.

In 1961, a research project was conducted in cooperation with the Tennessee Department of Public Health. In the 308 records of burns studied, 105 patients suffered injuries because their clothing caught fire.

Another study involved the evaluation of flame-retardant fabrics in two nursing homes in Arkansas. In these homes, one half of the sheets, pillowcases, bathrobes, blankets, bedspreads, drawsheets, and other cotton clothing and fabric items were treated with a flame-retardant chemical called APO-THPC.*

The principal finding in that study—and I consider this to be most important—was that there was no problem of acceptability of the texture, odor, or other physical or esthetic properties of the treated fabric.

At the University of Michigan, the U.S. Public Health Service is sponsoring a study of injuries from burns to obtain information regarding the cause, cost, and treatment of burns. This program was initiated in 1964 and, to date, we have processed and analyzed approximately 600 burn cases from Ann Arbor, Mich., Cincinnati, Ohio, Richmond, Va., and Chicago, Ill.

*Tris (1-aziridinyl) phosphine oxide and tetrakis (hydroxymethyl) phosphonium chloride.

Of the cases of severe burns studied, about 40 per cent involved the ignition of clothing.

In Birmingham, Ala., the Public Health Service and the Jefferson County Health Department are conducting a retrospective study of patients who suffered burns. In the 1,395 cases analyzed, 179 injuries from burns were attributed to ignited clothing.

Further analysis indicates that fires from ignited clothing caused the more serious burns. Of the 179 clothing ignitions, *37 per cent* required skin grafts and extensive surgery. Only *6 per cent* of those whose clothing did not ignite required extensive surgery and hospitalization.

What are we going to do to end such fires? Do we need a law? Frankly, I hope not. Cooperation is preferable to coercion. It should nevertheless be pointed out that in Great Britain, since 1964, it has been illegal to sell inflammable nightdresses for children.

Our own Congress has become increasingly concerned with consumer problems and with health problems. The election just past may have changed some of the faces in Congress, but I can say with certainty that the current deep concern for the health of the people of the United States will not change within the most influential and powerful legislative body in the world.

Congress has expressed considerable interest in the problem under discussion. This past summer, Warren G. Magnuson of the State of Washington, chairman of the Senate Commerce Committee, announced that the Federal Trade Commission would undertake a study of the problem of the flammability of clothing. A U.S. Public Health Service team is providing much of the information for this study from cases of burns caused by ignited clothing in Denver, Colo.

Senator Magnuson and Paul Rand Dixon, chairman of the Federal Trade Commission, agree that the problem relating to the flammability of children's clothing is "indeed a serious one" because "in its present form the Flammable Fabrics Act contains no requirements that clothing be flameproofed or that flame spread rate must be minimal." This last is a direct quotation from Chairman Dixon.

To quote Mr. Dixon more fully, he said: "It is our intention to initiate a study of the problem of the flammability of clothing, particularly clothing for use by children. In the course of such study, we shall most likely work closely with the Public Health Service, Division of Accident Prevention of the Department of Health, Education, and

Welfare, and with the Department of Commerce."

One of the physicians advising the Senate Commerce Committee on the problem of flame-retardant fabrics was Dr. Abraham B. Bergman, director of outpatient services, Children's Orthopedic Hospital, Seattle. Dr. Bergman was invited to be with us today.

I shall not dwell further on this interest in our common problem except to offer one direct quotation from Senator Magnuson, who emphasized to Dr. Bergman and Chairman Dixon that the Senate Commerce Committee—here I quote directly—"wants to have every possible safeguard for children as well as adults included in provisions adopted to strengthen the Flammable Fabrics Act."

Further powerful evidence of congressional interest in the subject of our conference was the passage by the Senate of a bill to establish a National Commission on Hazardous Household Products. The work of this commission would have included investigation of the use of flame-retardant fabrics. The House did not agree to this proposal, but suggested that existing agencies in the executive branch could perform this necessary investigation and analysis.

Senator Maurine B. Neuberger of Oregon introduced an amendment to strengthen the Flammable Fabrics Act during the session of Congress just adjourned, and while this amendment made little actual progress on the Senate calendar, it did attract more than sporadic interest. Senator Neuberger will not be a member of the 90th Congress convening next year, since she did not seek reelection, but two cosponsors of the proposal, Senator Magnuson and Senator Thruston B. Morton of Kentucky, will return.

Two new subcommittees—both exclusively concerned with consumers—came into being during the closing session of this past Congress.

The chairman of the Senate Commerce Committee designated a standing Consumer Subcommittee, while the chairman of the House Government Operations Committee named a special Consumer Subcommittee.

And so 1967—like 1966—may well be, at least in this respect, the "Year of the Consumer."

Let me quote briefly from President Lyndon B. Johnson's message to Congress of last March 21, in the transmittal of his "Proposed Programs and Legislation to Further Protect the Consumer Interests."

The opening four paragraphs of this statement read:

"The consumer's interest is the American interest.

"In guarding it, in promoting it, we improve the lives of every man, woman, and child in our Nation.

"Consumers are all the people—the worker, the farmer, the businessman, and their families.

"Every domestic program of the Federal Government in a very real sense is directed toward the consumer."

But, again, I urge your consideration of 1967 as the "Year of the Consumer," and ask that we consider our responsibilities here and now with great care.

As part of that consideration, I urge that we all remember the temper of the people and of the Congress as reflected in recent legislation on the safety and efficiency of drugs, the adequacy of water, the control of air pollution, and on the safety of our automobiles.

Let me remind you also that, with presidential and congressional concurrence, the Public Health Service has been reorganized, given a fresh mandate, and has been instilled with new determination to protect the public against preventable disease and preventable injury.

Sometimes members of the public do not focus very sharply on what they expect from government and industry, but at other times they and their elected leaders do—very sharply. It is clear, for example, that a national mandate to move ahead in protecting the consumer has been given to government agencies in the last 2 years.

We in the Public Health Service hope very much that we shall all be able to avoid future situations like those that brought forth the air pollution and automobile safety laws, in which national legislation seemed to be the only way to accomplish improvements for the public benefit.

Accordingly I urge that this conference explore with courage and complete objectivity all facets of the subject matter covered by the definitive title, "Conference on Burns and Flame-Retardant Fabrics." This should not be a forum for failure, but a springboard for action.

I ask that you do *not* let this conference deteriorate into a high-level, professional debating society but, rather, that you bring forth constructive determinations for future action; for this is our shared responsibility to nearly 200 million fellow citizens who, too long, have gone without the full measure of protection that we are capable of bringing to them.

# PRESENT STATUS OF THE TREATMENT OF BURNS*

Curtis P. Artz and Dabney R. Yarbrough, III

Department of Surgery
Medical College of South Carolina
and the
Veterans Administration Hospital
Charleston, S. C.

## Significance

Burns today continue to constitute a major health hazard in the United States. A major burn is one of the most severe forms of trauma to which man is subject. An extensive burn may be disastrous medically, financially, and psychologically. Major disabilities, as the result of a severe burn, are common, and rehabilitation may be discouragingly difficult. A high degree of motivation on the part of the patient is required for successful restoration of the individual to a relatively normal, productive place in society.

The average number of injuries from burns per annum is 1,973,000, according to data from the National Health Survey. These data from the years 1957 to 1961 reveal approximately 937,000 activity-restricting injuries from burns, of which 268,000 were classed as bed-confining injuries.

The most common cause of fatal accidents among children and the elderly is fire or explosions, according to the 1962 survey by the Division of Vital Statistics of the U.S. Public Health Service, U.S. Department of Health, Education, and Welfare. Data from this source reveal 7,534 deaths for that year, with a further 849 deaths attributable to accidents caused by electric current. Fire and explosion of combustible materials in that year resulted in a death rate of 4.1 per 100,000 population. Fatal injuries involved 4,421 males and 3,293 females. Approximately 7.5 persons per 1,000 population receive injuries from burns

*Based on a paper presented at the *Conference on Burns and Flame-Retardant Fabrics,* held at The New York Academy of Medicine, December 2 and 3, 1966. The conference was sponsored by: the New York and Brooklyn Trauma Committee of the American College of Surgeons, Chicago, Ill.; The National Fire Protection Association, Boston, Mass.; the Section on Plastic and Reconstructive Surgery of The New York Academy of Medicine; and the Division of Accident Prevention of the U. S. Public Health Service, Washington, D. C. The conference was held in cooperation with the American Academy of Pediatrics, Evanston, Ill.; the American Public Health Association, New York, N. Y.; and the National Safety Council, Chicago, Ill.; and was supported by a grant from the U. S. Public Health Service.

TABLE I.—INJURIES FROM BURNS REPORTED IN THE UNITED STATES IN 1962; ANALYSIS BY AGE

| | | | |
|---|---|---|---|
| Under 1 year | 264 | 35 to 44 years | 717 |
| 1 to 4 years | 1,082 | 45 to 54 years | 937 |
| 4 to 14 years | 726 | 55 to 64 years | 858 |
| 15 to 24 years | 318 | 65 to 74 years | 966 |
| 25 to 34 years | 505 | 75 years and over | 1,151 |

TABLE II.—REGIONAL NUMBER OF DEATHS AND RATES DUE TO BURNS REPORTED IN THE UNITED STATES IN 1962

| *Area* | *Deaths* | *Deaths per 100,000 population* |
|---|---|---|
| New England | 394 | 3.7 |
| Middle Atlantic | 1,144 | 3.3 |
| East North Central | 1,174 | 3.2 |
| West North Central | 543 | 3.5 |
| South Atlantic | 1,509 | 5.8 |
| East South Central | 901 | 7.5 |
| West South Central | 1,105 | 6.5 |
| Mountain | 225 | 3.3 |
| Pacific | 650 | 3.1 |

annually. Material from the same source reveals the breakdown by age of injuries from burns shown in Table I.

Twenty-nine per cent of the annual deaths from injuries from burns occur in children less than 15 years old. Twenty-eight per cent of deaths from burns and explosions occur in persons 65 and older. A regional preponderance is also noted with a higher rate of deaths resulting from injuries from burns occurring in the southern part of the United States. The regional number of deaths and rates due to burns are shown in Table II.

Moyer states that in 1940, accidents destroyed 17.04 years of human life for every 1,000 inhabitants of the United States. Only 15.5 years of life were destroyed by cancer per 1,000 population during that same year. He estimates that more than 6,000 hospital beds are occupied the year around by patients suffering from burns.

It is clear from the above that burns and related injuries exact a significant yearly toll of life and working years. This loss of working years is increased by the frequency of major disabilities resulting from severe injuries from burns. The loss of working years is further increased in relation to other major health hazards (heart disease, stroke, and cancer) because of the preponderance of injuries sustained by the younger age groups.

## Causes of Burns

The common cause of injury from a burn in the 0- to 3-year age group is scalds.[7] These injuries are usually the result of the overturning of containers of hot liquids by the inquisitive child and of bathtub accidents. In the 3- to 15-year age group, burns from flames predominate in the category of major injury from a burn, usually as a result of misuse of fire and matches. Gas stoves, open heaters, and space heaters also account for a high percentage of burns in this age group. In adults, burns are commonly the result of home and industrial accidents. Burns from flames resulting from the ignition of clothing generally produce the more extensive injuries. In the younger age groups, females are particularly prone to this extensive injury because of the nature and characteristics of their clothing.[5]

Burns in military personnel are quite common, and they result from a variety of causes. Burns due to flame throwers, vesicant gases, phosphorus, and aviation fuel account for a high percentage of burns in the military. These burns obviously are usually very extensive, and they result in relatively high mortality.

## Severity

Burns are usually classified etiologically as thermal (flame or scald), chemical, electrical, and radiation-induced. Thermal burns constitute the majority, while chemical, electrical, and radiation burns are usually the result of occupational hazards.[4] The severity of an injury from a burn is often related to the etiology; burns from flames are commonly more extensive.

The severity of an injury from burning with implied prognosis is generally judged by two criteria: extent and depth. The depth of a burn is usually categorized as first, second, or third degree. Any given injury from a burn will usually exhibit all three degrees of depth in varying proportion.

First-degree burns involve destruction of the outer layers of epidermis only. They are characterized by erythema and small, superficial blisters. Pain is usually minimal and of a burning nature. Edema is also minimal. This degree of burn is commonly seen with sunburn and with a brief flash exposure to flame. Pain usually subsides rapidly (in 24 to 48 hours), and healing takes place uneventfully in 3 to 6 days. Healing is usually associated with peeling of the devitalized superficial epidermis. Infection is not a problem in this superficial injury.[8]

A second-degree burn is a deeper injury associated with destruction of all the epidermis and much of the corium. Physical characteristics of second-degree burns include erythema, marked subcutaneous edema, and extensive fluid-filled blisters. Pain, tenderness, and sensitivity to pinprick are prominent in the early stages. The surface of the second-degree burn is visibly moist in contrast to the dry surface of the third-degree burn. A tough, brownish crust forms in 24 to 48 hours. Barring infection, healing should take place uneventfully beneath the crust in 14 to 21 days. Near the time of complete healing, the crust will peel away, revealing the pink, newly regenerated epithelium beneath. Serious infection is unusual in the properly managed second-degree burn, but may occur and may produce disastrous results. Conversion of second-degree burn to full-thickness injury, as well as invasive sepsis, may occur with severe infection. Collectively, first- and second-degree burns constitute a partial-thickness injury.

Third-degree burns or full-thickness burns are the most severe form of injury from burning. The entire dermis and corium, down to subcutaneous fat, are destroyed by coagulation necrosis. The surface of the third-degree burn presents a dry, insensitive, pearly white, or charred appearance. As all cutaneous nerve endings are destroyed, pain is not a prominent feature of this depth of injury from burning. Thrombosis and coagulation of blood in superficial vessels occur, and these appear as fine brown lines on the surface. Increased capillary permeability with subsequent edema is usually more prominent than in second-degree burns. A tough, brownish eschar forms over the burned surface in 48 to 72 hours. Over the succeeding 3 to 4 weeks, autolysis occurs beneath the eschar, resulting in separation. This process is usually accompanied by suppuration. In most cases, separation of the eschar will reveal a highly vascular bed of newly formed granulation tissue. Wound healing may then be completed by debridement of all eschar and the application of a split-thickness skin graft to cover the wound. In the absence of grafting at this stage, healing occurs slowly by the conversion of granulation tissue to excessive amounts of scar tissue with resulting severe contractures.[3]

The extent of an injury from burning is usually expressed as a percentage of total body surface area. Several different methods of assessing the percentage of body surface area involved by injury from burning are available to the physician.[6] The most accurate of these methods is the Lund and Browder chart.[9] This chart compensates for changes in the relative percentages of body surface area occurring from infancy through adulthood.

Another popular method for rapidly estimating extent of burn is the *Rule of Nines.* This rule, originally devised by Pulaski and Tennison, divides the body surface into 9 per cent areas or multiples of them. The rule states that the head and neck, and each upper extremity constitute 9 per cent of the total body surface area. The anterior trunk, posterior trunk, and each lower extremity constitute 18 per cent ($2 \times 9$) divisions of the body surface area while the perineum constitutes 1 per cent. This easily remembered rule is a good rough guide to the extent of a burn, but is not nearly so accurate as the Lund and Browder chart.

Minor burns include those partial-thickness burns that involve not more than 10 per cent of the body surface area. Full-thickness burns involving no more than 3 per cent of total body surface area and not involving certain critical areas (face and neck, joints, hands and perineum) are generally considered minor.

## Treatment of Burns

First aid in burns should be directed initially toward extinguishing flaming clothing. A person whose clothes are on fire should not run, as this only fans the flames and increases the severity of the burn. He should not remain standing, as this position may cause him to inhale the flames and smoke, or cause the hair to be ignited. Falling to the floor and rolling in a rug or blanket may put out the fire. Smothering the flames in any expeditious manner is desirable. Coats, towels, or bed clothing may be used. Water, if readily available in sufficient quantity, is ideal. Unidentified liquids should never be used to extinguish flames. Tragic accidents have occurred when buckets of kerosene, gasoline, or other flammable liquids, thought to be water, have been thrown on a person whose clothes were afire. Dirt and sand may be used to extinguish flames if no other suitable material is available.

Application of cold water or towels soaked in ice water will bring striking immediate relief of pain. Cold may have some value in arresting the effect of heat on tissues if used immediately. The application of cold by any convenient method immediately after the burn is the best first-aid measure known.

The wound from burning should be covered as soon as feasible. This minimizes contamination of the wound and decreases pain by preventing air from coming into contact with the injured surface. Any clean, dry cloth may serve as an effective emergency dressing. Salves, ointments, and materials other than soap or clean water should not be applied to the wound. Stimulants should be avoided. If medical care is available within several hours, oral intake should be curtailed. In the rare situation of mass casualties dilute solutions of salt and bicarbonate by mouth may be indicated. Any burn of a critical area, or involving more than 1 or 2 per cent of the body area, should be seen and treated by a physician.[2]

Chemical burns resulting from contact with acid or alkali should be irrigated immediately with large quantities of water. Any clothing soaked with the injurious agent should be removed. If a large quantity of chemical burning agent has come into contact with the skin, the patient should get into a bathtub or under a shower as soon as possible. The patient suffering respiratory arrest from the inhalation of smoke should receive artificial respiration by positive pressure, using the mouth-to-mouth technique.

If the wound from burning is minor it should be cleansed with soap and water and bandaged, using some type of lubricated gauze or anesthetic ointment. Larger burns or burns in the critical areas previously cited should be treated in a physician's office or a hospital emergency room. The patient may be taken to the physician at a normal and comfortable rate of speed with the exception of cases in which respiratory difficulty is a problem. In this context, it is well to note that burned patients being transferred from one hospital to another should not be transferred under emergency conditions in most cases. It is the referring physician's responsibility to see that the patient arrives at his destination in optimal condition. This should include an adequate airway, a stable route of intravenous administration (preferably in the form of a large-bore intravenous cannula), maintenance of intravenous fluid therapy en route, application of appropriate dressings and administration of tetanus prophylaxis. Gastric decompression by nasogastric tube should be instituted if indicated, and an indwelling urinary catheter inserted if possible. Intravenous narcotics in appropriate dosages should be given if necessary. A note citing the treatment given and any other pertinent information should be sent to the receiving hospital.

Major burns should always be treated in a hospital. The operating room or a specially equipped dressing room for patients suffering from burns, if available, is preferable for initial care. As in all massive traumatic injuries, attention should be directed first toward insuring an adequate airway. A large-bore venous cannula should then be inserted for the administration of colloid and electrolyte solutions in appropriate amounts and at proper rates of infusion. At this time, blood samples can be drawn for hematologic and chemical studies, as well as typing and cross-matching. Intravenous narcotics can be given at this point if required. Estimation of fluid requirements and rates of infusion can be made from several convenient formulas including the Brooke and the Evans. Necessary alterations in rate and quantity of fluid infused can be made according to the patient's response. An indwelling urinary catheter should then be put in place for the hourly monitoring of urinary output.

At this point it is well to complete the medical history and physical examination. Particular attention should be paid to the method of injury, allergies, status of tetanus immunization, present medications, and previous illnesses.

Appropriate tetanus prophylaxis should now be given and the wounds from burning cleansed with detergent, debrided, and dressed. Wounds may be managed subsequently by the open or closed method or by a combination of both methods. In general, wounds of the face and perineum are best managed by the open technique, while circumferential wounds and burns of the hands, feet, and joints are best managed by the closed method. The use of topical germicidal solutions and antibiotics, such as dilute solutions of silver nitrate and Sulfamylon, have been used extensively in recent years and show promise.

Management of a wound from a burn over the 3 to 4 weeks following injury should be directed toward early removal of eschar and closure of the wound by grafting. This should include frequent dressing changes, cleansing and debridement, and homografting where feasible. If homografts are available, they should be removed and fresh homograft applied at intervals no greater than 5 days. This technique results in many of the benefits of complete closure of a wound, maintains a clean bed of granulation tissue for autografting as soon as feasible, and obviates the prolonged period of rejection of homograft. A program of active physical and occupational therapy should be started as early as possible.

## Complications

Early complications in burns (within the first 72 hours) are usually related to respiratory tract damage and difficulties in resuscitation from shock.[10] Occasionally, multiple injuries may present complications as seen in victims of explosions and aircraft accidents.

Complications in the respiratory tract may be either obstructive or irritative. Obstruction of the upper respiratory tract is relatively uncommon, but it may result from massive edema of the neck and of oropharyngeal and laryngeal soft tissues after major burns of the head and neck. Obstructive problems are obviously best handled by prompt tracheostomy.

Inhalation of smoke and other irritating products of combustion can result in atelectasis, severe bronchospasm, and pneumonitis. Inadequate oxygenation is the inevitable result. Problems of this nature may require tracheostomy, intermittent positive pressure breathing, expectorants, maintenance of hydration with careful avoidance of fluid overload, bronchodilating drugs, and appropriate antibiotics.

The most common complications associated with resuscitation from shock are acute renal insufficiency resulting from poor renal perfusion and red cell hemolysis, and pulmonary edema as a result of fluid overload. Both of these complications should be rare in the patient whose resuscitation is monitored carefully by measurements of central venous pressure and hourly urinary output.

Complications that occur later in the treatment of the burned patient include sepsis in the wound, the most feared of all complications. Sepsis in a wound from burning is presently the single greatest cause of mortality in the burned patient.[11] The most common bacteriologic offenders are staphylococcus and pseudomonas.

Infections of the genitourinary tract and thromboembolism are also common late complications. Acute gastroduodenal ulceration with hemorrhage or perforation may occur in as many as 20 per cent of patients with major burns, and may require operation.[12]

Other late complications are related chiefly to scarring and prolonged immobilization, and they may include calculi, osteoporosis, calcification in and about joints with limitation of range of motion, atrophy and fibrosis of muscle from disease, contractures of scar tissues, and cosmetic deformities. Complications due to poor maintenance of nutrition are also quite common.

## *REFERENCES*


1. Artz, C. P. and Hardy, J. D. *Complications in Surgery and Their Management.* Philadelphia, Saunders, 1961.
2. Artz, C P. and Larson, D. L. Treatment ot burns, *Curr. Probl. Surg. 1*:40, 1965.
3. Artz, C. P. Thermal and radiation injuries, ch. 8 in: *Christopher's Textbook of Surgery,* L. Davis, ed., 8th ed., Philadelphia, Saunders, 1964.
4. Artz, C. P. and Reiss, E. *Treatment of Burns.* Philadelphia, Saunders, 1957.
5. Artz, C. P. Unpublished data.
6. Berkow, S. A. Method of estimating the extensiveness of lesions (burns and scalds) based on surface area proportions, *Arch. Surg. 8*:138, 1924.
7. Bleck, E. E. Causes of burns in children, *J.A.M.A. 158*:100, 1955.
8. Jackson, D. Diagnosis of the depth of burning, *Brit. J. Surg. 40*:588, 1953.
9. Lund, C. C. and Browder, N.C. Estimation of areas of burns, *Surg. Gynec. Obst. 79*:352, 1944.
10. Moncrief, J. A. Complications of burns, *Ann. Surg. 147*:433, 1958.
11. Order, S. E. and Moncrief, J. A. *The Burn Wound.* Springfield, Ill., Thomas, 1965.
12. Teplitz, C. and Moncrief, J. A. *Observations on the pathology and pathogenesis of gastroduodenal ulcerations in burns.* Annual Research Progress Report, U.S. Army Surgical Research Unit, Brooke Army Medical Center, Ft. Sam Houston, Texas, 1963.

# STATISTICS AND EPIDEMIOLOGY OF BURNS*

ALBERT P. ISKRANT

Chief, Epidemiology and Surveillance Branch
Division of Accident Prevention
U.S. Public Health Service
Arlington, Va.

ACCIDENTS caused by fire and explosion are the second leading cause of all nontransportation deaths in the United States (8,000 annually), a rate of 4 per 100,000 population. They are the leading cause of death from nontransportation accidents for age groups 1 to 4 years old and the second leading cause for persons 5 to 14 and 45 and over. Generally, death rates for accidents from this cause are higher for nonwhites than whites, and higher for males than females (Figure 1). More than 80 per cent of the deaths occur in the home (Figure 2); more than half from November through March. Geographically, the highest accidental death rate from fire and explosion occurs in the South and Southwest (Figure 3). Nonmetropolitan areas have higher death rates than metropolitan areas, possibly reflecting a lack of fire departments, local rather than central heating, and a shortage of emergency medical services in these areas.

While death rates from fire and explosion are highest for children 1 to 4 and persons 65 and over, the injury rates are lowest for these age groups. The National Health Survey estimates that 260,000 persons are injured each year from this cause, a rate of 1.5 per 1,000. Persons in the 15- to 24-year group have the highest injury rate, and the male rate is higher than the female (Figure 4). About 35 per cent of the injuries from fire and explosion occur in the home, and about 40 per cent are injuries sustained at work (Figure 5).

Improper use of a petroleum product to start a fire is the leading

*Based on a paper presented at the *Conference on Burns and Flame-Retardant Fabrics,* held at The New York Academy of Medicine, December 2 and 3, 1966. The conference was sponsored by: the New York and Brooklyn Trauma Committee of the American College of Surgeons, Chicago, Ill.; The National Fire Protection Association, Boston, Mass.; the Section on Plastic and Reconstructive Surgery of The New York Academy of Medicine; and the Division of Accident Prevention of the U. S. Public Health Service, Washington, D. C. The conference was held in cooperation with the American Academy of Pediatrics, Evanston, Ill.; the American Public Health Association, New York, N. Y.; and the National Safety Council, Chicago, Ill.; and was supported by a grant from the U. S. Public Health Service.

Since this conference was held the Division of Accident Prevention has become the Injury Control Program, National Center for Urban and Industrial Health.

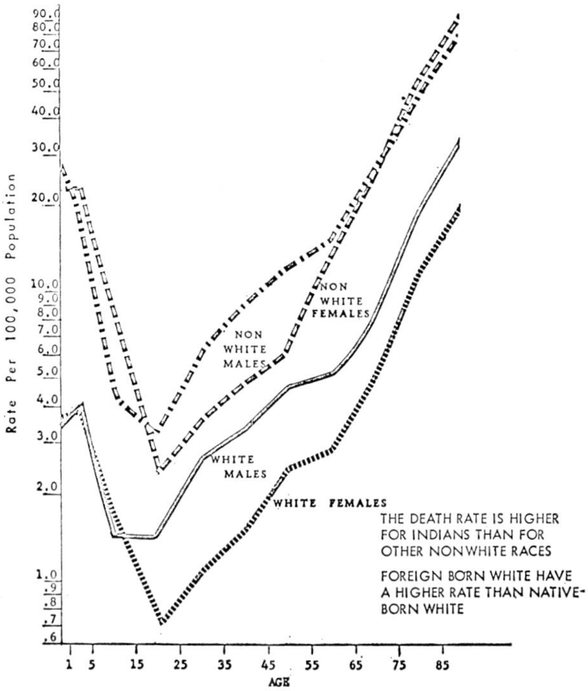


Fig. 1. Annual death rates from fire and explosion by age, color, and sex for the United States, 1959-1961.

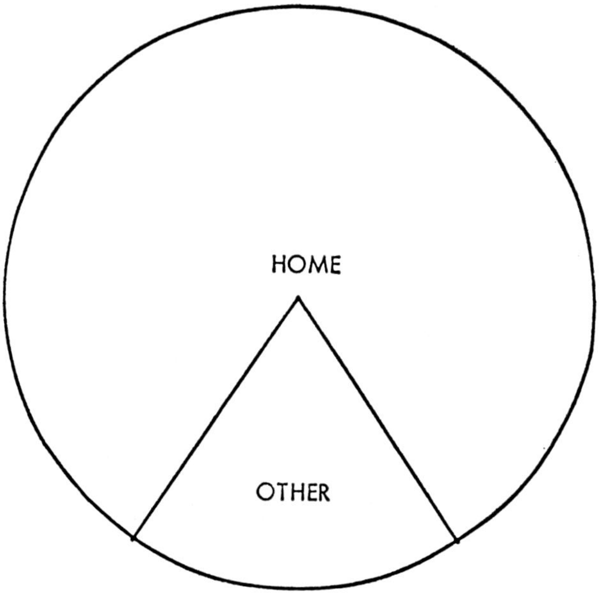


Fig. 2. Accidental deaths from fire and explosion by place of occurrence. Fatalities in the home comprise more than 80 per cent of all deaths from fire and explosion; they total 7,500 per year. Burns from hot substances cause another 400 deaths per year.

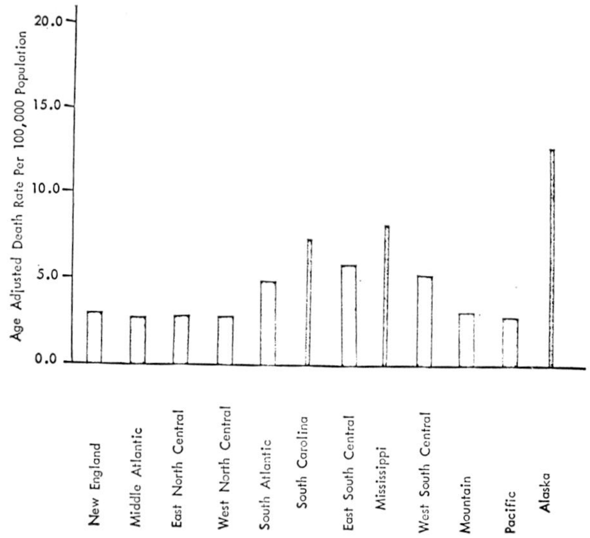


Fig. 3. Death rates for fire and explosion vary by state and geographic region. The South and Southwest have the highest rates for the country; Alaska, Mississippi, and South Carolina have the highest rate for states.

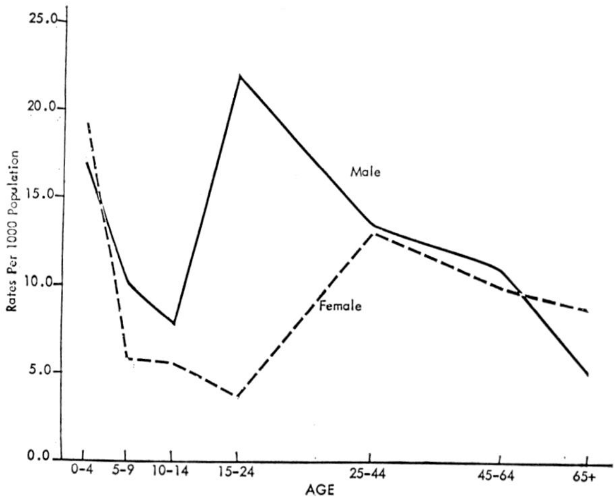


Fig. 4. Injury rates for all burns.

cause of conflagrations in the home that result in deaths and injuries to children; however, faulty wiring or fuses and defective stoves or flues are also contributing factors. More than one half of the injuries received by children in conflagrations in the home occur while they are alone in the dwelling; in many instances, the child has been injured in attempting to maintain a fire by using a petroleum product.

Of the estimated 2 million persons burned from all causes each year (seriously enough to require medical attention or to restrict their usual activity for a day or more), about 100,000 require hospitalization.

Burns caused by hot substances, corrosive substances, steam, or open flame account for only about 400 deaths per year and, again, are essentially a problem of preschool children and elderly persons. Rates are somewhat higher for nonwhite than white, and about three fourths of them occur in the home. More than 1.3 million persons are injured each year from contact with hot objects or open flame, a rate of 7.5 per 1,000. The rate of injury is higher for those with incomes under $4,000 and is higher in urban than rural areas. Burns from contact with open flames are more common in the South, and higher for females than males. Injuries and deaths from these causes occur approximately 75 per cent of the time in the home (Figure 6). The rate for burns in the home is much higher for children than for older groups, and is about twice as high for females as males.

Although burns are universal, the type of accident causing the burn varies with age, sex, culture, geographic location, weather, and the like. Burns from heating sources frequently involve burns from flame in open fireplaces and stoves in parts of the South, in floor grills in the West and in other parts of the United States, and space heaters in many rural and poorer urban areas. The problem of burns from hot water sustained by little children and elderly persons involves accidentally turning on showers and taps in bathtubs in some cultures, and falling into tubs of hot water in others. Other common causes of burns, also varying with culture and environment, include cook stoves, skillets (especially when they contain hot grease), electric appliances (including cords), electric wall sockets, trash burning, misuse of petroleum products, and matches.

A major problem involves the ignition of clothing, a particular problem of girls, especially in conjunction with open fires or flame. However, the ignition of clothing is common to both sexes, all ages,

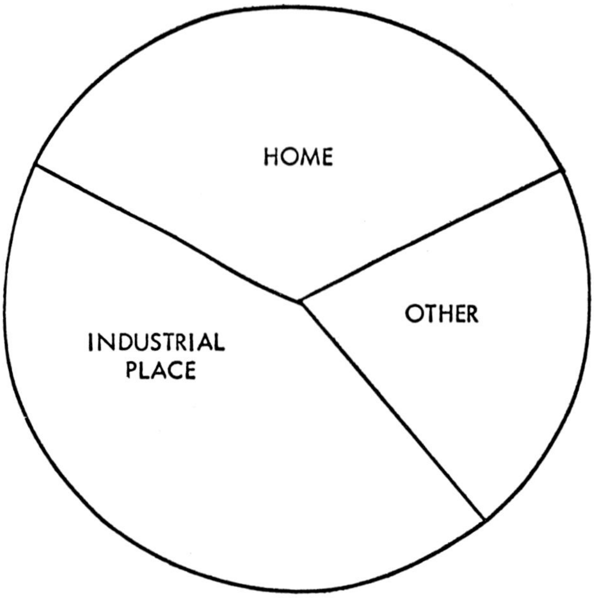


Fig. 5. Injuries from fire and explosion by place of occurrence. A total of 260,000 persons are injured each year by fires and explosions.

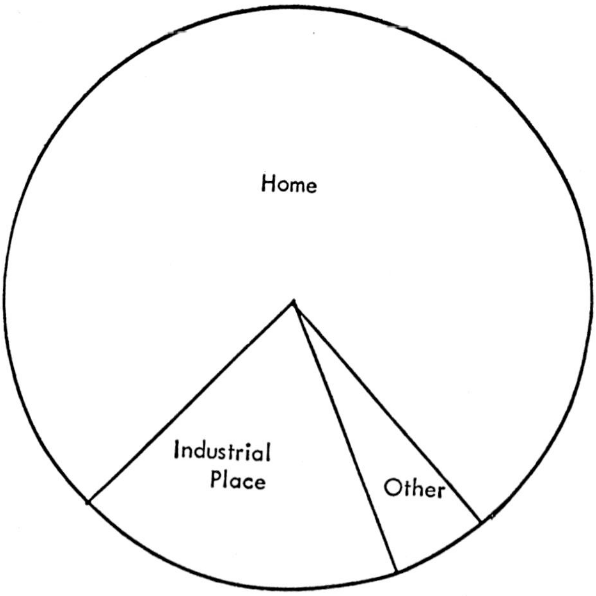


Fig. 6. Injuries from contacts with a hot substance or an open flame by place of occurrence. A total of 1.3 million persons are injured each year by such contacts. More than 75 per cent of such injuries occur in the home. An additional 400,000 persons suffer burns from other sources.

and in accidents that occur in both the home and at work.

Following is a description of some of the factors involved in injuries from burns affecting different age groups.

## Infants

Infants (age 1 and under) frequently are burned from climbing into containers of water left on floors, from being placed in extremely hot bath water, or from turning on hot water taps when left unattended while being bathed. Infants in the crawling stages suffer burns to hands, buttocks, and lower extremities from hot floor grates, or they are burned while using hot stoves and space heaters for support. Crawling children pull on cords of electric appliances, toppling over coffee pots, frying pans, irons, vaporizers, etc. This appears to be a major problem with infants, and they are burned most often from the contents of the electric appliance, i.e., hot coffee in coffee pots and water vaporizers rather than from the appliance itself. It matters little whether the child is walking, crawling, in a stroller, or in his mother's arms, the child still manages to grasp cords. Parents drink hot beverages while holding infants who get these liquids spilled on them or who pull on cups that contain them. Parents also frequently drop ashes from their lighted cigarettes on the children, or even allow them to come into contact with the burning tips.

Parents who are "safety conscious" may pull the cord from the appliance, but leave it plugged into the socket. Infants no longer can pull over the hot liquid or appliance, but can and do put these live cords in their mouths, suffering burns, and infants in their teething stage chew on extension cords or put the coupling into their mouths.

## Preschool Children

Burns to the preschool child (ages 1 to 5) involve many of the same agents of burning common to infants, but often the activity that is engaged in changes. For instance, these children usually fall onto floor grates, play on them, or back into space heaters, trip over cords of electric appliances (although from ages 1 to 3 they still seem to pull these cords), start to climb on stoves to reach cupboards, etc., or are burned while watching trash fires. Little girls' dresses ignite from sparks from trash fires, from the open flames of stoves, from unscreened fireplaces, or from contact with pilot lights of space heaters.

Perhaps these sources constitute the greatest single hazard for burns sustained by girls.

The preschool child frequently sticks any small metal object, particularly bobbypins, into wall sockets. Preschool children fall into containers of hot water left on floors, as do infants; play with taps, thereby turning on hot water; or jump into or fall into baths being drawn for other family members.

The misuse of matches is a serious problem with the preschool child, and improperly stored matches are readily available to the curious child, who plays with matches near paper and trash or often in combination with flammable liquids stored under the sink, in the garage, or in the basement. Matches and the misuse of flammable liquids are common causes of burns to boys, more so than to girls.

While infants pull on tablecloths, spilling hot liquids, foods, etc., onto themselves and have hot ashes and cigarettes dropped on them, the preschool child reaches and grabs for extended handles of cooking utensils such as pots and pans, cups containing hot beverages, and runs into lit cigarettes.

## Schoolchildren (6 to 17)

The problem of trash fires varies in different cultures from one age group and from one sex to another. Young schoolchildren (ages 6 to 10) are primarily burned around fires while watching them. Older schoolchildren may be given the task of starting and maintaining trash fires. However, in some cultures and in some areas of the country, these chores are assigned to younger children, as the male parent may be absent from home, the parents may be occupied with other chores, and some children, under such circumstances, may participate to a greater degree in home maintenance.

Flammable liquids used to aid or boost fires in cooking or heating stoves and trash fires contribute to the problem of burns in schoolchildren. The misuse of flammable liquids is more common in Southern areas because of the lack of central heating. Antiquated cooking stoves that require flammable liquids are also common in this area.

The problem of floor grates and space heaters also affects this age group. At the start of the heating season many forget about the high temperature of the floor furnace grates, and they are burned while walking barefoot over them. As in the case of preschool children, falling into and backing into space heaters is a problem, and frequently clothing is ignited.

Children going through puberty frequently suffer from skin conditions and, because they are more conscious of their appearance at this age, they use sun lamps. Often they are burned from prolonged exposure or burn their eyes when not using protective glasses.

When young girls start taking a more active role in the kitchen, they are victims of burns from grease, backflash and explosions when lighting the pilot lights of ovens, catch their loose clothing on open flames of stoves, and suffer burns from hot cooking utensils. Young girls also frequently ignite their clothing when warming themselves by heaters using wood, coal, or other fuel.

Another problem of schoolchildren, primarily boys aged 6 to 10, involves experimenting with matches and flammable liquids to build fires and "shooting" match guns made with rubber bands, while older boys more frequently are burned from fireworks and chemistry sets.

### Adults (18 to 64)

Because the kitchen is her domain, a woman is more frequently the victim of burns involving activities in the kitchen. Very often women are burned while lighting the ovens of stoves. Gas is turned on and the temperatures set high, allowing gas to accumulate and, when a match is lit, an explosion or backflash occurs. Often pilot lights go out, again accumulating gas, and when this is coupled with lack of ventilation, serious explosions can result even from a lit match, cigarette, or any source of flame. Faulty stoves, lack of knowledge or experience in operating procedures, or carelessness are the main causes of these explosions.

Burns caused by cooking utensils such as pots and pans are common and frequently involve hot handles, pouring grease from skillets with no pouring spout, and splattering grease. Often grease in skillets catches fire; and in an attempt to extinguish the flame by throwing the pan in the sink or out the door, more serious burns result. Pressure cookers cause steam burns when tops are removed too soon.

Many common household cleaning products can cause burns that, if not immediately treated, can cause infections. Lye, although it has been largely replaced by more modern cleaning agents, is still found in many homes—mainly in those of lower socioeconomic groups—and it is frequently a cause of burns according to more recent statistics.

Men are more frequently burned by backflash and explosion while attempting to light pilots of hot water heaters, furnaces, space heaters, and from using flammable liquids to start or boost fires in heating or cooking sources or while burning trash. Furnace explosions generally involve converted units or lack of knowledge or absence of directions regarding lighting and operating procedures. In some cases where directions are available, the lighting is poor or the directions are located in an inaccessible area.

Ignition from a carburetor and contact with hot radiator caps or hot car manifolds are but a few of the more common ways men get burned while working on cars. During the dismantling of junked cars, often sparks from acetylene torches ignite gas vapors in empty gas tanks. Such sparks can cause ignition when flammable liquids are spilled on clothing. Welding operations in conjunction with flammable liquids often result in serious burns; however, arc welders more frequently cause burns to the eye because of lack of protective goggles.

Sun lamps continue to be a source of burns to young adults. Older adults frequently sustain burns from sun lamps when using them for therapeutic reasons. This is also true for heating pads and hot-water bottles—though it is more of a problem to the elderly.

Smoking in bed and in overstuffed furniture begins to be a problem with older adults, particularly when combined with adverse physical conditions, drinking, or the use of drugs.

## Elderly (65 and Over)

Elderly people, who often live alone, are more susceptible to serious injuries of all types. Many are recluses from society because they have lost their mates or are separated from their families. Some of these elderly people are approaching senility, have delayed motor reflexes, or have suffered strokes and do not respond well to emergency situations.

Hot-water burns, a major problem for infants, are also a major problem for the elderly, who enter tubs of hot water and are unable to emerge, or they may have sensory deficiencies and do not realize that the bath water is too hot. Hot-water bottles that leak or are left on too long are also a problem to the elderly.

Smoking in bed and in overstuffed furniture is another major problem with the elderly, and very often the burns they receive under such circumstances are fatal. While the elderly also receive burns from sources common to other age groups, burns from heating pads are a particular problem. Elderly people use heating pads for therapeutic reasons, for example to stimulate poor circulation; and in so doing the heating pad is often set too high, and these patients, because of sensory deficiencies, do not realize that they are being burned.

People in this age group, like infants, have less resistance to injuries, and they suffer more serious burns that often result in death.

## Clothing Ignition

As already discussed, many sources of injury from burns are common to all ages and both sexes, but are *more* common to particular age groups or to either sex. Clothing ignition is common to both sexes, all ages, and in both home and work accidents. Burns are generally more serious when clothing is ignited. The amount of heat generated by the burning of any ordinary clothing fabric is sufficient to produce the most serious form of deep burning. Deep burns over large areas explain the clinical severity, prolonged hospitalization, and extremely high cost of treatment of such burns. However, in burns from scalding, where clothing does not ignite, it may, depending upon the fabric, protect the victim.

Ignition of clothing frequently occurs when flammable liquids are spilled and then ignited when close to the pilot lights of furnaces, to hot-water heaters, and to space heaters. This often happens to children while they are playing with improperly stored flammable liquids, and to both men and women who use these products for cleaning purposes.

*Note.* The illustrations accompanying this article were supplied by the Division of Accident Prevention, U. S. Public Health Service, and are reproduced by permission.

# SURVEY OF FATAL CLOTHING FIRES*

Ernest E. Juillerat, Jr.

Manager, Fire Record Department
National Fire Protection Association
Boston, Mass.

The National Fire Protection Association has collected statistics annually on fires that kill three or more persons. We know that these fires occur mostly in dwellings, and that they account for about 10 per cent of the annual death toll from fires. This year we decided to study the circumstances surrounding the one- or two-fatality fire, with special interest in the clothing fire. We began the survey February 1, 1966.

The several hundred fatalities reported in these few months will not seem a large number compared to the more than 2 million injuries from burns that occur in the United States each year. However, it is a significant number if one remembers that this particular survey involves only the fatal fires. We plan to continue this survey through 1967; by then we expect to have more than 2,000 cases on record.

Unfortunately, first notification of a fire fatality does not come to us until one to four weeks after the incident. We then send a questionnaire to the fire chief, coroner, police chief, or other person who conducted the investigation. Response to the questionnaires has been somewhat better than expected, but the portion of the questionnaire that deals with the details of the victim's clothing was in many cases left blank. This is because the investigating officer rarely notices these details; he is interested mainly in the cause of the fire and whether death was accidental or otherwise.

The two major considerations in this preliminary analysis of the survey are the single-fatality clothing fire and the single-fatality nonclothing fire. Under these two major headings, the data were tabu-

*Based on a paper presented at the *Conference on Burns and Flame-Retardant Fabrics,* held at The New York Academy of Medicine, December 2 and 3, 1966. The conference was sponsored by: the New York and Brooklyn Trauma Committee of the American College of Surgeons, Chicago, Ill.; The National Fire Protection Association, Boston, Mass.; the Section on Plastic and Reconstructive Surgery of The New York Academy of Medicine; and the Division of Accident Prevention of the U.S. Public Health Service, Washington, D.C. The conference was held in cooperation with the American Academy of Pediatrics, Evanston, Ill.; the American Public Health Association, New York, N. Y.; and the National Safety Council, Chicago, Ill.; and was supported by a grant from the U.S. Public Health Service.

lated to show, under various age groups, the sex of the victim, the cause of death, the occupancy in which the fire occurred, and any hindrance or physical or mental handicap that contributed to the victim's inability to escape. Fires classified as clothing fires were also tabulated to show the type of clothing worn by the victim, the type of fabric, and whether a flammable liquid spilled on the clothing was a factor.

By way of definition, we call a clothing fire one in which the destructive, or unfriendly, fire begins with the ignition of the victim's clothing: the clothing is ignited by a cigarette, by burning rubbish, by a cook stove, etc. The nonclothing fire is one in which the destructive, or unfriendly, ignition begins elsewhere, and the victim is unable to escape for one reason or another. These fires would include those in which the victim's cigarette ignites the bedding when he falls asleep, a handicapped person is unable to leave a burning apartment, etc.

The following is a summary of the tabulation of the first 650 one- and two-fatality reports received in the survey. Of the 650 victims, 6 were firemen on duty, 517 were civilians who died in nonclothing fires, and 127 were civilians who died in clothing fires. The clothing fires, therefore, caused little more than one fifth of the fatalities in the one- and two-fatality fire grouping. All the clothing fires were single-fatality fires. From these figures one can reasonably estimate that 2,100 to 2,200 deaths are caused by clothing fires annually.

Clothing fires struck the very young and the very old. Almost three times as many deaths occurred in the 0- to 5-year age group as in any other 5-year age group up to age 60. Past age 60, the number of incidents began to rise sharply, and the past-70 age group exceeded the 0-to-5 age group in number of clothing fire deaths.

The nonclothing fires took many more lives in the 0-to-5 age group: 4 times as many as any 5-year group from age 6 through age 40, and 3 times as many as the 5-year groups above age 40. Males outnumbered females about 2 to 1 in the 0-to-40 age group in clothing fires, but the ratio was about 1:1 above age 40. As children, boys play with matches and fire far more than girls. Psychologists tell us that the incidence of arson among girls is almost nil. In later years, both the male and the female seem to take up the bad habit of smoking in bed.

The cause of death of 20 of the 127 victims of clothing fires was reported as asphyxiation or smoke poisoning. The remainder of the deaths were from burns. The ratio was 1:1 in the nonclothing fires.

The great majority of the deaths occurred in and around the home. A few occurred in automobiles, industry, brush and grass areas, and in various other locations.

Fifty-nine, almost half, of the clothing-fire victims were in some way handicapped in helping themselves when the fire started. Thirteen were too young to act; 19 were physically handicapped; 3 were mentally ill or senile; 8 were intoxicated; 16 were asleep. Most of the physically or mentally handicapped were past 40 years old. More than half the victims were alone at the time the fire started: 7 children were unattended, and 66 adults were alone when the fire started. In the remaining 54 incidents, at least one other person was nearby, but the victim was fatally burned before he could be effectively aided. This gives some indication of the swiftness and intensity of clothing fires.

The predominant source of the ignition of clothing among adults was careless smoking. Running a far second was the cook stove, followed by the rubbish fire and the heating stove, in that order. With children, it was playing with matches first, followed by heating stoves and cook stoves.

Sixty-five, or half, of the 127 clothing-fire victims were wearing ordinary street clothing: 43 were wearing sleepwear; 7 were wearing only underclothing; 12 were wearing other types of dress. Unfortunately, fewer than half the reports specified the fabric of the clothing worn by the victim. Of those that did specify, 78 per cent listed cotton as the fabric ignited. The other 22 per cent was distributed fairly evenly among other natural fabrics, synthetics, and mixtures.

A flammable liquid spilled on the clothing was a factor in 25 of the 127 cases. The liquid was gasoline in 15 cases; lighter fluid, chemicals, and miscellaneous other liquids in the remaining 10 cases.

The foregoing figures are from a small sampling, but they tend to reconfirm much of what we already know. From now through 1967, we shall make an added effort to get more and better information on the fabrics involved and circumstances surrounding clothing fires among the reported fatalities.

# DEVELOPMENT OF CLOTHING FOR PROTECTION FROM HAZARDOUS THERMAL EXPOSURE*

R. E. Seaman

Textile Fibers Department
E. I. du Pont de Nemours & Co., Inc.
Wilmington, Del.

From time immemorial, man has been struggling to protect himself from the hazardous elements of his environment. During all this time, isolation from thermal radiation, particularly in the form of fire, has been a major problem. It remains so today, even though technological progress in developing heat barriers has now reached a high point, by using ceramics, metals, and other inorganic materials, we today can design an unlimited number of nonporous structures to isolate a fire while its useful energy is being harnessed.

This, however, is not the case when we reverse the situation and attempt to put a barrier (i.e., clothing) around man to protect him from open flames or other high-energy heat sources. In such a situation we at least do not want the clothing to contribute to a person's injury by extensive burning. The fabric worn should preferably be completely inert to flames. When you add other desirable parameters such as low heat transfer, durability, comfort, style, and pleasing appearance, the problem of designing an acceptable clothing system does not lend itself to an easy solution. Furthermore, except in specific cases such as military clothing or sophisticated systems used in hazardous industrial situations, you cannot force a person to wear clothing that is not comfortable or does not, for some other reason, appeal to him.

About 3 years ago we set out to attack this problem. The incentive to do so came from the availability of a high-temperature resistant nylon fiber that we have trademarked Nomex. Because of the present high price of this material relative to other textile fibers, we have thus far

*Based on a paper presented at the *Conference on Burns and Flame-Retardant Fabrics,* held at The New York Academy of Medicine, December 2 and 3, 1966. The conference was sponsored by: the New York and Brooklyn Trauma Committee of the American College of Surgeons, Chicago, Ill.; The National Fire Protection Association, Boston, Mass.; the Section on Plastic and Reconstructive Surgery of The New York Academy of Medicine; and the Division of Accident Prevention of the U.S. Public Health Service, Washington, D.C. The conference was held in cooperation with the American Academy of Pediatrics, Evanston, Ill.; the American Public Health Association, New York, N. Y.; and the National Safety Council, Chicago, Ill.; and was supported by a grant from the U.S. Public Health Service.

TABLE I.—CLASSIFICATION OF THERMAL HAZARDS

1) Fabric is the hazard
2) Hazard is external
   a) Convective heat
   b) Conductive exposure
   c) Radiant energy

TABLE II.—TRUE PROTECTION PHILOSOPHY

I) *Conditions of exposure*
   a) Classification
   b) Magnitude
   c) Duration
II) *Test method*
   a) Conditions and procedures to simulate anticipated exposure
   b) Analysis of results to yield practical significance
III) *Design wearable protective clothing*
IV) *Limit the use of clothing worn*

TABLE III.—FABRIC REQUIREMENTS FOR USE IN HYPERBARIC CHAMBERS

1) Flame-retardant at elevated air pressure
2) High ignition temperature under conditions of flammability
3) Low flame propagation rate
4) Low release of energy during combustion
5) Minimum liberation of noxious gases

confined our study to military and specialty civilian clothing systems where the improved performance justifies the initial expense.

We directed our attention first to the nature of the thermal environment. Thermal hazards may be separated into two broad categories to identify uses where the clothing or fabric itself is the major hazard (i.e., it is readily combustible in the presence of even a small flame) as opposed to circumstances in which the hazard is mainly external and, therefore, requires that the clothing insulate the wearer from the deleterious effects of heat. We then classified the latter group by the type of exposure (Table I). These classifications include the thermal sources of convective heat, as in the flames of a flash solvent fire, conductive heat transmitted from a hot surface, and radiant energy emitted from industrial furnaces. As we shall see, the type of clothing required for each category and classification is not necessarily the same; only through an appropriate study of the environment involved can satisfactory clothing systems be designed.

The next problem we encountered was the inadequacy of the testing procedures available to evaluate heat transferred through a fabric system. A useful test method must controllably simulate or duplicate the anticipated hazard and yield data that can be used to evaluate the fabric variables under study. In addition, analysis of the results must be in practical form, so that the ultimate user is given an understanding of the degree of protection provided by a specific design.

We have used these requirements as the basis for developing an over-all concept we term "true protection philosophy" (Table II). The first concern in such a concept involves the condition of exposure, i.e., the classification, magnitude, and duration of exposure. Next, proper testing methods must be included, followed by application of the data to design a wearable clothing system that provides protection from a specific thermal exposure. The final requirement is that clothing developed for a given exposure be limited to its designed use. This last point is very important to avoid presenting a false sense of security to the wearer. No single system can possibly handle all potential hazards without turning into a "man-from-Mars" suit.

Using this philosophy, and with the cooperation of various industrial concerns, we began to evaluate our Nomex fiber in the indicated exposures.

An example of a condition where the fabric itself is a hazard is found in hospital clothing worn by bedridden patients. We are cooperating in a program with the Veterans Administration in the wear-testing of pajamas by such patients. Important requirements in this use are permanent flame resistance for the life of the garment plus comfort, durability, and launderability.

A special problem area within a hospital is the hyperbaric chamber. Here the oxygen pressure can be increased to three times normal; under these conditions, conventional cotton clothing is quite susceptible to

TABLE IV.—PROTECTION FROM CONVECTIVE HEAT

| *Fabric* | *Thickness in mils* | *Total fabric weight oz./sq. yd.* | *Time (seconds) to transmit heat to cause* | |
|---|---|---|---|---|
| | | | *Pain* | *Blister* |
| Glass fabric (5 oz./sq. yd) | 6 | 5 | <1.0 | 2.4 |
| Durable flame-retardant cotton (11 oz./sq. yd.) | 24 | 11 | 1.0 | 2.6 |
| Nomex nylon (5 oz./sq. yd.) | 15 | 5 | 1.7 | 4.4 |
| 11 oz. flame-retardant cotton plus thermal knit of cotton (13.4 oz./sq. yd.) | 114 | 24.4 | 2.2 | 5.6 |
| 5 oz. glass outer layer plus thermal knit of Nomex (7.1 oz./sq. yd.) | 108 | 12.1 | 3.7 | 9.4 |
| 5 oz. Nomex outer layer plus thermal knit of Nomex (7.1 oz./sq. yd.) | 118 | 12.1 | 6.6 | 17.0 |

rapid, almost explosive burning if ignited. The flammability characteristics of fabrics of Nomex and both untreated and flame-retardant-treated cotton have been studied under actual hyperbaric conditions. The desirable fabric requirements for this environment were found to be those indicated in Table III. The fabric should maintain flame-retardant properties with increased pressure of air and concentrations of oxygen. If the concentration of oxygen reaches a level where flammability does develop, the fabric-ignition temperature should be as high as possible, the flame-propagation rate low, and the amount of energy released on burning at a minimum. Finally, combustion should not release noxious gases. Fabrics of Nomex were found to fulfill these requirements to the highest degree of those tested.

When the hazard is external to the clothing and the fabric barrier is expected to be not only flame-retardant but to provide protection from the external hazard, additional problems must be solved. The approach we have adopted in studying this type of hazard is demonstrated in our work on convective heat exposure. An understanding of the magnitude of the hazard was obtained through actual burn tests conducted at the Daytona Speedway in Florida. Dummies were dressed in various protective uniforms and placed in a car containing high-test racing fuel that was then ignited. Recorded temperature measurements under the fabrics and a study of the damage to exposed "skin" were used to indicate the amount of injury suffered under these exposure

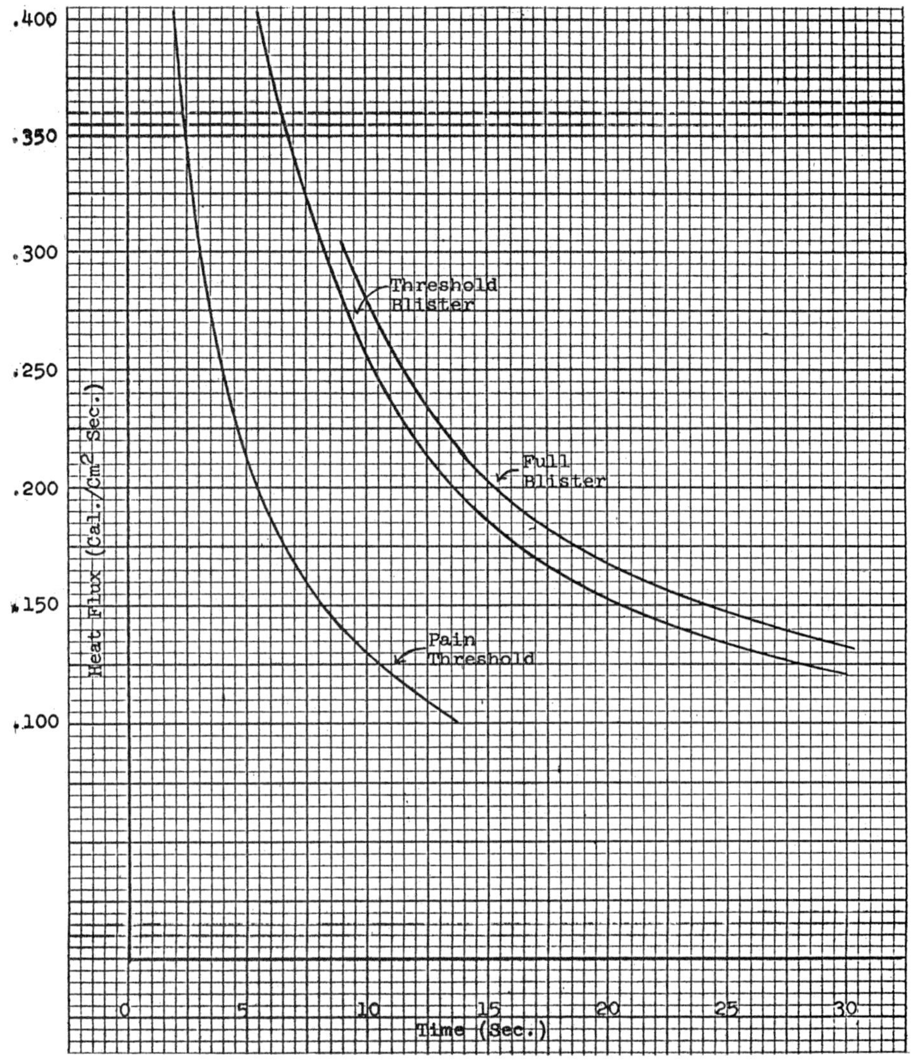


Fig. 1. Heat flux versus time of exposure to threshold pain and blistering.—United States Navy Air Development Center, Johnsville, Pa.

conditions. These practical tests, while they provided insight into the problem, proved difficult to analyze and indicated the need for a laboratory test that could be used to characterize various protective fabrics.

The laboratory test that we developed uses a 2,500° F. flame as the heat source and measures the amount of heat blocked from a sensing disk, as a function of time, by the clothing under study. These measure-

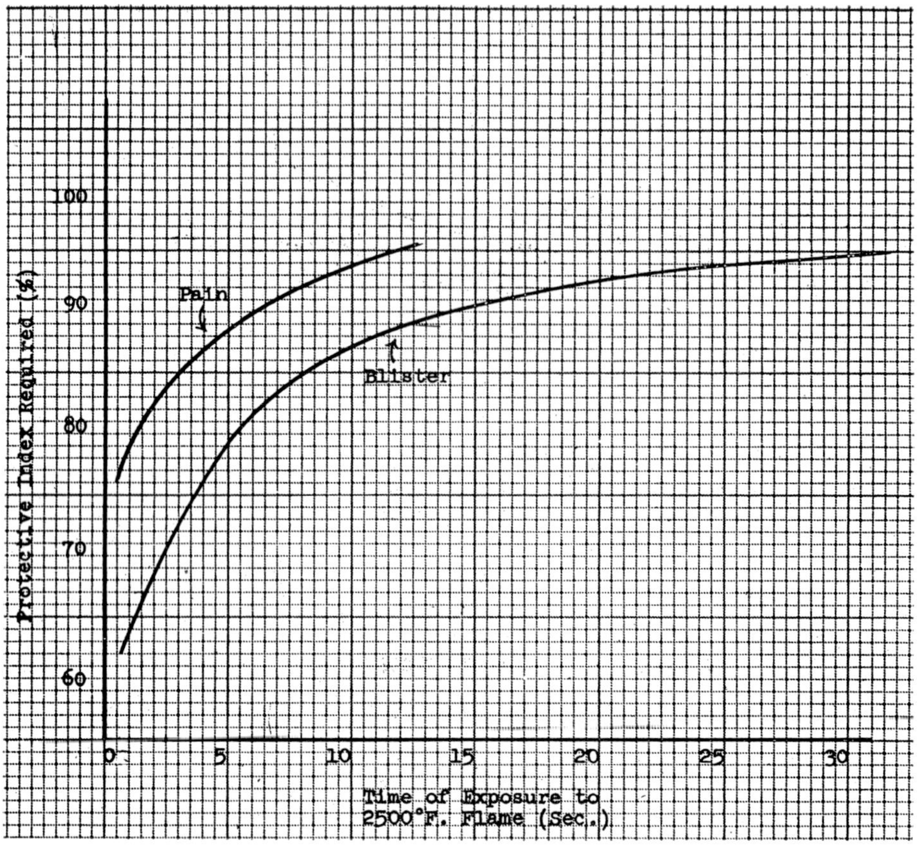


Fig. 2. Protective index required versus exposure time for pain and blister thresholds.

ments are then used to rate its effectiveness. In addition, the heat that is transmitted can be compared with the heat that can be tolerated by human tissue before injury occurs, and a protection time can then be established, as shown in Table IV. This table details the type of information obtained from laboratory measurements of fabrics of Nomex, permanent flame-retardant cotton, and glass fiber. Both single and multilayer systems are included. You will note that a high fabric-insulation value yields longer times of exposure before pain or blister occurs. When a layer of underwear is added to the outer layer, the time of protection is greatly increased. This results from the increased mass of material that must be heated by the thermal source, and from the large quantity of air trapped between the layers, which provides added thermal insulation. The difference in heat capacity of the individual fibers is evident from a comparison of the last two fabrics cited in the table. This parameter dominates both total fabric weight or thickness in these fabrics. The data also show the importance of multiple-layer fabrics if an extended time is necessary for the wearer to react and escape from the vicinity of the heat source.

The last two columns in Table IV referred to the time it takes to pain or blister, using a specific clothing barrier. These data are obtained by first measuring the rate at which heat must be applied to skin to cause damage (Figure 1). This graph shows these data as developed by the U.S. Navy. It demonstrates that high-heat fluxes, such as would occur in a flash fire, can obviously be tolerated for only very short periods of time. Second, by using our laboratory test, we calculate a "protective index" by establishing the amount of available heat that the fabric blocks as a function of time. Third, combining these data with the naval information, we can relate the protective index to the time it takes to cause pain or blistering as shown in Figure 2. This graph is particularly useful from two points of view. First, if the time of exposure is known, or can be estimated, one can design clothing to provide the desired protective index associated with this time interval. It also shows that for even very short exposure times, a high percentage of heat must be blocked or tissue damage will occur. One practical application of this work has been the development of a two-layer uniform that was worn by all but one of the drivers at the Indianapolis 500 race this year.

We are currently extending this work to include the effects of convective and radiant heat. Although the work is not complete, we believe we shall be successful in defining the conditions required to protect a person from these energy sources.

To summarize, I should like to emphasize that it is possible today to "protect" a person from fire with correctly designed clothing using any fiber. The degree to which such attire can be made lightweight, comfortable, durable, and appealing depends on the fiber and finishing procedures used. Adoption of such fabric will in turn depend on the desire of the consumer to accept thermal protection as one of his needs.

# FLAME RETARDANTS AND THEIR APPLICATION TO TEXTILES*

George L. Drake, Jr.

Southern Utilization Research and Development Division
Agricultural Research Service
U. S. Department of Agriculture
New Orleans, La.

Fire is constructively involved in some way in almost everything we do. This is truly paradoxical. We should not have the high standard of living that we now enjoy were it not for combustion. Yet fire, uncontrolled, destroys millions of dollars of property annually.[1]

There is no estimate of the extent of personal injuries and losses that are due to the ignition of textiles, but the figure is certainly very high. Fire prevention is the positive approach to reduction of these injuries and losses. A number of organizations have been active in the search for flame retardants for cellulosic fibers that would be both effective and durable for the useful life of the fabric.

Efforts to make textiles flame-resistant are not new,[2] but early research investigations were limited to the use of water-soluble compounds. For example, such substances as borax, boric acid, diammonium phosphate, and ammonium sulfamate impart resistance to flame but, because they are water soluble, the fire retardant finishes are removed by washing. Several such treatments[3] are still valuable for domestic use where nondurable flame resistance is sought for such items as curtains, draperies, potholders, and upholstery padding. For example, one effective domestic treatment uses 7 ounces of borax and 3 ounces of boric acid dissolved in 2 quarts of hot water. Cotton items are thoroughly wetted with the solution and dried by any convenient means.[3] Given this or similar treatment, cotton will be flame-resistant until wet or washed.

The most widely used flame-resistant finish for cotton in industrial

*Based on a paper presented at the *Conference on Burns and Flame-Retardant Fabrics,* held at The New York Academy of Medicine, December 2 and 3, 1966. The conference was sponsored by: the New York and Brooklyn Trauma Committee of the American College of Surgeons, Chicago, Ill.; The National Fire Protection Association, Boston, Mass.; the Section on Plastic and Reconstructive Surgery of The New York Academy of Medicine; and the Division of Accident Prevention of the U. S. Public Health Service, Washington, D. C. The conference was held in cooperation with the American Academy of Pediatrics, Evanston, Ill.; the American Public Health Association, New York, N. Y.; and the National Safety Council, Chicago, Ill.; and was supported by a grant from the U. S. Public Health Service.

applications is of the antimony oxide chlorinated paraffin type; vinyl chloride is sometimes added. A combination of such chemicals is applied to tents, tarpaulins, and other outdoor products, and is durable throughout the service life of these products. It is known as FWWMR (flame, water, weather, and mildew resistant) treatment. This finish adversely affects the "hand" (or feel), the drape, flexibility, and the color of the fabric, since additions up to 60 per cent are required in many cases to obtain adequate durability of the flame-resistant treatment.

The task of developing an effective durable flame-retardant finish for cotton is difficult because of the many requirements the finish must meet. To be satisfactory for most uses, a flame retardant must: 1) be easy to apply, preferably with existing finishing equipment from a water solution; 2) be effective with few additives to avoid excessive increases in weight; 3) produce a finish durable to laundering and dry cleaning; 4) leave the fabric air-permeable; 5) be physiologically inactive; 6) render the fabric resistant to afterglow; 7) not stiffen the fabric appreciably; 8) cause little or no loss in strength; and 9) be reasonable in cost.

The products and potential markets for flame-resistant fabrics are large and varied. In 1963, a total of 19 million pounds of cotton was utilized in fabric with flame-resistant finishes, both durable and nondurable. Of this, approximately one half of the finish was FWWMR. An annual potential for fire-resistant finishes on woven cotton fabrics has been estimated as equivalent to 354 million pounds. Since only 19 million pounds were actually finishes, this leaves an unfilled potential of 335 million pounds of cotton. In addition, if cotton were to capture some of the market now held by synthetics, possibly another 422-million pounds could be finished.[18]

The largest estimated potential market of 551 million pounds is for household items, such as bedding, blankets, sheets, curtains, drapes and slip covers. Industrial uses, estimated at 172 million pounds, are for such items as automobile covers, upholstery, tops, awnings, tents, mail bags, umbrellas, and other products requiring heavy textiles. The apparel market, estimated at 52 million pounds, is composed primarily of night wear, dressing gowns, work clothes and uniforms. This market potential is for the consumption of cotton in uses in apparel whose flame resistance is desirable with no increase in cost. The potential market for apparel falls off very rapidly with increasing cost; adding the flame retardants makes some of the changes in properties of fabrics unacceptable. However, the fire-resistant finishes of today are more effective, more durable, and better suited to the entire market than were the finishes of the past.[18]

The major breakthrough in the development of a satisfactory, durable, flame-retardant finish for cotton was made at the Southern Regional Research Laboratory about 1950 when tetrakis (hydroxymethyl) phosphonium chloride, known as THPC, was used. Reeves and Guthrie[4] found that THPC would react with and make aminized cotton flame retardant. Later the reaction of cotton with THPC and other substances, such as melamine urea, was studied in an effort to eliminate the aminization of the cotton. It was found that THPC reacts and polymerizes with methylolmelamine as well as with many other substances, and can form insoluble polymers inside the cotton fibers to produce good flame-resistant finishes. Simultaneously, this process involves some cross-linking of the cellulose chains in cotton.

A typical formulation that gives satisfactory results on 8-ounce fabrics contains 16.4 per cent THPC, 3.0 per cent triethanolamine, 9.4 per cent trimethylolmelamine, and 9.8 per cent urea based on the total weight of the solution. The treatment can be applied with standard chemical-finishing equipment. The solution is applied to fabric with a padder, using a tight squeeze-roll pressure. The fabric is then dried, cured at an elevated temperature, and washed by any of the usual washing procedures. A softener used to reduce stiffness and improve strength may be applied with the treating formulation or applied as a separate step in treating the fabric. This process was commercialized in 1956; several finishing mills in the United States and England are now using processes based on it for making fire-resistant cotton fabric. Much of the durable flame-resistant cotton fabric produced in the United States contains the THPC-amide finish or some modification of it. This finish is effective on most cotton fabrics of loose weave, and on heavier fabrics, that is, fabrics weighing 6 ounces or more per square yard. It is also satisfactory on some fabrics of lighter weight and of loose construction: for example 3/3 steep twill of about 4 ounces per square yard. Typical additives range from 18 per cent to 28 per cent, depending upon fabric weight, the resin system used, and the durability required. THPC resin systems are amenable to vat-dyed fabrics and may be used as the bonding agents for pigment-dyed fabrics. A textile treated with this finish withstands laundering and, in addition to being flame-resistant, is glow-resistant and imparts considerable resistance to rot and mildew. The main disadvantages of the process are cost, stiffness imparted to some fabrics, and formaldehyde odors liberated during the curing operation. Treatment of fabric with a wash-wear finish prior to treatment with this flame-retardant finish may improve the efficiency of the process and the hand of the fabric.[5]

It was determined later that the chemical fixation of a water-soluble precondensate of THPC and amides in cotton fabric with ammonia and ammonium hydroxide has certain advantages. This technique, referred to as the ammonia cure method, tends to reduce loss of the strength of a fabric associated with the heat-cure method. The improved strength imparted by this method may be due to less cross-linking of the cellulose and, to a lesser extent, to the lower temperature of resin, as compared to the heat cure method. A THPC finish using ammonia cure is in commercial production in England under the name of Proban.[6, 7] It has been reported that an improved precondensate can be obtained by incorporating diammonium sulfite monohydrate and sodium acetate in the formulation and then drying the wetted fabric and fixing the finish in ammonium hydroxide.[18]

According to the literature the disadvantages of stiffness and loss of strength in fabrics treated with the THPC formulation can be reduced by adding a methylol-substituted triazone or triazine or a cyclic ethyleneurea and also by adding a polyvinyl chloride resin with a softening point of between 170° to 200° C. A typical formulation is: 6 to 20 per cent THPC, 3 to 12 per cent of the methylol compound, 1 to 4 per cent tertiary amine, 3 to 12 per cent urea, 7 to 25 per cent PVC resin and water added depending upon the solids content desired. The solution is applied to cotton by a padding technique, and the cotton is then dried and cured for 10 seconds at 370° C. and afterwashed.[8, 9]

In October 1956, scientists of the Southern Utilization Research and Development Division announced one of the most effective and durable flame retardants: APO-THPC. APO is the abbreviation for tris (1-aziridinyl)phosphine oxide. The polymer from APO-THPC imparts a very durable flame-resistant finish with an additive relatively low in resin, and is satisfactory for use on all-cotton fabrics with the exception of tightly constructed lightweight fabrics and those weighing less than about 3 ounces per square yard. There still exists a need for an adequate flame retardant for lightweight fabrics such as sheers and nets. The APO-THPC finish is best on fabrics weighing 6 ounces per square yard and heavier. It is somewhat less than completely satisfactory on print cloth and other lightweight goods weighing less than 4 ounces per square yard. Satisfactory flame resistance can be obtained with comparatively little resin additive (8 to 12 per cent) to heavier fabrics, but more (15 to 18 per cent) is required for lighter fabrics which stiffen and weaken in the process. The finish is effective also on rayon, wool, and silk, and on blends of these fabrics, but not on cellulose acetate, nylon, or polyester fibers.[10, 11, 12, 13]

This treatment can be applied readily to cotton by use of commercial equipment. Essentially the treatment consists of padding the fabric through an aqueous solution of APO-THPC, drying at a relatively low temperature, curing it at an elevated temperature to form a highly cross-linked resin within the fibers, and then washing and drying the cotton.

APO-THPC-treated fabrics with approximately 15 per cent additive withstand repeated laundering and dry cleaning. Char length in the standard vertical flame test is about 3 inches for most fabrics.[16] Treated fabrics pass the 180° strip angle flame test[14] before and after washing. After softening, the fabric retains about 90 per cent of its breaking strength and a high percentage of its tearing strength. Treated fabrics continue to offer protection, even after exposure to fires and high-temperature irradiation, by the formation of a relatively tough and pliable carbonaceous fabric structure after being charred.

A new flame retardant based on APO and thiourea has recently been found to be successful for use on cottons.[17] A typical treating solution consists of 25 per cent APO, 15 per cent thiourea, a wetting agent, and 3 per cent polyethylene softener. Fabric is treated by the conventional pad-dry-cure technique. The flame resistance is excellent, and remains durable under laundering and dry cleaning. The finished fabric is also rot- and mildew-resistant and has some crease resistance.

APO is initially toxic and must be handled with care, but once the material is polymerized the end products are reported to be harmless.[17]

Techniques have been developed for imparting durable flame resistance to the surfaces of cotton textiles of low density such as cotton pile and napped fabrics. A spray technique has been used to apply the

THPC-based flame retardants. The chemical cost is reduced by using this technique, and the treated material retains its tensile and tear strength. In addition, the textile surface fibers are made more resilient.

Flame-retardant fabrics with better hand and strength result if the fabric to be treated is free of starches or sizes and is absorbent. Failure to eliminate starch causes increased stiffness and reduced wash fastness of the finish. Fabrics treated on a continuous basis are better than those produced in batches. To prevent migration of solution and stiffening of the treated fabrics, the least amount of tension possible should be applied to the fabric as it comes from the pad. Treating solutions must be kept cool, and padding must be done with a heavy squeeze-roll pressure to assure complete penetration of the fiber. Drying, which is probably the most critical operation in applying flame-retardant finishes, should be carried out below 212° F. to prevent the surface from curing before the inside of the yarn is dry. A high drying temperature causes stiffness of fabric and low tearing strengths. High air velocity also causes migration. The fabric must be dry before curing, and curing must be done immediately after drying.

What is new on the horizon? Research is continuing on the development of flame-retardant finishes with a higher phosphorus: nitrogen ratio which should improve efficiency in the process of imparting them and should be adaptable to fabrics of all weights.

Arthur[15] has shown that a free-radical mechanism is involved in the pyrolytic degradation of cotton cellulose and that, by the attachment of certain groups (aromatic) to cellulose, there is a decrease in free-radical formation. Reduction of free-radical formation should increase the flame resistance of cellulose. This fundamental information may be a lead to the development of new and better flame-retardant finishes for cotton.

## *REFERENCES*


1. *Accident Facts.* Chicago, Nat. Safety Council, 1962.
2. Speel, H. C. and Schwarz, E. W. K., eds. *Textile Chemicals and Auxiliaries,* 2d ed., New York, Reinhold, 1957, pp. 466-90.
3. Reid, J. D., Reeves, W. A., Frick, J. G., Jr. *Making Household Fabrics Flame-Resistant,* U.S. Department of Agriculture Leaflet No. 454. Washington, D.C. Govt. Print. Off., 1959.
4. Reeves, W. A. and Guthrie, J. D., *Textile World 104* (2):101, 176-82, 1954.
5. British Patent 884,785.
6. Reeves, W. A. and Bourdette, V. R. *Textile Industries 128:*105-06, 109, 1964.
7. Drake, G. L., Jr., Reeves, W. A. and Perkins, R. M., *Amer. Dyestuff Reporter 52:*603-11, 1963.
8. British Patent 975,095.

9. British Patent 973,355.
10. Reeves, W. A., Drake, G. L., Jr., Chance, L. H. and Guthrie, J. D., *Textile Res. J. 27*:260-66, 1957.
11. Fisher, C. H. and Perkerson, F. S. *Textile Res. J. 28*:769-78, 1958.
12. Drake, G. L., Jr., Beninate, J. V. and Guthrie, J. D., *Amer. Dyestuff Reporter 50*:27-32, 1961.
13. Drake, G. L., Jr. and Reeves, W. A., *Natl. Safety News 90* (1): 58, 135-136, 1964.
14. Reeves, W. A., McMillan, O. J., Jr. and Guthrie, J. D., *Textile Res. J. 23*: 527-32, 1953.
15. Arthur, J. C. Jr. and Hinojosa, O., *Textile Res. J. 36*:385-87, 1966.
16. U.S. Federal Supply Service. *Textile Test Methods.* Fed. Specifications CCC-T191b, Method 5902, Washington, D.C. U.S. Govt. Print. Off., 1951.
17. LeBlanc, R. B. *Textile Res. J. 35*: 341-46, 1965.
18. Hall, A. J. *Textile World 116*:98-100, 102, 1966.

# PILE FABRICS AND THEIR FLAMMABILITY*

Harry A. Freedman

Product Development Manager
Borg Fabrics
Delavan, Wis.

Initially the title of this presentation was to be "Blending of Natural and Synthetic Fibers." As you will see from the following discussion, there are many interrelated important factors that affect the flammability of pile fabrics. To discuss any one factor without consideration of the others would result in a situation similar to that in the story of the blind man and the elephant. Certainly the first blind man was not completely wrong when, after feeling the animal's trunk, he described the elephant as long and snakelike. Similarly, in discussing the flammability of pile fabrics, the three major subjects of fiber blends, fabric construction, and chemical finishes must all be considered not separately, but as a total concept.

The words "pile fabric" may be broadly interpreted as meaning any type of fabric from suedes through velours and furlike construction to very deep pile construction up to 10 inches and 12 inches in depth. For the purpose of simplicity I shall limit my discussion to those fabrics that have a napped or raised surface in excess of one eighth of an inch. Fabrics that fall into this category are: 1) brushed knits, such as brushed mohair sweaters; 2) napped knits such as fleece and constructions up to about one half of an inch in height of the pile; 3) napped or brushed woven and tufted fabrics; and 4) sliver knit, or the "deep-pile" furs.

In almost every one of these categories, very definite technical differences distinguish the fabrics, but they may all be classed as pile fabrics for apparel. In addition to the apparel grouping, other categories such as toys, throw rugs, carpeting, upholstery fabric, etc., should be considered. In these additional categories will be found such constructions as knit, woven, and tufted fabrics of cut and uncut loops as well

*Based on a paper presented at the *Conference on Burns and Flame-Retardant Fabrics,* held at The New York Academy of Medicine, December 2 and 3, 1966. The conference was sponsored by: the New York and Brooklyn Trauma Committee of the American College of Surgeons, Chicago, Ill.; The National Fire Protection Association, Boston, Mass.; the Section on Plastic and Reconstructive Surgery of The New York Academy of Medicine; and the Division of Accident Prevention of the U.S. Public Health Service, Washington, D.C. The conference was held in cooperation with the American Academy of Pediatrics, Evanston, Ill.; the American Public Health Association, New York, N. Y.; and the National Safety Council, Chicago, Ill.; and was supported by a grant from the U.S. Public Health Service.

as the conventional, brushed, napped, and furlike finishes.

The major significant factors affecting the flammability of pile fabric are fiber blends, chemical finishes, and the construction of fabric. Almost all common textile fibers known today are used in pile fabrics in one form or another. The practice of blending types of fiber to achieve improved performance, appearance, or economy has resulted in the development of an indefinite number of fabrics, each designed for a particular use.

The major domestic categories of man-made fibers used in pile fabrics today are acrylic, cellulosic, modacrylic, polyamide, polyester, and olefin. In apparel-type fabrics, as in toys and in many floor coverings, the acrylic and cellulosic fibers are those most commonly used. This is dictated by the performance, esthetics, and economics of these two fibers. Unfortunately, both fibers have a propensity toward flammability under certain conditions. While the acrylic fibers are considerably less prone to be flammable than the cellulosics, improper construction of acrylic fabrics can result in potentially dangerous pile fabrics. While polyamide, polyester, and olefin fibers are not considered flammable fibers, they do not have any flame-inhibiting properties that would aid in retarding the flammability of fabrics in which they might be blended with acrylic or cellulosic fibers.

The two modacrylic fibers currently being produced in this country, Verel* and Dynel,** are nonflammable. Not only are these fibers flame-resistant in themselves but, when properly used in blends, they aid in inhibiting the flammability of other fibers. In pile fabric blends, it is a rule of thumb that a modacrylic fiber will not have any significant flame-inhibiting properties below a 25 per cent level. In otherwise potentially flammable fabrics, the addition of 30 to 35 per cent modacrylic fiber to the blend will generally result in giving the fabric sufficient flame resistance to render it safe for use in apparel (Figure 1). Polyvinylchloride fibers commonly used in pile fabrics in Europe have a somewhat similar flame-inhibiting tendency.

With few exceptions, fiber blends in themselves are not entirely responsible for dictating the degree of flammability of a fabric. Relatively flame-resistant pile fabrics can be produced even from 100 per cent rayon, provided the fabric construction is correct and the proper chemical finishes have been applied.

*Registered trademark, Tennessee Eastman Company.
**Registered trademark, Union Carbide Corporation, New York, N. Y.

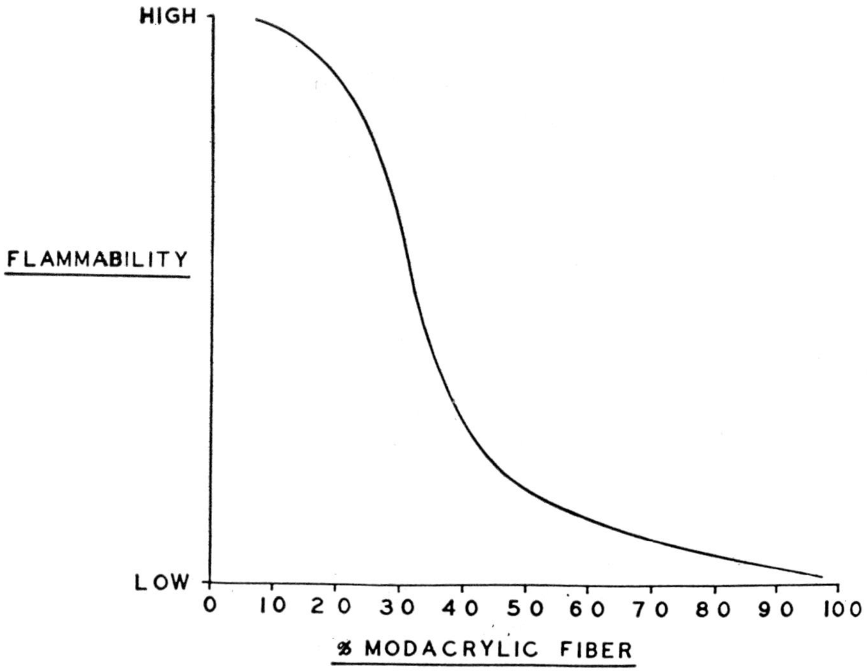


Fig. 1. Theoretical curve of a rayon-modacrylic blend fur fabric.

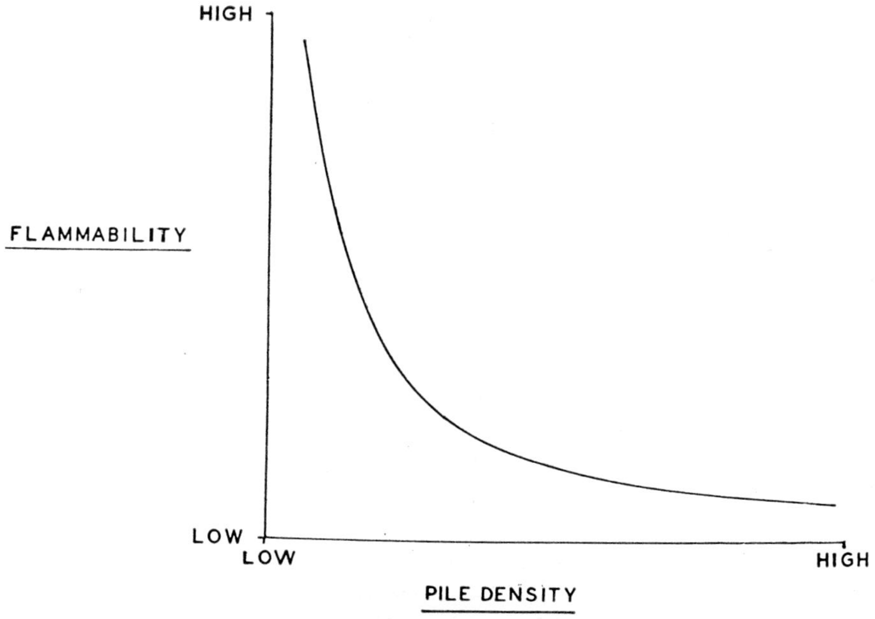


Fig. 2. Theoretical curve of pile density versus flammability.

The second major factor in the flammability of pile fabric, its construction, is probably the most complicated and variable of the three basic factors. In essence, the flammability of a fabric as related to its construction is an inverse function of the amount of surface of the fabric exposed to the air. In other words, the higher the density of a fabric, the lower its tendency to be flammable, and vice versa (Figure 2).

Under the heading of fabric construction, each of the following individual factors will play a role in determining flammability:

1) *Yarn twist.* In pile fabrics containing unopened yarns, the tighter the yarn twist the lower the tendency of the fabric to burn.

2) *Cut versus uncut loops.* In pile fabrics, cut loops will burn more readily than the uncut construction.

3) *Pile density.* As previously indicated, the weight per unit volume (not area) of pile is inversely proportional to the fabric flammability.

4) *Pile height.* Generally speaking, the shorter the pile the higher the pile density and the lower the danger of flammability (Figure 3).

5) *Uniformity of pile surface.* Generally, the more uniform the pile surface and the greater the pile surface density, the lower the tendency of the fabric to be flammable (Figure 3).

6) *Pile position.* Many lightweight fabrics that might normally have poor flammability if sold with the pile in an erect, open state become acceptable when the pile is flattened, effectively increasing the pile density (Figure 4).

7) *Fiber blend location.* If a multifiber pile fabric has the flame-retardant portion of the blend on the pile surface, its flammability will be inhibited, and vice versa (Figure 5).

While the preceding graphs and sketches depict theoretical situations, it should be appreciated that these theories are applied daily by designers and finishers of pile fabric. Adherence to these principles will assure the production of safe pile fabrics.

The third general factor affecting pile fabric flammability is the application of chemical finishes. The normal fiber finishes, such as softeners, bodying agents, lustering agents, etc., are normally used in such small amounts as not to have any effect on the flammability of a pile fabric.

Some types of pile fabrics may be treated with very effective flame-retardant chemicals. However, not all pile fabrics can be subjected to

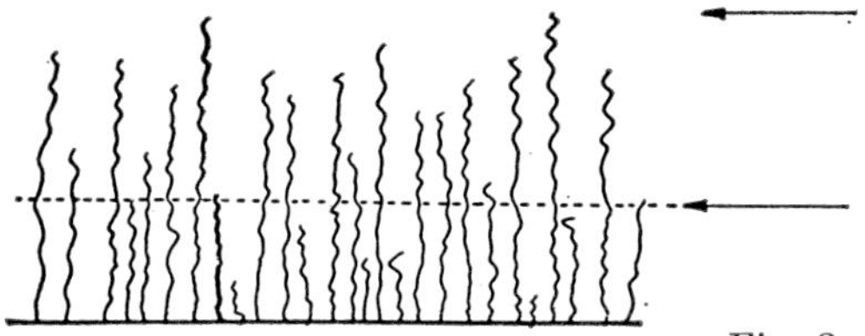


Fig. 3

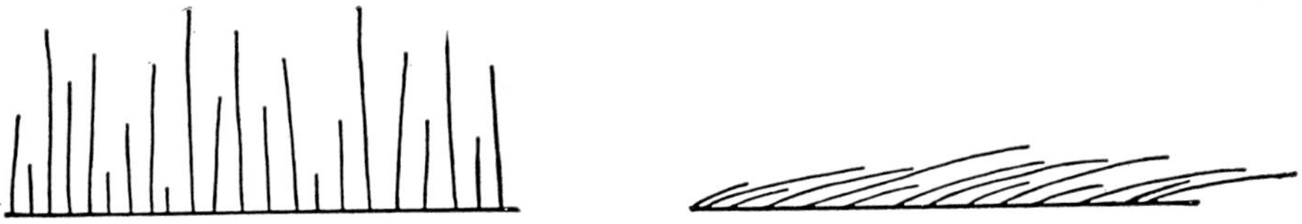


Fig. 4

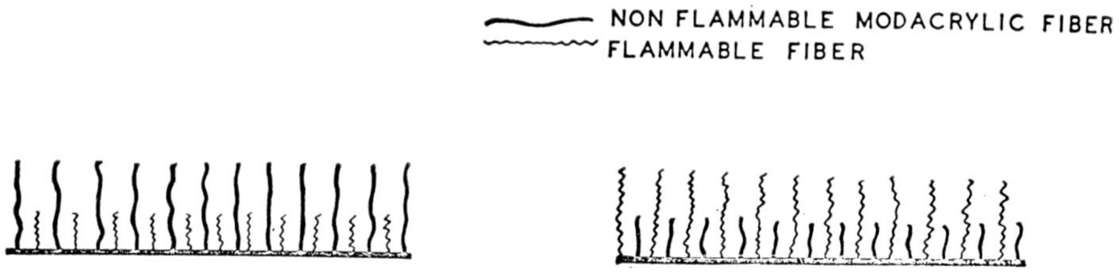


CONSTRUCTION vs. FLAMMABILITY

Fig. 5

this treatment. Additionally, most flame-retardant finishes adversely affect the properties of fabric, making their use impractical. The fabric may become stiff or harsh to the touch; a change in color is also common.

Even where flame-retardant finishes have been successfully applied, many of these finishes have not been resistant to removal by laundering or dry cleaning.

For many years, the major manufacturers of cellulosic and acrylic fibers have attempted to render their apparel fibers flame-retardant by incorporating chemicals within the fiber itself. To date, none of these efforts has proved commercially successful.

Intelligent application of the principles of fiber blend, fabric construction, and chemical treatment by the major pile fabric producers has produced, and can continue to produce, safe pile fabrics.

Above and beyond the production of safe pile fabric for use in apparel, manufacturers of pile fabric have produced fabrics designed to hasten the recovery of victims of burns. Borg Fabrics has on the market a polyester bed pad designed to be used by victims of burns or bedsores. When the patient is placed directly on this polyester-pile bed pad, the pad permits body fluids to drain away from the injury, allowing the air to reach the wound for rapid healing. Not only are the pads completely washable and stain-resistant, but they may even be autoclaved many times without loss of properties of the fabric. Additionally, there are pile fabrics specifically designed to protect fire fighters and pilots of jet fighters from the heat of a fire.

I hope that the preceding discussion has helped describe the parameters of a flame-retardant fabric. I believe I speak for all the major pile fabric manufacturers when I say we are willing and anxious to work toward producing safe pile fabrics, and we hope to assist in the formation of realistic codes and bylaws.

# APPLICATION AND DEVELOPMENT OF FLAME-RETARDANT FINISHES IN TEXTILE MILLS*

J. W. WEAVER

Manager, Research and Development Laboratory
Cone Mills Corporation, Greensboro, N. C.

My assignment on this occasion is to represent the textile industry of the United States on behalf of the American Textile Manufacturers Institute, Inc., New York, N. Y. This institute is the central trade association of the textile manufacturing and textile finishing industries in this country. The mills comprising this association produce and distribute the great bulk of the more than 13 billion yards of textiles made annually by this, the world's largest, textile manufacturing industry.

Representatives of the institute helped to create national textile flammability standards, were instrumental in enactment of the Federal Flammable Fabrics Act in 1954, and welcomed this law, which has removed dangerously flammable materials from commerce. Our firms also have devoted substantial effort to research in flame-retardant processes, and they actively market such products today wherever demand exists for them and the customer is willing to meet the price. We are as conscious as any industry of our public responsibilities. We desire safety in our products, and we are close students of all valid accident records. Therefore we welcome this opportunity to tell you where this industry stands today in the area of flame retardancy, with which you are concerned.

For the purpose of this discussion let me direct our consideration to a specific portion of our annual production of 13 billion yards.

Suppose that because of education or legislation it would be desirable to consider making all nightwear and related garments flame-retardant.

*Based on a paper presented at the *Conference on Burns and Flame-Retardant Fabrics,* held at The New York Academy of Medicine, December 2 and 3, 1966. The conference was sponsored by: the New York and Brooklyn Trauma Committee of the American College of Surgeons, Chicago, Ill.; The National Fire Protection Association, Boston, Mass.; the Section on Plastic and Reconstructive Surgery of The New York Academy of Medicine; and the Division of Accident Prevention of the U.S. Public Health Service, Washington, D.C. The conference was held in cooperation with the American Academy of Pediatrics, Evanston, Ill.; the American Public Health Association, New York, N. Y.; and the National Safety Council, Chicago, Ill.; and was supported by a grant from the U.S. Public Health Service.

By nightwear and related garments, I mean nightgowns and pajamas, negligees, housecoats, smoking jackets, and related items, for both sexes and all ages. By "flame-retardant" I mean that the fabric used is able to pass the Vertical Flame Test designated by the American Association of Textile Chemists and Colorists as "Fire Resistance of Textile Fabrics" 34-1966; by the American Society for Testing Materials as "Fire-Retardant Properties of Treated Textile Fabrics" D626-55T; and as Federal Specification CCCT 191b "Flame Resistance of Cloth: Vertical" Method 5902.

Our supposition requires that we know the size of this market; that data from the United States Department of Commerce and the National Cotton Council of America show that it consumes 180 million pounds of fiber annually, providing 300 million garments that have a retail value of almost 1 billion dollars.

Three fourths of this 180 million pounds of fiber is cellulosic, that is, cotton or rayon. Ninety per cent of this is woven fabric and the remaining 10 per cent knitted.

Restricting ourselves to the woven cellulosic materials, we are talking about an annual market for about 200 million garments made from 400 million yards of cloth weighing about 120 million pounds.

But we are realistic enough to recognize that all textile fibers suitable for apparel are susceptible to fire, and that, although none of our common fabrics in use for many years can be called "dangerous," we agree that under certain circumstances it may be desirable to render these fabrics more flame-retardant.

As we explore this market, one of the first questions we encounter is why the cellulosic fibers comprise so large a part of our nightwear product.

The first element of public acceptance of these goods is unquestionably price.

The prices of fibers currently available for use in this specialized market are cited in the accompanying table.

Looking a bit further into price, we may note that a typical cotton flannelette for nightwear use, made of cotton that costs about 22¢ a pound, currently sells in the markets at approximately 27¢ a yard, or $1.00 a pound, and becomes children's sleepwear garments retailing at $1.98 or $2.98. It requires no special knowledge of the markets to note that were the mill to use a fiber that cost two or three or four times as

PRICES OF FIBERS

| *Fiber* | *Price per pound* |
|---|---|
| Cotton | $0.22 |
| Rayon | 0.28 |
| High modulus rayon | 0.36 |
| Cellulose acetate | 0.41 |
| Polyester | 0.72 |
| Acrylic | 0.77 |
| Nylon | 0.78 |
| Modacrylic | 0.78 |

much, the price of the cloth would be substantially higher, the garment manufacturer's costs would be correspondingly higher, and the consumer would be paying more for the end product.

A second reason why the public demands these cellulosic products is "comfort." There is no question that the moisture-absorption characteristics, the drape and feel, or "hand" as it is known, of cotton are preferred for garments worn next to the skin. Rayons have been engineered to imitate cotton as closely as possible in these properties, and they too are acceptable.

There is not now any single fiber that is inherently flame-retardant and that is acceptable to the consumer in price, comfort, and general satisfaction.

There are self-extinguishing or flame-retardant synthetic fibers, such as Dynel and Verel, which are available, but when used alone in wearing apparel they are not acceptable because of cost, discomfort, and loss of esthetic properties, including the variety of color that the public demands.

Compromises are possible by blending these unacceptable flame-retardant fibers with acceptable conventional fibers. This makes the blend more comfortable and more acceptable, but simultaneously renders it less flame-retardant. The amount of flame-retardance desired must be established before any such blend can be properly designed.

Since we lack a breakthrough that would give us an ideal fiber combining the elements of price, comfort, and consumer satisfaction with inherent flame retardancy, the best approach now appears to be a chemical treatment that can be applied to cotton or rayon or some unknown blend, so that the mass market may be supplied from conventional equipment now turning out these 400 million yards a year. But the chemical treatments available today for making these fabrics flame resistant or self-extinguishing also make them unacceptable to the public for nightwear, because of increased cost, decreased comfort, and loss of hand and drape.

Most of the fabric now used in the market is dyed and chemically finished on what we call "continuous systems" where the preparation, dyeing, finishing, and washing are carried out on an endless piece of cloth. Only in this way can we dye and finish great quantities of fabric rapidly and economically and bring them to market attractively priced.

Progressive mills in our industry have looked carefully into available chemical treatments, such as the finishes based on tris (1-aziridinyl) phosphine oxide (APO) and tetrakis (hydroxymethyl) phosphonium chloride (THPC), and many of them have conducted plant production runs that use all practical flame-retardant systems on this continuous equipment.

We have found no significant market acceptance from our efforts. We do find acceptance in the limited area of industrial protective garments, where the user compromises on desirability of fabric qualities to offset exposure to occupational hazards, and where the extra cost of protection is willingly accepted, and in nonapparel uses where bodily comfort and hand do not apply.

But these treatments are unacceptable for normal apparel including the nightwear we are considering. Their cost is high. For the nightwear flannelette previously mentioned, selling for about 27¢ a yard, we estimate an added cost for fire retardancy of 20¢ a yard or more. The higher costs of cloth, the higher costs of manufacturing garments from such goods, all accumulate, so that the child's sleeping garment that now retails at $1.98 would be $3.98 and the $2.98 garment would move at least to $4.98. Multiply these prices by 200 million garments a year and you have some idea of the increase in the public's annual clothing bill for nightwear alone. The increased cost would fall most heavily on persons who have large families and who probably are least able to bear the added expense.

Because of these difficulties we who are engaged in research and development are continuously seeking better chemical treatment than we now have.

We are emphasizing improvements in the finishing of lightweight nightwear fabrics that today require proportionately more chemical add-on than heavier fabrics. Less than half the weight of these added chemicals actively promotes flame retardancy, while more than half is "binder" to achieve "life-of-garment" durability of the finish. Ways are sought to reduce this excessive weight, which in turn destroys the hand of the fabric. Emphasis must be given to reduce this stiffness and boardiness for such goods used as apparel.

Producers of synthetic fibers also are attempting to reduce this excess weight by putting the flame-resistant material inside the fiber; this would eliminate the need for a "binder" for a durable finish. Existing patents (British patent 958,120 and U.S. patents 2,816,004; 2,953,-463; and 3,266,918) suggest ways to do this. The approach is on sound theoretical ground and we await developments. But no such fibers are being produced in commercial quantities today.

We have pointed out that high add-on of expensive chemicals and limited production today dictate costs for fabrics with flame-retardant treatment approximately double those of untreated fabrics. We could normally contend that the costs of new products are usually high, and that normally, in time, they come down. But this may be oversimplification if cost is not the only determining factor. Great Britain has had more than two years' experience with a law on children's nightwear garments that exempts yard goods, and it may be appropriate to quote briefly from a recent statement of the Federation of Piece Dyers and Finishers, Manchester, as follows:

> It is believed that there has so far been considerable reluctance on the part of the public to buy flame-resistant winceyette [cotton flannel], primarily no doubt on account of the additional cost, which has the effect of making the price per yard of treated winceyette in the region of that of plain brushed nylon material. It may perhaps be assumed that those who buy material in the piece, to make up at home, do so for reasons of economy. The majority of these customers, therefore, are not likely to regard as a good buy winceyette which may cost 2 shillings [28¢] to 3 shillings [42¢] more per yard than the ordinary untreated material. . . . It is believed that there is a certain amount of hesitancy by the public in buying chemically treated fabrics because of the "harsh feeling" as against untreated material.

In summary, we must admit that we are not satisfied with the present state of flame-retardancy as it applies to the nightwear industry, or to other areas of the apparel industry with the exception of those industrial safety clothing items cited. We cannot tell you that we can see a new fiber or a new chemical process or any other solution that would provide flame retardancy with the elements of price, comfort, and consumer satisfaction that the public gains from existing products.

Sound theoretical foundations have been constructed in this area. Some excellent basic research has been performed. We have made test runs and we have sought practical results. We have offered treated goods to some segments of the market. But we who are in the production area cannot yet write all the specifications for the kinds of finishes that would do the job for the mass markets. And although there has been an occasional public interest in fire-retardant goods, such demand has been conditioned on retention of low price and retention of qualities of comfort that no present flame-retardant finish affords. The industry meantime continues to devote extensive research effort to the study of flame-retardant processes, and has made such processes available where conditions of exposure to hazard has invited them, and where the substantially increased costs involved could be borne.

On behalf of the textile industry I want to emphasize our keen interest in problems of flammability and our conviction that the present Flammable Fabrics Act has proved its value. It successfully removed garments of real danger from the markets. It has permitted those fabrics and garments that have been in common use for generations to remain on the markets and to continue to give consumer satisfaction at reasonable cost. In view of the billions of garments distributed and the countless days and weeks and months of their useful and satisfactory service, we doubt that any evidence can be produced in any area that would convincingly or reasonably suggest a need for closer regulation.

# DEVELOPMENTS IN THE COTTON INDUSTRY*

WILLIAM M. SEGALL

National Cotton Council of America
Washington, D. C.

We are here on this occasion to review the progress that has been made in the prevention of accidents that occur through the flammability of fabrics. And although there may be some who view the situation with alarm, and insist that not enough progress has been made, I should like to state at the outset my feeling that, within the framework of the free-enterprise system under which we live, definite strides have been taken in the past 25 years toward minimizing—although admittedly not eliminating—this kind of accident. And I should like further to call attention to the role of the cotton industry in the progress that has been made in this respect.

The cotton industry has made significant contributions to the development of fire-resistant finishes. Representatives of the cotton industry helped to perfect the clothing-flammability test without which there would be no legislation on the flammability of textiles. The industry cosponsored and supported the Flammable Fabrics Act; today, people of the cotton industry are participating actively in every effort to provide consumers with greater protection from the dangers of fire.

This problem of fire safety has three separate aspects that I should like to have you think about with me for a little while. The first of these is the situation involving unusually hazardous fabrics: such items as brushed-rayon torch sweaters, cowboys' chaps on playsuits, nitrocellulose-coated fabrics, filmy nettings, etc. These are fabrics that are so dangerous that they should be eliminated from the market. The proscription of these fabrics was the task that Congress set itself in 1953. Let me quote to you a portion of Report No. 425 of the House

*Based on a paper presented at the *Conference on Burns and Flame-Retardant Fabrics,* held at The New York Academy of Medicine, December 2 and 3, 1966. The conference was sponsored by: the New York and Brooklyn Trauma Committee of the American College of Surgeons, Chicago, Ill.; The National Fire Protection Association, Boston, Mass.; the Section on Plastic and Reconstructive Surgery of The New York Academy of Medicine; and the Division of Accident Prevention of the U. S. Public Health Service, Washington, D. C. The conference was held in cooperation with the American Academy of Pediatrics, Evanston, Ill.; the American Public Health Association, New York, N. Y.; and the National Safety Council, Chicago, Ill.; and was supported by a grant from the U. S. Public Health Service.

of Representatives on H. R. 5069, the bill that later became the Flammable Fabrics Act: "The major problem in formulating legislation to control the use of dangerously flammable textiles is to discriminate between the conventional fabrics that present moderate and generally recognized hazards and the special types of fabrics which present unusual hazards and are highly dangerous." This, in essence, is the philosophy of the Flammable Fabrics Act: "... to discriminate between ... conventional fabrics ... and fabrics which present unusual hazards. ..." And in this the Flammable Fabrics Act has done its job admirably.

The second aspect of safety from fire with which we should be concerned is that involving hazardous, or potentially hazardous, situations or occupations, such as those of steel workers, military pilots, and others. Here we have a somewhat different and much more complicated problem. The danger from a hazardous *fabric* such as a "torch sweater" is that an accident can be caused by a tiny flame or other minor source of ignition. In a hazardous occupation a relatively slow-burning fabric would not necessarily prevent an accident, because the source of ignition could be overwhelmingly large or long-continuing. Thus for protection we require not merely nonpropagation of flame, we need also a barrier that will protect a man from a flame or source of ignition that may well impinge on him for a long time. The best answer to this problem is cotton treated with fire-retardant finishes. This treatment ensures not only that the fabric will not support combustion but that it will maintain a barrier of char for protection of the substrate–in this case a human body. And there has indeed been increased use in recent years of durably treated cotton fabrics used in protective clothing.

The third aspect of this whole problem of fire safety involves the extension of protection to clothing and fabrics considered to be of normal flammability and used under normal circumstances but which, through an element of carelessness, may still cause accidents. This is a problem still unsolved: one that will require more research and close cooperation between safety-minded organizations and the textile industry.

Almost all textile fibers are combustible to some degree and, if exposed to flame through carelessness, may cause injury by burning or melting. And although the Flammable Fabrics Act has been entirely successful in eliminating from the market particularly hazardous fabrics such as those used in torch sweaters, there are certain inadequacies to the test method as presently used.

In the first place, the test suffers from lack of *precision*. While it is perfectly capable of differentiating between fabrics that differ widely in their flammability characteristics—and this, to be sure, is what the test was designed to do—its ability to make finer distinctions is subject to question. The inherent variability in the test method and in the fabrics themselves can lead to erroneous conclusions.

There is also some question about the *validity* of the test, i.e., are we measuring in all cases what we think we are measuring? Fabrics that in everyone's opinion are completely safe are sometimes eliminated from commerce because of the failure of the test to provide adequate discrimination of flame intensity. For example, I am aware of instances in which two lightweight fabrics both burned rapidly—one with a small flame in less than 3½ seconds, the other with a large flame in slightly more than 3½ seconds. The latter was undoubtedly a more dangerous fabric, but it passed the flammability test.

Conversely, the lack of a method for testing narrow fabrics and loose fibrous materials may well allow some dangerous materials to be used. These shortcomings are now under study. New procedures for testing narrow fabrics and loose fibrous materials have been devised, and they are now being evaluated. Some research has also been done by the National Bureau of Standards on the measurement of flame intensity, but this is a complicated subject, and we are far from a solution for it.

Another shortcoming of the test method is its failure to take into account elements of hazard other than flaming. There are certain fabrics that resist flame propagation; but they do it by melting and falling away. It can easily be seen that such a thermoplastic fabric could lead to serious injury when used in apparel; burns occasioned by adherence to the skin of heated fibers could be as much hazard as flaming.

Now let us look at the subject of fire-retardant finishes. Chemical treatments to prevent the burning of textile fabrics have been with us for a long time. Simple nondurable treatments with such mixtures as borax and boric acid are still used today where properties such as hand and stiffness are not critical and durability is not needed. But it is obvious that for most textiles we need a treatment that is durable and that has no effect on other properties of the fabric or garment. The closest we have come to this is using organic phosphorus compounds such as THPC,* based on the work of U.S. Department of Agriculture scien-

*Tetrakis (hydroxymethyl) phosphonium chloride.

tists back in the early 1950's. And so, at present, we do indeed have finishes that are suitable for certain applications—outdoor fabrics, certain household fabrics, and a few specialized clothing items. But in general these finishes are deficient in hand, texture, absorbency, and other properties important in apparel. These deficiencies are particularly apparent when finishes are applied to lightweight fabrics in which the need is probably greater. Their effect on fabrics is to a large extent a result of the tremendous add-on (frequently 20 to 22 per cent) needed to produce resistance to flame, and this large add-on results also in high chemical cost, which makes the treated garments in many cases too expensive to be acceptable to consumers.

And so, although we have made some definite progress in protecting the public in the United States against injuries involving hazardous fabrics in normal situations, and normal fabrics in hazardous situations, we now must face the problem of normal fabrics in normal situations. What solutions can we offer? None, I am afraid. About all we can do at this time is to list what we might need in order to find the solution: information, education, and research.

First, there is a great dearth of factual information on the subject of injuries from burns involving clothing—and I want to stress my use of the word *factual!* There is entirely too much *mis*information being bruited about in the guise of fact. Unfortunately, the whole subject of injuries from burns is too fraught with emotion. There is no one, regardless of his private interests, who would not take any measures necessary to prevent a particular child from being injured in a particular accident. But at the risk of seeming insensitive, it behooves us to take a dispassionate look at the true facts about the flammability of fabrics.

Fabrics do burn. And people wearing garments made of fabrics do suffer injuries from burns. But whether a particular fabric, as used in a particular garment, bears any responsibility for the injury, is a much more complicated question. Statistics are cited on accidents "involving burning clothing." But "involving" cannot be taken as equivalent to "caused by." The person who is seriously burned because he was sprayed with flaming oil by an exploding heater would have been injured had he been wearing asbestos, or armor plate, or nothing at all.

For example, let me quote from a study made several years ago of accidents involving burns. This was "An Investigation of Fabrics Involved in Wearing Apparel Burns, by the Committee on Accident Prevention, American Academy of Pediatrics, and the Committee on Wearing Apparel, National Fire Protection Association." Both these groups are sponsors of this conference. Case No. 5 states that a "slip being worn by 12-year-old girl while she lighted an oil-fired range ignited when range exploded"; Case No. 6 says, ". . . shirt tail of 44-year-old man became moistened with range oil while he was cleaning the kitchen range. Shirt tail ignited when he went to the basement and opened the door of coal-fired furnace"; and Case No. 56 describes how a "19-year-old girl spilled fuel oil on nightgown when she got up to light oil stove. Ignition occurred when she bent down with match to light stove."

Surely no one could honestly assume that the fabric—whatever it was—was at fault in these cases. And surely no investigation of these fabrics could produce any information that would be of much value in a study of injuries from burns involving textiles. And surely any compilation of injuries that included a significant number of cases like these would be a weak weapon with which to indict "hazardous" clothing textiles.

I understand that the Public Health Service of the U.S. Department of Health, Education, and Welfare is presently working on a study of injuries from burns in which an attempt will be made fully to assess the causes, major and minor, of these accidents. It is my fervent hope that from this study we shall be able to obtain information on which to base future work in this area.

The second major need that I cited is for education. Education of consumers directed at reducing the carelessness that causes accidents could undoubtedly reduce injuries and save lives; but it probably is not the ultimate solution to the problem of flammable clothing. And while this is an area in which the cotton industry cannot take the lead—there are other groups far better qualified—we certainly want to offer our cooperation to any of these groups in any of their activities.

The third great need is for research—to develop improved fire-resistant finishes, at lower cost, with minimum effect on other fabric properties and, if possible, with other added benefits that consumers find desirable. The cotton industry has definite plans for increased research in this direction. A decision has already been made by the Cotton Producers Institute of this city to place a large contract with a well-known research organization for the development of improved methods for producing fire-retardant cotton fabrics.

The U.S. Department of Agriculture has a long record of successful accomplishments in this area on behalf of cotton, and it will, I am sure, continue to produce significant advances.

It would seem that, in addition, the situation might offer an important opportunity for research by the chemical industry. If a treatment could be developed that would solve the problem of the flammability of fabrics, with no effect on other properties of fabrics and garments, and with an add-on of perhaps 5 per cent on the weight of the goods, the potential market might be as much as 2 billion yards a year—depending on the cost of the treatment—which would consume some 25 million pounds of chemical—a tidy market, I should think, for any company or group of companies.

The cotton industry stands ready to offer its full cooperation to the fire-safety groups represented here or to anyone else, in making any practical approach to the problem of providing greater protection to the public in the United States.

# AIDING FABRIC AND GARMENT DESIGNERS IN REDUCING FIRE HAZARD*

HERBERT J. WOLLNER**

President, ACH Fiber Service, Inc.
Boston, Mass.

DARE we ask how the apparel industry of the world would stand up under an investigation similar to that to which the automobile industry has recently been subjected? The hazard of flammability in clothing is not an isolated problem. It is not simple and cannot be dissociated from the human being, from his behavior, his use of fire whether for cooking or smoking, from the environment of his own creation. Just as it is impossible to provide automotive equipment that is foolproof—so it is likewise impossible to provide clothing materials that are absolutely fireproof. The problem is certain to become increasingly complex as industrial developments unfold before an increasingly complex society. Take the idea of paper clothing. Trade journals announce its imminent reality. What will be the over-all impact of this new arrival?

As we know, wool still is the most secure and safe fiber in wide use as apparel. Nevertheless the American Wool Council remains constantly alert to the problem of hazard from fire confronting the textile industry. For example, it recognizes that when wool is blended with other more readily ignitable fibers, the relative noninflammability of such a mixture could be seriously impaired.

Research is being conducted throughout the world in regard to such matters. In 1964 Simms, in England, writing in the *Wool Record,* broadly discussed the subject and touched upon those aspects of it to which we believe attention must increasingly be paid. The research directed toward modification of combustible fibers should not cease,

*Based on a paper presented at the *Conference on Burns and Flame-Retardant Fabrics,* held at The New York Academy of Medicine, December 2 and 3, 1966. The conference was sponsored by: the New York and Brooklyn Trauma Committee of the American College of Surgeons, Chicago, Ill., The National Fire Protection Association, Boston, Mass.; the Section on Plastic and Reconstructive Surgery of The New York Academy of Medicine; and the Division of Accident Prevention of the U. S. Public Health Service, Washington, D. C. The conference was held in cooperation with the American Academy of Pediatrics, Evanston, Ill.; the American Public Health Association, New York, N. Y.; and the National Safety Council, Chicago, Ill.; and was supported by a grant from the U. S. Public Health Service.

**Representing the American Wool Council, New York, N. Y.

but I believe that emphasis should now be directed, in addition, elsewhere.

In accepting the request of the American Wool Council to represent wool at this conference, I do so in the full realization that such contributions as might be made would have to grow from a broader base of concept than merely, shall we say, the promotion of wool as a fiber. Actually, there is not enough wool produced in the entire world to take care of merely the incidental clothing needs of mankind. In light of this fact, it is academic to talk about the very real advantages of wool fabric and wool clothing. To meet man's apparel and textile needs, fibers must be obtained from sources other than animal. These other sources are mainly vegetable and synthetic.

In view of this, it has seemed appropriate to reexamine the whole burden of the problem that confronts us and to seek some suitable suggestion that would help in clarifying the over-all need. The American Wool Council has shown in its film on the flammability of fabrics some of the simpler difficulties to which the clothing designer and the prudent housewife, not to mention the physician and the fire marshal, are subjected.

I now offer some ideas on immediate steps that might well be taken.

The large, well-staffed and well-directed research laboratories of the total fiber industry have contributed greatly in the past to our better understanding of the nature of fiber combustibility and, undoubtedly, they will do so in the future. It is to be expected that, as these findings from research are reflected in fiber modification, an important element in the resolving of the problem of flammability will be met.

This however is not the entire issue. One is persuaded that those who are responsible for the design of garments, the construction of draperies and the like, have very much to contribute toward solving the problem, and that not enough has been done in this area. Yet here in the intermediary position between fiber and fabric manufacturer on the one hand, and the retailer on the other, is a most essential part of the industry which, through its possible lack of discrimination in choice of fiber or fabric combinations, can hold the balance between success and failure. Very little organized knowledge is available about the circumstances that occasion and promote fire accidents involving garments and draperies and upholstery. This is regrettable.

It is my view that the first order of importance in any national effort should now be accorded a sound program for gathering information. This should be done for the purpose of demonstrably establishing, in terms of incidence, frequency, circumstances, etc., the kinds of fiber, fabric construction, and especially garment design associated with causing or promoting fires. Such data should be computerized, and this information should then be translated into meanings that will serve our great garment design and manufacturing industry. Our garment and drapery designers and manufacturers, in the presence of a competitive market, can be readily expected to use competent information when it is properly made available to them and translated into trade or commercial terms.

Such a system on a continuing basis would demonstrate its value by quickly pointing out areas of vulnerability as new products are brought on the market. Types of fabric construction most susceptible to hazard might then also become matters of immediate notice and interest to home economists, interior decorators, and architects.

I suggest that the U. S. Public Health Service prepare, with the aid of experts in these fields, a suitable and simple report form to be distributed to hospitals, fire departments, insurance companies, first-aid stations and the like in appropriately selected geographic sample areas. On these forms a detailed description in codified form would be made for return to a central office after each fabric-involved fire. It would list such definable matter as to how fabric appeared to be related to the cause or promotion of the fire and would include suitable descriptive details including, if possible, the country of origin of the garment. This information should be such as to help garment designers, interior decorators, and others in the conduct of their affairs. Let me repeat, these simple forms should be made out for transmission to a center equipped with computers where the data could be made quickly available for significant study. The information so derived, periodically distributed to interested groups such as designers and makers of garments, fabric manufacturers, and the like, can become an instrument for constructive recognition of sore spots and a ready index of areas where changes seem desirable.

A number of years ago a vogue for brushed sweaters of a flammable synthetic fiber resulted in injuries from burning incurred by some of those who wore them, for the sweaters caught fire from lighted cigarets and other such sources of ignition. Had a ready and rapid index of experience been available, much misery might have conceivably been averted.

The laboratories of the fiber producers should continue their very contributive effort along the lines that presently engage them. The time has arrived, however, when garment designers, retailers and others should have before them results of experience with the fibers in actual use. I am persuaded that they will take constructive advantage of any such development and that its results will be reflected in the development of products of a high level of security.

# FIBERGLAS: A TRUE FIRE-SAFETY FABRIC*

JOHN F. FERGER

Vice-President
Decorative and Home Furnishings Division
Owens-Corning Fiberglas Corporation
New York, N. Y.

THERE are two inherently fire-safe textile materials known to man, and both are derived from minerals: glass fiber and asbestos. One is glass; the other is rock. Both materials are inorganic, so neither will burn. Textile glass fiber (available under the trademark "Fiberglas") starts to soften at 975° F. and to melt at 1,500° F. It will *not* burn.

The big difference between the two materials is that glass fiber has great versatility as a textile for end products. In 1965—for the first time —production of glass-fiber fabrics surpassed woolen and worsted fabric output. Weavers produced a total of 280 million linear yards of glass-fiber fabrics in 1965.

The point here is that in glass fiber you have a *true* fire-safe commercial fabric, not a laboratory experiment—a material attractive to consumers and readily available in a variety of end products.

If we could sell Fiberglas textile materials in their unfinished state my speech would end now, for we should then have the ultimate in a noncombustible textile material. In order to turn greige goods into consumer products, however, organic resins and colorants must be added to achieve desirable esthetic effects. Selectively compounded and properly applied, these organic finishes do not detract from the fire-safety features of Fiberglas products. Improper selection and use of such materials can endanger the fire-safety characteristics inherent in the product, and great care is constantly taken to guard against such circumstances.

Our company's policy in this area is simply to do everything in its

*Based on a paper presented at the *Conference on Burns and Flame-Retardant Fabrics,* held at The New York Academy of Medicine, December 2 and 3, 1966. The conference was sponsored by: the New York and Brooklyn Trauma Committee of the American College of Surgeons, Chicago, Ill.; The National Fire Protection Association, Boston, Mass.; the Section on Plastic and Reconstructive Surgery of The New York Academy of Medicine; and the Division of Accident Prevention of the U. S. Public Health Service, Washington, D. C. The conference was held in cooperation with the American Academy of Pediatrics, Evanston, Ill.; the American Public Health Association, New York, N. Y.; and the National Safety Council, Chicago, Ill.; and was supported by a grant from the U. S. Public Health Service.

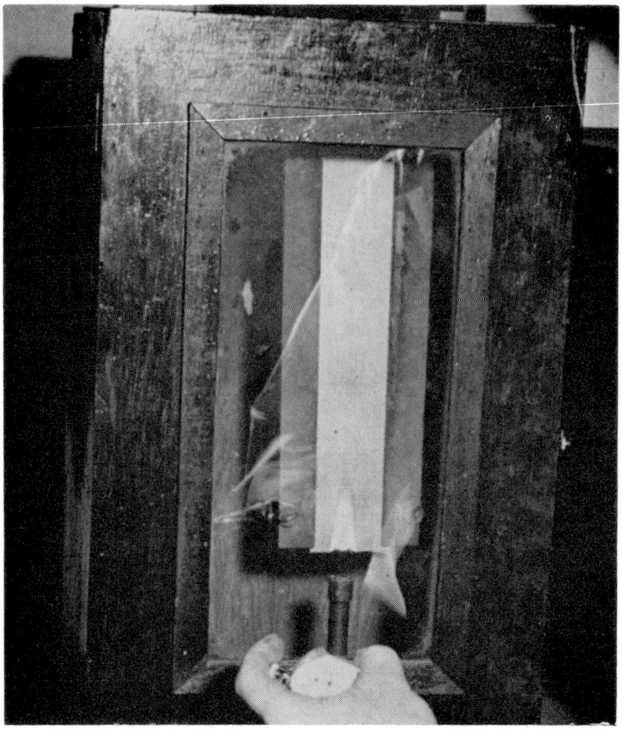

Fig. 1. A test, No. 34, of the American Association of Textile Chemists and Colorists (AATCC). A piece of fabric is held under a $1\frac{1}{2}$-in. flame for 12 full seconds. As may be seen, the finishing and coloring coating on the material (in this case mattress ticking) chars but does not burn (the glass fiber, of course can neither char nor burn). So far the fabric is acceptable.

power to maintain the integrity of Fiberglas. In this case we are talking about fire-safety, so we put our materials through a battery of fire tests from unfinished greige goods to end products.

The heart of our "integrity" program is a series of tests run on any new product marketed for the first time. We use standard tests of the American Association of Textile Chemists and Colorists along with more severe tests such as the series developed by the Boston and Los Angeles fire departments. We also modify standard tests to make them even more stringent. We feel that if a fabric supports combustion for any reason, it is considered combustible and not acceptable.

Some of the tests that we perform on fabrics and end products made of Fiberglas textiles are shown in Figures 1 to 8. The program is more extensive than many carried out by manufacturers of combustible

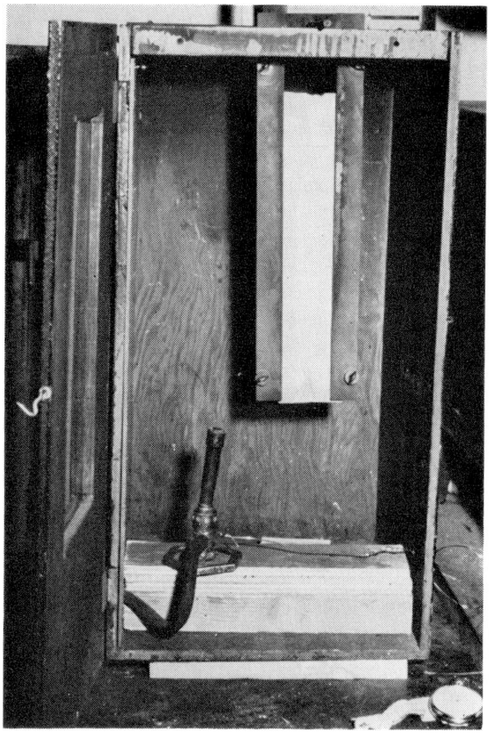

Fig. 2. In a modified AATCC test a $1\frac{1}{2}$-in. flame is held under the fabric shown in Figure 1 for 2 seconds and then removed. This is a more severe test and, this time, the coating on the fibers of the fabric burns all the way. We rate this ticking combustible and, therefore, unacceptable.

fibers because we want to be sure our material keeps its inherent fire-safe characteristics.

This testing, however, is only the first step in the program that ensures the integrity of our products. Once a fabric is rated as combustible we offer technical assistance to the weaver, finisher, or manufacturer to help him solve his flammability problems. We also request a corrected sample for retesting.

Our technical staff, working with weavers and converters, has solved numerous problems in finishing and coloring Fiberglas fabrics and in developing fire-safe blends and laminates. Recently, for example, we rated an acrylic-backed drapery as combustible. The weaver accepted our assistance, the product was modified, and recent tests show the fabric is now rated noncombustible.

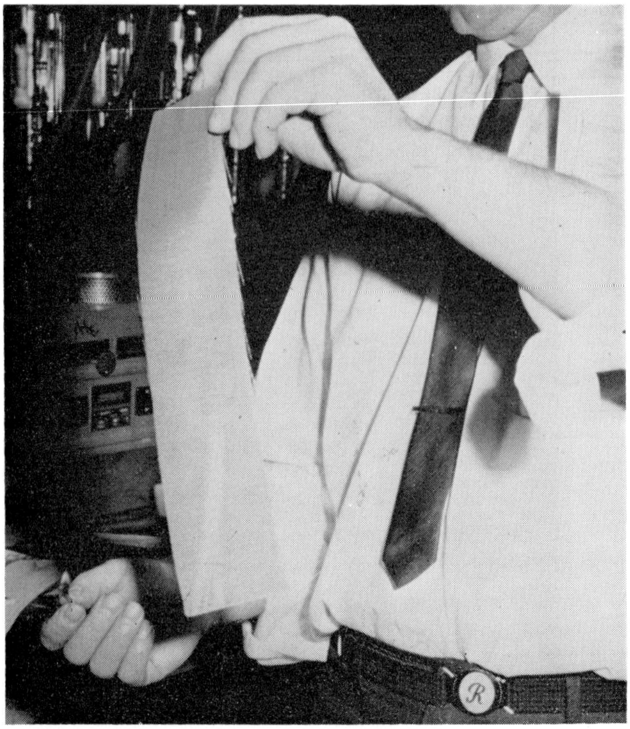

Fig. 3. The simplest test is the match test. Again, the coating on the ticking shown in Figures 1 and 2 burns and is rated combustible. The Los Angeles Fire Department has devised a mattress test that requires a burning cigarette to be placed on a simulated mattress. This mattress has Fiberglas ticking filled with urethane foam and cotton batting. This test has been modified slightly by substituting a methenamine tablet that gives a controlled 90-second burn for the cigarette.

If we find a company that will not accurately rate its fabrics, certain measures can be taken, such as withholding endorsement, merchandising support, and technical assistance. However, we have never had to do this.

The integrity program has proved so effective that all weavers volunteer their new fabrics for testing by Owens-Corning Fiberglas because they know that their customers—the manufacturers of draperies and bedspreads—will ask them what our testing has shown.

Going back to a point I made before: Fiberglas is not an experimental fabric. In the decorative area alone we are predicting that 183 million yards of glass-fiber fabrics will have been produced by the end of 1966.

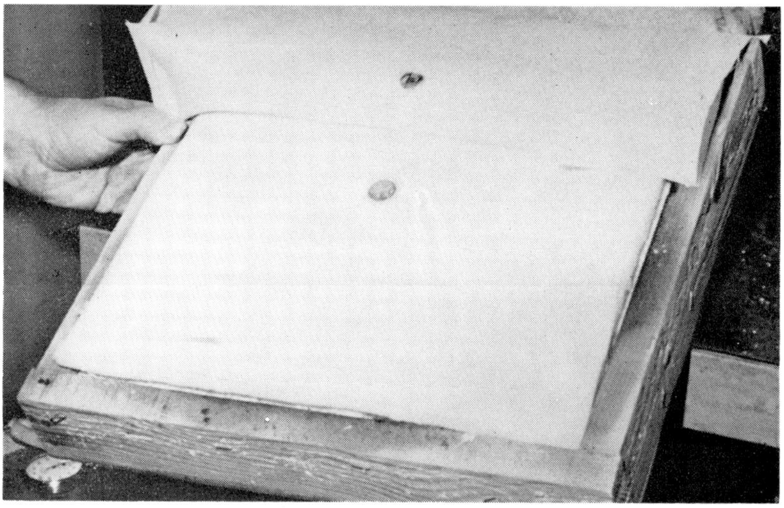

Fig. 4. Here the foam of the mattress cited in Figure 3 has melted but the cotton is not smoldering and the Fiberglas ticking appears charred but still intact.

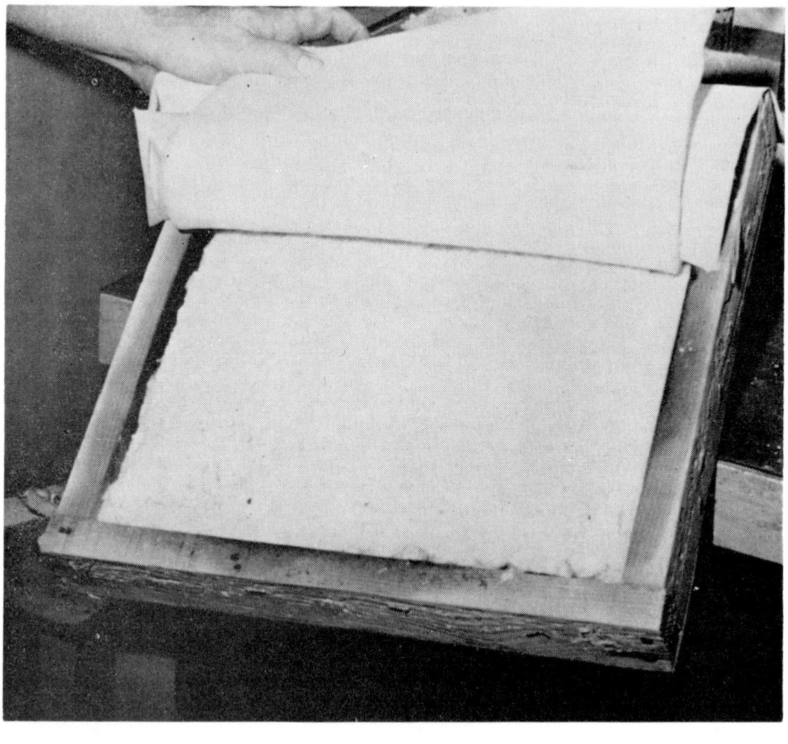

Fig. 5. The more severe version of the test cited in Figure 4 requires that a cotton sheet be placed on top of the bed to make conditions as realistic as possible.

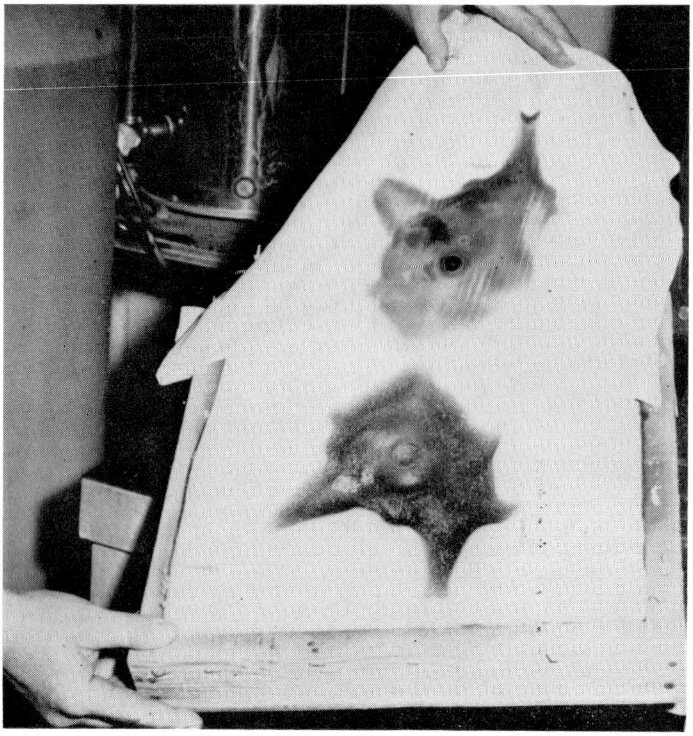

Fig. 6. Here the foam has melted again, but the cotton is safe and the Fiberglas ticking, although it appears charred, is intact. This ticking was rated noncombustible. The Boston Fire Department has developed its own stringent fire tests adapted from the AATCC versions. The major change is that the height of the flame is raised from one and a half to six inches.

Fiberglas is a great commercial success because it offers consumers a unique range of wanted features. Besides being fire-safe, Fiberglas fabrics resist rot and mildew, they always hold their original shape, they cannot shrink, they resist fading, and they are virtually maintenance-free. Fiberglas fabric is the original drip-dry, wrinkle-free, permanent-press fabric. To these desirable qualities the weavers, manufacturers, and finishers have added many new advances in styling.

Let us take a look at the areas in which Fiberglas fabrics are a major factor, and also at some imminent applications:

The biggest use for Fiberglas fabrics continues to be draperies. We enjoy a leading position in this market. Fire safety, of course, is an important property for draperies. Our company has received numerous

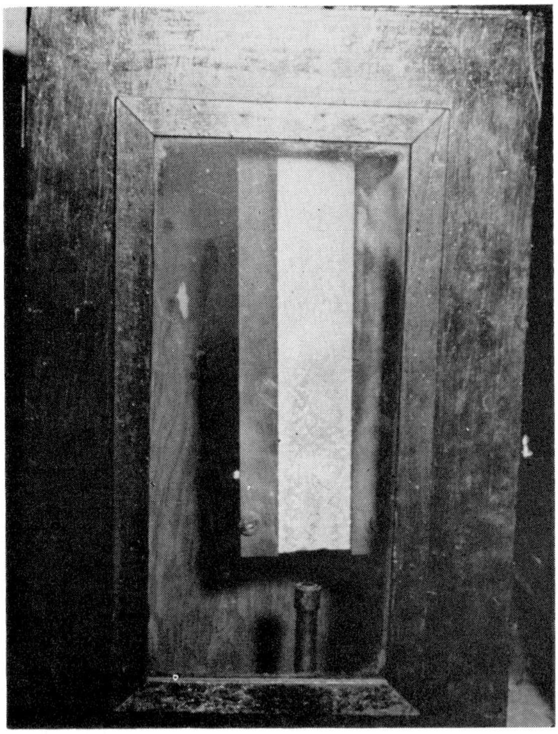

Fig. 7. Here a drapery fabric is undergoing the first Boston test. So far it is acceptable. Even after the more severe 2-second test the fabric does not burn.

letters from consumers stating that their houses have burned to the ground and the only things left intact were their Fiberglas draperies.

New curtains for hospital cubicles are now being tested, and users report a unique safety feature: in the event of an oxygen fire, the curtains can be thrown over the patient as a protective covering.

Window shades are coming back into favor, and Fiberglas textiles constitute worthy candidates for use in their manufacture.

Recently Fiberglas textile products have been making a move away from the windows to other portions of the home. This development was previously not feasible because of certain limitations in our fiber line. Problems of fiber-to-fiber abrasion, lack of softness, comfort, and flexibility all restricted Fiberglas to beautifying the window.

But with the development of Fiberglas Beta (Owens-Corning's trademark name for "B" size fiber), the finest commercially available

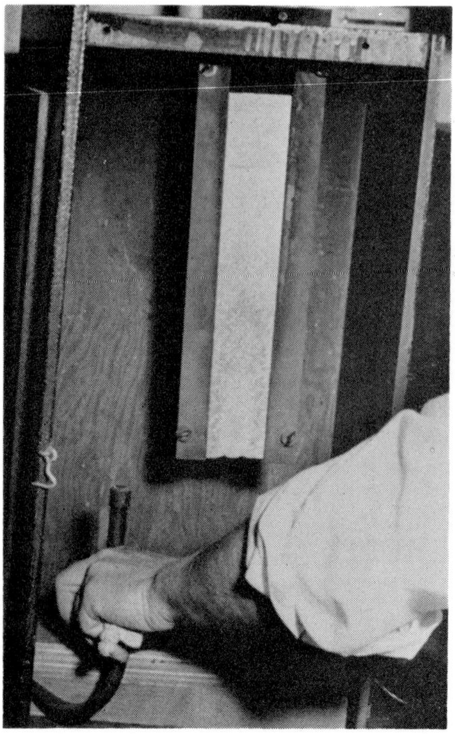

Fig. 8. The drapery fabric shown in Figure 7 passes the severe 2-second test. It also passed the match test and was accordingly rated noncombustible.

textile fiber known, glass-fiber fabrics offer the long-desired softness, pliability, and flexibility needed for other decorative applications of fabrics, such as bedspreads, table cloths, and mattress ticking. We are now cooperating with the quartermaster of the U.S. Army in testing and evaluating a fire-safe mattress ticking.

We are also experimenting with blankets containing 30 per cent Beta and 70 per cent acrylic yarns. Our tests show that Beta fibers give the blankets substantially increased fire retardance.

The concept of blending Beta with organic man-made fiber fabrics shows great promise and is an area we are exploring actively.

The fire-safety of Fiberglas has also helped to increase the production of industrial, commercial, and other hard-use glass-fiber fabrics to 134 million linear yards in 1965. Some typical applications are: filter bags, now used at temperatures as high as 700° F., inflatable buildings, such as the tennis dome at Forest Hills, awnings for home and commercial use, and protective clothing, such as auto-racing suits.

Looking into the future, we see other applications, as in slip covers and upholstery—all with the easy-care, fire-safe features of the Fiberglas textiles drapery, plus a permanent, uniform fit.

Still further ahead we see that the use of fire-resistant Fiberglas could mean a big increase in safety for apparel such as dresses, lounging robes, and rainwear.

Louis Segal, of the California State Fire Marshal's Office, has mentioned the problem of fire-retardant ready-to-wear apparel. He has pointed out that to satisfy the needs and demands of the public, clothing must have many attributes—style, comfort, wear, ease of maintenance, and resistance to spots and wrinkles. When present developments are completed we feel confident that Fiberglas will meet all these criteria.

As more and more Fiberglas products are accepted by the market—for reasons ranging from ease of care and high style to resistance to fire—it should be of some comfort to all of us to know that these products will be helping to reduce that terrible statistic—6,000 persons killed in domestic fires in 1965.

# THE USE OF SYNTHETIC MODACRYLIC FIBERS*

R. S. Brissette

Marketing Manager, Fibers and Fabrics Division
Union Carbide Corporation
New York, N. Y.

In presenting for your consideration an account of our experience in the use of synthetic modacrylic fiber I intend to describe the contributions that this fiber makes to the problem of producing flame-retardant fabrics. I wish also to point out, I hope realistically, the very real problems of developing and marketing such fabrics. Personal safety in the use of fabrics is a minor consideration for the consumer, as it is in regard to many other products. Most people put greater value on the glamour and esthetics of fabrics than they do on their own safety.

There are three natural divisions of the subject that I wish to cover: 1) what we are trying to accomplish in dealing with the problem of flammable fabrics and what the textiles are that we are using; 2) how to solve the problem of flame-retardant fabrics by exploiting the particular properties of modacrylic fibers; and 3) how these properties have been combined in such a way as to provide a salable, usable product, yet one that provides real safety from fire.

Textiles, perhaps more than any single category of products, are bought by the consumer primarily for esthetic reasons: for qualities of style, color, and design. The basic function of textiles—to cover someone or to keep him warm—is assumed by the customer to be inherent in the product he buys. A woman in buying a coat is not particularly worried in most instances as to whether it will keep her warm. She is more concerned about the style, the cut, the color, the trimming and, to some degree, about the label. This outlook applies to sweaters, dresses, stockings, and other such items. Some functional aspects of textiles used in clothing, home furnishings, blankets, carpets, or other such products *can* be promoted to some extent: for instance, the

*Based on a paper presented at the *Conference on Burns and Flame-Retardant Fabrics,* held at The New York Academy of Medicine, December 2 and 3, 1966. The conference was sponsored by: the New York and Brooklyn Trauma Committee of the American College of Surgeons, Chicago, Ill.; The National Fire Protection Association, Boston, Mass.; the Section on Plastic and Reconstructive Surgery of The New York Academy of Medicine; and the Division of Accident Prevention of the U. S. Public Health Service, Washington, D. C. The conference was held in cooperation with the American Academy of Pediatrics, Evanston, Ill.; the American Public Health Association, New York, N. Y.; and the National Safety Council, Chicago, Ill.; and was supported by a grant from the U. S. Public Health Service.

warmth without weight of synthetic fabrics and their durable creases, which make it easier for the housewife to take care of them. These promotional qualities of fabrics accord with the modern trend toward automated, easier living.

But there still remains the fundamental problem of always having to set first the design and the style in fabrics that are largely assumed to serve their basic functions. There is also in our technological age the automatic urge to develop more efficient manufacturing techniques to reduce prices and help expand markets. These techniques generally create opportunities for new design and styling and thus reinforce this aspect of the production and marketing of textiles. I mentioned a moment ago the development of the durable crease, which illustrates how necessary it is for these fabrics to be adaptable to present methods of laundering and dry cleaning.

I think the proliferation of basic fiber types further indicates the need for active consideration of style and design as they apply to the construction of textiles. There are, for example, the filament nylon fibers for upholstery, dress goods, and lingerie; the acrylic, modacrylic fibers for carpets and scatter rugs; the modacrylic fibers for pile coats and pile trim; a combination of polyesters with cotton for dress goods, slacks, and suits. Each one of these fibers has created for itself certain markets based on the purposes it serves best, but in almost every instance it is the prime function of the fiber to provide latitude for creativity and ease of care once the product is in the hands of the consumer.

It must be kept in mind that modacrylics, like other types of fiber, cannot solve all the problems of esthetics, processing, care in the home, construction of the fiber, etc. Modacrylics do provide a latitude in style in certain markets, as we shall see shortly, but if they are set aflame the fire is self-extinguishing. This fact will remain of minor importance to the consumer until he or she is specifically educated as to the value of this property in products and, more important, becomes aware that textiles made from these fibers are available and that they meet the criterion of flame retardancy.

The problem accordingly becomes one of development, of marketing and, primarily, of education: a product must be given style to meet demands in certain areas; it must be marketed in such a way that the consumer will recognize the need for their fire-retardant qualities; and, third, this characteristic must appeal to the consumer educated as to the value of having nonflammable products in her home. These considerations, then, constitute the problem. What does the modacrylic fiber contribute toward its solution?

## Solutions Through Modacrylics

Modacrylic fiber, as defined by the Federal Trade Commission, is one made from a copolymer resin that contains not more than 85 per cent of acrylonitrile, the remainder consisting of several resins such as vinyl chloride or vinylidene chloride. These fibers are primarily available in what is known as staple form, which is similar to that of cotton or wool, in that the fibers are short and can accordingly be processed into yarns for knitting, weaving, felting, tufting, and other such uses. The fibers when made into fabrics produce goods that are warm, soft, and generally characterized as having a wool- or furlike "hand" and appearance. The fibers are dyeable, they are basically and chemically inert and, most interesting to participants in this conference, they can be ignited but the fire is self-extinguishing when the source of the flame is removed.

I believe that it is important to note that the fibers, while burning, tend to shrink and contract but do not drip a hot melt that in some cases can be more of a problem than the burning fabric itself. The fact that fire ignited in modacrylics extinguishes itself is due primarily to the presence of vinyl chloride or the vinyl chloride copolymer, which is inherently nonflammable; a component that, moreover, under the temperatures of ignition, will release products that extinguish the flame when the source of it is removed. The presence of modacrylic fiber in blends in sufficiently high amounts will therefore act as a fire extinguisher for any more flammable component such as cotton or rayon. The ignition and burning of a fabric in actual service involves many factors, such as the temperature of the source of the ignition, the time of exposure, the angle at which the fabric is exposed, air currents in the area, density and distribution of fibers in the fabric, and many other variables.

A very real problem in developing suitable fabrics that are nonflammable is that there are four or five tests sponsored by the trade or required by the government that are used regularly, and none of these under the same circumstances will give the same results. At this point I think it will be well to consider some specific instances in which modacrylic fiber can definitely make a contribution to the safety of a textile composed of modacrylic alone or of blends containing it.

## Typical Applications

To illustrate what we are talking about in terms of esthetic construction and uses let me cite specific samples and demonstrations.

*Work clothing*. Fires ignited in garments made from 100 per cent modacrylic fibers are self-extinguishing. This fiber, moreover, provides a high degree of chemical resistance and cleanability in a soft, comfortable garment. A fire in a blended fabric of which one third of the composition is cotton in order to provide increased absorption of moisture displays the same self-extinguishing characteristics although it burns somewhat longer. More important, perhaps, there is no afterglow, since the afterglow of many cellulosic items can also contribute to a bad burn.

*Rugs*. A popular item in the home today is a loose, fluffy, lustrous scatter rug. In this product the fibers are loose and widely separated, and there is good air flow among them. If wrong fibers are used on the surface, the rug is highly flammable. A wholly modacrylic rug of this type, however, is hard to ignite and the fire is self-extinguishing. The ignition of hearth rugs caused by flying sparks from open fireplaces is not common in the United States but is prevalent in Europe, where these rugs are extremely popular. In England particularly this product, known as a hearth rug, is used in front of open fires where small children often play. The contribution made by nonflammable modacrylics in this area is of particular value.

*Blankets*. Of the many popular types of blanket on the market today there are two that are basically fire-resistant: the wool blanket and the modacrylic. In developing the modacrylic blanket it was necessary to build into it warmth, stability of color, washability, and hand, all at a price that the consumer would find attractive. The modacrylic blanket has inherently and for its complete life the characteristic of extinguishing any fire ignited in it. A burning match or any other source of flame, if dropped on a blanket composed of synthetics, starts a fire of a chemical type that may consume the entire blanket within a very short time. However a similar source of flame on a blanket of 100 per cent modacrylic fiber causes fire that is confined to the immediate area, and no further damage or ignition is possible. The public requires much education in this connection; and this education will become increasingly important as time goes on both for adults and children, and especially for the traveling public as it moves from one hostelry to another.

*Apparel pile fabrics.* A popular fabric today is that used in the coat of simulated fur, which can be made from a number of fibers or from fiber blends; in its most popular forms it generally contains modacrylics.

Wrongly selected surface fibers are subject to a flash fire across the surface of a pile that can produce burns about the face and hands before the garment can be taken off or before the fire can be extinguished. Modacrylic fibers contribute the necessary esthetic and wear characteristics to these fabrics and still provide a degree of fire retardancy when used in the proper proportions even where more flammable fibers are present.

*Hair goods.* Finally I should like to cite the characteristics of Dynel modacrylic in something that appeals to almost all women—and that is hair. Wigs and hairpieces of 100 per cent Dynel are available all over the world in great variety and are promoted as the realistic, practical substitute for real hair. Dynel can be curled, set, braided, washed and, if necessary, dry cleaned. One might say that since this fiber is produced in a continuous strand, we are selling beauty by the mile. Important, we think, but not of real interest to women, is the fact that a fire ignited in this fiber is self-extinguishing and that, if ignited, this fiber will not melt and drip. Human hair, as everyone knows, will flare dramatically when touched with a flame.

## Summary

This, then, has been a capsule review of my firm's Dynel modacrylic fiber and of the various textile and fiber products in which it is used. In making all possible products, from rugs to wigs, the same basic material is used, and this material has the basic property of being hard to ignite; moreover, any fire ignited in it extinguishes itself. Thus flame retardancy is already present in garments and other products based on Dynel—as I have tried to show. That the consumer is not often aware of this is in the end, I feel, primarily because she is more often motivated by esthetic considerations than by anything else. Safety from fire in apparel is an area in which more education of the consumer is required; and this goal is a continuing aim of our development and merchandising policies and programs.

# ROLE OF THE FIRE PROTECTION AGENCY*

LOUIS SEGAL

Fire Prevention Engineer
California State Fire Marshal's Office
Los Angeles, Calif.

I AM speaking to you today in a dual capacity, both as a representative of the State Fire Marshal's Office of California and as chairman of the Committee on Wearing Apparel of the National Fire Protection Association of Boston, Mass. This is quite appropriate, because in my admittedly biased opinion these two agencies have been by far the most active of all groups attempting to solve the clothing fire problem in behalf of the public.

In 1945 the State of California enacted the first legislation of its kind in this field. The legislature passed a law that expressed concern over the hazards of flammable clothing, and directed the state fire marshal to conduct research and establish reasonable regulations to protect the citizens of the state.

In undertaking this program of research, we found that the only group actively engaged in similar work was the American Association of Textile Chemists and Colorists. The AATCC, an industry-oriented organization, was most cooperative and helpful, and we worked closely with it in the development of our standards and regulations, which were put into effect on January 6, 1947.

These regulations, while of quite limited scope, were of inestimable value just 5 years later when the great so-called "torch sweater" uproar occurred. The extremely hazardous nature and the widespread sale of these sweaters were first discovered by our office in Los Angeles in December 1951.

At that time we were the only governmental agency in the country

*Based on a paper presented at the *Conference on Burns and Flame-Retardant Fabrics,* held at The New York Academy of Medicine, December 2 and 3, 1966. The conference was sponsored by: the New York and Brooklyn Trauma Committee of the American College of Surgeons, Chicago, Ill.; The National Fire Protection Association, Boston, Mass.; the Section on Plastic and Reconstructive Surgery of The New York Academy of Medicine; and the Division of Accident Prevention of the U. S. Public Health Service, Washington, D. C. The conference was held in cooperation with the American Academy of Pediatrics, Evanston, Ill.; the American Public Health Association, New York, N. Y.; and the National Safety Council, Chicago, Ill.; and was supported by a grant from the U. S. Public Health Service.

in a position to take direct legal action against the vendors, which we did with considerable success. However, our first and most vigorous response was to warn the public through all available news media regarding these dangerous articles. The resulting publicity soon reached nationwide proportions. Not only did this publicity greatly increase public awareness of the hazards of flammable clothing, but it also attracted the attention of Congress and was no doubt largely responsible for passage of the Federal Flammable Fabrics Act in 1953.

Meanwhile the National Fire Protection Association had been contemplating the formation of a Committee on Wearing Apparel, and had been actively interested in our work in California. Again, the sweater episode probably furnished the necessary impetus to hasten decision, and the committee was officially established early in 1952.

As with all committees of the National Fire Protection Association (NFPA), the Committee on Wearing Apparel is made up of persons providing a well-balanced representation of all the broad interests concerned with clothing-fire safety. Present membership includes four persons from the fire services, three from insurance companies, two from retail merchants or associations, five from the textile fiber or fabric industry, one each from the National Safety Council and the National Bureau of Standards, and two from the medical profession. The last are Dr. Carl A. Moyer of the Michigan Technological University, and Dr. Robert Trimby, representing the American Academy of Pediatrics.

Over the years, the Committee's work has been marked by some rather vigorous controversy and dissension. In 1953 the textile industry fostered the promulgation by the U.S. Department of Commerce of a Commercial Standard, CS 191-53, *Flammability of Clothing Textiles.* This later was incorporated as the reference standard in the Federal Flammable Fabrics Act.

The basic disagreement on the NFPA Committee has been primarily between industry and fire service representatives as to the adequacy of the Commercial Standard. Over objections made by industry, both in and out of the committee, NFPA Standard No. 702 was adopted in 1962, incorporating several significant differences from the Commercial Standard. The disagreement continues, but apparently we are no longer fighting a lonely battle. The federal law and the Commercial Standard are currently undergoing close scrutiny by both Congress and the U.S. Department of Commerce.

Initial activities of the committee stressed research on the burning properties of textiles and fibers, and the development of appropriate test methods and a recommended safety standard. We also endeavored to collect detailed information regarding clothing-fire incidents, and we compiled statistical data from many case histories.

Currently, the primary effort of our committee is to foster and encourage a vigorous program of public education regarding the hazards of flammable clothing. We are convinced that therein lies the only hope for an immediate, significant reduction in clothing-fire casualties. More restrictive legislation, even if attainable, can be of only very limited value in solving the over-all problem. There is much hope for the future in increased usage of existing or still-to-be-discovered inherently flame-resistant synthetic fibers, and in improved techniques for providing durable flame resistance by chemical processes. But for now, the immediate and tragic problem is that *the great bulk of our population simply is not aware that clothing can burn.*

The scope of the effort which any fire protection agency can devote toward reducing the number of clothing-fire casualties must depend of course on the size of the organization, available time, manpower, and budget. The problem is highly complex, and the scope of activities can be very broad. It is vitally important, however, that every fire protection agency of whatever size, even down to the one-man Volunteer Fire Department should try to do at least two things:

First, it should investigate all clothing-fire accidents. It is not enough for us to know just that the clothes people wear are catching fire. We need to know who, how, why, what, where, and when. More specifically, we need to know the age and sex of the victim, his physical and mental condition, detailed circumstances of the accident, the source of ignition, the type of fabric and style of garment, and what action was taken by the victim or others at the time. All remaining clothing of the victim should be retained for testing whenever possible.

Second, every agency should carry on a continuing and effective program of public education. We must succeed in making almost 200 million people much more aware than they are now that much of the common, everyday clothing in wide general use is readily flammable. This is a great challenge and a most difficult assignment, because there is tremendous competition for the public's attention. However, there is only one alternative, and I am sure you will agree that it is unacceptble. The alternative is to continue to tolerate about 2,000 fatalities annually from the ignition of clothing, and to continue to fill untold thousands of hospital beds with critically burned victims.

We in the fire service like to believe that we are making some progress in the field of fire prevention, but there are still far too many fire casualties, and our failures, when they survive, become your patients. Clothing fires account for thousands of these patients, and many of you have decided to practice preventive medicine by enlisting yourselves directly in this aspect of fire prevention work. We fervently welcome and applaud this decision.

# THE FEDERAL FLAMMABLE FABRICS ACT*

HENRY D. STRINGER

Director, Bureau of Textiles and Furs
Federal Trade Commission
Washington, D. C.

THE Federal Flammable Fabrics Act became effective on July 1, 1954. The purpose of the act was "To prohibit the introduction or movement in interstate commerce of articles of wearing apparel and fabrics that are so highly flammable as to be dangerous when worn by individuals, and for other purposes."

The law was enacted because of a rash of burnings resulting from the sale of so-called torch sweaters and from the use of nitrocellulose materials in clothing.

I want to emphasize that the act does not prohibit the sale of flammable clothing but only of those articles of apparel and fabrics that are unusually flammable, that is, those that ignite easily and burn with extreme rapidity.

Articles of apparel made from textiles are tested under Commercial Standard 191-53. The tests are performed in an apparatus described in the standard and under conditions prescribed in it. The specimens tested are each 2 by 6 inches. Preliminary tests are made to determine the direction of the fastest burning. Each specimen is placed in a holder, and is tested on a bone-dry basis. The specimen is placed in the apparatus at a 45 degree angle. A stop watch is used, and there is a flame impingement of 1 second. If the specimen ignites, it burns a stop thread on burning upward, and a dropped weight stops the timing mechanism. If, in the case of a fabric that has a plain surface, the average burning time is 3.5 seconds or more, the fabric is Class I: normal

*Based on a paper presented at the *Conference on Burns and Flame-Retardant Fabrics,* held at The New York Academy of Medicine, December 2 and 3, 1966. The conference was sponsored by: the New York and Brooklyn Trauma Committee of the American College of Surgeons, Chicago, Ill.; The National Fire Protection Association, Boston, Mass.; the Section on Plastic and Reconstructive Surgery of The New York Academy of Medicine; and the Division of Accident Prevention of the U. S. Public Health Service, Washington, D. C. The conference was held in cooperation with the American Academy of Pediatrics, Evanston, Ill.; the American Public Health Association, New York, N. Y.; and the National Safety Council, Chicago, Ill.; and was supported by a grant from the U. S. Public Health Service.

The views expressed in this paper are those of the speaker, not necessarily those of the Federal Trade Commission.

flammability. If the average burning time of 5 specimens is less than 3.5 seconds, then 5 more specimens are tested and the average of the 10 is taken. If the average time is less than 3.5 seconds, the fabrics are Class III: rapid and intense burning.

A fabric that has a raised fiber surface is tested in the same manner; however, it is necessary to have a base fabric ignition or fusing with an average timing of less than 4 seconds to have a Class III: rapid and intense burning.

The Commercial Standard also provides for dry cleaning and washing under certain circumstances.

Shortly after the act became effective we wrote the state fire marshals of all the states, asking them to advise us of burnings from ignited clothing and to furnish us with samples of the cloth if possible.

During the 12 years that the law has been in effect we have received information and samples in many cases of burns. In only one of the reported cases did the fabric fail the test prescribed under the Flammable Fabrics Act. In that case some well-meaning ladies of an auxiliary of a veterans' organization went into a retail store and bought cotton blankets that they made into bed jackets for patients in a veterans' hospital.

From all these facts one may conclude that the Flammable Fabrics Act has not prevented the sale of clothing and fabrics that burn and cause injuries and death. The act has removed from the market only those fabrics that are unusually hazardous.

Generally speaking, textiles that do fail the test are fabrics that have raised fiber surfaces and extremely sheer fabrics, particularly those made of fibers of the cellulosic family.

One cannot say on these grounds that the Flammable Fabrics Act has been a failure, for it was designed only to remove from the market fabrics that were unusually hazardous. But, as I have said before, it has not prevented people from receiving burns from ignited clothing.

I think one serious shortcoming in the Commercial Standard is the failure, in the case of plain surface fabrics, to take into account the intensity of the flame.

In our administration of this law, we have seen fabrics fail the test when the flame was of such low intensity that it could have been put out safely with a slap of the hand; yet it was replaced in end use with a fabric of heavier weight and made mainly of a cellulosic fiber that passed the test because of slower burning, yet with a flame that went to the top of the test apparatus. This is one of the anomalies of the law.

As to a solution for the problem of preventing burns from ignited clothing, I can speak only as a layman. As an administrator of the law I have listened to so many accounts of personal tragedies that I feel some solution must be found.

I have seen fabrics treated with a permanent fire-retardant or fire-resistant finish that would appear to be the answer for some fabrics but not for all. Some fabrics simply will not burn. The addition of these finishes do affect the "hand" of the fabric and are more expensive than conventional finishes. It is my understanding that the finish cannot be successfully applied to sheer fabrics such as lawns and organdies.

Safety is one of the hardest things there is to sell. I have heard that an experiment was made in a lady's dress department where the same dresses, some with a fire-retardant finish and others with conventional finish, were put on sale. The women were fully advised of the safety factor, yet they invariably bought the dresses with the conventional finish because they were cheaper. Such is human nature.

I understand that some research is being done on fabrics that are blends of flame-inhibiting fibers and the natural fibers. Perhaps from this research will come some sort of solution.

I have seen no statistics on the subject, but from observation I surmise that women are more likely to receive burns from ignited clothing than men, and this would be true from childhood through adulthood. This is because of the difference in clothing worn by members of each sex from childhood through their adult years. Perhaps women would be safer from burns if they dressed as men do and, of course, some now do so.

In conclusion: I believe the Flammable Fabrics Act has prevented many cases of burns by keeping off the market fabrics of an unusually hazardous nature; but it has by no means prevented burns from ignited clothing. The only solution to the whole problem, in my opinion, is the development and use of some method of treating fabrics that will prevent them from burning.

# U.S. DEPARTMENT OF COMMERCE AND THE FLAMMABILITY OF CLOTHING FABRIC*

A. F. Robertson

Chief, Fire Research Section
National Bureau of Standards
Washington, D. C.

The U.S. Department of Commerce is concerned about the tremendous suffering and waste resulting from accidental or "unwanted" fires. A monetary waste of roughly 1 per cent of the gross national product is not something to be complacent about. An assessment in dollar terms of the personal tragedy of the estimated 12,000 fire fatalities and 250,000 serious injuries from burns that occur each year would be very difficult to determine. The staggering loss is surely a burden for the public to carry. It seems appropriate, therefore, that attention should be directed to the causes of these injuries and fatalities. In this paper let us limit our interest to casualties associated with fires involving clothing.

## Size of the Problem

Although the National Fire Protection Association, the National Safety Council, and the Public Health Service publish information that may be used to estimate the over-all size of the problem, information on the circumstances leading to the accidents and the character of combustible material involved is, unfortunately, not available. However, experience in England, as well as fragmentary studies made in this country, suggest that these casualties involve clothing typical of that used by the population at large, and would be little influenced by other than major changes in the flammable character of materials considered acceptable for use in clothing. Again, by analogy with experience in

*Based on a paper presented at the *Conference on Burns and Flame-Retardant Fabrics,* held at The New York Academy of Medicine, December 2 and 3, 1966. The conference was sponsored by: the New York and Brooklyn Trauma Committee of the American College of Surgeons, Chicago, Ill.; The National Fire Protection Association, Boston, Mass.; the Section on Plastic and Reconstructive Surgery of The New York Academy of Medicine; and the Division of Accident Prevention of the U. S. Public Health Service, Washington, D. C. The conference was held in cooperation with the American Academy of Pediatrics, Evanston, Ill.; the American Public Health Association, New York, N. Y.; and the National Safety Council, Chicago, Ill.; and was supported by a grant from the U. S. Public Health Service.

England and Canada, we estimate that about one fifth of the fire fatalities, or about 2400 deaths, result from ignition of clothing each year. It seems likely that a much larger fraction, perhaps four fifths, or about 200,000, of the nonfatal fire injuries each year result from ignition of clothing. These are only approximations of course, but they provide a fair estimate of the size of the problem.

## Inadequate Experience Records

To the best of our knowledge, although the complete loss records are not available, these losses have shown only a modest increase over the years, reflecting mainly the increase in the total population. In the late 1940's and early 1950's, the appearance on the market of highly flammable sweaters and play cowboy suits caused such highly publicized accidents that Congress became alarmed and passed the Flammable Fabrics Act* in 1953. By this act, the Commercial Standards CS-191-53** and CS-192-53,† as promulgated by the secretary of the U. S. Department of Commerce, were designated as the official means for determining the flammability of materials used for clothing. By Section 4*b* of the act, the secretary of the department is charged with the responsibility of recommending changes in the act if at any time he finds that the tests specified by the Commercial Standards are inadequate for protection of the public. The responsibility has been delegated, in turn, by the U.S. Department of Commerce to the National Bureau of Standards.

The act was intended to prevent the commercial distribution of unusually flammable fabrics or films used for clothing purposes. We believe this objective has been achieved, but we have neither a record of the casualties resulting from the lack of control prior to the act, nor adequate fire casualty records to show present experience. We do know, however, that it is difficult in the retail trade to secure clothing material that fails to pass the standards established by the act. We also know, subjectively, that although many clothing fire accidents occur, there are few accounts that describe accidents similar to those previously experienced with the torch sweaters and cowboy chaps.

The experience reported in Britain, as mentioned earlier, suggests that people are being burned in the clothing they commonly wear.

*Public Law 88, 83d Congress, First Session; 15 U.S.C.A., par. 1191; 67 Stat. 111: June 30, 1953.
**Flammability of Clothing Textiles CS191-53, U. S. Department of Commerce, June 30, 1953.
†General Purpose Vinyl Plastic Film CS192-53, U. S. Department of Commerce, May 22, 1953.

Because of this, we have been reluctant to recommend changes in requirements on flammability that would modify significantly the types of clothing material available to the public, particularly since such changes might not reduce significantly the number or the severity of accidents from burning. Thus, at present, we have no basis for predicting a reduction in accidents from burning reported if, for instance, a decision were arbitrarily made to characterize as hazardous fabrics that burn in less than 20 seconds rather than the 3.5 seconds specified in the present federal law.

The annual national expenditure for clothing represents about 30.5 billion dollars, or about 7 per cent of the total for all personal expenditure. This large expenditure surely justifies a careful study of our casualties resulting from ignited clothing. Such a study should provide data on accidents from burns with adequate background data, not only on the nature and causes of them but also, to the extent possible, on the type of clothing involved and technical properties of the fabric, including its flammability. It also would seem appropriate to consider the social and economic costs imposed on the public by a severe change of flammability requirements. For the present, we hope industry will continue research on and the development of clothing made of flame-retardant materials that will be economically, esthetically, and usefully acceptable to the public.

## Work in Progress

Information on fire casualty experience is currently being secured with the cooperation of the U.S. Public Health Service, whose regional survey teams now operating in Denver and Boston are furnishing reports of great value. Our role in this work is to secure technical characterization of the clothing samples when these are available.

It will be some time, however, before anything like a national picture of the situation can be developed. The biases that can be introduced by localized reporting are evident from the limited study already made of the results obtained from Denver where, apparently, local collection of trash is not widely practiced. These results suggest that about 60 per cent of clothing-fire accidents result in one way or another from careless use of flammable liquids, usually gasoline which, in many cases, was being used for starting trash fires. Certainly, drastic changes in flammability of clothing fabrics would be necessary to influence significantly the record of injuries from burns under such circumstances.

Several groups have encouraged adoption of NFPA Standard 702* instead of CS-191-53. This standard makes use of the same test equipment as CS-191-53, but the test method differs primarily by application of the flame continuously to the edge of the specimen rather than for one second to the surface of the specimen. The National Bureau of Standards has explored the possible use of this procedure and the effect it might have on the type of fabrics now considered acceptable. The results were surprising in showing that perhaps as few as 1 in 50 fabrics might be classified differently, but the burden of testing would be seriously increased since by the NFPA method all fabrics would be forced to ignite. One advantage that might be achieved by use of the NFPA Standard is derived from the inclusion of a qualitative test method for materials other than textile. It is evident, however, that NFPA Standard 702 does not provide a useful basis for selection of fabrics of significantly less hazardous flammability. Indeed, we must await results of the survey of accidents from burns that is now in progress to determine whether any but a drastic change in the method of testing would be useful as a basis for achieving significant reduction in accidents from burns.

The National Bureau of Standards also has made recent studies of the test equipment and procedures called for by Commercial Standard CS-191-53. The standing committee has been reconstituted to consider recommendations that the Federal Trade Commission, the National Bureau of Standards, and the public have made for revision of this standard. The changes being considered, if adopted as the legal basis for rejecting unusually flammable fabrics, will be of a type that will define the test method more adequately and, thus, permit closer duplication of results between laboratories but will not necessarily provide any significant change in the potential hazard presented by clothing.

The National Bureau of Standards is also exploring new and improved methods for measuring the transfer of heat between fabric and skin. We plan to continue these studies as part of our work to achieve a better understanding of the hazards involved and thereby assist in reducing the tragedy of casualties from burns.

*Fire Tests: Flame-Resistant Textiles and Films, 1966, NFPA 702, National Fire Protection Association, Boston, Mass.

## SUMMARY

The U. S. Department of Commerce is concerned with the great national waste and suffering caused by unwanted fires. It is sensitive to the need for public safety, as evidenced by the Flammable Fabrics Act.

The National Bureau of Standards, under its delegated authority, has conducted studies of existing and modified test methods for measurement of flammable hazards associated with clothing fabrics. A cooperative program has been initiated recently with the Public Health Service to secure records of injuries from burns; these records should yield evidence on the type of fabrics currently associated with injuries from ignited clothing. This program is just starting, and we expect that it will be some years before a clear understanding of the national picture becomes available. However, when the results of this survey become available, we expect to have a better technical understanding of the causes of clothing-fire accidents and of ways of reducing them. To date there appears to be no technical evidence to show that a significant reduction in the number of accidents from burning clothing can be achieved without major changes in the flammable behavior of clothing fabrics. Thus, we hope that industry will continue the development of permanently retardant-treated fabrics that will be economically, esthetically, and usefully acceptable to the public. We believe, although we have no direct evidence, that such fabrics will significantly reduce, but not eliminate, clothing-fire injuries.

# CONTROLLING THE CLOTHING FIRE PROBLEM*

## OBSERVATIONS ON THE BRITISH EXPERIENCE

EUGENE L. LEHR

Deputy Chief
Division of Accident Prevention
U.S. Public Health Service
Arlington, Va.

THIS report will be based upon correspondence from official and nonofficial sources in Britain; conversations with Dr. C. A. Boucher of the British Ministry of Health; review of selected papers from British medical and industrial sources, and observations I made while in London and Birmingham in September, 1966.

Many of you here may be familiar with the British problem of clothing fire burns and efforts toward their control. Those who are not may be interested in a brief description of the factors leading to joint action by government and industry, and the present status of implementation.

### CLOTHING FIRE BURN PROBLEM IN BRITAIN

Deaths from clothing burns in homes and residential institutions in England and Wales ranged from a high of 329 to a low of 234 during the five years 1958 to 1962.[1] In 1964, there were 277 such deaths. The rate for females is about 4½ times the rate for males, for all ages. The highest number of deaths and the highest rate is in the elderly, particularly those 75 and over. The next highest rate is in children under 5 years of age.

Children's nightdresses and open fires have been identified as specific objects of concern by the Home Office, which has general responsibility for the safety of the home. Other organizations actively interested or involved include the Ministry of Health, the Royal Society for Pre-

*Based on a paper presented at the *Conference on Burns and Flame-Retardant Fabrics,* held at The New York Academy of Medicine, December 2 and 3, 1966. The conference was sponsored by: the New York and Brooklyn Trauma Committee of the American College of Surgeons, Chicago, Ill.; The National Fire Protection Association, Boston, Mass.; the Section on Plastic and Reconstructive Surgery of The New York Academy of Medicine; and the Division of Accident Prevention of the U.S. Public Health Service, Washington, D.C. The conference was held in cooperation with the American Academy of Pediatrics, Evanston, Ill.; the American Public Health Association, New York, N. Y.; and the National Safety Council, Chicago, Ill.; and was supported by a grant from the U.S. Public Health Service.

vention of Accidents, the Medical Research Council, the Textile Institute, the Furnishing Fabric Manufacturers' Association, and the Retail Trading-Standards Association.

The Industrial Injuries and Burns Research Unit at the Birmingham Accident Hospital has been responsible for making available extensive data on burn injuries. Dr. John P. Bull, director of the Unit, and his predecessor, Dr. Leonard Colebrook, have made important contributions not only in the field of burn treatment, but also in studies of the social, medical, and environmental factors related to this form of injury.

Dr. Bull has reported[2] that accidents in which clothes catch fire are the main cause (90 per cent) of fatal domestic burns. They account for just over one half of all inpatient admissions to the Birmingham Burns Unit. The total case mortality for clothing burns is about 23 per cent, as compared to 3 per cent for other burns. For the elderly, the mortality rate is 73 per cent.

## Preventive Measures

The British have developed three basic categories of preventive measures: 1) education (or propaganda as they describe it), 2) better guarding of open fires, and 3) the provision of flame-resistant clothing. In the latter two categories, the government, after consultation with trade associations, has taken direct but incomplete regulatory action under authority of the Consumer Protection Act of 1961. An earlier attempt at regulation by police power is reported to have been largely unknown by the public. The Children's and Young Persons Act made it an offense to leave a child up to 12 with an unguarded coal fire. The penalties were rarely invoked. Punitive measures against parents after death or serious injury of a child were ineffective.

## Regulations and Standards

The Consumer Protection Act of 1961 authorizes the Secretary of State to impose by regulation, on any prescribed class of goods, safety requirements that in his opinion are expedient to prevent or reduce risk of death or personal injury. In addition, he is authorized to prescribe the marking of goods with such warnings or safety instructions as he deems appropriate.

Previously a 1952 Heating Appliances Act required gas, electric, and oil-burning radiant heaters to be sold with protective guards. British standards for guards to cover coal fires were adopted in 1956. Dr. Bull reports that many families who most need them do not obtain effective guards. The difficulties range from cost considerations to lack of knowledge and lack of availability in retail outlets.

Early in 1964 the Home Office began consultations with consumers' safety organizations and trade associations about the possibility of regulating the flammability of children's nightwear. As a result, regulations regarding children's nightdresses were developed and came into operation in October 1964.

### Effectiveness of Legislation

Dr. Boucher evaluated effectiveness of the legislation in causing a reduction in burn morbidity in these words:

> It is probably too early to draw any conclusions, since the Children's Nightdresses Regulations only came into operation on 1st October 1964. Nevertheless, if two six month periods 1) October 1963 to March 1964 and 2) October 1964 to March 1965 are studied from the point of view of fatal clothing burns from nightwear in children under the age of fifteen, during the first period 10 girls died and, during the second period, only 4.

Dr. Bull, during our visit to his research unit in Birmingham, said it was his impression that the regulations on nightdresses were having a beneficial effect among infants. There have been no admissions for nightdress fires that have involved treated materials or flame-retardant synthetics. He emphasized that this was only an impression—that there were insufficient experience and data from which to determine a trend. Other variable factors, such as an increase in central heating installations in new homes might affect the rate of exposure. He also pointed out that the regulations covered finished garments; that many mothers made childrens' nightclothes at home, from yard goods that might or might not meet the standard for low flammability.

### Possible Expansion of the Regulations

Industry has expressed concern over the inadequacy of the regulations on nightdresses and of the testing standards. The Textile Institute points out that a fabric may have passed the test, but that the finished garment may have characteristics that would allow it to ignite and burn at a rate hazardous to a child.[3] Dr. A. R. Urquhart comments: "The more one knows about the subject the less happy one is likely to be about the present criteria for safety, for the existing standard of flame resistance was originally developed for nonthermoplastic fabrics, and is not satisfactory for synthetics. Medical and safety people are concerned because the regulation covers only part of the total hazard from clothing ignition, and completely misses the highest risk group—the elderly."[4]

Plans are now well advanced toward revisions that might expand the 1964 regulation. Dr. Boucher reports:

> A Working Party on Flammable Clothing was set up by the Home Secretary in May 1965 to consider the possibility of extending the scope of the Children's Nightdresses Regulations 1964; other kinds of children's clothing, old persons' nightwear and material sold in the piece were particularly in mind. The Working Party considers that the present requirements in the regulations relating to threads should be amended and the present exception in favour of infants' gowns should be limited to gowns having a specified chest measurement so that infants would not be able to wear such gowns from the age of about six months, when most children become mobile. The actual measurement has not yet been decided. The Working Party has also noted the high incidence of clothing burns involving the elderly and is considering the desirability of promoting regulations for safer clothing both for the elderly and the disabled.

## My Own Observations

It is dangerous to draw conclusions from very limited direct observation. My comments should be considered with that constraint in mind. It is my impression that the British have been progressive in government-industry cooperation in attacking the problem of regulation. It also appears from the literature that textile and retail groups have been imaginative in marketing techniques designed to make the customer aware of the importance of flame-retardant garments and in producing attractive types of garments beyond the scope of the regulation. A spot check of three representative department stores indicated that there is general compliance with the nightdresses regulations. Display stocks of apparel covered by the requirements were clearly identified as flame-retardant.

A senior buyer for one of the leading retail chains was quite frank in his appraisal of the current situation. Competition and the absence of a strong demand on the part of customers create a problem for even the highly motivated merchandiser who might like to promote the sale of low-flammability dresses, robes and other kinds of garments not subject to the 1964 regulations. Despite this, responsible retailers are experimenting with marketing new products, and making efforts toward consumer education.

In summary, it can be said the British have recognized that the combination of flammable clothing and unprotected heating appliances in so many homes has created a critical medical and an economic problem. The government has undertaken an admittedly limited approach to the control of that problem. They recognize the limitations, and are proceeding with some deliberation toward expanded regulations. The Home Office has involved affected trade groups in the process. The forthcoming expanded requirements are bound to reflect the collective knowledge and experience of these groups. An unanswered question is whether legal controls can be developed that will effectively protect all age groups, or whether a combination of consumer demand and the availability of a widespread, competitively priced product might accomplish the same result.

### *REFERENCES*


1. Bull, J. P., Jackson, D. M., and Walton, C. Causes and prevention of domestic burning accidents, *Brit. Med. J. 2*:1421-27, 1964.
2. *Ibid.*
3. Jones, E. B. *The Flammability of Clothing Fabrics.* Manchester, Textile Inst. and Industry, 1965.
4. Urquhart, A. R. *Performance Priorities of Textiles for Garment Manufacture.* Manchester, Textile Inst. and Industry, 1965.

# INDUSTRIAL EXPERIENCE IN THE USE OF FLAME-RETARDANT FABRICS*

Robert S. B. Holmes

Assistant Director of Safety
United States Steel Corporation
Pittsburgh, Pa.

"It takes all kinds of people to make a world," and to paraphrase this trite and timeworn expression, "it takes many kinds of fabrics to satisfy U. S. Steel's protective apparel requirements." Protective apparel has been used by U. S. Steel for many years. When I started with the corporation in July 1934 at Clairton Works, I was given protective apparel to wear over my work clothing. Prior to 1961, the corporation met its protective apparel requirements primarily from stock items of safety suppliers.

On April 1, 1961, as a result of considerable study by U. S. Steel's Applied Research Laboratory, the first move was made toward standardization of protective apparel. This standardization took place in blast furnace, foundry, and open-hearth operations, and established *basic protection* as durably treated, flame-retardant cotton. Please note this phrase basic protection, because for some jobs, such as tapping a furnace, additional protection of the type afforded by aluminized rayon or aluminized asbestos garments worn over this basic protection was, and still is, required.

One cause of burns in the steel industry is molten metal or slag splashes. Admittedly, open flames and ignition of combustible gases are potential burn hazards, but molten metal is the greatest burn potential. Therefore, an acceptable durably treated cotton garment must, above everything else, protect against molten metal.

To determine the ability of a durably treated, flame-retardant fabric to withstand splashes of molten metal or slag, a severe but simple test was devised. This test uses a rectangular frame approximately

*Based on a paper presented at the *Conference on Burns and Flame-Retardant Fabrics,* held at The New York Academy of Medicine, December 2 and 3, 1966. The conference was sponsored by: the New York and Brooklyn Trauma Committee of the American College of Surgeons, Chicago, Ill.; The National Fire Protection Association, Boston, Mass.; the Section on Plastic and Reconstructive Surgery of The New York Academy of Medicine; and the Division of Accident Prevention of the U. S. Public Health Service, Washington, D. C. The conference was held in cooperation with the American Academy of Pediatrics, Evanston, Ill.; the American Public Health Association, New York, N. Y.; and the National Safety Council, Chicago, Ill.; and was supported by a grant from the U. S. Public Health Service.

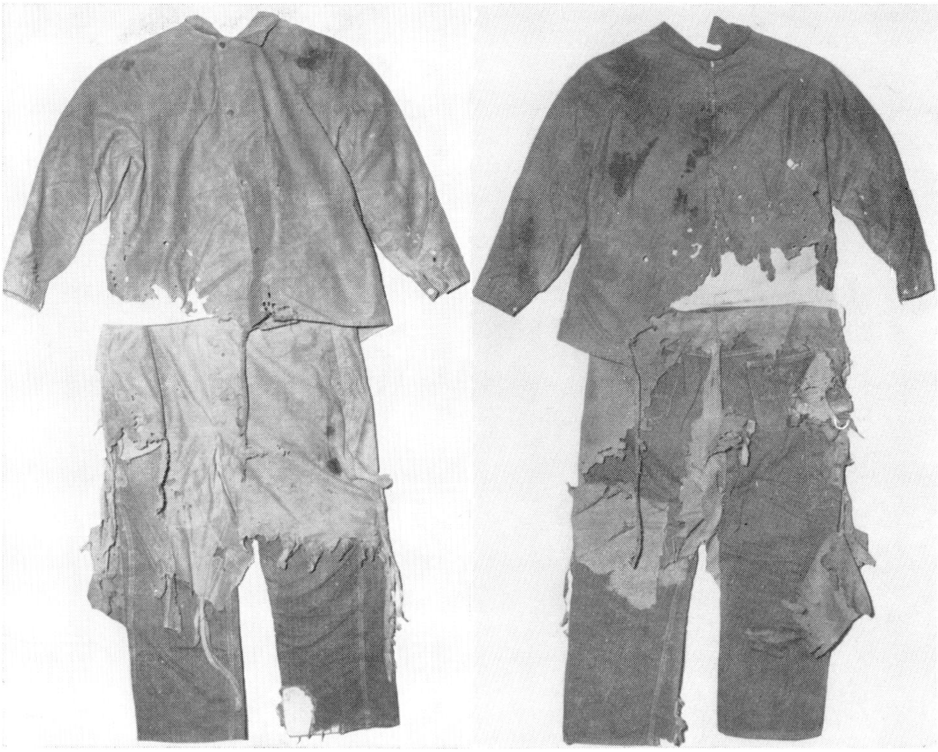

Fig. 1. Front. Fig. 2. Back.

9″ x 32″ constructed so that it is inclined 75° to the horizontal. A piece of the fabric to be tested is affixed to the frame. Underneath the test fabric is placed a Tex Trude polyethylene film 0.6 mils thick. This polyethylene film, when subjected to molten metal, reacts similarly to the human skin and permits a prediction of the burn potential to the wearer. Onto the inclined frame with its fabric and "synthetic skin" is splashed a small ladle of molten metal. Specific attention is paid to several things. Does the molten metal or slag adhere to the fabric or does it run off? Is the fabric consumed or to what degree is it damaged; and, most important, what happens to the "synthetic skin?" A fabric and its finish that have passed this "splash test" are then subjected to standard char, afterflame, and afterglow tests.

The protection provided by this fabric has been unbelievable in some cases, as shown by Figures 1 and 2. They show what remains of a

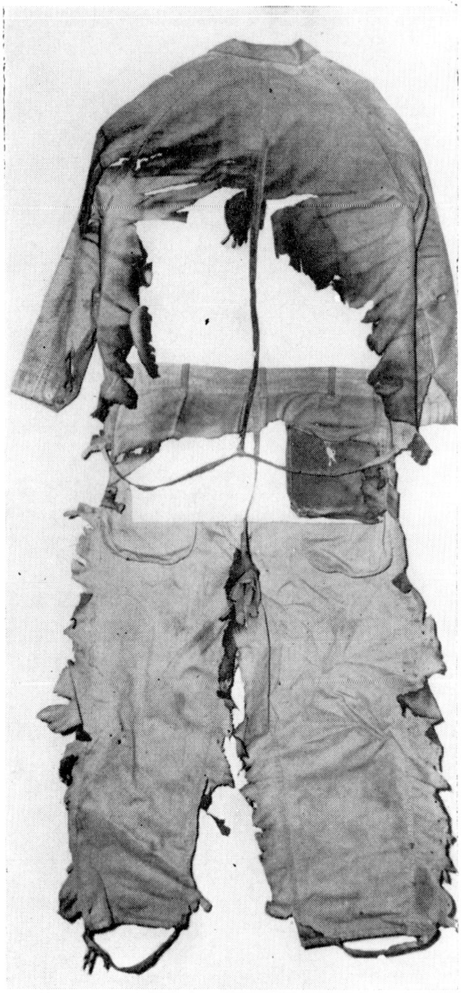

Fig. 3

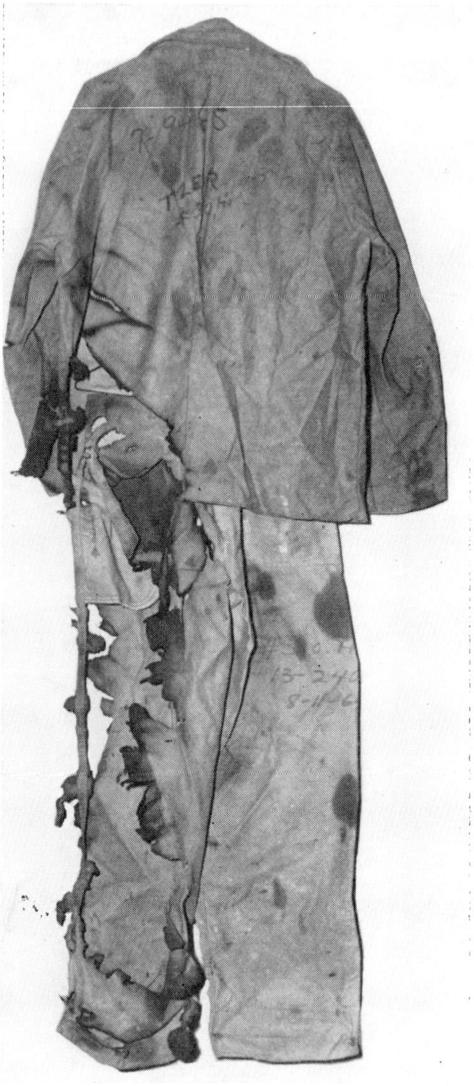

Fig. 4

jacket and pants which were splashed with molten metal at a temperature of about 2,500°F. Steel was being teemed into ingots when the ingot molds were inadvertently moved, causing the molten metal stream from the ladle to strike the top of the mold and spray the steel pourer. The "blue jeans" and cotton thermal underwear shown in the photographs are those worn by the steel pourer at the time of the incident. Notice particularly that there are no scorch or burn marks on them even though the protective jacket and pants are a total loss. This man sustained no body burns; the case, however, was a disabling injury because the man was not wearing gloves at the time and sustained burns of the hands.

Figure 3 shows another example. Here, too, the photograph tells the story. In this case, flames erupted from a furnace and engulfed the back of the charging machine operator—who was out of his cab at the time. You can see what happened to the protective apparel. The charging machine operator sustained no burns, and returned to his regular work immediately.

Figure 4 shows the result of an eruption in an ingot mold spilling about 3,000 pounds of hot metal and splashing the steel pourer—again no burns, and no loss of work time.

These three examples will permit you to make your own evaluation of our durably treated, flame-retardant cotton fabric's ability to provide protection against molten metal. This protection has been good—exceptionally good. Yet we have had our "troubles" with durably treated cotton apparel—these "troubles" have been in the area of service life. Some of these early garments lasted only a day, others a week, some a little longer. In fact, the service life of these garments 5 years ago was considered by operators to be about 4 weeks maximum. While the garments were providing adequate protection, they were "nickeling and diming us to death" from a cost standpoint. In trying to solve this service life problem, we also learned of the effects of radiant heat and how the treatment or finish affected the ability of the fabric to stand up under exposure to radiant heat. As you can appreciate, it took time to determine that the type of finish applied to a fabric can have a significant effect on that fabric's ability to withstand radiant heat. Fortunately, when durably treated cotton is exposed to radiant heat, it "fails safe," that is, it scorches, which can be visually detected by management and the garment removed and replaced. This is not the case with all fabrics; for instance, wool may be scorched by radiant heat, but the scorching is not readily determined visually and hence the garment may be continued in service beyond its safe period. To combat the effect of radiant heat, a change was made in the type of finish applied to the fabric that resulted in modifying U. S. Steel's specification from a thermal setting resin plus a polyvinyl chloride thermoplastic

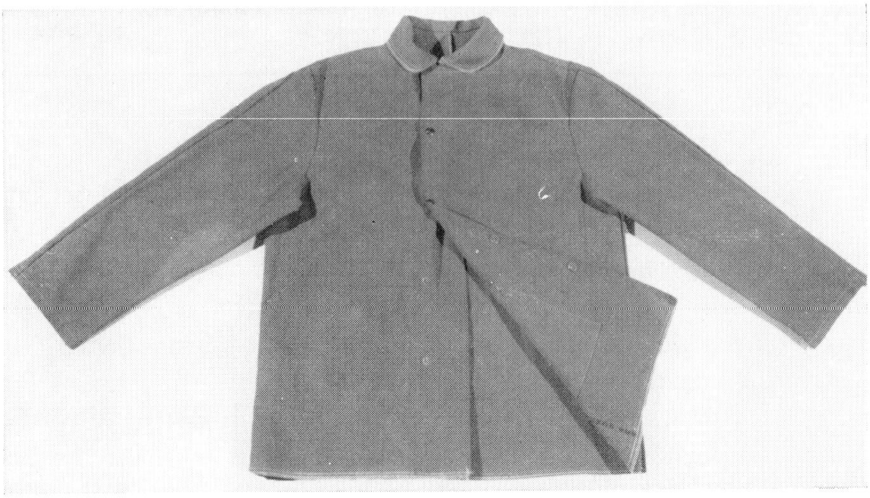

Fig. 5

extender to a thermal setting resin with a latex thermoplastic extender. This change gives a finish that resists radiant heat deterioration and does not weaken the fabric to the same degree as the original finish.

Having established the effect of use conditions, i.e., molten metal, radiant heat, and abrasion when encountered individually or in combination with each other, we wrote fabric and finish specifications based upon the conditions which this fabric and finish would encounter in actual use. This led to establishing 5 fabric types based upon 5 general areas of use. These we call USS 100, USS 200, USS 300, and so forth.

USS 100 fabric must be able to withstand exposure to extreme heat or open flame, as encountered in fire entry.

USS 200 demands a fabric that can withstand exposure to high radiant heat where little possibility of contact with heated metal, molten metal, or slag exists. While there will be massive areas of radiant heat, this fabric will experience relatively little exposure to sparks or metal globules.

USS 300 fabric must withstand exposure to high radiant heat while the employee is performing active physical work and with occasional exposure to sparks or globules of molten metal.

USS 400 fabric is the most widely used fabric. It must protect against exposure to some radiant heat but with frequent exposure to

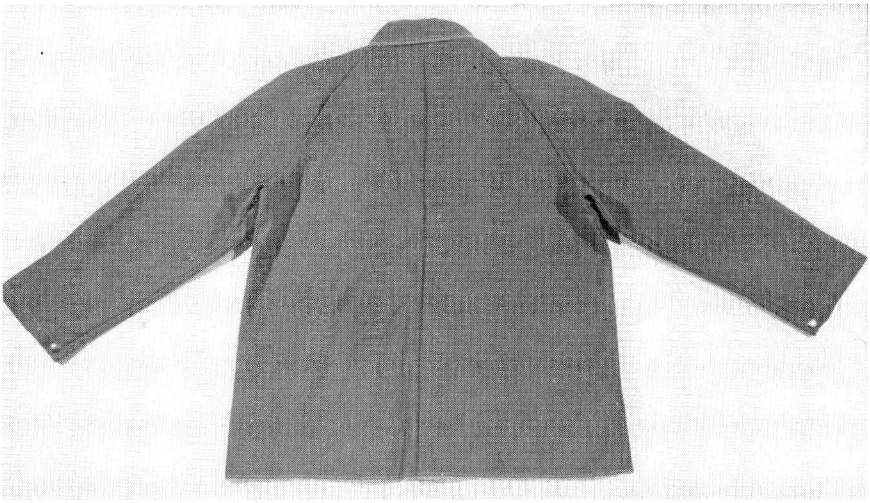

Fig. 6

sparks, molten metal, or slag globules, and active work conditions such as climbing and material handling.

USS 500 fabric involves abrasive wear, found in material handling but with little exposure to radiant heat and only rare or occasional exposure to hot metal splash or open flame.

Common to all five of these "use condition categories" are the problems of pattern design and garment manufacture. These aspects contributed to our service life problem. First, it is important to bear in mind that the garment in question is protective apparel, not work clothing. Protective apparel is worn over work clothing; hence its pattern design must provide for this bulk, otherwise binding occurs and sets up points of strain that result in tears, fabric wear, pulled seams, and reduced service life. Obviously a torn or ripped garment cannot provide full protection against metal splash.

The jacket in Figures 5 and 6 shows how pattern design is influenced by use requirements. It has a set-in sleeve front and raglan back. This is to provide a good fit, yet ample freedom for work movements. The collar closure is a Velcro fastener. This assures a tight, comfortable closure for all neck sizes and will prevent globules of hot metal from entering at the neck. The front closure has a 2″ overlap, so that no matter how an employee may stoop, squat, or kneel, the overlap prevents hot metal from entering the gap and causing body burns. The snaps used in the front closure are light-duty type. Heavy-duty snaps tend to tear out the fabric. At the bottom and leading edge of the jacket there is a minimum of exposed stitching, and only on the sleeve is there a turned seam. The reason is that a needle piercing the fabric makes holes much like the perforations along the edges of a postage stamp–it makes for needle cutting and creates a point of weakness for easy tearing or ripping. This is particularly true when seams are resewn to correct mis-stitching. In like manner, any time this fabric is turned it creates a point of easy tear or critical wear, much as does folding a piece of paper and creasing it with your thumbnail; you know how easily that will tear. The pocket, of course, is on the inside so that it will not catch and hold molten metal. The specifications for this jacket and the trousers that go with it comprise a 17-page specification known as USS 400. While this jacket may not be a thing of beauty, it is serviceable and it does protect. In closing, I emphasize that the wear characteristics of a treated fabric are significantly different from those of the same fabric in the untreated state, and that it is these treated characteristics that should be matched against requirements in use to determine pattern design and manufacturing specifications in order to assure maximum protection, optmium service life, comfort, and acceptable costs.

*Note.* The six illustrations accompanying this paper were provided by the United States Steel Corporation and are reproduced by permission.

# FLAME-RESISTANT TEXTILES*

THOMAS D. MILES

Fabric Engineering and Finishes Branch
Clothing and Organic Materials Division
U.S. Army Natick Laboratories
Natick, Mass.

ALL the commercially available flame-resistant materials that possess any potential for use as military protective clothing or tentage have been or are being evaluated. Synthetic fibers such as Dynel and Nomex, and new commercial finishes such as tris(1-aziridinyl) phosphine oxide-thiourea (APO-thiourea) for cotton are examples of flame-resistant materials currently undergoing evaluation. Flame-resistant textiles are used in large amounts by the military for tentage. During the past 2 years about 25 to 50 million yards of flame-resistant tentage materials have been procured. Other uses include flame-resistant protective clothing and flight clothing. Since other contributors to this conference are describing the properties and typical applications of Dynel, Nomex, and the commercially available flame-resistant finishes, this discussion will be limited to two aspects not covered in the general discussion of flame retardants.

The first is the flammability of flame-resistant materials in oxygen-enriched atmospheres.

Textile materials that are flame-resistant in atmospheres containing the amounts of oxygen present in the earth's atmosphere at sea level do not necessarily retain flame resistance when the oxygen content is increased. The flammability of a textile in high oxygen-content atmospheres is of interest in designing clothing for long-range space missions.[1]

Preliminary studies of the flammability of materials under zero gravity conditions[2] indicate that the products of combustion tend to subdue the flame because of the absence of convection in a weightless condition. However, weightlessness itself could not be relied upon as a

*Based on a paper presented at the *Conference on Burns and Flame-Retardant Fabrics,* held at The New York Academy of Medicine, December 2 and 3, 1966. The conference was sponsored by: the New York and Brooklyn Trauma Committee of the American College of Surgeons, Chicago, Ill.; The National Fire Protection Association, Boston, Mass.; the Section on Plastic and Reconstructive Surgery of The New York Academy of Medicine; and the Division of Accident Prevention of the U.S. Public Health Service, Washington, D.C. The conference was held in cooperation with the American Academy of Pediatrics, Evanston, Ill.; the American Public Health Association, New York, N. Y.; and the National Safety Council, Chicago, Ill.; and was supported by a grant from the U.S. Public Health Service.

means of eliminating flame hazard since the zero gravity condition would not be present at all times.

At present, methods of measuring the flammability of textiles in enriched oxygen atmospheres have not been standardized. Methods can be designed to answer a variety of questions:

1) How hazardous are textiles in enriched oxygen atmospheres? The measurement of burning rate would be of prime importance in any method designed to answer this question; the means used to ignite the textile would be of little interest.

2) How readily might textiles be ignited by a potential hazard such as overheated wires in electronic equipment? In this case, the ease of ignition would be of prime interest, and the means of ignition used in the test method should simulate the potential hazard. A glowing wire in contact with the textile would be a logical source of ignition to simulate the overheating of electronic equipment.

3) How flame-resistant (i.e., self-extinguishing) are textiles in enriched oxygen atmospheres? Contact of the textile with flame and measurement of the duration of flaming would be required in a method measuring flame resistance in enriched oxygen atmospheres.

Since resistance to flame rather than ease of ignition or rate of burning was our interest, a method was designed in which the textile material was brought into contact with flame, and the duration of the flaming, if any occurred, was timed. The sample of fabric (1¾ inch × 1 inch) was suspended on a platinum wire inside a sealed glass chamber containing a 30 per cent oxygen, 70 per cent nitrogen atmosphere. The source of the flame was a right triangle (1¼-inch sides) of black ignition paper placed under the sample of textile and ignited from outside the sealed chamber by infrared radiation. Samples were tested at a variety of pressures ranging from one atmosphere (14.7 psia) to one third atmosphere (4.9 psia).

It was found that the durable flame-resistant finishes that are commercially available did not make cotton self-extinguishing in the enriched oxygen atmosphere. Only the nondurable ammonium sulfamate made cotton fabrics self-extinguishing. A lightweight Nomex fabric (3 oz./sq. yd.) burned in enriched oxygen atmospheres regardless of the pressure, while a Nomex fabric of heavier weight (6.5 oz.) burned at one atmosphere and at two thirds atmosphere but became self-extinguishing at one half atmosphere. Inert materials such as fiber glass fabric and fabric made from carbon fiber did not burn or ignite under any of the test conditions. The effect on the flammability of two antibacterial finishes was also measured. These finishes are of interest in the problem of designing clothing that must be worn for extended periods of time. One finish, benzalkonium chloride, caused inert fabrics such as fiber glass to ignite and flame while the same inert fabric treated with neomycin sulphate did not ignite in the enriched oxygen atmosphere.

The other aspect of our work that may be of some interest is concerned with flame-resistant finishes for textiles. Some of the problems in finishing fabrics with laundry-durable flame retardants are: 1) there are no durable flame retardants for cotton-nylon blends containing a high nylon content; 2) durable flame retardants usually decrease tear strength by 30 to 50 per cent; and 3) there are no laundry-durable flame retardants that can be applied without curing the fabric at a high temperature.

Two of these problems are related to the fact that all durables are fiber-reactive. The high-temperature cure is required to force the reaction of the flame retardant with the fiber. The loss in tear strength is due to the decreased mobility within the fabric structure caused by cross-linking due to the reactive finish. We considered means of improving the durability of a nonreactive flame retardant that had shown some promise in making blends with a high nylon content flame-resistant. The nonreactive flame retardant is 2,3 dibromopropyl phosphate,[3] a fully brominated triallyl phosphate that is usually durable through only 1 to 3 accelerated launderings. It was found that, with the addition of a small amount of polyvinyl chloride resin, this retardant can be made durable through the required 15 accelerated washes. The application of the finish to the fabric is from a solvent. No cure is required, so that processing speeds can be much higher than that of aqueous applications, which require the fabric to be cured at high temperatures.

The finish, when applied to a 50 per cent cotton-nylon fabric in the range of 30 to 40 per cent add-on, will provide flame resistance durable through the required 15 accelerated launderings. The tear strength is good. An untreated 8-oz. 50 per cent cotton-50 per cent nylon sateen with a 6.3 lb. warp tear and 7.6 lb. tear strength across the fill, had a tear strength of 8.7 lb. in the warp and 10.0 lb. across the filling when treated. Cotton and cotton-Avril fabrics have also been treated. A 2-yd./lb. cotton sheeting, it was found, had a tear strength of 4.7 × 4.2

lb. before treatment and 4.3 × 3.9 lb. after flame-resistant finishing.

Since all previous durable flame retardants that have reduced tear strength have also reduced wear life in garments worn on the abrasion course at Fort Lee, Va., it will be interesting to see whether the retention of the high-tear strength of this treated nylon-cotton fabric will be accompanied by a retention of the good wear life that the untreated fabric has shown on the wear course.

## *REFERENCES*

1. C. Huggett *et al.* The Effects of 100% Oxygen at Reduced Pressure on the Ignitibility and Combustibility of Materials, *US Air Force Sch. Aerospace Med.*, December, 1965.
2. Kizmey, T. H. *Flammability in Zero Gravity.* Houston, Tex., NASA Manned Spacecraft Center.
3. U. S. Patent 3,046,297, Michigan Chemical Co., St. Louis, Mich.

# PROGRAM ACTIVITIES OF THE DIVISION OF ACCIDENT PREVENTION U.S. PUBLIC HEALTH SERVICE*

A. F. Schaplowsky

Chief, Community Services Branch
Division of Accident Prevention
U. S. Public Health Service
Arlington, Va.

The U.S. Public Health Service is the principal agency of the federal government that is concerned with the prevention of disease and injury and the general improvement of the health of the people of the Unted States.

The Division of Accident Prevention is the organizational unit of the U.S. Public Health Service that is primarily concerned with accidental trauma. The division's activities are of two general kinds—fact finding and a program of activities designed to prevent or minimize injury. The accompanying figure describes in a simple manner how the division functions.

Through research grants funds are made available to public and private nonprofit institutions and organizations to conduct research on the prevention of accidents. The Experimental Research Branch performs research directed by the division and conducted by division personnel with division facilities or by contracting with other research organizations. Information obtained by the Epidemiology and Surveillance Branch about accidental injuries and deaths from death certificates, from the National Health Survey, and from other sources is accumulated and analyzed in various ways to determine the extent and nature of the problems involved, and to determine hypotheses for

*Based on a paper presented at the *Conference on Burns and Flame-Retardant Fabrics,* held at The New York Academy of Medicine, December 2 and 3, 1966. The conference was sponsored by: the New York and Brooklyn Trauma Committee of the American College of Surgeons, Chicago, Ill.; The National Fire Protection Association, Boston, Mass.; the Section on Plastic and Reconstructive Surgery of The New York Academy of Medicine; and the Division of Accident Prevention of the U. S. Public Health Service, Washington, D. C. The conference was held in cooperation with the American Academy of Pediatrics, Evanston, Ill.; the American Public Health Association, New York, N. Y.; and the National Safety Council, Chicago, Ill.; and was supported by a grant from the U. S. Public Health Service.

Since this conference was held the Division of Accident Prevention has become the Injury Control Program, National Center for Urban and Industrial Health.

DIVISION OF ACCIDENT PREVENTION

| | |
|---|---|
| *Fact-finding* | |
| Research Grants Branch | |
| Experimental Research Branch | |
| Epidemiology and Surveillance Branch | |
| *Program* | |
| Community Services Branch | |
| Modification or control of agents | Information and education |
| Reduction of the environment's injury potential | Reduction of the seriousness or aggravation of injuries that occur |

countermeasures. This branch also contracts for special studies and investigations relating to injury control. Another activity involves the work of surveillance teams. These teams consist of a small number of individuals from various professional disciplines who investigate in depth the circumstances surrounding the causation of injuries.

The information from these fact-finding activities is utilized to develop program activities designed to prevent or minimize the injuries that occur as a result of accidents. In general the approaches taken in program activities are:

1) *Modification or control of agents of accidents and agents of injury.* Working with manufacturers in many instances has resulted in the modification of a product.

2) *Reduction of the injury potential of the environment.* The division has been instrumental in stimulating the need for and cooperating in the development of standards by the National Bureau of Standards, American Standards Association, and other agencies. The division encourages and assists in the development of protective community laws or ordinances.

3) *Information and education.* Education of the public about a particular injury problem and about the suggested behavioral or environmental changes required for control is accomplished through use of mass media and through the program activities of state and local health departments. These program activities include group meetings, education in schools, the showing of films, exhibits, and the injury-prevention aspects of other public health programs.

4) *Reduction of the seriousness or aggravation of injuries that*

*occur.* The division works with communities to improve their emergency medical services.

I should now like to mention the activities of the Division of Accident Prevention as they relate more directly to the subject being discussed at this conference.

One of the first research efforts of the division was to negotiate a contract with the Tennessee Department of Public Health for a study entitled "Accidental Injuries to Tennessee Children." The study consisted of household interviews of 383 families in which a child had had an accidental injury and had received service from the Crippled Children's Service of the State Department of Public Health during the two-year period 1959 to 1961. The study attempted to relate environmental, physical, sociological, and physiological factors to the causation of accidents in children. Of the 308 burn incidents studied, 105 patients had suffered burns in which their clothes caught fire.

Another project recently completed was an evaluation of flame-retardant fabrics in two nursing homes in Arkansas. In these nursing homes half of the sheets, pillowcases, bathrobes, blankets, bedspreads, drawsheets, and other clothing and fabric items were treated with tris(1-aziridinyl) phosphine oxide and tetrakis(hydroxymethyl) phosphonium chloride (APO-THPC) as a flame retardant. A small number of THPC-treated sheets was also supplied for staff use and evaluation. Conclusions indicate that there were no allergic reactions on the part of any of the patients that could be attributed to the use of fabrics with the flame-retardant finishes. Also there was no problem of acceptability of the hand, odor, or other physical or esthetic properties of the treated fabrics. Samples of materials used were pulled before the first washing, after 1, 5, and 10 washings, and at regular intervals thereafter for the life of the fabric for evaluation by the U. S. Department of Agriculture Laboratory in New Orleans, La. Sixteen different tests including flammability, rip test, tear strength, and many other tests were performed. Because of the short time involved in the project, definitive conclusions could not be reached regarding the retention of flame retardancy throughout the normal life of the treated materials and the differences in wear and tear qualities of treated and untreated materials.

We also conducted a search of the medical and legal literature for references to cases of burns involving the ignition of clothing. Abstracts of important papers are kept in the division's library.

A very important current piece of research involves the Burn Unit at the University of Michigan Medical Center. Here we are sponsoring a study on burn injuries (National Burn Information Exchange) to obtain information regarding the etiology and cost involved in burns and methods of treatment.

This project was initiated in 1964. Information is being obtained from Burn Units at the University of Michigan Medical School and at St. Joseph's Mercy Hospital, Ann Arbor, Mich.; the University of Cincinnati, Cincinnati, Ohio; the Medical College of Virginia and St. Philip's Hospital, Richmond, Va.; Cook County Hospital, Chicago, Ill.; the Medical College of South Carolina; the University of Texas School of Medicine at Galveston, and the Brooke Army Medical Center, San Antonio, Texas. These Burn Units include a high proportion of serious cases referred to them by private physicians and from other sources of treatment.

Of the cases studied at these special Burn Units (and bear in mind that these are *severe* burn cases), about 40 per cent are reported to have involved ignited clothing. An analysis was made of the type of clothing and fabric ignited from the reports of three of these units—the University of Michigan, the Medical College of Virginia, and St. Philip's Hospital. Of the 111 patients whose clothes ignited (burning 153 articles of clothing), 92 were reported to be cotton, 38 were unknown or not specified, and the remaining 23 articles were either cotton or a synthetic comprised of synthetics and silk or wool.

Other fact-finding activities of the division include the work of a surveillance team located at the Denver General Hospital in Denver, Colo. Here a five-man professional surveillance team investigates in depth the circumstances surrounding the occurrence of various types of injuries. This team has investigated a number of burn cases involving many different agents. A small number of burn cases involving ignited clothing have been investigated and, as part of the investigative procedure, pieces of the clothing that burned are obtained when possible. We are making copies of these reports available to the National Bureau of Standards for their work pertaining to fabric flammability. Our over-all plan is eventually to install 8 or 10 of these surveillance teams in various geographic areas of the country so that we may have a geographically representative sampling of injuries investigated in depth. Our second team now is being formed in Boston.

Our Program has included the Textile Flammability Conference held in Boston on October 2, 1962, under the sponsorship of the National Fire Protection Association and the Division of Accident Prevention of the U.S. Public Health Service. The proceedings of that conference were published by the National Fire Protection Association. A significant number of the published proceedings was purchased by the Division of Accident Prevention and distributed throughout the country and overseas. Since that meeting an exhibit has been developed, showing "concepts of preventing burn injuries" through the use of flame-retardant fabrics, materials, and clothing. Variations of this exhibit have been shown at 15 national, regional, and international meetings. These conferences have included the American Public Health Association, the American Society of Plastic and Reconstructive Surgeons, the American Academy of Pediatrics, the National Home Economics Association, the American Medical Association, the Greater Kansas City Home Show, the American Hospital Association, the American College of Surgeons, and many other organizations. More than 100,000 people in carefully selected audiences have been able to see that certain flame-retardant fabrics are now available in limited quantity, how they burn or do not burn, how they feel, how they look, and how they may be used. Excellent cooperation has been received from members of state and local health departments who have assisted in manning this exhibit. Local fire marshals and firemen have helped to arrange proper safeguards for this exhibit. Many United States industries have contributed materials for the exhibit and for distribution of copies of them to all participants. We plan to continue this kind of educational activity.

At the request of Al Higgins Productions, the division staff and representatives of the National Fire Protection Association served as technical advisors for the film *Your Clothing Can Burn*. This film has been promoted through our regional offices. Many state health departments have purchased copies of this production for use in their health education programs.

Through our direction of women's activities interest has been stimulated and education programs have been developed for the National Grange, the AFL-CIO Women's groups, the National Congress of Parents and Teachers, and other associations. Division staff members have assisted in the preparation of articles on clothing burns for many publications including *U.S. Medicine*, *The Reader's Digest*, and *Pageant*.

Internally, our division has been assisting the Bureau of Medical Services of the U.S. Public Health Service, the Veterans Administration, the Division of Indian Health, the Department of Defense, and many other governmental agencies, including the General Services Administration, by supplying technical material and information on injuries and deaths associated with clothing and burns.

I have abstracted five items from the summary of our recommendations to the Safety Officer of the Bureau of Medical Services of the Public Health Service: 1) all new mattresses, foam pillows, and bed pads should possess flame-resistant covers; 2) all new cubicle curtains, bedside screens, and draperies for patients' rooms should be flame-resistant; 3) all bedding in connection with oxygen tent service should be flame-resistant; 4) flame-resistant robes and pajamas should be available for high-risk smokers; 5) other bedding of flame-resistant materials should be purchased as money becomes available. These are but a few of the recommendations that are now being made throughout government circles to stimulate the purchase of flame-retardant clothing and fabrics that will reduce the incidence of burn injuries.

Last year a three-year burn control project was begun in Jefferson County, Ala. This is in a well-staffed, local health department situated in Birmingham, with established health programs throughout all communities in the county. The health department-medical complex in this county consists of a teaching hospital of the University af Alabama Medical College, a children's hospital, a veterans' hospital, and a rehabilitation center. Its first effort in determining the nature of the burns problem in that community was to conduct a retrospective study of patients with burns who were treated or hospitalized in five Jefferson County hospitals during a 5-year period beginning February 1, 1961, and extending through January 1, 1966. All injuries from burning included in this report occurred in the home or on the home premises. Reports on approximately 1,395 patients were analyzed. Of the total of 1,395 admitted, 179 were listed as having their clothing ignited; and 101 did not state whether or not the clothing caught fire. A further analysis indicates, however, that it is the burning clothing that contributes to the more serious burns that require lengthy hospitalization and extensive surgery. For instance, of the 179 whose clothing ignited, 37 per cent required skin grafts and extensive surgery, whereas only 6 per cent of those whose clothing did not ignite required extensive surgery and hospitalization. The relation of ignited clothing to the degree of burn indicates that 16 per cent of those whose clothing ignited received third-degree burns compared to 3 per cent of those whose clothing did not ignite. The report also shows that a greater number of days of hospitalization was required on a percentage basis for those whose clothing did not ignite. It is also apparent from this analysis that the per cent of the body area burned is much greater in the cases where the clothing ignites when compared to the cases where ignition of the clothing is not involved. The health department is now prepared to launch a very intensive community educational program to reduce the number of injuries from burns.

It might be well for you to know that we have conducted a number of other small pilot programs at the community level that are forerunners of the Birmingham Project. In Mississippi County, Ark., the focus was on the fires. Detailed investigations (with help from the county fire marshal) and analyses of the causative agents of the home fires were made. Tabulations were also made of the admissions for nonfatal burns in the local county hospital. An educational program was developed. It consisted largely of a visual demonstration that explained dramatically the properties of petroleum products and how electricity and home maintenance in general are involved in home fires. After this educational program was extensively used in the community for 1 year the incidence of nonfatal injuries from fire sustained by patients admitted to the local hospital was reduced by approximately 50 per cent. The fire-prevention kit developed here is now being produced commercially. It is being used in more than 35 states by health departments, fire departments, and others. Flame-retardant fabrics are always mentioned when this kit is used.

In Robeson County, N. C., a project was focused on the high-incidence group (which in this case was the nonwhite child under 10 years of age). The investigations revealed how he was burned, how he was treated, length of hospitalization, cost of hospitalization, and other related items. One of the most significant dividends from this study was our information on the emergency first-aid treatment of burns in this community. In some cases this involved the folklore of the Indian tribes and mixed racial groups. In many cases a minor burn was infected and compounded, which caused a severe injury requiring extensive plastic surgery and rehabilitation. Sometimes frog viscera, contaminated water, and horse manure were used in emergency treatment for burns sustained by children. The local health department initiated a comprehensive educational program on first aid for burns throughout the rural areas of the county.

Another pilot project that the division supported was in the State of Mississippi. It involved four counties near Jackson, where the focus was on injuries from burns as a *community problem.* This resulted in an extensive educational program.

One other pilot program involves the implementation of an inspection service for nursing homes and an educational program carried out by the State Health Department of Idaho, with heavy emphasis on efforts to prevent injuries to patients caused by fire.

From this résumé of activity, it should be apparent that public health officials are more than casually interested in the medical problems of burns and in their prevention and minimization.

We solicit the full cooperation of the textile industry, retail merchants, professional groups, and volunteer organizations throughout the United States to combine their talents and energies in order to improve the technology of, and to make more readily available, flame-retardant clothing, especially for children, for the aged, for the disabled, for those in special high-risk occupations, and for sportsmen who must protect themselves from serious and disabling burns.

The Public Health Service plans to continue its fact-finding efforts, and to work with industry, medicine, private organizations, and government agencies in seeking solutions to the problem. We shall continue to provide leadership for and encourage state and local health agencies in developing and conducting educational and informational programs to increase man's knowledge of hazards, his perception of the risk involved, and improve his ability to cope with situations that produce injuries.

# MERCHANTS' VIEWS ON FLAME-RETARDANT TEXTILES AND INJURIES FROM BURNS*

P. J. Fynn

Chairman, Technical Committee
Merchandising Division
National Retail Merchants Association
New York, N. Y.

Everyone here is participating in this conference because of an interest in reducing the toll in human life and suffering and in loss of property caused by fire; therefore my presence, in representing organizations and people who make available to the buying public the clothing and household textiles involved, makes it implicit that they too are interested in selling "safe" merchandise.

Discussions preceding mine have presented tragic results for persons who have been involved in fires that ignited their clothing, the technology available to render textiles nonflammable, and existing and proposed legislation for regulating the fire hazards of apparel produced by the textile industry.

Certainly no one can object to the intent of any proposed action, ruling, or law applied to the textile and garment industries that would eliminate a hazard to the life or limb of any person, but it is valid to question the effectiveness of any such measure and to examine any corollary effects to make sure that the proposals do not raise more problems than they solve. Some consideration should be given to the following points:

The Flammable Fabrics Act has been in effect for 13 years, and during this time there has been no recurrence of incidents similar to those that gave impetus to passage of the act. There had been a rash of accidents in which particularly flammable apparel had become ignited while worn by children, who died of the burns received. Present

*Based on a paper presented at the *Conference on Burns and Flame-Retardant Fabrics,* held at The New York Academy of Medicine, December 2 and 3, 1966. The conference was sponsored by: the New York and Brooklyn Trauma Committee of the American College of Surgeons, Chicago, Ill.; The National Fire Protection Association, Boston, Mass.; the Section on Plastic and Reconstructive Surgery of The New York Academy of Medicine; and the Division of Accident Prevention of the U. S. Public Health Service, Washington, D. C. The conference was held in cooperation with the American Academy of Pediatrics, Evanston, Ill.; the American Public Health Association, New York, N. Y.; and the National Safety Council, Chicago, Ill.; and was supported by a grant from the U. S. Public Health Service.

legislation has apparently been successful in excluding such hazardous materials from commerce.

In regard to proposals intended to enlarge the scope of the Flammable Fabrics Act as presently based upon the testing procedures of Commercial Standards 191-53: this cannot be done merely by changing or adding words intended to encompass fabrics other than those used for apparel. The tests in question, intended specifically for fabrics used in apparel, would not yield meaningful or realistic results if applied to materials intended for drapery or bedding. A new test technology will have to be evolved to yield results that correlate with other uses.

All textiles are consumed by fire, and most of them support combustion or contribute actively to any encompassing flames. Some fibers are difficult to ignite and, once ignited, will extinguish themselves upon removal of the igniting flame or will only smolder or burn slowly. Possible nonburning exceptions are metal fabrics, Fiberglas, and asbestos, and even these can melt or in other ways be destroyed as fabrics. This applies also to fabrics chemically treated to suppress combustion. There are no *fireproof* textiles nor are there any known means of rendering them *fireproof*.

As we have heard in detail, chemicals can be applied to many textiles to make them resistant to ignition and also self-extinguishing, but such chemicals, if they are to be durable enough to sustain washing and dry cleaning, will invariably affect the appearance, feel, or other aesthetic properties of the fabric in such a way as to render it unsuitable for many uses, especially in apparel. Also the chemical treatments have as yet unexplored potentials for causing allergic reactions and dermatitis.

Attempts to limit apparel or household textiles specifically to nonburning or slow-burning fibers or to fabrics chemically treated for fire-resistance will drastically limit the consumer's present wide freedom of choice in matters of color, texture, tactile qualities, style, and other esthetic properties presently available in a great variety of products. In addition to drastic restrictions in choice there would be unavoidable and considerable increases in cost to the consumer.

Any regulation of garment manufacturing intended to specify the fiber and chemical properties of garments manufactured for use in garments for children or for the aged could not control home-made items or the adapting by the consumer of other materials to such uses.

It is unfortunate that a certain number of individuals in every age group will die in any selected interval of time and that, whatever the circumstances, some deaths will be attributable to fire. Are there reliable statistics to support the view that the number of deaths caused by fire could be reduced significantly by using fire-resistant textiles? How often in cases of injury or death by fire has clothing been the sole or chief cause? Anyone involved in an encounter with fire may be seriously burned regardless of the nature of the clothing. How many deaths caused by fire could actually have been prevented if the victim had been wearing fire-retardant clothing? A single untimely death is one too many, but no regulation, however well-conceived and vigorously enforced, will prevent injury or death by fire. So—how far should regulation be carried in attempts to reduce deaths caused by flammable apparel when such regulation will reduce for the total population its capacity for living a life of free choice? Many untimely deaths result from what are normally such innocuous agencies as bees, mushrooms, and vaccinations. Must such agents then be eliminated? The U.S. Public Health Service, according to a public statement made by Dr. James Goddard, has statistics to show that death can result from the ingestion of a single tablet of aspirin and that, statistically, one child dies every 3 days from the effects of aspirin. Are these untimely deaths to be controlled by denying the entire population the choice of availing themselves freely of the undeniable benefits of a drug proved to be usually effective?

This oversimplified and perhaps not too apt parallel was drawn only to point out that records and statistics can dramatize a peril and stimulate a reaction that could be more detrimental to the community than the peril itself—the cure can be worse than the disease.

This is not intended to defend any practices in the textile industry that create a hazard to the consumer but only to point out that the elimination of death and injury resulting from clothing fires would not be accomplished immediately by persuading textile manufacturers to produce nonflammable goods only, and even if this ideal could be achieved would the public accept the restrictions on freedom of choice and the kind of textiles that would be the unavoidable concomitant?

For a merchant to exist in a free enterprise system he must be able to make a profit from supplying his customers with what they demand. Merchants of integrity try to the best of their ability and resources to do this while at the same time delivering honest values for money received and by refraining from selling merchandise having any concealed hazard. No merchant could retain the custom of his trade if he censored his wares and sold only what he thought was good for his customers.

For instance, there is an honest, legitimate market for such potential destroyers of life and health as shot-guns, axes, knives, dynamite, lye, deadly vermin exterminators, and poisonous chemicals of all sorts. There are many accidental deaths and injuries annually caused by such agents. Their very nature and reason for existence makes it impossible to render them "safe." Should merchants censor these items and refuse to sell them? The hazards inherent in the possession and use of such things are so obvious that the normal instinct for self-preservation is relied upon to motivate the use of proper knowledge and caution in their use. The key here is the fact that the hazard is obvious. In the case of fire hazards in the use of textiles the danger is not so apparent: the peril lies in the concealed hazard.

This brings up the matter of educating the consumer and the possible moral duty of the merchant in ensuring that the customer realizes all aspects of risk and hazard in the use and possible misuse of the merchandise. New substances and materials appear with increasing frequency in a host of new applications, and even the inventors and technical developers of these new items are not always aware of possible hazards to the public under all conceivable conditions of use. The larger retailers who can afford the talent have their own laboratories and technical staff to check on safety and suitability of new products in order to avoid booby traps. They make every effort to tell the customer just what he is buying and how to make the best use of it.

Any information or instructions given on labels must presuppose some background of knowledge on the part of the customer. It seems a little unnecessary, in light of the basic law of self-preservation, to inform a customer that clothing and textiles will burn when exposed to flame or high temperatures.

One of the larger merchandising organizations recently supplied a paper entitled "Textile Safety," which is available as Bulletin MP66-12 from the National Fire Protection Association, Boston, Mass. Because I have not had time to obtain the written consent of the author or of the Association I cannot quote it directly. But in essence it points out what is the common experience and view of merchants of clothing and textiles: namely, that fire-resistance or any other safety features of textiles have no appeal for customers at the point of sale, and that the standards of a product's performance set up by any group on the basis of an engineer's approach usually ignore the desires and demands of the consumer.

We have had experience in my own company in trying to sell to our own customers what was good for them. Some time ago, during a flare-up of nationwide publicity on cases of burns caused by ignited apparel, we created a particular garment in a flame-proofed version and promoted it vigorously with special displays that called attention to its nonflammable quality. Because of hard realities these garments were necessarily priced about one dollar higher than comparable nontreated garments. A few weeks later the special price was removed and the stock was mixed with the regular garments because no one was buying the safety garments at the premium price. Everyone probably figured: "It can't happen to me."

This whole problem of hazards from fire is a matter of public education. Modern conditions of living in our cities have produced several generations of children whose only experience with open flame is a match or cigarette lighter. Largely gone are bonfires, camp fires, pot-bellied stoves, fired kitchen ranges, open hearths, fireworks, and other factors that gave growing children experience with and exposure to fire, and exposure to a stream of parental admonitions on the perils and dangers of fire and the precautions necessary while in the vicinity of fire. Many people grow up unaware of the fire hazards in their surroundings, including their clothes.

The solution to the problem is not to limit all clothing and textiles to those that can be rendered fireproof. This would be a very confining limitation indeed and one that, I am sure, the consuming public, which includes each one of us, would not tolerate. Nor is the whole solution to be found in developing ways and means of rendering fireproof all articles, both existing and potential. The solution is in educating the public to an awareness of and respect for potential death in the flame of a match and the small glow of a cigarette.

Given the proper conditions, everything will "burn": even a steel and concrete structure.

# LEGAL ASPECTS OF THE CLOTHING FIRE PROBLEM*

ARNOLD B. ELKIND

American Trial Lawyers Association
New York, N. Y.

FROM a historical perspective we hope that this conference marks the opening of a new phase of the continually intensifying consumer revolution. This revolution unquestionably has real potential meaning to more citizens of the United States than the civil rights upheaval or the recent pronouncements of the Supreme Court on the rights of defendants in criminal cases. Except for the automobile safety legislation, it has been carried out with so little fanfare that the average citizen is unaware of the dramatic legal changes that have affected him in the past 20 years as a user of manufactured products.

When I came to the Bar in 1939 it could have truthfully been said for almost all practical purposes that "the injured user is just a loser." The consumer was the virtually unprotected dupe and victim for an economy intent on expanding its industrial power and commercial activity. This had been going on from colonial times. Four principal weapons have been used in dealing with this situation that, together with an improvement in general education, have affected the consumer revolution in the field of safety thus far. They are: 1) the jury system in civil trials; 2) a partisan Trial Bar that has made itself better informed; 3) a humanitarian judiciary; and 4) enlightened political leadership at the federal level.

This conference focuses on the right of the consumer to be clothed in fabrics that do not unreasonably expose him to the tortures of the flame. Let us examine the weapons of the consumer revolution in the law as they are brought to bear on textile manufacturers in order to vindicate and protect this important right.

*Based on a paper presented at the *Conference on Burns and Flame-Retardant Fabrics,* held at The New York Academy of Medicine, December 2 and 3, 1966. The conference was sponsored by: the New York and Brooklyn Trauma Committee of the American College of Surgeons, Chicago, Ill.; The National Fire Protection Association, Boston, Mass.; the Section on Plastic and Reconstructive Surgery of The New York Academy of Medicine; and the Division of Accident Prevention of the U.S. Public Health Service, Washington, D.C. The conference was held in cooperation with the American Academy of Pediatrics, Evanston, Ill.; the American Public Health Association, New York, N. Y.; and the National Safety Council, Chicago, Ill.; and was supported by a grant from the U.S. Public Health Service.

We start with the jury, which is available in civil cases under the Constitution, and offer for your consideration what amounts to a truism among knowledgeable trial advocates and insurance companies: the realization that a burned human has a better chance of receiving a large monetary award from a jury than a person who has sustained a comparably disabling injury in any other way. The reason for this begins with the fact that juries are always instructed by the judge to award damages for pain and suffering if there is fault and if any recovery is to be awarded to the injured person under the rules that apply. In the usual case the trial advocate for the injured individual is faced with the problem of bringing home to the jury what pain and suffering have meant to his client. Without that understanding the evaluation in terms of dollars is haphazard. Such understanding is not always easy to establish, for in the case of many injuries there is no subjective experience for the jury to use as a guide.

But all of us have experienced the exquisite anguish of a hot match or an overheated kitchen utensil, and we can readily understand, by magnification of that experience, the torture endured by one who has an extensive area of burn. Even more telling in terms of the receptivity of juries is the educational and religious experience common to so many jurors, in which burning is equated with the tortures of hell as the ultimate punishment for the most heinous offenses against God and man. Those childhood associations prepare the jury to come to terms easily with the enormity of the pain that a burned plaintiff has suffered through no fault of his own. Awards of $5,000 per day for such pain have been sustained in the courts. This past spring a textile manufacturer was ordered by a jury to pay a housewife $140,000 for burns that she sustained when her cotton pajamas brushed against a kitchen burner. The pajamas caught fire and burned her body.

This case illustrates the power of the second weapon, to wit: the partisan Trial Bar that has taken pains to become better informed. The American Trial Lawyers Association, a partisan Trial Bar representing injured people, makes it its business to be institutionally aware of the fact that our Federal Flammable Fabrics Act regulations have lagged. The lawyers discuss these matters at their postadmission legal education seminars and conventions. When we talk of the American Trial Lawyers Association we are speaking of about 20,000 lawyers from all over the country who customarily represent injured people. The reasonable probability today is that a serious burn case will eventually be entrusted to one of these trial specialists.

While the news media may not consider the gross inadequacy of the federal regulations on fabrics to be newsworthy, the fact is that the information exists in the circles where it can be meaningful in terms of consumer protection. The lawyers in question know about the English experience in fire-retarding clothing.* They know that the flammability tests now incorporated in the federal regulations fail to establish the fact that those same fabrics will not become torches under a variety of real environmental conditions. They have witnessed those inappropriate flame tests in a glass box and understand that the principal value is to the manufacturer, who can easily show compliance with the requirements of federal regulations.

So while the results of flammability tests may be admissible, the jurors can be told under the law that the manufacturer's duty to exercise reasonable care is not—I repeat, is not—satisfied by naked compliance with the Flammable Fabrics Act tests, and the verdict against cotton pajamas proves that when a jury is informed of the choices available to the manufacturer at the present stage of our technology, it will find industry at fault for producing a fabric for clothing that unreasonably endangers the wearer. And this must be so in this space age of scientific achievement.

In the well-tried case involving flammable fabrics the lawyer for the plaintiff will emphasize that the fabric was inappropriate for the user in terms of safety. This point is stressed because the judge will charge the jury that the standard of care to which the manufacturer is held is the standard of a reasonably prudent manufacturer. The plaintiff will argue that a reasonable prudent manufacturer should make inquiry and become informed as to the ultimate use to which the fabric will be adapted. Will this fabric be used in an infant's garment? Will it be used in hospitals or nursing homes where the aged and infirm are found? Will it be used by a housewife in the kitchen, where sources of combustion are ever present? The processor who is charged by law with knowledge of the combustible characteristics of his product can be held to a duty to make inquiry and suggestions as to what fabric should be used for a particular purpose. The failure to make inquiry and to

*The Consumer Protective Act of 1961 authorized the Home Secretary to regulate for any prescribed class of goods the safety requirements that in his opinion are expedient to prevent risk of death or personal injury. In 1964 the Home Office adopted regulations requiring flame-retardant nightwear for children.

recommend a fabric with better fire-retardant characteristics could be considered negligence.

Can manufacturers, converters, and finishers perpetually evade liability by disclaiming knowledge or by saying "I did only what I was told?" Will they be protected by adopting an ostrichlike attitude? Will the law pay a premium for ignorance? The answer will be "No." The test is not whether the manufacturer or converter actually knew to what use the fabric would be utilized. The test is whether, as a reasonably prudent manufacturer, he knew, or *should have known,* the use to which the fabric would be put, and the law presumes his knowledge of the flammable characteristics of his product. It would be for the jury to decide whether inquiry should have been made along each step of the way by the various processors in the manufacture of clothing as to what use will be made of the finished garment. With some reasonable degree of certainty we can predict that the continuance of present trends of liability will entail an obligation on the part of some processor before the retailer to ascertain whether the fabric for which he is responsible will be used in children's clothing, or in the kitchen, or in hospitals or nursing homes. My hope is that the industry will anticipate the legal duty of making such inquiry and will voluntarily adopt realistic standards and procedures in order to determine intentions as to the ultimate disposition of the product and to make recommendations.

Those representatives of the textile industry who are present may well be saying "that Elkind is trying to frighten us into assuming obligations to the consumer that the law does not require us to assume. There haven't been any new laws passed that affect us, and the regulations haven't been changed. The history of litigation in this field suggests that we stand fast." Let me therefore explain briefly why the past experiences in which so many lawsuits were successfully defended are inappropriate criteria for assessing what should be done in the future.

Under our jurisprudence most questions of fact are determined by juries. Questions of law are determined by the judges. There was a time when the judiciary, concerned primarily with encouranging the progress of the industrial and commercial revolutions, laid down legal principles that artificially insulated manufacturers, wholesalers, and middlemen from the claims of the consumer that he had sustained an injury because of a defective product. In order to safeguard the commercial and manufacturing community from being answerable to the public at large for delinquencies in the duty of care in connection with the design or manufacture of their product, the judges evolved a concept that they called "privity," and they insisted for almost 65 years, from 1842 on, that there be a contractual relation between an injured consumer and the delinquent manufacturer or wholesaler or distributor or retailer in order for the injured consumer to have a basis of claim.

In other words, we were so loaded against the consumer during the 65-year period that if someone were to have given me a garment that had been sized with nitrocellulose, and it were actually to have exploded into flame, causing me to sustain terrible burns, and if this had happened 60 years ago, there would have been no one whom I could have successfully sued. But if I had bought that coat from a retailer I could sue the retailer because of the contractual relation between us. The retailer in turn could sue his wholesaler who, in turn, might sue the contractor or converter who, in turn, could sue the finisher. You can readily see that this system was procedurally unsound, cumbersome, and patently unfair.

In the past 50 years there have been dramatic changes. These started by permitting the consumer to sue a manufacturer even though he had no contractual relation, provided he could prove some fault or negligence in the manufacturing process or inspection procedures. This obligation of proving fault, however, was onerous and extremely expensive for the injured consumer, since it generally required him to become familiar with and punch holes in the defendant's manufacturing and inspection procedures, necessitating usually that the injured man hire technicians and expert witnesses. Only those cases involving serious injuries would warrant the type of legal activity and expense necessary to present facts on fault to the court. When this inequity was recognized, the next step then was to impose on the manufacturer and retailer and distributor a commitment, as a matter of law, to the public, whereby the public is virtually guaranteed that the product, when used in the appropriate way, will not cause an unanticipated injury. This is a rule of strict liability that found full expression only in 1960. It is gradually being accepted as the law in almost every state of the Union. When judges make these changes in the common law you can be sure that they are expressing a genuine need based on human experience. The law is slow to respond to the needs of the community, but when the reforms begin the adaptation is inexorable. The reforms are under way.

You can easily see that under such a rule of strict liability a garment that a jury finds to be unreasonably flammable can be the vehicle whereby a manufacturer or a wholesaler or, in fact, anyone in the commercial chain, can be required to indemnify an injured individual for whatever damage that person sustains by virtue of the flammability of the garment.

At the risk of repetition, let me say again that compliance with the Flammable Fabrics Act does not automatically mean that industry is exonerated from liability to a consumer who sustains an injury as a result of the burning of a garment. The garment, even though it complies with the Flammable Fabrics Act, may have characteristics that make it inappropriate for use in a child's dress or suit, or in something that by design is to be used in the area of the kitchen stove or by the aged and infirm. The jurymen remain the judges of the facts in lawsuits, and they can still decide that the manufacturer of the garment did not exercise prudence in using the particular cloth for a given garment even though that cloth, as I say, was manufactured in such a way as to pass the Flammable Fabrics Act requirements set forth in its regulations.

How much clearer can I make the situation to you than by telling you that the converters were held liable in a case that involved ordinary cotton pajamas that caught fire in the kitchen. The jury felt that the manufacturer was negligent in distributing cotton pajamas. That jury felt that cotton should not be used for clothing unless it were fire-retarded, in the way that the English are fire-retarding their cotton clothing for certain groups and in line with the technological intelligence we acquired during and since World War II. You must anticipate that the responses of an increasingly large number of juries in the years ahead will be to condemn the use of cotton and to subject those using it to liability for the damage that results when the cotton burns while being worn.

Now manufacturers may feel that since this is an enterprise risk, they can protect themselves by carrying insurance or increasing their insurance limits, and that all responsible manufacturers will follow suit, so that the price of the garments and materials will reflect this increased cost, and will eventually be passed on to the public in any event. So we can go on making flammable garments, and those few unfortunates will be compensated by the few extra pennies that will be charged for each yard of fabric that we sell.

I submit to you that this response is shortsighted and immoral, and that it will eventually prove to be a stopgap. It is shortsighted because it does not answer the needs of the community and must therefore fall of its own weight. The cost of insurance premiums, which includes a profit to the insurance companies, will foreseeably grow and become increasingly oppressive as recoveries become more common.

It is immoral to use for increased insurance premiums money that could be used to make fabrics with much greater flame resistance.

What I have actually been doing here is to present the case for the consumer. I hope I have persuaded some of you that the wisest course in your business councils will be voluntarily to adopt manufacturing procedures and techniques and distribution norms that will substantially reduce the frightening statistic that 150,000 people are burned each year as a result of excessively flammable clothing. The proceedings of this meeting, I am told, will find their way into the literature of our intellectual community and will become part of our generalized knowledge. The standard of care in this bootstrap fashion becomes elevated to some degree by what has been done here in the last 2 days.

The final thought, however, with which I should like to sear your minds as you reconsider your responsibilities to the consumer, is to introduce to you the concept of punitive damages. In the days when the consumer had to be in privity with the defendant it could be said that he had nothing more than a slingshot to counterattack industry. The right to sue for negligence of the manufacturer armed him with a bow and arrow. With the warranties of the Sales Act the law gave him a rifle, and the rule of strict liability of the 1960's equipped the consumer with a cannon. With the right to sue for punitive damages the consumer comes into the atomic age.

Three weeks ago a jury in Westchester County, New York, awarded a woman a verdict against the Richardson-Merrell Company for wrongfully marketing an anticholesterol called MER/29. That verdict was $1,205,000, but of that amount $850,000 was awarded as punitive damages. This was the amount that the jury said had to be imposed as punishment to teach the Richardson-Merrell Company a lesson, and it was undoubtedly based on the economic structure of the company. In other words, the richer the company the more money it must pay in order to learn a lesson. There are approximately 500 suits pending against the Richardson-Merrell Company, and the outcome of those cases is going to be influenced by what happened in the Westchester case. So far the law appears to be that each consumer is entitled to punitive damages, for in an earlier case tried in the southern part of New York State about 6 months ago a jury had assessed Richardson-Merrell for approximately $100,000 as punitive damages.

It is doubted by at least some legal scholars that a company can ultimately insure itself against punitive damages. Courts have given conflicting answers to this question, but one argument advanced in the negative is that it is contrary to public policy to defeat by insurance the very purpose for which the principle of punitive damages was adopted. In other words, it is argued that the social purpose of punitive damages is to teach a delinquent a lesson, and that the social purpose would be frustrated if it became normal for the delinquent to purchase immunity in advance by means of an insurance premium.

The doctrine of punitive damages comes into play when there is a showing of a willful disregard of the rights of an injured person. I believe that if there were to be a repetition of the cowboy suit tragedies of the 1940's, or some similar situation in which a number of children or housewives were to be burned in epidemic fashion, and if there were to be a showing of a manufacturing and distribution philosophy that suggested a willful contempt of the interests of the consumer, you would have an excellent parallel and a predictable legal denouement in which punitive damages would be awarded in addition to compensatory damages.

Unfortunately, every man present knows that such an epidemic can occur again. Will it be a rayon fringe that fuzzes out in the washing machine and becomes a fuse to a cotton jacket or dress? Will it be a weave that loosens with use and cleaning and becomes readily combustible? And do not count on the statistical improbability of sources of ignition! Kitchens in the newer apartments are scarcely larger than closets in the houses in which we were raised, and a moment of inattentiveness in such a kitchen can provide a source of ignition.

The clothing industry's problem is genuine; it is of this moment. The industry has a great opportunity to take a positon of leadership on consumer safety. I know I express the sentiment of every lawyer who has vicariously experienced the torture of a burned client when I wish you unbounded success on a course toward eliminating flammable fabrics. I urge you to fire-retard garments: particularly those that can be sold to children and that our wives and daughters may use in the kitchen. The doctors and lawyers who get into this act will applaud and support the effort. If the effort bogs down—if the desirable ends cannot be reached voluntarily—the doctors and lawyers will do their best to alleviate the distress and to prevent the exposure of others to injury.

# ACTION AND PROGRAM FOR THE FUTURE*

GEORGE F. CRIKELAIR

Professor of Surgery
and Director of Plastic Surgery Service
Columbia-Presbyterian Medical Center
New York, N. Y.

SEVERAL years ago, as many of you know, I became interested in flame-retardant clothing after two child patients of ours died; both were severely burned because their clothing had caught fire. At that time there seemed to be a paucity of information and interest regarding the subject and it was difficult to obtain assistance.

Thanks to the encouragement of Dr. Alexander Garcia, then chairman of the New York Regional Committee on Trauma of the American College of Surgeons, and to Dr. Robert Kennedy, Director, Field Program, Committee on Trauma, of the American College of Surgeons, the search has been most profitable. The serious work and interest of government agencies, private industry, medical and other organizations too numerous to mention have added to our knowledge. An incidental but most delightful part of the search has been the addition of many new friends in varied disciplines—friends who are superbly motivated to help their fellow men.

In particular, I am indebted to the members of my committee who have done all the work in setting up this most stimulating meeting, and I should like to now extend thanks from all of us to Mr. William White, Chief, Liaison Services, Division of Accident Prevention, U.S. Public Health Service; Mr. A. Schaplowsky, Chief, Community Services Branch, Division of Accident Prevention, U.S. Public Health Service; Mr. Sidney Ascher, Regional Accident Prevention Consultant, U.S. Public Health Service; Dr. Robert Kennedy, Director, Field Program, Committee on Trauma of the American College of Surgeons; Mr. James Sibbison, Chairman, Chief Information Services, Division of Accident

*Based on a paper presented at the *Conference on Burns and Flame-Retardant Fabrics,* held at The New York Academy of Medicine, December 2 and 3, 1966. The conference was sponsored by: the New York and Brooklyn Trauma Committee of the American College of Surgeons, Chicago, Ill.; The National Fire Protection Association, Boston, Mass.; the Section on Plastic and Reconstructive Surgery of The New York Academy of Medicine; and the Division of Accident Prevention of the U. S. Public Health Service, Washington, D. C. The conference was held in cooperation with the American Academy of Pediatrics, Evanston, Ill.; the American Public Health Association, New York, N. Y.; and the National Safety Council, Chicago, Ill.; and was supported by a grant from the U. S. Public Health Service.

Prevention, U.S. Public Health Service; and Mr. Chester Babcock, Assistant Technical Secretary, National Fire Protection Association.

I should also like to thank The New York Academy of Medicine for its interest and hospitality—and I direct these words to Dr. Howard Reid Craig in particular.

Speaking for all doctors, may I repeat the words I spoke several years ago to the American Association of Textile Chemists and Colorists here in New York City, to whom I said that we in the medical profession should be delighted to lose business in that the care of burned patients is our business. We shall be happy to give up this business to all of you who are dedicated to the development of permanently flame-retardant fabrics.

As our knowledge increases, as industry becomes more proficient at developing clothing that is permanently flame-retardant, as the teaching being done by all of you and your organizations spreads to more and more people, as there is increased interest throughout the country stimulated by meetings such as this, we hope the problem of burns caused by burning clothing will be solved. In solving this problem, there are some areas in our discussions and thinking that must be clarified. Clothing does burn despite the fact that it meets the present standards established in 1953; it depends on the circumstances. We have heard criticism of the effort to make clothing permanently flame-retardant—criticism that suggests that it is the action taken after the clothing catches fire, such as running instead of rolling, that is responsible for the injury; criticism that suggests that cigarette lighters and matches are left for children to play with, so—why blame the clothing? I think we must face realities: that if a child reaches over a stove, the clothing will burn, and the child will run. Our aim should be directed not at doing away with stoves or the normal reactions of children but to offer them protection, as much as we can, from these realities of existence.

Where do we go from here? Do we go home to hope and to teach some more? Do we go home to wait for national legislation? Do we go home knowing or at least hoping that our children or relatives won't be burned because their clothing catches fire? One thing is certain: we go home knowing that we have accomplished a great deal by talking with each other these past 2 days; that we have all increased our own knowledge; that we can take this information to the organizations we represent; that the papers presented here will reach many people by publication in the *Bulletin of The New York Academy of Medicine.*

But is that enough? I think not.

We know that our legislators in Washington, D.C., are looking into this problem and that their investigations may be costly and time-consuming. If we did the investigating for them, they could use their time and our money more profitably in solving other problems.

Therefore, I propose that we help solve the problem for the people in this country and for our legislators. How can this be done?

1) By establishing today a new organization entitled "Flame-Retardant Clothing Association."

2) By electing today a chairman, a secretary, and an executive committee to set up our rules, regulations, by-laws, and constitution.

3) By establishing committees within this Association; a committee on statistics, a committee on cotton, a committee on man-made fabrics, a committee on medicine, a committee on governmental agencies, a committee on retailers, a committee on membership, a committee on education, and a committee on safety. The chairmen of these committees will constitute the Executive Committee.

4) By having an annual meeting at which each committee could meet and spend time at work by itself, at which each committee could report progress, formulate future plans, and make suggestions to the membership of the other committees.

The purpose of the Association would be to develop clothing that is permanently flame-retardant, to educate the public in its availability and desirability, and to further the exchange of knowledge by all disciplines concerned. I suggest that there should be financial profit from the development of flame retardant clothing by all parties except medicine and government. By this I mean that industry should not be penalized financially, since financial gain on its part adds to the well-being of our country.

We can envision workshops, study groups, exhibits, and scientific sessions at the annual meetings. We can perhaps hope that this group eventually will affect national legislation if such legislation is needed.

I solicit your comments on these suggestions in the general discussion to follow in the hope that we can take some formal action now.

In closing, may I thank the chairman, the speakers and all of you for your interest and participation in this meeting.

# CONFERENCE ON BURNS AND FLAME-RETARDANT FABRICS*

## General Discussion

WILLIAM G. JOHNSON, *Chairman*

General Manager
National Safety Council
Chicago, Ill.

HERBERT J. WOLLNER, LOUIS SEGAL, A. F. ROBERTSON, ALBERT P. ISKRANT, PAUL V. JOLIET, JOSEPH R. PALMER, HARRY A. FREEDMAN, GEORGE L. DRAKE, JR., R. BRUCE LEBLANC, GEORGE S. BUCK, JR., H. C. HOTTEL, PERCY BUGBEE, JOHN L. SEVERANCE, JOHN APPEL, P. J. FYNN, PHIL DYKSTRA, DONALD A. DUKELOW

MR. WILLIAM G. JOHNSON: I should like to call for discussion of Dr. George F. Crikelair's specific suggestions as to forming a new organization on flame-retardant clothing. However, I have some questions on cards, and I should prefer to finish the questions first. But I know from meetings of this sort that we shall have comments also. Let me remind you that Dr. Kennedy stated in the introductory session that any comments would be limited to two minutes until we have heard from everyone who wants to talk. Then, if it is not yet 4 o'clock, and anyone has more to add, we shall hear him.

*Held at The New York Academy of Medicine, December 2 and 3, 1966. The conference was sponsored by: the New York and Brooklyn Trauma Committee of the American College of Surgeons, Chicago, Ill.; The National Fire Protection Association, Boston, Mass.; the Section on Plastic and Reconstructive Surgery of The New York Academy of Medicine; and the Division of Accident Prevention of the U.S. Public Health Service, Washington, D.C. The conference was held in cooperation with the American Academy of Pediatrics, Evanston, Ill.; the American Public Health Association, New York, N.Y.; and the National Safety Council, Chicago, Ill.; and was supported by a grant from the U.S. Public Health Service.

Participants and their affiliations: Herbert J. Wollner, president, A. C. H. Fiber Service, Inc., Boston, Mass.; Louis Segal, fire prevention engineer, California Fire Marshal's Office, Los Angeles, Calif., and chairman, Committee on Wearing Apparel, National Fire Protection Association, Boston, Mass.; A. F. Robertson, chief, Fire Research Section, National Bureau of Standards, Washington, D.C.; Albert P. Iskrant, chief, Epidemiology and Surveillance, Injury Control Program, National Center for Urban and Industrial Health, U.S. Public Health Service, Arlington, Va.; Paul V. Joliet, chief, Division of Accident Prevention, U. S. Public Health Service, Arlington, Va.; Joseph R. Palmer, men's underwear buyer, Sears Roebuck & Co., Chicago, Ill.; Harry A. Freedman, product development manager, Borg Fabrics Division, Amphenol Corporation, Delavan, Wisc.; George L. Drake, Jr., Southern Utilization Research and Development Division, Agricultural Research and Development Division, Agricultural Research Service, U.S. Department of Agriculture, New Orleans, La.; R. Bruce LeBlanc, senior textile specialist, Technical Service and Development, Dow Chemical Co., Midland, Mich.; George S. Buck, Jr., National Cotton Council, Memphis, Tenn.; H. C. Hottel, Massachusetts Institute of Technology, Cambridge, Mass.; Percy Bugbee, National Fire Protection Association, Boston, Mass.; John L. Severance, American Textile Manufacturing Institute, New York, N.Y.; John Appel, Safety Division, Commonwealth Edison Co., Chicago, Ill.; P. J. Fynn, chairman, Technical Committee, Merchandising Division, National Retail Merchants Association, New York, N.Y.; Phil Dykstra, manager, Home Department, National Safety Council, Chicago, Ill.; Donald A. Dukelow, assistant director, Health Education of the Public, American Medical Association, Chicago, Ill.

Here is a written question for Mr. Wollner: "What has been your experience with fires caused by washing and tumble-drying textiles that are combined with natural rubber products?"

MR. HERBERT J. WOLLNER: I was asked that question this morning. I have had no immediate experience with such mixtures of fabric and natural rubber but I have had experience with some experiments of tumble-drying certain unidentified plastic materials of a resilient character that did overheat when temperature controls got out of hand, especially under certain conditions of limited ranges in humidity. I am not prepared to extrapolate beyond that.

MR. LOUIS SEGAL: It is a well-known fact that rubber is subject to spontaneous heating at elevated temperatures above approximately 200° F. People who commonly launder or dry clean clothing are very well aware of this; they used to have fires continuously until they learned. We shall probably still have fires in the home because the public is not very well informed of this.

But if, for instance, you put a throw rug with a rubber backing in a drier and the temperature reaches 200° F. you may very well have a fire; also in the case of any article of clothing that has rubber in it.

MR. JOHNSON: Thank you, Mr. Segal. Here is a question for Dr. Robertson: "Please list the natural and synthetic fibers in order of their flammability."

DR. A. F. ROBERTSON: I really think that I had better not try to do that at this point in the meeting.

MR. JOHNSON: It might be in order, if you have such a list, to give it to the staff for the permanent record, so that anyone who wants such information may seek it for himself.

UNIDENTIFIED SPEAKER: I think we ought to comment on that question. I don't believe anyone can list fibers in the order of their flammability if he takes into consideration all the factors of flammability. Do you agree, Dr. Robertson?

DR. ROBERTSON: Yes. I should expect that the flammability ranking of the different textile fibers would depend on the construction of the fabric involved, on the nature of the source of ignition, and the characteristics of the method used for measurement.

MR. JOHNSON: A question for Mr. Iskrant: "Would it be possible to obtain a set of the charts you used to illustrate the burn cases? And am I correct in believing that these charts will be in the proceedings?"

MR. ALBERT P. ISKRANT: They will be, and they are also available to anyone here.

MR. JOHNSON: "Wouldn't a sampling of injuries and fatalities from burns prepared by doctors or hospitals be very helpful in pinning down more specific needed information? Let us sharpen our statistics. Get type of garment or house furnishings and identification." This is a question for Dr. Joliet. It seems to me that the epidemiological team of the Public Health Service is trying to do this. The question here is should the doctors and the hospitals collect this information.

Let me comment on that. We have made many efforts to persuade hospitals to tabulate more data than they do, and it seems economically and administratively difficult, if not impossible. We receive one-sentence descriptions.

It seems clear at present that if data are to be collected in the emergency room it must be done through some kind of funded project, perhaps of the type that the Public Health Service has at Denver, or through any other type of funded undertaking, because the doctor cannot take the time and the nurse usually won't or can't obtain a factual account. Somebody else usually has to do it. Is there anybody who feels differently about that?

MR. JOSEPH R. PALMER: A point I should like to make is that if we can get data for a broad geographic cross-section, not just for one area, the information will be more meaningful and more of a true sampling.

MR. JOHNSON: We agree with you, and we have supported legislative appropriations for the Public Health Service to try to get such data. But we need more support in terms of public support, legislative support, for appropriations when a governmental project is in question.

Here is a query for Dr. Richard A. Prindle. "On what basis was the 40 per cent estimate of modacrylic content made? Is this blend effective with all fibers or dependent upon the flammability of the other fiber?"

[Dr. Prindle was not present at this point.]

MR. HARRY FREEDMAN: I think I can answer that, at least partly. A 40 per cent blend of modacrylic is effective as far as upgrading a relatively flammable fiber—shall we say, a fiber that will not pass a flammable fabrics test—to the point where it will pass the test.

In answer to the second part of the question, the degree of the effect of flame retardancy of the modacrylic is dependent upon the flammability of the other flammable portion of the fabric. The percentage of modacrylic in it, of course, could be lowered with a less flammable fiber, so that if you have a relatively nonflammable fiber as the other portion of the blend you might have an acceptable 25 per cent modacrylic level.

With a very flammable fiber conceivably you might have to use more than 40 per cent, but in the majority of cases 40 per cent is a reasonable amount that will make an acceptable, safe garment.

MR. JOHNSON: The next question is: "Does the durable press process affect the flammability of fabrics? And if so, how?" Can anybody answer that?

MR. GEORGE L. DRAKE, JR.: It does not usually increase the flammability.

MR. JOHNSON: It does not affect it.

MR. DRAKE: I might add one statement here. Most permanent press resins contain nitrogen. We have found that nitrogen in the presence of phosphorus acts synergistically to improve the degree of flame resistance. Therefore permanent press resins might even improve the degree of flame resistance of a fabric.

MR. JOHNSON: A question for Mr. Drake. "You mentioned a flame temperature of 400° F. for cotton and afterglow temperature of 650° F. Is there an error here?"

MR. DRAKE: No, there is no error. As you know, cellulose is composed of carbon, hydrogen, and oxygen. When a flame-retardant finish is applied to cotton we think it imparts flame resistance by the formation of Lewis acid and dehydration of the cotton, theoretically to form carbon and water. Flame retardants are not this efficient; thus flame-retardant fabrics in contact with a flame do not produce carbon and water only. Some carbon monoxide and dioxide are produced. A flaming cellulose is a reducing flame. The heat of formation for producing carbon dioxide (the cause of afterglow) is much higher than the heat of formation for carbon monoxide. In fact, three to four times as many kilocalories are involved in producing carbon dioxide. This makes a big difference in the glowing temperature.

MR. JOHNSON: Another question: "Why not obtain statistics on burns from the doctors who treat the victims? Request cooperation via the American Medical Association and use standard questionnaires made available to all hospitals. A one-year report should be sufficient." Would you comment on that.

MR. ISKRANT: Yes. Burns comprise a relatively small proportion of the injuries occurring in the United States. I should like to obtain complete reporting of all injuries, but I must say that the facilities available to me are such that I could not possibly handle reporting from all physicians of all injuries because that would be approximately 40 million a year.

If there is a special emphasis on burns and some facilities are made available to me to install nation-wide reporting from physicians, I believe I could handle the reports. I have done so with other diseases. But with my present resources I could not possibly handle the reports on burns also.

MR. JOHNSON: Another question: "Do they require labeling of yard goods in England, e.g., 'suitable for children's sleeping garments' or 'unsuitable'?" Can anybody answer that question?

UNIDENTIFIED SPEAKER: No, not yet.

MR. JOHNSON: I have a note here. Do you have a comment, Mr. Segal, that you wanted to make on labeling?

MR. SEGAL: Yes, if there aren't any other questions.

MR. JOHNSON: I have two other comments, but no more questions.

MR. SEGAL: First, I should like to thank the National Fire Prevention Association publicly for making it possible for me to be here. I don't want you to think that the State of California is so rich it can send its employees all the way across the country every time there is a meeting. It can't, but the NFPA felt strongly enough about my being here that they picked up the larger part of the expenses.

And along that line: if any of you who are interested genuinely in fire prevention activities are not members of the NFPA, may I urge you to consider joining it. That's partial payment.

My principal comment, though, is this: you may have heard me ask Mr. Elkind about this matter of the legality of labeling garments that are capable of causing burns, and I was very encouraged by his answer because I think this is a possible direction we should be exploring. I advocate that we get or try to get a national law requiring that any fabric that can reasonably be expected to contribute to an injury from burns must say something on a permanently attached label to the effect, not necessarily that this is a highly flammable garment, but perhaps, at least, that it should be kept away from open flames.

We have all agreed here there are directions in which to go, but there are problems connected with all of them. It has been my opinion for many years that because of these problems the immediate necessity is to educate our public. I can't think of a more direct or effective way of doing this than by a warning label right on the garment.

As an inducement to people to do better than they are doing now, you could exempt those garments that wouldn't need such a label: for instance, wool or an adequately treated garment or something made of the modacrylics. This would create some problems of defining what would need the label and what would not, but these are not unsurmountable problems, and I hope that the textile industry, after hearing what Mr. Elkind had to say, might consider this as one way out of their dilemma.

MR. R. BRUCE LE BLANC: Whether a fabric is flammable or not is hard to say. It is difficult to specify the flammability or nonflammability of a textile fiber. It depends on particular circumstances in which the fiber is used.

The British law is a good example of legislation that requires the use of fire-retardant fabrics. The legislation requires that children's nightdresses be flame-retardant, and the law specifies a test that must be passed.

This British test was designed for treated cotton. Nylon, as Dr. Crikelair's film showed (I think it was a nylon slip in that dress) was burning and dripping, and it caused the burns on the leg of the little girl.

Nylon is very flammable, but it passes the British test and it is used. I estimate that probably 75 per cent—probably more—of the nightdresses for children up to the age of 14 covered by the law are of brushed nylon. The way the manufacturers got around the problem of cost was to make a fabric that is very, very light, about 2 ounces per square yard. This fabric is brushed nylon; it is cheaper because it is very light in weight and can compete with treated cotton.

So this business of the flammability of a fabric is something for which you would have to specify a test, and the test would have to be applicable to the particular fiber. Our present tests are not good for synthetic fibers.

MR. SEGAL: May I answer that briefly? I was careful not to relate this to fabric flammability. I said fabrics that can be capable of causing a burn injury, and I meant to include synthetics that might be somewhat flame-resistant in some tests.

I am well aware that nylon doesn't burn too readily but that it can be a serious contributor to burn injuries.

MR. LE BLANC: Nylon burns very readily.

MR. SEGAL: Not necessarily. It depends on what it has on it or in it, but it can be quite flame-resistant too.

I also realize that there could be problems in this connection, but I foresee other problems that will be more difficult than that of making some distinction between a garment that will need such a label and one that will not. I don't think that this question is unimportant.

MR. GEORGE S. BUCK, JR.: I think, Mr. Segal, that your idea really is totally impractical, partly for the reasons given by the last speaker. You know that there are involved in the possibility of an accident not only the fiber, but the construction of the garment, the manner in which it is worn, and the manner in which it is used. It would be impossible in any way of which I can conceive to obtain agreement among textile producers, manufacturers, and retailers as to which garments possess any potential hazard and which ones don't. Obviously many people would be saying that their particular fiber and their particular fabric and their particular garment did not pose any hazard, and then the whole thing would break down into a great big competitive snarl.

Now I hope that we can set in motion at this meeting some plans that will prove truly constructive, and I want to speak to that point when the opportunity arises, but I don't think that this is the time.

MR. JOHNSON: Let me now redirect your attention to the specific proposal that Dr. Crikelair made. Have you any questions to ask him concerning it?

MR. JOSEPH R. PALMER: I should like to ask Dr. Crikelair if there should be a committee on testing. I think Mr. Segal will confirm the fact that testing is very sophisticated because of the differences in fiber that have been pointed out. Every fabric, every weave, every synthetic, every blend is almost a different animal.

Another problem lies in our words, our terminology. Flame-resistant and flame-retardant are two different words, and one is almost more powerful than the other. But we need clearly understood words and universally understood words, so that we shall be talking the same language all over the country. Whether one is a doctor or a safety man or a retailer, this dictionary of ours must be right from the beginning.

MR. JOHNSON: You think we need a committee on vocabulary, do you?

MR. PALMER: On vocabulary, especially on semantics.

MR. BUCK: May I comment on Dr. Crikelair's proposal?

MR. JOHNSON: Surely.

MR. BUCK: I think Dr. Crikelair has made an important proposal here, one that we ought to consider carefully.

As some of you know, I have been in this field for a long while—I think about 31 years—working with flame-resistant treatments, flammability of textiles, and on every one of the committtees that has been concerned with this subject.

And for too many years this matter has been breaking down into a conflict between the medical people and the health people on the one hand and the textile industry on the other. It shouldn't be that way because we in the textile industry have exactly the same interest.

We should like to see this problem solved. There is a problem. We don't think it is a problem that can correctly be applied to our products any more than it can be applied to combustible housing or to many other products that are involved in accidents. But if there is a possibility of a solution, we are interested in working toward it.

And when I read the abstracts of the papers to be presented here, and read Dr. Crikelair's proposal, it seemed to me that this might be a key opportunity to build on that proposal something constructive and effective that would take us toward the goal we want to reach. I made a few notes on the proposal.

As you know, we have been interested in fire-resistant finishes for many years and have made partial progress toward obtaining some that can be widely adopted. I think that probably the only final solution to the problem lies in improved fire-resistant finishes. I think education can help. Maybe labeling could help somewhere if it were practical. There are other things we might do—certainly we need information. But we ought to work as hard as we can toward obtaining better fire-resistant finishes.

We ought to work on improved methods of testing because we do not have any really adequate measure of what it is in a textile product that constitutes hazard under various conditions. We all know the flammability test in the federal law is inadequate in many ways; it is inadequate in that it screens out only the really hazardous textiles. But it is also inadequate in that—in some cases—it categorizes fabrics as hazardous that are completely normal in their performance.

The test doesn't take into account the hot melting effects associated with some thermoplastic fibers which, as medical people certainly ought to know, are accountable for some very deep and serious burns—yet this factor is not considered in this test method.

As I said, there are many things we could do: secure selected adoption of new finishes; conduct research to see how to stimulate demand for fire-resistant finishes; collect information on accidents; educate the public; and then, when eventually we have the right finishes, we should be able to promote their use because, without promotion, I don't believe people will pay for the cost of these finishes.

So I fully endorse Dr. Crikelair's suggestion. I think if we can arrange to follow it up we shall have made the most important constructive move that has ever been made in flame safety.

I didn't know everything Dr. Crikelair was going to suggest from his notes when I saw them in New Orleans. I thought perhaps we ought to have a national committee for safe clothing. This organization, in my opinion, might start informally; later on it might be given some formal basis. It should be endorsed by the textile people, by the chemical industry that furnishes chemicals for fire-retardants, by the medical people, by the fire safety people. I hope they will all indorse such a move.

This committee should represent those interests. It ought to represent, by all means, the medical profession. It ought to represent the National Fire Protection Association, the National Safety Council, the Underwriters Laboratories, and other similar groups.

It ought to represent industry, and by industry I mean primarily the textile industry and the producers of fibers, the chemical industry, which is also involved, and, let us hope, informally or otherwise, that it will represent the government agencies also.

I think the scope and purpose of such a permanent committee ought to include the following main points:

First, research. We do not have the finishes we must have to provide the public with maximum protection. We do not yet have satisfactory treatments, but I think it is entirely practical that, with enough effort, we could get them, and if the government and public agencies want to make the maximum contribution they can toward safety, then *they* ought to help us with this research job.

By and large that research has been carried out, either carried out or stimulated, up to now, entirely by industry. I include the Department of Agriculture, which has done such important work. That research, incidentally, was stimulated and encouraged by the cotton industry.

The second biggest job is information. This committee could help us organize a way to obtain information on burns, on accidents, on the circumstances related to them. That is needed.

The third job is education. We have all talked about that. The committee could do that.

The fourth job is coordination.

Now if we can take up these points at this meeting and build on them, I think that we shall soon begin to show progress and that, eventually, we shall have a solution. I urge that such a committee be formed properly, with one representative and one alternate from the key associations representing these different interests; that we have a meeting of this committee not later than January of next year; and that at that meeting we proceed to elect the officers suggested by Dr. Crikelair, lay out a program, and start implementing it. I can think of no better man to be chairman, if I might anticipate that meeting, than Dr. Crikelair himself.

MR. JOHNSON: I think those were excellent comments, and we appreciate having them. Is there anybody else who wishes to comment briefly on Dr. Crikelair's proposal?

MR. H. C. HOTTEL: I detect a sensitivity to various kinds of interests. I am wearing a wool suit and cotton shirt and underwear and, as a college professor, I am doing no consulting in the textile industry; but I am chairman of the National Academy Committee on Fire Research, a committee that is distressed with the status of fundamental understanding of fire in this country. I know we offend quite a few persons in saying we think the British understand fire better than we do and in expressing our distress at the absence of equivalent concern here.

Several times this matter of validity of testing has come up. Sometimes it seems to have been presented as on the edge of being an excuse for absence of action; at other times as an absolutely valid reason for protesting legislation, because legislation in the absence of understanding is a very dangerous thing.

My own personal research area is combustion, and so I am familiar with flame and industrial furnaces generally. I can think of nothing more complex than to combine the complexity of fabric with the complexity of flame in arriving at an empirical test of inflammability. The point has been made that we don't know what flammability means. I don't think the point has been adequately made yet that when one subjects a material to an empirical flame test, he does it because he does not know enough about the problem to define a better test. One should recognize the fact that flame has two different characteristics. One is supplying heat, and the other is supplying chain carriers at a level of energy that guarantees ignition.

Any empirical test is bound to bias the testing of some fabrics that were not in the group of materials considered when the test was established. A textile representative is justifiably concerned over the fact that a test was not designed to show his fabric to be safe, and he can be partly and sometimes wholly right. A major area that needs attention is the examination of the mechanism of ignition and propagation in fabrics by an agency that is disinterested enough to minimize the suspicion that the test is being rigged in favor of the other fellow. I can think of no better place for such research than the Bureau of Standards, where some fire research is being done, where there is some knowledge of flammability. Thermal effects and ignition effects and flame propagation effects in fabrics must be separated in a very much more sophisticated way than has been done.

MR. JOHNSON: You are speaking of the need for research in that area. The previous speaker called attention to the need for this proposed association to promote research. So I take it then that your comment was in favor of this proposal as one helpful way to get that work done in the Bureau of Standards?

MR. HOTTEL: Of this general proposal to organize something?

MR. JOHNSON: Yes.

MR. HOTTEL: I think anything that stimulates some good effort is worthwhile.

MR. JOHNSON: Very good. Any other comments?

MR. PERCY BUGBEE: I should be glad to make a comment on this proposal. We have been interested in this subject, of course, for many, many years and had a committee working on it for more than 20 years.

I think we perhaps have overlooked the fact that the situation that we are talking about and the magnitude of it would be very much worse if much weren't being done by the 20,000-odd fire departments around the United States in visiting homes and educating people and talking about these things. I am sure you will never get a figure that will measure the results of this activity but I know a great deal of it is going on and that it helps to make this problem not as big as it otherwise would be.

I think the suggestion that the medical profession, the Public Health people, the fire protection people, and the industry form a conference committee of some kind that will recognize the interests of all these groups and get together to discuss them on a regular basis and that will develop further the thinking of this conference is a good one. I am sure you will find the fire protection people ready and anxious to participate.

MR. JOHN L. SEVERANCE: I should like to ask Mr. Buck whether he would put his suggestion for the establishment of a committee in the form of a motion.

MR. JOHNSON: I was going to come to that. Let me see if I can get any other comments, for a reason that I shall explain in a moment. Any other comments?

MR. JOHN APPEL: I think this committee you are talking about should include representation from some of the high-risk industries in which fire-retardant work clothing is necessary or desirable.

MR. JOHNSON: I take your motion, sir, in this light. I think in meetings of this type there is always the question of who is bound and in what way is he bound.

For example, I here represent the National Safety Council. So I should like to take your motion in the broad sense that it is or it is not—as it will turn out by a show of hands—the consensus of those present here as individuals, not as organizations. Is what I have said, is my understanding of the proposed action, consistent with your proposed motion?

MR. SEVERANCE: I was just going to second George Buck's proposal if he had put it in the form of a motion.

MR. JOHNSON: Well, is my statement of the question satisfactory? Is that satisfactory to you, sir? Is my statement of the proposition satisfactory to you, George, based on what is in the record of your statement and what Dr. Crikelair proposed?

MR. BUCK: It is to me, and I put it in the form of a motion if that is what you would like.

MR. JOHNSON: The reason I wanted to state it as a consensus of those present is that you always have a rather delicate question of binding organizations, and I have seen conferences of this type in which somebody raised procedural questions. Am I now speaking for the whole National Safety Council? No, I am talking as Bill Johnson, General Manager of the Council. So I am trying to get around that procedural problem.

MR. BUCK: I think you are entirely correct. I think that if we agree here that this is a good thing to do, and by some such mechanism as you propose, we could go back and those of the national organizations which have an interest in this will arrange to send a representative.

MR. JOHNSON: Very good. Is there any further discussion of the proposal?

Then may I see a show of hands of all those who favor this proposal?

[Show of hands]

MR. JOHNSON: I shall not count the showing of hands for the moment. It is pretty heavy.

Now, if I may see hands of those who are opposed to this action.

I see no opposition. I gather you are applauding your own statesmanship.

Anything further?

MR. P. J. FYNN: I should like to call attention to the fact that in a number of the areas where it has been suggested that subcommittees or working groups be formed, there is a long history of activity in other organizations. Care should be taken not to duplicate effort or, shall we say, "reinvent the wheel" on a lot of these things.

MR. JOHNSON: I assume, sir, that if people such as yourself would help in the formation of this committee there would not be duplication. Certainly we don't want duplication. Any further comments?

MR. SEGAL: There have been some indications that maybe we have been trying to oversimplify this problem. The question has been raised about needing much more information and much more research on technical questions.

I should like to argue in opposition to this. I think we are in danger of overcomplicating the problem, too.

I don't want this to go on for many more years while nothing is done. I am concerned about the material that is going to be sold tomorrow and next year, and I think we know enough to say this much: there are a lot of fabrics on the market now that ignite readily and burn fast. There are other textiles that melt and cause serious injuries. It doesn't take any scientific genius to recognize their simple evident properties, and I think we can do something about these problems right now without any further great effort to find out many underlying, highly technical complex properties that aren't really that germane to the issue.

To become even more blunt about it, I am going to come right out and say that cotton and its derivatives are the greatest offender. This is not the fault of the industry or the fault of cotton, which just happened to be born that way. It is a marvelous fiber in every respect, and that's why it is so popular. That's why it is so widely used and that's why it is so much involved in our clothing fire problem because it also, unfortunately, happens to be damned flammable.

You don't need any more tests or methods or refinements to find that out.

If we can't do anything, then I think we should admit it and just say we are going to wait until we come up with some answers 10 or 15 or 20 years from now. I don't want to wait that long.

MR. LE BLANC: I am Chairman of the American Association of Technical Chemists and Colorists' Committee on Fire-Resistant Test Methods. We are working on test methods at present to try to apply these fire-resistant methods to all fabrics. This is not an easy job.

MR. JOHNSON: I appreciate what you are saying. I should also remind you of my introductory remark, that I think more and more people are looking to all of us as technicians to progress in our technical work at a little faster pace than was adequate 10 or 20 years ago.

MR. SEGAL: I hope I made it clear that what I, for one, am advocating is that we must make the public more aware of the problem: first, because the other solutions under discussion are going to take a long, long time to arrive and, as I said a moment ago, I don't want to wait.

If we can save 100 out of these 2,000 lives, I don't think this is a trivial goal and I think we might be able to do that if we increase our efforts before the technical solutions come along.

Just a few moments ago a very excellent point was made: that we do have a large segment of the population that probably cannot be reached by education, and this is why I advocate the possibility of putting a label right in the garment that everyone would see. I think it is worth considering.

MR. PHIL DYKSTRA: I think the action taken here this afternoon—the proposed organization of a permanent committee—is most commendable. However, unless such a committee receives adequate financial support, it will be seriously handicapped in its efforts.

I propose to the fabric industry, especially to all the representatives of that industry in attendance at this conference, that such support logically seems to be primarily their responsibility. If industry is genuinely sincere about finding a solution to the problem of preventing burns from clothing—and their past actions indicate that they are—it might well use as a gauge for its financial support for research, advertising, public information, etc., contributions comparable to the monies its companies have devoted to the promotional and developmental activities of sanforization, perma-press, and similar processes.

DR. DONALD A. DUKELOW: I have been much interested and stimulated by the discussions we have had over these two days, particularly since, about three years ago, the House of Delegates of the American Medical Association gave a specific charge to our staff. We, the staff, were directed to make certain investigations and to make whatever efforts could be made for promotion of activities that would reduce both the hazard and the frequency of burns from clothing fires.

From the small inquiry we were able to make we found that it would be frustrating to try to publicize to any extent materials that didn't exist or, as it has just been pointed out, exist for institutions only and in very limited supply even for them.

So we have been quite unhappy with our health education activities and with the promotion of the safety concepts that are involved in prevention of fires from ignited fabrics.

I am happy to see we are moving forward. I can assure you that when we reach the stage where we can incorporate this into our health and safety educational activities, not only among the physicians of the country but among the public that they serve, we shall be only too happy to join with you in every way possible.

MR. JOHNSON: Any further comments? Then before turning the chair back to Dr. Joliet for adjournment, I should like to say that I think this has been a wonderful meeting, not only in a technical and informative sense, but as a really good example of democracy in action, the sort of thing of which this country can be proud.

# A ROMAN EXPERIENCE WITH HEAT STROKE IN 24 B.C.

The caloric annoyance visited upon most of the United States each summer scarcely requires anything by way of special comment, since the subject is thoroughly presented in newspapers and is endlessly reiterated in radio broadcasts. The physician is aware of the burden that the heat inflicts on his more fragile patients, especially on those who already are troubled by circulatory or psychic disease. It is also observable that persons who come to the United States *from the tropics* sometimes find our summer climate intolerable and retreat to equatorial regions for relief. Despite its promoters, New York is not necessarily a "summer festival."

But if our thermal history has been intermittently grievous, we may reflect that others have had it worse. In the year 24 B.C. Aelius Gallus conducted a military campaign in Arabia. The following is a concise summary written by Dio Cassius* (ca. A.D. 150-235), an industrious Roman lawyer, senator, and historian.

> While this was going on, another and a new campaign had at once its beginning and its end. It was conducted by Aelius Gallus, the governor of Egypt, against the country called Arabia Felix, of which Sabos was king. At first Aelius encountered no one, yet he did not proceed without difficulty; for the desert, the sun, and the water (which had some peculiar nature) all caused his men great distress, so that the larger part of the army perished. The malady proved to be unlike any of the common complaints, but attacked the head and caused it to become parched, killing forthwith most of those who were attacked, but in the case of those who survived this stage it descended to the legs, skipping all the intervening parts of the body, and caused dire injury to them. There was no remedy for it except a mixture of olive oil and wine, both taken as a drink and used as an ointment; and this remedy naturally lay within reach of only a few of them, since the country produces neither of these articles and the men had not prepared an abundant supply of them beforehand. In the midst of this trouble the barbarians also

*Dio, (*Roman History*) LIII.29.3-8. Loeb Library ed., transl. by E. Cary, vol. 6, pp. 269-71. Reprinted by kind permission of the Harvard University Press.

fell upon them. For hitherto they had been defeated whenever they joined battle, and had even been losing some places; but now, with the disease as their ally, they not only won back their own possessions, but also drove the survivors of the expedition out of the country. These were the first of the Romans and, I believe, the only ones, to traverse so much of Arabia for the purpose of making war; for they advanced as far as the place called Athlula, a famous locality.

The identity of Aelius Gallus, leader of the heat-struck military expedition described by Dio Cassius, is not entirely clear. Max Wellmann, writing in the Pauly-Wissowa *Real-Encyclopädie der Classischen Altertumswissenschaft,** vol. 1, p. 493, says that Gallus the soldier is very probably identical with one Marcus Aelius Gallus, a pupil of Asklepiades. This Gallus, a physician, is repeatedly mentioned by Galen and is said to have devised a theriac useful against scorpion stings.

S. J.

*Stuttgart, Metzler, 1894. See also Schiller, Hermann: *Geschichte der Römischen Kaiserzeit.* Gotha, Perthes, 1883-1887, vol. 1, pp. 198-202. A more recent treatment of the Arabian expedition will be found in Cook, S., Adcock, F. and Charlesworth, M. P.: *The Cambridge Ancient History.* Cambridge Univ. Press, 1944, vol. 10, pp. 247-254.

# TELEVISED CLINICAL SCIENCE SEMINARS

**Tuesday Evenings, 8:30-9:30 P.M.**

STATION WNYC—TV UHF—CHANNEL 31

**August 8, 1967**

## HYPERTHYROIDISM

KENNETH STERLING
Chief, Medical Section
Bronx Veterans Administration Hospital
Assistant Clinical Professor of Medicine
Columbia University College of
Physicians and Surgeons

SIDNEY C. WERNER
Professor of Clinical Medicine
Columbia University College of
Physicians and Surgeons

**August 15, 1967**

## STROKES

CLARK H. MILLIKAN
Chief of Section on Neurology
Mayo Clinic, Rochester

JULIAN R. YOUMANS
Associate Professor of Neurosurgery
Medical College of South Carolina

C. THORPE RAY
Professor of Medicine
University of Missouri
School of Medicine

DALE GROOM, *Moderator*
Director of Postgraduate Medical Education
Medical College of South Carolina

*Program Courtesy of*
*Medical College of South Carolina*

**August 22, 1967**

## DIGITALIS AND DIURETICS

C. THORPE RAY
Professor of Medicine
University of Missouri
School of Medicine

LAMAR CREVASSE
Associate Professor of Medicine
Chief, Division of Cardiology
University of Florida College of Medicine

THOMAS KILLIP
Associate Professor of Medicine
Chief, Division of Cardiology
Cornell University Medical College

DALE GROOM, *Moderator*
Director of Postgraduate Medical Education
Medical College of South Carolina

*Program Courtesy of*
*Medical College of South Carolina*

**August 29, 1967**

## ANGINA PECTORIS

C. HILMON CASTLE
Assistant Professor of Medicine
University of Utah College of Medicine

CAMPBELL MOSES
Associate Professor of Medicine
University of Pittsburgh School of Medicine

DALE GROOM
Director of Postgraduate Medical Education
Medical College of South Carolina

GEORGE ROBERTSON
Assistant Professor of Medicine
Tufts Medical School

*Program Courtesy of*
*Medical College of South Carolina*

BULLETIN OF
THE NEW YORK ACADEMY
OF MEDICINE

VOL. 43, NO. 9 SEPTEMBER 1967

# THE PATHOLOGY AND PATHOGENESIS OF DIABETIC NEUROPATHY*

C. L. DOLMAN

Pathologist, Vancouver General Hospital
Clinical Associate Professor of Pathology
University of British Columbia
Vancouver, Canada

THE earliest accounts of the pathology of diabetic neuropathy go back to the turn of the century when Auché[1] and Fraser and Bruce[2] described degeneration of the peripheral nerves, and Pryce,[3] Leichtentritt,[4] and Williamson[5] described demyelination and gliosis of the dorsal columns of the spinal cord in diabetics. In 1929, in an often quoted article, Woltman and Wilder[6] published their findings in 10 cases of diabetic neuropathy (4 postmortems and 6 amputated limbs), and summarized the literature. Subsequently only sporadic case reports appeared, until the last decade, when several systematic investigations of the lesions were attempted, with the particular objective of elucidating the pathogenesis.[7-10] Newer tools such as the electron microscope, which are just beginning to be applied in this field, are hampered by the difficulty of obtaining suitable biopsy specimens. A full review of the whole subject of diabetic neuropathy with 206 references was published last year by Colby.[11]

*Presented at a meeting of the Clinical Society of the New York Diabetes Association, held at The New York Academy of Medicine, January 26, 1967.

First I propose to discuss the lesions on an anatomical basis in the light of my own observations and of reports from the literature. Then I shall review current hypotheses bearing on the pathogenesis of these lesions. Let me here interject that, in order to appraise the whole picture, it is necessary to integrate the experiences of many authors. The fact that one worker has not been able to find lesions of a kind noted by another does not necessarily refute the latter's claim, but is more likely due to the chance selection of material, or sometimes to the methods of study.

## The Lesions

*Brain.* There is no specific encephalopathy. Diabetics are often hypertensive and tend to have severe atheroma. They are therefore more prone to suffer cerebral infarcts and hemorrhages, and to do so at an earlier age than the average person. These lesions do not differ in any respect from those incurred by nondiabetic subjects and therefore need not be discussed further.

*Cranial nerves.* The majority of the cranial nerves have shown dysfunction clinically. Unfortunately, pathological observations are almost nonexistent. I have never seen any lesions myself. The only relevant pathological report in the literature is by Dreyfus *et al.*[12] In a patient who died during an attack of oculomotor paralysis, one of the third nerves showed a fusiform swelling with destruction of myelin sheaths and axis cylinders, and retrograde changes in the proximal portions of the nerve and its nucleus.

*Spinal cord.* The spinal cord, like the brain, may be the seat of infarcts due to vascular insufficiency. An example of this change was described by Ellenberg and Krainer.[13] The spinal cord may also undergo a variety of more specific degenerations, of which the most frequently encountered involves the dorsal columns. As already noted, this was one of the earliest to be described pathologically. It is probably the form that gives rise to the clinical picture of pseudotabes. In the majority of such cases the most extensive damage is found in the lumbosacral region where the dorsal columns, with the exception of the funiculi proprii, are diffusely demyelinated. This degeneration either does not rise to higher levels or is confined there to the funiculi graciles. Occasionally the upper segments of the cord are selectively affected. In some such instances, the changes undoubtedly represent a

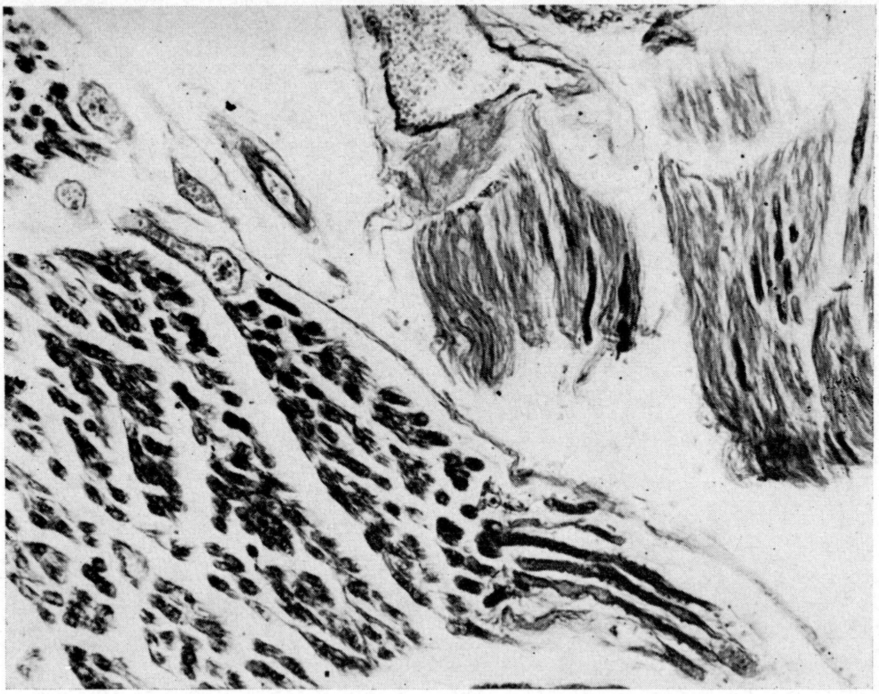

Fig. 1. Severely demyelinated posterior roots to right, in contrast to fully myelinated anterior root at left. The intraneural vessels are normal in both. Luxol-fast-blue—periodic acid Schiff. ×167.

Wallerian degeneration from foci of myelomalacia below; in others, they appear to be primary lesions. In the portion of the dorsal columns involved, myelin sheaths are lost as well as, to a lesser extent, axis cylinders. Frequently large numbers of fine unmyelinated axons persist. The process must be a slow one since, in contrast to what is found in infarcts, macrophages and catabolic products are usually absent; but in severe cases astrocytes proliferate and fibrous gliosis results.

The dorsal roots not only participate in this process but are often more severely demyelinated. Axis cylinders again are less affected. Occasionally, fibrosis has been noted, but it is usually not prominent. The severely demyelinated dorsal roots may provide a striking contrast to the normal anterior roots (Figure 1). The dorsal horns are normal. In the dorsal root ganglia, various degenerative changes varying from peripheral vacuolization to complete dissolution of neurons has been reported, with resultant loss of axons and proliferation of the capsule cells. These lesions are minor and they are greatly overshadowed by the root lesions.

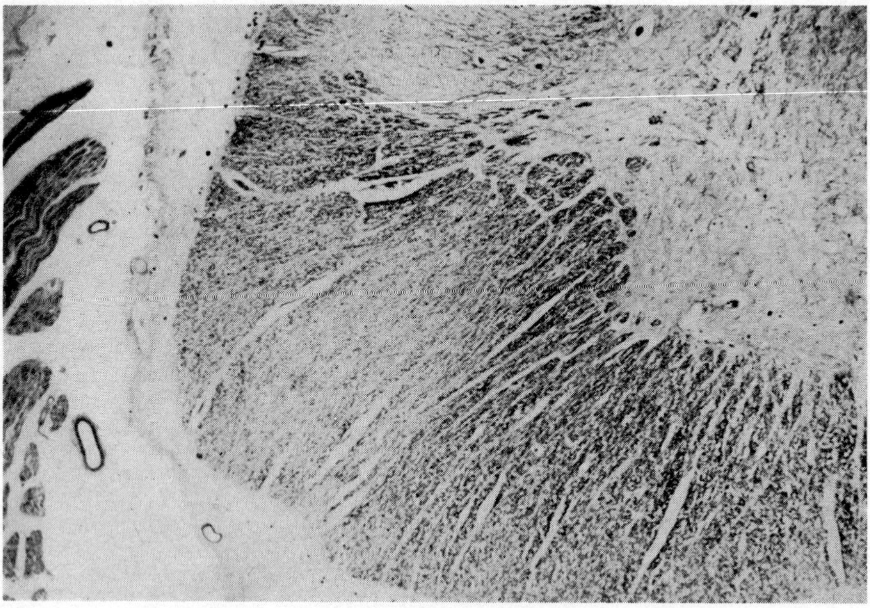

Fig. 2. Spinal cord. Degeneration of lateral column. This was bilaterally symmetrical and combined with degeneration of the dorsal columns. Luxol-fast-blue—periodic acid Schiff. ×34.

Less common than dorsal column degeneration is dorsolateral sclerosis of the cord.[14] The pathological features here are identical with those in the dorsal columns (Figure 2). Causes other than diabetes for the degeneration have not always been excluded with certainty.

Diabetic amyotrophy has formed the basis of many clinical investigations. One of the chief authors in this field is Garland, who considered initially that at least part of the lesion was situated in the spinal cord.[15] Marked loss of ventral horn cells has indeed been reported in one instance,[9] but usually only the occasional nerve cell is lost or may show an axon reaction.[8,16]

*Peripheral nerves.* The most frequently noted and severest damage is found in the peripheral nerves. The lesions are usually fairly symmetrical, are often most extensive in the distal portions, and particularly affect the sciatic nerves and their branches. The descriptions and interpretations of these lesions have varied. For example, Greenbaum *et al.*[9] felt that large fibers suffered most and that axons degenerated to the same degree as myelin sheaths, and concluded that the process was essentially a primary neuronal degeneration. My own observations led me to believe that patchy demyelination was the major feature, although

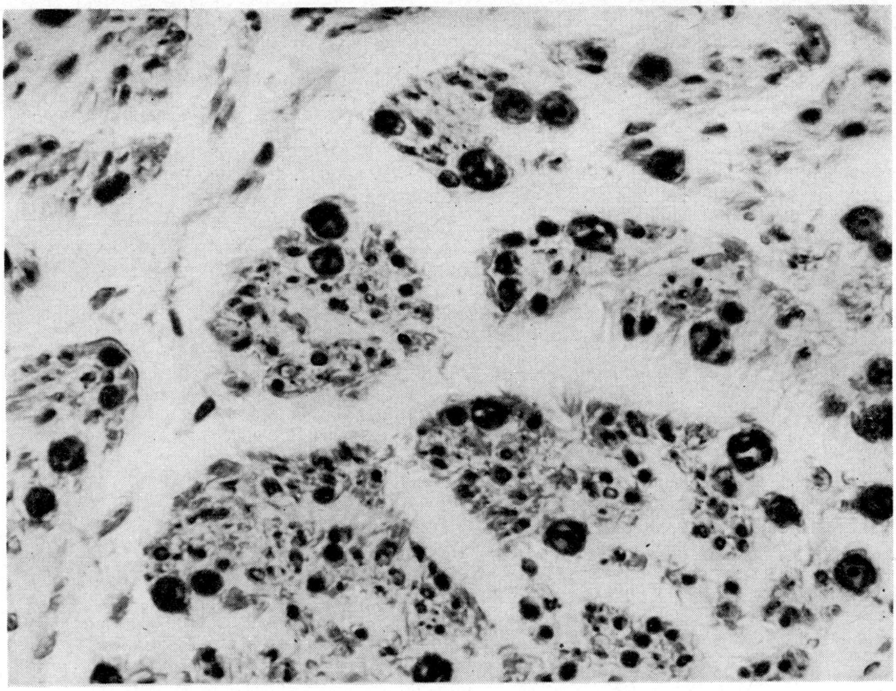

Fig. 3. Sciatic nerve. Naked axis cylinders persist between large and smaller myelinated fibers. Luxol-fast-blue—Holmes. ×585.

undeniably axons also were lost (Figure 3). Thomas and Lascelles[10,17] confirmed this claim by finding segmental demyelination and remyelination in teased-out isolated fibers of diabetic sural and radial nerves. In a few fibers, axonal degeneration had occurred. Many fibers, however, were intact and showed only myelin loss, some only at the nodes of Ranvier, others over one or more internodal segments. Frequently the internodal lengths were shortened.

Electron microscopic studies by Sarah Luse[18] also demonstrated focal segmental demyelination. In addition to this, Luse observed loss of unmyelinated axons, revealed by an accordionlike folding of the Schwann cytoplasm after disappearance of the "C" fibers. Peripheral nerve conduction studies tend to support the importance of demyelinization in diabetic neuropathy.[19] The presence of motor fiber degeneration was established by means of the intravital methylene blue technique by Woolf and Malins,[20] who noted transformation of the normal petaled, flowerlike terminal arborizations of motor end plates into single "balloons" and "soap bubbles." Further, Coërs and Hildebrand[21] found marked collateral sprouting of motor fibers in both diabetics and alcoholics, the sprouting being a regenerative phenomenon after axonal damage. Schwannian proliferation, sometimes very marked, accompanies the degeneration of nerves, while true fibrosis is seen less often.

*Autonomic nervous system.* The autonomic nervous system, which is clinically so often severely affected in diabetes, is unfortunately a difficult field to investigate pathologically. Berge[22] examined postmortem bowel specimens and was unable to notice any difference between the ganglion cells and vessels of three groups of patients—diabetics with diarrhea, diabetics without diarrhea, and normal controls. In a recent peroral jejunal biopsy studied with the electron microscope,[23] the vessels were reported as normal, but no mention was made of the nerves and ganglion cells. In my own series of 20 sympathetic trunks and ganglia, I was not convinced of any definite pathological changes.[8] However, Appenzeller and Richardson[24] recently described giant neurons, about twice the normal size, exhibiting severe degenerative changes and even dissolution in the sympathetic ganglia of four out of five diabetics and three out of four alcoholics. These cells did not display the conventional axon reaction. No lesions were seen in postganglionic fibers. Such observations are difficult to interpret since, according to Herzog,[25] swelling and degenerative changes in the neurons of sympathetic ganglia are found not only in a great variety of diseases, but are encountered occasionally in ganglia of apparently healthy subjects. Further studies are needed, and it is hoped that electron microscopic examination of surgically excised sympathetic ganglia and of postganglionic fibers may shed some light on this field.

*Muscles.* Small foci of typical neurogenic atrophy are often seen in the muscles, particularly of the foot and leg, of diabetics. These exceed in frequency those found in normal controls and tend to occur at an earlier age. Clinically, weakness and atrophy have often been most pronounced in proximal muscles, particularly in the thighs, and in the pelvic and shoulder girdles.[15, 26, 27] But Feller and Szyrynski[28] described 14 patients with distal muscle involvement, often in the hands, and Ellenberg[29] had previously reported a similar case. Locke *et al.*[27] studied 17 biopsies of muscles of diabetics. They drew attention to "single fiber atrophy"—i.e., single small fibers scattered among healthy ones—that preceded the usual unit pattern of neurogenic atrophy (Figure 4). This placed the lesion at the level of the single fiber and its end plate.

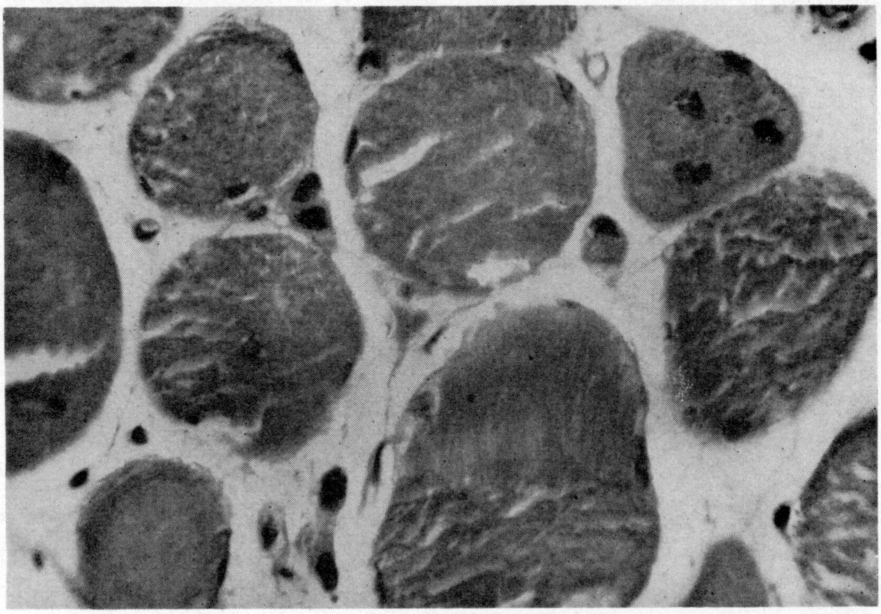

Fig. 4. Muscle. Small atrophic fibers lie between large normal ones. One fiber contains several central nuclei. Hematoxylin and eosin. ×585.

Coërs and Hildebrand[21] emphasized that this single fiber atrophy, which they also found in alcoholics, is not myopathic, but is due to degeneration of single terminal motor fibers that later spreads to the main axon and results in the familiar picture of neurogenic atrophy. Many so-called myopathic features, such as swelling and centralization of nuclei, are undoubtedly characteristic of the early phases of neurogenic atrophy.

*Joints.* Charcot joints, particularly affecting the tarsal and proximal metatarsal joints, but occasionally the ankles, knees, and spine, may be a troublesome complication of diabetes. In x-ray studies of one series,[30] the overgrowth of bone has been notably absent, but in other cases studied histologically, fibrosis, granulation tissue, and overgrowth of bone were present, sometimes to a very marked degree.[31-33]

*Summary of pathological changes.* Except for obvious vascular accidents, the most commonly encountered lesions are degeneration of the peripheral nerves, with segmental demyelination, some loss of axons (probably both "A" and "C" fibers), and degeneration of terminal motor axons and end plates. The cell body takes comparatively little part in this process. Demyelination of sensory roots and tract degeneration may occur in the spinal cord, mainly in the dorsal columns, sometimes as combined dorsolateral sclerosis. Denervation phenomena are found in joints and muscles.

## Pathogenesis

The hypotheses about the pathogenesis of diabetic neuropathy can be divided into two broad groups; one postulates an underlying angiopathy and the other a metabolic defect.

Diabetics have always been known as subject to severe premature arteriosclerosis. Woltman and Wilder,[6] who found marked sclerotic changes in the leg arteries of all their cases, attributed the lesions in the nerves to vascular insufficiency. Objections were raised to this conclusion on the grounds that neuropathy may exist in the absence of appreciable peripheral vascular disease while, on the other hand, persons with nondiabetic atherosclerosis or even thrombosis of the leg arteries, had healthy nerves. Attention then shifted to vessels of smaller caliber. Goldenberg *et al.*[34] found, in the amputated legs of diabetics, lesions that differed from those usually encountered in ordinary arteriosclerosis. In small arteries there was thickening of walls and endothelial proliferation, whereas the arterioles and capillaries showed hyaline thickening of the walls, with marked affinity for the periodic acid Schiff reagent. Agenaes and Moe[35] described changes in dermal capillaries in diabetes, comparable to the vascular lesions found in the kidneys and in the eye. Despite many investigations in this field, the facts are not yet indisputably established. For example, during the past year three electron microscopic studies were published. One group reported significant thickening (by measurement of the basement membrane) of diabetic dermal capillaries;[36] a second claimed that the lesions consisted of collagen deposition rather than basement membrane thickening;[37] and a third was unable, in a blind study, to distinguish diabetic capillaries from normal controls.[38]

Fagerberg[7] examined histologically a large number of diabetic sural nerves, mainly obtained by biopsy. He was impressed by the arteriolar thickening in the nerves, which was present in both young and old subjects. Further, he found a high correlation between the presence of diabetic disease in the nerves, kidneys, and eyes. He concluded that arteriolar disease was responsible for the demyelination. This is a unifying and therefore attractive theory. However, there are several points against its acceptance. If one examines larger areas of the nervous system, it becomes apparent that very often it is not possible to relate abnormalities in the vasa nervorum to the state of the nerves. In other words, normal arterioles and capillaries may be in badly demyelinated segments while, by contrast, hypertensive patients whose arteriolar lesions closely resemble those of diabetics may have almost obliterated intraneural vessels accompanying normal nerves. Moreover, occlusion of vasa nervorum with resulting nervous damage, as exemplified by periarteritis nodosa, usually leads to infarcts of the nerves rather than demyelination. Again, the lesions of diabetic neuropathy follow a definite anatomical pattern, e.g., the posterior roots may be severely damaged while the anterior ones are spared, which is easier to explain by selective vulnerability to a general metabolic disorder than by a structural alteration of vessels. Furthermore, the lesions resemble those encountered in metabolic disorders and intoxications. For example, in investigations such as those by Coërs,[21] findings have run parallel for alcoholics and diabetics; and, in plumbism, the lesions consist of segmental demyelination with isolated axon degeneration and destruction of end plates.[39]

We do not yet know the exact nature of the metabolic derangement in diabetic neuropathy. Nutritional disorders have been ruled out by the lack of response to therapy. Recent work by Field and his coworkers[40, 41] has demonstrated abnormalities in the fat and carbohydrate metabolism of diabetic nerves and spinal cord. Greenbaum[42] believes that symptoms are due to poor diabetic control, but this opinion is not shared by others.[43, 44] Thomas and Lascelles[10, 17] suggested as the basic fault an abnormality of the metabolism of Schwann cells that leads to myelin breakdown.

## Conclusion

There is one very large gap in knowledge of the pathology and the pathogenesis of diabetic neuropathy. All the lesions described are those seen in patients with a chronic, usually mild, clinical neuropathy. Such patients characteristically display amazingly slight neurological disabilities in view of the severe degrees of degeneration of the nerves. The really troublesome neurological manifestations, particularly those associated with pain, are often transient, so that there is little opportunity for histological study of the nervous system. Greenbaum[42] claims that there is one single diabetic neuropathy, which may show many clinical variants. The only pathological report available on a transient mononeuropathy, that by Dreyfus *et al.*[12] on an oculomotor nerve, showed a lesion that differed from that usually seen in nerves by being focal and by producing a swelling. Although the authors attributed it to vascular insufficiency, no occluded vessels were seen. Careful histological studies of further cases of this kind must be awaited before any definite conclusions can be drawn about the uniformity of the neuropathies.

Finally, I draw your attention to a penetrating comment by Theobald Smith, the famous American microbiologist and comparative pathologist. In a letter sent to Simon Flexner nearly 50 years ago, after criticizing a paper which had been submitted for publication in a well-known journal, Smith writes as follows: "Pathology, being practically the last synthesis of a large number of coordinated and subordinated factors, must actually be studied before these other factors have been cleared up, and as a result pathology must be more or less descriptive; but insofar as it is descriptive it must not claim more for that description than the evidence warrants."[45]

## REFERENCES


1. Auché, F. Des altérations des nerfs périphériques chez les diabétiques, *Arch. Méd. Exper. et Anat. Path. 2*:635, 1890.
2. Fraser, T. R. and Bruce, A. On a case of diabetic neuritis with a description of the postmortem examination of the nerves and muscles, *Edinburgh Med. J. 42*:300, 1896.
3. Pryce, T. D. On diabetic neuritis, with a clinical and pathological description of 3 cases of diabetic pseudo-tabes, *Brain 16*:415, 1893.
4. Leichtentritt, H. Erkrankung peripherer Nerven und des Rückenmarks bei Diabetes mellitus. Diss., 32 pp. Berlin, G. Schade, 1893.
5. Williamson, R. T. Changes in the spinal cord in diabetes mellitus, *Brit. Med. J. 1*:122, 1904.
6. Woltman, H. W. and Wilder, R. M. Diabetes mellitus. Pathologic changes in the spinal cord and peripheral nerves, *Arch. Int. Med. 44*:576, 1929.
7. Fagerberg, S. E. Diabetic neuropathy. *Acta Med. Scand. 164* (Suppl. 345): 80, 1959.
8. Dolman, C. L. Morbid anatomy of diabetic neuropathy, *Neurology 13*:135, 1963.
9. Greenbaum, D. *et al.* Pathological observations on six cases of diabetic neuropathy, *Brain 87 (2)*:201, 1964.
10. Thomas, P. K. and Lascelles, R. G. Pathology of diabetic neuropathy, *Quart. J. Med. 35*:489, 1966.
11. Colby, A. O. Neurologic disorders of diabetes mellitus. *Diabetes 14*:424 and 516, 1965.
12. Dreyfus, P. M. *et al.* Diabetic ophthalmoplegia, *A.M.A. Arch. Neurol. Psychiat. 77*:337, 1957.
13. Ellenberg, M. and Krainer, L. Diabetic neuropathy, *Diabetes 8*:279, 1959.
14. Griggs, D. E. and Olsen, C. W. Changes in the spinal cord in diabetes mellitus, *Arch. Neurol. Psychiat. 38*:546, 1937.
15. Garland, H. and Taverner, D. Diabetic myelopathy, *Brit. Med. J. 1*:1405, 1953.

16. Muri, J. Diabetic arthropathy and intercapillary glomerulosclerosis, *Acta Med. Scand. 135*:391, 1949.
17. Thomas, P. K. and Lascelles, R. G. Schwann cell abnormalities in diabetic neuropathy, *Lancet 1*:1355, 1965.
18. Luse, S. A. and Moon, T. R. Ultrastructural study of peripheral nerves in human diabetes mellitus and in steroid-induced hyperglycemia in the rabbit, *Anat. Rec. 154*:380, 1966.
19. Gilliatt, R. W. Nerve conduction in human and experimental neuropathies, *Proc. Roy. Soc. Med. 59*:989, 1966.
20 Woolf, A. L. and Malins, J. M. Changes in the intramuscular nerve endings in diabetic neuropathy; a biopsy study. *J. Path. Bact. 73*:316, 1957.
21. Coërs, C. and Hildebrand, J. Latent neuropathy in diabetes and alcoholism, *Neurology 15*:19, 1965.
22. Berge, K. G. *et al.* Intestinal tract in diabetic diarrhea, a pathologic study, *Diabetes 5*:289, 1956.
23. Mitgaard, K. Diabetic visceral neuropathy, *Diabetes 15*:43, 1966.
24. Appenzeller, O. and Richardson, E. P. Jr. Sympathetic chain in patients with diabetic and alcoholic polyneuropathy, *Neurology 16*:1203, 1966.
25. Herzog, E. In: *Handbuch der Speziellen Pathologischen Anatomie und Histologie.* Henke, F., Lubarsch, O. and Rössle, R., eds., vol. 13. Würzburg, H. Stürtz, 1955, p. 414.
26. Garland, H. Diabetic amyotrophy, *Brit. J. Clin. Pract. 15*:9, 1961.
27. Locke, S. *et al.* Diabetic amyotrophy, *Amer. J. Med. 34*:775, 1963.
28. Feller, J. and Szyrynski, V. Motor neuropathy in diabetes mellitus, *Med. Serv. J. Canada 18*:433, 1962.
29. Ellenberg, M. Diabetic neuropathy presenting as the initial clinical manifestation of diabetes, *Ann. Int. Med. 49*: 620, 1958.
30. Bailey, C. C. and Root, H. F. Neuropathic foot lesions in diabetes mellitus, *New Eng. J. Med. 236*:397, 1947.
31. Foster Major, D. B. and Bassett, R. C. Neurogenic arthropathy (Charcot Joint) associated with diabetic neuropathy, *Arch. Neurol. Psychiat. 5*:173, 1947.
32. Zucker, G. and Mader, M. J. Charcot spine due to diabetic neuropathy, *Amer. J. Med. 12*:118, 1952.
33. Degenhardt, D. P. and Goodwin, M. A. Neuropathic joints in diabetes, *J. Bone Joint Surg. 42B*:769, 1960.
34. Goldenberg, S. *et al.* Nonatheromatous peripheral vascular disease of the lower extremity in diabetes mellitus, *Diabetes 8*:261, 1959.
35. Agenaes, O. and Moe, H. Light and electron microscopic study of skin capillaries of diabetics, *Diabetes 10*:253, 1961.
36. Pardo, V. *et al.* Electron microscopic study of dermal capillaries in diabetes mellitus, *Lab. Investig. 15*:1944, 1966.
37. McMillan, D. E. *et al.* Forearm skin capillaries of diabetic, potential diabetic and nondiabetic subjects, *Diabetes 15*: 251, 1966.
38. Friederici, H. H. R. *et al.* Observations on small blood vessels of skin in the normal and in diabetic patients, *Diabetes 15*:233, 1966.
39. Meyer, A. In: *Greenfield's Neuropathology,* 2d ed. London, Edward Arnold, 1963, pp. 268-270.
40. Field, R. A. and Adams, C. C. Insulin response of peripheral nerve II. Effects on lipid metabolism. *Biochim. Biophys. Acta 106*:474, 1956.
41. Gabbay, K. H. *et al.* Sorbitol pathway presence in nerve and cord with substrate accumulation in diabetes, *Science 151*:209, 1966.
42. Greenbaum, D. Observations on the homogeneous nature and pathogenesis of diabetic neuropathy. *Brain 87(2)*: 215, 1964.
43. Ellenberg, M. Diabetic neuropathy. A consideration of factors of onset, *Ann. Int. Med. 52*:1067, 1960.
44. Mulder, D. W. *et al.* Neuropathies associated with diabetes mellitus. A clinical and electromyographic study of 103 unselected diabetic patients, *Neurology 11*:275, 1961.
45. Letter from Theobald Smith to Simon Flexner, dated June 1, 1920. From the Flexner papers in custody of the American Philosophical Society Library, Philadelphia.

# AXONS, SCHWANN CELLS, AND DIABETIC NEUROPATHY*

SIMEON LOCKE

Assistant Professor of Neurology
Harvard Medical School
Boston, Mass.

DISCUSSIONS of diabetic peripheral neuropathy have often had the implicit suggestion of a unitary process—a single disorder with a single underlying pathogenetic mechanism. This has led to the unresolved controversy between proponents of a vascular and a metabolic etiology. Surely the clinician cannot help but be aware that the postulation of a unifying mechanism of production of the peripheral neurological concomitants of diabetes is a naive oversimplification. Some disorders, as the isolated mononeuropathy of sudden onset, circumscribed duration, and complete recovery, must be of vascular origin. Others reflect the increased susceptibility of the peripheral nerves of patients with diabetes to focal trauma.[1] In each, large fibers are often preferentially affected, while signs and symptoms are restricted to the distribution of a major nerve trunk. The more usual peripheral polyneuropathy, characterized by a distal affection of overlapping terminals of long nerves, with decreased appreciation of pain and temperature—the modalities mediated by smaller fibers—is thought to be of metabolic origin. Perhaps a better understanding of the possibilities of metabolic derangement can be obtained by a review of the dynamic relations between a peripheral nerve and its environment.

Peripheral nerve trunks consist of large and small sensory and motor fibers collected in bundles. Longitudinal collagen fibers that have a diameter of 700 to 850 Å. surround these bundles as the epineurium.[2] Each nerve bundle is surrounded in turn by concentric lamellated, flattened endothelial type cells of the perineurium. Delicate fibers of the endoneurium extend into the bundles between the myelinated and unmyelinated nerves. The collagen of the endoneurium, 500 to 600 Å. in diameter, is arranged in two layers: an outer layer of longitudinal fibers is the sheath of Key and Retzius. An inner collection of

*Based on a paper presented at a meeting of the Clinical Society of the New York Diabetes Association, held at The New York Academy of Medicine, January 26, 1967.

longitudinal, oblique, and circular fibers corresponds to the sheath of Plenk and Laidlaw.[3] Endoneurial collagen is formed by endoneurial fibroblasts[4] and perhaps by Schwann cells.[5] All axons, myelinated or not, are in intimate relation with Schwann cells.[6,7] The Schwann cell is surrounded by a basement membrane that separates it from the endoneurium. The so-called neurilemma, or sheath of Schwann cells, should be distinguished from the axolemma, or true sheath of the axon.[8]

Normal myelinated fibers are interrupted at a regular interval by annular constrictions known as the nodes of Ranvier. Between the nodes, the internodal segment of myelin is formed by the spiral wrapping of an individual Schwann cell.[9] The length of the internode depends upon the "stretching" produced by the growth of the axon. Early myelination produces long nodes.[10] Internodal length varies directly as the diameter of the fiber,[11] although after the age of 65, irregularities of length are common.[10] Interruption in the internodal myelin is produced by the Schmidt-Lantermann incisures. Schwann cell cytoplasm lies in these clefts.[12] Immunologic studies[13, 14] indicate a distinction between myelin of the peripheral and central nervous system.

An axon, often extending thousands of times the diameter of the nerve cell body, is dependent upon the perikaryon for axoplasm, which is elaborated in the nerve cell body and flows into the fiber.[15] Following section of a nerve, outflow of axoplasm occurs at the cut end, which becomes covered by myelin. The myelin, distended by axoplasmic flow, ultimately bursts and the process recurs.[16] Apparently axoplasm can exist in a sol as well as a gel state.[17] Increase of axoplasmic mitochondria occurs at the node of Ranvier,[18] where the axon is constricted to less than one half its diameter at the internode.[8] The two opposed Schwann cells of adjacent internodes extend fingerlike processes of about 500 Å. in diameter which interdigitate at the node, leaving a 150 Å. gap as a possible pathway for ionic current.[19] Schwann cell mitochondria are concentrated at the node,[8,20] where the collar of the Schwann cell has a close apposition to the axolemma (of the order of 20 Å.) and an increase of electron density at the point of contact.[20] The dimensions of the proximal paranodal bulb are greater than those of the distal. Myelin in the paranodal region is crenated and the underlying axon fluted,[21] apparently increasing surface relations. The possibility of an intimate metabolic interrelation between Schwann cell and axon has been suggested,[21,22] with the node behaving as a point of energy exchange. Schmitt[23] points out that an important evolutionary advance from unicellular to multicellular organisms, with the associated need for rapid communication over long distances, may have depended on solving the problem by local metabolic energy supplied by satellite cells. This intimate dependence between contiguous cells should not be surprising in light of transneuronal degeneration that occurs in visual,[24] auditory,[25] and other neuronal systems. Indeed, the outcome of the historical debate on continuity versus contiguity of cells may require some reinterpretation in light of the recent demonstration[26] not only of propagation of tracer elements from nerve cell body into axon but, more important, ultimate transsynaptic appearance in the muscle innervated by the nerves with tagged axoplasm.

The dependence of Schwann cells on the axon they surround is well demonstrated in Wallerian degeneration. Following section of the fiber, the distal axon degenerates, the Schwann cells remove axonal remnants and myelin debris,[27] and proliferate to form the bands of Büngner.[28] Widening of the incisures has been reported in states of deterioration.[17] Activity of the Schwann cell is prominent in the peripheral stump, with central activity confined to a few millimeters adjacent to the section and never exceeding 10 per cent of that in the peripheral stump.[28] The myelin internode proximal to the section degenerates if the Schwann cell nucleus has been involved by the section. When the nucleus remains proximal to the damage, retrograde degeneration does not occur, but the terminal internode is short.[29] The stimulus for nuclear proliferation induced by Wallerian degeneration may be the degenerating myelin, for the larger the fiber the greater the increase of nuclei.[30] Degeneration and regeneration, of course, go on actively and simultaneously.[31] Regenerated nerves have a higher cell population than normal,[32] and the normal linear relation between fiber diameter and internodal length disappears,[33] to be replaced by short internodes.[10] Not only do regenerating nerve fibers suppress the migration of Schwann cells,[34] but the nature of the peripheral stump has bearing on the final axonal diameter. Sectioned medullated spinal nerves sutured to a nonmedullated postganglionic autonomic trunk produce marked decrease in myelin formation.[35] Even connections with the periphery are influential, for the decrease in size of the fiber in the central stump —affecting axon proportionally more than myelin—remains present until peripheral connections are established.[36, 37] Finally, the plasticity of the

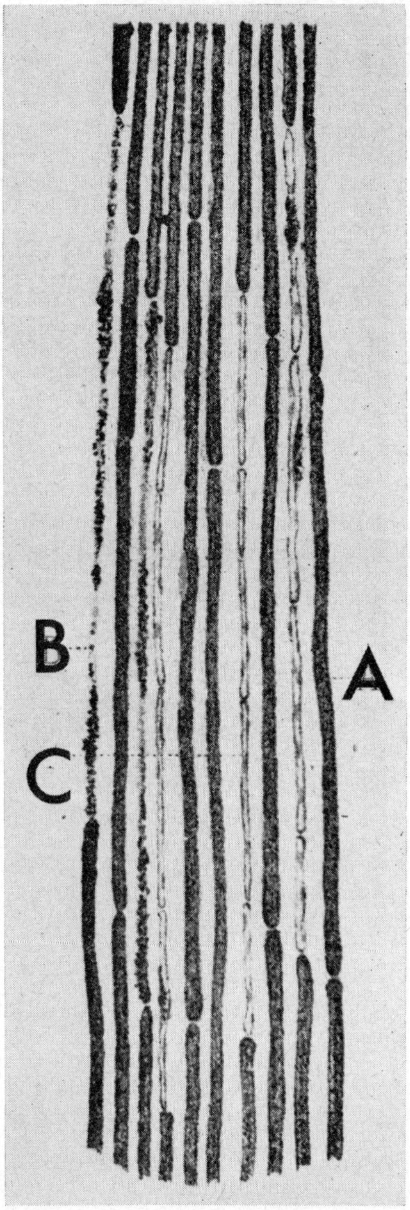


Fig. 1. Experimental segmental demyelination. Nerve stained with osmic acid and picrocarmine. *A*. Normal fiber; *B*. degenerating segment; *C*. internodal segment replaced by a series of short and narrow segments limited by well-marked nodes during the period of regeneration. Reproduced from Gombault.[42]

regenerative process is indicated by proximal collateral nerve sprouts that invade adjacent regenerating Schwann cell sheaths[38] in a manner reminiscent of the distal collateral regeneration in partially denervated muscles.[39]

A peripheral nerve, then, is not a simple structure vulnerable in only one way and with a single stereotyped reaction. The response of the soma, axon, and myelin to toxins differs.[40] Wallerian degeneration affects the axon primarily. Toxins, such as diphtheria, affect the individual Schwann cell. The demyelination associated with involvement of individual Schwann cells is designated segmental, with the implication of relative preservation of axon. "The occurrence of segmental demyelination suggests that individual Schwann cells are randomly attacked and that myelin degeneration occurs when the normal metabolic functions of the Schwann cell are disturbed."[41] This segmental demyelination of Gombault is discontinuous; it spares the axis cylinder, may be followed by recovery or by Wallerian degeneration, does not result from a tropic change in spinal centers, and in man "appears to play an important role in certain disorders of peripheral nerves where, until now, only the characteristic lesions of Wallerian degeneration have been described."[42] Fibers that have undergone segmental demyelination manifest marked variation of internodal length.[43] Although it has been argued that the conduction velocity of nerve action potential is related to myelin sheath thickness and not to internodal length[44] as had been previously claimed,[11] the fact is that in experimental segmental demyelination a decrease in conduction velocity is observed,[45] presumably because the decreased myelin thickness results in decreased resistance, increased capacitance, current leakage, and resultant decrease of current density at the node.[45, 46] This decreased density of current delays the regenerative action potential, decreasing the rate of saltatory conduction.

The usual suggestion for the mechanism of the peripheral distribution of signs and symptoms in diabetic polyneuropathy relates to the elaboration of axoplasm in perikaryon and propagation into the axis cylinder, with failure of function of axoplasm before it reaches the distal nerve terminals.[47] Demonstration by standard histological techniques of patchy demyelination in diabetic neuropathy[48] and delineation of segmental demyelination in single fiber preparations[49] raises the possibility that the site of abnormality is the Schwann cell rather than the axis cylinder. The distal distribution of the abnormality would be attributed to the demonstrated decrease in lipogenesis and oxygen uptake from proximal to distal part of the nerve. "A depressing influence acting on the nerve as a whole might cause greater and earlier damage (i.e., demyelination) at the distal tip, where lipogenesis is lowest."[50] The difficulty of distinguishing the axonal and Schwann-cell vulnerability to metabolic impairment is emphasized by the slit sheath preparations in which, following extrusion of axoplasm, the respiratory rate is of the same order as that in the intact fiber. In addition, sheath cells maintained high potassium, low sodium, and similar enzymes to those of axoplasm.[23] Destruction of axis cylinders with attendant Wallerian degeneration in severe cases of diabetic neuropathy[51] is quite concordant with Gombault's original description, and the demonstration of large and small internodes correlates well with the reduction of motor nerve conduction velocity present in patients with diabetes even in the absence of overt manifestations of clinical neuropathy.[52]

Not only is the question of a vascular or metabolic etiology of diabetic neuropathy still unresolved, but the possible sites of metabolic impairment are not yet delineated. It appears with increasing knowledge that the mechanism of production of the disorder, like its clinical manifestations, is really multiple. Perhaps, then, it is best to speak of the neuropathies of diabetes.

## *REFERENCES*


1. Mulder, D. W., Lambert, E. H., Bastron, J. A. and Sprague, R. G. Neuropathies associated with diabetes mellitus, *Neurology 11*:274-84, 1961.
2. Thomas, P. K. Connective tissue of peripheral nerve: an electron microscope study, *J. Anat. 97*:35-44, 1963.
3. Thomas, P. K. Changes in endoneurial sheaths of peripheral myelinated nerve fibers during Wallerian degeneration, *J. Anat. 98*:175-82, 1964.
4. Denny-Brown, D. Importance of neural fibroblasts in the regeneration of nerve, *Arch. Neurol. Psychiat. 55*:171-215, 1946.
5. Nathaniel, E. J. H. and Pease, D. C. Collagen and basement membrane formation by Schwann cells during nerve regeneration, *J. Ultrastructure Res. 9*: 550-60, 1965.
6. Gasser, H. S. Properties of dorsal root unmedullated fibers on the two sides of the ganglion, *J. Gen. Physiol. 38*:709-28, 1955.
7. Causey, G. and Hoffman, H. Relation between the Schwann cell and the axon in peripheral nerves, *J. Anat. 90*:1-4, 1956.
8. Hess, A. and Lansing, A. I. Fine structure of peripheral nerve fibers, *Anat. Rec. 117*:175-99, 1953.
9. Geren, B. B. Formation from the Schwann cell surface of myelin in the peripheral nerves of chick embryos, *Exp. Cell Res. 7*:558-62, 1954.
10. Lascelles, R. G. and Thomas, P. K.

Changes due to age in internodal length in the sural nerve in man, *J. Neurol. Neurosurg. Psychiat. 29*:40-44, 1966.
11. Hursh, J. B. Conduction velocity and diameter of nerve fibers, *Amer. J. Physiol. 127*:131-39, 1939.
12. Webster, H. deF. Some ultrastructural features of segmental demyelination and myelin regeneration in peripheral nerve, *Progress Brain Res. 13*:151-74, 1964.
13. Waksman, B. H. and Adams, R. D. Comparative study of experimental allergic neuritis in the rabbit, guinea pig and mouse, *J. Neuropath. Exp. Neurol. 15*:293-334, 1956.
14. Waksman, B. H. and Adams, R. D. Allergic neuritis: An experimental disease of rabbits induced by injection of peripheral nervous tissue and adjuvants *J. Exp. Med. 102*:213-37, 1955.
15. Weiss, P. and Hiscoe, H. B. Experiments on the mechanism of nerve growth, *J. Exp. Zool. 107*:315-95, 1948.
16. Lubinska, L. Outflow from cut ends of nerve fibers, *Exp. Cell. Res. 10*:40-47, 1956.
17. Lubinska, L. Physical state of axoplasm in teased vertebrate nerve fibers, *Acta Biol. 17*:135-40, 1956.
18. Causey, G. *The Cell of Schwann.* Edinburgh, Livingstone, 1960.
19. Finean, J. B. and Robertson, J. D. Lipids and the structure of myelin, *Brit. Med. Bull. 14*:267-73, 1958.
20. Landon, D. N. and Williams, P. L. Ultrastructure of the node of Ranvier, *Nature 199*:575-77, 1963.
21. Williams, P. L. and Landon, D. N. Paranodal apparatus of peripheral myelinated nerve fibers of mammals, *Nature 198*:670-73, 1963.
22. Smart, I. Myelinization as the establishment of a counter-current exchange mechanism, *J. Anat. 97*:480, 1963.
23. Schmitt, F. O. Axon-satellite cell relationships in peripheral nerve fibers, *Exp. Cell. Res. (Suppl.) 5*:33-57, 1958.
24. Matthews, M. R. Further observations on transneuronal degeneration in the lateral geniculate nucleus of the Macaque monkey, *J. Anat. 98*:255-63, 1964.
25. Powell, T. P. S. and Erulkar, S. D. Transneuronal cell degeneration in the auditory relay nuclei of the cat, *J. Anat. 96*:249-68, 1962.
26. Korr, I. M., Wilkinson, P. N. and Chornock, F. W. Axonal delivery of neuroplasmic components to muscle cells, *Science 155*:342-45, 1966.
27. Nathaniel, E. J. H. and Pease, D. C. Degenerative changes in rat dorsal roots during Wallerian degeneration. *J. Ultrastruct. Res. 9*:511-32, 1963.
28. Abercrombie, M. and Johnson, M. L. Outwandering of cells in tissue cultures of nerves undergoing Wallerian degeneration, *J. Exp. Biol. 19*:266-83, 1942.
29. Lubinska, L. Region of transition between preserved and regenerating parts of myelinated nerve fibers, *J. Comp. Neur. 113*:315-36, 1959.
30. Joseph, J. Changes in nuclear population following twenty-one days degeneration in a nerve consisting of small myelinated fibers, *J. Anat. 82*:146-52, 1948.
31. Nathaniel, E. J. H. and Pease, D. C. Regenerative changes in rat dorsal roots following Wallerian degeneration. *J. Ultrastruct. Res. 9*:533-49, 1963.
32. Abercrombie, M. and Santler, J. E. Analysis of growth in nuclear population during Wallerian degeneration, *J. Cell Comp. Physiol. 50*:429-50, 1957.
33. Vizoso, A. D. and Young, J. Z. Internode length and fiber diameter in developing and regenerating nerves, *J. Anat. 82*:110-34, 1948.
34. Abercrombie, M., Johnson, M. L. and Thomas, G. A. Influence of nerve fibers on Schwann cell migration investigated in tissue culture, *Proc. Roy. Soc. B. 136*:448-60, 1949.
35. Young, J. Z. Functional repair of nervous tissue, *Physiol. Rev. 22*:318-74, 1942.
36. Sanders, F. K. Thickness of the myelin sheaths of normal and regenerating peripheral nerve fibers, *Proc. Roy Soc. B. 135*:323-57, 1948.
37. Aitken, J. T. and Thomas, P. K. Retrograde changes in fibre size following nerve section, *J. Anat. 96*:121-29, 1962.
38. Causey, G. and Hoffman, H. Axon sprouting in partially deneurotized nerves, *Brain 78*:661-68, 1955.

39. Wohlfart, G. Collateral regeneration in partialy denervated muscles, *Neurology 8*:175-80, 1958.
40. Peterson, E. R. and Murray, M. R. Patterns of peripheral demyelination *in vitro, Ann. N. Y. Acad. Sci. 122*:39-50, 1965.
41. McDonald, W. I. Effects of experimental demyelination on conduction in peripheral nerve: A histological and electrophysiological study, *Brain 86:* 481-500, 1963.
42. Gombault, A. Contribution à l'étude anatomique de la névrite parenchymateuse subaiguë et chronique—névrite segmentaire péri-axile, *Arch. Neurologie* (Paris) *1*:11-38, 177-90, 1880.
43. Fullerton, P. M., Gilliatt, R. W., Lascelles, R. G. and Morgan-Hugites, J. A. Relation between fiber diameter and internodal length in chronic neuropathy, *J. Physiol. 178*:26P-28P, 1965.
44. Sanders, F. K. and Whitteridge, D. Conduction velocity and myelin thickness in regenerating nerve fibers, *J. Physiol. 105*:152-74, 1946.
45. McDonald, W. I. Effects of experimental demyelination on conduction in peripheral nerve: A histological and electrophysiological study, *Brain 86:* 501-24, 1963.
46. Kaeser, H. E. and Lambert, E. H. Nerve function studies in experimental polyneuritis, *Electroenceph. Clin. Neurophysiol.* (Suppl.) *22*:29-35, 1962.
47. Locke, S. Peripheral nervous system in diabetes mellitus, *Diabetes 13*:307-11, 1964.
48. Dolman, C. L.: Morbid anatomy of diabetic neuropathy, *Neurology 13*:135-42, 1963.
49. Thomas, P. K. and Lascelles, R. G. Schwann cell abnormalities in diabetic neuropathy, *Lancet 1*:1355-57, 1965.
50. Manjo, G. and Karnovsky, M. L. Biochemical and morphologic study of myelination and demyelination, *J. Exp. Med. 107*:475-96, 1958.
51. Thomas, P. K. and Lascelles, R. G. Pathology of diabetic neuropathy, *Quart. J. Med. (NS) 35*:489-509, 1966.
52. Lawrence, D. G. and Locke, S. Motor nerve conduction velocity in diabetes, *Arch. Neur. 5*:483-89, 1961.

# ATHEROSCLEROSIS: THE FACTS AND THE MYSTERIES*

WILLIAM DOCK

Chief, Medical Service
Veterans Administration Hospital
Brooklyn, N. Y.

IN the worry and strain of modern life arterial degeneration is not only very common, but develops often at a relatively early age. For this I believe that the high pressure at which men live and the habit of working the machine to its maximum capacity are responsible. Angiosclerosis is the Nemesis through which Nature exacts retributive justice for the transgression of her laws."**

When Virchow's pupils studied the arterial lesions of men, they revised Lobstein's endarteritis nodosa to arteriosclerosis nodosa, and finally Felix J. Marchand suggested that they stop talking about atheromalike arteriosclerotic lesions and simply say atherosclerosis. Atheroma was the medical term for wen or sebaceous cyst, and is still defined as such in our medical dictionaries. While the material in wens and in arterial atheromas is grossly similar, we now know that the histologic and chemical structure of arterial atheromas is much closer to xanthomas of skin and tendons than it is to sebaceous cysts, which contain sebum secreted by epithelial cells. Xanthomas and atherosclerotic plaques contain material chemically close to beta-lipoprotein of plasma and quite different from the lipid in wens, in platelets, or red cells, and significantly different from the alpha lipoprotein of plasma (T. D. V. Lawrie, cited in Dock[1]). As Wilens has shown, such lipid accumulates in arterial walls when plasma is allowed to percolate through the wall under pressure in excised vessels.[2] It has also been shown that when animals develop these lesions in consequence of dietary change, with or without hypothyroidism, lesions grow faster in hypertensive than in normotensive rabbits, chickens, or dogs.

In man the pulmonary arteries usually are free of lesions when systemic arteries are severely involved. However, severe atherosclerosis

*Presented at a meeting of the Rudolf Virchow Medical Society in the City of New York, held at The New York Academy of Medicine, January 9, 1967.
**Osler, W. *N.Y. Med. J. 64*:797-806, 1896.

is seen in persons who experience the early onset of pulmonary hypertension, as in congenital left-right shunts and mitral stenosis. The pulmonary arteries have blood containing slightly more platelets and lipid than systemic blood, they have similar velocity and volume flow, and they have the same hemodynamic shear force and turbulence at bends and bifurcations. But as long as pulmonary arterial pressure is normal, i.e., below 60 mm. Hg even during exercise, no atheromas form even in familial hyperlipemia, with xanthomas and severe systemic atherosclerosis. The facts of human pathology, obvious even in Virchow's day, thus indicate that percolation pressure is critical for the development of atherosclerosis. Neither platelet stickiness, hyperlipemia, thrombocytosis, nor the stresses produced by the rapid flow of blood around the curving walls cause these lesions where pressure is below 60 mm. Hg.

Once pressure is at that level, rapid flow does accelerate atherogenesis, as we see in the femoral artery leading to an arteriovenous fistula. Similar lesions never occur in veins, even in portal hypertension, even in thick-walled varicose veins. It is a fact that the deposition of plasma lipids percolating through the intima fits the facts of human and experimental pathology, while the mural thrombosis theory is in conflict with these facts. The theory of formation in situ is supported only by the fact that isotopic precursors of cholesterol can be detected in cholesterol formed by bits of arterial intima growing in cultures. But since all body cells can synthesize cholesterol and all intimal tissue contains living cells, this does not prove anything. It certainly fails to explain the absence of atheromas in pulmonary arteries and in veins.

The localization of atheromas in the systemic vessels is related to the pulse pressure and to innate intimal thickness, or that developed as a result of arteritis or, in experiments, of intimal regeneration after injury. Also the rate of atherogenesis, at any given level of plasma lipid or arterial pressure, is faster in young or fast-growing succulent intima than in the aged relatively static tissue. Thus lipid droplets can be seen accumulating in the intima of the aorta and coronary arteries in suckling humans and suckling rabbits. Here arterial pressure is relatively low, and lipid, though high compared to that at birth or after weaning, is much lower than in dietary atherosclerosis of rabbits or the plasma of most adults in the United States. In the rabbits the lipid droplets reabsorb on weaning. Humans who received no dairy products after being taken off the breast also quickly lose the "*Säuglings-Cholesterolosis*," as Virchow's pupils named this infantile atherosclerosis.

It is not known whether the composition of the intimal ground substance is an important factor in lipid decomposition. G. Manley (cited in Dock[1]) has given data on the relative amount of chondroitin sulphate, heparatin, and hyalouronate, from fetal life to the senium in aorta, pulmonary artery, iliac, and radial arteries. Hyalouronate is more abundant, chondroitin less, in the pulmonary artery. The chondroitin percentage also falls from aorta to radials, rises in aging vessels, and is higher in severely atherosclerotic than in normal iliacs. But this difference may be a result, not a cause, of the atheroma formation. Ground substance and inner elastic lamellae have been given, even in Virchow's writing, as "the cause" of arteriosclerosis, and this conjecture is still urged by Moon and by Holman. The mystery is why degeneration occurs in certain sites and on certain diets.

It now seems well established that the beta-lipoprotein levels in plasma are higher in animals or men with atheromas than in controls of same age and sex, and that they are higher in young men than young women. But by the time thrombosis and clinical disease occur, cholesterol or beta-lipoprotein levels in many populations are relatively less elevated in coronary cases than are the plasma triglyceride levels. The latter affect platelet stickiness, fibrinolysin, and plasma clotting times more than do the beta-lipoproteins. Another mystery is that the sex difference in lipids, coronary disease, and thromboembolic disease, which is so striking in white people, is absent or, at early ages, reversed in the United States Negroes. Thus sex hormones, genetic background, and diet all play important roles in determining plasma content of the lipids that are deposited in atherosclerosis and that accelerate thrombosis. In white people, the diet of young men and women is very different just at the time when adolescent boys are rapidly developing plaques in the aorta and the coronary arteries but we have no reports on diet, hormone levels, or paths of hormone degradation in Negro women as compared with whites.[3]

So far as relation of diet to plasma lipids is concerned, we have plenty of facts. Individuals and species vary enormously in sensitivity to cholesterol, to saturated fats, to sucrose,[4] and even to high calorie intake of unsaturated fat and starch. In people with xanthomas and high lipids, alcohol and saturated fats raise levels, while diets low in calories, but with a high ratio of polyunsaturated fat to calories may strikingly reduce triglycerides and beta-lipoprotein, as well as cholesterol in plasma. The diets that raise lipids and cause atherosclerosis in birds and animals, the diets consumed by populations with high rates of coronary disease and thromboembolism, are also diets that raise lipid levels in patients with coronary disease when such diets are resumed after they have been on therapeutic trials of diets normal for primates—fruit, vegetables, grain, fish, lean meat, and oils pressed from seeds. Caffeine and nicotine, which raise lipid levels of coronary patients, apparently act like catecholamines, emotional stress, or hypothalamic stimulation of rabbits, all of which raise lipid levels in those on atherogenic diets.

Last, let us turn to the theories on mural thrombosis, intimal hemorrhage, and the ulceration of atheromas that so often triggers thrombotic occlusion. Carl von Rokitansky and other early observers thought the plaques might be organized mural thrombi, and this thesis has been espoused recently by J. B. Duguid in Britain. It ignores the absence of similar lesions in veins and pulmonary arteries, and the mural injury that might initiate thrombosis and become "the" original cause. The opposite view was given in detail in 1938 by Milton C. Winternitz.[5] His monograph gives an excellent review of earlier studies of the arterial vasa vasorum and of intimal hemorrhages. To Winternitz purpura from the rare normal vasa entering the intima could initiate the formation of plaque, or by damaging or rupturing the surface could cause mural thrombosis, leading to further vascularization and larger hemorrhages or occlusive thrombosis.

Lately Friedman[6] has urged the "paucity" of intimal vessels, even when plaques have been formed due to lipid infiltrate from the plasma. He feels that mural hemorrhages are extremely rare, while J. C. Patterson in Canada, and Milton Helpern in New York regard them as frequent and occasionally large enough to cause stenosis and myocardial infarction without luminal rupture and thrombosis. Like M. Friedman, S. Wilens (cited in Dock[1]) is impressed by rarity of vascularization of the plaques and considers this the main reason they become necrotic. Winternitz' beautiful illustrations of vessels in early lesions, both in the aorta (see his Figure 82), and in coronary arteries (his Figures 77, 83, 84), seem to have been overlooked by Friedman. On the other hand, we do not know how rare or common such lesions are when sought by the injection and clearing technique used by the Yale group. We can accept as facts that plaques ulcerate and cause thrombosis, that undermining at sites of ulceration can simulate mural hemorrhage, but just how ulceration occurs and whether hemorrhage into plaques is very rare, occasional, or frequent remains a mystery.

From the standpoint of Virchow, who thought of morbid anatomy only as a small part of the picture of disease and of the far greater spectacle of human suffering, the most important fact is that arteriosclerosis flourishes best on our curious diet, a product of wealth and our industrial production of eggs, dairy products, and stall-fed swine and cattle, as well as of sucrose, nicotine and caffeine. These latter items were exotic or unknown to Western Europe before the 16th century. The foods were daily items of diet only for the most prosperous people until the 20th century. Frustration, hostility, anger, all raise blood lipid levels, but in animals or men on physiologic diets the effects on the vessels are minimal.

The next most important fact is that patients and doctors would rather risk shortening their lives than give up customary pleasures. Most men and women will reject the notion that diet can cause disease, although they will usually attribute the pain at onset of coronary disease to some item in the last meal they ate. In 1916 William Ophüls, professor of pathology at Stanford University, began to teach medical students that diet was an important and perhaps the only controllable factor in atherosclerosis. T. Leary at Boston University followed in 1934. But none of their students believed a word of it. Today only a minority of physicians accept this in principle, fewer still in practice or in their own way of life. Man not only fails to burn up cholesterol and saturated fat as do the carnivores, but fails to face the facts of life, in pathogenesis as in politics. Machiavelli remarked that "a man would sooner forgive the murder of his father than the theft of his patrimony." As long as men will sooner forgive the loss of their lives than the loss of new-found foods and drugs inhaled or ingested all day long, there will always be a high death rate from atherosclerosis and from bronchial cancer.

## *REFERENCES*

1. Dock, W. Confusion in coronary lesions compounded, *Amer. J. Cardiol. 18*:150, 1966 (13 references).
2. Wilens, S. T. and McClusky, R. T. Permeability of excised arteries and of other tissues to serum lipids, *Cir. Res. 2*:175-82, 1954.
3. Dock, W. Why are men's coronary arteries so sclerotic? *J.A.M.A. 170*:152, 1959 (17 references).
4. MacDonald, I. and Braithwaite, D. M. Influence of dietary carbohydrate on the lipid pattern in serum and in adipose tissue. *Clin. Sci. 27*:23, 1964.
5. Winternitz, M. C., Thomas, R. M. and Le Compte, P. M. *Biology of Arteriosclerosis.* Springfield, Ill., Thomas, 1938.
6. Friedman, M. and van den Bovenkamp, G. The pathogenesis of coronary intramural haemorrhages, *Brit. J. Exper. Path. 47*:347, 1966.

# BRIEF PSYCHOTHERAPY AND THE EXISTENTIAL SHIFT

*The Annual Schilder Memorial Lecture**

JAN EHRENWALD

President, the Schilder Society
New York, N.Y.

I FIRST met Paul Schilder when I was a third-year medical student in Vienna. The vaulted auditorium of the Psychiatrische Klinik was crowded with students from all faculties attending the young professor's Saturday evening lectures on psychoanalysis. The date was the winter of 1922, a year before the publication of Freud's *The Ego and the Id*. Schilder's discourse was still largely steeped in Freud's discovery of infantile sexuality; of the mechanisms of resistance and repression; of sexual symbolism in dreams and neurotic symptoms. These lectures were my first introduction into the field—a field full of fascination, wonderment, and doubt. Schilder, at the time, appeared to me as the authoritative spokesman of psychoanalysis, an inspiring guide who led the novice into unknown territory and promised dark and dangerous sights—and insights—at the end of the road.

In the ensuing years Schilder's position in regard to Freudian orthodoxy underwent many revisions. By classical psychoanalytical standards his approach might well be described as eclectic, incorporating, as it did, Adlerian, Rankian, Reichian and, in the end, Sullivanian concepts. Schilder was a therapeutic activist, like Stekel or Ferenczi, when an active, directive technique was called for. He pioneered in group therapy when this was desirable, and he used hypnosis and narcoanalysis, as well as drug treatment, when drugs were indicated. Above all, he was fully aware of both the scope and the limitations of classical psychoanalysis as a therapeutic tool, and he resisted the temptation to be drawn by his compulsive patients into the interminable analyses that Freud had cautioned against.

Can Schilder therefore be legitimately described as an advocate of brief psychotherapy? It all depends on what we mean by the term.

*Presented at the Schilder Memorial Meeting of the Schilder Society, held at The New York Academy of Medicine, January 26, 1967.

There is an unconfirmed story about a woman afflicted with hysterical urinary retention who was presented to Schilder during one of his rounds at Bellevue Hospital. He curtly introduced himself and shot a simple question at the young woman: "I am Dr. Schilder, Mrs. Jones. Why can't you pee?" The woman was so shocked by this informal approach that she instantaneously wet her bed then and there. It is improbable that Schilder's intervention was of lasting benefit to the patient, but it is a graphic—though fictitious—example of quick symptom removal that can be accomplished by "brief" psychotherapy.

The fact is that brief psychotherapy has a long and checkered career. It has ranged all the way from primitive healing to the short-term analytic psychotherapy of our day; its history has run the whole gamut from uncritical acceptance to unconditional rejection. There still are critics who regard brief psychotherapy as a rudimentary if not corrupt version of classical analysis, an inferior substitute for the real thing to meet the poor man's need. But clinical experience over the past five decades with various methods of treatment, short-term and long-term, supported by the records of about two millennia of prescientific psychotherapy, suggests that virtually all methods—from magic and faith healing to Freudian analysis and Pavlovian conditioning—have been effective in their own right. It is true, we are still at a loss to distinguish genuine therapeutic results from so-called spontaneous remissions. We are still having difficulties in supplying statistical proofs of the superiority of one rival school over the other.

Still, it is one of the paradoxes of the history of our subject that a wide variety of approaches have been capable of meeting the patients' needs while at the same time they seemed to bear out the validity of their respective therapists' theoretical propositions—Freudian, Jungian, Adlerian, Sullivanian—as the case may be.

Elsewhere I have tried to account for this state of affairs.[1] I noted that one of the hallmarks of the unfolding doctor-patient relation is the patient's tendency to confirm with his productions the therapist's conscious or preconscious wishes and theoretical expectations regarding the validity of his doctrine or of the school of thought to which he owed allegiance. This is what I have described as *doctrinal compliance*.

It goes without saying, however, that doctrinal compliance alone cannot explain the therapeutic efficacy, real or apparent, of an inert placebo, a magic ritual, or of an assortment of mutually conflicting—or patently false—dynamic interpretations. Nor am I satisfied that the usual references to suggestion, transference, or transference cures can tell the whole story.

It is true that suggestion and transference are ever-present ingredients of the therapeutic situation. But critical study of the pertinent literature, from Ferenczi and Freud to Ida MacAlpine, T. X. Barber, B. Wolstein, or L. Wolberg, shows that more often than not transference is apt to be explained in terms of suggestion, and suggestion in terms of transference. In short, we are taken through the paces of circular reasoning and still left at a loss to find the effective principle in the broad spectrum of therapeutic transactions from prescientific psychotherapy to the most sophisticated analytic techniques.

What, then, is the key to our puzzle? I propose to show that it can be found in the opening phases of the therapeutic process, psychoanalytic or otherwise. The opening phase in virtually all forms of treatment is characterized by a pattern of feedback operating between therapist and patient. Virtually all patients who seek help from a professional healer do so with the hope and expectation that they will be helped. And all practitioners—from the untutored magician to the scientifically trained therapist of today—approach their task with varying degrees of conviction that they are indeed capable of helping their patients. Given a favorable cultural climate these reciprocal attitudes tend to reinforce one another: the patient's trusting, hopeful response to his therapist reinforces the latter's therapeutic motivations; and the therapist's motivation to help, his show of confidence in the efficacy of his approach, tends to reinforce the hopeful expectancy of the patient. I have been able to show elsewhere that the resulting pattern of circular feedback is characteristic of virtually all forms of psychotherapy.

Needless to say, such complementary and mutually reinforcing pairs of attitudes are by no means confined to the doctor-patient relation. They can be discerned in the relation between the leader and his followers; between the prophet and his disciples; between the myth-maker and the myth-taker or recipient of his message. Indeed I have pointed out that the same formula accounts for the effectiveness of what theologians described as the *effective myth*. But here, again, merely pointing to this aspect of the therapeutic situation and to its resemblance to the dynamics of the effective myth begs the issue. It fails to account for the effectiveness of an individual therapist's "effective myth" or for the charismatic healer's *charisma*. It does not explain the dynamics of the occasional striking improvements seen in brief psychotherapy of all denominations. Positive transference tells only part of the story. What is the other part? What are the factors that provide the momentum for the opening phase of the treatment process?

Let us look at the traditional set-up of the psychoanalytic situation as it evolved at the turn of the 19th century. The analytic patient, instead of being confronted with a stern, judgmental, authoritarian figure haranguing him with the usual exhortations and admonitions, found himself in the presence of an unobtrusive, silent, nondirective listener, whose only demand was for the patient to give free reign to his thoughts and fantasies, to say everything that came to his mind, regardless of the conventional taboos current in his time. All this, it should be noted, took place with the patient in a recumbent position, with the analyst sitting behind the couch, relieving him of the impediments of the customary face-to-face confrontation. It is readily understood that this radical change in the habitual pattern of communication between patient and doctor is in itself apt to shift the relationship into a new gear. The novelty of the setting and its contrast to traditional modes of communication is even more striking if we bear in mind the *Zeitgeist*—the spirit of the time—when the psychoanalytic movement was launched.

Viewed in historical perspective, a more or less dramatic change in the circumstances surrounding the therapeutic situation has always been an important feature of the healing approach. To be more precise, every new departure in theory and practice has sought to enhance the impact of the new by making use of the time-honored ingredients of success salvaged from the past.

The seeker of help, consulting a medicine man or entering the precincts of a Greek temple or a sacred Christian shrine, leaves behind the hustle and bustle of the market place. The magic rites of the shaman or of the *curandero*, or the solemn rituals of the officiating priest, transport the believer into a spiritual climate worlds apart from his ordinary mode of existence. At the same time, he is brought closer to the divinity worshiped by his ancestors or to revered ancestral figures represented by the deity itself. Stated in the terms of Mircea Eliade, it is a shift to the *sacred* from the *profane*.[2]

A latter-day clinical example of a comparable shift can still be seen in the abrupt transformation of the contemporary psychotherapist donning the mantle of the hypnotist, regressing, as it were, to the role of a magician possessed of supposedly infinite powers. The transformation is a two-way process in which the regressive trend—the "regression in the service of treatment"—is shared by patient and therapist alike.[1]

Yet here, again, it is interesting to note that abrupt changes of this order are by no means confined to the doctor-patient relation. Such changes may be seen in modern man's uneasy metaphysical posture, which wavers between a wholly pragmatic scientific outlook and his lingering tendency toward superstitious beliefs and practices, especially when he is under stress or in the throes of emotional conflict. Indeed, modern man shares these two contrasting attitudes with his preliterate cousins and precursors. We know that preliterate man, even under most primitive conditions, by no means lives by magic alone; he is only a part-time primitive. B. Malinowski,[3] in his much-quoted study of the Trobriand Islanders, describes in great detail the magic rituals that permeated their daily lives. But when going out on a fishing expedition they also made sure to check their fishing gear, to overhaul their canoes, to avoid the reefs, and to negotiate the shallows. To be on the safe side they "praised the Lord" but also passed the ammunition; they subscribed to what amounts to a dual orientation toward the world: one pragmatic, the other magical. This is what Evans-Pritchard described as the philosophy of *dual causality*.[4]

The scientifically oriented hypnotherapist and his hypnotic subject, regressing as they do "in the service of treatment," are graphic illustrations of the same point. So is the psychoanalyst who adheres to the principle of strict psychic determinism while he tries, at the same time, to change his patient's personality in apparent contradiction to the principle of determinism. So is the natural scientist or positivistic philosopher of our day, who alternates between the inner certainty (or illusion) of freedom and the compelling evidence to the contrary supplied by his daily experience in the laboratory. The dichotomy between the *sacred* and the *profane;* between a person's membership in a group and his role as an independent, self-directed individual, reflects the same polarity. So do the periodic interruptions of his workday routine by spells of religious dedication, followed in turn by traditionally condoned Bacchanalian revels, siestas, or carnivals. Indeed, existential shifts including ecstasies and possessions, from "below" as well as from "above," are part and parcel of the varieties of religious experience.

In the rarefied air of esthetic experience the existential shift occurs in more subtle ways but in virtually unlimited shades, gradations, and existential modalities. The actor who impersonates a stage character and the audience that responds to his performance are transported into worlds of their own—heroic, farcical, surrealistic, absurd—as the case may be. The viewer of an early Renaissance painting may find himself enveloped in the luminosity of an Umbrian landscape, the dwelling-place of ethereal beings, all stillness, translucent color, and measured repose. Or else he may find himself face to face with the tortured canvases of Picasso's Guernica series, substituting jarred, broken, and distorted forms for animate or inanimate objects. He may be exposed to the turbulent splashes of action painting or drawn into the dizzying vortex of contemporary op art—if not into the outpourings of a schizophrenic artist *manqué*.

Some of these deviations from our standard way of experience may indeed be little more than pathological aberrations, sound and fury signifying nothing. They may be due to psychological entropy, to the encroachment of sheer randomness upon the basic trend for order and lawfulness that patterns organic life and human affairs in general. But these deviations too are indicative of man's craving for ever-recurrent changes of his posture in the universe—even though the notes sounded may be jarring and the new posture found may bring only temporary relief.

The variety of existential shifts occurring in the psychotherapeutic situation is perhaps more limited, but they are capable of penetrating into much deeper levels of personality. The shifts may range from the base line of secondary process functioning to primary process functioning; from inhibition to "dis-inhibition"; from the supremacy of the ego to the supremacy of the id. They may involve abrupt swings from a person's habitual level of psychological adaptation to a new baseline, as in the case of hypnosis, waking suggestion, or I. H. Schultz's autogenous training. Shifts of this order may thus include both vegetative regulatory functions and alterations of psychological ego defenses.

Strictly speaking, it is this total reshuffling and reorganization of a person's external adaptations and inner experiences, affecting all levels of his orientation in the world and the whole repertoire of behavioral responses to his environment that is here described as the *existential shift.* It goes without saying that in the course of routine psychotherapeutic or analytic practice such dramatic changes are few and far apart. They may manifest themselves merely as *formes frustes* of the total experience. They may be fleeting and transient, or else they may usher in a lasting departure from previous faulty patterns of adaptation. They may be subtle and barely perceptible to the naked eye, or they may initiate radical changes of personality, comparable to the molting of a snake or the emergence of a butterfly from its chrysalis stage.

Viewed in this light it is readily understood that existential shifts occurring in the opening phase of the treatment are of crucial importance for the further course of psychotherapy, analytic and otherwise. By accident or by design, whether deliberately pursued or merely as incidental by-products of the therapeutic situation, they may jolt the patient out of his faulty level of functioning and help him to attain a new, more appropriate level of adaptation. The existential shift, followed by methodical analysis of resistances, of the transference relationship, by the attainment of dynamic insight and the necessary period of "working through," may thus constitute a decisive step toward ultimate recovery.

How, then, does the existential shift come about? In the field of religious experience it has long been sought by diverse rituals, ascetic practices, ablutions, and spiritual disciplines. In the world of esthetic experience it may be the gift of the creative artist to a receptive audience. If we focus on psychotherapy proper, we can discern four major triggering factors.

The first is largely situational. It is derived from the psychological impact of a celebrated (or well-publicized) healing shrine or institution; from an "effective" myth—or a cluster of such myths—shared by therapist and patient, and the culture in which they are immersed.

The second factor is constituted by the external paraphernalia of the therapeutic situation combining, if possible, the virtues of both old and new fads and fashions of the healing art. These virtues range from the time-honored rituals of the temple sleep or the hypnotic trance to the analytic couch; to Moreno's psychodramatic stage; to Reich's Orgone box or to Wolpe's techniques of experimental conditioning.

A dynamically more significant factor is the patient's confrontation with whatever insights can be opened up for him in the course of analytic psychotherapy. Insight of this order may be the genuine article. Alternatively, it may be largely due to the patient's doctrinal compliance with the ideas of his therapist. It may merely be indicative of the operation of his positive transference. But in either case it may be accompanied by the shock of recognition and may set in motion a therapeutically desirable chain of events. This is what Franz Alexander described as the "auspicious," in contrast to a vicious cycle.[5] It may mobilize the patient's recuperative and regenerative powers, to which Joost Meerloo has recently called attention.[6]

A fourth factor that may trigger off an existential shift is closely akin to the patient's confrontation with new analytical insight. It can be described as the *value shock*. The value shock is in effect a familiar feature of the classical analytic situation in which the analyst refrains from assuming a moralistic, judgmental position even in the face of the patient's offensive behavior, of his poorly controlled instinctual drives, his incestuous or pregenital impulses. I noted that the shock effect of such a neutral attitude had been even more pronounced in the repressive climate of the Victorian era. But a therapist, deliberately reversing the role of the authoritarian, compulsive, inconsistent, or "double-binding" parent, may still take by surprise a rebellious adolescent of our day. A value shock is likewise involved in the planned role reversals practiced by the psychodramatist or in the techniques of so-called "paradigmatic" psychotherapy advocated by B. Nelson, Marie Coleman, and others.

It should be noted, however, that in some of the detached, alienated, and ideologically confused youngsters of our time the value shock may have to be applied in the opposite direction. The therapist may be called upon to put before them a new, humanistic, religious, or even authoritarian system of values that had been absent in their early conditioning, leaving them aimless, adrift, and perplexed in their later years. Under otherwise favorable circumstances sudden confrontation with a novel system of values may then provide a salutory shock of its own. If so, it too may be attended by an existential shift and serve as the nucleus for the formation of a new superego and as a point of departure for further maturation of the personality as a whole. It is apparently the need for this type of "rebound" experience to which the diverse existential therapies owe their current popularity.

Viewed in this light, the manipulation of values emerges as an important tool of the therapeutic approach. Yet for precisely this reason any rigid, normative position is apt to impair the therapist's usefulness in meeting the idiosyncratic needs of a wide variety of patients. The moral therapist of a past age who had his hands tied by a ready-made system of values and the old-fashioned clergyman of today who still feels duty-bound to subscribe, ex officio, to fixed, unalterable rules of conduct, may find themselves in the same predicament.

The modus operandi of the existential shift is another matter. In the field of psychotherapy proper it is triggered off by the power of words and other forms of symbolic communication. We are here confronted with a graded scale of what can be described as psychophysiological *leverage effects*. Clearly, the leverage effect of the equation $3 \times 4 = 12$, is infinitesimal. Except for some hidden numerological meaning, it provides a point of rather redundant information. But Goethe's Faust was overawed by the sight of the pentagram on the threshold of his study. His latter-day descendant, Professor Jung, attached profound archetypal significance to the figure *four*, and considered the *mandala* a symbol of deep spiritual revelation. Viewed in this context, the *experiential* (or emotional) significance of the numerals 3, 4, or 5, is far in excess of their *referential* (information-carrying) connotation. This is still more true when the symbol is primarily of an experiential nature: when the Star-Spangled Banner or the Union Jack flutters in the breeze; when the Nazi swastika offends my sensibilities; or when Camus' version of the myth of Sisyphus presses home to me the tragic aspects of the human situation. Thus my response to the spoken or written word; the impact of symbol, metaphor, or myth ranges all the way from insight and edification to the inner stirrings of affect and its psychosomatic corollaries; from goose pimples to palpitations; from tears to twinges of intestinal discomfort. There is, behavioristically speaking, a *gradient* of leverage effects possessed by a broad system of symbolic or communicative behavior. The smallest leverage is attached to verbal cues whose effect is confined to cortical neurons and synapses. Their effect increases with the overspill of affective responses in various autonomic centers and from there into the viscera, smooth muscles, and endocrine glands.

If this is true, the existential shift triggered by the therapist's personal impact upon his patients—in conjunction with the patient's corresponding hopes and expectations—may well account for the crucial importance of the opening phase of psychotherapy, both prescientific and scientific. Above all, it may be responsible for at least part of the successes of brief psychotherapy. Viewed from this angle, brief psychotherapy may indeed be regarded as a *forme fruste* of long-term analysis. It could also be stated, however, that by the same token, long-term analysis derives a considerable part of its momentum from the leverage effects touched off in its opening phase. This is also borne out by the observation that patients who have failed to respond to analytic insights offered in the course of years may suddenly be able to reactivate—and utilize—the insights gained when they change to a new therapist who succeeds in bringing about a belated existential shift.

It would be tempting to document by illustrative case histories the four major factors involved in the triggering of such shifts. But two condensed case reports must suffice in the present context. My first case illustrates the part played by the value shock and the existential shift in brief psychotherapy—actually the "briefest" in my files.

*Case 1.* Charlie B. is a baby-faced young man of 23. He has been married for 1½ years but stayed away from his wife several nights a week to drink and play cards with his buddies. He was a law student but became hopelessly bogged down in his academic work and admitted he had only "stuck it out" because of pressure from his father. The older Mr. B. is a self-made man, anxious to see his son "making good" in a professional career. He was a controlling authoritarian personality who ruled his family with an iron hand. Charlie never dared to rebel openly against his father and his drinking was an indirect expression of protest against him. At the same time it helped Charlie to escape from his wife who, he felt, had likewise become a controlling and demanding figure in his life. He felt guilty for his misdemeanors, drank more to allay his guilt feelings, and became increasingly contrite, lachrymose, and depressed.

He was sullen and uncommunicative during his first interview. Faced with a new doctor of his father's choosing and his father's age, he took it for granted that he would once more be put through the third degree of harangues and exhortations, followed by an ultimatum to mend his ways or forfeit his father's financial support.

The therapist's unexpectedly permissive, nonauthoritarian, laissez-faire attitude took Charlie completely by surprise. The sudden reversal of the original parental role projected into the transference relationship effected precisely the value shock which was required to prepare the ground for a total reorientation of Charlie's attitude toward his work and family. It soon became evident that Charlie was not cut out for a professional career. He wanted to work as a carpenter, to tinker about the house and have a good time with his buddies. In addition, he obviously had an unresolved Oedipal conflict and a latent homosexual trend. Yet his whole background, his limited intelligence and lack of motivation made him ineligible for psychoanalysis. Nevertheless, the initial momentum gained by the leverage effect of the value shock, and the explicit approval of his dropping out of college—concurred in by the older Mr. B.—brought about a prompt improvement in the clinical picture. Treatment was terminated after four sessions.

Charlie's case is a typical example of "brief" psychotherapy, leading to quick symptom removal triggered off by the dynamics of an existential shift and leaving the rest to the individual's innate adaptive and recuperative potential. Given such recuperative potential, the patient may indeed reach a new level of adaptation enabling him to use more adequate ego defenses than before. Brief psychotherapy, viewed in this light, in effect amounts to an induced "spontaneous" remission presided over by a therapist, aware of the existing psychodynamics and of the patient's personality resources.

My second illustrative case history takes us to a dynamically more involved situation.

*Case 2*. Robert M. was referred to me by his general practitioner and a surgical consultant. A strapping six-footer, aged 19, he was a student at an Ivy League college. Yet for the last year he had been suffering from persistent abdominal pain with occasional severe exacerbations. At times he felt dizzy and came close to fainting. Diagnostic study, including GI series, x-ray examination of the gastrointestinal tract and gallbladder, showed no abnormalities. Neurological findings, EEG, CSF, vestibular reactions, were likewise normal. In his first psychiatric interview, Robert was noncommittal. He had nothing to complain about, shrugged his shoulders with each half-finished sentence accompanied by an embarrased smile. It soon transpired that he had never been able to communicate—to finish a sentence—with his cold, rejecting mother or his domineering, authoritarian father, a wealthy stockbroker. An older sister, he stated, was the apple of their eyes. Robert, in turn, withdrew from his family into a position of silent, sullen, cynical rebellion, trying to control his rage lest he incur even more of his parents' disapproval. He failed at school and escaped into a world of daydreams, books, and esoteric artistic interests.

On discovering that the new therapist was ready to ally himself with Robert's need to break away from his domineering father and his "materialistic" values, he loosened up. He brought up his conflict about a girl of whom his parents disapproved, etc. In the further course he openly vented his anger against his mother and sister and admitted being terrified of his father. He produced a line drawing representing an enormous boot with which a "giant" crushed his hand. (His father was of Prussian origin.) In another drawing Robert depicted himself the size of a Kafkaesque insect cowering in an enormous box. By that time he had become fully aware of the origin of his difficulties. The insight gained was accompanied by a dramatic relief of all his psychosomatic symptoms, including his pains and dizziness.

Thus Robert's condition showed marked symptomatic improvement after less than four months of analytically oriented psychotherapy. Here, again, the improvement was touched off by a value shock, brought to bear, however, on a more abstract level of leverage than in the previous example.

I need not remind you that classical analysis is not satisfied with mere symptom removal, transference cures, or existential shifts of this order. It sets its sight on major changes and reconstruction of personality. Still, I have learned from experience—from my own as well as that of my colleagues—that even long-term analysis that fails to bring about an existential shift, falls short of its objective. Brief psychotherapy may well be little more than a *forme fruste* of long-term analysis. But by the same token it could be stated that long-term analysis derives a considerable part of its momentum from the leverage effects touched off by existential shifts effected in its opening phase. Failing this, time remains an uncertain ally, and all analytic insight, resistance analysis, and "working through" is apt to be a lost labor of love—or of fruitless technical proficiency.

Let me add one more comment. Both the efficacy and the limitations of brief psychotherapy show a close resemblance to the pharmacodynamics of palliative treatment with our modern psychotropic drugs. In fact, what I described as the psychophysiological leverage effect applies with equal strength to both the physiological and to the psychological ends of the therapeutic spectrum. The fact is that our familiar tranquilizers and energizers circumvent the magic of words and symbols. They reach their target by the same "final common pathway" as do the messages conveyed to the patient by "effective myths," by inert placebos, or by purely verbal means. Drugs, on the other hand, try to make a shortcut toward this objective. Apart from the imponderables of the prescribing doctor's personal impact, they dispense with the paraphernalia of the affective overspill or neurohumoral synaptic transmission proceeding over the whole network of the central and vegetative nervous system. Drugs go—or are claimed to go—straight to the raw nerve endings, chemoreceptors, or brain cells, skipping the intermediary steps that verbal cues or other symbolic messages must travel to reach the same goal.

This may be the reason why the advocates and enthusiasts of psychotropic drugs or, for that matter, of electric or insulin shock treatment, insist that the leverage effects of such physical interventions can well be compared with the psychophysiological concomitants of what I described as the existential shift. Such procedures too may jolt the patient out from his pathological baseline of adaptation. But I submit that here, too, we are dealing merely with the opening phase of the treatment process. Only man, through the healing encounter with his fellow man—only the patient's personal experience, psychoanalytic, existential, or otherwise—can consolidate the gains achieved by the leverage effect of whatever words, symbols, or psychotropic drugs are brought to bear on him in his hour of crisis.

## *REFERENCES*

1. Ehrenwald, J. *Psychotherapy: Myth and Method.* New York, Grune, Stratton, 1966.
2. Eliade, M. *The Sacred and the Profane.* New York, Harper, 1961.
3. Malinowski, B. *The Argonauts of the Western Pacific.* New York, Dutton, 1932.
4. Evans-Pritchard, E. E. *Witchcraft, Oracles and Magic Among the Azande.* Oxford, Clarendon Press, 1937.
5. Alexander, F. Psychoanalytic Contributions to Short-Term Psychotherapy. In: *Short-Term Psychotherapy.* Wolberg, L., ed. New York, Grune, Stratton, 1965.
6. Meerloo, J. A. M. *Illness and Cure.* New York, Grune, Stratton, 1964.

# THE PHYSIOLOGICAL SIGNIFICANCE OF FIBRILLATION ACTION POTENTIALS*

JOSEPH GOODGOLD
Associate Professor of Rehabilitation Medicine

ARTHUR EBERSTEIN
Assistant Professor of Rehabilitation Medicine

Electrodiagnostic Section
Institute of Rehabilitation Medicine
New York University Medical Center
New York, N. Y.

THE interpretation of electromyographic records is a quest common to all electrophysical investigation—the problem of translating the vertical oscillations, *amplitude*, temporal variations, *duration*, and wave-form configuration of the oscilloscopic tracing into meaningful clinical information. It would be ideal if classification of the patterns of amplitude, duration, and wave form would suffice to identify particular lesions but, unfortunately, electromyographic specificity does not pertain. Electrical potentials with the same parameters may be present in quite dissimilar neuromuscular diseases. Fibrillation action potentials of muscle fall into this category.

Indeed there is a twofold problem: 1) the practical consideration of distinguishing fibrillations from other similar spontaneous discharges that have no pathological implication, and 2) the theoretical consideration of establishing the pathophysiological significance of fibrillation action potentials.

It is the purpose of this presentation to report on current concepts related to both of these questions.

## DIAGNOSTIC CRITERIA

Fibrillations are spontaneous muscle-action potentials of short duration associated with fine twitching that is not visible at the surface of

*Presented at a combined meeting of the Section on Physical Medicine and Rehabilitation, with the New York Society of Physical Medicine and Rehabilitation, held at The New York Academy of Medicine, October 5, 1966.
The work described in this paper was supported by Grant 8-0162-814 from the John A. Hartford Foundation, Inc., New York, N. Y.

the skin. They may recur rhythmically and arrhythmically. Fibrillation potentials are not exclusively indicative of disease of the lower motor neuron but are encountered as follows:

1) Approximately 10 per cent to 15 per cent of otherwise normal muscles show an isolated area where fibrillation potentials may be recorded. Muscles that are most prone to trauma, such as the extensor digitorum brevis, or gastrocnemius are most suspect. For this reason spontaneous activity in skeletal muscle with the characteristics of fibrillation potentials are not considered significant unless identified in at least three different sites of electrode exploration.

2) In primary myopathic diseases: the occurrence of fibrillation potentials in lesions other than neuropathies was vehemently denied by many investigators during the early years of electromyography. As recently as 1957 Buchthal[1] noted that fibrillation potentials were rare and occurred only in severe myopathies; in a more recent publication, the same investigator[2] reported an incidence of approximately 30 per cent in progressive muscular dystrophy (in 29 of 76 patients, or 34 of 108 muscles). The experience in our own laboratory shows a somewhat lesser incidence, approximately 15 per cent.

3) In affections of the lower motor neuron: fibrillations are not uniformly present in denervated muscle but in fact may be recorded in only 25 to 30 per cent of examinations. Landau[3] observed exposed muscle and noted visually that only a small percentage of the total population of denervated muscle fibers actually fibrillate.

4) Potentials indistinguishable from fibrillations have also been described in *a*) collagen diseases[4]–i.e., polymyositis, scleroderma, rheumatoid arthritis, *b*) botulinum intoxication,[5] *c*) hyperkalemic periodic paralysis,[6] *d*) acute renal insufficiency.

Fibrillations are diminished by lowering the local tissue temperature and are augmented by mechanical irritation. They are never observed in atrophy due to inactivation.

What are the physical measurements that characterize fibrillation? The answer to this question depends on the authority referred to and, perhaps, also to the year of citation. Table I presents a compilation of some typical values reported during 1938 to 1966 inclusive.

The amplitude of fibrillations is apparently related to the type and lead-off area of the recording electrode. Li, Shy, and Wells[11] reported data on the denervated skeletal muscle of the rat in which

PARAMETERS OF FIBRILLATION ACTION POTENTIALS

| | *Denny-Brown and Penny-backer,*[7] *1938* | *Feinstein et al,*[8] *1945* | *Golseth,*[9] *1947* | *Buchthal,*[1] *1957* | *Richard-son,*[10] *1964* | *Buchthal,*[2] *1966* |
|---|---|---|---|---|---|---|
| Freq./sec. | 2 | 2-10 | 2-30 | 2-10 | 2-20, 30 | 13 irregular no regular (63 patients) |
| Duration msec. | — | 1-2 | 1-2 | 0.5-3 | 1-1.5 | 1-5 av. 2.7± .1 |
| Amplitude mv. | 1-3 | 3-100 | 10-100 | 50-200 | 20-300 | 100-300 mv. conc. needle elect. lead-off area |
| Config. | diphasic rarely triphasic | monodi-phasic | mono- or diphasic | triphasic, 3d phase very small | di- or triphasic | of 128 patients: 36 triphasic 6 complex |

extracellular recordings were made with glass microelectrodes. The fibrillation voltages ranged up to 3 mv. Buchthal and Rosenfalck[2] reported that 50 per cent of the voltages recorded with concentric needle electrodes (lead-off area 0.03 $mm^2$.) measured 100 to 300$\mu$v while with the 50 $\mu$ lead-off area of a multielectrode, voltages up to 8.5 mv. were obtained.

An important characteristic in identification of fibrillation potentials involves careful observation of the polarity of the wave form.[2] When recorded outside the end-plate zone the initial deflection is invariably positive; if recorded within the innervation area, the potentials are initially negative. The zone of innervation of muscles varies so that geographically it may extend as a band over the middle 10 per cent of one muscle (e.g., biceps brachii)[12] while in another the innervation zone is widespread (30 per cent), e.g., in a short muscle with varying fiber length such as the opponens digiti quinti.

With regard to potentials recorded in the end-plate zone the question of differentiating the action potential of fibrillation from normally occurring spontaneous activity becomes important since the most common masquerader of fibrillation may be referred to as end-plate activity that manifests itself in several ways:[13]

1) The least confusing is a barely perceptible base line disturbance associated with a hissing sea shell sound, "end-plate ripple." Frequently this phenomenon is much more evident audiometrically rather than visually on the oscilloscope.

2) Easily identifiable potentials of approximately 50 to 100 μv. amplitude, irregular in rhythm and characteristically monophasic negative, with a slow return of the potential to baseline. Electrically, these bear strong resemblance to the normally occurring miniature end-plate potentials (m.e.p.p.). The difference in voltage (1 mv. versus 100 μv.) reflects the fact that the m.e.p.p. are recorded with microelectrodes and the end-plate noise detected with large macroelectrodes commonly employed in electromyography. Like m.e.p.p. these negative discharges are localized nonpropagated electrical events.

3) A third variety of end-plate activity appears as a diphasic potential of negative-positive polarity of average amplitude of 150 μv. This activity is frequently associated with sensation of sharp pain by the subject during the insertion of a needle. This variety of spontaneous activity was identified as originating from intramuscular nerves by Jones *et al.*[14] This view of its origin is disputed by Buchthal and Rosenfalck[2] on the basis of occurrence in totally denervated muscles and the disparity between the amplitude of 150 μv. and the average amplitude of 45 μv. recorded by Buchthal and Rosenfalck from the nerve terminals in the normal end-plate zone.

The essential point, however, is that fibrillations and spontaneous, normal, propogated potentials that arise in the zone of innervation are difficult to differentiate and must be evaluated by reference to: 1) incidence of fibrillation potentials in the total samplings, 2) recording from areas outside the innervation zone, and 3) their relation to the total electrodiagnostic picture.

Because these potentials have the same significance as fibrillations it is pertinent to consider briefly another abnormal spontaneous potential that is referred to as a positive sharp potential or positive sharp wave. This potential is most often observed in severely involved muscles in association with fibrillations. Its duration and amplitude are frequently greater than fibrillation potentials. The monophasic configuration may originate in a manner similar to the demarcation or current of injury; propagation ceases at the margin of damaged tissue.

As with fibrillations, it is significant that positive sharp potentials are not exclusively indicative of lower motor neuron lesions (denervation) but have been recorded and reported in myopathies (Lambert, Norris *et al.*, Buchthal *et al.*). In our own laboratory they are encountered much more frequently in denervation.

## Physiological Consideration of the Action Potentials of Fibrillation

Within the framework of the preceding discussion it can be said that fibrillation potentials are the most prominent electrical feature of denervated muscle. The equally prominent physiological change in denervated muscle is the hypersensitivity that the muscle membrane develops toward acetylcholine. How are these two events linked?

In 1936 Brown, Dale, and Feldberg clearly elucidated the mechanism of normal neuromuscular transmission in demonstrating that intra-arterial injections of minute quantities of acetylcholine (ACh) evoked muscle contraction equivalent to that observed following maximum nerve stimulation. In 1937 Brown[15, 16] made further observations on the effect of ACh on denervated muscle and reached the following conclusions:

1) The configuration of fibrillation potentials and the diphasic potentials recorded from single muscle fibers in response to stimulation with ACh were sufficiently similar to consider that fibrillation represented single muscle-fiber potentials.

2) Denervated muscle becomes hypersensitive to ACh so that application of 1/100 dilute ACh results in a fivefold increase in the duration of contraction as compared to normal muscle. Brown also observed that fibrillation activity was potentiated by ACh.

In 1943 Kuffler[17] applied droplets of ACh to muscle fibers and localized the site of hypersensitivity to the end-plate zone in both normal and denervated frog muscle. Kuffler concluded that the distal (i.e., away from end-plate) region of the normal muscle fiber was relatively insensitive. In denervation, however, the whole fiber sensitivity was increased $1 \times 10^5$ times.

Axelsson and Thesleff[18] applied minute quantities of ACh by electrophoresis through micropipettes to discrete areas of the muscle membrane. They found that in the normal muscle the sensitive area was localized to the end plate over a distance of 0.1 mm. In the denervated muscle of the cat, however, the receptor area enlarged progressively to involve the entire length of the muscle membrane.

Does increased sensitivity to ACh invariably involve the occurrence of fibrillations? The answer is a negative one based on studies provided by Towers *et al.*[19] in 1941, by Solandt and Magladery[20] in 1942, and substantiated by Johns and Thesleff[21] in 1961. The essential methodology involves inactivation of the limbs by section of the spinal cord plus unilateral transection of the motor nerve (e.g., sciatic). Comparison was made of the incidence of fibrillation and ACh sensitization. The denervated limb presented fibrillation potentials and hypersensitization to ACh. Fibrillation was not seen in the inactivated limb. There was, however, an increase of ACh sensitivity to a lesser degree than through inactivation alone.

Some investigations have been carried out in order to define the relation between area of membrane sensitivity and level of secretion of ACh itself. In 1960 Miledi[22] studied the effect on hypersensitivity of normal and denervated muscle that had been excised and maintained in a medium of either Ringer's or ACh solution. Miledi demonstrated that increased sensitivity developed to the same degree in the denervated muscle without regard to the concentration of ACh in the environment. He concluded, therefore, that the deprivation of ACh was not a factor in the development of sensitivity.

Thesleff[23] considered the same problem but administered botulinum toxin in order to inhibit the liberation of ACh. In direct contradiction to Miledi, Thesleff demonstrated that the effect of deprivation was the development of sensitivity along the entire length of the membrane similar to that observed in denervated muscle. In effect, therefore, the lack of transmitter substance determined the presence and extent of chemosensitivity.

With regard to botulinum toxin the paralysis of muscle function appears to be accomplished at the presynaptic level uniquely. It is widely accepted that the presynaptic vesicles randomly liberate quantities of ACh that give rise to the m.e.p.p. as described by Katz, Fatt, Del Costillo, and others. A large synchronous discharge of the quanta is sufficient to produce a critical end-plate potential. Botulinum toxin blocks the presynaptic mechanism so that quanta of ACh are not released and the m.e.p.p. cease.

In 1959 Katz and Miledi[24] studied the effects of denervation on the m.e.p.p. and demonstrated that after section of the nerve the m.e.p.p. persist, then disappear for several days to reappear again but at slower frequency. Katz and Miledi concluded that a possible source of ACh packets (and the resultant m.e.p.p.) in the denervated muscle were the Schwann cells that were observed to overgrow and fill the troughs in the synaptic clefts. Miledi reported that the m.e.p.p. that reappeared could be recorded only at the end plate even though the ACh hypersensitivity could be demonstrated along the entire length of the muscle fiber. The persistence of m.e.p.p. in the immediate period following denervation has been reconfirmed during the current investigation in our laboratory. In addition it was observed that the mean amplitude and frequency of the m.e.p.p. of fast fibers of semitendinous muscle of the frog almost doubled in magnitude during the first hour following transection of the motor nerve.

It is of interest to note that Thesleff reported that m.e.p.p. that reappeared after denervation were unaffected by botulinum toxin.

In 1962 Diamond and Miledi[25] studied foetal albino rats and recorded m.e.p.p. but of a slower frequency than in the adult. The rat muscle membrane was also shown to be of greater sensitivity to ACh than adult muscle. As normal development progressed there was a recession of sensitivity from the distal ends to remain only at the end-plate area. Diamond and Miledi also reported the occurrence of "fibrillationlike" potentials in the foetus that sometimes persisted up to one week after birth. It is interesting to speculate that increased hypersensitivity and fibrillation potentials contain some features of regression to a lesser stage of neuromuscular maturity.

In summary, then, there are two realities encountered in study of muscle fibers whose nerve supply has been compromised: 1) denervated skeletal muscles fibrillate, and 2) denervated muscles are hypersensitive to ACh.

How and if these factors are causally related remains an unsolved and interesting area of investigation deserving of further study.

## *REFERENCES*


1. Buchthal, F. *An Introduction to Electromyography.* Scandinavian Univ. Books. Copenhagen, Gyldendal, 1957.
2. Buchthal, F. and Rosenfalck, A. Spontaneous electrical activity of human muscle, *Electroenceph. Clin. Neurophysiol. 20*:321-36, 1966.
3. Landau, W. M. Synchronization of potentials and response to direct current stimulation in denervated mammalian

muscle, *Electroenceph. Clin. Neurophysiol. 3*:169, 1951.
4. Lambert, E. H., Sayre, G. P. and Eaton, L. M. Electrical activity of muscle in poliomyelitis, *Trans. Amer. Neurol. Ass. 79*:64, 1954.
5. Peterson, I. and Broman, A. M. Electromyographic findings in a case of botulism, *Nord. Med. 65*:259-61, 1961.
6. Morrison, J. B. Electromyographic changes in hyperkalemic familial periodic paralysis, *Ann. Phys. Med. 5*:153-55, 1960.
7. Denny-Brown, D. and Pennybacker, J. B. Fibrillation and fasciculation in voluntary muscle, *Brain 61*:311-34, 1938.
8. Feinstein, B., Pattle, R. E. and Wedell, G. Metabolic factors affecting fibrillation in denervated muscle, *J. Neurol. Neurosurg. Psych. 8*:1-11, 1945.
9. Golseth, J. G. and Fizzell, J. A. Electromyographic studies on cats after section and suture of the sciatic nerve, *Amer. J. Physiol. 150*:558-67, 1947.
10. Richardson, A. T. Clinical Electromyography. Chap. 23, 536-55, in: Walton, J. N. *Disorders of Voluntary Muscle.* Boston, Little, Brown, 1964.
11. Li, C.-H., Shy, M. and Wells, J. Some properties of mammalian skeletal muscle fibers with particular reference to fibrillation potentials, *J. Physiol. 135*:522-35, 1957.
12. Christensen, E. Topography of terminal motor innervation in striated muscle of stillborn infants. In: *The Innervation of Muscle,* Bowman, H. D. and Woolf, A. L., eds. Baltimore, Williams, Wilkins, 1960, pp. 17-29.
13. Buchthal, F. Spontaneous and voluntary electrical activity in neuromuscular disorders, *Bull. N. Y. Acad. Med. 42*:521-50, 1966.
14. Jones, R., Lambert, E. and Sayre, G. Source of a type of insertion activity in electromyography with evaluation of a histological method of localization, *Arch. Phys. Med. 36*:301-10, 1955.
15. Brown, G. L., Dale, N., Feldberg, W. Reactions of the normal mammalian muscle to acetylcholine and to eserine, *J. Physiol. 14*:394-423, 1937.
16. Brown, G. L. Action of acetylcholine on denervated mammalian and frog's muscle, *J. Physiol. 89*:220-37, 1937.
17. Kuffler, S. W. Specific excitability of the end-plate region in normal and denervated muscle, *J. Neurophysiol. 6*: 99-110, 1943.
18. Axelsson, J. and Thesleff, S. Study of supersensitivity in denervated mammalian skeletal muscle, *J. Physiol. 149*:178-93, 1957.
19*a*. Towers, S., Howe, H. and Bodian, D. Fibrillation in skeletal muscle in relation to denervation and to inactivation without denervation, *J. Neurophysiol. 4*:398-401, 1941.
*b*. Towers, S. S. Persistence of fibrillation in denervated skeletal muscles and its nonoccurrence in muscle after tenotomy, *Arch. Neurol. Psychiat. 42*:219-23, 1939.
20. Solandt, D. Y. and Magladery, J. W. Comparison of the effects of upper and lower motor neurone lesions on skeletal muscle, *J. Physiol. 5*:373-80, 1942.
21. Johns, T. R. and Thesleff, S. Effects of motor inactivation on the chemical sensitivity of skeletal muscle, *Acta Physiol. Scand. 51*:136-41, 1961.
22. Miledi, R. Acetylcholine sensitivity of frog muscle fibers after complete or partial denervation, *J. Physiol. 151*:1-23, 1960.
23. Thesleff, S. Supersensitivity of skeletal muscle produced by botulinum toxin, *J. Physiol. 151*:598-607, 1960.
24. Katz, B. and Miledi, R. Spontaneous subthreshold activity at denervated amphibian end plates, *J. Physiol. 146*:45-46, 1959.
25. Diamond, J. and Miledi, R. Study of foetal and new-born rat muscle fibers, *J. Physiol. 162*:393-408, 1962.

# COMPREHENSIVE APPROACH TO A CHILD WITH A BIRTH DEFECT*

MYRON WINICK

Assistant Professor of Pediatrics
Director, Birth Defects Clinic
New York Hospital-Cornell Medical Center
New York, N. Y.

RECENTLY an 11-year-old boy was referred to our clinic for examination and treatment. He is a bright youngster who is quite aware of his problem: just how aware did not become obvious to me until he allowed me to read parts of a diary he has been keeping since he was nine. With his permission I quote the opening paragraph.

> I was born at 11:00 p.m. on December 27, 1956, at Brooklyn Hospital. I was almost like any other child except four things that were not right on me. The first two things that are not right is that my forehead is pointed instead of round and that my arm is curved instead of straight. The second two things that were not right on me is that my fourth toe is missing on both feet. I hope when I grow up I will have an operation to fix the accident.

The opening paragraph in this diary says in a few simple words what psychologists and physicians are just beginning to understand. It says: "I am different. I don't want to be different. Change me so that I can be like the others." Even when the malformation is only cosmetic, this urgent need to belong can have devastating effects on the development of a child.

Superimpose on this a functional handicap, sometimes severe—the inability to walk without crutches and braces; the passing of urine into a bag; poor bowel control—and one can see a second, perhaps even greater problem with which the child is faced—an inability to do, to share, to partake in the normal activities of life: schooling, employment, sports, games—all the things that go with normal growing up.

Starting then with a problem that involves multiple handicaps, the child embarks on a long and arduous road. First and foremost is medical

*Presented at a meeting of the Section on Obstetrics and Gynecology of The New York Academy of Medicine, February 28, 1967.

rehabilitation: not cure—this can rarely be achieved—but rehabilitation.

In addition to his handicap is the need for hospital care, visits to the clinic, diagnostic procedures, operations, appliances. The child who is born with a meningomyelocele may have five major operations in the first year of life, perhaps six months in the hospital, weekly visits to the clinic, fittings for braces, kidney studies every three months, and daily medication for urinary tract infections.

Then there are special problems. Some of our patients are unable to move their bowels adequately because the anal sphincter is paralyzed. These children may need daily enemas or actual manual removal of feces by the parent. One mother asked me, "How can we expect him to achieve any real independence when I must help him eliminate every day?" The road to rehabilitation presents its own consequences and leaves its own scar, independent of the disease.

Can these children grow up normally? No. Anyone dealing with this problem can assure you that there is nothing normal about an environment of clinics, hospitals, operating rooms, and special schools.

Our aim is to see first that these children *will* grow up; second, to see that they learn to accept and live with their handicap; third, to teach them to function up to their maximum potential and, finally, to help them to a pleasurable and useful utilization of their leisure time.

The impact of a birth defect on a child, as we see, is catastrophic. It is upon this child that major rehabilitative efforts must be focused. No one can do this alone. In fact, one cannot even begin to help him without the assistance of the child's family, for it is the family that must bear the major part of the burden.

What about the parents? What emotions are churned up by the birth of a malformed child? After the stunning shock and incomprehension—"Why me? What have I done?"—there follow feelings of guilt over somehow being involved in the genesis of the tragedy—"If only I had had German measles as a child. Was that really a cold in the first trimester? Should I have taken that aspirin?" Little things that might cause birth defects and that can pass unnoticed in the normal pregnancy hit with devastating force when a malformed infant is born.

These fears must be dispelled. Parents must be helped to accept, for acceptance is a prerequisite to family harmony. This is easy to say but difficult to achieve. One study indicates there is a breakup of more than 50 per cent of families where a severely malformed child is involved.

The effect of such a disruption on the child is obvious. With all his other problems the child finds himself the "cause" of breaking up a family, and he reaps the results of a broken home life.

When one begins to realize the total scope of this problem, one can see that our patient is not simply the child with a birth defect. The problem involves the entire family constellation and the pressures exerted on it. This includes the young girl who has become a mother for the first time, the young man who suddenly faces awesome responsibilities, the grandparents who in their desire to protect their own children offer poorly thought-out advice, and all the other relatives and friends who have definite ideas on management. The obstetrician, entirely well-intentioned, may minimize the defect—because he does not want to alarm the patient and subconsciously because he will not be involved in the future. The pediatrician, because of limited previous experience, may direct the parents to do nothing because "the child will die." Time passes and the child does not die but emerges a hopeless physical and mental invalid for whom little can be done. This is the family, and these are some of the initial pressures to which it is exposed.

A comprehensive approach to the management of a child with a birth defect begins with the family. The parents are met first. Their attitude, their strength or weakness can alter the entire plan of treatment. They must be told the truth—objectively and candidly. They must be told, but not overwhelmed.

Possible causes must be explored but if, as in most cases, none is found, the parents must be assured that nothing they did caused the abnormality. The nature of the defect should be explained and its consequences examined, the over-all treatment should be discussed and, finally, the prognosis should be outlined. Questions should be answered. If the answers are unknown this should be made clear—what is said on this occasion may come back to one 10 years later.

Once the parents understand the consequences of the defect, treatment can begin. A plan of management must be worked out. This may involve several physicians, nurses, therapists, psychologists, social workers, and other persons; but the responsibility, the final decisions, must rest solely on the physician who, being experienced in these problems, can relate to the parents and to the child. This then is the basic premise upon which the entire concept of comprehensive care rests—centralization of responsibility and a team approach.

There are numerous ways in which such a program can be organized. At The New York Hospital a child with a birth defect is first seen in the general pediatric clinic, where a full medical evaluation is made. If, for example, he has a meningomyelocele, he is referred to the Birth Defects Clinic, which is supported by the March of Dimes, at our hospital. Here a complete history is taken and a physical examination is made; certain diagnostic tests are done.

The problem is then discussed by a panel consisting of a pediatrician, neurosurgeon, urologist, orthopedist, nurse, physical therapist, social worker, and psychologist. Together they evolve a plan of management.

This plan must take into consideration both medical and social factors. It must not only suggest treatment but it must suggest the proper sequence—the proper timing. Timing is exceedingly important. An attempt to increase any function before a child is ready for it may actually cause harm.

At times medical management may have to be deferred because of overwhelming social problems. Hospitalization may be extended because of conditions at home. An operation may be performed not strictly for medical reasons but to make the child socially acceptable. A child, unable to control his bladder, may dribble urine continually. This means diapers. In school this presents a socially unacceptable situation; therefore one might decide to operate on the urinary tract so that it can empty into an external receptacle. The child remains dry but wears a bag in which the urine is collected. This poses its own problem —for, as was pointed out at the onset—now he is different. All this must be considered as this child's plan of rehabilitation evolves.

The physician in charge is responsible for implementing the plan of treatment of the child with all his complications and defects. This type of follow-up offers certain advantages. The parents have one physician responsible for the care of their child to whom they can go to discuss their problems. The various specialists involved are available at all times. Each specialist is aware of what the other is doing; a coordinated plan of management can be thus evolved.

Special facilities should be available to the clinic or associated with it. Genetic counseling is of extreme importance in certain cases, and trained persons should be on hand to counsel parents about future pregnancies. Because analysis of chromosomal patterns will sometimes yield important information, facilities for making such studies should be available. Our center includes a cytogenetic unit that performs both of these valuable functions. In addition, we hold a clinic in conjunction with the genetics clinic once a month when children with malformations involving genetic abnormalities are seen.

Another person who should be an integral member of any team administering a birth-defects program is the social worker. All patients at our Center are studied by the social worker, who makes and helps implement recommendations for assistance to the family.

The role of the social worker continues to assume greater and greater proportions as we gather more experience. This functionary is not merely a source of referral to agencies although this is an important part of her work. She is a family counselor, an interpreter to the family of the doctor's wishes, and a shoulder to lean on when the feeling of being overwhelmed begins.

The social worker must keep the team constantly aware of the current socioeconomic condition of the family. She must concern herself with problems that on the surface may not appear germane to the child's illness but that in reality may be a cause of great concern to the child and his family. Weekly visits to the clinic for physical treatment are useless unless the child keeps the appointments. What about transportation or baby-sitting for the other children in the family? The social worker has become the link between the physician and the social agencies capable of implementing some of the physician's recommendations. It is she who arranges for state aid, for city programs, school placement, institutionalization, and payment for braces or other appliances. The more we learn of the complexities of total care the more we must rely on the social worker to implement that care.

The public health nurse, another important member of the team, provides continuity of care—a bridge from clinic to home. She is the link between the sheltered environment of the hospital and the realities of the outside world—she serves as both medical observer and practical counselor. She must be alert to danger signs and at the same time must reassure the family when things are under control.

The public health nurse serves the family not only by carrying out the decisions of the medical panel, but by instructing the parents in methods of caring for their child. She serves the medical team by providing valuable data and by suggesting practical means of implementing the program that has been proposed. She serves the community in helping to rehabilitate a child so that he may take his place as a useful member of society.

The impact of birth defects on the family cannot be ignored. As mentioned earlier, one of the physician's most difficult tasks is to tell the parents that their child has been born defective and to try to help them accept the reality. This is only the beginning, for the initial shock soon changes to a sustained ever-present problem, a problem that does not cease when the child goes home from the hospital. In fact, as the child begins to grow and develop, the handicap becomes more noticeable, more socially unacceptable, and therefore more difficult to cope with. The problem is always there.

Comparison of the child's progress with that of normal children will lead only to a parent's feelings of frustration and defeat. It is far better to draw attention to individual development, to observe the incredible progress some of these children make in spite of their handicaps, the mastery of brace- and crutch-walking, the pride in the face of a four-year-old as he maneuvers his own wheel chair, the blind child who learns to read Braille, the gradual assumption of responsibilities no normal child will ever have to assume. Such children are learning to cope with their handicaps and are learning to function within society.

This painful but progressive mastery of a handicap should also be a source of great pride to parents, pride in their child and pride in themselves, for their patience and understanding will have been largely responsible for the progress. It is not enough then to change feelings of guilt and frustration to those of passive acceptance. What is needed is a realistic understanding of the capabilities of the child, of the road to the achievement of those capabilities, and of the amazing progress he can make within the limits of his handicap.

For the father there are all these problems. There is one additional problem: money. What is this going to cost, doctor? What is the cost of rehabilitating a multihandicapped child? A child, for example, with meningomyelocele? Two major neurosurgical operations, one major urologic operation, three or perhaps four orthopedic operations, special tests, months of hospitalization, years of medical supervision, of physical and occupational therapy, special educational facilities, recreational facilities—$50,000? Or $100,000?

The figures are unreal for most people. The cost of such care can rarely be met by a single individual. This must be pointed out to the father at the onset. Management entails a coordinated effort of pooling community, voluntary, and governmental resources. These resources must be constantly increased at every level. The government will usually contribute in areas of proved value; until it does, the community must bear the burden. The voluntary agencies, for example the March of Dimes, have at least two important functions: pioneering new approaches to treatment, and supporting research in causes and care.

The child's father cannot be expected to bear the cost of the medical catastrophe alone. If he is, he may soon destroy himself and his family in the attempt. Even if the parents are able to adapt and to help their child toward maximum rehabilitation, they must do this without seriously neglecting their normal children. It is no success if the maximum potential for a handicapped child is attained while two siblings become seriously disturbed.

Again, one should attempt to turn this tragedy into something positive. The normal child should gain certain experiences from growing up with a handicapped brother or sister. This can best be achieved by including him as an active member of the family team caring for this child. Slowly the sibling will learn certain kinds of responsibility and self reliance. He will eventually emerge a stronger and a more secure individual.

The normal child can not only adapt to the new situation, but can develop increased sensitivity as a result of growing up with a child who has a malformation.

In spite of all possible efforts the problem is sometimes too great for the physician and the family. This may be anticipated early in some cases. In others, one can just wait and see. When such a situation occurs, it must be faced squarely. The aim is still to do the most for the child and the family. Sometimes only minimal change is achieved in the child while the whole family is destroyed. This is the result of creating false hope.

The problem of institutionalization is very complex. It must be considered in the context of each family. First, as to the child—will he be able to function better in a sheltered environment? Can he live happily there? Second, as to the siblings—will they suffer irreparable emotional damage if the child is kept at home?

Finally, as to the parents. Can they cope with the handicap and still preserve their family and themselves? If all the answers point in one direction, the decision is simple. For example, a handicapped child who can function within society, in a family where the siblings have accepted and indeed concerned themselves with the problem under careful parental guidance—in such a family, institutionalization will be untenable, and probably should never be considered.

Conversely, one might have a hopelessly retarded, frequently convulsed, constantly screaming child, who takes the mother's every minute and causes her to neglect her other children. If the father comes home to such an environment each day and wishes he could retreat to the comparative peace of his office, there is little question here either. It is in the in-between situations that difficulty arises.

Generally, the family itself will come to a decision in these circumstances. Unless the family decision is obviously bizarre, the physician should respect it and reinforce it. This is exceedingly important; for when a decision is made to institutionalize a child, it is not made easily. One misplaced word by a physician who has become the family counselor could destroy that decision. The positive aspects of the decision should be emphasized.

The feeling of relief over avoiding certain problems at home, on realizing that increased specialized care is available within an institution, the fact that the parents can still visit the child and can still contribute to developing whatever potentials are there—all of these things will help the parents without developing more feelings of guilt and inadequacy.

One must continually remember that when a child is born with a birth defect, he is born into a family. In his early helplessness and dependence, in his later triumphs and failures, that family can be the handicapped child's greatest asset or an overwhelming liability. The task of all concerned is to assure this child a happy and responsible family and to help the family in molding an adult: a handicapped person, to be sure, but one able to function within the limits of that handicap and to take his place as a responsible member of society.

This consideration leads to the inevitable conclusion that the child with a birth defect poses a problem not only to himself and his family but also to society in general.

Fifty years ago many of these defective children might have wound up in a sideshow. Even today the achondroplastic dwarf, the "rubber man," the "walking skeleton" are seen as attractions in a circus. And

250 years ago, within our own culture, both the mother and child might have been burned alive.

Earlier civilizations attached omens to certain malformations. Still earlier, malformations were believed to result from human matings with animals or gods. These superstitions, which are part of the literature of our culture, have been handed down from generation to generation. Even today we have mothers who caution their pregnant daughters to keep their minds clear of bad thoughts and not look at ugly things.

Subconsciously people tend to distrust or even fear a child or an adult with a malformation. This social conditioning makes the problem much more complex, perhaps, than most other handicaps. Should we save these children from death and habilitate them so that they will be able to function as productive human beings, only to send them into a world that would prefer to deny their existence? Anyone who deals with birth defects must concern himself with the social problem for, unless it is mastered, the fruits of his work are lost. Indeed he is making things worse by increasing the number of handicapped people who must face intolerable social pressures.

The solution of the problem of persons with birth defects lies in education of the public through informative programs. The public must understand the problem. It must become aware of what is being done. It must be exposed to people who have birth defects. Segregating handicapped persons in special schools with special recreational facilities, providing them with special sheltered living and with special working conditions protects them from a world that they must face sooner or later.

A sheltered environment shuts them out from a world that is unable to understand and assimilate them. Handicapped children, whenever functionally possible, should study, play, and mingle with children who are normal. This will prepare them for life as it must come. It will also, I suspect, dispel within the normal child the fears and superstitions that his elders often display toward the handicapped.

How many of us, when we see a handicapped person, know how to act? With all our good intentions, our supereducations, our 20th-century sophistication, we are not sure whether to push that wheel chair up the hill or let the person struggle. What is more, we are embarrassed to ask. Subconsciously, we should prefer not to be exposed to such a problem. This, I submit, is the result of many years of subtle conditioning. Perhaps it is too late for us, perhaps not. But our children can be conditioned differently. They can see others handicapped by malformations, learn about them, play with them and, in that way, allay the superstitions of the past.

In summary then: the comprehensive approach to a child with a birth defect involves numerous facets: 1) the family must be supported; 2) the child must be medically rehabilitated, properly educated, taught to enjoy his leisure time, and placed in a rewarding and productive vocation; 3) society must be prepared to accept more and more children and adults with congenital malformations.

Birth defects constitute a group of mishaps caused by a multitude of agents most of which are as yet unknown. It may take many years to discover and eradicate them. The consequences, meanwhile, must be controlled. Herein lies a major task: one that entails a whole new concept of combined medical and social action aimed at making the child a productive citizen and a happy, satisfied person.

# FACTORS AFFECTING THE SURVIVAL OF PATIENTS WITH OVARIAN CARCINOMA*

ALLAN B. WEINGOLD
SANFORD SALL AND MARTIN L. STONE

Department of Obstetrics and Gynecology
New York Medical College-Metropolitan Hospital Center
New York, N. Y.

## INTRODUCTION

THE ovary is the site of more varieties of new growth than any other structure in the body. It is a frequent site for both primary and secondary tumors. Approximately 15 per cent of ovarian tumors are carcinomas, and these account for 20 per cent of all gynecological cancers. Ovarian carcinoma presents a constant challenge. Therapeutic results are no better today than in past decades. The advances in diagnosis and treatment that have led to improved survival rates for other gynecologic cancers are apparently not applicable to cancer of the ovary. The problem is further compounded by the increased incidence of ovarian cancer that is associated with the increase in life expectancy. About 10,400 women die each year as a result of this disease.

The results of treatment are notoriously poor; the five-year survival rates is only 15 to 20 per cent. Cancer of the ovary ranks fourth among neoplasms causing death in women over 40 years of age. Poor therapeutic results and the high death rate may be due to a greater malignancy inherent in ovarian cancer, but they are more probably secondary to the difficulty in early diagnosis.

## EPIDEMIOLOGY

The average age at the time of diagnosis is 53.2 years. The peak incidence is the sixth decade (Figure I). Two hundred and eighty-two females per 100,000 have ovarian carcinoma after 45 years of age as compared with 30.4 per 100,000 before 45.[1]

Approximately 45 per cent of patients with ovarian carcinoma are

*Presented at a meeting of the Section on Obstetrics and Gynecology, The New York Academy of Medicine, March 22, 1966.

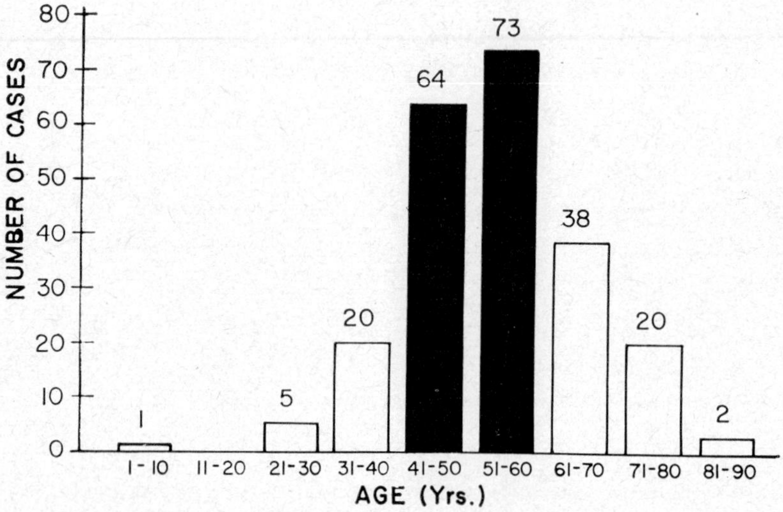


Fig. 1. Age distribution of 223 patients who have ovarian carcinoma. Mean age: 53.2 years.

nulliparas. This figure is considerably higher than the 20 per cent nulliparity rate given for the general population.

## Classification and Pathology

There are many types of ovarian carcinoma classified on a histogenetic or embryological basis. Of clinical importance is the fact that the most common forms are cystadenocarcinomas that arise from a benign counterpart—the cystadenomas, either pseudomucinous or papillary serous. The latter have the highest malignant potential and are bilateral in 50 per cent of cases. The frequency of malignant change or development justifies the concept of precancerous lesion for these benign cysts and affords a basis for early diagnosis and preventive care. The diagnosis and surgical management of the benign stage obviates the malignant phase.

Ovarian cancer spreads by implantation on adjacent serosal surfaces with peritoneal and omental involvement in 85 per cent. In advanced cases this leads to adhesions and fixation. The opposite ovary is commonly affected even if this is not grossly evident. The uterus is frequently involved by lymphatic spread. Distant metastases involve liver, lungs, and long bones. The spread of cancer of the ovary can be divided into four stages: 1) confined to ovary, 2) pelvic involvement, 3) abdominal involvement, and 4) involvement of lower pleural sacs.

## Symptoms

Except for the very interesting but comparatively rare endocrine tumors, early cancer of the ovary has no pathognomonic symptoms. For this reason, cancer of the ovary is often referred to as a silent cancer. Its onset is insidious, and in the early stages it is asymptomatic and undetectable. More than one half of the cases are inoperable when first seen. When more advanced, the cancer may give rise to a palpable mass and to pressure symptoms. Other findings that may be present include abdominal discomfort, ascites, and the complications of torsion or rupture. Ascites is not specific for ovarian cancer since it occurs with benign lesions, such as fibromas, as well. All types of cancer of the ovary show the same end picture: peritoneal involvement with ascites and cachexia.

The initial presenting symptom is abdominal pain in 36 per cent of patients, abdominal swelling or the presence of a mass in 34 per cent.[2] Ten per cent of the patients with ovarian carcinoma first present themselves with intestinal obstruction secondary to extensive peritoneal involvement. Approximately 15 per cent of the patients are first seen with abnormal uterine bleeding; only half of these are specifically related to functional tumors.[3] This bleeding may result from coexisting uterine disease, fluctuating estrogen levels due to cortical stromal activity, pelvic hyperemia, or uterine metastases (Figure 2). Bleeding occurs frequently enough with ovarian carcinoma for the latter to be considered in any differential diagnosis of unexplained metrorrhagia.

The average duration of symptoms prior to diagnosis is at least four months. A significant factor in diagnostic delay on the part of both patient and doctor is the protean nature of the symptoms in ovarian carcinoma.

## Diagnosis

Ovarian cancer is usually diagnosed only when it reaches a size or stage to be clinically evident. This may be dependent on the occurrence of pressure symptoms or on incidental findings during routine pelvic examination or examination for a nonrelated complaint.

Diagnostic aids include a thorough general physical examination,

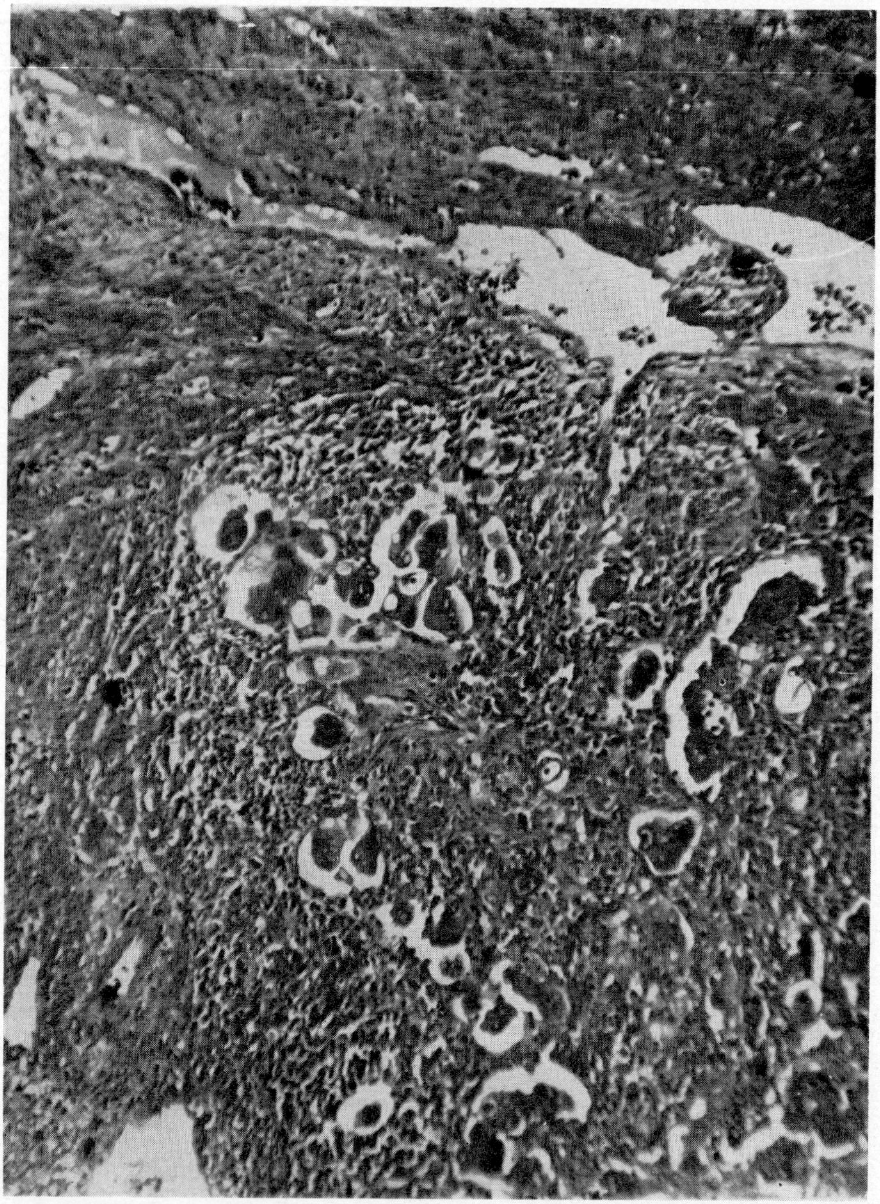

Fig. 2. Endometrial metastases of ovarian carcinoma. Note psammoma bodies adjacent to the myometrium above. ×100.

x-ray studies for evidence of a soft tissue mass or calcification, cytologic examination of the ascitic fluid and, in selected cases, culdoscopy. In many cases, diagnosis will not be made until an exploratory laparotomy is performed.

When ovarian cancer is suspected, the patient should be examined for the possibility of a primary growth elsewhere, particularly in the gastrointestinal tract.

## Therapy

*Preventive.* In view of the silent and insidious nature of cancer of the ovary, prevention and early detection assume paramount importance. Careful evaluation and treatment of the benign cystic precursors will do much to enhance early diagnosis and treatment with resultant improvement in over-all results. This necessitates annual pelvic examination to detect asymptomatic cysts. The cost of routine pelvic examination is small compared to that involved in the treatment of established carcinoma of the ovary. We cannot overstress the importance of early detection of the benign counterparts or the incipient malignancy. It affords us an opportunity that must be realized.

Laparotomy is indicated for all tumors larger than 6 cm., for all solid tumors, and for all in postmenopausal women. This permits specific diagnosis and proper surgical treatment predicated on correct diagnosis.

The value of "prophylactic" ovarian surgery incidental to other pelvic surgery is no longer debatable. Removal of the ovaries is indicated when pelvic operations are carried out in the patient past 40 years of age. Available evidence of detrimental effects on the vascular system is not conclusive. If such symptoms of deprivation are apparent, the exogenous replacement of hormone is simple and effective.

*Active.* The generally accepted therapeutic regimen for ovarian carcinoma is total abdominal hysterectomy, bilateral salpingo-oophorectomy, and postoperative external radiation. Preferences of individual physicians, extent of the disease, operability, age, and pervious operations are some of the factors that account for variations from this accepted and recommended treatment.

Nowhere else in medicine is a thorough knowledge of gross pathology so important to the operating surgeon. This knowledge is essential to prevent needless castration as well as to insure adequate operations when indicated. All ovarian tumors should be sectioned at the table so that further information is made available to plan the extent of the surgical procedure. Important considerations to be evaluated at the time of operation include: 1) unilateral or bilateral, 2) cystic or solid, 3) free or fixed, 4) presence of implants or papillations, 5) ascitic fluid–hemorrhagic or not, and 6) presence and integrity of capsule.

In advanced cases we are dealing with a single disease, and operation as complete as possible is carried out. This includes total hysterectomy and bilateral salpingo-oophorectomy. Omental resection is carried out as indicated. If adhesions and fixations are marked, as much of the bulk of the tumor is removed as is possible. Excision of the primary mass and omentum is advantageous though by no means curative. It reduces intra-abdominal pressure and the extent of the secretory surfaces.

X-ray treatment is indicated for all ovarian cancers, since some are especially radiosensitive; there is no way of determining in advance which tumor will respond. While roentgen therapy may not be curative, it may lead to a decrease in the amount of ascitic fluid. Therefore, if there is no contraindication, x ray is given for two purposes: 1) to retard the formation of fluid, and 2) to cause regression to make an inoperable case operable. It may take as long as a year to obtain the maximum effect.

Recently, chemotherapeutic agents have been applied extensively in ovarian carcinoma. Nowhere in gynecology is the need for additional therapeutic modalities greater than in this disease. Most frequently the carcinoma has progressed beyond curative resectability at the time of diagnosis. The agent of choice for adjuvant and palliative chemotherapy of ovarian carcinoma at the New York Medical College-Metropolitan Hospital Center is chlorambucil (Leukeran). This is a variant of the polyfunctional alkylating group.[4] It is an oral preparation that is given in doses of 0.2 mg. per kilogram of body weight per day. Our results are somewhat better than those obtained in earlier attempts with other drugs. An excellent or good response defined as the disappearance or considerable decrease in size of the tumor and an associated resolution of major symptoms is obtained in about 40 per cent of the patients. Happily, we have noted a relatively small number of severe toxic reactions. Our present principle of management in these cases with a limited prognosis indicates continuous intermittent chemotherapy.

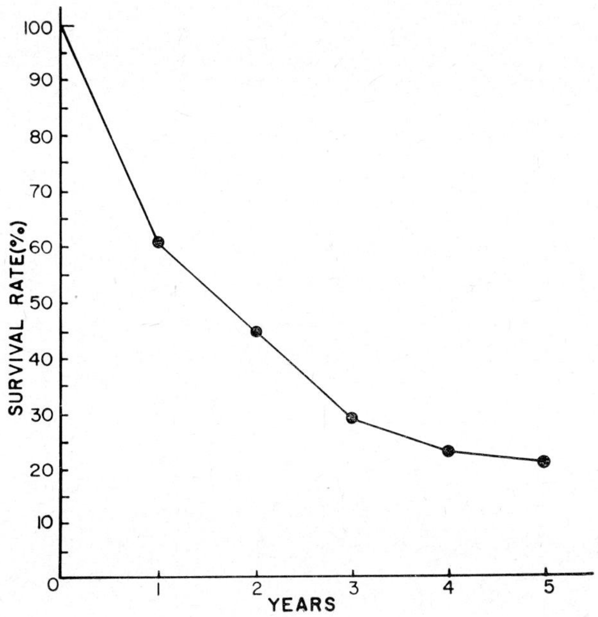


Fig. 3. Five-year survival curve of patients who have ovarian carcinoma.

## Factors Affecting Survival

A survival curve for 223 patients treated during a five-year period at the New York Medical College-Metropolitan Hospital Center is indicated in Figure 3 and is typical of the therapeutic results in this disease. The five-year figure of 20.6 per cent is consistent with the majority of reports in the recent literature although there are a number of series with considerably higher survival rates.[5-7]

Statistics on ovarian carcinoma have been notoriously unreliable, and perhaps for that reason they have been a source of continuous frustration to gynecologists. The problem of finding a classification that will set up homogeneous groups within which the method of treatment is the only variable is especially difficult. Three variants that are illustrative of the heterogeneous nature of ovarian cancer are: 1) histogenetic origin of the tumor, 2) histologic degree of tissue dedifferentiation, and 3) clinical stage of the disease. These are more variable from one clinic to another in cancer of the ovary than they are for any other kind of gynecologic cancer.

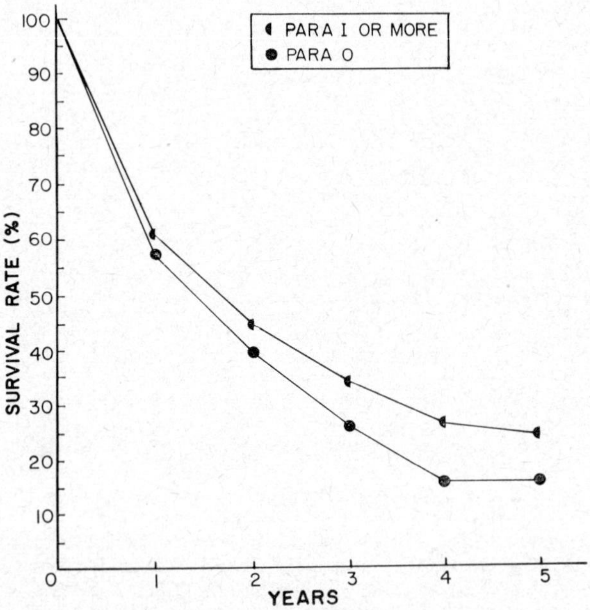


Fig. 4. Factors affecting survival in ovarian carcinoma: parity. Decreased survival in the nulligravida.

The percentage of survival is higher for patients under 40 years of age. This is apparently true irrespective of pathologic types and is in conflict with the frequently voiced clinical impression that cancer in older patients grows more slowly and is more benign in its effects. The rate of survival is higher in parous women than in nulliparas. This is demonstrated in Figure 4.

One possible explanation for this finding is the presence of an inherent defect in the ovarian germ plasm leading to ovarian dysfunction and sterility, neoplasia, and poorer response by the host to a biologically unfavorable tumor.

A correlation of the duration of symptoms prior to diagnosis and survival usually shows no significant differences. It is possible that a longer duration of symptoms may reflect a more slowly growing carcinoma of lower biologic activity. The patient who has more serious and earlier symptoms that cause her to visit the doctor sooner may have a more virulent tumor that is associated with a higher rate of metastasis.

This concept is also at variance with the more orthodox teachings that relate short duration of symptoms with better survival in patients

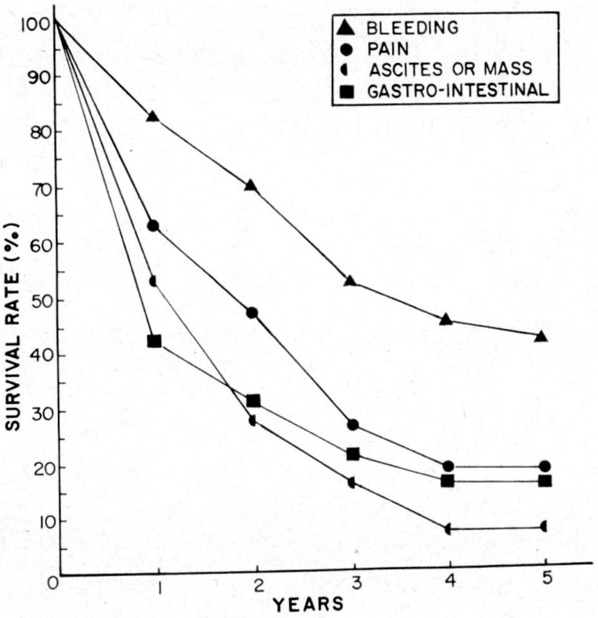


Fig. 5. Factors affecting survival in ovarian carcinoma: presenting symptom. Increased survival with vaginal bleeding.

with cancer. The type of symptoms in relation to survival is illustrated in Figure 5. It is noted that the most favorable prognosis is associated with vaginal bleeding. This may be accounted for by the frequent association of bleeding with granulosa cell tumors, in which the overall outcome is better than in other ovarian carcinomas. In addition, the occurrence of bleeding, frequently unrelated to the carcinoma, is apt to result in an early visit to the doctor with consequent early diagnosis and treatment.

Survival rates, when analyzed by pathologic type, show remarkable variation throughout the country. Except for the high survival rate for granulosa cell tumors and the uniformly poor results in solid ovarian cancer, there is little agreement in the series reported during the past 20 years.

When analyses of series of similar racial type, age, and pathological type produce widely divergent results, the initial areas of investigation must be: 1) therapy, and 2) criteria of diagnosis. Unfortunately, the number of patients who are amenable to curative operation at the

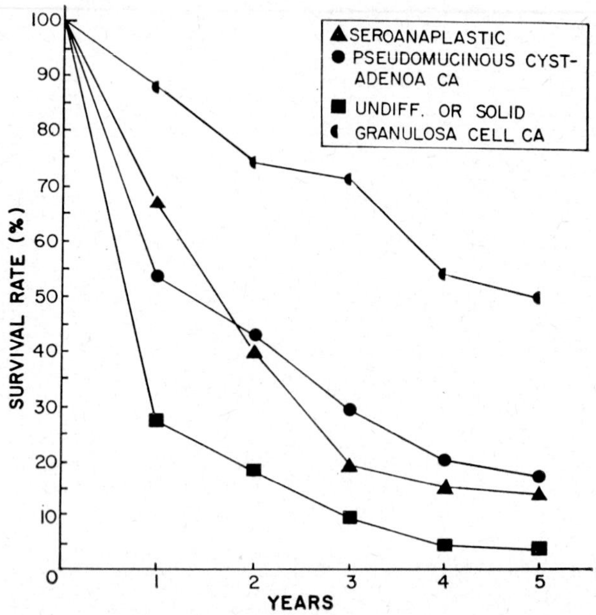


Fig. 6. Factors affecting survival in ovarian carcinoma: pathologic type.

time of diagnosis of ovarian carcinoma is consistently small enough to make its treatment a much less significant variable than in other gynecologic neoplasms. These differences are based on variations in classification and, more significantly, variations in histologic criteria for the diagnosis of malignancy. The precise survival figures reported in any article were at least as dependent upon the pathological criteria for malignancy and the categories included as upon any actual or claimed excellence of treatment.[8]

The biologic activity of a neoplasm, although not an infallible criterion, is a reliable sign of the benign or malignant nature of that tumor. We do not imply that those series in which low survival figures are reported represent more accurate histologic diagnosis, but the disparity in survival would seem to be related to strictness of criteria of malignancy in establishing the diagnosis of ovarian carcinoma. Typical survival curves of the four major pathologic types are illustrated in Figure 6.

When the type of treatment is studied in relation to five-year end results, it is apparent that incomplete operation, used primarily for what appeared to be localized unilateral disease, is associated with a lower survival rate than the recommended total hysterectomy and bilateral salpingo-oophorectomy. The fact that radiation therapy does not seem to have a beneficial effect on survival in most centers may be explained by the fact that radiation is more frequently given to patients in whom gross spread has already been noted at the time of operation.

## Discussion

It is discouraging to note that there is apparently no significant correlation between survival and most of the factors usually considered important in prognosis. This is particularly true for the frequently emphasized factors of diagnostic delay, symptoms, and methods of treatment.

The other factors analyzed, including age, parity, and pathologic type and stage of tumor, may have some effect on survival insofar as they play a role in the relation between tumor and host. The increased survival rate for younger patients is not completely understood. One might postulate that the general constitutional and hormonal status in this age group affects the biologic activity of the tumor.

The adverse effect of nulliparity on both incidence and survival may be evidence of an underlying biologic defect accounting for the infertility, the neoplasia, and the poor response on the part of the host.

Pathologic type is a factor affecting survival. In addition to the analytic and statistical influence of criteria for the diagnosis of malignancy and classification, there is an actual variation in biologic activity as evidenced by the granulosa cell tumor group. There did not appear to be a relation between the stage of the disease and survival. Such findings parallel observations that have been made on various types of cancer. The question that is raised is whether localized cancers are associated with a better prognosis because they were treated when still localized or whether cancers are localized because of particular tumor-host factors that determine both localization and a more indolent biologic course. The former postulate assumes a biologic uniformity of all cancers of the same type, the only variable being the duration of the disease. It does not recognize factors other than the time of therapy as being of importance. The later postulate assumes biologic variability among cancers of the same site of origin and does not exclude a time-progression relation.

TABLE I—NUCLEAR DIFFERENTIATION AND LYMPHOID INFILTRATION IN OVARIAN LESIONS OF PATIENTS SURVIVING FIVE YEARS
Structural Criteria: Five-Year Survivals

| *Nucl. grade* | *Lymphoid Infiltration* 0-1 | 2 | 3-4 |
|---|---|---|---|
| 0-1 | 2 | | |
| 2 | | 3 | |
| 3-4 | 2 | 2 | 1 |

It has been noted in the present study as well as in other reports that prolonged survival is not equivalent to eradication of disease, that is, cancer may behave as a chronic disease and may be associated with prolonged survival despite persistence of cancer tissue. Such findings cannot be reconciled with the orthodox concept that cancer progresses in linear fashion with time and that only therapeutic interruption of this progression can bring about prolonged survival or clinical cure.

On the other hand, the clinical behavior of cancer is consistent with the thesis that there is decided heterogenicity in the tumor-host relation in individual cases of homologous cancers. It is therefore pertinent to inquire as to what objective evidence there is that would give substance to such a concept.

Previous studies by Black and Speer[9] at this center have suggested that certain structural characteristics of the primary tumor and regional lymph nodes could be correlated with the biologic behavior of mammary and gastric carcinomas. Those features included the degree of nuclear differentiation and lymphoid infiltration of the primary tumor as well as histiocytic reactivity in the sinuses of the regional lymph nodes. In view of such reports we have compared the structural features of long- and short-term survival in cases of ovarian carcinoma. Since regional lymph nodes are not as available as are the specimens of resected ovarian cancers, no evaluation could be made on the structure of the lymph nodes in ovarian carcinoma.

The pertinent structural and biologic features of the ovarian carcinomas in 10 patients who survived for more than 5 years have been reviewed. All of these carcinomas were of the papillary serous or seroanaplastic type; in three of the patients regional metastases were present at the time of the original diagnosis. Microscopic examination of these cancers revealed a tendency toward nuclear differentiation and lymphoid infiltration (Table I) of a degree not found in a series of

TABLE II—NUCLEAR DIFFERENTIATION AND LYMPHOID INFILTRATION IN OVARIAN LESIONS OF PATIENTS DYING UNDER TWO YEARS
Structural Criteria: Dead Under Two Years

| *Nucl. grade* | *Lymphoid Infiltration* 0-1 | 2 | 3-4 |
|---|---|---|---|
| 0-1 | 12 | 1 | |
| 2 | 7 | | |
| 3-4 | | | |

similar types of ovarian cancer in which the patients died within two years of diagnosis (Table II). It would appear from these observations that survival in patients with ovarian carcinoma is related to intrinsic features of the tumor-host relation. Although the small size of these samples makes such a conclusion less than absolute, it is in keeping with previous studies of prognostic factors in mammary and gastric carcinoma.

The most conservative interpretation of the available data would suggest that survival in patients with ovarian carcinoma involves factors other than therapeutic intervention. We are expanding these clinicopathologic correlations in the belief that the ultimate control of this disease will come from such knowledge rather than from the application of either more extensive surgery or more radiation therapy.

## Summary and Conclusions

1) Two hundred and twenty-three cases of ovarian carcinoma have been analyzed for factors affecting the survival rate.

2) At the New York Medical College the five-year survival rate was 20.6 per cent. A review of the literature reveals similarly poor results in most series.

3) Standard indices for prognosis including duration of symptoms, character of symptoms, and method of treatment could not be correlated with the survival rate.

4) Age, parity, and pathological type and stage of the tumor apparently can influence the survival rate.

5) The survival rate was increased in patients who were less than 40 years of age and was decreased in nulliparas.

6) Patients with granulosa cell tumors have the highest five-year survival rate.

7) Series showing unusually high five-year survival rates may indi-

cate less rigidity in establishing criteria for diagnosis of malignancy.

8) Localization is associated with high survival rates irrespective of the duration of the disease.

9) It is postulated that survival in patients with ovarian carcinoma involves factors other than time and type of treatment.

10) Experimental evidence suggests that the most significant factors affecting survival are the biologic activity of the tumor and the host-tumor interrelation.

## *REFERENCES*


1. Randall, C. L. and Hall, D. W. Results of the treatment of ovarian malignancies, *Amer. J. Obstet. Gynec. 63*:497, 1952.
2. Stone, M. L., Weingold, A. B., Sall, S. and Sonnenblick, B. Factors affecting survival of patients with ovarian carcinoma, *Surg. Gynec. Obstet. 116*:351, 1963.
3. Sall, S., Weingold, A. B., Sonnenblick, B. and Stone, M. L. The effect of vaginal bleeding on survival in ovarian carcinoma, *Surg. Gynec. Obstet. 117*:5, 1963.
4. Weingold, A. B. and Stone, M. L. Cancer chemotherapy in gynecologic malignant conditions, *New York J. Med. 62*: 2654, 1962.
5. Cutler, S. J., Ederer, F. C. and Greenberg, K. A. Survival of patients with ovarian cancer, *J. Nat. Cancer Inst. 24*:541, 1960.
6. Allan, M. S. and Hertig, A. T., Carcinoma of the ovary, *Amer. J. Obstet. Gynec. 58*:640, 1949.
7. Turner, J. C., Remine, W. H. and Dockerty, M. B. A clinicopathologic study of 172 patients with primary carcinoma of the ovary. *Surg. Gynec. Obstet. 109*:198, 1959.
8. Dougherty, C. M., Ancoin, R. and Cotten, N. Diagnosis of cystadenocarcinoma of the ovary, *Obstet. Gynec. 18*: 81, 1961.
9. Black, M. M. and Speer, F. D. Lymph node reactivity in cancer patients, *Surg., Gynec. Obstet. 110*:477, 1960.

# HEALTH SERVICES IN NEW YORK CITY*

Report by

The Committee on Public Health

The New York Academy of Medicine

## I. Municipal Hospitals in New York City

In a recent report on the municipal hospitals in New York City, the Committee on Public Health pointed out that the present system appears to have outlived its original function and should be replaced by one that meets the present needs of the community more adequately.

The report cited three elements that combined to cause the present difficulties: 1) inappropriate administrative procedure and practice, 2) budgetary restrictions, and 3) limitations in the personnel system.

These elements are both restrictive and self-defeating, the Committee noted, and have prevailed for many years. Thus, it may be seen that the present state of obsolescence affecting the municipal hospitals has a long, unfortunate history.

A drastic overhaul is necessary to remedy the situation, the Committee believes. In this light, the Committee strongly recommends that:

1) The status of each municipal hospital should be reviewed on the basis of its age, condition, capacity, and location in order to determine whether it should be retained in operation, renovated, or discontinued when feasible, according to a master plan.

2) Those hospitals that are to be retained should no longer be municipal institutions but should be converted into autonomous community hospitals. These autonomous community hospitals should be open institutions capable of providing progressive care, including long-term care.

3) With the conversion of municipal hospitals to autonomous community hospitals, the need for a municipal Department of Hospitals and a Board of Hospitals would no longer exist and they should therefore be abolished.

4) The transition of the municipal to autonomous community hospitals should be accomplished in orderly progression.

5) Each municipal hospital that is converted to an open autonomous community hospital should be controlled and operated by a trusteeship. The trustees should be public-spirited, knowledgeable citizens drawn from the immediate community.

6) A Hospital Authority should be created over all these newly established community hospitals upon their conversion from municipal status.

7) The present state of affiliation should be reviewed. For the future, any contemplated affiliation should be highly selective and not necessarily permanent.

---

*Approved by the Executive Committee of the Committee on Public Health, March 27, 1967. Approved by the Committee on Public Health, April 3, 1967.
This report does not necessarily represent the opinion of the Council of The New York Academy of Medicine.

8) Under the proposed system the present new unit of health services in the city government created by executive order in the mayor's reorganization plan would be unnecessary.

In contrast, any plan to modify the present municipal hospital system is not likely to achieve the desired objective of improving the situation, the Committee on Public Health believes. Indeed, it should be emphasized that with the enactment of Medicare and Medicaid, there no longer is any social or medical reason for the continuance of the municipal hospital system of New York City. Since it may be presumed that there will be no more medical indigency, the reason for the existence of the municipal hospital system will be removed. That is why the Committee on Public Health recommended in its report that the system should be abolished.

Actually, the only reason for the continuance of the system is political, involving as it does the authority and control over federal funds. The New York Times recognized this fact in an editorial, saying: "Politically, this [the Committee's] proposal will have little appeal in a period when so much of the revenue to support all hospitals is coming from public sources."

The present sorry plight of the municipal hospital system is the result of "an ill-fitting administrative system; rigid and unwieldy financial restraint; and a vise-like civil service." Bureaucracy and red tape brought the system into decline. Ironically, the safeguards were created to keep the administration honest and fair. Now so cramping, they were designed to prevent the kind of political pillage that was a feature in other areas of city administration.

In truth, government has little to choose between two operational systems. In one, there is strong central authority as against a large measure of local autonomy. With respect to finances, it may have either strict and detailed control with a line budget or latitude with an operational performance budget. As for policy in personnel, it is almost certain that a bureaucracy will be created in either case: one based on civil service, the other on the patronage system.

Thus, it appears that the body politic has the choice of equally undesirable eventualities: paralysis or weakness and anemia. Each system has its defects; these become especially observable in a hospital system comprised so much of services and accommodations. The larger the system, the more complex are its shortcomings.

The present situation exemplifies vividly how overcentralization in administration, line budgets, and civil service lead to trouble. Yet past experience shows that sooner or later the alternative of more flexible budgets, patronage and delegated authority in government along with decentralization and individual autonomy have led to abuses and irregularities and produced a situation that is even worse than the paralysis induced by centralized authority, line budgets, and civil service.

After rejecting the Committee's recommendation that the city dispose of its municipal hospitals, the city administration disclosed a plan to retain the present system in a modified form. Under this plan, five new departmental sections or bureaus would be added to the Department of Hospitals. If there is one sure way of defeating decentralization, it is either to retain or create bureaus, the Committee believes.

Again, according to the announced plan, each hospital administrator would have autonomy, budget freedom, purchasing and construction power, and exemption of personnel from civil service. All of this has a familiar ring. Such a program is not only vulnerable to bringing hospitals under political influence with its inefficiency and worse, it is, in fact, an invitation to the use of power with loose control. To attempt to overcome hampering restrictions of civil service and a line budget by exemptions and exceptions is simply to exchange one set of weaknesses for another.

In the view of the Committee on Public Health, the function of government is to do those things which citizens cannot do for themselves or do so well or as easily. On its part, the city government is clearly incapable of operating effectively a municipal system of general care hospitals. But on the other hand, the record shows abundant evidence that private citizens can do a better job of running their hospitals than can the city.

That is why the Committee on Public Health strongly reaffirms its recommendation that the city government should take immediate steps to convert the municipal hospitals into autonomous community facilities, controlled and operated by public-spirited citizens drawn from the local area.

## II. Health Services Administration

In its report on the municipal hospitals of New York City, the Committee on Public Health pointed out that if the city hospitals were converted to open autonomous community hospitals, if both the Board and Department of Hospitals were abolished, and if a Hospital Authority were established, the present Health Services Administration in the city government, created by executive order, would be unnecessary. If there is no useful purpose in retaining the municipal hospital system, the need for the new Health Services Administration as created by executive order is even less defensible.

The declared purpose of a health services administration is to bring together related services provided by the Department of Hospitals, the Department of Health, the Community Mental Health Board, and the Medical Examiner's Office, into one large agency. Among the reasons advanced in support of this move are increased economy and greater efficiency through the coordination of similar services in various departments.

Yet, the Committee notes, the Health Services Administration does not include the medical components of the Departments of Welfare and Education. A very large segment of health services is carried on under Welfare in the Medicare and Medicaid programs. There is a large and important part of the population, the youths, to be covered by health services in the schools. Even the federal government has recognized the interconnection between Health, Education, and Welfare by placing them all under one tent.

The fundamental question is whether the Health Department, the municipal hospital system, if it is retained, the Community Mental Health Board, and the Medical Examiner's Office, to say nothing of Education and Welfare, can be coordinated successfully. The second related question is whether such coordination of similar services in these departments will achieve the increased economy and greater efficiency that is claimed. In answering these questions, it is important to differentiate health services from personal health services. Health services is the broader term, including impersonal as well as personal services. Also in providing health services there are two different approaches and modes of operation. One is essentially preventive; the other curative. Then, there is the fundamental difference between the aforementioned departments in the areas of health and disease covered. In sum, each department differs in its area of activity and in its proportion of personal and impersonal services as well as of preventive and curative approaches. By and large among these departments the dissimilar outweigh the similar services. When the whole complex is considered, the interdepartment duplication of services is not large. In addition, the rationale underlying the original division of health services with subsequent growth of separate departments, now entrenched by time, does not make one sanguine about the probability of harnessing them by administrative fiat in a significant and effective way to achieve in the future the avowed goals. For all these reasons, it is difficult to become optimistic that the Health Services Administration would succeed in effecting greater economy and efficiency.

Worse, the Health Services Administration under the reorganization plan, besides not accomplishing what is wanted, may produce what is not wanted. Following an application of Parkinson's law, it creates in actuality a superstructure with yet another executive layer. Thus, it adds a top administrator of the newly-created agency to a deputy mayor, already supposedly responsble for health matters.

As created, the Health Services Administration is highly autocratic. It almost seems as though in the attempt to escape the paralyzing effect of over-restraint, the reorganizers have moved to the other extreme of underrestraint. Government does not function as a corporation. Experience has shown the advisability for a democratic government to have its controls and restraints.

The Committee is convinced that it is possible for city departments to work together on important projects without an expensive and elaborate overlay. In recent years, the Health Department has extended much-needed help to the Welfare Department and as much help as it was permitted to the Department of Education.

In the light of the foregoing, the Committee on Public Health concludes that a health services administration of the type produced by the reorganization plan is not needed.

## III. Organization of Personal Health Services

Although not approving of the creation of the existing Health Services Administration, the Committee on Public Health would point out the desirability, indeed need, of an over-all city-wide organization of personal health services.

Over the last two decades medicine has been undergoing profound and vast changes in a number of ways, some actuated from within the discipline. But changes in response to outside developments have also occurred. Through enabling legislation the government has taken more and more responsibility in making it possible for everyone to obtain essential medical and hospital services. While bringing benefit to the public, the latest acts in the sequence, Medicare, Medicaid, and Regional Medical Centers, suddenly imposed a large responsibility that was a challenge to it. These developments directed attention to the present system of health care.

This legislation affects both the purveyor and the recipient. That is to say, it concerns personal health services based upon a doctor-patient, one-to-one, relation in the broadest sense, including paramedical personnel. As a general term it covers services rendered under the auspices of government or by private enterprise. In the latter they may be with or without profit. Included in the term are various types of service: preventive, diagnostic, therapeutic, and rehabilitative.

All these services are performed by a vast array of personnel, much of it specialized, and their efforts are directed toward the entire gamut of diseases. As for the sites of personal health services, they take place in the main in the home, the physician's office, or the hospital. In addition, they are conducted in clinics of the health department, school, and industry. There are several ways in which, on the one hand, the services are financed; on the other hand, the physician is compensated.

To say that the enabling legislation changes the complexion of health services would be an observation of surface or appearance. A vital substance called money is to be pumped into the blood stream of health services. This economic support may well bring, along with transformation, a change in the foundation, structure, and function of delivery of health services.

Far-reaching in breadth and depth are the effects of this legislation for both the purveyor and recipient of personal health services. Three effects should be mentioned:

1) Lack of funds will be no barrier to seeking needed medical care. This provision is not new. It has always been true. The new feature is who bears the cost. For a long time it was charity by hospital and medical profession. At its peak it furnished the best of medical care. But through a train of events it has been gradually diminishing and is now coming to a close. All this will be a thing of the past. It is the end of an era. Charity has given way to welfare and social security, in which government has acknowledged that it has a responsibility for the unfortunate.

There is another new and important difference flowing from the recent legislation. There will be no more nonpaying patients. All patients will be alike in one respect: they will be paying patients. All will therefore be private patients. For that reason they will be entitled to equal treatment and accommodations. Ability to pay for health care will no longer be a basis for classifying patients or for providing different accommodations. It is the hope, indeed anticipation, that at the point of receipt of medical care, the distinction between private and welfare patients will disappear.

2) When everyone is a paying patient, the class system in hospitals will end. No longer will there be hospitals for the indigent; nor will there need to be. Distinctions between types of hospitals based on the patient's financial capabilities and resources will be removed. Accommodations in all hospitals will have fewer levels and the lowest will be raised. In all probability there will be no wards in the hospital of the future.

Although there will be equality of a paying status, social and economic differences as well as class distinctions will remain among patients. Hence it is likely that there will always be those who will want and can afford to pay for special accommodations.

Nevertheless, in the future the larger number will have adequate quarters with all essentials at hand. More attention will be paid to planning a functional hospital and less to separation on an economic basis.

3) With financial provision, the volume of health services is expected to expand. This anticipated expansion raises several considerations. Foremost always is the concern that the medical care be adequate and of uniformly high quality. Then too, adequate manpower and facilities will be needed. Still another important point has to be taken into account. Over recent years the cost of medical care,

especially hospitalization, has been mounting. So high has it become that there is a common phrase, catastrophic illness, which describes the financial blow.

All government health services have ultimately cost more than originally estimated. Already president Lyndon B. Johnson has delivered a plea to cut the cost of medical care. Waste and inefficiency are never justifiable, and they become intolerable if excessively burdensome or perilous. So economy and efficiency seem certain to be watchwords that will be heard and goals that will be sought.

All this raises the question how well is New York City prepared to render personal health services to all its citizens under the new financial arrangement in an orderly, economic, and efficient manner.

In part apologetically, in part boastfully, it has been said many times in health circles that New York City is unique, a law unto itself. There is nothing else like it. Here is a large, concentrated population with a vast array of independent health agencies of all varieties. There are departments in government with official, public administration. Abounding among them are many privately owned or operated, nonofficial, mostly nonprofit agencies. With this complex of resources, public and private agencies divide responsibility for health services.

In structure and function this vast heterogeneous complex is a fragmented agglomeration of independent, autonomous, uncoordinated components. That is not to say that there are no good units. Some are quite good; others less so. But there is no central head, no over-all organization, no master plan.

Indeed, the city has never had an over-all organization of all health services, or a master plan that carried authority. The history of Health Councils in New York City is dismal and disappointing. Despite several earnest efforts they did not become the potent force desired, expected, and necessary. Self-interest and lack of authority were too great to overcome. As for the Hospital Council and its valiant years with an unenforceable master plan, not until recently did it gain some measure of limited authority.

Surely the present health services carrying the handicap of lack of organization and system cannot be expected to meet this new challenge with maximum economy and effectiveness.

To obtain unification with leadership, organization, and system with these many different agencies, some official, some not, it is obvious that certain arrangements must be avoided, certain desirable, indeed essential, features must be sought. Not wanted are overcentralization, civil service system, and overly detailed budgetary control. Similarly to be avoided are waste from duplication, overlapping, and inefficient operation. On the positive side, what is desired and needed is a flexible organization with authority that can embrace both public and the many private, nonprofit agencies. Each individual agency should have autonomy over and responsibility for its own operation while being a member of the larger organization and operating according to its policies.

Three principal functions of the over-all organization should be fiscal authority and responsibility; policy making; and planning. The organization would therefore act as a public corporation with the necessary financial power to discharge its responsibilities. Adequate, high-grade service with solvency would be its goals. Performance budgeting with an enlightened personnel system would be the preferred mode of operation.

The over-all organization would be the one agency that would view the city as a whole and its various constituent areas in determining its needs in personal health services. Out of these overviews would come policy and planning. These decisions would have to be backed by factual material. Parenthetically, it should be noted that Congress underlined the utility and significance of preparation when it recently enacted what some believe to be one of the most important pieces of legislation on health—provision for comprehensive health planning.

Only one type of organization avoids all the drawbacks and fulfills all these desiderata. It would have to be a new organization in health services. Certainly no agency already in existence should be raised to a supreme position over the others. None could meet all the specifications and requisites. Rather, a Personal Health Services Authority to include all the various individual agencies should be created.

The Hospital Authority containing all hospitals, recommended by the Committee on Public Health in a previous report, could be the forerunner or first step toward the larger organization. It could be duly expanded to include all the personal health services, with a change of its name to Health Services Authority. Or from the beginning the establishment of a Health Services Authority might be undertaken.

By whichever procedure, the Committee on Public Health strongly recommends the creation of a Health Services Authority. Such an authority offers most promise of meeting the needs of the people of New York City.

# HOMICIDE BY MEANS OF PLAGUE BACILLI

It is widely rumored that medicine is no longer a learned profession and that the physician, especially in the United States, is not to be regarded as an intellectual or even as a cultivated man. He goes to the opera under conjugal pressure only, he spurns the ballet, he detests Picasso, and he reads little. Instead of giving his days and his nights to the volumes of Addison, as a hypochondriac sage advised, he is content with detective stories.

Against these charges, especially the last-named, he is not utterly defenseless. If our profession has produced countless handbooks of morbid anatomy, it has also produced the creator of Sherlock Holmes. Hence we have the right to choose.

That detective stories are not limited to the world of fiction may become apparent to the doctor as early as the time of his internship, especially if he has done ambulance duty or emergency service. Here he learns that anything may happen—and almost everything does.

For a strong dose of true-life detective romance that equals the most extravagant clinical reminiscence, we may recommend an article by Dr. D. P. Lambert, M.D., D.T.M. & H., and captain in the famous Indian medical service. The paper is titled The Pakur* Murder and was published in the *Medico-legal and Criminological Review*, vol. 5, pp. 297-302, 1937.

Two half-brothers named Benoyendra and Amarendra Pandey were joint heirs of a family estate. Benoyendra soon showed clinical evidence of being a bad egg, i.e., he was prodigal of rupees, he consorted with dancing girls, and he sent false telegrams for nefarious purposes.

One day Amarendra was in a crowded railroad station in Calcutta; the wicked Benoyendra came to see him off, a courtesy inconsistent with his previous behavior. Amarendra was jostled by someone and felt a puncture in his arm. Three days later he visited a physician, who found a mark resembling a needle puncture. On the next day the patient had fever, pain in the axilla, and a small wheal near the puncture. A blood culture was taken. The patient now began to have high fever, axillary

*Pakur does not appear in ordinary atlases. From indirect evidence it must be in or near Bengal.

adenopathy, and signs in the lungs. The puncture wound became ulcerated. On about the eighth day Amarendra died and was cremated in accordance with Hindu custom. On the next day plague bacilli were found in the blood culture. There had been no plague in the vicinity for three years.

A private investigator discovered that the bad Benoyendra was friendly with a bacteriologist named Taranath. This malefactor, it was learned, had telegraphed to the Haffkine Institute in Bombay and had requested a live culture of plague bacilli. Unsurprisingly, the request was refused. Later Dr. Taranath convinced a Calcutta physician that he had devised a cure for plague, which he wanted to test against live cultures. In this way he gained access to a laboratory but the cultures there did not survive. After further intrigue in Bombay Dr. Taranath again obtained live bacilli. Meanwhile Benoyendra attempted to insure Amarendra's life by a noncancellable policy for 51,000 rupees; this negotiation failed.

Ultimately Benoyendra and Dr. Taranath were arrested and put on trial. The jury found both defendants guilty of conspiracy to murder. The judge sentenced both men to death but the Calcutta High Court reduced the sentence to transportation for life.

S. J.

# OFFICERS AND STAFF OF THE ACADEMY

1967

*President*
PRESTON A. WADE

*Vice Presidents*
JOHN L. POOL
FRANK B. BERRY
FREDERICK R. BAILEY

*Treasurer*
JAMES E. THOMPSON

*Recording Secretary*
CHARLES A. R. CONNOR

*Trustees*
J. BURNS AMBERSON
HOWARD REID CRAIG
FRANK GLENN
MILTON J. GOODFRIEND
SAMUEL W. LAMBERT, JR.
ROBERT L. LEVY
ASA L. LINCOLN
JOHN L. MADDEN
DICKINSON W. RICHARDS, JR.
ROBERT H. WYLIE

*Council*
The President
The Vice Presidents
The Trustees
The Treasurer
The Recording Secretary
The Chairmen of the Standing Committees

*Director*
JAMES E. MCCORMACK

*Librarian*
GERTRUDE L. ANNAN

*Executive Secretary*
*Committee on Public Health*
H. D. KRUSE

*Executive Secretary*
*Committee on Medical Education*
ROBERT S. GOODHART

*Executive Secretary*
*Committee on Special Studies*
HARRY BECKER

*Business Manager*
ROBERT M. BRERETON

*Legal Counsel*
DAVIS POLK WARDWELL SUNDERLAND & KIENDL

*Library Consultants*
JANET DOE CURT PROSKAUER

## STANDING COMMITTEES OF THE ACADEMY—1967

The President of the Academy is an ex officio member of all committees except the Nominating Committee

### COMMITTEE ON ADMISSION

IRA SNOW JONES, *Chairman*
FRANCIS G. GEER, *Secretary*

SIDNEY BLUMENTHAL
JOHN W. V. CORDICE, JR.
WILLIAM J. EISENMENGER
LEO B. HALLERAN
BARBARA FURMAN LIPTON
JAMES JOSEPH O'ROURKE
S. FRANK REDO
ISADORE MAX TARLOV
HARVEY J. TOMPKINS
PHILIP D. WILSON, JR.

### NOMINATING COMMITTEE

GEORGE H. HUMPHREYS, II, *Chairman*

CHARLES E. KOSSMANN
WALSH MCDERMOTT

### COMMITTEE ON LIBRARY

BRONSON S. RAY, *Chairman*

FRANK B. BERRY
PAUL F. CRANEFIELD
GEORGE E. DANIELS
NORMAN DEANE
V. KNEELAND FRANTZ
EDWARD F. HARTUNG
SAUL JARCHO
SAMUEL W. LAMBERT, JR.
ALBERT S. LYONS
JOHN M. MCLEAN
WILLIAM B. OBER
COLTER RULE
MORTON D. SCHWEITZER
RICHARD B. STARK
HILTON H. STOTHERS
JOSEPH A. TAMERIN

GERTRUDE L. ANNAN, *Librarian*

### COMMITTEE ON PUBLIC HEALTH

ARTHUR A. FISCHL, *Chairman*
BERNARD J. PISANI, *Vice Chairman*

J. BURNS AMBERSON
GEORGE E. ANDERSON
HENRY ARANOW, JR.
*GEORGE BAEHR
FREDERICK R. BAILEY
HENRY L. BARNETT
OTTO E. BILLO
ABRAM BLAU
WILLIAM H. BUTTON, JR.
MCKEEN CATTELL
E. CRAIG COATS
WILLIAM J. EISENMENGER
HENRY I. FINEBERG
ALFRED E. FISCHER
MILTON J. GOODFRIEND
ARTHUR VOSE GREELEY
LOUIS M. HELLMAN
WILLIAM M. HITZIG
WILBUR B. HURLBUT
HENRY L. JAFFE
OSWALD R. JONES
MILTON D. KLEIN
MARCUS D. KOGEL
*SHEPARD KRECH
ROBERT W. LAIDLAW
RACHMIEL LEVINE
*ASA L. LINCOLN
HAROLD W. LOVELL
NORTON M. LUGER
S. W. MOORE
HARRY MOST
EQUINN W. MUNNELL
THEODORE W. OPPEL
JEAN P. PAPPS
*HOWARD A. PATTERSON
PAUL I. ROBINSON
GEORGE M. SAYPOL
BEVERLY CHEW SMITH
PHILIP M. STIMSON
HARVEY J. TOMPKINS
MAXIMIN DEM. TOUART
PETER VOGEL
*I. OGDEN WOODRUFF

H. D. KRUSE, *Executive Secretary*

*Emeritus Member

## COMMITTEE ON MEDICAL EDUCATION

M. Ralph Kaufman, *Chairman*
George G. Reader, *Vice Chairman*

Alfred A. Angrist
Rudolf L. Baer
Albert M. Betcher
John Z. Bowers
J. Robert Buchanan
Edward C. Curnen
Michael M. Dacso
Clarence E. de la Chapelle
J. Frederick Eagle, Jr.
Edward E. Fischel
Edward W. Hook, Jr.
Robert S. Hotchkiss
Richard C. Karl
Charles E. Kossmann
George James
Henry D. Janowitz
William S. Langford
David Lehr
Leo Mayer
Marsh McCall
Rustin McIntosh
Peter Marshall Murray
Carl Muschenheim
Edmund D. Pellegrino
John L. Pool
Milton J. Raisbeck
Paul Reznikoff
Albert C. Santy
Aura E. Severinghaus
Isidore Snapper
Theodore H. Spaet
Lester R. Tuchman
William I. Wolff
Harry M. Zimmerman

Robert S. Goodhart, *Executive Secretary*

## COMMITTEE ON SPECIAL STUDIES

Byard Williams, *Chairman*

Harry S. Altman
Norton S. Brown
Martin Cherkasky
Anthony C. Cipollaro
Duncan W. Clark
William Cooper
John M. Cotton
Edwin F. Daily
Murray Dworetzky
William W. Field
Carl Goldmark, Jr.
Irving Graef
Sidney M. Greenberg
August H. Groeschel
Harold D. Harvey
Louis Leiter
Mack Lipkin
David Lyall
Henry B. Makover
Arthur M. Master
George W. Melcher, Jr.
Rowland L. Mindlin
James A. Moore
Joseph Post
Willard C. Rappleye
J. Beall Rodgers
Peter Rogatz
Leonard S. Rosenfeld
Frank A. Seixas
Solomon Silver
Carl H. Smith
Samuel Standard
Milton Terris
Lewis Thomas
Edward Tolstoi
Aaron O. Wells
George M. Wheatley
Herbert B. Wilcox, Jr.

Harry Becker, *Executive Secretary*

## COMMITTEE ON SECTIONS

John L. Pool, *Chairman*

The Chairmen and Secretaries of the 16 Sections of the Academy

Robert S. Goodhart, *Secretary*

## Other Committees Appointed Annually by the President—1967

### EDITORIAL BOARD — ACADEMY BULLETIN

CHARLES E. KOSSMANN, *Chairman*

GERTRUDE L. ANNAN
MARGARET BEVANS
RALPH W. GAUSE
CHARLES A. RAGAN, JR.

SAUL JARCHO, *Editor*

### COMMITTEE ON ART

ALBERT C. SANTY, *Chairman*

JOHN J. CONLEY
MEYER M. MELICOW

### COMMITTEE ON REVISION OF BY-LAWS

JOHN L. MADDEN, *Chairman*

RUSTIN MCINTOSH
DICKINSON W. RICHARDS, JR.
G. JARVIS COFFIN
FRED A. METTLER
JAMES J. SMITH

### JOINT CONFERENCE COMMITTEE WITH THE MEDICAL SOCIETY OF THE COUNTY OF NEW YORK

*From the N.Y. Academy of Medicine*
PRESTON A. WADE
JOHN L. POOL
JAMES E. MCCORMACK
CHARLES A. R. CONNOR

*From the N.Y. County Society*
JOHN A. LAWLER
C. JOSEPH DELANEY
RICHARD D. BRASFIELD
WILLIAM L. WHEELER, JR.

### COMMITTEE ON HONORARY FELLOWSHIP, MEDAL AND PLAQUE

GEORGE A. PERERA, *Chairman*

GEORGE BAEHR
E. HUGH LUCKEY
ALEXANDER T. MARTIN
WM. BARCLAY PARSONS
HAROLD A. ZINTEL

### GIBBS PRIZE COMMITTEE

ROBERT F. LOEB, *Chairman*

ARTHUR M. FISHBERG
WILLIAM GOLDRING
ROBERT S. HOTCHKISS
JOHN K. LATTIMER
VICTOR F. MARSHALL

Other Committees Appointed Annually by the President—1967 (*Continued*)

### BERNARD S. OPPENHEIMER FUND COMMITTEE

SOLOMON SILVER, *Chairman*

JAMES E. MCCORMACK
CLARENCE E. DE LA CHAPELLE
ROBERT S. GOODHART
GEORGE G. READER

### LOUIS LIVINGSTON SEAMAN FUND COMMITTEE

WILLIAM H. SEBRELL, JR., *Chairman*

HENRY B. MAKOVER
BERWYN F. MATTISON
NATHANIEL H. COOPER
WALSH MCDERMOTT
HARRY MOST

### COMMITTEE ON PHYSICAL FACILITIES

ROBERT L. LEVY, *Chairman*

GEORGE BAEHR
FRANK B. BERRY
HOWARD REID CRAIG
FRANK GLENN
SAMUEL W. LAMBERT, JR.
JAMES E. MCCORMACK
JOHN L. POOL
JAMES E. THOMPSON

### COMMITTEE ON DENTISTRY (Interprofessional Relations)

*From the N. Y. Academy of Medicine*
BEVERLY CHEW SMITH, *Chairman*
FRANK B. BERRY
GEORGE CHRISTAKIS
JOHN CONVERSE
ROBERT S. GOODHART
STUART STEVENSON

*From the N. Y. Academy of Dentistry*
MALCOLM W. CARR, *Chairman*
EDGAR BACON
RALPH T. BOWMAN
WALTER MOSMAN
HOMER VAUGHAN
SAMUEL WALD

---

## OFFICERS OF AFFILIATED SOCIETIES

| | *1966-1967* | *1967-1968* |
|---|---|---|
| THE HARVEY SOCIETY | ABRAHAM WHITE, *President* | RACHMIEL LEVINE, *President* |
| | RALPH L. ENGLE, JR., *Secretary* | RALPH L. ENGLE, JR., *Secretary* |
| NEW YORK PATHOLOGICAL SOCIETY | CHANDLER A. STETSON, *President* | JAMES BERKMAN, *President* |
| | DONALD G. MCKAY, *Secretary* | ROBERT MCCLUSKEY, *Secretary* |
| NEW YORK ROENTGEN SOCIETY | HARRY Z. MELLINS, *President* | MILTON ELKIN, *President* |
| | ARNOLD L. BACHMAN, *Secretary* | DAVID BAKER, *Secretary* |
| SOCIETY FOR EXPERIMENTAL BIOLOGY AND MEDICINE (New York Section) | FREDERICK S. PHILIPS, *Chairman* | FREDERICK S. PHILIPS, *Chairman* |
| | LOUIS J. CIZEK, *Secretary* | LOUIS J. CIZEK, *Secretary* |

# OFFICERS OF SECTIONS

| 1966-1967 | 1967-1968 |
| --- | --- |
| **ANESTHESIOLOGY AND RESUSCITATION** | |
| Louis R. Orkin, *Chairman* | Louis S. Blancato, *Chairman* |
| Louis S. Blancato, *Secretary* | Francis F. Foldes, *Secretary* |
| **DERMATOLOGY AND SYPHILOLOGY** | |
| Frank E. Cormia, *Chairman* | Anthony N. Domonkos, *Chairman* |
| Anthony N. Domonkos, *Secretary* | Helen O. Curth, *Secretary* |
| **HISTORICAL MEDICINE** | |
| Gregory I. Altschuller, *Chairman* | J. Edwin Drew, *Chairman* |
| J. Edwin Drew, *Secretary* | Blair O. Rogers, *Secretary* |
| **MEDICINE** | |
| Saul J. Farber, *Chairman* | Saul J. Farber, *Chairman* |
| Rachmiel Levine, *Secretary* | Rachmiel Levine, *Secretary* |
| **MICRO- AND MOLECULAR BIOLOGY** | |
| Morris Schaeffer, *Chairman* | Morris Schaeffer, *Chairman* |
| Victor J. Cabasso, *Secretary* | Victor J. Cabasso, *Secretary* |
| **NEUROLOGY AND PSYCHIATRY** | |
| Arnold P. Friedman, *Chairman* | Arnold P. Friedman, *Chairman* |
| Arthur Zitrin, *Secretary* | Arthur Zitrin, *Secretary* |
| **OBSTETRICS AND GYNECOLOGY** | |
| Seymour L. Romney, *Chairman* | Edward A. Graber, *Chairman* |
| Edward A. Graber, *Secretary* | Bernard J. Pisani, *Secretary* |
| **OCCUPATIONAL MEDICINE** | |
| Norbert J. Roberts, *Chairman* | Norvin C. Kiefer, *Chairman* |
| Norvin C. Kiefer, *Secretary* | Robert E. Eckhardt, *Secretary* |
| **OPHTHALMOLOGY** | |
| Donald M. Shafer, *Chairman* | Goodwin M. Breinin, *Chairman* |
| Edward A. Dunlap, *Secretary* | Richard C. Troutman, *Secretary* |
| **ORTHOPEDIC SURGERY** | |
| Hudson J. Wilson, Jr., *Chairman* | James A. Nicholas, *Chairman* |
| James A. Nicholas, *Secretary* | Monroe Schneider, *Secretary* |
| **OTOLARYNGOLOGY** | |
| Daniel C. Baker, Jr., *Chairman* | Franz Altmann, *Chairman* |
| Franz Altmann, *Secretary* | Max L. Som, *Secretary* |
| **PEDIATRICS** | |
| Sidney Blumenthal, *Chairman* | Laurence Finberg, *Chairman* |
| Laurence Finberg, *Secretary* | Stuart S. Stevenson, *Secretary* |
| **PHYSICAL MEDICINE AND REHABILITATION** | |
| Joseph B. Rogoff, *Chairman* | Arthur S. Abramson, *Chairman* |
| Arthur S. Abramson, *Secretary* | Joseph Geo. Benton, *Secretary* |
| **PLASTIC AND RECONSTRUCTIVE SURGERY** | |
| Richard B. Stark, *Chairman* | Richard B. Stark, *Chairman* |
| Joseph A. Tamerin, *Secretary* | Joseph A. Tamerin, *Secretary* |
| **SURGERY** | |
| William I. Wolff, *Chairman* | Joseph M. Ford, *Chairman* |
| Joseph M. Ford, *Secretary* | |
| **UROLOGY** | |
| Edward A. Brady, *Chairman* | William J. Nelson, *Chairman* |
| William J. Nelson, *Secretary* | R. Keith Waterhouse, *Secretary* |

BULLETIN OF
THE NEW YORK ACADEMY
OF MEDICINE

Vol. 43, No. 10 October 1967

# A STUDY OF LEE HARVEY OSWALD: PSYCHOLOGICAL CAPABILITY OF MURDER*

David Abrahamsen

Member of the Board of Governors
Center for the Study of Violence
Brandeis University
Waltham, Mass.
Psychiatric and Medical Director
Foundation for the Prevention of Addictive Diseases
New York, N.Y.

The assassination of President John F. Kennedy in Dallas on that grim day in history, November 22, 1963, was only an hour and a half old when Lee Harvey Oswald was captured. Several hours later he was charged with the murder of the president and of J. D. Tippit, police officer, and, in the next 24 hours, he was tried and convicted by the news media and the public itself. His execution was equally swift, at the hands of his self-appointed executioner, Jack Ruby, in an unexpected, split-second shooting.

Throughout Lee Oswald's brief two-day imprisonment he relentlessly professed his innocence. During visits from his wife, his mother, and his brother Robert, his story remained unchanged. And even under intensive interrogation by the police—which lasted intermittently

*Material from the forthcoming book *The Violent Society* by David Abrahamsen, to be published by Random House, Inc. Part of this paper was presented at a meeting of the Association for the Advancement of Psychotherapy, New York, N. Y., at The New York Academy of Medicine, March 31, 1967.

for 12 hours, although there is no trace of its having been recorded—Oswald steadfastly denied he had shot President Kennedy or Officer Tippit.

Oswald wanted to—and did—take his secret to the grave. Such was his nature. In spite of the overwhelming accumulative evidence, nobody was going to learn from him whether he was truly the murderer. This is in contrast to assassins of previous presidents of the United States—Lincoln, Garfield, and McKinley—each of whom readily admitted his deed. As a matter of fact, each openly publicized his murderous act. Most well known in this respect is John Wilkes Booth who, after having shot President Lincoln, leaped to the stage and exclaimed: "*Sic semper tyrannis!*"[1]

But not Lee Harvey Oswald. Oswald's behavior after the assassination differed markedly in one respect from that of the other three assassins. No confession, no written statement was forthcoming from him to testify to any motive or responsibility on his part in killing President Kennedy.

The doubts created by the absence of a confession are manifold. Nurtured by worldwide controversy and emotional reactions to the death of a president, they have thrown a shroud of mystery around President Kennedy's murder and on the question of whether Oswald committed the crime—despite the Warren Commission's findings that he *was* the assassin and that he acted without assistance. This paper will show that if there were any conspiracy involved, Oswald was a conspirator against his own parents, his own family—against himself.

Although strong circumstantial evidence does seem to indicate Oswald's guilt, this claim should be substantiated by evidence of his psychological motivation and capability of murder, based upon our understanding of human behavior obtained through psychoanalytic knowledge. Here, however, I should like to cite Freud's reminder that we must "fix the limits of what psychoanalysis can accomplish in biography in order that every omitted explanation should not be held up to us as a failure."[2] From psychoanalytic experience we know that if we can uncover a person's early psychological motivations and their influence upon his character and personality structure, we are able not only to construct a meaningful picture of the forces shaping his past and present behavior, but also to predict some aspects of his possible future behavior.

This paper is therefore a study of Lee Harvey Oswald's instinctual and emotional development, his life experiences and behavior and, specifically, his psychological capability of murder in the light of what we already know of murderers in general and of Oswald in particular.

The goal of any psychoanalytic inquiry is to illustrate the connection between the person's external experiences and reactions to them and his behavior in the light of the instinctual vicissitudes and characterologic development. Even though a person does not admit to an act, criminal or otherwise, we may use our understanding of his instinctual and emotional make-up in determining whether the act in question lies within the realm of probability for him to commit.

As early as 1906 Freud pointed out, in a paper entitled "Psychoanalysis and the Ascertaining of Truth in Courts of Law," one of the differences between a criminal and a hysteric: "In the case of the criminal it is a secret which he knows and hides from you, but in the case of a hysteric it is a secret hidden from him, a secret he himself does not know."[3] Freud, more than anyone, however, was aware that both the neurotic and the criminal may unconsciously withhold information as a form of resistance against conscious awareness of the true meaning of the aggressive impulse and the object: as, for example, the criminal who may have killed a person representing his unconscious homosexual attachment to his parent of the same sex.

Using later corroboration of Freud's studies, we may say that ascertaining the tie-in between the criminal's personality structure and his deed is often further complicated by conscious elements as well. As I pointed out in 1944 in my paper, "The Dynamic Connection Between Personality and Crime,"[4] the criminal's act is repudiated and disowned, either wholly or in part, by his ego defenses, the ego repudiating a part of its own id as it does in all conflict situations. But in addition, even though the criminal is not psychotic, he frequently feels so consciously justified in his act that he denies it because he believes the punishment resulting from admission would be totally undeserved.

From my studies of the psychopathology of numerous murderers, I have observed that homicide is due not so much to murderous impulses per se, as to the *persistent, intense conflict* between the person's instinctual urges and his environment, which gives rise to these homicidal inclinations.

This conflict, due to serious early traumatic situations, is rooted primarily in childhood–in preoedipal fixations, particularly during the latter phase of oral development, with inability to withstand frustration and with impulsive hostile acting out.

This is seen in aspects of the character structure of many criminals who show heightened passivity–frequently an oral clinging with dependency reactions and, at the same time, impulsive or deliberate acting out of murderous rages when they have been disappointed because a superior or an equal has let them down, although these let-downs are often more fantasy than fact. In criminal gangs and in the Mafia, the oral inhibitions (not "squealing" on each other even in extreme circumstances) suggest the profound oral-dependent fixations as well as their great dependency upon one another. This mutual dependency in living and verbalizing is, in fact, stressed more heavily in the criminal society or organization than in any other group.

In studying the experiential factors in murders, one finds considerable evidence of sexually overstimulating experiences, including observation of parents' sexual intimacy (primal scene), in the development of profound psychosexual disturbance. The struggle against passivity frequently results in feelings of helplessness, often alternating with the defense against that helplessness, namely, hostile acting out and the consequent feeling of omnipotence.

Interestingly enough, we often find in murderers visual hypersensitivity and difficulties in speech and spelling as a result of a distorted relation between speech and the related process of thought in early childhood, a point in general emphasized by Dr. Phyllis Greenacre in the genesis of acting out.[5]

We are all aware that the manifestations of conflicts found in various types of criminals are also found in all forms of psychic disease. However, it is by the enlarged constellation and marked intensity of certain of these features that we may distinguish the murderer and the potentially dangerous person.

Research into murderers discloses that every homicide is unconsciously a suicide, brought about by the murderer's sudden and sharply increased loss of projected "self-esteem." This is of interest since, in a sense, every suicide is considered psychologically a homicide. The person is killing the introjected parent.

As a result of the impoverishment of his ego, there is a withdrawal of emotional interests, feelings, and concern–libidinal cathexes–from the outside world, as seen in depressed patients as well as in criminals. Here we find a mobilization of regressed fantasies centering fundamentally around feelings of vengefulness against the father in the oedipal situation.

An extreme case of vengefulness, narcissistic withdrawal, and fantasies of grandiose accomplishments is the 27-year-old man who, on three separate occasions during the course of a single week, killed a total of three people, ostensibly in order to rob them. Although of superior intelligence, he had had a severely disturbed childhood and a long criminal career prior to these murders.

To my question, "Did you feel guilt or remorse?" he answered: "To me, authority means nothing." Asked how he felt when he killed, he replied: "It doesn't bother me to kill. It doesn't result in emotions. It's like an animal instinct." And when I continued with, "You said you didn't care whom you killed. How about your wife and child?" his response was: "Oh, no. I wouldn't kill them because they are me"—seemingly an ego-ideal expression, but in actuality reflecting his primitive narcissism.

So distorted was his viewpoint that when he was asked, "Do you consider yourself a criminal?" he answered: "From society's standpoint, yes! A rebel against modern times." This distortion is also reflected in the fact that even while in prison facing a death sentence, which he finally received but which was later commuted, he still had fantasies about getting back at the district attorney, telling me, "I want to have my sweet revenge." Despite the fact that he was in a supreme state of passive helplessness—confined behind bars in a prison ensuring maximum security—he imagined himself as having the power to strike back.

It is surprising to note the relatively little attention accorded by criminologists, penologists, and law authorities to the relation between certain psychological elements and the criminal's behavior. When he commits his crime, it is invariably founded on his feeling that *he MUST show his mother that he is not insignificant and is able to take revenge upon her for rejecting him.* Indeed, it is the feeling of helplessness behind his acting out that is the most striking phenomenon. The self-betrayal that the criminal frequently exhibits by revisiting the scene of his crime stems not only from his unconscious need for punishment but also from his unconscious need *to proclaim that he is not helpless to strike back*. He must show his power by striking back—there is no other way out. He must show that this act of revenge belongs to him *alone*. These feelings are grouped around his oedipal helplessness—"the struggle against passivity,"[6] as Freud termed it—and his attempt to restore his narcissistic self-esteem.

In contrast to the openly hostile murderer, we have those in whom all hostility is disguised—often termed the "model child" type—and where there is an overwhelming emotional involvement with the victim.

A prime example is the 57-year-old unmarried woman who killed her 95-year-old mother. When I was called in to examine her at the prison ward of the psychiatric hospital, I learned that for 30 years she had held the same job, living with and supporting her aging mother and masochistically sacrificing her own desires in favor of her mother's demands. Only in the last few years had she openly exhibited her diverted hostile feelings by becoming suspicious and critical toward her co-workers.

Four months before the murder, her mother had suffered a broken hip and had become bedridden. With this staggering prospect of increased emotional, physical, and financial strain, the daughter became depressed and suicidal and sought the help of a psychiatrist, apparently in vain. Early one morning, as she watched her sleeping mother, she was overcome by confusion and hopelessness. Using a hammer she had covered with cloth to soften the blows to the skull, she clubbed her mother, who died the following day.

After receiving a suspended sentence, she came to me for treatment, during which she related a dream: "I was in a big spider web which covered the length of the bed. I must have moved to get out, but I woke up."

In her free associations, she said: "I think of my mother, the good times we had, of Christmastime, what we would have been doing—I have not gotten rid of mother, which is not the way things should be. I was caught in a web. I must have felt I was in her web."

This dream was her first realization of being ensnared by a devouring mother and her own flylike insignificance and helplessness. The web covering a bed suggests feelings of being seduced into submission, of a need for embryonic protection and growing awareness of her dependency and, perhaps most important, being forcibly prevented from having a sexual life of her own.

The fact is, she had remained a virgin and had had no romances because, in her own words, "I never had the time." Yet the major part of her sessions revolved around remembrances of how good her mother was, which revealed the continued inability to recognize the hostile feelings that had resulted in her reactive overdependence that eventually led her to murder. While her superego retained only the introject of her overwhelmingly demanding mother, in a masochistic way she created the image of a good mother who deserved obedience and love—the ego-ideal being made up of imaginary positive maternal components.

The prime mark of the murderer is a sense of helpless impotence and a preoccupation with revenge, carried over from early childhood. Intertwined with this nucleus of feelings, which color and distort his view of life and all his acts, are certain other traits characteristic of the actual or potential killer. If we observe such a person closely, we can detect many of these traits.

Perhaps most obvious is his irrational hatred for others, his suspiciousness and hypersensitivity to injustices or rejection. Hand in hand with these go his self-centeredness and inability to withstand frustration, so that he is given to frequent, uncontrollable emotional outbursts and impulsive indulgence in hostile acts as an expression of his need to retaliate and destroy.

We recognize these symptoms more readily in the person who kills in a fit of passion, who is so unable to bear the intensity of his tortured feelings that he must discharge them immediately. But the same current of twisted feelings, though much more disguised, is nevertheless operative in murderers who seem more withdrawn, self-centered, and calculating.

When he is unable to curb his hostile aggressive tendencies, the disruption of the ego defenses permits the emergence of murderous acting-out impulses. Through repressing any awareness of his intolerable reality situation, he avoids experiencing the real emotional content of his feelings. The danger level is reached when all former outlets for his hostile aggression have been exhausted. If he fails to find new outlets, and gratification in some form becomes impossible, his locked-in emotions are apt to burst through and engulf him.

In summing up, then, we may try to set down, *as an orientation only*, some distinguishing characteristics of the murderer (Table I).

We are now faced with the question: Does Lee Harvey Oswald's

Table I—SOME DISTINGUISHING CHARACTERISTICS OF THE MURDERER

1. Intense vengefulness and withdrawal due to feelings of helplessness, insignificance, and distrust related to preoedipal and also oedipal fixations.
2. Primal-scene experiences and sexually overstimulating situations.
3. Extreme regressive fantasy life, such as fantasies of grandiose accomplishments, which may facilitate acting out of hostile impulses.
4. Errors of speech or spelling related to possible disturbances during the preoedipal period.
5. Tendency toward plasticity in identification.
6. Inability to withstand frustration and to find sufficient gratification for the discharge of hostile aggressive drives through constructive outlets.
7. Inability to transform primitive narcissism into healthy ego-ideal and superego elements, with dependency expressed in subservience to or contempt for authority.
8. Suicidal tendencies with wide mood swings.
9. Victim often constitutes composite picture of murderer's self-image.
10. Previous antisocial, delinquent, or criminal acts accompanied by actual or threatened violence.

personality structure and behavior, so far as we can determine, give us distinct clues that fit him within the framework of a murderer?

As the basis for my study of Oswald I have studied his "Historic Diary," his letters to his mother, wife, and brother, extensive magazine and newspaper reports, the exhaustive Warren Commission hearings with the psychiatric examination of him at the age of 13, and material received through personal communication with others who have studied his and his family's background and life. Space permits me, however, to cover only the most salient aspects of life experiences which, to my mind, have had a crucial bearing upon his early development.

The many million words in the 26 volumes by the Warren Commission containing 552 witnesses' testimony related to President Kennedy's death include an exhaustive inquiry into Lee Harvey Oswald's life, behavior, and family background. Unfortunately, little of his early development was probed, and there are a great many contradictions, especially in the testimony of his mother, Marguerite Claverie Oswald, who had the most sustained contact with him. But although the information disclosed is spotty,* a picture of Lee Harvey Oswald's personality, with definite character traits, emerges.

One of the traits that stands out most consistently in the memories of those who knew Lee Harvey Oswald is that he was withdrawn and lonely.

*A great deal of material about Oswald's early childhood is also given by, among others, his aunt and mother's sister, Mrs. Lillian Murret; his mother's friend of some 25 years, Mrs. Myrtle Evans; his half-brother, John Pic; his brother, Robert Oswald; his wife, Marina Oswald; and many of his former schoolmates, teachers, and neighbors. Information about his adolescence and early adulthood is given by the aforementioned as well as by men who served with him in the United States Marines, and by Mrs. Ruth Paine and others who befriended Lee and Marina Oswald.

Mrs. Murret, the aunt with whom he lived on and off as a small child, states: "He would just rather stay in the house and read or something. . . . He wouldn't go out and play, and he just wanted to be in that room all the time, and he wouldn't even talk to the other children. . . ."[7] His mother says: "Lee was a very quiet and studious boy. . . . The children were always more or less home. And particularly Lee. . . . He was a normal boy. . . . He could keep himself occupied. . . ."[8] Mrs. Evans, close friend and landlady of Marguerite Oswald, says that "he didn't bring boys in the house . . . he would always seem to prefer being by himself . . . the way he kept to himself just wasn't normal, I think. . . ."[9] And Edward Voebel, a former junior high school classmate of Lee Oswald, states: "He didn't make friends. . . . People and things just didn't interest him generally. He was just living in his own world. . . . Lee didn't go out and look for friends. He didn't seem to care about having friends. . . ."[10]

Although his brother Robert states that he considered Lee to be normal in every way,[11] the impression of Lee as lonely, uncommunicative, and unfriendly or even hostile is also confirmed by almost everyone who knew him, including his wife and his fellow Marines.

The details of Lee's infancy and early childhood indicate that he was predisposed to becoming severely disturbed emotionally. His problems began early, in a sense before he was born. His father's sudden death two months before Lee's birth in New Orleans on October 18, 1939, and his mother's subsequent financial difficulties were the beginning of a disrupted infancy and childhood that were to have far-reaching consequences. As with many children faced with the same circumstances, Lee's inability to understand his father's death may have made him imagine that his father had not cared about him, that he had thought of him as a burden or had deserted him for being "bad." The passing of the father and his own uprooting not only deprived Lee of the influence of a father with whom he could identify and of a mother's consistent care, but also robbed him of a home and family life with constant parental figures.

Lee stayed in his aunt's house with his mother, his five-year-old brother Robert, and eight-year-old half-brother, John Pic, for one or two months, until Mrs. Oswald began to go to work.[12] The family was then split up; Mrs. Oswald went back to her home with Lee, while his two brothers were put in a Lutheran boarding home. The neglect in his early childhood is shown inadvertently by his mother's own testimony: "I let a couple have my home, plus $15 a month in order to care for Lee while I worked, and this couple after about two months' time had neglected Lee and so I had to put them out of the house and there again I had to quit a job, and take care of Lee until I could make arrangements and my sister could help me with it." [13] Myrtle Evans says that neighbors told Marguerite Oswald that ". . . when Lee was in the high chair . . . he used to cry a lot, and they thought they were whipping little Lee, so she came home unexpectedly one night, and the child had welts on his legs, and she told them to get out and get out now."[14]

There were many different people who took care of Lee—an aunt, maids, couples, baby-sitters. It is reported that one baby-sitter who lived with the Oswalds for 14 days in the middle of 1942, when Lee was two-and-a-half years old, had said that "she couldn't take it any longer . . . he wouldn't listen and he was bad. He had a little toy gun, and he threw it after her and broke the chandelier in the bedroom. . . . He threw it at her when he got mad, and she had an awful time with him. . . ."[15] The many difficulties his mother had are again shown by her own testimony: "So when Lee was three years old, I was having it very difficult with Lee, because of the different people to take care of Lee, and the different jobs I had to give up."[16]

Unable to cope with her situation with Lee, she put him in the same boarding home as his two brothers—on the day after Christmas in 1942. But this place, too, was a transitory one, since she took him out from time to time for varying periods. This fact made it difficult for Lee to be close to anyone, not only because of the great age difference between him and his brothers but also because his mother, whenever in the mood, insisted upon having him stay with her, an impression we find confirmed in various testimony.

The circumstances following the death of Lee's father were such as to prevent Lee's formation of adequate identifications and, thus, of sound ego and superego development. It may be added that, according to various reports, his mother had wanted a girl when Lee was born. This, no doubt, aroused in her feelings of guilt toward Lee for which she tried to compensate by smothering him with love. We may also assume, on the basis of the data, that her intermittent overindulgence of Lee could be further related to her feelings of guilt over boarding him out and her identification with him as an orphan, Lee's mother having herself been a semiorphan. Her mother had died in 1911, when Marguerite Claverie Oswald was four or five years old[17] and, like Lee, she too had been raised by relatives and housekeepers her father had engaged.[18]

Marguerite is described in her youth as having been a "very beautiful girl,"[19] gregarious, talented, and "money conscious."[20] In making a living for herself she was ingenious. Her tongue was sharp; "she was a person that kept to herself."[21] Proud and independent, wanting the best for her children, she was quick to pretend in a moment of anger she needed no one; yet her ambivalence came to the fore in that she showed strong dependency and self-pity in accepting money and other favors from her sister. Because of her narcissistic self-esteem she used terms such as "people of our caliber" and took it for granted that help should be given her, although she resented any inference that she would accept charity.

Mrs. Murret, her eldest sister, relates that "if you disagreed with her or if you expressed an opinion that she didn't agree with then she would insist that you were wrong. . . . She would do things at the spur of the minute . . ." and was impulsive. . . . "She would just act right now regardless of the consequences once she made up her mind." She was also unforgiving. Easily offended, she would walk off in a huff and not talk to the person for months. Then, when she needed something, she would come back as if nothing had ever happened.[22] And Lee, in many ways, showed very similar behavioral traits, as we shall see later.

If Lee's life was to be dramatic, so was his mother's. Three months pregnant, she left her first husband, Edward John Pic, Jr.; then she married Robert Edward Lee Oswald, who died; and in July 1943 she met Edwin A. Ekdahl, whom she married in 1945 after an intermittent courtship. After three years of arguments, separations, reconciliations, and new arguments, they were divorced in 1948, the jury finding that Marguerite was "guilty of excesses, cruel treatment or outrages" unprovoked by Ekdahl's conduct.[23]

In Marguerite Oswald's emotional make-up we find many of Lee's traits, in particular her rigidity, unrealistic and narcissistic self-idolatry and attention-seeking, withdrawal, hypersensitivity, possessiveness, disrespect for authority, false pride, exploitation of people, cruelty, impulsiveness, and acting out regardless of consequences. In Lee, however, these traits were more sharply delineated, in particular his tendency toward acting out, withdrawal, sadism, desire to be in the limelight, and contempt for authority.

We have relatively little information about the first 18 months of Lee's life. Indirectly, though, we can surmise that there was considerable disturbance during this phase, since he was unmanageable, as we have seen. And later, in his early teens, according to Mrs. Evans:

"He would come home, and he would get his books and his music, and then when he wanted supper, or something to eat, he would scream like a bull. He would holler, 'Maw, where's my supper?'. . . . Her whole life was wrapped up in that boy, and she spoiled him to death. Lee was about 13 about that time. . . .[24] The main thing that seems to stand out in his conduct was the way he demanded to be fed when he would come from school. Margie would be downstairs maybe, talking to me or something, and he would come to the head of the stairs and yell for her to come up and fix him something to eat. He would just stand up there and yell, 'Maw, how about fixing me something to eat?' and she would jump up right away and go running upstairs to get something for him. . . .[25] Lee had reached the point where he was noisier and more determined with his mother, and it was getting a little unbearable. . . . It seemed to be a situation that was getting worse all the time. . . ."[26]

Lee's persistent oral demands were associated with an inability to tolerate not only direct oral frustration but all frustration of derivative oral strivings.

Although we also have no specific information about Lee's development from 18 months to 3 years of age, the impressions of his half-brother John Pic from the years in the children's boarding home are interesting: ". . . Robert and I enjoyed Bethlehem. . . . Things for myself became worse when Lee came there. . . . They had a ruling that if you had a younger brother or sister there and they had bowel movements in their pants the older brothers would clean them up, and they would yank me out of classes in school to go do this and, of course, this peeved me very much. . . ."[27]

At the age of almost three-and-a-half, Lee was either not yet toilet-trained or frequently regressed to soiling himself. His later parsimony and cruelty are suggestive of problems and fixations related to his anal phase of development and the traits of the so-called anal character.

Of special significance also is the fact that throughout most of his childhood Lee slept in the same bed with his mother, as revealed in his half-brother's testimony: "Lee slept with my mother until I joined the service in 1950. This would make him approximately ten, well almost eleven years old. . . . In the same bed. . . ."[28]

We are all well aware of the feelings of guilt, revulsion, and fear of being devoured that are elicited through such intimacy.

Mrs. Evans' testimony further reveals Marguerite Oswald's excessive attachment to Lee: "She dumped all her love on Lee. . . .[29] She kept Lee with her all the time (during her marriage to Edwin Ekdahl and possibly for a period preceding it) so that they would all be together on these business trips he had to take. . . . He was her baby, and she loved him to death . . . and she spoiled him to death. . . . I don't think that she ever parted with Lee for a minute. . . . She just poured out all her love on him, it seemed. . . ."[30]

Keeping Lee close to her all the time may well have exposed him to his mother's intimate sexual experiences and to sexual overstimulation which, during his oedipal stage, would have reinforced his affection and hatred for the intruder, and stirred up considerable castration anxiety and fear in him. His strong ties to his mother, which may have reinforced his "femininity" and undoubted castration fears, showed up later in his pronounced shyness with girls, his attempts to belittle other men, his interest in uniforms and guns, and his loss of sexual interest, ending in impotence, during his marriage. Only for a short time, while in the Marines and in the Union of Soviet Socialist Republics, did he exhibit interest in girls, apparently because he was outside his mother's domain. But once he was back in the United States, his need for maternal dependency came through again in his relation both with his mother and with his wife.

Most important for our probing of his disturbed psychosexual development, however, is his having slept with his mother for so many years and his probable exposure to his mother's and stepfather's sexual intimacy—primal scene—further stimulating his infantile anger and increasing his already severe frustrations. Such sexual overstimulation, in combination with his heightened orality, narcissism, and decreased tolerance for frustration, may well have elicited scopophilic acting-out tendencies that he partially gratified through incessant reading, through

Table II—EXAMPLES OF SPELLING ERRORS IN LEE HARVEY OSWALD'S WRITINGS

| | | | |
|---|---|---|---|
| Complusery | Compulsory | Opions | Opinions |
| Kicten | Kitchen | Esspicialy | Especially |
| Yonuge | Young | Jelous | Jealous |
| Exalant | Excellent | Conservorie | Conservatory |
| Tehniction | Technician | Aquiataces | Acquaintance |
| Sptacular | Spectacular | Domatory | Dormitory |
| Divocied | Divorced | Cimima | Cinema |
| Oppossition | Opposition | Arrestled | Arrested |
| Enviorments | Environments | Disire | Desire |
| Permonet | Permanent | Reture | Return |
| Admiriers | Admirers | Understade | Understand |
| Habituatated | Habituated | Admirares | Admirers |
| Quiality | Quality | Freiend | Friend |
| Patroict | Patriotic | Marraige Beaure | Marriage Bureau |

watching television all day and, later, through observing and investigating. For example, in a letter he sent from the Soviet Union to his brother Robert, November 26, 1959, he wrote: "I have been a pro-communist for years and yet I have never met a communist, instead I kept silent and observed. . . ."[31] And a former Marine acquaintance also confirmed that "it (meaning Oswald's going to Russia to investigate Communism personally rather than simply joining the American Communist Party) seemed to fit his personality."[32] This scopophilic acting out later was transformed into exhibitionistic acting out. He identified with dictators such as Fidel Castro, which allowed him to act out in an exhibitionistic way by imitation of the dictator as well as to identify with the aggressor. This he ultimately carried to a peak where, secretly, he became the arch aggressor through a criminal act.

Exhibitionism associated with childhood disturbances may manifest itself in a variety of ways, among them delayed speech and poor spelling. Although Oswald may have had impediments in speech, we have no information about them. But we do know that his ability to spell was greatly impaired. The record shows that in the third grade he received *A*'s in all subjects but *D* in spelling. His fourth-grade "IQ was recorded at 103; on achievement tests in each of the three years (fourth, fifth, and sixth), he twice did best in reading and twice did worst in spelling."[33] In 1952 his IQ on the Wechsler Intelligence Scale for Children was 118, indicating, the psychologist noted, "a present intellectual functioning in the upper range of bright normal intelligence."[34]

The numerous errors of spelling in his "Historic Diary," letters, and notes are striking (Table II).

These errors express onomatopoesis—the making of a name or word from a sound. His extensive writing as well as his continual need to expound his political views verbally served more as a means of exhibiting himself than of communication. Listening to a phonograph record I received of his radio interview in New Orleans about Castro during early autumn in 1963, I received the distinct impression that Oswald was merely talking, without giving any deeper meaning to what he was saying. It seemed that instead of communicating he was exhibiting himself.

His misspellings originated from the same root as his craving to be in the limelight, to be dramatic, the center of attraction. His narcissistic desire was to call attention to himself, to pose and display himself and others, to appear more than he was. The manifestation of the childhood disturbances in association with this hysterical form of exhibitionism is a common attribute of schizophrenic conditions.[35]

His need to call attention to himself was also vividly manifested in other areas of his short life. In his earlier years he tried to amuse people by clowning. For example, he made a joke of his ill-fitting shirt by saying, "Ma bought 'em big. She thought they'd shrink."[36] A photograph of Lee in the classroom at the age of 15 shows the entire class paying serious attention to the teacher except for Lee, who is facing the photographer in the rear of the room, pointing to himself and mugging for the camera.[37] His clowning, we may assume, was also a defense against his feelings of insignificance. Lee went to Moscow secretly, thus increasing the element of shock in his defection. There, he walked into the United States embassy and threw his passport on the desk, declaring he was through with America. And later, according to his "Historic Diary,"[38] he went to the Soviet embassy and offered to reveal everything he knew of Marine Corps operations, certain that this would impress his Soviet hosts and coerce them into accepting his application for citizenship. When he returned to the United States in 1962, he

TABLE III—DELINQUENCY AND VIOLENCE IN LEE HARVEY OSWALD

1) 1948—Chased half-brother, John Pic, with a knife and threw it at him.[40]
2) 1952—Threatened John Pic's wife with pocket knife during a quarrel.[41]
3) 1952—Struck his mother during same quarrel (second reported incident of his having hit her).
4) 1952—Extensive truancy. Of 64 school days, he was "present on 15 full and 2 half days. . . ."[42]
5) 1953—Remanded to Youth House for 3 weeks (April 16 to May 7, 1953) and then put on probation.
6) 1955—Wrote and signed note to his school, under his mother's name, falsely stating he must leave school because they were moving out of town, although his plan was to join Marine Corps.
7) 1956-1959—Court-martialed twice in Marine Corps (once for insubordination, once for illegal possession of a gun).
8) 1956-1959—Shot himself in the hand "accidentally" while in Marines.
9) 1959—Attempted suicide in the U.S.S.R.
10) 1962-1963—Used aliases and falsified his identification card.
11) 1962-1963—Struck his wife on a number of occasions.[43]
12) 1963—Shot at General Edwin A. Walker.

was disappointed because "there were no photographers present when he arrived. . . ."[39]

Connected with his need to show off and shock people, which turned his neurotic tendencies into acting out, we see his antisocial, delinquent, and criminal activities before he was accused of assassinating President Kennedy (Table III). It would be wrong, though, not to include the minor delinquencies displayed by his mother, who may have unwittingly reinforced Lee's own criminal propensities (Table IV).

In Lee's case, his acting-out impulses reflected an organized activity rooted in an inability to withstand frustration connected with unconscious fantasies related to the primal scene–frustrations producing helpless impotence and a preoccupation with fantasies of revenge.

His wish to show off, though, was ambivalently tinged, counterbalanced by withdrawal (possibly a narcissistic withdrawal) and by his desire for revenge that he wanted simultaneously to proclaim and yet to keep secret. This secret was kept alive in his fantasies, the range of which may indicate their seriousness:

In a report by the psychiatric social worker at New York City's Youth House for Boys, to which Lee was remanded from April 13

TABLE IV—DELINQUENCY IN MOTHER, MRS. MARGUERITE OSWALD

1) 1945—Changed Lee Harvey Oswald's birth date from October 18, 1939 to July 9, 1939, to get him into elementary school earlier.[44]

2) 1947—Exposed 16-year-old son, John Pic, to stepfather's infidelity by having him and his young friend accompany her to the other woman's home, where the friend posed as Western Union messenger so that Mrs. Oswald could force her way into the apartment.

3) 1948—Falsely swore John Pic was 17, so that he could join Marine Corps Reserves to supplement family income. Disapproved of his going back to finish school, which compelled him to sign her name to report cards and excuse notes.[45]

4) 1953—Without notifying authorities, when Lee was on probation as a truant, she left New York City with him and moved back to New Orleans.

5) 1955—Arranged with lawyer for papers showing Lee's age as 17 instead of 16, so that he could join Marine Corps, although authorities discovered his true age and refused the application.

to May 7, 1953, because of truancy, it is stated that "he admitted to fantasies about being powerful and sometimes hitting and killing people, but refused to elaborate on them."[46] Lee was then 13 years old.

The psychiatrist's report from the same institution says of his fantasies: "Lee has vivid fantasy life turning around the topics of omnipotence and power through which he tries to compensate for his present shortcomings and frustrations."[47] This same report also states that "Lee has to be diagnosed as a personality pattern disturbance with schizoid features and passive-aggressive tendencies."[48] Nowhere does the report state, as erroneously reported in news media, that Lee was considered potentially dangerous and suffering from schizophrenia. However, as we can see from his later fantasies and behavior, in all probability he was already at least borderline paranoid.

At the age of 16 he worked out a plan to steal a pistol displayed in a store window by using a glass cutter to cut the window and by using a plastic pistol to threaten any intruders. His classmate, to whom he had divulged the plan, says: "It was just a fantastic thing he got in his mind."[49] Lee never carried out the plan.

His wife, Marina, describes Lee in one respect as different from other people: ". . . at least his imagination, his fantasy, which was quite unfounded, as to the fact that he was an outstanding man . . . he was very much interested . . . in autobiographical works of outstanding statesmen of the United States and others . . . I think that he compared himself to these people."[50] Indicating that the prospect of helping Cuba seemed to quicken his hopes of fame, she further testified: "He was even interested in the airplane schedules, with the idea of kidnapping a plane. I talked him out of it."[51] And in another segment: "He very much wanted to go to Cuba and have the newspapers write that somebody had kidnapped an aircraft. . . . He said that after 20 years he would be prime minister. I think that he had a sick imagination—at least at that time I already considered him to be not quite normal—not always, but at times. . . ."[52]

The lack of a permanent father, and the trauma of Ekdahl's all too short-lived presence, were Lee's greatest narcissistic personal, emotional injury. This, in addition to the many substitute father and mother figures in his childhood, made the boundaries of Lee's ego fluid and, at the same time, made possible his different identifications —a plasticity of identification such as we find in the schizophrenic or even the homosexual person, or in the criminal where lack of identification with father-law-authority is so conspicuous as not to require elaboration. The weakness of Lee's ego due to his narcissistic disposition also resulted in clinging yet fluctuating relations built on infantile dependency or on a narcissistic object choice—that further led to unstable identification and dread of emotional involvement.

One of the most striking examples of his inability to be emotionally involved occurred in 1959 as Oswald was nearing the end of his duty with the Marines in California. His mother, ill and apparently unable to work because of a nasal injury, persuaded Lee to obtain a release on grounds of hardship so that he could return home to support her. But after barely three days at home he insisted upon leaving again. According to his mother . . . "he wanted to work on a ship in the import and export business" because he felt that was the only way he could earn enough money with his lack of skills and training. Despite her pleading with him to remain, on the third day . . . "he came with his suitcase in the room and said, 'Mother, I am off.' So since his mind was made up, I told him goodbye."[53]

Although apparently he had saved $1,600 while in the service, his mother states that all he gave her was $100 to tide her over until her insurance claim was settled. Quite obviously, he had used her illness as a means to his own narcissistic ends, to hasten his long-planned defection to the Soviet Union. He had in fact obtained his Soviet visa in Los Angeles shortly before returning home. So obsessed was he with his own immediate gratification that he could not postpone his desires even when his mother seemed to need him most.

On September 19, 1959, two weeks after leaving his mother, he wrote her the following brief letter from New Orleans:

> Dear Mother:
>
> Well, I have booked passage on a ship to Europe. I would of had to sooner or later and I think its best to go now. Just remember above all else that my values are very different from Roberts or your's. It is difficult to tell you how I feel. Just remember this is what I must do. I did not tell you my plans because you could harly be expected to understand.
>
> I did not see Aunt Lillian while I was here.
>
> I will write again as soon as I land.
>
> Lee.[54]

On the surface, the letter seems no more than a cryptic apology. But reading between the lines reveals a great deal more. The entire tone is accusing yet wistful, almost resigned; determined, yet pleading for acceptance. He intimates that his mother approves more of Robert because his brother shares her attitudes, and he is helpless in trying to be like them. He has despaired of making her understand his feelings and must therefore keep them to himself—in order to be free of her control, he must be secretive.

The letter gives us an inkling of his jealousy, of his sense of isolation, of his intense narcissism, and of his fear of involvement with her.

Significant also in these brief lines is his unexpressed hostility toward his mother, a "You never loved me so I may as well do what's good for me!" There is not so much as perfunctory concern for her health or finances. He left her to discover his true intentions from newspaper reporters some weeks later, hung up on her in November when she phoned him in Moscow, sent her a note in December asking for money without even knowing whether she could afford it, and then wrote her and Robert in January, 1960, to the effect that "I do not wish to ever contact you again. I am beginning a new life and I don't want any part of the old."[55] He never wrote her again until about two years later, in 1961, when all his attempts to get out of the Soviet Union had been unsuccessful and he obviously needed her help once more. We see here behavior that is not only regressive in character;

rather his whole behavior is anaclitic in the sense that as long as his mother can do anything for him, he is good to her. But if she is unable to help him, he loses all interest in her—and in all values.

His desire for revenge, presumably against only the depriving mother, was also unconsciously directed against the missing father whom he had wished, at the same time, to replace—all bringing about unconscious feelings of guilt that demanded punishment. His image of father and mother became intertwined, a confusion of giving and withholding that he projected into others. The world became nothing but an endless procession of people tantalizing him, holding things out to him on a string—giving and punishing.

Nowhere more than in Lee's attitude toward the United States and the Soviet Union did he express so symbolically his fantasy wish for the all-giving father-mother, the death wish against the abandoning father and seductive-rejecting mother, and his desire to lash out and punish them both by rejection. When the United States failed to fulfill his expectations, he deserted, pinning all his hopes on finding his Utopia in the Soviet Union. But there was also disillusionment there, and he soon moved toward rejecting again.

Lee's feeling of rejection first hit a low point when, five days after he had arrived in Moscow, the police telephoned. Since his visa had expired that day, they said he must leave the country within two hours. This was a crushing blow. For years he had lived in the fantasy that the country would welcome him with open arms, like a good parent and, instead, they were rejecting him outright, as if he were an orphan. Lee's reaction was immediate and violent. He slashed his wrist in a suicide attempt. A person with a sound mind would have reacted less hysterically, but to Lee Oswald, remaining in the Soviet Union was truly a matter of life and death.

Again the manifestation of secret exhibitionism had come to the fore. His attempt at suicide suggests a violent acting out of a rejection fantasy and perhaps a reenactment of past violent reactions to imagined or real rejections. His intent in committing suicide—the wish to be dead—signified an unconscious identification with his dead father, a point so well demonstrated by Freud in "Dostoyevsky and Parricide."[56] But the attempt also served to put Lee in the limelight.

Only the quick action of a girl who had befriended him saved his life. Waking up in the hospital ward for the insane was a shock to

Lee. Seeing the other mentally ill patients frightened and upset him. No doubt it was like looking in a mirror, and he cringed from his own reflection. After much insistence and complaining, he was moved, after a few days, to the regular ward. In his "Historic Diary" he commented that the nurses there were suspicious of him. He did not recognize the extent of his own emotional sickness–the threatening disintegration of his personality structure.

His despondency was soon offset, however, by the attention he gained. Not only was he released from the hospital and his visa extended, but the Soviet Union gave him financial subsidy, an apartment in Minsk, and a job at which he earned a good salary. Women flocked around him, and for a while he could feel superior to other men. He was in high spirits now.

But soon everything changed. He grew disenchanted with the Soviet system, the discipline, and the party rules and restrictions. His dissatisfaction reached a peak, it would seem, when the girl with whom he fell in love refused his proposal of marriage. Now, when the Soviet Union offered him citizenship, he turned it down, reverting to his old pattern of rejecting everyone whenever he felt rejected. He applied at the United States embassy for return to the United States.

In the light of his past withdrawal from close emotional relations, Lee Oswald's marrying Soviet-born Marina Nicolaevna Pruskova and having two children with her is surprising. But this, too, was part of his need for revenge. He had married her on the rebound, to hurt the girl who had turned him down. Although he eventually felt he loved Marina and did bring her to the United States with him, his narcissistic pattern nevertheless ran true to form; she and the children were primarily sources of *self-gratification,* his own needs taking precedence over theirs. He would leave home and return according to the pressure of his own compulsive drives. Although he could seldom provide them with even the barest of necessities because of difficulty in finding and holding jobs, he nevertheless indulged himself with such personal extravagances as having his notes on the Soviet Union typed professionally, buying a rifle, and having circulars printed for his activities in the committee on Fair Play for Cuba. All too often his family's comfort depended upon the kindness of Marina's Russian-speaking friends. Yet their efforts were usually rewarded with Lee's jealous resentment rather than gratitude.

Although sometimes affectionate toward his wife, for the most part he was domineering and possessive, punishing, and castrating. Marina admitted that Lee had struck her on a number of occasions and that he was quick to rebuke her harshly for such trifles as being five minutes late with dinner or forgetting to serve the butter. Although she was a stranger in a foreign country, he refused to help her learn English because *he* wanted practice in speaking Russian. And he seemed determined to keep her from having friends, in fact drove away any except those who could overlook his arrogance and sullenness.

Once rejected, Lee never forgave. In his paranoid-tinged obsession, anyone who opposed him loomed as an authority and a threat to his masculinity. This feeling may also have derived from an unconscious homosexual conflict that became heightened by his impotence. In the past, Lee's defense had been withdrawal, which had served a dual purpose: he could ward off rejections and inflict them simultaneously. Thus self-preservation and revenge had been interlocked. No one could hurt him, but he could hurt them. He was in control—superior and safe.

This defense, however, no longer brought him gratification. His self-regard was, as in others with similar character structure, intimately connected with his narcissistic libido. The greater the loss of genuine self-esteem, the more he withdrew from the outer world.

But loneliness and feeling left out were not in themselves enough to turn Lee into a murderer. It was the accumulation and relentlessness of the rejections he experienced and the way he reacted to them. It was his inability to appraise himself and others realistically, the degree to which he felt unjustly persecuted. It was the feeling that he must refrain from making any demands and that he dared not express any anger over his frustration. Above all, it was the hopelessness that resulted from his still unexpressed anger and, consequently, the extent to which he had to withdraw into his fantasies to find satisfaction.

Because of his primitive narcissism, it became impossible to deflect gratification into personal, social, or altruistic values.

His egocentricity having remained on a pregenital level, he had failed to develop what later should have become a mature ego-ideal. What he projected ahead of him as his ego-ideal was only a substitute for the narcissistic gratification he had lost in his childhood, exactly in the period of his life when he was his own ideal. The libidinal object remained principally homosexual, as evidenced by the way he related to strong masculine figures and his attempt to act out this strength by imitation. In his relations with his mother and wife he took on the role of dictator, but on a childish–preoedipal–level. On the oedipal level, however, he had to act out the unconscious impulse to kill the strong person.

By early autumn, 1963, Lee's feelings of rejection and frustration were reaching a new peak. The Soviet Union had disappointed him, he had failed to reverse the undesirable discharge issued by the Marines, and he was losing job after job in the United States. Now Lee was in a fury, obsessed with vengefulness and with proving his own power. He would show the Soviet people what a mistake they had made in waiting so long to accept him. He would show *everyone* that he could not be humiliated, pushed around like an insignificant child. His feelings of persecution became magnified. He saw all men as wielders of power, always standing in his way, a constant threat to his having whatever he wanted. These men were authorities he had to combat.

Although Lee Oswald had great hostility toward women, his hatred for men was far deeper and more consuming. He felt both rejected and overwhelmed by them. They stimulated his feelings of helplessness and doubts about his own masculinity, which he had to conceal in order to maintain his own sexual identity. There was only one way he could assuage these fears–by showing contempt for men and remaining aloof from them. He dared not come close to them for fear of being exposed and rejected. His withdrawal and reticence served a dual purpose: he could ward off rejections and inflict them simultaneously. Thus self-preservation and revenge were interlocked, as mentioned before. He felt no one could hurt him, but he could hurt them.

Now, however, this defense no longer brought enough satisfaction. He had to show his power more directly. But, as in childhood, he was biding his time. He kept his every move secret. That way he could look down on them as he felt they had looked down on him. He could enjoy the feeling of knowing something they did not know–that he was as powerful as they. And one day he would shock them all by proving it. Secretly, and under a false name, A. Hidell, he bought a rifle and practiced at a firing range. His use of the name Hidell is interesting, since it starts with the same letter as his real middle name, indicating that for narcissistic reasons he could not give up the first letter of his real name even in falsification—he could not completely give up his own identity. In this connection it is worth mentioning that the main reason Heinrich Himmler, chief of the Nazi Gestapo, was caught by the British Intelligence Service at the end of World War II was that he had taken on a pseudonym that began with the same letter, *H*, as his real name. Himmler, too, could not completely give up his own self.

In Oswald's case, the gun, a symbol of masculinity, bolstered and reinforced his feeling of manliness and power. One night he had taken a shot at General Edwin A. Walker, a man who was against all social progress that would give people the "fair share" to which Lee Oswald felt entitled. Once again he had failed, and this no doubt redoubled his need to make himself felt.

In his paranoid-schizophrenic state of mind and exalted opinion of himself, he was indignant and enraged at the world that refused him the recognition he felt was his due. Although he concealed it well, he was in a state of frantic desperation. Now he knew what he wanted to do and proceeded with a one-track mind. All his thoughts and acts revolved around his only goal: proving his worth and power. He worked out his scheme with singular secretiveness. The same deception he had used all his life to hide his fears he now transplanted to calculating his plans for revenge.

On or about September 23, 1963, he deceived his wife by telling her that he was going to Houston to look for a job. He sent her from New Orleans to Dallas with a friend, and he himself disappeared the following day from his cheap lodging without paying his bill. Instead of looking for a job, he went to Mexico City on September 24; he conspired to obtain a visa back to the Soviet Union via Cuba. His request was for himself *alone*. When he was told at the Cuban consulate that he needed a visa from the country of destination before they could do anything for him, Lee flew into a rage and slammed out of the place. Adding insult to injury, the Soviet embassy told him it would take four months before they could act on his application. Again men in authority stood in his way. But now there was no holding him back; he was determined to win out over them. In a mood of rejection and defiance, Oswald finally had to go back to Texas on October 3, 1963.

Exactly what his motives were in wanting to return to the U.S.S.R. is not completely clear, but conjecture offers a number of possibilities. It may have been his old pattern of rejecting the United States because he had again been rejected by her. More likely, though, it was a way of insuring his escape once he had murdered someone who opposed all that the Soviet Union represented; he could then return in triumph to that country, where they would acclaim him as their hero.

The night before President Kennedy's assassination was a tumultuous one for Oswald. He had been living in a room in Dallas, to be closer to his new job at the Texas School Book Depository, and now spent only weekends with Marina and the children, who were staying with a friend in nearby Irving. But that Thursday he returned unexpectedly, ostensibly to patch up a quarrel with his wife. She had been angry with him after discovering he had rented his room under an assumed name, and hardly talked to him. He tried to placate her, but she remained cool and aloof, although she testified later that she had not been as angry as she had pretended. Marina stated that Lee was upset and went to bed before her; she thinks he did not sleep much that night. When she awoke the next morning he was gone, and she later discovered he had left his ring and $170 in a dish on a dresser—possibly as a symbolic goodbye, since he had taken his rifle with him at that time.

Marina's inconsistent, submissive-rejecting behavior merits attention here because it is similar to that of the wives of many sex offenders. As disclosed in a research project I conducted a number of years ago, these women are often basically masculine types who compete with men; frequently they unconsciously provoke their husband's rape of another woman by being seductive and then rejecting.[57] In Marina's case, her masochistic submissiveness covered over the masculine and aggressive attitudes by which she attempted to deny her femininity. But her ability to control Lee was a threat to his masculinity and no doubt revived his childhood (the oedipal) helplessness he had felt toward his mother. Marina's rejecting and hostile attitude that evening may therefore have been acting as an added precipitant in his determination to carry out his secret plans.

In his paranoid-schizoid state of mind and deflated opinion of himself, his regressed fantasies of proving his power by taking revenge became imperative.

Obviously Lee Oswald was no ordinary killer. He would not have chosen his victim at random; in that sense he was special. Lee Oswald chose a victim that was all he had ever wanted to have and be but could not–someone who could command attention and control others as he himself wished so desperately to do. President John F. Kennedy fitted well within that frame. He was the composite of all Lee's yearnings and frustrations. John Kennedy belonged to a close family, he had a father who protected him, and John Kennedy had power and authority. He was commander-in-chief of the armed forces, including the Marines. As president, he represented all the United States–the United States Lee now hated more than ever for belittling and degrading him as long as he could remember.

Perhaps most significant, President Kennedy was a father, the father of the country and the father of two children toward whom he showed great love.

Lee's old narcissistic hurt–abandonment by his father and deprivation by his mother–was being revived. His disrupted family life had made him turn to the Marines, where he had hoped to find masculine identification, gratification for his dependency needs, and yet an escape from the greatest menace, his mother. But not only were these unrealistic expectations not fulfilled during his service in the Marines; later the Marine Corps had even refused to rescind his undesirable discharge. All this led Oswald to see the Marines as the frustrating object. His anger at this frustrating object underwent a change–a displacement toward the government of the United States, followed by its being focused toward the president, who was the embodiment of the government. His desperate need to identify with Marxism was an unconscious rejection of his own parents–as represented by the government of the United States.

President Kennedy was the composite of Lee's parental images, fundamentally a mother figure with a superimposed father figure from whom he ambivalently expected either total help or punishment–or both. The murder was both an act of self-punishment and of revenge–castration of himself as punishment for his death wish against a hated mother and father, as well as castration of the man who represented those powerful figures and a proclamation to his mother that he was strong—a man. But in killing John F. Kennedy, Oswald also unconsciously expressed his deep longing for death. His homicide was unconsciously a suicide—signifying his identification with his dead father—a death that he craved and that was so ironically fulfilled.

In view of Lee Harvey Oswald's highly disturbed early childhood emotional development, the distortion of his character that resulted in the lack of superego and ego-ideal formation, his inability to withstand frustration and his hostile acting out, his displaced anger toward men and his lack of masculine identification, his withdrawal, his narcissistic core that led him to feelings of being insignificant and powerless and to excessive feelings of revenge and fantasies of grandiose accomplishments, his previous delinquent acts and his previous violent act representing desires to harm a person seriously, we find an intimate connection between his personality structure and a motivation and capability of homicide. Therefore, in conclusion, I find that Oswald was psychologically capable of murder.

Oswald's predominant motive was revenge, and he carried it even beyond the murder. Denying the crime increased his sense of power and intensified the gratification he derived from his revenge. Like the secret of sexual intimacy his mother once kept from him, he now had a secret of his own. He alone knew the answer that no one else knew. In the words of Shakespeare, "The rest is silence."

## *REFERENCES*


1. Weissman, P. Why Booth killed Lincoln, A psychoanalytic study of a historic tragedy. In: *Psychoanalysis and the Social Sciences,* vol. 5. New York, Int. Univ. Press, 1958, p. 100.
2. Freud, S. *Leonardo da Vinci, A Study in Psychosexuality.* New York, Random House, 1947, p. 118.
3. Freud, S. Psychoanalysis and the ascertaining of truth in courts of law. In: *Collected Papers,* vol. 2. London, Lund Humphries, 1924, p. 18.
4. Abrahamsen, D. The dynamic connection between personality and crime and the detection of the potential criminal illustrated by different types of murder, *J. Criminal Psychopathol. 5*:482, 1944.
5. Greenacre, P. *Trauma, Growth and Personality.* New York, Norton, 1952, p. 227.
6. Freud, S. Analysis terminable and interminable. In: *Collected Papers,* vol. 5. London, Hogarth, and Inst. Psychoanal., 1950, p. 355.
7. *Hearings Before the President's Commission on the Assassination of President Kennedy.* Washington, D.C., Govt. Print. Off., 1964, vol. 8, p. 122.
8. *Ibid.,* vol. 1, pp. 231-32.
9. *Ibid.,* vol. 8, pp. 51, 52.
10. *Ibid.,* vol. 8, pp. 7, 13.
11. *Ibid.,* vol. 1, p. 311.
12. *Ibid.,* vol. 8, p. 47.
13. *Ibid.,* vol. 1, p. 254.
14. *Ibid.,* vol. 8, p. 47.
15. *New York Times,* Sept. 28, 1964, p. 38A. Also, *Hearings . . . ,* vol. 1, p. 37.
16. *Hearings . . . ,* vol. 1, p. 254.
17. *Ibid.,* vol. 8, p. 95.
18. *Ibid.,* vol. 1, p. 252.

19. *Ibid.*, vol. 8, p. 98.
20. *Ibid.*, vol. 1, p. 145.
21. *Ibid.*, vol. 8, p. 42.
22. *Ibid.*, vol. 8, pp. 98-99.
23. *New York Times,* Sept. 28, 1964, p. 39A.
24. *Hearings . . .* , vol. 8, pp. 51-52.
25. *Ibid.*, vol. 8, p. 55.
26. *Ibid.*, vol. 8, p. 57.
27. *Ibid.*, vol. 11, p. 17.
28. *Ibid.*, vol. 11, p. 75.
29. *Ibid.*, vol. 8, p. 48.
30. *Ibid.*, vol. 8, pp. 50-55.
31. *Report of the Warren Commission on the Assassination of President Kennedy.* New York, McGraw-Hill, 1964, p. 368.
32. *Hearings . . .*, vol. 11, p. 94.
33. *Report of the Warren Commission . . .*, p. 601.
34. *Ibid.*, p. 357.
35. Abrahamsen, D. *Mind and Death of a Genius.* New York, Columbia Univ. Press, 1946, p. 156.
36. Private communication.
37. Jackson, D. The evolution of an assassin, *Life,* Feb. 21, 1964, pp. 70-71.
38. *Report of the Warren Commission . . .*, pp. 369-70.
39. *Hearings . . .*, vol. 1, p. 331.
40. *Report of the Warren Commission . . .*, p. 601.
41. *Ibid.*, p. 602.
42. *Ibid.*, p. 603.
43. *Hearings . . .*, vol. 8, p. 353.
44. *Report of the Warren Commission . . .*, p. 599.
45. *Ibid.*, p. 353.
46. *Ibid.*, p. 356.
47. *Hearings . . .*, vol. 8, p. 223.
48. *Ibid.*, vol. 8, p. 224.
49. *Ibid.*, vol. 8, p. 9.
50. *Ibid.*, vol. 1, p. 23.
51. *Ibid.*
52. *Ibid.*, vol. 1, p. 22.
53. *Ibid.*, vol. 1, p. 212.
54. *Ibid.*, vol. 1, p. 201. Also, *New York Times,* Sept. 28, 1964, p. 40A.
55. Oswald, L. H. Historic Diary, *Life,* July 10, 1964, p. 29.
56. Freud, S. Dostoyevsky and parricide. In: *Collected Papers,* vol. 5. London, Hogarth, and Inst. Psychoanal., 1950, p. 229.
57. Abrahamsen, D. *The Psychology of Crime,* 2d printing. New York, Columbia Univ. Press, 1967, pp. 164-65. Also, Palm, R. and Abrahamsen, D. A Rorschach study of the wives of sex offenders. *J. Nerv. Ment. Dis. 119:*167-172, 1954.

# THE PROBLEM OF FEVER OF UNKNOWN ORIGIN*

EMANUEL APPELBAUM

Professor of Clinical Medicine
New York University School of Medicine
New York, N. Y.

DESPITE advances in knowledge and the development of many new diagnostic techniques, one still encounters instances of fever that cannot be readily explained. These cases, generally referred to as FUO or fever of unknown origin, constitute a challenging problem to the clinician. It is my purpose to discuss briefly the more important diseases and entities to which the physician must be alerted when faced with a problem of unexplained fever. As suggested by Beeson,[1] the diseases to be considered may best be grouped under four headings: infections, neoplasms, collagen diseases, and miscellaneous.

## INFECTIONS

*Tuberculosis.* One of the most important diseases requiring consideration in cases of fever of unknown origin is tuberculosis, particularly the miliary form, which is often difficult to diagnose. It is well known that in miliary tuberculosis a roentgenogram of the lungs is frequently nonrevealing until late in the course of the disease, when tubercles or effusions may appear. In the more chronic forms of miliary tuberculosis, in which the infection is more indolent and lesions are less widely disseminated, the patients may remain asymptomatic for a long time. It is also well to bear in mind that a tuberculous infection may be localized predominantly in an extrapulmonary organ or system, as the liver, the meninges, or the genitourinary tract.

In view of the paucity of clinical findings in many instances of miliary tuberculosis it is frequently necessary to resort to a variety of laboratory studies for the purpose of establishing a diagnosis. These include roentgenograms of the lungs and other organs, careful search for tubercle bacilli in the sputum, in gastric washings, stools, urine, and other secretions, and various biopsy examinations. Of par-

*Presented at a meeting of the American-Hungarian Medical Association, New York, N. Y., held at The New York Academy of Medicine, April 14, 1967.

ticular importance is the performance of biopsy of the bone marrow and of the liver, with diligent examination for the presence of tubercles. In an excellent study on miliary tuberculosis of the liver, Terry and Gunnar[2] noted that in miliary infection the tuberculous process within the liver is frequently massive and may produce a variety of tubercles: caseating, noncaseating, and granulomatous forms. At times a pleural or pericardial biopsy may prove helpful. On occasion, the bone marrow culture may be positive for tubercle bacilli. On the other hand, it is very difficult as a rule to demonstrate bacillemia. The tuberculin test is not helpful, since a positive reaction does not prove active infection, and a negative result does not exclude with certainty the diagnosis of tuberculosis. It is of interest that, while the liver function tests not infrequently yield an abnormal result, the level of alkaline phosphatase is rarely elevated.

*Histoplasmosis.* This fungus infection is prevalent in some parts of the eastern and midwestern United States. It may appear in an acute disseminated form, with severe systemic symptoms, including fever, hepatosplenomegaly, and lymphadenopathy, or as a chronic disease, simulating cavitary pulmonary tuberculosis. Diagnosis can be made by isolating the fungus in cultures of the blood, bone marrow, sputum, and urine, or in biopsy material. The organism may also be found microscopically in specially stained tissue sections. Changing complement-fixing antibody titers and a histoplasmin skin test converted from negative to positive may be considered as evidence in support of the diagnosis of histoplasmosis. A single positive skin test, however, indicates only exposure to this infection.

*Coccidioidomycosis.* This fungal infection is prevalent in several areas of the western United States. The disease appears in several forms, which may resemble tuberculosis or histoplasmosis. The diagnosis is made by the isolation of the fungus in culture or by the microscopic demonstration of characteristic spherules in properly stained tissue sections. The coccidioidin skin test and the complement-fixation test may be used only as supportive evidence for a clinical impression. It may be noted that cultural isolation of the organism is regarded as hazardous to laboratory workers.

*Malaria.* Although malaria had almost disappeared from the continental United States by mid-1940, it has remained a highly prevalent disease in certain areas of the world, particularly in Asia and Africa. The incidence of this disease is relatively high in southeast Asia, where many of our military personnel are stationed. It is therefore necessary to consider malaria in persons who have returned from visits to endemic areas. A diagnosis of malaria depends on recognition of the parasite in a stained blood smear.

*Schistosomiasis.* This disease is prevalent in Asia, Africa, the Philippines, South America, and the Caribbean Islands. Patients from an endemic area who have a history of intestinal disease, hepatic involvement, ascites, splenomegaly, and eosinophilia should be suspected of having schistosomiasis. The specific diagnosis is based upon finding the eggs in feces, urine, or in biopsy material obtained from lesions in the colon, rectal mucosa, or the liver.

*Amebiasis.* Contrary to the general impression, amebiasis is not limited to the tropics and is present throughout the United States. It appears at times in sizable epidemics. The most common serious complication of amebiasis is liver abscess, which is generally accompanied by persistent fever. This complication may occur in patients who have no previous history of intestinal disorder. The diagnosis is established by demonstrating the presence of *Endamoeba histolytica* in the stools. Repeated stool examinations are frequently necessary. In some cases it is not possible to find the parasite, especially if antimicrobials have been used. In these instances a response to specific therapy may be regarded as supportive evidence for the diagnosis of amebic infection. While the complement-fixation test is almost always positive in cases of amebic liver abscess, it is rarely used as a diagnostic procedure, largely because of the frequency of false-positive reactions.

*Brucellosis.* This disease is characterized in the main by fever, sweats, weakness, and various pains, which may continue unabated for weeks or months. Contrary to the general impression, the fever is usually not undulant but rather intermittent. Occasionally, sustained fever may be present. It may be well to remember that brucellosis is primarily an occupational disease and occurs most often in farmers, livestock producers, meat packers, and veterinarians. The diagnosis can be definitely established by cultural isolation of the Brucella from the blood or bone marrow. The agglutination test also provides a dependable laboratory method for diagnosis, especially if the titers are high. On the other hand, the Brucella skin test merely indicates past invasion of the body by the organisms, but it does not mean that active disease is present.

It may be noted that leukocytosis is most unusual in this disease.

*Subacute bacterial endocarditis.* In the majority of instances, subacute bacterial endocarditis is readily diagnosed on the basis of typical symptoms and positive blood cultures. There are, however, cases in which the disease is missed for many weeks and months. It is common knowledge that bacterial endocarditis is frequently overlooked in the elderly, who may present a confusing and atypical picture, suggesting the presence of psychosis, renal insufficiency, or gastrointestinal malignancy. In these patients the presence of a slight heart murmur and low-grade fever are frequently disregarded. It may also be noted that in right-sided endocarditis cardiac murmurs, peripheral embolic phenomena, and splenomegaly are often absent. The possibility of bacterial endocarditis should therefore be considered in every patient who has a prolonged fever and a heart murmur, and a series of several consecutive aerobic and anaerobic blood cultures should be done promptly. It is, of course, recognized that blood cultures are negative in about 15 per cent of cases; in some of these a bone marrow culture may yield positive results.

*Salmonellosis.* In recent decades there has been a marked decline in the incidence of large epidemics of typhoid fever. The disease, however, still occurs in sporadic form, with cases appearing singly or in small groups. The incidence of human Salmonella infections other than typhoid fever is unknown, but in recent years there have appeared reports of many cases of salmonellosis following ingestion of contaminated food products. Some of these patients presented typhoidlike symptoms, including sustained fever. In a case of obscure fever it is therefore necessary to consider the possibility of Salmonella infection and to perform cultures of the blood, stool, and urine, as well as agglutination tests.

*Obscure intra-abdominal infections.* In this category may be included occult biliary tract infection, localized suppurations and fistulae resulting from perforations in the gastrointestinal tract or in other viscera, suppurative pylephlebitis with multiple liver abscesses, and pelvic thrombophlebitis. These cases may be very puzzling and may frequently require repeated radiologic, bacteriologic, and biochemical studies. A clue to the diagnosis may at times be obtained from one of the tests or from a revealing detail in the history. In some instances a laparatomy is essential for definite diagnosis.

*Viral infections.* A considerable number of the acute febrile diseases fail to reveal any evidence of bacterial, fungal, or parasitic infection. Most of these illnesses are very likely of viral etiology. In this category may also be included cases with a clinical picture of infectious mononucleosis lacking laboratory confirmation. While recent advances in virology have been enormous, it is still difficult to apply the newer knowledge routinely to clinical material. On occasion, however, the patient will reveal symptoms suggestive of a specific virus disease, which will lead to the performance of cultures of pharyngeal and fecal material and to early- and late-phase serologic tests. This may result in a definite diagnosis.

## Neoplasms and Tumors

*Carcinomas.* It has long been known that neoplastic diseases may be associated with various gradations of fever and, at times, also with chills, mimicking an infectious disease. These symptoms have been observed not infrequently in patients with carcinoma of the lung, stomach, colon, pancreas, liver, or adrenal gland. Israel[3] in 1896 was the first to emphasize the importance of fever in the presence of renal neoplasm. Since then, many authors have directed attention to fever as a predominant symptom of hypernephroma. In any case of unexplained fever it is therefore important to perform appropriate radiologic studies, particularly pyelography and renal arteriography. Other pertinent tests include microscopic examination of exfoliated cells and of biopsy material, and radioisotope scanning.

*Lymphomas.* Fever is one of the predominant symptoms of lymphomas, particularly Hodgkin's disease. Of special interest is the Pel-Ebstein type of fever, noted in some cases of Hodgkin's disease. In these instances, the fever occurs in irregular waves of several days' duration separated by periods of remission. Positive diagnosis of the lymphomas depends upon microscopic examination of tissue, and biopsy of one of the enlarged lymph nodes is extremely important. On occasion a laparotomy appears justified for the purpose of diagnosis.

*Atrial myxomas and ball-valve thrombi.* Benign myxomas and ball-valve thrombi present a similar clinical picture, with symptoms resembling those of mitral stenosis and, at times, with symptoms related to obstruction of cardiac blood flow. In addition, the patients have intermittent fever and also, occasionally, embolic phenomena. As noted by Ross *et al.*,[4] a mistaken diagnosis of bacterial endocarditis is frequently made in these cases. The most important diagnostic clue in intracavitary tumors of the heart is the variation of signs and symptoms with changes in the position of the body. The diagnosis can be established by means of angiocardiography.

## Collagen Diseases

*Acute rheumatic fever.* This disease often presents great diagnostic difficulties, since no specific test is available for its diagnosis. Articular manifestations, erythema marginatum, subcutaneous nodules, fever, signs of progressive heart failure, and prolongation of the PR interval in the electrocardiogram constitute the leading evidences of rheumatic activity. Except for the fever, these definite signs of rheumatic activity are frequently lacking. In some instances of rheumatic heart disease the fever is due to pulmonary embolization and infarction. These cases often require long periods of study and recourse to therapeutic trials of various drugs, as salicylates, corticosteroids, and anticoagulants, before a diagnosis is made.

*Juvenile rheumatoid arthritis.* It has long been known that in juvenile rheumatoid arthritis, fever alone can precede the rheumatic manifestations by weeks, months, or even years. The febrile patterns are variable and have been the subject of study by several investigators.[5, 6] These cases usually require long periods of observation before the diagnosis of rheumatoid arthritis can be made on the basis of the characteristic clinical picture and the roentgenographic and serologic findings. It is important for clinicians to be alerted to the possibility of rheumatoid disease in children who have prolonged or frequently recurring fever.

*Systemic lupus erythematosus.* Fever is one of the predominant symptoms of disseminated lupus, which progressively involves the musculoskeletal, mucocutaneous, renal, cardiovascular, pleuropulmonary, gastrointestinal, neurologic, and hematologic systems. Of great importance is the presence in the patient's serum of a great variety of autoantibodies, including the antinuclear factors, one of which can induce the formation of the lupus erythematosus (L.E.) cell. The diagnosis of systemic lupus is suggested if the patient has a false-positive serologic test for syphilis, a positive Coombs test, or any one of the antinuclear factors. The presence of a positive L.E. cell test is generally regarded as confirmatory of the disease. However, failure to find these cells does not rule out the diagnosis of lupus erythematosus.

*Dermatomyositis.* This condition requires consideration in patients, particularly those past middle age, who have fever and pain or weakness in muscles, especially those of the girdle, the neck, and proximal parts of the extremities. There may or may not be involvement of the skin. The diagnosis is made by biopsy of affected areas of skin and muscle. It is of interest that in about 20 per cent of the cases there is an associated neoplasm of some type.

*Periarteritis nodosa.* Fever may be a dominant manifestation of periarteritis nodosa, which is a disease of diversified symptomatology. Manifestations that should arouse suspicion of this disease include: 1) cachexia and anemia, 2) polyneuritis and polymyositis, 3) abdominal symptoms, 4) signs of renal involvement, 5) hypertension, 6) signs suggestive of infection, as fever and leukocytosis, 7) eosinophilia, 8) bronchial asthma or focal pulmonary infiltrates, 9) skin lesions, such as nodules, purpura, bullae, or ulcers, and 10) signs of acute vascular involvement of the heart, mesentery, or brain. The diagnosis can be made by biopsy of skin and muscle or of an affected artery.

Cranial arteritis in elderly individuals may be placed in the same category. This condition may cause fever, headache, and leukocytosis. When the temporal artery is involved, the diagnosis can be made readily by biopsy of this vessel.

## Miscellaneous

*Cirrhosis of the liver.* It is well recognized that cirrhosis of the liver may cause considerable temperature elevations, possibly as a result of tissue destruction. Beeson[1] suggests also that patients with cirrhosis may have episodes of chills and high fever, due to an associated Gram-negative bacillus bacteremia. A diagnosis of hepatic cirrhosis can usually be made on the basis of the clinical picture, the course, and the laboratory findings of hepatocellular dysfunction. Occasionally liver biopsy is essential for diagnosis.

*Regional ileitis and ulcerative colitis.* On occasion fever is the principal symptom in these related diseases. The fever is a manifestation of toxicity. In some cases, a prolonged fever results from complications of perforation, such as localized peritonitis, abscess, or fistula. The diagnosis of the primary disease and the complications is usually made by x-ray examination of the gastrointestinal tract and by endoscopy. Occasionally a laparotomy is essential for diagnosis.

*Recurrent pulmonary embolism.* This condition may cause a pro-

FEATURES DIFFERENTIATING FAMILIAL MEDITERRANEAN FROM ETIOCHOLANOLONE FEVER*

| | *Familial mediterranean fever* | *Etiocholanolone fever* |
|---|---|---|
| Ethnic background | Mediterranean ancestry | Northern and eastern European ancestry |
| Periodicity | Attacks at irregular intervals | Regular cyclic episodes |
| Biochemical findings | Hyperfibrinogenemia<br>Proteinuria | Elevated plasma and urinary etiocholanolone |

*Adapted from a table by Cohn, G. L., in: *Cecil-Loeb Textbook of Medicine,* Beeson, P. B. and McDermott, W., eds., vol. II, Philadelphia, Saunders, 1963, p. 1276.

longed fever due to pulmonary infarction, pleuritis, or bronchopneumonia. The emboli originate in right-sided heart lesions or in thrombi of the peripheral veins of the extremities or pelvis. The source of the thrombi may remain obscure for a long time, leading to diagnostic difficulty. In all cases of unexplained fever it is well to bear this clinical entity in mind and to search repeatedly for evidence of peripheral thrombophlebitis. The newer procedures of pulmonary angiography and photoscanning are valuable diagnostic aids.

*Blood diseases.* In some forms of leukemia, hemolytic anemia, and other blood dyscrasias, fever is a dominant symptom and may greatly confuse the diagnosis. However, careful hematologic and bone marrow studies will generally lead to a solution of the diagnostic problem.

*Drug fever.* Febrile reactions to antibiotics and other chemotherapeutic agents constitute the main source of confusion, particularly hypersensitivity reactions to penicillin. Occasionally a persistent fever is due to the prolonged use of a certain drug. The diagnosis is confirmed by the defervescence that follows discontinuation of the suspected drug.

*Periodic fever.* Reimann[7] has called attention to an unusual group of cases in which there were febrile episodes at intervals of 7 to 10 days, continuing for periods of months and even years. These are sometimes associated with leukopenia or abdominal or thoracic pain. The reason for the periodicity of the fever is unknown. The syndrome comprises several etiologic entities, two of which, etiocholanolone fever and familial Mediterranean fever, appear to be hereditary metabolic disorders. Although these two diseases have common clinical findings, they can be distinguished, largely by certain ethnic and biochemical features shown in the accompanying table.

*Factitious fever.* Occasionally, fever is observed in an individual who shows no other signs of illness. If malingering is suspected, the temperature should be checked in the presence of a physician or nurse.

* * *

There is no special formula for the study of problems of fever of unknown origin. The clinical investigation should comprise a careful history, a complete examination of the patient, and a selection of appropriate laboratory tests. In the examination particular attention must be given to the search for tender areas, masses, enlarged lymph nodes, and various cutaneous and mucosal lesions, especially petechiae. A diligent search should be made for heart murmurs, with the patient in different positions. Proper appraisal of the size of the liver and spleen is of paramount importance. The fundi must be checked carefully for the presence of hemorrhages, papilledema, and choroidal tubercles. The physical examination should be thorough, with emphasis on signs frequently present in the more common diseases associated with prolonged fever.

The role of appropriate laboratory studies in making a diagnosis hardly needs comment. The pertinent tests have been mentioned already, but several of the procedures require some amplification and emphasis. Blood cultures should be taken in series of four or five successive tests at intervals of one culture every four to six hours. As previously noted, a culture of the bone marrow may occasionally yield a positive result when cultures of the blood are negative. The blood cultures should be made on aerobic and anaerobic media. The significance of a serologic test depends on the height of the positive titer and on the changing of titers during the different phases of a disease. The value of biopsies of the various tissues in making a diagnosis cannot be overemphasized. At times decisive help is obtained from the application of the technique of exfoliative cytology or of special biochemical or hematologic studies. It is, of course, frequently necessary to do various roentgenographic studies, including the special procedures of tomography, angiography, lymphangiography, and radioisotope scanning.

As previously mentioned, laparotomy may be indicated for diagnosis. In a recent report by Keller and Williams[8] on laparotomy in 46 cases of pyrexia of unknown origin, the cause of the fever was established by the operation in 38 patients, 35 of whom benefited from the surgical intervention.

It is, of course, realized that in many cases a correct diagnosis cannot be made, even after the most comprehensive study. In some instances fever and other manifestations subside without the benefit of a diagnosis. This probably applies to 50 per cent of the patients, in some of whom the febrile course is relatively short. In about 40 per cent of the cases a definite or presumptive diagnosis results from the use of laboratory tests, from the gradual evolution of typical symptoms, from laparotomy, or from the patient's response to some therapeutic procedure, such as the administration of certain antibiotics, salicylates, or other drugs. However, a response to a therapeutic trial cannot be regarded as absolute proof of a diagnosis. There remains an undiagnosed group of about 10 per cent of the patients in whom the unexplained fever continues.

## Summary

In this presentation I have discussed briefly the more important clinical entities that require consideration in the differential diagnosis of fever of unknown origin. Attention has been directed to pertinent laboratory tests and other procedures that may be of diagnostic aid. It has been noted that in many instances the fever subsides spontaneously without the benefit of a diagnosis, that following study and the application of certain procedures a diagnosis can be achieved in a fairly high percentage of the cases, and that only in a relatively small number of patients does the problem remain unsolved.

## *References*

1. Beeson, P. B. Fever of obscure origin, *Vet. Administ. Tech. Bull.* 5 (Ser. 10): 72, 1951.
2. Terry, R. B. and Gunnar, R. M. Primary miliary tuberculosis of the liver, *J.A.M.A. 164*:150-157, 1957.
3. Israel, J. Ueber einige neue Erfahrungen auf dem Gebiete der Nierenchirurgie, *Deutsch. Med. Wschr. 22*:345-49, 1896.
4. Ross, R. S., McKusick, V. A. and Harvey, J. C. The problem of fever in patients with valvular heart disease, *J.A.M.A. 165*:1-7, 1957.
5. Ansell, B. M. and Bywaters, E. G. L. Diagnosis of "probable" Still's disease and its outcome, *Ann. Rheum. Dis. 21*: 253-62, 1962.
6. Calabro, J. J. and Marchesano, J. M. Fever associated with juvenile rheumatoid arthritis, *New Eng. J. Med. 276*: 11-18, 1957.
7. Reimann, H. A. Periodic disease: Periodic fever, periodic abdominalgia, cyclic neutropenia, intermittent arthralgia, angioneurotic edema, anaphylactoid purpura and periodic paralysis, *J.A.M.A. 141*:175, 1949.
8. Keller, J. W. and Williams, R. D. Laparotomy for unexplained fever, *Arch. Surg. 90*:494-98, 1965.

# GRANULOMATOUS COLITIS

*A Panel Discussion**

Introductory Remarks

*Henry D. Janowitz* . . . . . . . . . . . 900

Clinical Features

*Arthur E. Lindner* . . . . . . . . . . . 901

Surgical Treatment

*S. Arthur Localio* . . . . . . . . . . . 906

Roentgen Features

*Richard H. Marshak* . . . . . . . . . . 910

*Presented at a combined meeting of the New York Academy of Gastroenterology and the New York Chapter of the American College of Gastroenterology, held at The New York Academy of Medicine, October 10, 1966.

# INTRODUCTORY REMARKS*

HENRY D. JANOWITZ

Head, Division of Gastroenterology, The Mount Sinai Hospital
Clinical Professor of Medicine, Mount Sinai School of Medicine
New York, N. Y.

In this age of molecular biology it is consoling to know that there is still much to be learned from the natural history of disease. It is sobering, however, to realize that good clinical observations are equally difficult to make.

The subject of this symposium is nonspecific granulomatous disease of the colon, granulomatous colitis. Many of us find it hard to realize that the clinical entity of regional enteritis was clearly demarcated only about 35 years ago. Most of us still find it difficult to understand why it has taken clinicians so long to recognize that this same disease process, known very early in its study to involve the stomach, duodenum, and jejunum, may be present in the colon as well.

Before we turn to the clinical presentation of this colonic entity, it is interesting to speculate on the cause of this delay in clinical recognition. I do not believe that the semantic problem was terribly important, although a wide variety of terms has been used to denote the same pathologic entity. Rather, two stereotypes of thinking have interfered. First was the tacit assumption that all inflammatory disorders of the colon of nonspecific or unknown origin were of unitary nature. "Ulcerative colitis" covered the entire clinical spectrum. Second was the explicit assumption, mainly of pathologists, that the ileocecal valve acted as a kind of barrier, regional enteritis remaining confined proximally, ulcerative colitis distally, although occasionally each could inch over the borderline. In retrospect, both assumptions, of course, were inadequate.

The danger at present is that we shall divide disease of the colon into two kinds: granulomatous and ulcerative, where before we assigned all "colitis" to one entity. However, good observers are already recognizing that other varieties of segmental colitis exist, especially those of vascular origin. It is to be hoped that our successors will not wonder why we were so slow to recognize these differences.

*Presented at a combined meeting of the New York Academy of Gastroenterology and the New York Chapter of the American College of Gastroenterology, held at The New York Academy of Medicine, October 10, 1966.

# CLINICAL FEATURES OF GRANULOMATOUS COLITIS*

ARTHUR E. LINDNER

Assistant Professor of Medicine
New York University School of Medicine
New York, N. Y.

FOR many years a physician could confidently make a diagnosis of ulcerative colitis when a patient was found to have chronic nonspecific inflammatory disease of the colon. (The term "nonspecific" assumes that the known infectious causes, such as amebiasis, bacillary dysentery, and tuberculosis have been ruled out.) In recent years, however, it has become apparent that there is a differential diagnosis of chronic nonspecific inflammatory disease of the colon and that such disease may be granulomatous rather than ulcerative in origin.

It was about 35 years ago—in 1932—that B. Crohn, Leon Ginzburg, and Gordon Oppenheimer first described the granulomatous inflammatory disease of the small bowel that has been called regional enteritis. It was their original concept that this was a disease of the small bowel that stopped abruptly at the ileocecal valve, since such was the finding in the patients described in their original report. Only 2 years later, however, R. Colp reported the case of a 22-year-old medical student who had granulomatous disease involving the ileum and the cecum. This was the first reported case of granulomatous colitis. It did not involve much of the colon—just the cecum—but this was sufficient to demonstrate that the ileocecal valve is no barrier to development of disease in the colon. Soon it became apparent that regional enteritis, although it commonly does involve the terminal ileum, can be found in any part of the gastrointestinal tract from stomach to anus. When granulomatous disease involves the colon, either alone or in association with disease in the ileum, it must be distinguished from ulcerative colitis.

The colon may become involved in the granulomatous process in one of several ways:

*Presented at a combined meeting of the New York Academy of Gastroenterology and the New York Chapter of the American College of Gastroenterology, held at The New York Academy of Medicine, October 10, 1966.

1) The colon alone may be the site of granulomatous disease. The entire large bowel may be involved, but usually the distribution of disease is segmental and right-sided, sparing the rectum and sigmoid.

2) Both the colon and the small bowel may be involved in granulomatous disease. In patients who have this disorder the disease seems to begin simultaneously in the two areas—at least both the small bowel and the colon are involved when the patient is first examined radiologically. Combined disease in the small bowel and the colon has been termed granulomatous ileocolitis.

3) The colon may become involved with granulomatous disease only after an operation has been performed for treatment of regional enteritis of the small bowel. The diseased segment of colon is usually immediately adjacent to an ileocolic anastomosis.

4) Finally, the colon may be involved directly by the formation of a fistula from an adjacent loop of the diseased small bowel. Such fistulae do not usually lead to granulomatous colitis; the lesion does not appear to spread, and the area in the colon heals when the diseased small bowel has been removed and the fistula closed.

Thus the colon alone can be involved in a granulomatous process, or both the colon and the small bowel, usually the ileum, can be the site of granulomatous disease. We believe that regional enteritis of the small bowel and ulcerative colitis do not occur in the same patient except, perhaps, rarely and by chance.

Granulomatous colitis and ileocolitis tend to begin in young adult life. Most patients acquire the disease in their late teens or early twenties. Patients complain of abdominal cramps, diarrhea, and sometimes fever. Gross blood in the stool is unusual, even in patients with protracted diarrhea and, when bleeding does occur, it is usually intermittent and not a prominent feature of the clinical course. In our experience, patients with gross rectal bleeding are usually those with involvement of the rectum and sigmoid.

Fistulae are common in granulomatous colitis, just as they are in regional enteritis. About half the patients with granulomatous disease that involves the colon develop fistulae; commonly these are perianal and perirectal. Internal fistulae generally arise from the small bowel and are thus unusual in the absence of small bowel disease. Extracolonic manifestations, such as arthritis and skin lesions, are less common than in ulcerative colitis.

Sigmoidoscopy is often normal in granulomatous colitis, and the finding of a normal-appearing rectum in a patient with clinical or roentgen evidence of inflammatory bowel disease immediately suggests the possibility of a granulomatous process. This is true, of course, because —unlike ulcerative colitis—granulomatous disease tends to spare the rectum. When the rectum *is* involved in the process, the sigmoidoscopic appearance resembles that of ulcerative colitis, although H. Lockhart-Mummery and B. Morson, of St. Mark's Hospital in London, suggest that in granulomatous disease the mucosa has a patchy cobblestonelike character, with islands of normal tissue intervening. Biopsy of the involved rectal mucosa and submucosa may reveal the presence of granulomas and thus establish the diagnosis.

## Pathology

The pathology of granulomatous colitis is similar to that of regional enteritis. There is a chronic inflammation that extends through the entire wall but it involves especially the submucosa. The bowel wall is thick and rigid with narrowing of the lumen, sometimes so advanced that a stricture forms. Several areas of disease ("skip lesions") may be present in the bowel, separated by lengths of normal-appearing gut. Ulcers are deep and they tend to be present as long linear ulcerations intersecting deep transverse ulcers or fissures. The intervening mucosa is red and swollen, and the luminal surface has a coarsely nodular appearance that has been compared to a cobblestone road. Involvement of the bowel wall itself may be asymmetrical rather than circumferential. Loops of involved intestine may become adherent to one another or to loops of normal bowel. Fistulae between loops of bowel or to other viscera may occur, and intra-abdominal abscesses may be present. Free perforation of the colon into the peritoneal cavity is rare. The mesentery is thickened and the mesenteric lymph nodes are enlarged. Carcinoma of the colon has thus far not been reported in association with granulomatous colitis.

Histological examination shows a chronic inflammatory reaction, most prominent in the submucosa but extending through the bowel wall, with edema and fibrosis. The ulcers are deep and they extend through the serosa as sealed-off perforations to which adjacent viscera may adhere. The characteristic histological feature is the presence of noncaseating granulomas with Langhans' giant cells and epithelioid cells

Granulomas may be scanty or absent, especially when ulceration is severe, but a diagnosis of granulomatous disease is warranted if the other pathological features are present. Regional lymph nodes on section may show characteristic granulomas.

## Prognosis

Paradoxically, perhaps, the prognosis in granulomatous colitis seems to be dictated largely by the status of the small bowel. Patients who have granulomatous disease confined to the colon seem to do relatively well. They often come to operation earlier than patients with ulcerative colitis, and their course may be more chronic and unremitting. Desperate acute episodes, such as toxic dilatation and free perforation, however, do not occur. The indication for operation is usually incomplete obstruction caused by stricture. Patients do well after segmental resection of the colon and they do not tend to develop recurrences of their disease. When ileostomy and total colectomy are performed for granulomatous colitis, spread of disease into a previously normal small bowel, although occasionally reported, is unusual.

When the ileum is involved in the disease, however—that is, in granulomatous ileocolitis—a different prognosis is encountered. The disease tends to be more severe than when only the colon is involved, and infection, abscesses, and fistulae are common indications for operation. Gastroenterologists generally feel that operation should be avoided as long as possible in ileocolitis because resection and anastomosis tend to spread the disease in both ileum and colon. Sometimes, of course, operation simply becomes mandatory. It is interesting that linear spread of granulomatous disease in either the large or small bowel is unusual in the absence of operation.

## Medical Treatment

The goal of medical treatment in granulomatous colitis is to induce a full remission or, failing this, to provide symptomatic and supportive treatment, make the patient as comfortable as possible, and keep him functioning in everyday life despite the activity of a chronic disease. Medical treatment is indicated: 1) for the uncomplicated case of granulomatous colitis; 2) for diffuse involvement of the small bowel, with disease so extensive that operation cannot be performed; and 3) for recurrent disease following surgical operation.

A number of regimens for the medical treatment of granulomatous colitis are available, the choice depending upon the severity of the symptoms and upon the preference of the physician. Supportive treatment includes dietary manipulation, rest, sedation, correction of anemia, and—probably as important as any of these—supportive psychotherapy by the internist or gastroenterologist. Antibiotics appear to be of little value in the treatment of granulomatous colitis itself and usually are reserved for the management of infectious complications, such as the formation of abscess. The insoluble sulfa drugs, such as sulfathalidine, are sometimes useful in treatment, as is salicylazosulfapyridine (Azulfidine).

We have the impression that ACTH and the corticosteroids are in general less effective in granulomatous than in ulcerative colitis and that they are less likely to induce a remission. Nevertheless, the hormones are often useful in the management of symptoms. When the disease is of moderate severity, prednisone or related oral compounds are administered; when the patient is severely ill intravenous ACTH may be the treatment of choice, as in ulcerative colitis. Again as in ulcerative colitis, if the rectum and sigmoid are involved, rectal instillations of steroids, either alone or in conjunction with administration of systemic steroids, may be of benefit.

One leaves a discussion of medical treatment with the disquieting feeling that the physician may relieve symptoms for the patient and make life in general more comfortable for him but that medical treatment may not alter at all the natural course of granulomatous disease.

# SURGICAL TREATMENT OF GRANULOMATOUS COLITIS*

S. Arthur Localio

Professor of Clinical Surgery
New York University School of Medicine
New York, N. Y.

The surgeon's concept of medical-surgical disease is limited by his opportunity to see and follow early disease and to be part of the medical triumphs. He is necessarily biased by observations drawn predominantly from medical failures. There is little doubt that for many patients afflicted with granulomatous disease of the colon medical management results in satisfactory remission and protracted control.

Hard statistical data are lacking regarding the need for surgery during the natural course of granulomatous colitis. Bryan Brooke, quoting B. Crohn, has stated that 80 per cent of patients with granulomatous disease of the small intestine ultimately require surgical operation. This figure may not be excessive for the large intestine.

The concept that granulomatous colitis is part of a pathologic entity that can affect any area or multiple areas of the gastrointestinal tract is now established. The clinical, radiographic, and operative differentiation of granulomatous colitis from ulcerative colitis is essential to proper surgical management. Ulcerative colitis is limited to the large intestine and is cured by total colectomy. The so-called "backwash ileitis" disappears after colectomy and ileostomy, as we know from observations made on the exteriorized ileum. The long-term prognosis of patients who have undergone operation for granulomatous colitis must be guarded, for even the most favorable follow-up statistics reveal recurrence rates of 16 per cent to 23 per cent. The patient, however, may be afforded years of improvement free of major disability and may again enjoy relief following intensive medical treatment, reoperation, or both.

My colleagues on this panel have covered the historical, clinical, and radiographic differentiation of granulomatous colitis and ulcerative

*Presented at a combined meeting of the New York Academy of Gastroenterology and the New York Chapter of the American College of Gastroenterology, held at The New York Academy of Medicine, October 10, 1966.

colitis. I should like to emphasize the fact that a preoperative biopsy taken from a rectum that appears grossly normal may prove valuable if the specific granuloma is identified microscopically. At exploration the presence of internal fistulae, skip areas in the small intestine, large succulent mesenteric lymph nodes, and a firm, rubbery, thick-walled, hose-like intestine are hallmarks of granulomatous colitis. In granulomatous disease the bowel, unlike ulcerative colitis, lends itself to safe primary anastomosis, and resection and primary anastomosis, even of the mildly inflamed rectum, are the surgical order.

The indications for operation are varied and overlapping, and they must be considered in the light of surgical urgency and the response to medical management. Although bleeding is not a prominent feature of granulomatous colitis, occasionally massive hemorrhage will occur and require urgent or emergency operation. We have among our 30 cases one example of massive uncontrollable hemorrhage in a patient with long-standing, right-sided disease; this condition required emergency intervention.

Obstruction is rarely complete in the large bowel, but the very character of the pathologic process with a rigid thickened wall and edematous mucosa leads to partial obturation of the lumen, cramps, diarrhea, and proximal distention in varying degree. If the symptoms are disabling, uncontrollable, and associated with chronic hypovolemia and disordered electrolytes, operation is indicated.

Internal fistulae occur in 15 to 20 per cent of the patients and may be colo-colic, colo-ileal or -jejunal, colo-vesical or colo-vaginal. They may be associated with intra-abdominal abscess, mass, spiking fever, and sepsis. Fistulae may extend outward through the abdominal wall, usually at the site of a preexisting incision or may proceed along the rectum to the perianal area.

Indolent, painful, infected perianal fissures, fistulae, abscesses, ulceration, and anal strictures are common complications of granulomatous colitis and occur in about 80 per cent of patients sometime during the disease. Anal complications may be a prominent and sometimes an early feature of the disease, even in the patient with minimal rectal involvement. These lesions tend to remain active until the colonic disease is brought under control. Anal disease concomitant with minimal involvement of the rectum does not constitute an indication for resection of the rectum unless the anal sphincter has been destroyed.

Perforation into the free peritoneal cavity with spreading peritonitis as seen in ulcerative colitis is very rare. Although it is occasionally reported, we have not seen this complication and, if we did, we should question the diagnosis of granulomatous colitis. Perforation with walled-off abscess and without internal or external fistulae does, however, occur and it requires operation.

Chronic invalidism, sepsis, anemia, malaise, weakness, and hypoproteinemia may or may not be associated with other problems, such as diarrhea and perianal disease, and they should be considered as indications for operation. We have avoided the words intractability and disability, for these may be too subjective to define.

Carcinoma is a definite threat in ulcerative colitis; it is almost unknown in granulomatous colitis. We have a single patient with granulomatous colitis who had an abdominoperineal resection for carcinoma of the rectum; five years later he had resection of the remainder of the colon for persistent symptomatic disease.

The surgeon should expect that many of his patients will be chronically ill, depleted, septic, and on steroid therapy. In spite of this, surgical mortality and morbidity are low with good preparation, steroid support where needed, and a high degree of technical skill. The Lahey Clinic mortality for resection in more than 300 patients with granulomatous disease in various areas of the gastrointestinal tract, including reoperations, is less than 2 per cent. We agree with most authors and favor resection. We believe it can be done with acceptably low morbidity and mortality.

If the entire colon is involved and the rectum cannot be salvaged because of extensive disease, destruction of sphincter or extensive fistulae, total colectomy and ileostomy are performed. For segmental disease, resection and end-to-end anastomosis are done. We have a patient with disease of transverse colon, splenic flexure, and descending colon with a gastrocolic fistula. He is well and free of disease more than 10 years after operation. For right-sided disease, with or without involvement of the terminal ileum, right colectomy and ileocolic anastomosis are performed. For disease affecting an unsalvageable rectum and left colon, abdominoperineal resection and permanent colostomy are indicated. Wherever possible, we try to preserve the rectum, even if it is mildly diseased, and perform ileorectal or colorectal anastomosis.

Sufficient time has not elapsed to give accurate information regarding recurrences following resection for granulomatous colitis. Brooke reports two instances of disease of the small intestine after total colectomy for granulomatous colitis. This does not occur following resection for ulcerative colitis. We have had 5 recurrences in 30 patients, an incidence of 17 per cent. Four of these required reoperation. One patient underwent subtotal colectomy and resection of several feet of ileum, repair of a rectovaginal fistula, and ileoproctostomy for extensive primary diseases; she required rectal resection and permanent ileostomy two years later. One patient had a small bowel recurrence following total colectomy and has been treated medically. Two patients with right-sided granulomatous colitis, one with extensive disease and multiple external abdominal fistulae and one with more localized disease, developed recurrence at the ileocolic anastomosis and required additional reresection. The fifth patient is mentioned above under carcinoma. Undoubtedly we can expect our recurrence rate to rise as the series increases in age. We suspect that the extent of the disease and the completeness of the resection, including diseased lymph nodes, have a bearing on the recurrence rate.

In summary, the surgeon must have a clear concept of the differences between granulomatous colitis and ulcerative colitis. He will be called upon to treat the complications of granulomatous colitis surgically. He should do this by resectional therapy with anastomosis where feasible with some hope of a permanent good result, with a reasonable mortality, and with the thought that because of of the recurrence rate he may, in a fair number of patients, be supplying a holding action that will give years of comfort and improvement in a disease that may again require intensive medical management or reoperation.

# ROENTGEN FEATURES OF GRANULOMATOUS COLITIS*

RICHARD H. MARSHAK

Clinical Professor of Radiology
Mount Sinai School of Medicine
New York, N. Y.

THE roentgen characteristics of granulomatous colitis, as seen on barium enema examination, are substantially those observed in regional inflammation of the small bowel. They include skip lesions (Figure 1), longitudinal ulcerations, transverse fissures, deep ragged ulcerations, eccentric involvement of the wall, pseudodiverticula, pseudopolypoid changes producing a coarse cobblestone mucosal pattern, and internal fistulae and sinus tracts.

The earliest roentgen features we have observed are small irregular nodules along the contours of the bowel, associated with slight rigidity and thickening of the haustral markings (Figure 2). These minimal findings usually extend over a short segment or are seen in the form of skip lesions. On occasion the process is diffuse. Spasm and irritability are present but are less marked than in ulcerative colitis, and the bowel is more easily filled.

Overfilling and distention of the colon may obscure the slight irregularity of the contour described above. The mucosal pattern disclosed after evacuation is helpful in these cases, as it may reveal thickening or nodularity of the mucosa with an irregular ropelike appearance (Figure 3). Although small areas of ulceration may be difficult to identify, their presence may be suggested by straightening or rigidity of a segment or by the presence of pseudodiverticula on the opposite wall. This is due to the fact that ulceration produces spasm and contraction and the opposite uninvolved wall becomes folded. On occasion tiny ulcers are seen extending perpendicularly from the contour of the colon or as tiny specks within the lumen. Pathologic examination of tissue at this stage reveals mucosal edema, submucosal infiltration, and small irregular ulceration. The small ulcers combine to pro-

*Presented at a combined meeting of the New York Academy of Gastroenterology and the New York Chapter of the American College of Gastroenterology, held at The New York Academy of Medicine, October 10, 1966.

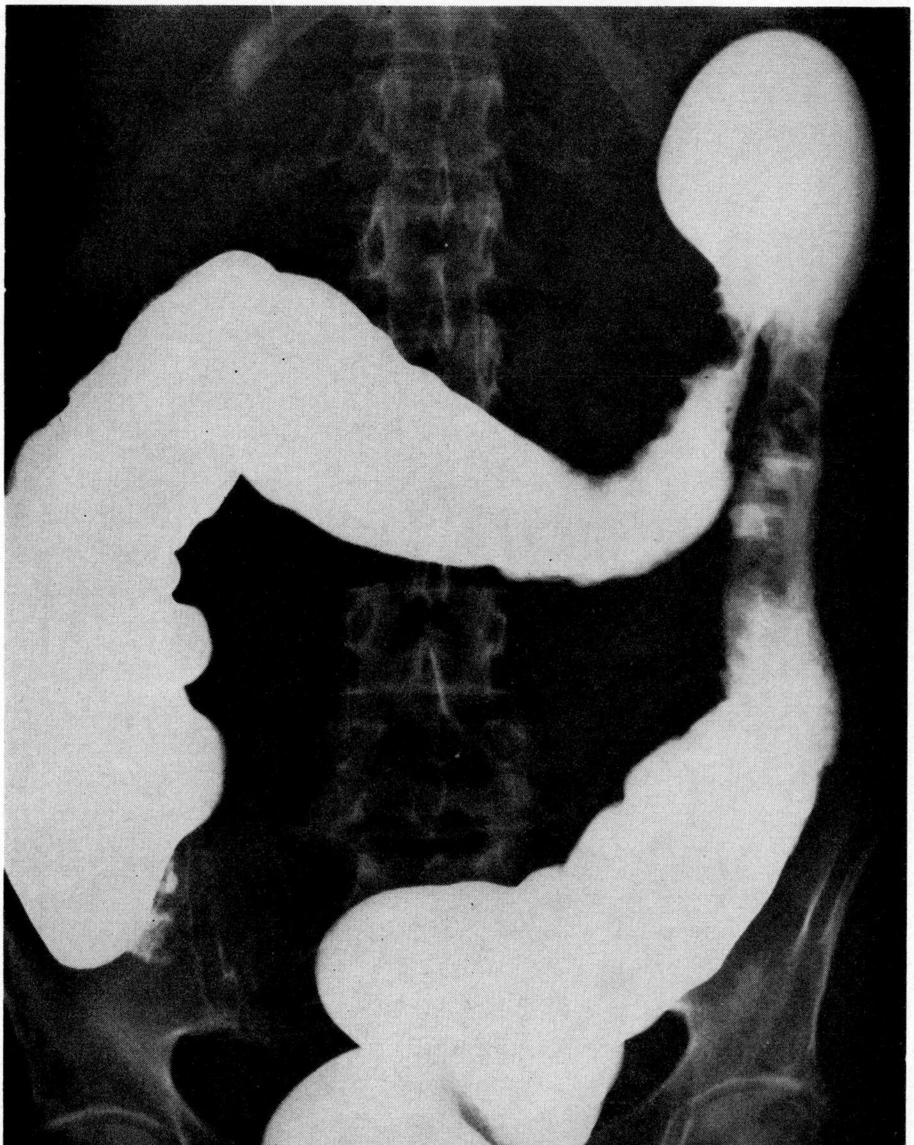

Fig. 1. Granulomatous colitis. There are two skip lesions; one in the distal transverse colon, and the second in the proximal descending colon. The intervening bowel is normal. There is marked irregularity of the contour, and large inflammatory polyps are present. The remainder of the colon is normal.

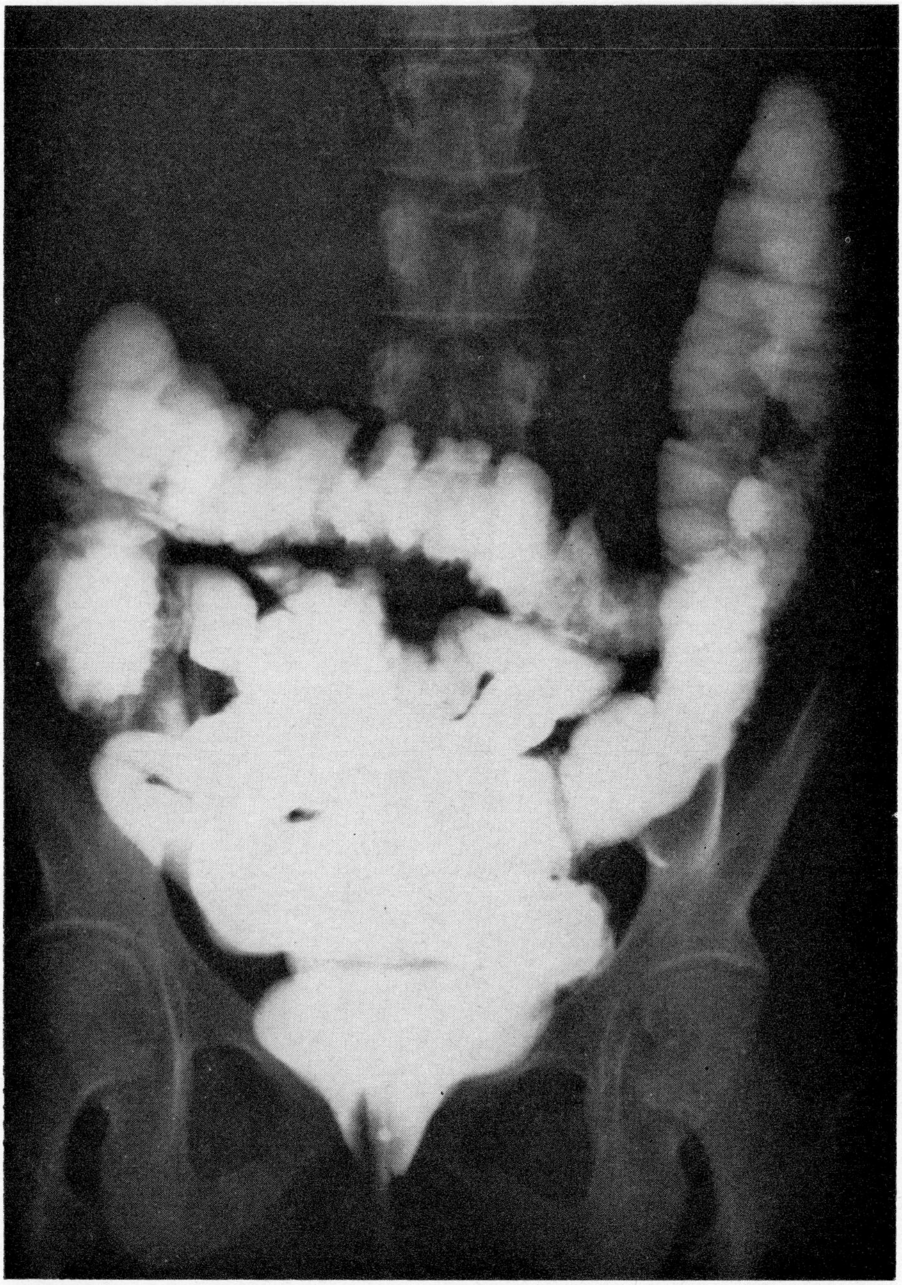

Fig. 2. Granulomatous colitis. There is minimal involvement of the right side of the colon to the mid-descending colon with irregularity of the contours and small nodular defects. The findings are more marked in the distal transverse colon. There is some rigidity and lack of distensibility.

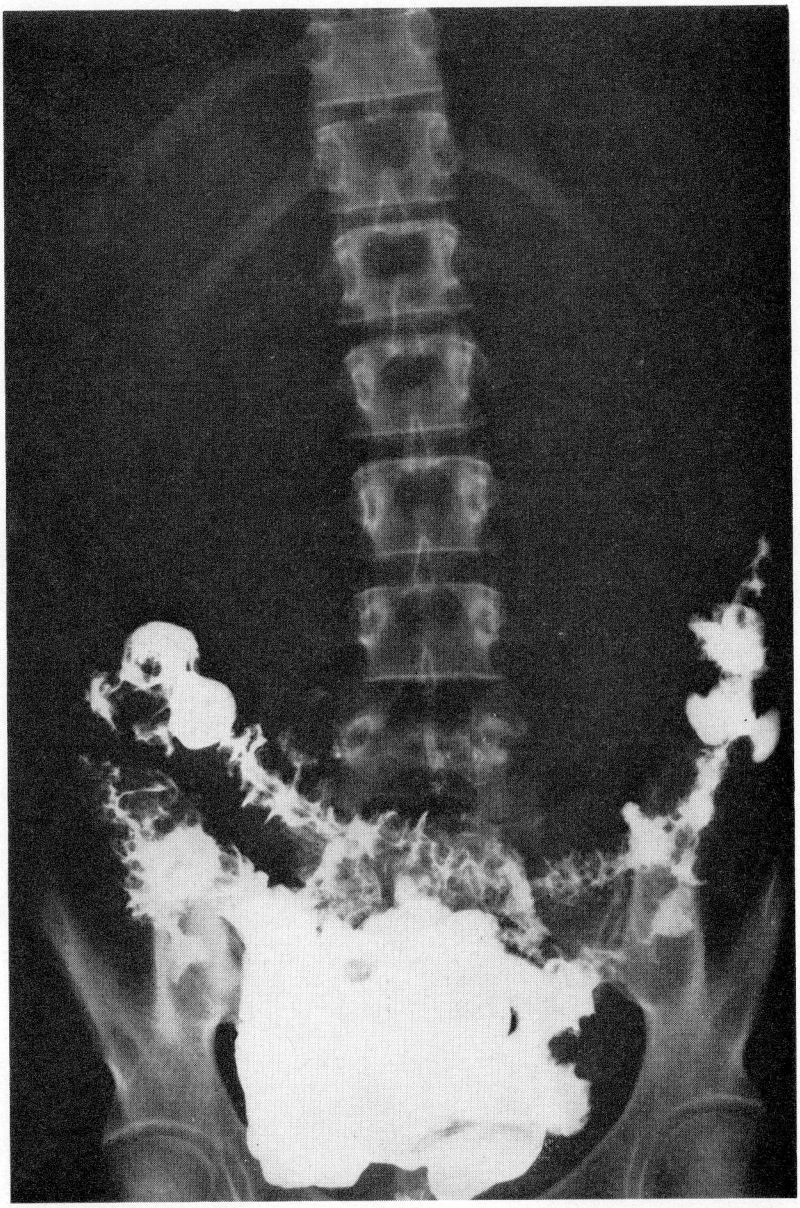

Fig. 3. Same case as in Figure 2, evacuation film. Mucosal pattern has an irregular cobblestone appearance. Several small skip lesions, indicated by the pseudodiverticula, are identified.

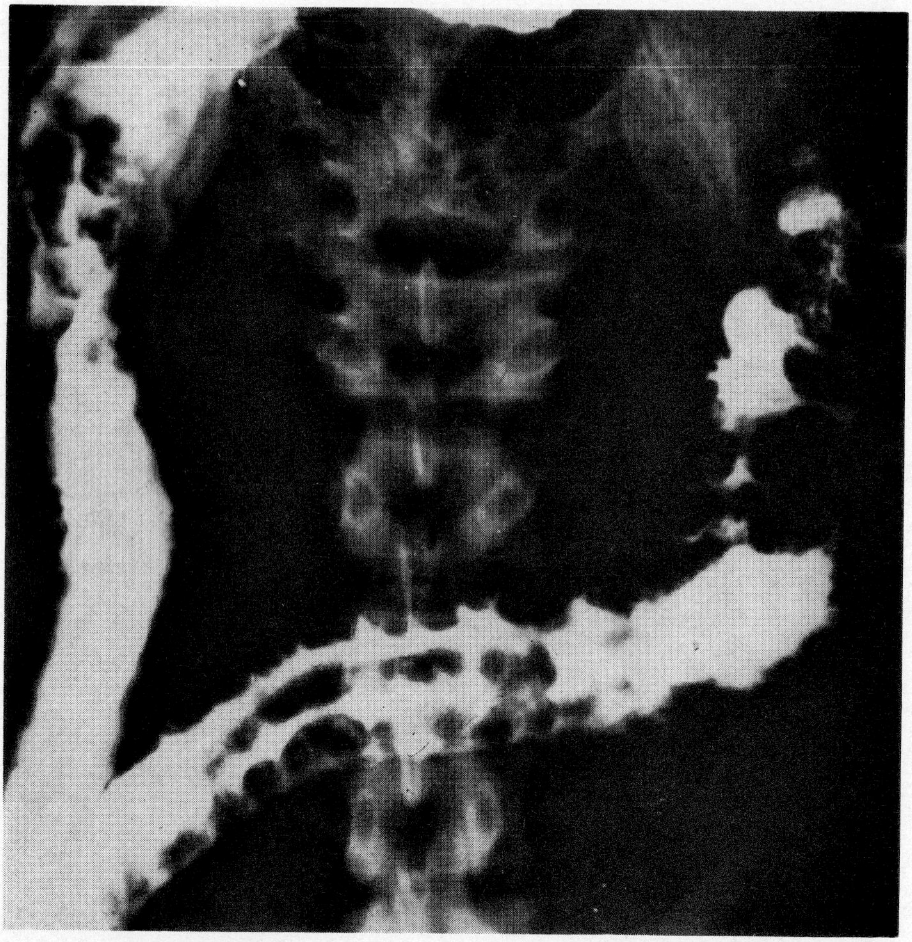

Fig. 4. There are marked longitudinal and transverse ulcerations.

duce large longitudinal ulcerations or gutters that are frequently multiple (Figure 4). When this is associated with transverse linear ulcerations (Figure 5), it produces the characteristic cobblestone pattern (Figure 6). Transverse ulcers may penetrate beyond the contour of the bowel so as to present in profile as numerous long spicules (Figure 5) perpendicular to the long axis of the bowel or as sinus tracts. At times they ultimately lead to intramural abscesses that may be large, producing marked irregularity of the contour of the bowel (Figure 7). When they penetrate into adjacent loops a fistula is formed (Figure

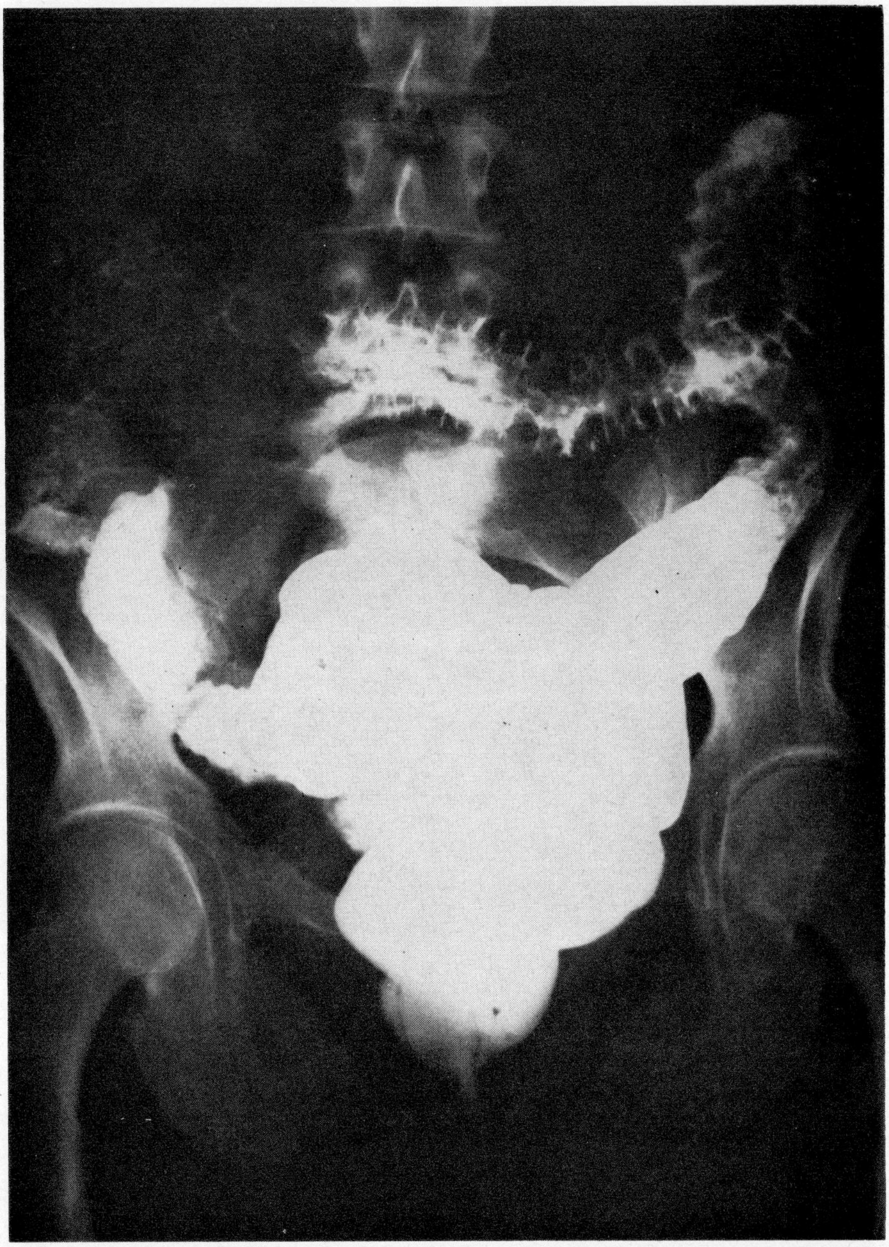

Fig. 5. Same case as in Figure 4 one year later. There is extensive ulceration of the transverse colon with numerous and marked transverse ulcerations. The terminal ileum is also involved. The rectum, sigmoid, and lower descending colon are normal.

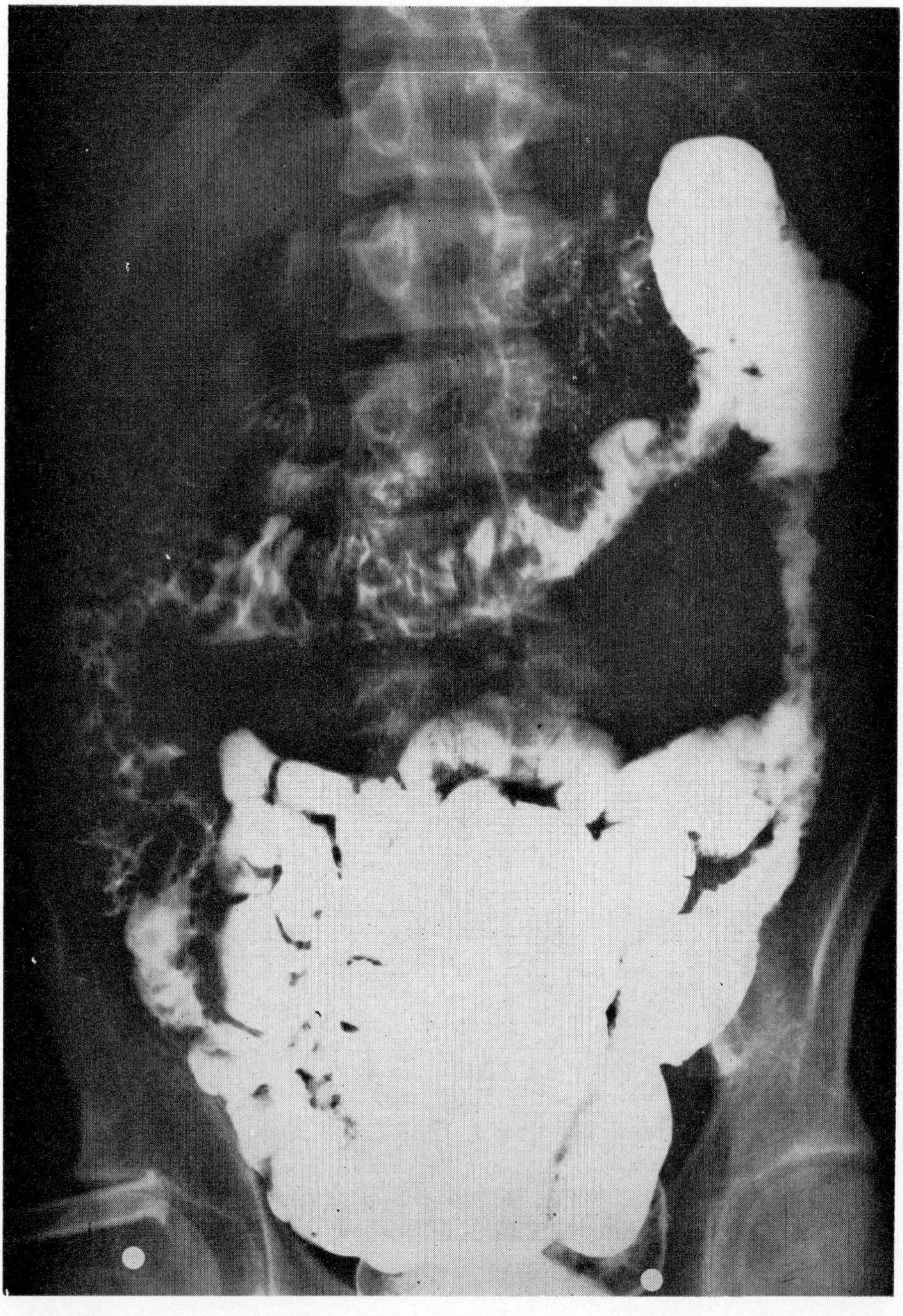

Fig. 6. Granulomatous ileocolitis. Marked cobble-stoning, produced by the longitudinal and transverse ulcerations, with narrowing and rigidity of the colon. The rectum is normal. The involvement of the ileum was seen simultaneously with the involvement of the colon. This has been true in most of our cases.

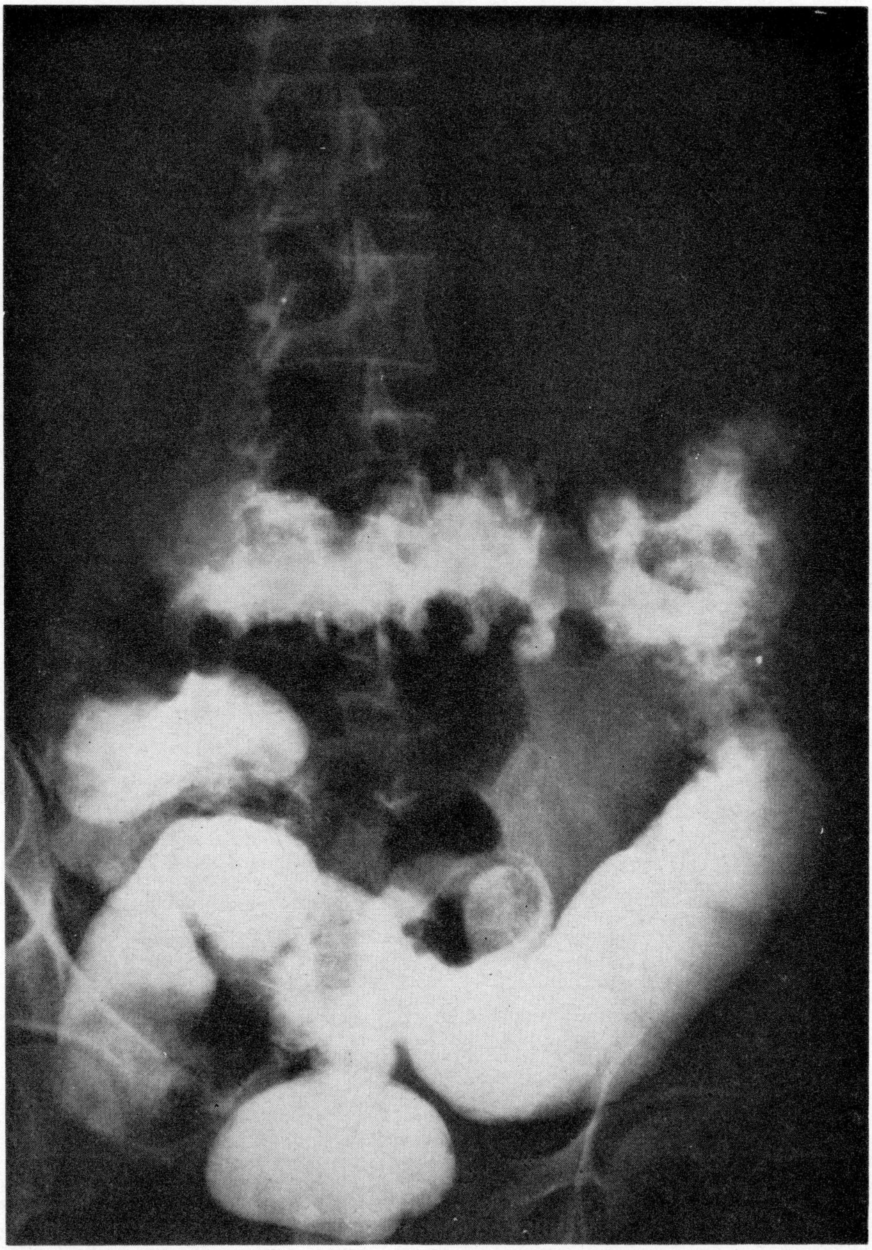

Fig. 7. Granulomatous colitis. Marked irregularity of the contours due to numerous large saclike ulcerations. The left side of the colon is normal.

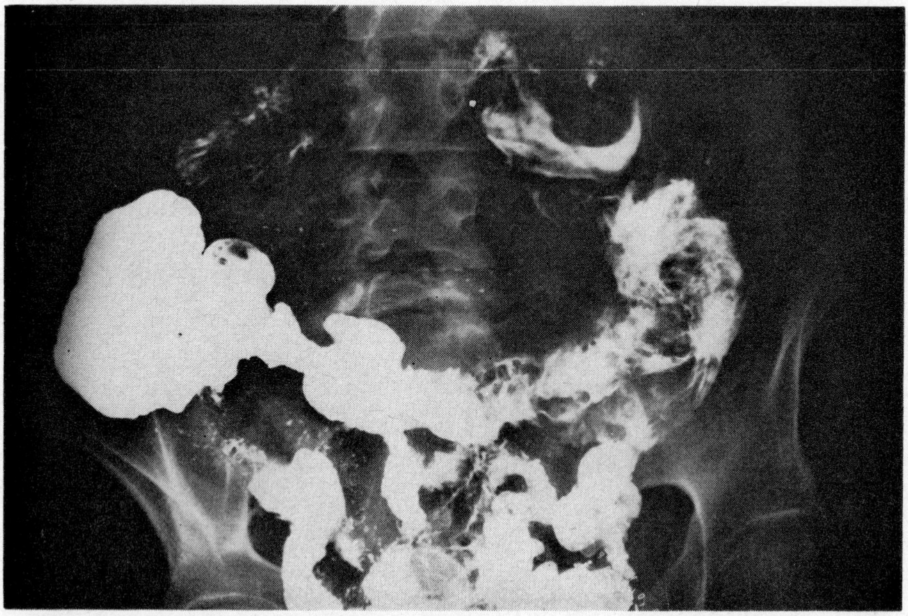

Fig. 8. Same case as in Figures 5 and 6. There is more extensive involvement, with a fistulous communication between the splenic flexure and the stomach. The distal transverse colon is markedly ulcerated, with gross irregularity and distortion of the contour.

8). Fistulae, however, are less common than in regional enteritis. In later stages of the disease the entire mucosa may be sloughed off because of diffuse ulceration. In those cases in which the bowel is diffusely and symmetrically involved and there are no typical features of granulomatous disease, differentiation from ulcerative colitis may be impossible, especially in the absence of characteristic features in the small intestine (Figure 9).

In some instances larger, irregular, nodular contour defects with hazy margins are seen. These are primarily due to mucosal and submucosal edema. Although ulceration is frequently present at this time ulcers can rarely be demonstrated roentgenologically in these defects. When the ulcers are large, circumferential narrowing of the bowel wall due to spasm occurs, and carcinoma is simulated.

Marked thickening of the bowel secondary to intramural fibrotic changes is common in granulomatous colitis; it produces irregular, stenotic segments and strictures (Figure 10). Occasionally granulomatous colitis presents as a single stricture of the colon. When this stricture

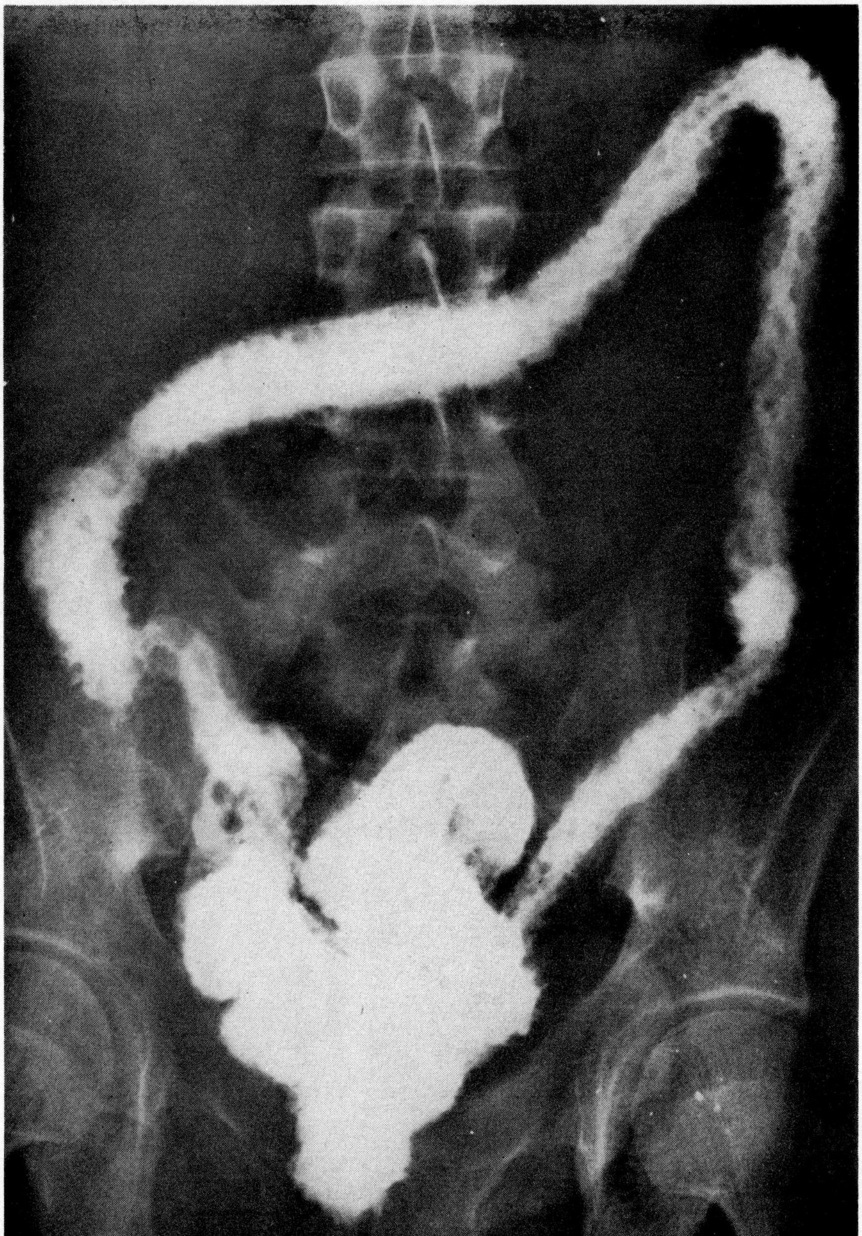

Fig. 9. Granulomatous ileocolitis. Moderate degree of narrowing and rigidity of the entire colon with ulceration of the mucosa and numerous small inflammatory polyps. This type of diffuse involvement can be seen in both ulcerative and granulomatous colitis. Involvement of the terminal ileum with typical regional enteritis enables the radiologist to make a diagnosis of granulomatous ileocolitis.

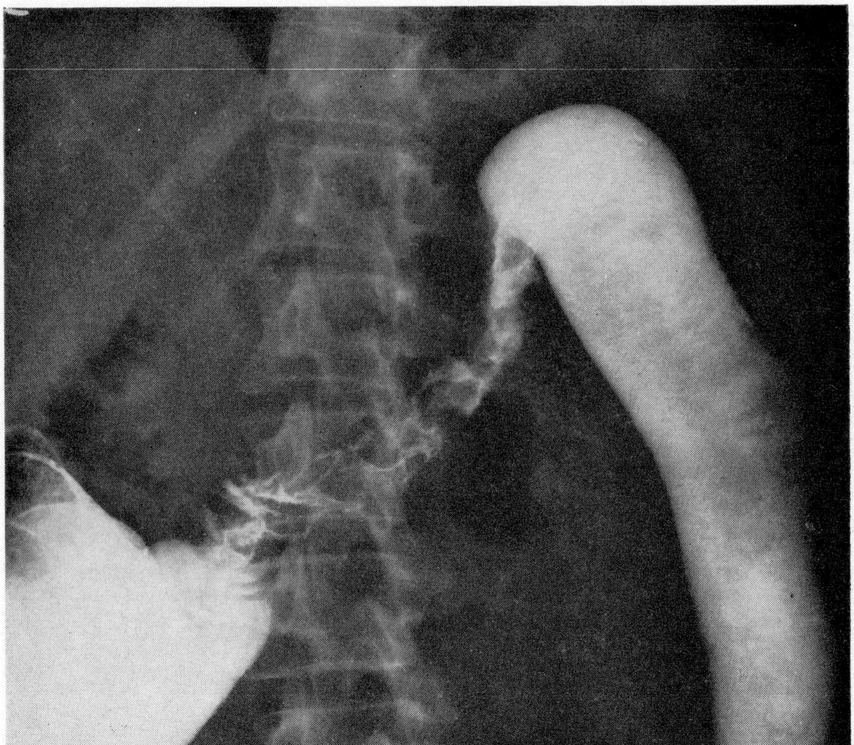

Fig. 10. Granulomatous colitis. The distal half of the transverse colon is narrowed. Another short segment of narrowing is seen in the mid-descending colon. In the absence of granulomatous disease elsewhere, differentiation of the latter lesion from carcinoma would be difficult.

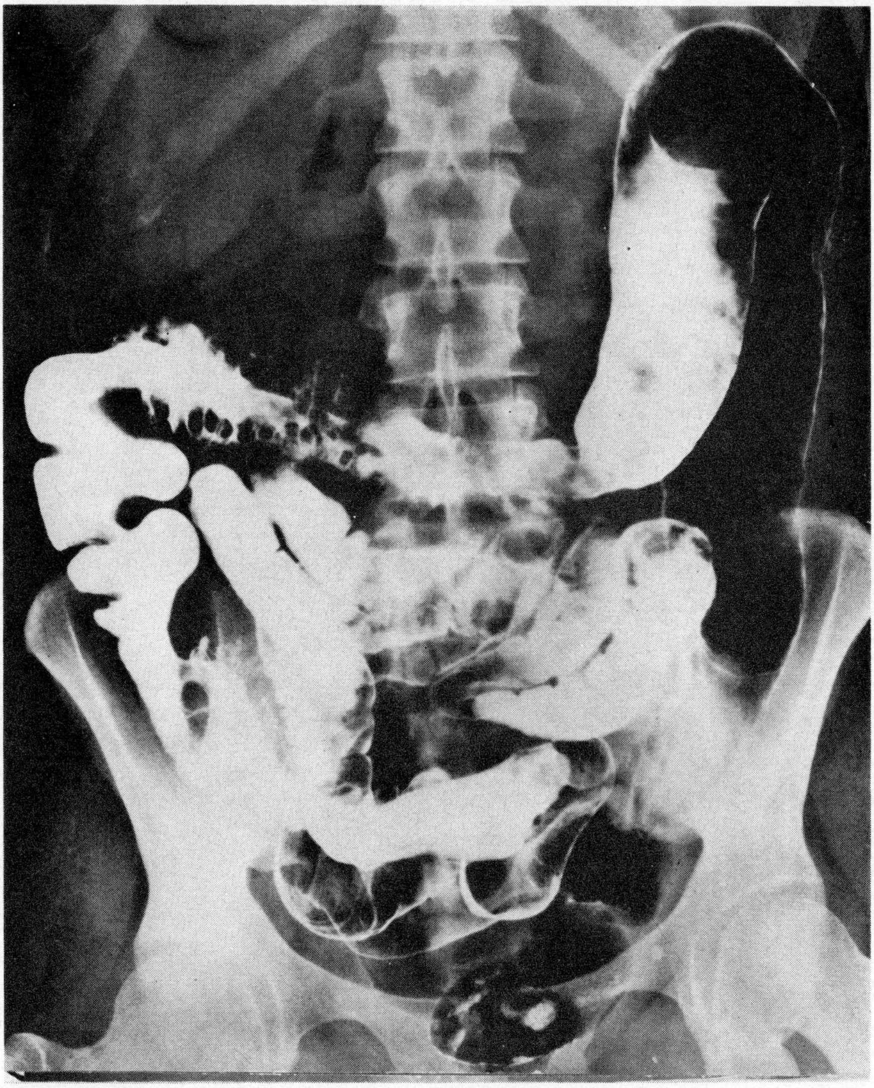

Fig. 11. Granulomatous ileocolitis. The findings are severe in the descending colon where there are narrowing, rigidity, and marked ulceration. The inflammatory process is segmental. The unevenness of involvement is another characteristic feature of granulomatous disease.

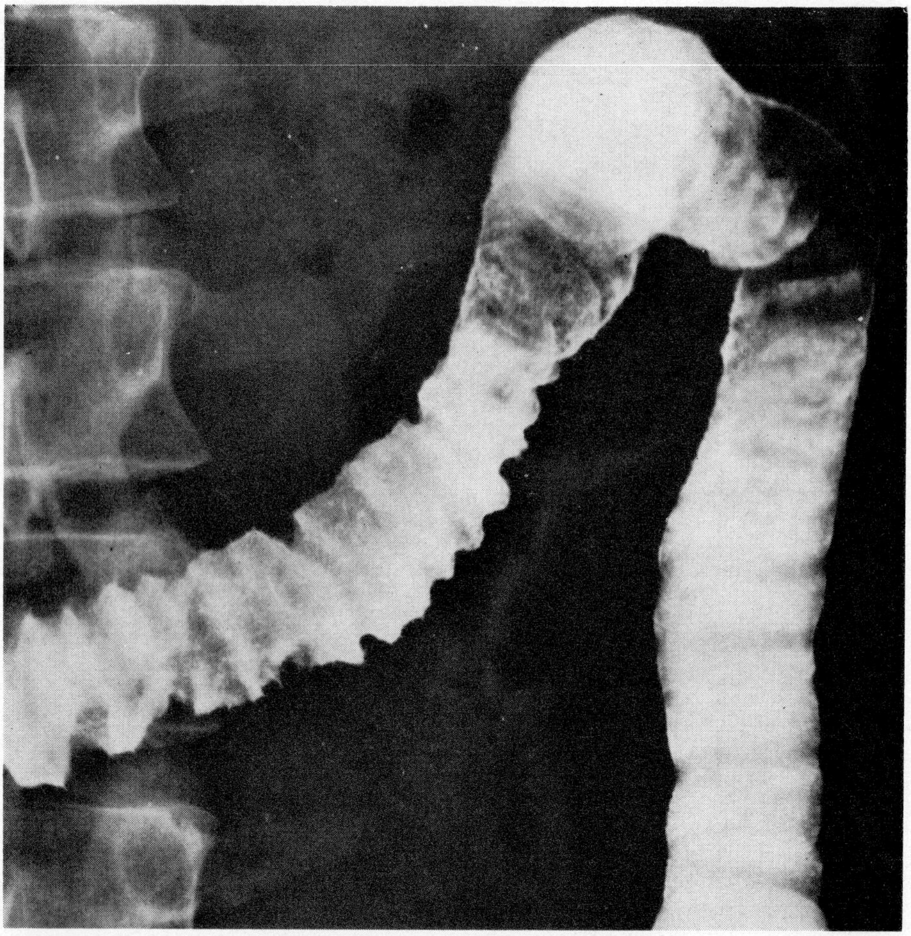

Fig. 12. Magnified view of distal transverse colon demonstrating numerous tiny spicules and a granular appearance of the barium due to small ulcerations. In this case the filled colon showed narrowing of the cecum and terminal ileum; the remainder of the colon appeared normal. Only the evacuation film demonstrated the extent of involvement.

is eccentric and associated with overhanging edges, differentiation from carcinoma may be impossible. In most cases, however, there is further evidence of involvement of the bowel in the form of skip lesions, strictures, or other identifying features of granulomatous disease.

Linear extension of the disease in granulomatous colitis, as in regional enteritis, is uncommon in the absence of surgical operation, but normal areas between skip lesions may become involved. A minimally involved colon with multiple skip lesions may become severely and diffusely ulcerated in a short period of time.

There are no specific roentgen features of granulomatous ileocolitis except for the anatomical distribution (Figure 11). In the small bowel the characteristic findings of regional enteritis are not affected by concomitant inflammatory disease of the colon. In the majority of these cases the inflammatory process in the small bowel is confined to the distal ileum, but at times long segments of small bowel are involved.

Granulomatous ileocolitis must be distinguished from so-called backwash ileitis (ulcerative colitis with involvement of the terminal ileum). In the latter cases, narrowing of the intestinal lumen is usually minimal and the length of ileum involved is small. Sinus tracts, skip areas, and fistulae are not seen, and the mucosa is only slightly altered with minimal thickening of the folds. In a rare case differentiation is impossible. Involvement of the colon in patients with ileocolitis most frequently occurs in continuity with the disease in the ileum. Segmental involvement of the colon is more common than diffuse involvement of the entire large bowel.

In those cases in which the radiologic findings of granulomatous disease of the colon are subtle, a motility follow-through film of the colon performed as part of a small-bowel examination may be helpful. Tiny ulcers, which may be the earliest roentgen manifestation of granulomatous colitis, are best seen in the evacuation films of the barium enema examination (Figure 12).

# A HISTORY OF THE LEGAL REGULATION OF MEDICAL PRACTICE IN NEW YORK STATE

John Barry Bardo

Yale University, New Haven, Conn.*

Regulation of the practice of medicine in New York was recognized as necessary early in the history of the colony and state. A colonial law in 1684 prohibited the practice of medicine "without the advice and consent of such as are skillful in the said Arts." In 1760 another colonial law provided for the regulation of medicine in New York City through the examination and licensure of candidates by specified magistrates. After the Revolution, examination by a magistrate was made contingent on the possession of certain educational qualifications. Legislation enacted in 1797 provided a measure of regulation of medicine; it permitted magistrates to license individuals by indorsing certificates of study issued by reputable physicians and surgeons.

The law of 1760 had not been retroactive, and the irregular practitioners already in the city were therefore unaffected by it, but the laws of 1797 required that:

> ... no person practicing physic or surgery at the time of the passage of the Act should continue to so practice without satisfactory proof to the Chancellor, a judge of the Supreme Court, a master in chancery, or a Judge of the Court of Common Pleas, that he had practiced for two years . . . or had studied that time with a reputable physician or surgeon, and had filed a certificate to that effect with the County Clerk.

The act further required that no other person should practice physic or surgery without a certificate from one or more physicians or surgeons that he had studied medicine for four years under the preceptors signing it, and that he was qualified to practice.[1] Applicants were not required to pass examinations. Legislation passed in 1806 made the pro-

*Presently at the Tufts University School of Medicine, Boston, Mass.

fession itself responsible for the regulation of "physic and surgery."[2] The law permitted incorporation of medical societies in each county and authorized the officers of the county and state societies to examine and license candidates. Candidates for licensure could appeal the decisions of local bodies. This law, the object of which was to obtain incorporation for a medical society for "the suppression of empiricism and the encouragement of regular practitioners,"[3] was intended to secure independence for the State Medical Society and the county medical societies, while the newly incorporated State Medical Society was recognized as the more important body insofar as it could pass on the refusal of a county society to grant a medical license to a properly qualified student, and could grant this privilege in countermand to the action of the county societies.[4] In subsequent years laws were enacted requiring the registration of practitioners with the county clerk, and penalties were imposed for the illegal practice of medicine.

An important step in the regulation of medical practice occurred when the University of the State of New York, through its Board of Regents, was authorized in 1809 to incorporate colleges, and empowered such colleges to grant the degree of doctor of medicine without examination by the censor. This degree constituted a license to practice. Incorporated colleges with the approval of the regents could also endorse degrees conferred by colleges outside the state.

The period from 1806 to 1872 appears to have been a difficult one for the regulation of medical practice; three forces then contended for control of the power of licensure. These were the organized medical profession, the medical colleges, and the University of the State of New York, acting through its regents. Under the law of 1806, the only penalty for practicing without a license was the inability to collect fees by action at law. A further revision of this law in 1813 omitted all penalties for practicing without authority. The Revised Statutes of the State, passed in 1827, were designed to

> forbid the practice of physic and surgery to any one not a member of a county society, and not only to regulate the licensing of practitioners, but to provide for the good behavior of licentiates by prescribing a legal method of expelling members of county societies for forfeiting their right to practice medicine for gross ignorance or misconduct in his profession or immoral conduct or habits.[5]

Under this law no one could practice unless he had a license or a diploma from an incorporated medical society of the state or had the degree of M.D. from a university. If he was authorized to practice in another state or country and had a license or diploma from a medical society in such a state or country he was required to file a copy of his license or diploma with the county clerk, and to give the medical society of the county satisfactory proof of his having followed the plan of study prescribed for students in New York State.[6]

Further confusion arose when the penal clause of the 1827 statutes, which make an unlicensed practitioner guilty of a misdemeanor, was repealed.

The laws became even more inefficient and confused. An act passed in 1844 made it a misdemeanor to practice without a license in cases of gross ignorance, malpractice, or immoral conduct.[7]

In 1872 the regents were first empowered to appoint "one or more boards to consist of not less than seven members who shall have been licensed to practice physic and surgery in this State."[8] Under the law three separate boards of examiners were appointed to examine and license candidates in the schools of medicine then in existence. Although this law first established the principle that licenses should be granted by a state department and not by those engaged in teaching and practicing medicine, the principle was limited in application, and the other sources of licensure—the medical societies and the colleges—continued to hold their powers. By an 1880 statute, however, the societies were divested of their legal right to issue licenses, and that power now was divided between the regents and the colleges. Further streamlining of regulations came in 1890, when the medical degree no longer sufficed as a license to practice and the power to grant licenses was granted solely to the regents. Candidates for licensure were required to have specified preprofessional education and to have attended only medical schools registered by the University. Another significant provision of this law created a Board of Medical Examiners that represented the regular medical profession, the homeopathic, and the eclectic schools; these boards were charged with the responsibility for examining and licensing candidates.[9]

In 1893 the laws relative to medical practice were consolidated into the Public Health Law. The next major statutory change occurred in 1907 when the three separate boards of examiners were replaced by one board that was made responsible for medical licensure and of the enforcement law. To assist the board, the regents were empowered to appoint a secretary.[10] The same statute for the first time recognized osteopathy as one of the schools of medicine.

After 1907 there were still provisions in the law that permitted various kinds of medical sects. Still prevalent, according to J. J. Walsh, were sellers of false cures and remedies: "We still permit the compounder of medicine, even more impudent in his ignorance and almost without pretense of knowledge of his avocation, just as he did in the eighteenth century."[11]

Between 1893 and 1926 charges of illegal practice were commonly prosecuted by counsels for the various medical societies and, pursuant to the Public Health Law,[12] fines imposed for convictions were paid to the county medical societies, which in turn used these fines to pay their lawyers. Defense lawyers protested that the prosecuting attorneys were motivated to conduct successful prosecutions more by prospective fines than by an intention to maintain high standards of medical practice. An outcry arose demanding prosecution of such cases by public attorneys and, in practice, the New York County Medical Society, which had made it a policy to refuse fines from convictions for illegal practice, began to use the services of the district attorney of New York County in such prosecutions. This practice was based on the fact that violation of statutes of the Public Health Law regarding medicine constituted a misdemeanor and that, as such, it should be prosecuted by the law officers of each county, namely the district attorneys. This practice became so widespread that a demand arose for intervention by the attorney general.[13]

Between 1907 and 1927, the statutory responsibility for professional licensure and law enforcement was vested in the New York State Board of Medical Examiners. This Board hired medical investigators, who supervised the licensing examinations prepared and rated by the Board; these investigators were charged with the responsibility for enforcement of medical professional laws. They gathered evidence based on complaints submitted to the secretary of the Board who, if the evidence seemed sufficient, referred it to attorneys who instituted criminal prosecution of the alleged violators.[14]

However, as indicated by the prosecution of cases of illegal practice by lawyers from county medical societies, the burden of professional law enforcement became too great for the limited agency of the Board of Medical Examiners.

Inadequate enforcement of the Public Health Law and of the Education Law[15] that related to medicine resulted in a convocation of doctors and lawyers representative of the several county medical societies of New York State. The purpose of this meeting, held at The New York Academy of Medicine in 1926 and 1927, was to obtain repeal of the medical regulatory statutes of the Public Health Law and to draft the so-called Medical Practice Act, Article 131 of the Education Law.

The Medical Practice Act prohibits the practice of medicine or the use of the title of doctor by an unlicensed individual.[16] Illegal practice constitutes a misdemeanor. The attorney general and, in some instances, the district attorney, are required to prosecute such cases in courts of specified jurisdiction. Under the Medical Practice Act no license is required of an intern or member of the resident staff of a legally incorporated hospital or of any resident physician serving in a state institution or in an institution of political subdivisions of the state, provided the physician has completed specified courses in a registered medical school in the United States or Canada, or in a foreign medical school that has maintained standards not lower than those prescribed for medical schools in New York State.[17]

The 11 articles of the Education Law that establish minimum requirements for entrance into the professions also postulate certain standards for professional conduct on the part of licensed practitioners. Violation of these statutory prohibitions may result in the revocation or suspension of a license or in a censure or reprimand. The final authority for the imposition of these sanctions, as established in the Education Law, is the Board of Regents. Section 211 of the New York State Education Law establishes the Board of Regents as the executor of all determinations regarding the discipline of violators. As prescribed by the Medical Practice Act, grounds for initiation of disciplinary proceedings are: fraud or deceit in admission to practice; conviction of a crime; failure to register where failure is not satisfactorily explained; fraud or deceit in practice; unprofessional conduct; immoral conduct; failure to become a citizen within a specified period; advertising for patronage by means of handbills, posters, circulars, letters, stereopticon slides, motion pictures, radio, or magazines; the use of secret methods, cure, or treatment in practice; criminal abortion or complicity in it; fee-splitting; alcoholism; drug addiction; and insanity.[18]

The Medical Practice Act authorized the action of the attorney general in enforcement.[19] The act specifically imposed upon the attorney general the duty of prosecuting all illegal practitioners of medicine. At the time the Education Bureau of the Department of Law (the attorney general) estimated on the basis of investigation that "of every four individuals practicing medicine within New York State, at least one was an unqualified charlatan."[20] The Department stated:

> An integral part of the proper administrative machinery for clearing the state of illegal quacks and charlatans is the assignment of a deputy attorney general to devote his entire time to the important work of prosecuting these cases on behalf of the citizens of the state.[21]

And while providing for prosecution of unlicensed individuals under the Education Law, the Medical Practice Act also created a Medical Grievance Committee separate from the Board of Medical Examiners. This Committee was charged with the duty of conducting hearings involving disciplinary charges against licensed practitioners. It was formed:

> To eliminate this licensed unethical group. This committee . . . modeled upon the grievance committee of the Bar, for the discipline of licensed physicians . . . has authority to investigate all charges of unprofessional conduct on the part of practicing physicians and to recommend to the Board of Regents the revocation of a physician's license, and the annulment of his registration or any other form of discipline.[22]

The Medical Practice Act provided: a means for uniform criminal prosecution of illegal practitioners, standards for entrance into the profession for professional conduct, and a mechanism by which those statutory standards might be enforced. Also it designated the Board of Regents of the University of the State of New York as executors of decisions in cases involving charges made against a doctor in regard to the legality of his licence.

While this most important statutory change promised increased effectiveness in professional law enforcement, such a condition was not immediately forthcoming. Although the attorney general of the State of New York had been made responsible for prosecutions of illegal practice of medicine, as already mentioned, the investigative body for professional law enforcement was still the State Board of Medical Examiners, whose funds for operation, in fact, came from the yearly registration fees paid by licensed doctors in the state. And the institution of the separate Medical Grievance Committee charged with the duty of hearing disciplinary cases did little to ease the burden carried by the investigators of the Board of Medical Examiners.[23]

In 1938 an investigation focused upon abortion rings and on the effectiveness of the State Education Department in dealing with them. Disciplinary action was instituted in Kings County under the direction of John Amen, an assistant attorney general. Preliminary findings of this investigation disclosed a discouraging picture of disciplining abortionists who were physicians. Statistics showed that during the entire existence of the Medical Grievance Committee, 52 of 77 formal charges involving abortion or attempted abortion were dismissed. In the 25 cases in which guilt was found, 7 licenses were revoked and 14 suspended; 4 physicians were censured.[24]

Until the fall of 1938 responsibility for the investigations of violations of the professional statutes rested on both the Division of Professional Education and the secretaries of the professional Boards of Examiners in medicine, dentistry, and pharmacy, who were under the direct supervision of the associate commissioner for Higher and Professional Education. These secretaries reported the results of their investigations to the assistant attorney general assigned to the department, who then instituted and conducted formal hearings before these bodies, including the Medical Grievance Committee.

At that time the regents created a new position bearing the title of executive secretary of the Division of Professional Conduct. The duties of this functionary included responsibility for investigation of all complaints, of all unprofessional conduct or illegal practice in any of the licensed professions and, as well, of supervision of the New York office responsible for the administration of laws that dealt with the professions. The intent to provide the public and the professions with more efficient and systematic enforcement of the acts that dealt with professional practice was further implemented in 1940, when the regents established the Division of Law Enforcement. The regents attached all professional investigators and inspectors to this division and installed the executive secretary of the Division of Professional Conduct as director. This newly established division was mandated to secure evidence stemming from complaints and to prepare cases based upon such complaints.[25]

The secretaries of the medical and dental boards were administratively divested of all responsibility in relation to investigations and the gathering of evidence, despite their objections. The statutes that fixed responsibility for investigations on these secretaries remained unchanged.

The associate commissioner for Higher and Professional Education reported: "one of the outcomes of this new procedure has been the striking increase in the number of cases prepared and presented to the Medical Grievance Committee."[26]

The second major administrative change that took place during this period occurred in 1941 when, the statute notwithstanding, the function of registering physicians, osteopaths, and physiotherapists was transferred from the secretary of the State Board of Medical Examiners to a central registration unit.

Although there was subsequent modification of the machinery for enforcing the laws relating to the professions, including medicine, the objectives of the Division of Law Enforcement (now called the Division of Professional Conduct) have remained the same; these are to suppress the practice of professions by unlicensed and unregistered individuals and to prevent the violation of professional laws by licensed practitioners. The policy of the division, since its inception in 1940, has been to obtain voluntary compliance with the Education Law and to educate both licensed and unlicensed persons as to the provisions of regulatory statutes.[27] And while disciplinary action against professional practitioners is the most severe form of action and is taken, in most cases, as a last resort, it is significant to the history of the regulation of medical practice in New York State to understand the aims of the machinery of the New York State Education Department and of allied officials and organizations.

In order to curtail and suppress the unlawful practice of medicine by unlicensed and unregistered persons and to prevent and detect the violation of the statutes by licensed and registered practitioners, the Division of Professional Conduct performs the following functions: 1) it investigates complaints alleging violations of the professional laws; 2) it dismisses complaints lacking merit; 3) it appears at hearings of the professional boards and grievance committees; and 4) it supplies stenographic assistance to the assistant attorney general and to the hearing boards and grievance committees.[28]

The objective of the assistant attorney general in the Bureau of Education is to assist in the enforcement of the laws that deal with the professions and to suppress illegal practice and unprofessional conduct. The assistant attorney general evaluates investigations made by the Division of Professional Conduct and prosecutes disciplinary and criminal cases. When satisfied as to the adequacy of evidence gathered by the Division of Professional Conduct, the assistant attorney general prepares formal charges and initiates the administrative hearings. He acts as legal adviser to the Division of Professional Conduct and is, in turn, dependent upon the effectiveness of the Education Department in obtaining evidence with which he can proceed with successful prosecutions and thus discharge the responsibility given him by the statute.

The disciplinary mechanism is set in motion by complaints from patients or physicians or from other sources. Complaints of illegal or unprofessional conduct are commonly made in writing to the offices of the New York State Education Department, the office of the attorney general, or to the offices of the state or county medical societies. After referral to the Division of Professional Conduct, all complaints are reviewed, investigated, and either dismissed or acted upon in the following ways:

In disciplinary cases, the assistant attorney general in the Education Bureau prepares formal charges against the practitioner after he is satisfied with the evidence against the alleged violator. The charges specify the provisions of the Medical Practice Act allegedly violated, and itemize the violations in detail. Arrangements for hearing of the case before a subcommittee of the Medical Grievance Committee are made in conjunction with the director of the Division of Professional Conduct. At hearings of the subcommittee, the assistant attorney general presents the evidence to sustain the charges. During the course of the hearings, the assistant attorney general does not participate in deliberations of the hearing body, but is consulted in connection with the findings of the hearing body, and he prepares the findings and recommendations of the grievance committee pursuant to its instructions. In medicine he appears informally before the full Grievance Committee only to read and explain the findings and recommendations of the subcommittee. Where the full grievance committee rejects a finding of guilty, the case comes to an end. The assistant attorney general has no power to appeal to the regents. Where the finding of guilt is affirmed by the full Grievance Committee, the assistant attorney general and the respondent appear before the Regents' Committee on Discipline.

The objective of the hearing body in medical disciplinary proceedings is to protect the public by eliminating unprofessional and unethical conduct. To achieve this objective it hears charges and makes recommendations to the Board of Regents with regard to revocation of licenses or other disciplinary action.

In formal hearings held before the Medical Grievance subcommittee or the full Committee, the accused practitioner has the right to appear in person or by counsel, to cross-examine witnesses, and to question the evidence. The evidence for the case is first presented by the assistant attorney general, then by counsel for the respondent. Then witnesses are examined and cross-examined. During the hearing the assistant attorney general may be called upon to advise members of the Grievance Committee or subcommittee as to the admissibility of evidence and motions, and to give legal advice to members of the hearing body if necessary. The findings of the subcommittee are then submitted to the secretary of the full Medical Grievance Committee, which meets quarterly. In medicine, a finding of guilt may result only from a unanimous vote of the 16 members of the committee. The respondent is not present, and no testimony is taken at the meetings of the full Medical Grievance Committee. The full Committee has available a transcript of the record of the hearing held before the subcommittee. In addition to the record, it is customary procedure for the full Committee to question the subcommittee and the assistant attorney general. The full Committee usually follows the recommendation of the subcommittee. The minutes of the subcommittee hearing, as transcribed by the hearing reporter provided by the Division of Professional Conduct, are sent by the assistant attorney general to the assistant commissioner for Professional Education in Albany, who then sends the complete record and a memorandum for each case, including a brief biographical sketch of the alleged violator, to the three members of the Regents' Committee on Discipline. The Committee is sent the case record and the memorandum including a brief biographical sketch of the accused doctor and verbatim excerpts from the charges, findings, and recommendations of the Medical Grievance Committee. At hearings of the Regents' Committee on Discipline, the respondent and his counsel, the assistant attorney general, the director of the Division of Professional Conduct, the assistant commissioner for professional education and the secretary of the Medical Grievance Committee are present. Following deliberations by the Regents' Committee on Discipline, in which only the members participate, the commitee instructs the assistant commissioner for Professional Education to prepare its report and recommendations for the full Board of Regents. The members of the Committee then sign this report and submit it, through the assistant commissioner for Professional Education, to the secretary of the Board of Regents.

The full Board of Regents hears each case on the basis of a copy of the report of the Regents' Committee on Discipline and a copy of the assistant commissioner's memorandum on the accused practitioner citing the charges, findings, and recommendations. The record of the hearing by the subcommittee is submitted to the regents who, by formal vote, approve, modify, reject, or remand the report of the Committee on Discipline and empower and direct the Commissioner for Professional Education to execute an order carrying out their decisions. The order is prepared by the departmental counsel and served by the Division of Professional Conduct. An order becomes effective only when served personally on the accused; this is by departmental policy, not by law.

A physician may appeal from any disciplinary penalty imposed by the regents through the medium of a judicial review under the provisions of article 78 of the Civil Practice Law and Rules. In recent years the possible scope of judicial review has been expanded to include the severity of the penalty imposed, and a review of judicial determinations has indicated that in a few instances the courts have felt that the quantum of punishment assessed by the regents has been too severe. Appeals taken from final action of the regents must be brought in the Appellate Division of the Supreme Court, Third Judicial Department, in Albany. Since the attorney general conducts the hearings upon which disciplinary penalties are predicated, the Appeals Bureau of the Department of Law argues all the appeals under Section 78 of the *Civil Practice Law and Rules*.[29]

We may summarize the life history of a complaint by listing sequentially the steps involved:

1) Formal complaint received at offices of Division of Professional Conduct.

2) Investigation ordered by director of the Division of Professional Conduct, who makes recommendation as to necessity for further action, dismissal of complaint, or formal disciplinary proceedings.

3) Subcommittee of Medical Grievance Committee designates cases in which formal charges are to be presented, based upon facts revealed in investigation and after recommendation from the director of the Division of Professional Conduct.

4) Assistant attorney general prepares charges.

5) Subcommittee of Medical Grievance Committee holds hearings, makes recommendations to the

6) Medical Grievance Committee, which makes its decision based on subcommittee recommendation.

7) Assistant attorney general sends case record to assistant commissioner for Professional Education, who then sends case record and memorandum to the

8) Regents' Committee on Discipline, which makes its recommendations, sending them through the

9) Assistant commissioner for Professional Education to the

10) Board of Regents, who approve, modify, reject or remand the report of the Committee on Discipline. The decision of the Board of Regents is carried out by the

11) Commissioner of Professional Education, who acts through the Division of Professional Conduct.

12) Possible judicial review in the Appellate Division, Third Department, argued by the Appeals Bureau, Department of Law.

It is of interest to note, after delineating the process of formal medical disciplinary proceedings, that hearings on charges are held before members of the medical profession, so composed on the assumption that only members of the profession are qualified to understand and judge the technical facts presented. However, *most* questions presented before the Medical Grievance Committee are issues of simple fact and are not really complicated technical questions. Even questions involving abortions and drug addiction ultimately rest on an issue of fact: whether something that is contrary to the provisions of the law has or has not been done.[30]

Although external to the mechanism of the New York State Education Department, the various county medical societies in the state play an important adjunctive role in investigation of complaints against doctors. The county medical societies attempt to resolve complaints lodged by patients or other physicians against member physicians.

Grievance committees of the societies function primarily to adjust complaints of negligence or excessively high fees. Such complaints, commonly based on inadequate physician-to-patient communication, are mediated by the grievance committees of county medical societies.

The county medical societies' boards of censors act upon complaints of violation of medical ethics.

These committees of county medical societies act to maintain the code of ethics of the society and to maintain good physician-patient relations. Furthermore, the vigilance of these bodies may serve to deter doctors from possible legal action when charges that question the validity of the medical license, not solely the privileges of medical society membership, would be involved.

While the actions of committees of county medical societies are limited to members of a particular society, and while their authority is limited to censure and to suspension or revocation of society membership, such committees assist in the legal regulation of medicine, as such, by providing records and testimony helpful in obtaining prosecution through the Division of Professional Conduct of the New York State Education Department for professional misconduct.[31]

A criticism of the system within the State Education Department was that of the time-lag in prosecuting cases. In 22 medical cases studied from 1945 to 1947 the average lapse of time between preferment of charges and their eventual resolution was 411 days; the median time lapse was 352 days.[32] This delay may have reflected the point raised earlier, that disciplinary proceedings are held before a body of busy physicians. The determination of many cases may not require the medical knowledge of the Medical Grievance Committee, although it is for those cases in which a professional judgment is required that the body exists. No complete solution to the problem of delay has yet been proposed by doctors, lawyers, or members of the State Education Department.

However, despite an increasing professional population, the State Education Department facilities for enforcement have kept pace with the growing number of professionals and with the concomitant increase

TABLE I.*

| | Disciplinary complaints received by Division of Professional Conduct | | Cases closed By Division | | By Board of Regents | |
|---|---|---|---|---|---|---|
| | Total | Medical | Total | Medical | Total | Medical |
| 1965-1966 | 3836 | 193 | 4353 | 553 | 83 | 29 |
| 1962-1963 | 1289 | 909 | 521 | 112 | 66 | 38 |
| 1959-1960 | 701 | 144 | 817 | 91 | 50 | 24 |
| 1956-1957 | 1168 | 247 | 1096 | 278 | 47 | 23 |
| 1953-1954 | 696 | 118 | 644 | 148 | 59 | 27 |
| 1950-1951 | 448 | 96 | 268 | 62 | 34 | 20 |
| 1947-1948 | 190 | 63 | 198 | 91 | 49 | 34 |
| 1944-1945 | 469 | 96 | 529 | 148 | 58 | 32 |

*From records of the Division of Professional Conduct, New York State Education Department, Albany, N. Y.

in the bases of disciplinary and criminal action relating to the professional statutes. An increasing case load achievement of the Division of Professional Conduct has been attained through: 1) improvement in administrative procedures, including a 1961 increase from 10 to 20 investigators; 2) centralization of investigation; 3) pooling of investigators for service in all professions; and 4) increased field work. For a brief statistical sketch of the total and medical case loads of the Division of Professional Conduct and the Board of Regents since 1944 see Table I.[33] Medical disciplinary cases recorded from July 1, 1965, to June 30, 1966, appear in Table II.

While no determination of the average or median time lapse has been made in recent years, the lapse has been greatly reduced from that earlier mentioned. The increased case load achievement and decreased time lapse have been achieved in the face of a professional population that has grown from approximately 140,000 licensed persons in 1940, including roughly 35,000 medical practitioners, to 340,000 total professional licensees, including 42,000 licensed practitioners, in 1966.[33]

Regulation of medical practice has retained the character of supervision by legislation. The 19th century conflict regarding the seat of authority for licensure resulted in the establishment in 1890 of the principle that medical licenses be granted by the Board of Regents of the University of the State of New York. The Medical Grievance

TABLE II.*

| Received by Division | | Closed by Board of Regents | |
|---|---|---|---|
| Disciplinary | 167 | *Disciplinary:* | |
| Probation | 24 | Censure and reprimand | 10 |
| Restoration | 2 | Revocation | 3 |
| | 193 | Suspension | 6 |
| | | Resignation accepted | 1 |
| Investigation | 209 | Revocation stayed—probation | 9 |
| | 402 | | 29 |
| | | *Investigation* | |
| *Closed by Division* | | Restoration denied | 2 |
| Disciplinary | 553 | License restored | 3 |
| Investigation | 236 | Revocation stayed—probation | 1 |
| | 789 | | 6 |

*From records of the Division of Professional Licensing Services, New York State Education Department, Albany, N. Y., as of August 1, 1966.

Committee invoked the use of a panel of physicians in disciplining other physicians. Criminal prosecution of the unlicensed practitioners, previously the domain of district and other attorneys, became the responsibility of an assistant attorney general attached to the State Education Department. The investigative function now lies solely with the Division of Professional Conduct which, together with the assistant attorney general, is responsible for enforcement of the professional statutes.

Presently the provisions of the Education Law provide standards of qualification for practice, methods of examination, certification, registration of candidates, grounds for illegal practice, penalties, and disciplinary hearing proceedings. The procedures described above are the means by which the provisions of the law are enforced.

## *NOTES AND REFERENCES*

1. Provisions of act quoted from Walsh, J. J., *History of Medicine in New York,* 5 vols. New York, Nat. Americana Soc., 1919, vol. 1, p. 82.
2. *Laws of the State of New York,* 29th session. An act to incorporate Medical Societies for the purpose of regulating the practice of physic and surgery in this state. Albany, Barber, 1806, chap. 138.
3. Shaftel, N. History of the Medical Society of the State of New York, 1807-1957, *New York J. Med. 57*:446-47, 1957.
4. *Ibid.,* p. 447.
5. Purrington, W. A., quoted in Walsh, J. J., *op. cit.,* vol. 1, p. 85.
6. *Ibid.,* p. 86.
7. *Ibid.*
8. *Laws of the State of New York,* 95th session. An act relating to the examina-

tion of candidates for the degree of doctor of medicine. Albany, Brown, 1872, Chap. 746.

9. *Laws of the State of New York,* 113th session. An act to establish boards of medical examiners of the State of New York for the examination and licensing of practitioners of medicine and surgery; to further regulate the practice of medicine and surgery. Albany, Bank Bros., 1890.
10. *Laws of the State of New York,* 130th session. An act to regulate the practice of medicine, and to repeal Article 8 of Chapter 661 of the laws of 1893 and acts amendatory thereof. Albany, Lyon, 1907.
11. Walsh, J. J., *op. cit.,* vol. 1, p. 92.
12. Public Health Law of 1893. In: *Laws of the State of New York,* 116th session. Albany, Lyon, 1893, vol. 1, chap. 661, sec. 153.
13. *Ibid.;* and from conversations with Reed Dawson, legal counsel for the New York County Medical Society, held November 30, 1965, and August 21, 1966.
14. This and further discussion of the function of the State Board of Medical Examiners was supplemented by conversation with J. McCullough, senior investigator of the Division of Professional Conduct of the New York State Department and one of five medical investigators for the New York State Board of Medical Examiners, February 1933 to January 1937. Conversation held November 23, 1965.
15. The Education Law of 1910, sec. 1263, contained provisions that paralleled those relating to medicine in the Public Health Law of 1893, sec. 153.
16. Methods of obtaining a medical license in New York State as established by the Medical Practice Act of 1927 (art. 131, Education law): 1) passed by a state licensing examination prepared by the Board of Medical Examiners; 2) by the endorsement of a license issued by another jurisdiction; 3) by passing an examination given by the National Board of Medical Examiners; and 4) by acceptance by the Board of Regents of the applicant's "conceded eminence and authority" in his profession.
17. Prior to 1958 the standards of foreign medical schools were deemed unacceptable by an examining committee that made visits to foreign medical schools. This committee was composed chiefly not of doctors but of nonmedical educators, who returned to New York and printed lists of "approved" foreign medical schools. Since 1958, however, 40 of the 55 state and territorial jurisdictions in the United States have required that physicians trained in foreign countries other than Canada pass an examination given by the Educational Council for Foreign Medical Graduates as a prerequisite to admission to their licensing examinations.
18. *Report of the Temporary State Commission on Coordination of State Activities.* Albany, Williams, 1948, appendix D, pp. 414-15; and the *New York State Education Law,* sec. 153, in: *The Consolidated Laws of New York,* annotated, Eldridge, H. N. and Bronaugh, M., eds. Northport, N. Y., Thompson, 1928.
19. *New York State Education Law,* sec. 6513, subdiv. 5.
20. *Annual Report of the New York State Education Department,* 1927, p. 79. Albany, Univ. State of N. Y., 1928, p. 79.
21. *Ibid.,* p. 82.
22. *Ibid.*
23. *Laws of the State of New York,* 150th session, Albany, Lyon, 1927, chap. 85; an act to amend the education law to conform to the state department's law, in relation to the practice of medicine, dentistry, veterinary medicine and surgery, pharmacy, nursing and trained attendance, chiropody, optometry, engineering and surveying, architecture, public accounting and shorthand reporting, and repealing articles 8, 9, 10, 11, 12, 13 and 15 of the public health law and articles 4A, 7A, 8 and 8A of the general business law relating thereto; Article 8: Practice of Medicine, secs. 140 to 153; and from a conversation with J. McCullough.
24. Amen, J. H. *Report of the Kings County Investigation, 1938-1942,* p. 82.

25. *Thirty-sixth Annual Report of the State Education Department, 1940.* Albany, Univ. State of N.Y., 1941, vol. 1, p. 173; and *Thirty-seventh Annual Report of the State Education Department, 1941,* Albany, Univ. State of N.Y., 1942, vol. 1, pp. 186, 226-27.
26. *Thirty-seventh Annual Report of the State Education Department, 1941,* Albany, Univ. State of N.Y. 1942, vol. 1, p. 186.
27. The professions regulated by the Division of Professional Conduct now include: architecture, landscape architecture, certified shorthand reporting, chiropractic, dentistry, dental hygiene, osteopathy, physiotherapy, nursing (registered and practical), ophthalmic dispensing, optometry, podiatry, psychology, veterinary medicine, and social work.
28. *Report of the Temporary State Commission on coordination of State Activities, Second Interim Report.* Albany, Williams, 1948, p. 109.
29. *New York State Education Law,* sec. 6515, subdiv. 5.
30. From conversations with Reed Dawson.
31. From conversations with Reed Dawson.
32. *Report of the Temporary State Commission on Coordination of State Activities,* Table 24, p. 151.
33. From records of the Division of Professional Licensing Services, New York State Education Department, Albany, N.Y., as of August 1, 1966.

# THE LONGEVITY OF THE ANCIENT GREEKS (HAWKINS, 1829; ANGEL, 1947-60)

In 1958 Richard S. Stewart* wrote: "It is a curious and suggestive fact that the early history of classical Rome is better understood by modern scholars than by any historian of the time of Caesar Augustus." This surprising fact is the result of 19th and 20th century scholarship, exemplified by the researches of Theodor Mommsen (1817-1903), which were extended by countless successors. To the work of historians and classicists much has been added in recent decades by archaeologists and anthropologists. What is true of the Romans and their deeds is also true of the Greeks, so that we need not scruple to acknowledge that Herodotus, Polybius, and Thucydides have been outdone, though not displaced.

Lest these contentions appear brash or arrogant, we subjoin a series of excerpts by which the reader can see for himself what scholarship has accomplished during the last 150 years. These excerpts are limited to a single aspect of Greek history, viz. longevity.

"No documents remain to inform us of the rate of mortality, or of longevity, amongst the Greeks."

Hawkins, F. B. *Elements of Medical Statistics.* London, Longman, 1829, p. 5.

". . . there has been no inquiry into the possible increase in longevity, with attendant social problems, which the rise of civilization in ancient Greece may have produced. Such a study must be based largely on skeletal material, since no written data have been handed down from prehistoric Greece. . . .

From the third millennium B.C. to classical times (650-150 B.C.), longevity in ancient Greece increased slightly but significantly, as shown by study of skeletal remains. The data are too scanty to determine the exact change in life expectancy, since skeletal remains of really old people and of children are extremely inadequate in number. However, the change in age composition of the popula-

* Stewart, R. S.: Theodor Mommsen's *History of Rome, Harvard Library Bull. 12*:161-195, 1958.

TABLE—AVERAGE AGE AT DEATH OF MALE ADULTS*

| *Period* | *Date* | *Age* | *No. of specimens* |
|---|---|---|---|
| Neolithic-Early Bronze | 4000-2000 B.C. | 33.2 | 40 |
| Middle Bronze | 2000-1500 | 36.7 | 105 |
| Late Bronze | 1500-1150 | 39.3 | 164 |
| Classic | 650-300 | 44.5 | 82 |
| Roman | 120-600 A.D. | 39.4 | 62 |
| Turkish | 1400-1800 | 33.9 | 29 |
| Modern Greece | 1928 census | 56.1 | 30,873 |

* Aged 15 or older.

tion was not great enough (nor life expectancy of the historic period near enough to that of today) for social problems of old age to arise in modern form. The aged continued to participate in the life of the community, through the respect attached to their judgment and opinions."

Angel, J. L. Length of Life in Ancient Greece, *J. Gerontol. 2*:18-24, 1947.

". . . I have been able to repair and study over 600 skeletons and 1200 skulls dating from Neolithic times (pre 3000 B.C.) down to the 19th Century A.D. . . .

". . . It is natural to find a steady association between level of culture and average age at death of adults. This shows a change of about 10 years with rise and fall of culture. Perhaps more critical than this change in the average adult life span, with its increase of time for creative leisure, are the high infant and child death rates. At Middle Helladic Lerna we observe that at least 55% of 239 Bronze Age deaths are those of infants and children and 15% over 45; by classical times 49% of skeletons are those of children and infants and almost 25% are over 45, compared with the U.S.A. in 1900 where 35% of deaths were of infants and children and 42% over 45."

Angel, J. L. Physical and Psychological Factors in Culture Growth. In: Wallace, A.F.C., ed. *Selected Papers of the Fifth International Congress of Anthropological and Ethnological Sciences.* Philadelphia, Univ. of Penna. Press, 1960, pp. 665-670.

From a supplemental tabulation very kindly submitted by Dr. Angel, author of the two preceding passages, the accompanying table has been excerpted. Its data are based on work done by him in 1957-60. The increase of the age at death is clearly apparent.

It is understood that Dr. Angel will soon publish additional statistics that present the results of his most recent observations. These promise to be extremely instructive.

S. J.

THE NEW YORK ACADEMY OF MEDICINE

## TELEVISED CLINICAL SCIENCE SEMINARS

**Tuesday Evenings, 8:30-9:30 P.M.**

STATION WNYC—TV UHF—CHANNEL 31

**October 3, 1967**

### MALABSORPTION SYNDROME

MARVIN H. SLEISENGER
Chief, Department of Gastroenterology
Professor of Medicine
Cornell University Medical College

GRAHAM H. JEFFRIES
Associate Professor of Medicine
Cornell University Medical College

ELLIOT WESER
Assistant Professor of Medicine
Cornell University Medical College

**October 10, 1967**

### FUNDAMENTALS OF FLUID AND ELECTROLYTE BALANCE—PART I

HENRY T. RANDALL
Memorial Hospital
Professor of Surgery
Cornell University Medical College

PARKER VANAMEE
Associate Attending Physician
Memorial Hospital
Associate Professor of Medicine
Cornell University Medical College

**October 17, 1967**

## FUNDAMENTALS OF FLUID AND ELECTROLYTE BALANCE — PART II

HENRY T. RANDALL
Memorial Hospital
Professor of Surgery
Cornell University Medical College

PARKER VANAMEE
Associate Attending Physician
Memorial Hospital
Associate Professor of Medicine
Cornell University Medical College

**October 24, 1967**

## MANAGEMENT OF LYMPHOMAS

DAVID A. KARNOFSKY
Associate Professor of Medicine
Cornell University Medical College

JAMES J. NICKSON
Professor of Radiology
Cornell University Medical College

HENRY RAPPAPORT
Professor of Oncology
Chicago Medical School

**October 31, 1967**

## THE MANAGEMENT OF RESPIRATORY INSUFFICIENCY

EDWARD H. BERGOFSKY
Assistant Professor of Physiology
New York University School of Medicine

ROBERTA GOLDRING
Assistant in Medicine
Columbia University College of
Physicians and Surgeons

GUSTAVE A. LAURENZI
Associate Professor of Medicine
New Jersey College of Medicine and
Dentistry

# *NOTICE*

## PROGRAMS OF MEETINGS AT THE ACADEMY

The New York Academy of Medicine does not print or publish—either in the *Bulletin* or the Grey Folder—programs other than those arranged by its own sections or affiliated societies. The Academy does not assume responsibility for the printing or distribution of programs of other medical organizations or groups that meet regularly or occasionally in the Academy building. *Use of the Academy's facilities for meetings does not include publication of programs.*

The Academy's program booklet (*Grey Folder*) is free to Fellows and is available to others by subscription at $2.00 for eight issues, published from September through May. The *Grey Folder* contains *only* programs of the Academy's sections and affiliated societies. For subscription, write to *Grey Folder*, Room 60, at the Academy.

The *Bulletin of The New York Academy of Medicine*, which is sent gratis to Fellows only, is available by subscription at $10.00 per year for 12 issues, from:

**Stechert-Hafner Service Agency**
**21 East 10 Street, New York 10003**

BULLETIN OF
THE NEW YORK ACADEMY
OF MEDICINE

VOL. 43, NO. 11 NOVEMBER 1967

# INTERACTIONS BETWEEN IMMUNOCOMPETENT CELLS AND TARGET CELLS OR ANTIGENS*

JOHN R. DAVID

Assistant Professor of Medicine
Harvard Medical School
Robert B. Brigham Hospital
Boston, Mass.

As the interaction of immunocompetent cells with target cells or antigen is a broad subject, this brief review is limited to certain *in vitro* studies of the problem. The first part will be devoted to the destruction of target cells or tissues by the addition of immunocompetent lymphoid cells. The second part will deal with the stimulation and blast formation of lymphocytes by phytohemagglutinin and antigen, and the third with the inhibition of cell migration by antigen. As the symposium is concerned with cellular factors in autoimmunity, I shall try to discuss these three parameters of cellular behavior as they relate to one model of autoimmune disease, namely experimental allergic encephalomyelitis.

In models of target cell destruction by sensitive cells, such as those

*Presented as part of a symposium on *Cellular Factors in Autoimmunity*, held at a combined meeting of the Academy Section on Micro- and Molecular Biology with the New York Pathological Society, December 8, 1966.
This study was supported in part by Public Health Service Grant AI-07685 from the National Institute of Allergy and Infectious Diseases.

of Rosenau and Moon,[1, 2] Wilson,[3] and others, animals of one strain are sensitized with tissues from another strain. Lymphoid cells from the sensitized animals are placed on top of monolayers of target cells obtained from the same strain as that used to sensitize. Using this type of experiment, many workers have obtained similar results. The lymphoid cells from sensitive animals, but not those from normal controls, first aggregate about the target cells, a process that usually takes several hours. Cytotoxic changes are then observed after 12 hours; they reach their peak at 24 to 48 hours. The reaction occurs without the addition of complement, and thus far no complement has been detected in lysates of the sensitive cells (although the test used, the lysis of erythrocytes, would require the complete complement system and would not detect the presence of a few components).[3] In these studies it is necessary that the sensitive cells be alive, otherwise the effect is not produced. Wilson was able to suppress the cytotoxic action of sensitive cells with Imuran, using doses that inhibited certain metabolic activities of the lymphocytes without killing them.[4] Wilson's quantitative studies suggest that only 1 to 2 per cent of the lymphocytes actually lyse target cells. By using irradiated target cells, he also showed that the sensitive lymphoid cells were not just preventing target cell growth. Although Rosenau and Moon demonstrated that the reaction they were observing was immunologically specific,[5] most workers have compared the effect of sensitized cells with normal, unsensitized cells and not with the effect of cells sensitized to an unrelated antigen. Further, a few workers have been able to simulate the toxic effect of sensitive cells by adding large quantities of normal cells. Recent studies suggest that such sensitivity can be transferred to normal lymphocytes with RNA[6] or ribosomes[7] from sensitive lymphoid cells.

Most investigators believe that the sensitive lymphoid cells, in order to exert cytotoxic action, must be in intimate contact with the target cell. This is based on experiments such as those of Rosenau and Moon, and of Wilson, all using millipore chambers. When sensitive lymphoid cells were separated from the target cells by a millipore filter, there was no longer any destruction of the target cells. One objection may be raised to the conclusions drawn from these experiments. Contact between sensitive cells and target cells at some time may be necessary; however, these experiments do not rule out the possible mediation of cell destruction by a soluble material. It would, for example, be of great interest to determine whether lymphoid cells are stimulated by target cells on the *same* side of a millipore chamber to produce material that would be cytotoxic for the target cells on the other side.

In many but not all of the studies on target cell destruction, it was also found that sera from sensitized animals were cytotoxic for the target cells.[2] This reaction, however, was found to be complement-dependent and to occur more rapidly, usually in one hour. Except for one experiment, to be discussed later, such sera were not able to sensitize normal lymphoid cells to lyse target cells. Indeed, in experiments such as Moller's, sera from sensitized animals inhibited the cytotoxicity of sensitized cells.[8]

Similar studies have been applied to experimental allergic encephalomyelitis (AE). Bornstein and Appel showed that sera from animals with AE were capable of demyelinating cultures of rat cerebellum.[9, 10] The effective material in the sera was $\gamma$-globulin, and the reaction was complement-dependent and reversible. Of interest is the finding by these workers that sera from patients with multiple sclerosis as well as certain other neurologic diseases also demyelinated brain cultures.[11] Lamoureux *et al.* have found recently that cerebrospinal fluid from monkeys with AE as well as from patients with multiple sclerosis was capable of demyelinating cultures of brain tissue.[12, 13] It should be noted that sera from two monkeys that were sensitized with brain but did not develop the disease inhibited the cytotoxic action of sera from monkeys with the disease.[12] This is reminiscent of the finding of Paterson that certain antibodies from animals with AE will actually protect against the disease.[14] The presence of a cytotoxic material in cerebrospinal fluid from other neurologic diseases, especially in certain viral diseases such as infection with Coxsackie $B_2$ virus, may limit to some extent the primary etiological role of such factors.[13]

Studies by Koprowski and Fernandes and by Winkler demonstrated that sensitive cells from animals with AE can kill glial cells and demyelinate cultures of nervous tissue.[15, 16] Winkler found that lymphoid cells could do this at a time when sera did not.[16] Winkler and Arnason have further investigated the mechanism of this reaction. Since it was known that thymectomized animals as well as patients with ataxia telangectasia had decreased delayed hypersensitivity and showed decreased IgA in their serum, these workers attempted to block the action of sensitized cells with antibody to IgA. They found that the demyelination of rat trigeminal ganglion by sensitive rat lymphoid cells was blocked when rabbit antibody to rat IgA was added to the cultures, but not when rabbit antibody to rat IgM or IgG was added.[17] This suggested the possibility, among others, that lymphocytes might act either by secreting or having on their surfaces some material similar to IgA. The unique finding in Koprowski's study was the observation that serum from sensitized animals, while not toxic itself, would sensitize lymphoid cells obtained from animals sensitized with complete Freund's adjuvant, but without brain antigen. The possibility that in this case antibody sticks the lymphoid cells to the target tissue and that then the lymphoid cells kill the target cells leads to another group of experiments concerning this *in vitro* model.

Briefly, Holm and Perlmann[18] and Moller[19] showed that normal lymphoid cells were cytotoxic to allogenic cells if they were stuck to these by phytohemagglutinin or by antisera to the lymphoid cells. This cytotoxicity occurred only when lymphoid cells and target cells were antigenically histoincompatible. However, Moller found that cells from $F_1$ hybrids, which should not be able to recognize parental cells as foreign, nevertheless were capable of killing target cells of parental origin. Such lymphoid cells were active after they had been irradiated. Moller has suggested that this reaction is due to differences in cell surface structure, possibly unrelated to histocompatible antigens. The recent observation by Moller that in human cell systems it is possible to observe cytotoxicity with autologous cells on autologous targets complicates the interpretation of this phenomenon.[20] It should be recalled that both phytohemagglutinin and antibody do more than glue the lymphoid cell to the target. Both these materials are capable of stimulating and transforming lymphocytes.[21, 22] Further, Rosenau has reported that, if lymphoid cells from a nonsensitive animal were stuck to allogenic target cells with polylysine, they did not cause any target cell damage.[2] Thus the reaction involving "normal" cells with phytohemagglutinin or antiserum may not simply occur with normal cells but with cells that have been artificially stimulated to differentiate; this phenomenon may be different from the reaction of specifically sensitive cells with target cells that was discussed earlier.

Do the sensitive lymphocytes die in the cytotoxic process? Rosenau, who observed cultures with cinematography, thought they did.[2] However, in most systems this has not been specifically studied. It would be quite interesting, for instance, to see whether thymidine-labeled sensitive lymphocytes released label into the media after contact with target cells. Before leaving the subject of target cell reactions, it should be pointed out that macrophages have also been shown to exert cytotoxic effects on target cells.[23, 24]

The second model to be discussed, the stimulation of lymphocytes by antigen, is proving to be one of the most useful tools available for the study of immune cells in man. The early findings of Nowell[21] on the transformation of lymphocytes by phytohemagglutinin, and those of Permain *et al.*[25] and Hirschhorn *et al.*[26] on the stimulation of these cells by specific antigen have led to many interesting clinical observations. It has been shown, for instance, that anergic patients, such as those with Hodgkin's disease and sarcoidosis, have lymphocytes that respond poorly to phytohemagglutinin and other antigens.[27, 28] In this context, it is of note that Holm and Perlmann reported that lymphocytes from patients with Hodgkin's disease were less cytotoxic to allogenic target cells when stuck to these with phytohemagglutinin than were normal lymphocytes.[29] These workers also observed that this finding correlated with lack of transformation of the cells by phytohemagglutinin. Smithwick and Berkovich recently found that lymphocytes from tuberculin-positive patients were unresponsive to tuberculin during measles, and that measles virus, when added directly to PPD-sensitive lymphocytes, depressed stimulation by PPD (but not, interestingly enough, stimulation by phytohemagglutinin), suggesting a mechanism for the anergy often observed during the course of measles.[30] Of special importance is the recent finding by Fowler, Morris, and Whittley that lymphocytes from six patients with multiple sclerosis were stimulated to transform by autologous or homologous cerebrospinal fluid, whereas cells from nine control patients were not.[31] It will certainly be of great interest if such cells are also found in patients with viral encephalitis or if the phenomenon is specific for multiple sclerosis.

The exact relation of lymphocyte stimulation to delayed hypersensitivity is still not completely understood, and further study is necessary before we can say without question that it is a specific manifestation of delayed hypersensitivity.

The third model, inhibition of cell migration by antigen, first described by Rich and Lewis,[32] is one we have been studying during the past few years in the hope of learning more about sensitive cells.[33] The technique, based on the method of George and Vaughan,[34] consists, first, of placing peritoneal exudate cells obtained from animals with delayed hypersensitivity in capillary tubes. The cells then migrate out of the tubes onto glass coverslips in culture chambers. This migration is inhibited when specific antigen is in the media, and such inhibition can easily be quantitated. The reaction is immunologically specific. Furthermore, cells from animals making antibody but not exhibiting delayed hypersensitivity are *not* inhibited by antigen, and normal cells are not sensitized by incubation in sera from sensitized animals.[33]

Since this phenomenon appeared specific for delayed hypersensitivity, a study was carried out in collaboration with Dr. Philip Paterson to determine whether guinea pigs with AE might yield cells specifically sensitive to the encephalitogenic antigen. We found that peritoneal cells from guinea pigs with AE were indeed inhibited by extracts of guinea pig brain.[35] This appeared to be an organ-specific reaction. Guinea pig kidney extract, for example, did not inhibit the migration of these cells. Reports that neonatal brain does not produce either clinical or histologic evidence of AE and thus lacks the encephalitogenic antigen were confirmed in our experiments by means of neonatal rat brain. The absence of the encephalitogenic antigen in neonatal brain made it possible to determine whether cellular sensitivity in AE is directed specifically to the encephalitogenic antigens and not to other components in brain unrelated to the disease. It was found that neonatal rat brain did not inhibit the migration of cells obtained from guinea pigs with AE. In contrast, adult rat brain and guinea pig brain, which readily produce the disease, did inhibit the migration of such cells. These findings indicate that the cellular sensitivity is directed against a component that appears in the maturing nervous tissues parallel with the appearance of the encephalitogenic antigen—if indeed it is not the encephalitogenic antigen itself. The finding that cells from animals with AE are specifically sensitive to the antigens known to produce AE suggested strongly that cells of such specific sensitivity might well play an important role in the pathogenesis of the disease.

In light of the findings of Koprowski, we also tried to see whether sera from guinea pigs with AE, whose own cells had been inhibited by brain extract, could confer such sensitivity upon cells from animals sensitized with complete Freund's adjuvant but without brain. These experiments were uniformly negative. We were unable to sensitize such cells with sera.

Further studies on the inhibition of cell migration have shed some light on its mechanism, and some conclusions from these studies may be extended to the general problem of delayed hypersensitivity. Early in the course of our studies we found that only a few sensitive cells need be present for the whole population to be inhibited by antigen. By mixing cells from sensitive animals with cells from normal animals, we found that as few as 2.5 per cent of cells need come from the sensitive animals for inhibition to be observed.[36] The sensitive cells had to be alive for this to take place. Puromycin prevented the reaction.[37] These findings are consistent with the studies of McCluskey *et al.* and others who showed that most of the cells at the skin test site following passive transfer of delayed hypersensitivity were nonsensitive host cells.[38]

In an attempt to determine what cell type was the sensitive cell, we obtained cell preparations from lymph nodes of highly sensitive animals; these preparations contained about 95 per cent lymphocytes. Such cells were *not* inhibited by specific antigen, but when they were added in small numbers to normal peritoneal exudate cells, the resulting population *was* inhibited by antigen.[39] Bloom and Bennett demonstrated that sensitive peritoneal cells freed of lymphocytes were no longer inhibited by PPD, while the lymphocytes, when added to normal peritoneal cells, would cause inhibition by antigen.[40] It has been shown by Bloom and Bennett and by results from our laboratory that the lymphocytes act by producing a soluble material that inhibits the migration of normal peritoneal cells, presumably the macrophages. For instance, if lymphocytes from a guinea pig sensitive to ovalbumin are incubated for 24 hours with ovalbumin, the cell-free supernatant, when added to normal cells, inhibits cell migration. These same lymphocytes, when incubated in antigen-free medium or with an unrelated antigen such as bovine $\gamma$-globulin, do not form the active material. If puromycin is added to the mixture of sensitive lymphoid cells and antigen, the lymphoid cells no longer yield an active supernatant. The active substance is macromolecular, i.e., it is nondialyzable; it is heat-stable to 56° C. for 30 minutes.[36] We are presently attempting to characterize the material. The data available suggest an explanation for the phenomenon of inhibition of cell migration by antigen. The first event may be the reaction of specific sensitive lymphocytes with antigen.

This interaction results in the production of substances that either alone or in combination with antigen affect the remaining nonsensitive cells, presumably macrophages. The detection of material with these biological properties raises interesting questions as to its nature: whether continued presence of antigen is required for its effect, its relation to known immunoglobulins, and its relevance to *in vivo* events of delayed hypersensitivity.

Each of the three models discussed measures a different parameter of lymphocyte behavior in response to antigens. The first demonstrates the cytotoxic action of sensitive lymphocytes on target cells and may yield valuable information on the exact mechanism by which lymphocytes destroy target cells. This model may be directly related to the role that such cells play in homograft rejection, to tissue destruction by lymphocytes in certain autoimmune diseases, and to tumor immunity. The second model, the transformation of lymphocytes by antigen, focuses directly on the lymphocyte itself. How this transformation affects the function of the lymphocyte is not yet known. Although this phenomenon appears to be an immune reaction, the relation of lymphocyte transformation to antibody formation and delayed hypersensitivity remains to be determined. The third system described measures the presence of cells reflecting delayed hypersensitivity. It is presently of use in characterizing the soluble material which sensitive lymphocytes produce when stimulated by antigen. This material, *in vitro,* affects the behavior of nonsensitive macrophages, and may play a similar role *in vivo*. Such a material may also be involved in target cell reactions. It is not known at present whether these different models are measuring different functional parameters of the same cell, i.e., whether the same lymphocyte may be stimulated to transform, or make a soluble material that can affect normal macrophages, or can be cytotoxic when specifically sensitive to a target cell. It is possible that different groups of lymphocytes are involved in each of these reactions. It has been suggested that lymphocytes should not be considered as one type of cell; indeed, it appears that they may be a group of cells with differing life spans and differing functions.[41, 42] It remains to be determined in what manner these various models involving lymphocytes are related to each other.

### *REFERENCES*


1. Rosenau, W. and Moon, H. D. Lysis of homologous cells by sensitized lymphocytes in tissue culture, *J. Nat. Cancer Inst. 27*:471, 1961.
2. Rosenau, W. Interaction of lymphoid cells with target cells in tissue culture. In: *Cell-Bound Antibodies.* B. Amos, H. Koprowski, eds. Philadelphia, Wistar Inst. Press, 1963, p. 75.
3. Wilson, D. B. Quantitative studies on the behavior of sensitized lymphocytes *in vitro.* I. Relationship of the degree of destruction of homologous target cells to the number of lymphocytes and to the time of contact in culture and consideration of the effects of isoimmune serum, *J. Exp. Med. 122*:143, 1965.
4. Wilson, D. B. Quantitative studies on the behavior of sensitized lymphocytes *in vitro.* II. Inhibitory influence of the immune suppressor, imuran, on the destructive reaction of sensitized lymphoid cells against homologous target cells, *J. Exp. Med. 122*:167, 1965.
5. Rosenau, W. and Moon, H. D. Specificity of the cytolytic effect of sensitized lymphoid cells *in vitro, J. Immunol. 93*:910, 1964.
6. Wilson, D. B. and Wecker, E. E. Quantitative studies on the behavior of sensitized lymphoid cells *in vitro.* III. Conversion of "normal" lymphoid cells to an immunologically active status with RNA derived from isologous lymphoid tissues of specifically immunized rats, *J. Immunol. 97*:512, 1966.
7. Gerughty, R. M., Rosenau, W. and Moon, H. D. *In vitro* transfer of immunity by ribosomes, *J. Immunol. 97*: 700, 1966.
8. Moller, E. Antagonistic effects of humoral isoantibodies on the *in vitro* cytotoxicity of immune lymphoid cells, *J. Exp. Med. 122*:11, 1965.
9. Bornstein, M. B. and Appel, S. H. Application of tissue culture to the study of experimental "allergic" encephalomyelitis. I. Patterns of demyelination, *J. Neuropath, Exp. Neurol. 20*:141, 1961.
10. Appel, S. H. and Bornstein, M. B. Application of tissue culture to the study of experimental allergic encephalomyelitis. II. Serum factors responsible for demyelination, *J. Exp. Med. 119*: 303, 1964.
11. Bornstein, M. B. and Appel, S. H. Tissue culture studies of demyelination. *Ann. N. Y. Acad. Sci. 122*:280, 1965.
12. Lamoureux, G., Boulay, G. and Borduas, A. G. Cytotoxic antibody for cultured nervous tissue in serum and cerebrospinal fluid from Rhesus monkeys with allergic encephalomyelitis, *Clin. Exp. Immunol. 1*:307, 1966.
13. Lamoureux, G. and Borduas, A. G. Immune studies in multiple sclerosis. *Clin. Exp. Immunol. 1*:363, 1966.
14. Paterson, P. Y. Cells, Antibodies and Auto-immune Disease. In *Cell-bound Antibodies,* B. Amos, H. Koprowski, eds., Philadelphia, Wistar Inst. Press, 1963, p. 101.
15. Koprowski, H. and Fernandes, M. V. Autosensitization reaction *in vitro, J. Exp. Med. 116*:467, 1962.
16. Winkler, G. F. *In vitro* demyelination of peripheral nerve induced with sensitized cells, *Ann. N. Y. Acad. Sci. 122*: 287, 1965.
17. Winkler, G. F. and Arnason, B. G. Antiserum to immunoglobulin A: Inhibition of cell-mediated demyelination in tissue culture, *Science 153*:75, 1966.
18. Holm, G., Perlmann, P. and Werner, B. Phytohemagglutinin-induced cytotoxic action of normal lymphoid cells on cells in tissue culture, *Nature 203*:841, 1964.
19. Moller, E. Contact-induced cytotoxicity of lymphoid cells containing foreign isoantigens, *Science 147*:873, 1965.
20. Moller, G., Beckman, V. and Lundgren, G. *In vitro* destruction of human fibroblasts by non-immune histoincompatible lymphoid cells, *Inform. Exch. Group 5,* Sci. Memo 235, 1966.
21. Nowell, P. C. Phytohemagglutinin: initiator of mitosis in cultures of normal human leukocytes, *Cancer Res. 20*:462, 1963.

22. Sell, S. and Gell, P. G. H. Studies on rabbit lymphocytes *in vitro. I.* Stimulation of blast transformation with an antiallotype serum, *J. Exp. Med. 122:* 423, 1965.
23. Granger, G. A. and Weiser, R. S. Homograft target cells: specific destruction *in vitro* by contact interaction with immune macrophages, *Science 145:* 1427, 1964.
24. Granger, G. A. and Weiser, R. S. Homograft target cells: contact destruction *in vitro* by immune macrophages, *Science 151:*97, 1966.
25. Permain, G., Lycette, R. R. and Fitzgerald, P. H. Tuberculin-induced mitosis in peripheral blood leucocytes, *Lancet 1:*637, 1963.
26. Hirschhorn, K., Bach, F., Kolodny, R. L., Firschein, I. L. and Hashem, N. Immune response and mitosis of human peripheral blood lymphocytes *in vitro, Science 142:*1185, 1963.
27. Hirschhorn, K., Schreibman, R. R., Bach, F. H. and Siltzbach, L. E. *In vitro* studies of lymphocytes from patients with sarcoidosis and lymphoproliferative diseases, *Lancet 2:* 1964, p. 842.
28. Hersh, E. M. and Oppenheim, J. J. Impaired *in vitro* lymphocyte transformation in Hodgkin's disease, *New Eng. J. Med. 273:*1006, 1965
29. Holm, G., Perlmann, P., and Johansson, B. Impaired phytohemagglutinin-induced cytotoxicity *in vitro* of lymphocytes from patients with Hodgkin's disease or chronic lymphatic leukemia, *Inform. Exch. Group. 5,* Sci. Memo 273, 1966.
30. Smithwick, E. M. and Berkovich, S. *In vitro* suppression of the lymphocyte response to tuberculin by live measles virus, *Proc. Soc. Exp. Biol. Med. 123:* 276, 1966.
31. Fowler, I., Morris, C. E. and Whittley, T. Lymphocyte transformation in multiple sclerosis induced by cerebrospinal fluid, *New Eng. J. Med. 275:*1041, 1966.
32. Rich, A. R. and Lewis, M. R. The nature of allergy in tuberculosis as revealed by tissue culture studies, *Bull. J. Hopkins Hosp. 50:*115, 1932.
33. David, J. R., Al-Askari, S., Lawrence, H. S. and Thomas, L. Delayed hypersensitivity *in vitro.* I. Specificity of inhibition of cell migration by antigens, *J. Immunol. 93:*264, 1964.
34. George, M. and Vaughan, J. H. *In vitro* cell migration as a model for delayed hypersensitivity, *Proc. Soc. Exp. Biol. Med. 111:*514, 1962.
35. David, J. R. and Paterson, P. Y. *In vitro* demonstration of cellular sensitivity in allergic encephalomyelitis, *J. Exp. Med. 122:*1161, 1965.
36. David, J. R., Lawrence, H. S., and Thomas, L. Delayed hypersensitivity *in vitro.* II. Effect of sensitive cells on normal cells in the presence of antigen, *J. Immunol. 93:*274, 1964.
37. David, J. R. Suppression of delayed hypersensitivity *in vitro* by inhibition of protein synthesis, *J. Exp. Med. 122:* 1125, 1965.
38. McCluskey, R. T., Benacerraf, B. and McCluskey, J. W. Studies on the specificity of the cellular infiltrate in delayed hypersensitivity reactions, *J. Immunol. 90:*466, 1963.
39. David, J. R. Delayed hypersensitivity *in vitro:* its mediation by cell-free substances formed by lymphoid cell-antigen interaction, *Proc. Nat. Acad. Sci. 56:*72, 1966.
40. Bloom, B. R. and Bennett, B. Mechanism of a reaction *in vitro* associated with delayed-type hypersensitivity, *Science 153:*80, 1966.
41. Gowans, J. L. and McGregor, D. D. Immunological activities of lymphocytes, *Progr. Allerg. 9:*1, 1965.
42. Volkman, A. and Gowans, J. L. Origin of macrophages from bone marrow in the rat, *Brit. J. Exp. Path. 46:*62, 1956.

# PROBLEMS IN THE DEVELOPMENT OF A TNM SYSTEM OF STAGING FOR CANCER OF THE HEAD AND NECK*

JOSEPH NEWALL

Director, Department of Radiotherapy
St. Vincent's Hospital and Medical Center
Associate Clinical Professor of Radiology
New York University School of Medicine
New York, N. Y.

WITHIN recent years there has been a generally increased awareness within our profession of the need for a true evaluation of therapeutic methods. An appreciation of the interpretation of statistics and of the problems involved in the planning and conduct of clinical trials is a necessary accomplishment of every thoughtful physician.

The problem of the relative merits of surgery and radiotherapy, of course, is not new, but with the introduction of modern, elaborate, costly, and potentially dangerous forms of radiation therapy and the acceptance of increasingly radical surgery, it has become even more necessary to obtain an assessment of their real value. The publication of survival figures from series treated by different modalities in different institutions is of limited use as a means of comparison. The main reason for this is the relative numbers of patients in each individual series with advanced or localized disease. A series containing a relatively high proportion of patients in good condition with limited cancer will have a better survival rate than one in which the patients have more advanced disease or are in poor general health, even though the therapeutic methods used are of equal value. In 1961 Dr. Arthur James, acting for the American Cancer Society, collected from a broad review of the literature the survival figures following treatment by radiation and by surgery for cancer at the various sites.[1] One of the avowed purposes of the publication was that it should act as an encyclopedia of end results in cancer and as a reference for the student, intern, resident, and clinician. At every site, with the exception of the floor of the mouth, the results of surgical operation were better than those of radiotherapy. Yet this is not necessarily true, and a therapeutic

*Presented at a meeting of the New York Roentgen Society at The New York Academy of Medicine, January 16, 1967.

policy based on these figures would be wrong, for the very reasons outlined above. The obvious method to overcome this problem is to group patients with a similar extent of disease and then to compare the methods of treatment in each group. This—the definition of a set of standards whereby we may compare series of patients treated by different methods—is the main purpose of any system of staging.

Such a system for cancer of the cervix was originally developed by the League of Nations and has been in use since 1929; it has received international acceptance. It is only recently, however, that an attempt has been made to adopt similar policies for other sites, in particular for cancer in the head and neck.

In 1953 in Copenhagen a joint meeting of the Committee on Tumor Nomenclature and Statistics, of the International Union against Cancer (IUCC), and the Committee on Stage-Grouping in Cancer and Presentation of the Results of Treatment, of the International Congress of Radiology, invited the IUCC to continue investigations into the general techniques of staging with particular reference to cancer of the breast, cervix, and larynx. Such proposals were published by the IUCC in 1958 and in them the TNM System was adopted.[2] Two basic principles are involved in this method:

1) Cases comprising the group under study are identified by assigning to each certain symbols denoting the size and local extension of the primary tumor (T), the state of the regional lymph nodes (N), and the presence or absence of distant metastases (M).

2) Once these factors have been identified, conventional stages can then be defined usually by grouping various combinations of the alloted symbols. For example, in the International System a primary breast cancer of 2 cm. or less is denoted by the symbol T1. When it measures 2 to 5 cm. it is denoted as T2. The presence of palpable mobile nodes in the axilla is given the symbol N1. If there are no distant metastases, the symbol Mo is used. The two primary tumors above with palpable axillary nodes but no distant metastases may be described briefly therefore as T1N1Mo and T2N1Mo. Both are included as Stage 2 of the International Staging System. The various stages indicate the progression of the lesion and at each site they can be planned to indicate any peculiar clinical behavior on the part of the tumor.

It is, of course, the exact definition of the T, N, and M symbols that is of cardinal importance in the system. This implies careful examination and recording; to ensure accuracy this must be done at the time of the initial examination. Retrospective review of a series of cases will confirm this contention. The importance of accurate examination and description before treatment is started cannot be overemphasized. As an example one might consider the situation in which two identical sites are treated by methods of equal value and inevitably, therefore, have the same over-all survival rates (that is, assessing all patients together). Once they are analyzed by stage, differences can arise. In any system so far devised there are difficulties in determining with accuracy the exact staging in a number of cases. If we consider a hypothetical classification involving three stages, then if in the first medical center, the borderline cases between stages 1 and 2 are assigned to the more advanced stage and, in the second center, to the earlier stage, then the survival figures of Stage 1 in the first center will be better because of the exclusion of these borderline more advanced patients. If the same steps are adopted between Stages 2 and 3, the first center will again have a better survival figure in Stage 2 because of the exclusion of the more advanced patients and the inclusion of doubtful cases between Stages 1 and 2. Parodoxically, Stage 3 in the first center will still do better than in the second center because of the inclusion of the rather less advanced borderline cases between Stages 2 and 3.

Because of the critical nature of the original clinical examination, it has been suggested by nihilists that no system of staging can ever be accurate and that any attempt to define one is fruitless. This is, however, a confession of failure; any attempt at analysis and comparison of therapeutic methods is surely better than none. Quite apart from its main purpose, the adoption of a system inculcates not only the habit of careful examination but also the exact reporting of findings.

If we accept the need for accuracy, other factors must be considered before the system can be of universal value.

1) The system must be clinical. Where radiotherapy is the treatment an operative specimen other than biopsy will not be available; therefore operative and pathological findings cannot be used except as a means of establishing diagnosis. It is, of course, generally accepted that the inclusion of such data would increase the accuracy. To include them in a surgically treated series but not in a radiotherapeutic series would at once bias results in favor of the former.

TABLE I—PRIMARY TUMOR: GENERAL PRINCIPLES OF T CLASSIFICATION

| | |
|---|---|
| T1 | Tumor strictly confined to the organ of origin and of relatively small size. |
| T2 | Tumor limited to the organ of origin but of relatively large size or with limited extension beyond the original organ. |
| T3 | Tumor with wide infiltration reaching neighboring organ. |
| T4 | Tumor with considerable involvement of adjacent tissues and spread to neighboring organs. |

2) The basic principles, that is, the same number of T, N, and M factors, each showing a similar degree of extension, should be applicable to all sites. A system that adopts, for example, different criteria for lymph node staging has little chance of acceptance. It is sad but true that if the physician must refer to a set of reference charts each time a patient is staged, the system will not be used. The adoption of this principle has been one of the basic problems involved in the staging of head and neck cancer, as will be seen later.

3) All centers reporting results must adopt the same criteria even though they do not necessarily agree with its minutiae. Any modification will invalidate comparison with data derived from other centers.

With these basic factors in mind further attention can now be given to the various factors of the TNM System in relation to the head and neck and the difficulties that have been encountered in their elucidation and adoption.

It has been observed that the criteria for each factor can be adopted only in the light of the knowledge of the past behavior of the tumors and that the stages should be selected in such a way that a gradation between the results of present methods of treatment for each stage can be recognized. In other words, Stage 1 should carry an 80 per cent survival figure; Stage 2, 60 per cent; Stage 3, 30 per cent, and so on. The general principles of the T classification for all sites as originally proposed are seen in Table I.

The first proposals for a system of staging in cancer of the head and neck—in this case the larynx—were published by the IUCC in 1958.[2] In 1962 general agreement was reached on these proposals; also, systems were adopted for staging cancer of the buccal cavity, the pharynx, and the larynx.[3] The suggestion was made that the systems be put to clinical trial beginning on January 1, 1963. For various rea-

TABLE II—LYMPH NODE STAGING: IUCC 1958

| | |
|---|---|
| N0 | — No regional lymph nodes palpable. |
| N1 | — Regional lymph nodes palpable and movable. |
| N2 | — Regional nodes partially or completely fixed. |
| Nx | — Regional nodes not accessible and not visualized. |

TABLE III—LYMPH NODE STAGING: IUCC 1962

| | |
|---|---|
| N0 | — No palpable lymph nodes. |
| N1 | — Movable homolateral lymph nodes. |
| N2 | — Movable contralateral or bilateral lymph nodes. |
| N3 | — Fixed homolateral or bilateral lymph nodes. |

sons the proposals, although constituting a step forward, have not been found generally acceptable. For example, the classification for oral cavity, nasopharynx, and larynx contains four levels of T grading, while for oropharynx and hypopharynx only three groups are recognized. As a result, the T3 stage in larynx and in hypopharynx represents large differences in the extent of the disease. The original criteria for staging of nodes as proposed in the original proposals in 1958 are seen in Table II. By 1962, however, the classification had been modified to include all fixed nodes in a separate category (Table III). The size of the nodes was not considered.

But the IUCC was not the only body in the field by this time. The Committee for Radiation Therapy Studies (CRTS) proposed a definition of N staging that is different from that of the International Union; it is summarized in Table IV. The dominant features are those of size, multiplicity, bilaterality, and fixation of the lymph nodes. To reach agreement on each and all of these points has been the difficult factor that each committee has encountered in formulating proposals as to any staging system. The CRTS has also proposed T values for various sites within the head and neck—a typical example being that for the oral part of the tongue (Table V). The proposed T values for each of the sites considered in the head and neck by the CRTS are usually uniform, and the same basic values are considered in each.

Various committees representing other subspecialty groups have also

TABLE IV—LYMPH NODE STAGING: CRTS

| | |
|---|---|
| N0 | No clinical evidence of lymph node metastasis. |
| N1 | A single clinically positive node less than 3 cm. in diameter, not fixed, and interpreted as clinically containing metastatic disease. |
| N2 | A single node, not fixed, greater than 3 cm. in diameter, or ipsilateral multiple nodes not fixed. |
| N3 | Fixed, bilateral, or contralateral nodes, clinically containing metastatic disease. |

TABLE V—T STAGING: ORAL TONGUE: CRTS

| | |
|---|---|
| T1 | Tumor measuring 2 cm. or less in its largest diameter. |
| T2 | Tumor measuring from more than 2 cm. and to 4 cm. in its largest diameter, with minimal infiltration in depth. |
| T3 | Tumor measuring from more than 4 cm. in its largest diameter to one half the tongue with or without limited tension to the floor of the mouth. |
| T4 | Tumor measuring more than one half the tongue or massive extension to the floor of the mouth, with or without involvement of the mandible. |

been actively concerned with the problem but no formal proposals have been published. The final group concerned with the problem—the one that will undoubtedly be the major influence in national policy—is the American Joint Commitee for Clinical Staging and End Result Reporting. This Committee was organized in 1959 with the purpose of developing systems of staging for various sites. The development and organization of this group have been described by Copeland.[4] Representatives were appointed from the American College of Surgeons, the American College of Radiology, the College of American Pathologists, the American College of Physicians, the American Cancer Society, and the National Cancer Institute. Subcommittees designated as Task Forces were then appointed to consider each individual anatomical site. Proposals for the larynx were published in 1962[5] and for the Pharynx in 1965;[6] the Task Force for Oral Cancer reached some final agreement in December 1966.

The real contribution of the Joint Committee has been that for the first time an attempt has been made to produce a system based on an analysis of results in the light of clinical factors. This is in contrast to the IUCC and the CRTS Systems, which were obtained by discussion based on personal experience, opinion, and impression, but those, however valuable, can at times be notoriously misleading. Protocols were completed by various cooperating centers after review of the records of patients previously treated. The results were then collected and analyzed by the chairman of the appropriate Task Force and made available to the various members before each meeting.

The Task Force for cancer of the oral cavity reached its final conclusions in December 1966; it would be wrong to anticipate the findings. The proposals of the Group for Larynx and Pharynx, however, have met with fairly general criticism. Their lymph node staging differs from that suggested by the other bodies in that mobile nodes are grouped in one stage irrespective of whether they are ipsilateral, contralateral or bilateral. In addition, they continue the practice of the IUCC in that four T stages were adopted for larynx but only three for hypopharynx.

There remains lack of agreement on the staging for lymph nodes between the IUCC, the Joint Committee's proposals for larynx and pharynx, and the CRTS; undoubtedly it will be necessary to reach a compromise in these fields as well. For this reason too the findings and proposals of the Task Force on oral cavity cancer are awaited with considerable interest.

Amidst all this confusion and disagreement it is at least comforting to report general agreement on the consideration of metastases. Mo means no metastases; M1, metastases present.

At this point the matter rests—there are still conflicting principles in that the IUCC, the CRTS, and the Joint Committee's ideas do not coincide. In addition, the Joint Committee's standards regarding the head and neck differ, although it is to be hoped that some agreement will be reached ere long in this direction. Until some general agreement is reached on the T and N groupings, it will be pointless to consider dividing the groupings into progressive stages. Until this is done it will remain impossible to compare methods of treatment in head and neck, and any attempt to do so will be invalid. Some progress has been made, however, and we are already a long step in the right direction of knowing that a carcinoma of the tongue T1N1Mo treated in Aberdeen, Scotland is the same lesion as one similarly defined in Aberdeen, Idaho, or in Aberdeen, New South Wales.

### *REFERENCES*

1. James, A. G., ed. *Cancer Prognosis Manual.* American Cancer Society, 1961.
2. *Malignant Tumors of the Breast and Larynx—Proposal.* Paris, International Union Against Cancer, 1958.
3. *Malignant Tumors of the Buccal Cavity, the Pharynx and the Larynx.* Paris, International Union Against Cancer, 1962.
4. Copeland, M. M. American Joint Committee on Cancer Staging and End Results Reporting, *Cancer 18:*1637, 1965.
5. *Clinical Staging System for Cancer of the Larynx.* American Joint Committee, 1962.
6. *Clinical Staging System for Cancer of the Pharynx.* American Joint Committee, 1965.

# THERAPEUTIC AND INVESTIGATIONAL POTENTIAL OF HETEROLOGOUS LIVER PERFUSION*

JOHN C. NORMAN†
WILLIAM G. HARDISON and WILLIAM V. McDERMOTT, JR.

Departments of Surgery and Medicine, Harvard Medical School
Fifth (Harvard) Surgical Service and Second and Fourth (Harvard) Medical Services
Sears Surgical and Thorndike Memorial Laboratories, Boston City Hospital
Boston, Mass.

ACUTE hepatic failure with coma is a condition with high mortality and no satisfactory treatment. A retrospective survey by a group of gastroenterologists revealed that mortality was approximately 90 per cent in patients with hepatic coma from acute viral or toxic liver disease without cirrhosis.[1] Recently several groups have been investigating the possibility that the isolated pig liver, perfused with the blood of a patient with acute hepatic failure, might substitute for the patient's liver long enough to allow regeneration.[2, 3] The experience gained indicates that such perfusions are practical, physiologically sound, and capable of yielding clinical improvement. These observations, and the lack of evidence that the procedure is intrinsically harmful, have encouraged continuation of studies on the therapeutic potential of the ex-vivo perfused pig liver. During these studies certain aspects of hepatic physiology have been investigated. This report presents data concerning the potential of the perfused pig liver both as treatment for hepatic failure and as a preparation for the study of selected aspects of hepatic physiology.

## PERFUSION SYSTEM AND FUNCTION OF THE PERFUSED LIVER

The experimental and clinical perfusion systems have been described in detail in previous reports.[4, 5] Briefly, the experimental system employs arterialized, nonpulsatile, gravity inflow to the portal vein through the isolated organ to the suprahepatic inferior vena cava. The clinical

*Presented as part of a symposium on *Recent Advances in Hepatic Surgery,* held by the Section on Surgery of The New York Academy of Medicine, January 17, 1967.
†Markle Scholar in Academic Medicine.
This investigation was supported in part by Public Health Service Research Grants AM08681, AM10517, AM5413, AM09115 from the National Institute of Arthritis and Metabolic Diseases, Research Grant HE10539 from the National Heart Institute, and Research Grant FR0076 from the Division of Research Facilities and Resources, Bethesda, Md.

TABLE I—CHANGE IN HEPATIC CONCENTRATION OF ATP AND IN THE CONSUMPTION OF OXYGEN BY TISSUE SLICES, WITH HEPATECTOMY, ISCHEMIA, AND PERFUSION

| | *At laparotomy* | *Posthepatectomy* | | | *Post-four-hour perfusion* |
|---|---|---|---|---|---|
| | | *0 time* | *1 hour* | *2 hours* | |
| ATP ($\mu$M./gm. protein) | 3.1±.51 | 1.1±0.20 | 0.63±0.08 | 0.33±0.09 | 2.8±1.3 |
| Oxygen consumption $\mu$l/100 mg./hr. | 181±8.9 | 117±11.8 | 87.4±12.5 | 84.4±7.8 | 162±9.2 |

system employs an indwelling Scribner shunt in the patient for an inflow to the organ and for venous return. In both systems provisions are made for varying perfusate flow, temperature, *p*H, $pO_2$, $pCO_2$, and humidity within the perfusion chamber.

Maintenance of viability of the isolated liver in this perfusion system has been tested by measurements of hepatic adenosine triphosphate (ATP) concentration and of the consumption of oxygen by tissue slices. ATP concentration and the consumption of oxygen by livers subjected to graded periods of ischemia without perfusion dropped progressively. In comparison, after four hours of perfusion, ATP concentration and the consumption of oxygen by the livers were nearly as high as these measurements *in vivo* (Table I). These observations imply maintenance of viability by perfusion.

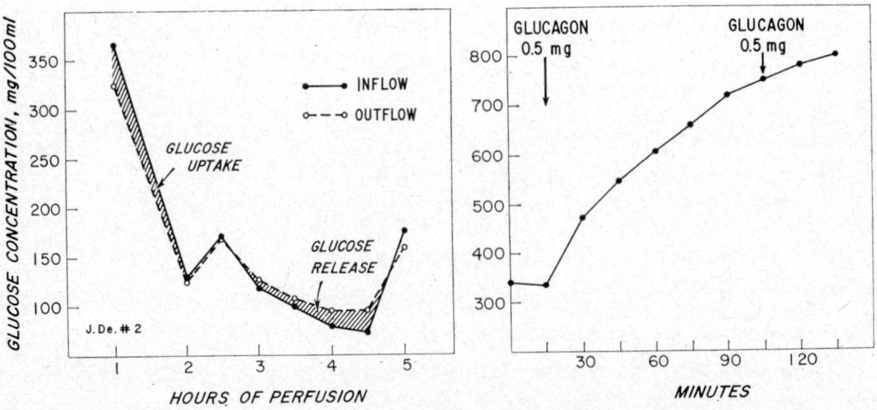


Fig. 1*a*. Inflow and outflow perfusate glucose concentrations during clinical perfusion. At concentrations over 150 mg./100 ml., the liver removes glucose from the perfusate; at concentrations less than 150 mg./100 ml., it releases glucose into the perfusate.

Fig. 1*b*. Effect of glucagon on perfusate glucose concentration during experimental perfusion. Glucagon causes a prompt rise in perfusate glucose concentration.

TABLE II—REPRESENTATIVE SIMULTANEOUS CONCENTRATIONS OF BILIRUBIN, BSP, AND BILE SALTS IN PIG BILE AND IN SERUM OF PATIENTS UNDERGOING PIG LIVER PERFUSION

| *Bilirubin (mg.%)* | *Patient serum* | *Bile* |
|---|---|---|
| J. De T. | 11.5 | 264 |
| W. M. | 26.0 | 236 |
| J. D. | 22.4 | 246 |
| *BSP (mg.%)* | | |
| A. G. | 5.6 | 365 |
| W. M. | 5.6 | 196 |
| E. H. | 4.0 | 190 |
| *Total Bile Salts (mg./ml.)* | | |
| J. De T. | 0.014 | 8.0 |

During perfusion the isolated liver also metabolizes substances appropriately. The ability of the liver to take up or release glucose in response to the concentration of glucose in the perfusate during chemical perfusion is shown in Figure 1*a*. At concentrations of glucose above 150 mg. per cent, the isolated liver removed glucose from the perfusate; at concentrations below 150 mg. per cent, the liver released glucose into the perfusate. In separate experiments, injection of glucagon* after four hours of perfusion caused a prompt and sustained rise in the concentration of glucose in the perfusate, indicating that the glycogenolytic mechanisms of the livers were intact (Figure 1*b*). Further evidence of the functional integrity of the perfused liver during clinical perfusion is given in Table II. High concentration gradients from patient plasma to pig bile for bilirubin, total bile salts, and bromsulfothalein occured. These data demonstrate that the hepatocytes of the perfused pig liver maintain their ability to clear, concentrate, and extrete substances appropriately.

The alkaline bile stimulated by secretin probably originates from the epithelium of the biliary tract.[6] Injection of secretin** into the perfusate of the isolated liver caused brisk flows of bile containing

*Glucagon, U.S.P. Eli Lilly and Co., Indianapolis, Ind.
**Boots Pure Drug Co. Ltd., Nottingham, England.

TABLE III—REPRESENTATIVE CHANGES IN CONCENTRATION OF BICARBONATE IN BILE (mEq./l.) AFTER INJECTION OF SECRETIN

| *Dose secretin* | *$HCO_3$ before secretin* | *Maximum $HCO_3$ after secretin* |
|---|---|---|
| 1 μ | 27 | 69 |
| 10 μ | 24 | 94 |
| 50 μ | 22 | 91 |
| 100 μ | 22 | 80 |

high concentrations of bicarbonate (Table III). When the increase in the flow of bile was plotted against the logarithm of secretin dose per kg. of liver, the resultant curve was consistent with the straight line relation described by Jonson *et al.* in the intact dog (Figure 2).[7] These observations indicate that the function of both hepatocytes and biliary epithelial cells of the perfused liver approximates that found *in vivo*.

## EXCRETION OF HUMAN BILE SALTS BY THE PIG LIVER

The major human bile salts are cholic, deoxycholic, and chenodeoxycholic acids. The major bile salts of the pig are hyocholic, hyode-

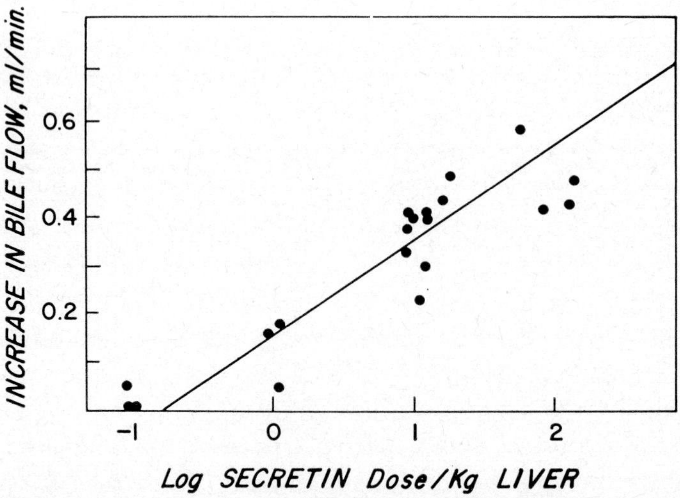


Fig. 2. Secretin dose-response relationship of the perfused liver. The increase in bile flow rises linearily with the logarithm of the secretin dose per kg. of liver.

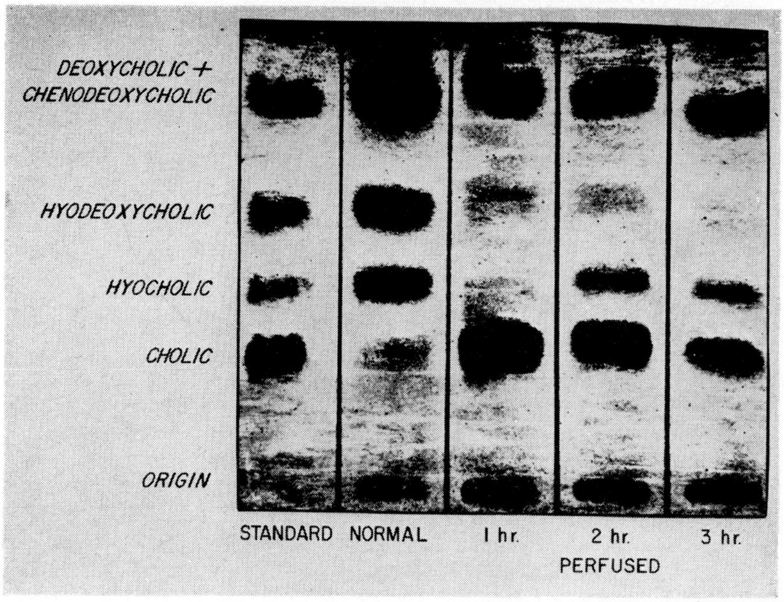


Fig. 3. Thin-layer chromatogram of bile salts from normal pig hepatic bile, and pig bile during clinical perfusion. Standard bile salts are included for reference. Cholic acid, present only in traces in normal pig hepatic bile, is present in large amounts in perfusion bile specimens.

oxycholic, and chenodeoxycholic acids. Cholic and deoxycholic acids do not appear to any appreciable extent in the pig. Hyocholic and hyodeoxycholic acids do not occur in man; i.e., two of the three major bile salts are different in the two species. Clinical perfusion of the isolated pig liver offered a unique opportunity to investigate cross-species metabolism of bile salts. Analysis of bile salts in the bile produced by pig livers during clinical perfusions indicated that the liver of the pig promptly concentrated and excreted the human bile salt, cholic acid. Figure 3 shows the thin-layer chromatogram of the hydrolyzed bile salts from normal porcine bile and from bile produced by the isolated porcine liver during clinical perfusion. A column containing bile salt standards is included. The chromatograms from each perfusion sample contained a prominent cholic acid band. Normal pig bile contained only a trace of cholic acid. Moreover, the perfused liver concentrated these predominantly human bile salts. Total bile salt concentration in bile from clinically perfused livers, 10.0 mg./ml., approximated that in bile produced by the intact animal, 10.7 mg./ml.

## Immunological Considerations

One theoretical objection to clinical *ex vivo* pig liver perfusion is the possibility that patients may become sensitized to pig protein and suffer immune reactions during perfusion. This problem was studied in five patients during 15 clinical perfusions. All patients underwent 2 or more perfusions and one was perfused 5 times over 18 days. After the perfusions, pig albumin and globulins were found in the patients' sera. However no antipig antibodies were detected by immunochemical, immunodiffusion, and tanned red blood cell techniques.[3] It is possible that immune reactions could occur, particularly if perfusions were performed infrequently over a span of many weeks. These data do indicate, however, that repeated perfusions over an 18-day period resulted in no severe immunological reactions.

## Experiences in Patients

Pig liver perfusion has usually yielded clinical and laboratory improvement in the patients perfused. In three of our five patients, hepatic coma cleared within 12 to 36 hours after perfusion. However, coma recurred despite further perfusions. These observations are in keeping with the report by Eiseman *et al.*, who noted temporary clinical improvement in seven of eight patients.[2] In each of our patients, perfusion consistently caused a decline in serum bilirubin, a substance known to require the liver for excretion. Yet we found that perfusion resulted in no change in the concentration of serum glutamic-oxaloacetic transaminase (SGOT) but caused inconstant changes in the concentration of alkaline phosphatase in the serum; these two substances are not known to be excreted solely by the liver (Table IV). Interpretation of serum values is difficult because of the uncertain amount of dilution that occurs when the patient's blood mixes with priming volumes and plasma expanders administered during perfusion. Estimation of substances excreted in the bile from the perfused liver, however, gives an assessment of the amount of these substances cleared from the patient without regard to dilution by normal blood or plasma expanders. The total amount of bilirubin and cholic acid excreted by the pig liver during a three-hour clinical perfusion was 160.4 mg. and 127 mg. respectively. The clearance of cholic acid was especially high. Utilizing serum concentration of cholic acid before perfusion, the number of liters of plasma cleared were calculated and compared

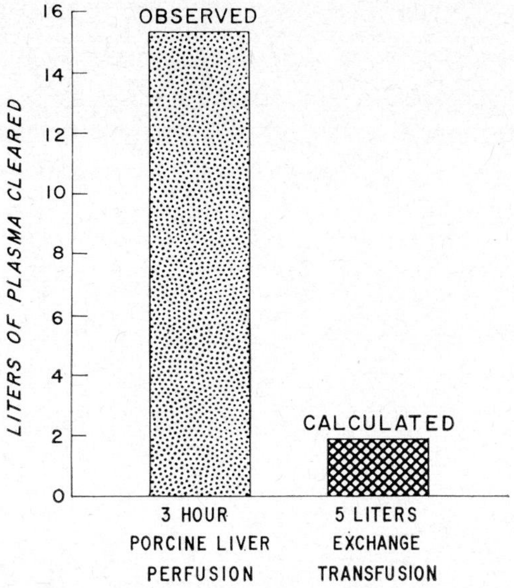


Fig. 4. Observed plasma cholic acid clearance during perfusion compared with theoretical clearance obtained by one blood volume exchange transfusion.

with the theoretical clearance obtained by a five-liter (one blood volume) exchange transfusion. Figure 4 shows that this perfusion was more efficient in clearing cholic acid than a theoretical exchange transfusion of one blood volume.

The improvement in laboratory values and the demonstrated clearance of bile salt and bilirubin are encouraging but not conclusive evidence that the factors causing death in hepatic failure are being treated effectively. At present it is not known whether death in hepatic failure is caused by an excess of harmful substances or by a deficiency of essential substances produced by the normal liver. Conceivably both factors are involved. Until more information is available, reliance must be placed upon clinical observation and upon the known indices of liver function as measures of therapeutic success.

The very high mortality associated with these procedures, although discouraging, must be interpreted with regard to the types of patients studied. Eiseman has reported only two survivors in the 20 known to him,[8] and we have had none. However, without exception the patients were near death before perfusion. The acute liver failure has usually been accompanied by advanced age, chronic alcoholism, or other com-

TABLE IV—REPRESENTATIVE VALUES FOR SERUM BILIRUBIN, ALKALINE PHOSPHATASE, AND GLUTAMIC-OXALOACETIC TRANSAMINASE IMMEDIATELY BEFORE AND AFTER CLINICAL PERFUSION IN FIVE PATIENTS

| | *J. De T.* | *E. H.* | *W. M.* | *J. D.* | *A. G.* |
|---|---|---|---|---|---|
| *Bilirubin* | | | | | |
| Before perfusion | 28.4 | 28.6 | 28.0 | 18.0 | 43.5 |
| After perfusion | 7.1 | 12.4 | 21.0 | 11.5 | 31.4 |
| *Alkaline Phosphatase* | | | | | |
| Before perfusion | 1.3 | 6.0 | 3.4 | 2.4 | 2.9 |
| After perfusion | 2.0 | 1.3 | 1.5 | 1.5 | 2.9 |
| *SGOT* | | | | | |
| Before perfusion | 174 | 170 | 160 | 276 | 734 |
| After perfusion | 172 | 180 | 280 | 270 | 640 |

plications. Of our five patients, all comatose when perfused, two were over 65 years of age, one had a probable midbrain hemorrhage before perfusion, and one was a severe chronic alcoholic. Of the eight patients reported by Eiseman *et al.*, seven had alcoholic cirrhosis and were bleeding from esophageal varices.[2] Only two of the reported patients were relatively young and were suffering from an acute circumscribed hepatic insult. The type of patient perfused is important when ultimate survival depends upon the regenerative capacity of the diseased liver.

## INVESTIGATIONAL POTENTIAL

The isolated perfused liver offers advantages for study of selected aspects of hepatic physiology. In contrast to the intact experimental preparation with operative endogenous influences, both neurogenic and humoral, the isolated organ is free from extraneous effects. This situation has proved valuable for the investigation of intrahepatic circulation. A correlation has been demonstrated between increasing flow, whole-organ oxygen consumption, and sinusoidal cross-sectional area.[9] In addition, the effects of various physical and pharmacologic agents on hepatic vascular resistance have been studied. Most of these experiments and their relations to clinical perfusions have been described in previous reports. Briefly, induced hypothermia during experimental perfusions increased transhepatic vascular resistance and decreased gravity-dependent flow rates. Low flow rates were associated with decreasing *p*H in the perfusate and increasing resistance, both of which could be temporarily reversed by elevation of the *p*H in the perfusate. Hemodilution and hemoconcentration of circulating perfusates during perfusion produced a prolonged decrease and increase respectively of transhepatic vascular resistance with proportional variations in gravity-dependent flow rates. These changes have been attributed to the viscosity of the perfusate. Epinephrine produced a marked immediate increase in resistance and a subsequent more gradual increase. The polypeptides Pitressin* and glucagon and the steroid methylprednisolone produced similar effects in reducing resistance and increasing flow rates.

Perfusion of porcine livers with human blood has also provided a unique opportunity to investigate the origin of certain biliary proteins. Rosenthal *et al.* have shown, using $I^{131}$-labeled human albumin in human subjects, that albumin in bile originates from circulating albumin rather than from synthesis by the hepatocyte *de novo*.[11] Our findings confirm his. Immunoelectrophoresis of the proteins in the pig bile from a clinical perfusion showed no pig protein. There were bands corresponding not only to human albumin, but also to human $\alpha$, $\beta$, and $\gamma$ globulins. These proteins could have been derived only from the patient's circulation.

## Comments

Investigations of pig liver perfusion as a potentially useful form of treatment have provided insights into hepatic function. The hemodynamics of the liver can be monitored and studied without interference from endogenous influences operative in the intact animal. Similarly, bile flow can be studied in the isolated preparation without interference from extrahepatic factors. It has been demonstrated that the bile flow of the perfused pig liver responds normally to secretin and bile salts, and it is expected that further investigations will yield information about qualitative and quantitative regulation of biliary flow.

Evidence thus far accumulated indicates that pig liver perfusion is a physiologically reasonable and potentially useful form of treatment for acute hepatic failure. Mortality has been high, but only patients near death have been considered for perfusion. Most have had under-

*Vasopressin, Parke, Davis and Co., Detroit, Mich.

lying liver disease, which might have prevented normal regeneration of the diseased organ had they survived. It is hoped that as further experience is gained, knowledge will permit extended observations upon patients who, despite a poor prognosis with conventional treatment, will nonetheless be salvageable.

## *REFERENCES*


1. Chalmers, T. C. Personal communication.
2. Eiseman, B., Liem, D. S. and Rafucci, F. Heterologous liver perfusion in treatment of hepatic failure, *Ann. Surg. 162*:329, 1965.
3. Norman, J. C., Saravis, C. A., Brown, M. E. and McDermott, W. V., Jr. Immunochemical observations in clinical heterologous (xenogeneic) liver perfusion, *Surgery 60*:179, 1966.
4. Norman, J. C., Brown, M., Ackroyd, F. W. and McDermott, W. V., Jr. Effect of increasing outflow occlusion on the rate and composition of ascites formation by the isolated perfused porcine liver, *Surg. Forum 16*:276, 1965.
5. Norman, J. C., Franco, F. O., Brown, M. E., Saravis, C. A., Ackroyd, F. W. and McDermott, Jr., W. V. Techniques of obtaining and preparing the porcine liver for experimental and clinical temporary ex-vivo perfusion. *J. Surg. Res. 6*:117, 1966.
6. Wheeler, H. O. Inorganic ions in bile. In: *The Biliary System,* W. Taylor, ed., Philadelphia, Davis, 1965, pp. 481-493.
7. Jonson, G., Sundman, L. and Thulin, L. The influence of chemically pure secretin on hepatic bile output, *Acta Physiol. Scand. 62*:287, 1964.
8. Eiseman, B. Personal communication.
9. Hardison, W. G., Greene, E. A. and Norman, J. C. Viability and effect of flow upon function of the ex-vivo perfused pig liver, *J. Lab. Clin. Med. 69*:245, 1967.
10. Norman, J. C., Covelli, V. H., Hardison, W. G. and McDermott, Jr., W. V. Experimental studies related to clinical xenogenic liver perfusion. *Transplantation.* (In press.)
11. Rosenthal, W. S., Kubo, K., Dolinski, M., Maxino, J., Mersheimer, W. L. and Glass, G. B. J. The passage of serum albumin into bile in man. *Amer. J. Dig. Dis. 10*:271, 1965.

# THE UMBILICAL VEIN IN DISEASES OF THE LIVER*

RICHARD E. KESSLER

Department of Surgery, New York University School of Medicine
Surgical Service, Manhattan Veterans Administration Hospital
New York, N. Y.

## INTRODUCTION

DURING the clinical study of patients with cirrhosis and suspected portal hypertension, it is often necessary to measure the portal pressure and visualize the portal venous system by angiography. To date, percutaneous splenoportography has been the method most widely used for this purpose. Unfortunately, splenic puncture is not possible after splenectomy, it is contraindicated in the presence of ascites and hemorrhagic diathesis, and it frequently fails to visualize the portal vein.[3] In the hands of the occasional practitioner splenic puncture is dangerous and the technical failure rate high.

In 1959 Gonzales,[4] by research on infant cadavers, developed a technique whereby the portal venous system could be entered by catheterization of the remnant of the umbilical vein. In 1964 Bayly[1] reported five years of clinical experience with this technique.

We have evaluated this technique in terms of simplicity, safety, and clinical application during 100 consecutive attempts to catheterize the remnant of the umbilical vein in adults.

## METHOD

The umbilical venous remnant exists as a cordlike structure that passes from the umbilicus to the porta hepatis in the free edge of the falciform ligament. It is approached through a small, vertical, midline incision in the epigastrium. The remnant of the vein is dissected extraperitoneally, hemitransected, and its pinpoint lumen opened and gradually dilated with Bake's common duct dilators down to the point where it communicates with the portal venous system. A 14F polyethylene catheter is then inserted through the vein into the portal venous system.

*Based on a paper presented at a meeting of the Section on Surgery, The New York Academy of Medicine, January 17, 1967.

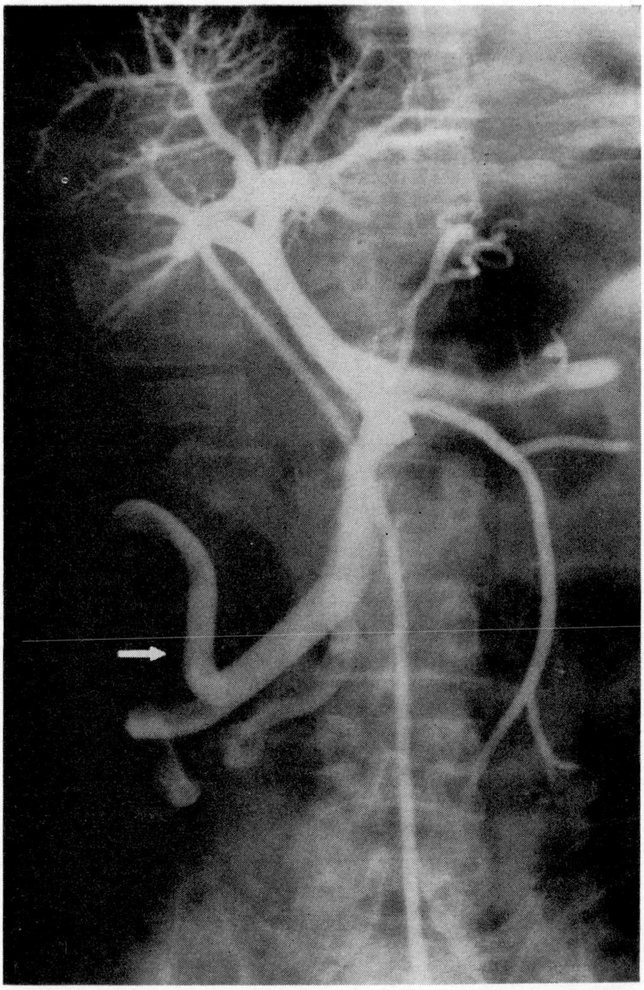

Fig. 1. Umbilical vein portogram from patient with cirrhosis and bleeding esophageal varices. Note the patent portal vein, gastroesophageal varices and large venous collaterals originating from the right colic branch of the superior mesenteric vein (*arrow*).

We use this approach to the portal venous system whenever splenic puncture fails to demonstrate a patent portal vein or cannot be performed because of contraindications, technical difficulties, or prior splenectomy. Catheterization of the umbilical vein is also performed in patients with proved liver metastases in order to obtain serial hepatograms as a means of measuring the therapeutic efficacy of anticancer drugs.[6] In patients with cirrhosis of the liver and bleeding esophageal

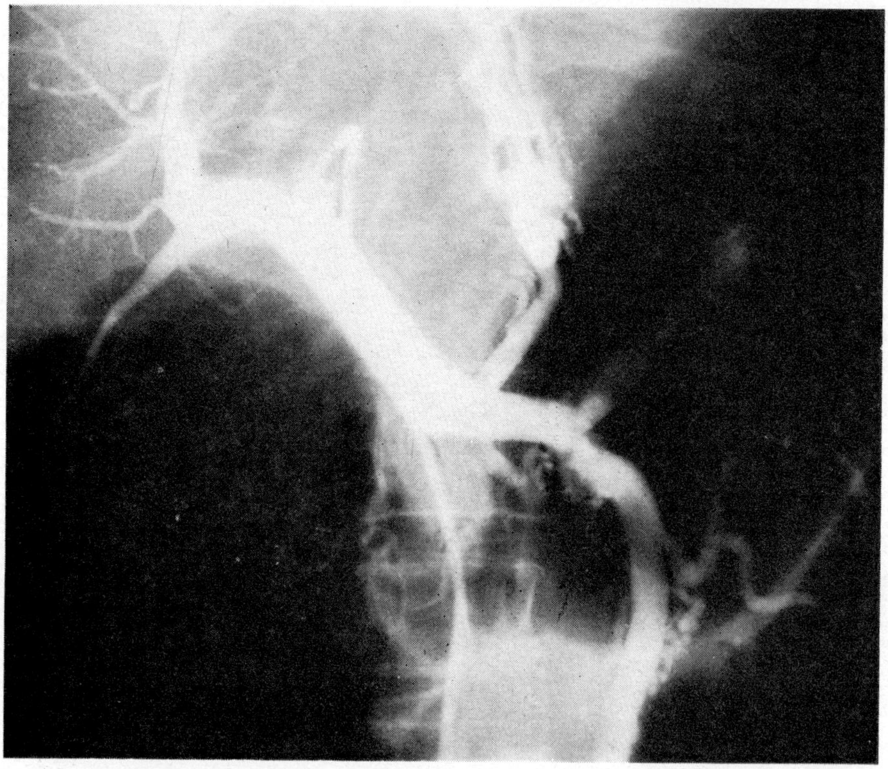

Fig. 2. Umbilical vein portogram from patient with cirrhosis, ascites, and bleeding esophageal varices. Note the large esophageal varices and runoff into the inferior mesenteric vein.

varices who are not candidates for a major surgical procedure, an umbilical vein catheter is used to study the response of the portal pressure to conservative modalities such as vasopressin, thoracic duct lymph drainage, and gastric hypothermia.

## Results

This technique is very accurate for monitoring the portal pressure over extended periods of time. We have measured the portal pressure more than 300 times in a single patient during an 11-day period while observing the response of the portal pressure to drainage of lymph from the thoracic duct.

When a contrast material is injected through an umbilical vein catheter, excellent portohepatograms are obtained. Figure 1 demon-

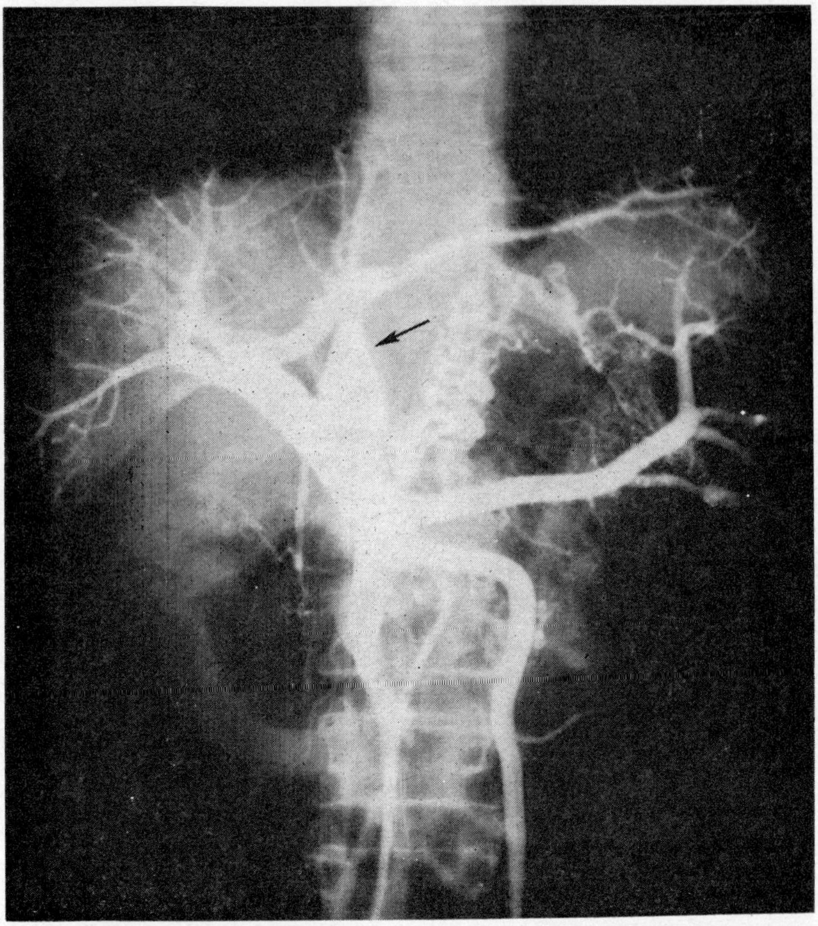

Fig. 3. Umbilical vein portogram from patient with cirrhosis and upper gastrointestinal bleeding of unknown cause. Note the gastroesophageal varices. Note ballooning of the umbilical vein indicated by the arrow.

strates the quality of the angiograms that can be obtained in this way. In patients who have cirrhosis of the liver, the contrast material passes down the portal vein and frequently fills the splenic and mesenteric veins and various venous collaterals. In patients who do not have cirrhosis, the dye rarely goes down the portal vein but progresses cephalad throughout the liver. Figure 2 demonstrates a portogram obtained in a patient with cirrhosis, ascites, and bleeding esophageal varices. Despite the large runoff through the coronary and inferior mesenteric veins, which might have prevented visualization of the portal vein on a

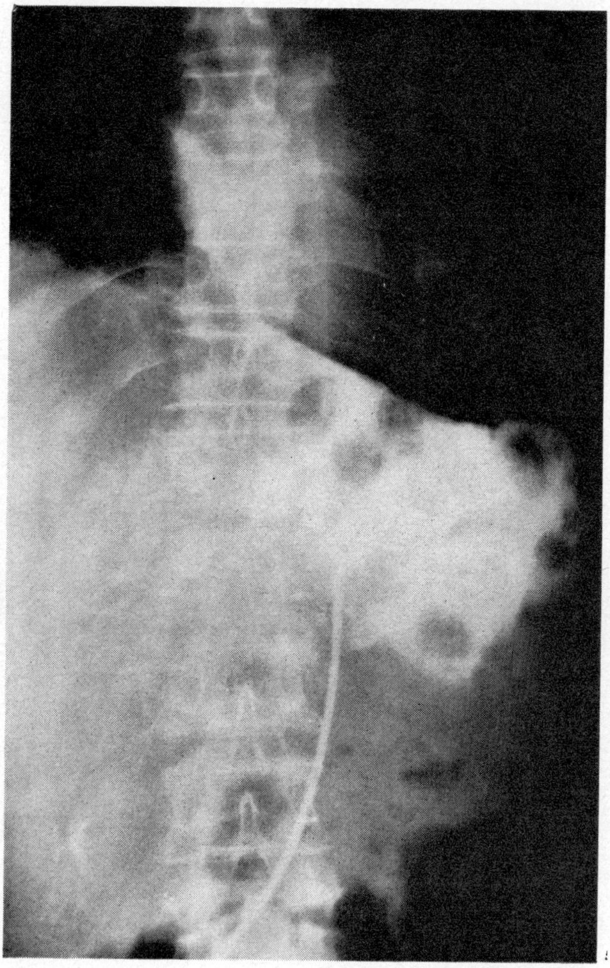

Fig. 4. Umbilical vein hepatogram from patient with proved liver metastases. Note the multiple radiolucent areas throughout the left lobe; these represent metastases.

splenic venogram, umbilical venography has demonstrated a patent portal vein and an excellent hepatogram phase as well. Figure 3 illustrates the value of umbilical vein catheterization in patients with upper gastrointestinal bleeding of undetermined cause in whom splenic puncture is contraindicated because of ascites. This portogram was obtained from a patient with cirrhosis and ascites in whom roentgenograms of the upper gastrointestinal tract and endoscopy had failed to reveal the source of the bleeding. This angiogram demonstrates the portal, splenic,

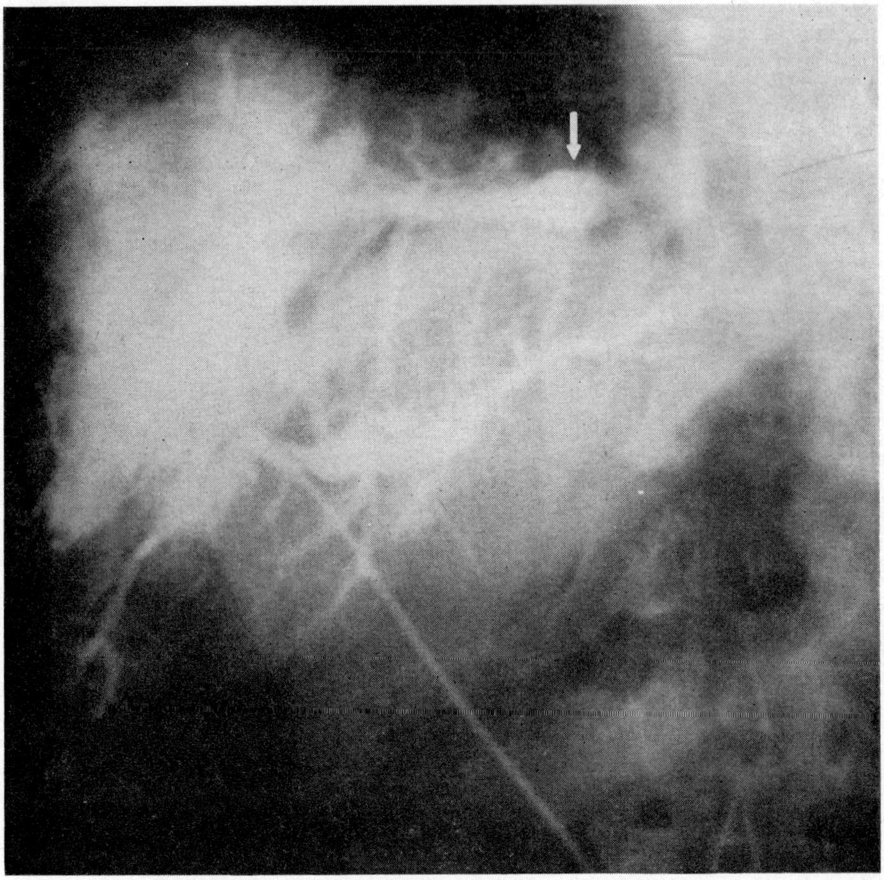

Fig. 5. Umbilical vein hepatogram demonstrating a right hepatic vein (*arrow*) entering the suprahepatic vena cava.

and mesenteric veins, and gastroesophageal varices.

If the umbilical vein catheter is not advanced through the umbilico-portal junction, the injection of a contrast material will result in ballooning of the umbilical vein. This may not prevent a successful angiogram and does not result in any complication. Figure 3 demonstrates this problem.

Hepatograms obtained several seconds after the injection of a contrast material result in dense, homogeneous opacification of the liver. In patients with space-occupying lesions of the liver, the lesions are demonstrated as radiolucent areas that can be accurately measured. Serial hepatograms obtained at weekly intervals permit an objective appraisal of anticancer drugs. Figure 4 illustrates a hepatogram obtained from a patient with proved liver metastases secondary to carcinoma of the sigmoid colon. This x-ray film demonstrates multiple radiolucent areas throughout the left lobe of the liver that failed to change in size after three weeks of 5-fluorouracil therapy. None of these lesions was evident on a scintoscan.

Whenever the umbilical vein catheter is advanced into the periphery of the liver, the contrast material is forced through the liver in sufficient concentration for radiographic visualization of the hepatic veins. Figure 5 demonstrates the catheter entering the right portal vein. The contrast material has opacified a right hepatic vein, which can be seen entering the suprahepatic vena cava.

In our first 100 attempts at catheterization of the umbilical vein, there were 9 failures, 5 of which occurred during our first 25 attempts. Thus, our over-all success rate is 91 per cent. There were only 4 failures in the last 75 attempts; this gave a success rate of 95 per cent. The failures were due to obliteration of the umbilical vein by metastatic invasion of the falciform ligament and to technical inability to enter the original lumen of the umbilical vein. Once mastered, this technique is simple and can readily be accomplished under local anesthesia in 15 to 30 minutes. It is also possible to recatheterize the umbilical venous remnant at a later date, provided this is done cephalad to the level of the previous catheterization.

There have been five complications observed in this study. Wound infections have not been observed. There were two minor episodes of bleeding into the incision, necessitating reopening of the wound for hemostasis. There was one case of dehiscence of the linea alba requiring secondary closure. There was one episode of bleeding caused by perforation of the umbilical vein with a small, firm catheter, which necessitated opening of the peritoneum for suture ligation of the proximal end of the umbilical venous remnant. Since that time we have used a soft, large polyethylene catheter without this complication. There was one major complication. This occurred in a patient who had cirrhosis of the liver and partial thrombosis of the portal vein demonstrated by umbilical vein angiography. Eight days after catheterization the patient died of hepatic failure. An autopsy revealed complete thrombosis of the portal vein. We have accepted this as a complication and believe that the umbilical vein catheterization may have contributed to propagation of the existing thrombus. In patients without cirrhosis the catheters have been left in situ for as long as five weeks without complication.

## Discussion

The technique of umbilical vein catheterization provides a safe and simple method for accurately measuring portal venous pressure and visualizing the portal system by angiography without the hazards and high technical failure rate of splenic puncture and despite the presence of ascites or prior splenectomy. It should be emphasized that successful catheterization of the umbilical vein is tantamount to successful angiography. This is in striking contrast to the results obtained with splenoportography. Furthermore, the research potential of a catheter located directly in the portal vein stimulates the imagination of the hepatologist.

The presence of a measurable lesion is essential for an objective appraisal of anticancer drugs. There are several methods currently used for detecting space-occupying lesions of the liver.[2, 5, 9] However, these techniques are difficult and time-consuming, or they fail to demonstrate hepatic tumors accurately. Umbilical vein hepatography permits precise measurement of hepatic tumors and may demonstrate lesions as small as 0.5 cm. in diameter.[7, 8] This is of considerable usefulness when evaluating the therapeutic efficacy of anticancer drugs at a time when the tumors are most vulnerable.

### *REFERENCES*


1. Bayly, J. H. and Gonzales, O. C. The umbilical vein in the adult: Diagnosis, treatment and research, *Amer. Surg. 30*:56, 1964.
2. Bonte, F. J., Kromer, J. S., Elmendorf, E., Presley, N. L. and Andrews, G. L. Scintillation scanning of the liver. II. Clinical applications, *Amer. J. Roentgen. 88*:275, 1962.
3. Burchell, A. R., Moreno, A. H., Panke, W. F. and Rousselot, L. M. Some limitations of splenic portography: I. Incidence, hemodynamics and surgical implications of the nonvisualized portal vein, *Ann. Surg. 162*:981, 1965.
4. Gonzales, O. C. A preliminary report of a new technique via the umbilical vein, *Clin. Proc. Child. Hosp. (Wash.) 15*: 120, 1959.
5. Hahn, R. G., Hodgson, J. R., Moertel, C. G. and Reitemeier, R. J. The use of tomography following thorium dioxide infusions to demonstrate malignant lesions in the liver, *Mayo Clin. Proc. 40*: 456, 1965.
6. Kessler, R. E. and Ramos-Yordan, F. Evaluation of anticancer drugs by umbilical vein hepatography, *Cancer 20*: 319, 1967.
7. Kessler, R. E. and Zimmon, D. S. Umbilical vein angiography, *Radiology 87*: 841, 1966.
8. Kessler, R. E. and Zimmon, D. S. Umbilical vein catheterization in man, *Surg. Gynec. Obst. 124*:594, 1967.
9. Nebesar, R. A., Pollard, J. J. and Stone, D. L. Angiographic diagnosis of malignant disease of the liver, *Radiology 86*:284, 1966.

# IMPLICATIONS OF UNTOWARD REACTIONS TO HALLUCINOGENS*

EDWIN ROBBINS, LILLIAN ROBBINS, WILLIAM A. FROSCH,
AND MARVIN STERN

Department of Psychiatry
New York University Medical Center
New York, N. Y.

SINCE the discovery of LSD in 1938 by A. Stoll and A. Hofmann, interest in this substance has grown so markedly that it has become one of the most discussed drugs in the United States. The history of the drug may be divided briefly into three phases.

The first, ushered in by Hofmann's accidental ingestion of some LSD in 1943, coincides with the period of increased research in neurochemistry and physiology and with the introduction of the tranquilizers. LSD was studied in one way by exploring its role as a psychotomimetic agent. It was hoped that a temporary and artificial induction of symptoms by means of it would lead to greater understanding of the nature of schizophrenia. However, a major breakthrough in this use of LSD did not occur, for the symptoms produced by it differed in many ways from those of functional psychoses. Clouding of the sensorium often accompanied the use of LSD, as contrasted with the clear state of consciousness observed in schizophrenia; moreover the hallucinations were mainly visual rather than auditory. The symptoms were found to be secondary to use of the drug, were limited in duration, and were not accompanied by the conviction of reality so typical of schizophrenia. Toward the termination of this early period some investigators began to discover that the hallucinogens had other properties, which led them to study their effects at first hand.

The psychedelic movement was given impetus when Aldous L. Huxley, introduced to mescaline by Osmond, glowingly described his experiences.[1, 2] Most of his observations have become the model for others who have used the hallucinogens. A number of intellectuals, artists, ministers, and psychotherapists began to follow Huxley's lead in

*Based on a paper presented at a meeting of the American-Hungarian Medical Association, New York, N.Y., at The New York Academy of Medicine, February 10, 1967.
This work was supported in part by Public Health Service Research Grant MH-08618 from the National Institute of Mental Health.

the hope that they, too, would have their conciousness expanded. From California came the "game" theme developed to a great degree by Leary and his followers at Harvard University. These persons, by proselytizing, created a movement for use of the drug among college students and also among nonstudents. In 1961 the Food and Drug Administration (FDA) carried out its first investigation of the nonmedical and illegal uses of LSD.[3] By this time LSD was more widely used by members of the community than by research workers. The emphasis on self-enlightenment that had been the initial rationale for its ingestion began to fade. This was caused partly by its more indiscriminate use by a larger number of people than were directly reached by leading proponents of the drug, and partly by the publicity given to wild LSD parties, which were described in feature articles in national magazines. As the drug became used for "highs," it was mixed with other substances, such as alcohol, or followed by marihuana or amphetamines in order to prolong its effect. Some LSD Centers had been established in California in the hope of administering the drug under controlled conditions.[4] However, in many of these centers there arose dissension, and struggles for power took place. By the time changes in the law impelled them to close, little useful information concerning the drug had been reported.

Although adverse reactions to LSD had been noted,[4-7] they were overshadowed by the attention devoted to the wonders of the psychedelic experience. Emphasis was centered on expanding consciousness, and on the ultimate good to come to mankind as a result of "turning on." Psychotic aftermaths to LSD were denied in many quarters and, in others, these reactions were considered temporary, reversible results of an unfortunate "trip."

As the frequency of self-administration increased, patients began to come to hospitals in larger numbers, and it soon became apparent that free access to LSD did not always have a benign outcome.[8] Tighter federal controls were established in order to gain a broader perspective of the issues involved, and the third phase, that of watchful waiting, was entered. A spokesman for Sandoz Pharmaceuticals concluded that it was unjust to "expect a house to maintain a preparation whose therapeutic usefulness is open to question, to risk its good name, and to carry the problem of distribution in the context of increasingly widespread misuse."[9] The existing supply of the drug was given to the FDA,

TABLE I—TYPES OF RESPONSES TO LSD RECORDED AT BELLEVUE HOSPITAL

| | *Group 1* *Early 1965* | *Group 2* *Early 1966* | *Total* |
|---|---|---|---|
| Type of reaction: | | | |
| Acute | 7 | 11 | 18 |
| Recurrent | 3 | 8 | 11 |
| Prolonged | 3 | 8 | 11 |

where it is now held pending distribution to approved researchers. As additional data are gathered and as the issues and controversies become more clearly identified, the laws pertaining to the use of hallucinogens may become redefined, particularly in view of increasing middle-class interest in a wide variety of drugs—tranquilizers as well as the illicit hallucinogens. In the 1930's and 1940's, for example, the smoking of marihuana was associated with musicians, with such communities as Harlem and Greenwich Village in New York City, and with criminals. Today there is uncertainty about the extent of the use of marihuana and LSD on college campuses. Some students have joined in a campaign to legalize the use of hallucinogens.

After it became apparent several years ago that the number of admissions to Bellevue Hospital because of LSD was rising, we began to tabulate the rate. A zenith was reached in 1966, when four people per week were hospitalized as a result of using the drug. This is a large number; it totaled more than 200 patients a year from just one cause. To date, three groups of patients have been studied in detail, approximately a year apart (Table I).[10, 11] Our findings have been consistent over time, and have accorded with data reported elsewhere.[12, 13] For the sake of clarification, we have divided the reactions into three major groups. Each is further subdivided into two parts.

## ACUTE REACTIONS

*Panic.* Patients in this category have most often been self-referred; they have come for treatment because they have become overwhelmed by some aspect of their reaction to LSD—usually depersonalization, loss of control, homosexual panic, or a paranoid reaction. Feeling unable to cope with their anxiety, and losing sight of the fact that the LSD reaction is limited in time, they have come to the hospital for termination of the experience. Reassurance frequently has sufficed. If not, tranquilizers have been used to take the edge off the feeling of anxiety, even though the LSD reaction continued. Although the majority of panicky subjects were using the drug for the first time, some guides or others who had taken a number of uneventful trips before also ran into trouble and sought help.

*Confusion.* This is in many ways similar to the pathological intoxication of the alcoholic or the marihuana user. There is an acute brain syndrome often characterized by delusions of grandeur and poor judgment—the patient attempts to fly, or walks into a moving car—sometimes with fatal results.

## Recurrence of Symptoms

*Early.* These reportedly occur within a short time, up to 72 hours after the drug is ingested, but the visual and other phenomena are less intense, as a rule, than at the height of the experience. Patients have not come to the hospital seeking help for a reaction of this type.

*Late.* The spontaneous return of symptoms has occurred as long as one year after the last use of the drug. The reasons for the reappearance of symptoms similar to those experienced with LSD are not clear. As far as we can tell, this syndrome develops both in psychotic and nonpsychotic people. For the former, it is not always possible to distinguish between symptoms of a continuous acute schizophrenic episode and those prompted by the administration of LSD. Reappearance of the symptoms may be associated with a feeling of pleasure, or of great anxiety—depending to some extent on the basic personality of the subject. Although it is suggested in some circles that recurrences should be enjoyed when they take place, this may not always be feasible, since the symptoms appear unpredictably and may occur at inconvenient times.

## Prolonged Reactions

*Psychotic.* The subjects we have examined in this group have come to the hospital voluntarily after the ministrations of friends, including additional doses of the drug, have failed. We have tried to be as accurate as possible in assessing the role of LSD in the development of a psychosis. Details of past life have been obtained from family and friends as well as from the patients. Eight of the first 11 psychotic persons we interviewed had been considered psychotic before coming to the hospital in an acute emergency. Only two had previously been to a mental hospital. The three nonpsychotic patients had been functioning marginally.

How can one evaluate the role of LSD in this group? It may be argued that the people who were "borderline" or already psychotic would have come to the hospital for treatment whether or not they had taken LSD. But the fact remains that they had been functioning well enough not to require professional attention until they took a trip. Hospitalization occurred when it was realized by their friends and associates that there was a deficit in their functioning after taking the drug, and that continued support of these people outside of a hospital was not possible. Duration of hospitalization ranged from one to nine months.

At present there is a great deal of uncertainty about the effects of LSD on the population at large. Unfortunately, comprehensive data are not available since the literature of the psychedelic movement, in recording the greatest experiences with the drug, has tended to minimize or suppress reports of adverse reactions. It was only when hospitals reported that the incidence of psychotic reactions was rising that informal, most often unpublished, acknowledgments began to be made by members of the psychedelic movement. Blum was among the first to note that psychotic reactions were not restricted to persons administering LSD to themselves.[4] He estimated a rate of 20 to 33 per 1,000 for the selected persons who took the drug under supervision in the psychedelic centers in California. Today, as the psychedelic movement has gained momentum there, an increasing number of young people who had been considered normal prior to taking LSD, have been requesting help because of psychotic reactions.[14] In a small series of hospitalized schizophrenic patients treated with LSD, the number of prolonged adverse reactions was quite low.[15] In one series of patients receiving LSD therapeutically under medical supervision no major adverse reactions have taken place.[16]

*Chronic anxiety*. This reaction develops in some persons who have taken LSD, and it can apparently continue for considerable periods of time. The anxiety can be explained by the ability of LSD, as well as of other substances that produce an acute brain syndrome, to alter psychological defences rapidly. Possibly it occurs more frequently in younger people or in those who do not have a well-defined self-esteem. While changes in psychological defences may be valuable therapeutically, disastrous as well as salutory effects may take place when the drug is ingested in the absence of external support. For example, a female graduate student, married for four years, took LSD at the instigation of her husband, and had a pleasant trip in which she focused her attention on feelings of depersonalization and color changes. In a second trip, again with her husband, she still felt apprehension initially, but ultimately was enormously pleased to find that long-present feelings of homosexuality were relieved. Her third trip, begun with hopefulness, was reportedly a good one, but has been horrifying in its aftermath. She became afraid of dying and for the past year has been apprehensive about falling asleep.

We attempted to compare the experience of users of the drug in the community with that of the Bellevue Hospital patients in order to see if any differences existed. Volunteers from the community were sought. Since many were reluctant to talk with us about their experiences with LSD, the sample was small. This group, however, was comparable to the hospitalized users of the drug in that neither group was composed of the lowest strata of society, nor of the most disturbed. In general, these users of the drug were younger and better educated, and their economic level was above that of the average Bellevue patient. Surprisingly, few reported taking LSD for their edification. "Kicks," rather than expansion of consciousness was the prime reason given. Following the typology of assumed gains implicit in the psychedelic literature, we asked questions about improvement in several areas.[17] Most were surprised that we wanted to know how taking LSD had brought about positive effects. They nevertheless tried to answer. Twenty per cent felt worse—more depressed and more suicidal than ever. Forty per cent could not see that it had made them feel different in any way. In the remaining forty per cent it was possible to find some feeling of gain, even though we had to make great allowances at times to score responses as positive.

The religious experiences associated with LSD are highly esteemed by some prominent people. Clergy given psilocybin during chapel exercises have reported mystical experiences.[18] It was hard to find objective evidence from the patients in our sample that went beyond "feeling at one with the world" or the "oneness" and "suchness" of things that led them to feel there must be a God. Masters and Houston, who have great interest in the evocation of religious imagery and feeling, found that only six of their 206 subjects, on taking the drug, had a truly religious experience.[19] None of our sample would meet their criteria. Those who reported feeling somewhat more religious did not behave in any more religious fashion subsequent to taking LSD.

Enhanced feelings of friendliness were often reported. Unfortunately, these feelings, which are a frequent concomitant of experience with LSD, rarely persisted long after the termination of the trip. Insight and self-knowledge are also considered to be accompaniments of expanded consciousness. For one woman, there was some genuine insight into her relations with men. For another, there was a realization under the influence of LSD that the police were tipped off to her prostitution ring by her telephone answering service.

Intellectual capacity was felt by some to be enhanced. One man said he became incisive and could immediately see to the heart of a problem. After using LSD, facts became an unnecessary and restrictive encumbrance. His grandiosity was untouched by any confrontation with reality. Some felt aesthetic awareness to be enhanced. One musician reported that her playing had improved and that her musical ear was keener. For an artist, the taking of LSD was coupled with a period of intensive work. She felt that her painting had become better, but she required hospitalization because of her continuing psychosis. Aesthetics was also approached on a different plane. One man became enamored of the flashing purple lights on the back of garbage trucks and reported being quite enthralled as he stood watching them.

Our estimate of the patients' subjective statements was that there was little of positive value for most, and some prolonged loss of self-esteem for several. Yet even the fact that they were in a mental hospital and knew this to be the result of taking LSD did not alter the view of many that the drug had been beneficial in some ways that could not be well defined. The optimism of the user of LSD has been commented upon by Blum, who also could not see the improvements that were reported to him.[4] In many instances the drug user's friends could not see them either.

It is of interest in this connection that the therapeutic value of LSD has not yet been unequivocally demonstrated.[20-22] Results are hard to evaluate because of the difficulty of planning and executing controlled studies and also because of the paucity of valid criteria for assessing psychotherapy in general. The value of LSD in the treatment of alcoholism, which has been widely hailed as of great potential, also is uncertain at the present time. Blum, for instance, stated that a thorough review of the literature on alcoholism led him to conclude that he was not as enthusiastic about its efficacy as some of his colleagues.[24] Dr. Ruth Fox, who has treated alcoholics with LSD, was initially optimistic,[25] but ultimately felt that the drug was not the prime determinant in bringing about recovery. She felt that factors such as contact, interest, and time spent with the patient played an equal role.[26] Furthermore, some of the "cures" initially attributed to the administration of LSD could not, in final analysis, be ascribed to the drug—as in the case of one person who remained sober because he was jailed, and as in the case of another, who stopped drinking after electroconvulsive therapy was used to offset an LSD-induced depression. Similarly, a follow-up of the prisoners whom Leary *et al.* reported as being helped by psilocybin[27] showed that the rate of return to prison four years after the experiment was begun was no different than for the control group.[28] It is possible that the initially lower rate of recidivism was influenced by the prisoners' knowledge that they had "buddies" at Harvard University to whom they could turn in time of stress.[5, 28]

In experiments in which the subject was unaware of receiving LSD, psychedelic experiences did not occur.[5, 29] Instead, there was confusion and, secondarily, fright.[5] Some people have been hospitalized after receiving LSD without their knowledge, and have been badly frightened by the experience. In one instance there was a prolonged psychosis. Parenthetically, it should be noted that many schizophrenic patients are attributing the onset of their illness to LSD administered without their knowledge.

What are the long-range effects of using these drugs? The data are not yet complete. It is a pity that the people who have administered the hallucinogens to the greatest number of subjects under a variety of conditions have not seen fit to report their results, both on a short-range and long-term basis. Some observers have felt that deterioration of personality takes place—and that long-term users are thought to function more poorly by people who have known them for years—

but this is impossible to substantiate. Thus far we have not seen any instance of permanent damage to the brain that can be attributed to LSD.

It is no longer possible to discuss LSD without considering the problem of the abuse of the drug in a broader context. At present, we should like to make some brief comments about marihuana since the two drugs are often used by the same people and pose similar social problems. The use of marihuana has increased considerably in the past few years, possibly because LSD has been so widely proselytized. The users of marihuana, who have been coming to the hospital in increasing numbers, have been admitted not because they have suffered adverse reactions but for other reasons. They have primarily been light-to-moderate users, and have shown no detectable physical damage as a result of their addiction.

There is a great deal of unanimity in the descriptions of the effects of smoking marihuana in the form called pot. Aside from the fact that smoking pot requires some degree of learning to appreciate the changes associated with being "high," several observations that are usually minimized should be made. One is that some degree of loss of control occurs during the period of intoxication. Psychological testing of subjects under the influence of marihuana has shown that there can be definite impairment in the capacity to perform more complex tasks,[30] so that driving a car, for example, may become hazardous. Although marihuana is smoked in groups, most users at the height of the high withdraw into their own fantasy world, so that ultimately the experience becomes asocial, rather than social. Some students have refrained from smoking pot because eventually they have seen friends who previously had enjoyed being high respond, instead, with dulling of attention and feelings of lethargy and depression.

With marihuana, as with alcohol, it is not the low doses that create social havoc, but excessive use in the higher dose range.[31, 32] Although it is possible to collect a series of papers that are essentially favorable to the widespread use of marihuana,[33] a better understanding of its effects may be obtained from reports from countries where, as a substitute for alcohol, use of the drug is unrestricted.[32] Extensive studies have shown that a mass addiction to marihuana has developed among the Moroccan urban proletariat.[34] Those using it in limited dose in India reportedly have felt themselves unharmed, but those taking larger doses have felt themselves harmed yet powerless to stop using it.[35] In this respect, habituation and dependence, as in the case of alcohol, can be postulated. With LSD also, some have experimented or thought of experimenting with sustaining highs by taking frequent doses.[36] This is reminiscent of the binge of the periodic alcoholic. We have observed an increase in the number of patients who have raised the dose for successive trips.

Murphy summarizes the comparison between alcohol and marihuana in the following fashion: "Both in the complexity of its effects and in more specific characteristics (it) is much closer to alcohol than to the opiates or to cocaine. Like alcohol, it appears to have no deleterious effect on the moderate user, who knows the correct amount for obtaining relaxation or euphoria without additional effects. As with alcohol, single doses given to naive, unstable subjects can produce an acute confusion, perhaps with violence, while the long-term use of heavy doses can probably lead to partial dementia or an organic reaction type psychosis."[32]

Amplification is necessary here since there have been no autopsy reports that show brain damage similar to that seen in chronic alcoholics. It is quite possible that biochemical or electroencephalographic alterations will be found as the chronic user is studied in greater detail.

Murphy further notes that marihuana, ". . . like alcohol is alleged to carry no danger for the stable personality, but to attract the neurotic and psychopathic, who are also the people that tend to take the heavy doses. Neither drug has a significant tendency to produce dependence; neither drug leads to withdrawal symptoms under normal conditions; and in neither case does desired dosage tend to increase with time. . . .

"There are differences of course. Cannabis in large doses may be more poisonous, and in small doses it has a more distorting effect on certain mental functions. It . . . is more likely to lead to an asocial passivity."

It is this last point that is most relevant for many of the people in our culture who are attracted to LSD and marihuana. There is a tendency to withdraw from the activities of society and to become more interested in contemplation of self and drugs. Among the collegiate users of drugs there has been a trend toward becoming more discouraged about achieving goals, toward giving up in advance rather than trying to improve conditions that are objectionable.[37] It is

TABLE II—HISTORY OF THE USE OF DRUGS BY GROUP 2

*Frequency of Use of Drugs in Addition to LSD*

| *Drug* | *Female (N=6)* | *Male (N=7)* |
|---|---|---|
| None | 1 | 2 |
| Marihuana | 5 | 5 |
| Barbiturates | 5 | 2 |
| Amphetamines | 3 | 2 |
| Opiates | 3 | 1 |
| Hallucinogens | 0 | 1 |
| Cocaine | 1 | 0 |
| Patent cough syrup | 1 | 0 |
| *Totals* (drugs used) | 18 | 11 |

*Number of Patients Using Additional Drugs*

| *Drugs* | *Female* | *Male* |
|---|---|---|
| None | 1 | 2 |
| One | 0 | 3 |
| Two | 0 | 0 |
| Three | 3 | 1 |
| Four | 1 | 1 |
| Five | 0 | 0 |
| Six | 1 | 0 |
| *Totals* | 5 | 5 |

quite likely that many adolescents and young adults who adopt this philosophy will never be able to regain the ground lost, and that ultimately its use will lead to less productive and satisfying lives than they might lead otherwise.

LSD may pose additional risks for the group in which the ego has not been solidly developed. Since the drug is supposed to bring out the "essence" of the personality, it requires a certain degree of self-understanding and knowledge to determine if the ideas that appear under its influence are accurate and relevant. For adolescents and young adults who have not been able to formulate a clear opinion about themselves, it is possible to accept incorrect ideas as meaningful and valid.

Considerable interest in the drug movement of today has centered on the rights of persons to do whatever they wish in the privacy of their own homes—even to engage in an activity that might potentially injure them. (This point is elaborately discussed by Comber in Blum.[4]) While this argument is felt by many to have merit, it is one that is difficult to justify in this connection, since society must bear the brunt of the failures, either by treating victims in hospitals, supporting them and their families, or by losing the potential production, of persons who are unable to function as well as before. From this standpoint, it should be emphasized that our function has been primarily to make people aware of the risks that certain drugs may pose for them, particularly since others have chosen to minimize or ignore them. People have not been rushing to buy thalidomide on the black market.

We have been struck by the number of users of LSD who have also been taking other drugs. In studying the second group of patients, it was quite apparent that most were deeply involved in the use of drugs; the women even more than the men (Table II). Frosch extended this work and surveyed the general and psychiatric population of Bellevue Hospital; he found that the users of LSD experimented more with drugs than the users of marihuana, but that the difference was not great. However, comparable data on the use of drugs by college students are not yet available, but surveys are being made. At Brooklyn College a preliminary survey revealed that 78 of 1200 respondents admitted using drugs.[36] The most popular drug was marihuana (53); next, barbiturates (10); only 2 reported using LSD and other hallucinogens. The rest reported using a scattering of drugs. Certainly these college students have not experimented as widely as have the patients in Bellevue.

The Brooklyn findings are in line with our hypothesis that the typical hospitalized user of drugs at the present time is more concerned with experiences and highs than with change in personality or with religious meditation. The over-all data, we feel, supply an answer to the question of whether the widespread use of drugs, which have some relatively high potential of harm, either direct or indirect, should be encouraged by legalizing their indiscriminate use in the community, particularly for those segments of the population that rely on intellectual activity for their functioning.

In summary, we should like to reaffirm the fact that we are not interested in intensifying any hysterical outburst against the use of marihuana or LSD, and that we are particularly interested in the continuation of research on use of the psychedelic drugs. At the same time, we have felt it important to publicize rather than suppress the risks attendant on the unsupervised use and abuse of the drugs, particularly since some of the people most likely to develop difficulties may have been lulled into a false sense of security by previous reports that emphasized only alleged benefits and ignored potential difficulties and their long-term gravity. As many as 200 people a year have come to our hospital because of adverse reactions to LSD. Approximately one third required more than a cursory period of hospitalization, and many functioned less well on leaving than they had before taking the trip that brought them there.

There are no data available on the extent of adverse reactions to LSD, and our figures are probably an understatement, since many who develop serious difficulties would rather turn to their friends than to authorities, for a variety of reasons.

In the past, when the use of LSD was more restricted, it was possible to contain many of the psychotic reactions within the LSD movement itself and to keep them from public attention. In recent years this has not been feasible, even though efforts are still made to prevent adverse reactions from being publicized. The rate of hospitalization has ranged between two to four cases per week over the past two years. This may be the result of several factors: less unsupervised taking of LSD because of publicity regarding untoward effects; greater awareness of the possibility of panic reactions by users and friends—hence, greater ability to cope with them; and increased sophistication by users of drugs and individual physicians as to the effective "antidotes" available in times of difficulty.

The philosophy that advocates "dropping out" in order to meditate, or to live in small autonomous groups, overlooks both the realities of having to provide materially for the group members in some way, and the pleasures of meeting challenges successfully. The few who have been able to "drop out" at a high level have worked hard at learning previously, and have been able to obtain outside financial support for their activities. For persons able to get others to support them, or who are willing to live on this basis, which occasionally means adopting a lower standard of living than the average college student takes for granted, nothing more need be said. For the majority, who may not be aware of what they are giving up, both in terms of responsibilities and satisfactions, "dropping out" prematurely may mean the permanent closing of doors that they themselves would want to keep open.

*REFERENCES*


1. Huxley, A. L. *The Doors of Perception. Heaven and Hell.* New York, Harper, Row, 1963.
2. Huxley, A. L. Mescaline and the "Other World." In: *Lysergic Acid Diethylamide and Mescaline in Experimental Psychiatry.* Cholden, L., ed. New York, London, Grune, Stratton, 1956.
3. *Organization and Coordination of Federal Drug Research and Regulatory Programs: LSD.* Hearings before the Subcommittee on Executive Reorganization of the Committee on Government Operations, U.S. Senate. May 24, 25, and 26, 1966. Washington, D.C. Gov. Print. Off., 1966.
4. Blum, R. H., ed. *Utopiates: The Use and Users of LSD 25.* New York, Atherton, 1964.
5. Cohen, S. *The Beyond Within.* New York, Atheneum, 1965.
6. Cohen, S. and Ditman, K. S. Prolonged adverse reactions to lysergic acid diethylamide, *Arch. Gen. Psychiat. 8*:475, 1963.
7. Rosenthal, S. N. Persistent hallucinosis following repeated administration of hallucinogenic drugs, *Amer. J. Psychiat. 121*:238, 1964.
8. Frosch, W. A., Robbins, E. S. and Stern, M. Untoward reactions to lysergic acid diethylamide (LSD) resulting in hospitalization, *New Eng. J. Med. 273*:1235, 1965.
9. Christen, J. P. Letter to Editor, *Brit. Med. J. 1*:1540, 1966.
10. Robbins, E., Frosch, W. A. and Stern, M. Further observations on untoward reactions to LSD, *Amer. J. Psychiat.* In press.
11. Frosch, W. A. Patterns of response to self-administration of LSD. Presented at the *5th Annual Meeting of American College of Neuropharmacology,* Dec. 7, 1966.
12. Ungerleider, J. T., Fisher, D. D. and Fuller, M. The Dangers of LSD, *J.A.M.A. 197*:389, 1966.
13. Fink, P. J., Goldman, M. J. and Lyons, I. Morning glory seed psychosis, *Arch. Gen. Psychiat. 15*:209, 1966.
14. Cohn, A. Y. Personal communication.
15. Fink, M., Simeon, J., Hague, W. and Itil, T. Prolonged adverse reactions to LSD in psychotic subjects, *Arch. Gen. Psychiat. 15*:450, 1966.
16. Pahnke, W. Personal communication.
17. Frosch, W. A., Robbins, E., Stern, M. and Robbins, L. Motivation for self-administration of LSD, *Psychiat. Quart. 41*:56-61, 1967.
18. Pahnke, W. Drugs and mysticism, *Int. J. Parapsychol. 8*:295, 1966.
19. Masters, R. A. L. and Houston, J. *Varieties of Psychedelic Experience,* New York, Holt, Rinehart, Winston, 1966.
20. Crocket, R., Sandison, R. A. and Walk, A., eds. *Hallucinogenic Drugs and Their Psychotherapeutic Use.* London, Lewis, 1963.
21. Abramson, H. A. *Uses of LSD in Psychotherapy and Alcoholism.* Indianapolis, Bobbs-Merrill, 1967.
22. Dahlberg, C. C. See ref. 3, above, p. 98.
23. Solursh, M. D. and Rae, J. M. LSD, suggestion, and hypnosis, *Int. J. Neuropsychiat. 2*:60, 1966.
24. Blum, R. H. See ref. 3, above, p. 120.
25. Fox, R. Is LSD of Value in Treating Alcoholics? See ref. 21, above.
26. Fox, R. Personal communication.
27. Leary, T., Metzner, R., Presnell, M., Weil, G., Schwitzgebel, R. and Kinne, S. A new behavior change program using psilocybin. *Psychotherapy: Theory, Res., Pract. 2*:61, 1965.
28. Freeman, S. Personal communication.
29. Gershon, S. and Olariu, J. JB 329—A new psychotomimetic. Its antagonism by tetrahydroaminacrin and its comparison

with LSD, mescaline, and sernyl, *J. Neuropsychiat. 1*:283, 1959-60.
30. Wallace, G. *The Marihuana Problem in the City of New York.* Lancaster, Cattell, 1944.
31. Watt, J. M. Drug dependence of the hashish type. In: *Hashish: Its Chemistry and Pharmacology.* Wolstenholme, G. E. W. and Knight, J., eds. Boston, Little, Brown, 1965.
32. Murphy, H. B. M. The cannabis habit: A review of recent psychiatric literature, *Bull. Narcot. (UN) 15, 1*:15, 1963.
33. Solomon, D., ed. *The Marihuana Papers.* Indianapolis, Bobbs-Merrill, 1966.
34. Benabud, A. Psychopathological aspects of the cannabis situation in Morocco; statistical data for 1956, *Bull. Narcot. (UN) 9, 4*:1, 1957.
35. Chopra, R. N. and Chopra, G. S. The Present Position of Hemp-Drug Addiction in India. *Indian Med. Research Memoirs 31:* (July) 1939. See ref. 32, above.
36. Alpert, R., Cohen, S. and Schiller, L. *LSD.* New York, New Amer. Library, 1966.
37. Block, J. H., Haan, N. and Smith, M. B. Draft Chapter for *Contributions to the Understanding of Adolescence,* Adams, J. F., ed. In preparation.
38. Pearlman, S. Drug use and experience in an urban college population. *Amer. J. Orthopsychiat. 37*:297-99, 1967.

# THE EVOLUTION OF GENDER IDENTITY*

Harry Gershman

Attending Psychoanalyst
Karen Horney Clinic

Dean, American Institute of Psychoanalysis

New York, N. Y.

The original title of this paper was "The Evolution of the Sexual Image." Upon reflection I became increasingly dissatisfied with the term "sexual image." Both words seemed too constricted. The word sexual, in spite of Freud's attempt to broaden its meaning to include almost all feelings, continued to be synonymous with genital, whereas the word image gives the connotation of a fixed concretized symbol, devoid of the dynamism that I feel is its most important element. What I have in mind concerns itself with the feeling of being masculine or feminine, with all its nuances and ramifications, in addition to sexual implications. The term gender connotes, for me, psychological aspects of behavior related to masculinity and femininity. It does not have the same meaning as sex. A person's sex is the result of a number of factors —chromosomal, external and internal genitalia, hormonal states, and secondary characteristics produced by estrogens. Sex is biological and gender is social. For a person to function and to be either masculine or feminine, there must be a congruence between the biological and the social. Since my interest is in the domain of the psychological, I feel that the words gender and identity are closer to what I wish to express.

I use the term identity as synonymous with self as Horney[1] conceived of it—as a dynamic composite of the idealized self, actual self, and real self. I also use the term as Erikson[2] saw it in the developing child, as it moves through a series of self-concepts and developmental levels. At each level the self-concept differs from the previous one, and the critical issues that must be solved also change with time. The person passes through a series of identities. The processes are not completed with the oedipal resolution, as Freud suggested. Important preadolescent and adolescent experiences must also be integrated into the personality

*Presented at a meeting of the Association for the Advancement of Psychoanalysis, New York, N. Y., held at The New York Academy of Medicine, February 15, 1967.

before maturity is attained in the social and sexual sphere. While the development of an identity is an example of a true continuum within an individual, I believe that the core is crystallized very early. All periods of life provide experiences that contribute to a sense of identity. The evolution of identity is continuous, although there are points where the pace and even the direction may change sharply. A gender role is not established at birth, but results cumulatively from experiences encountered and transacted through explicit instructions, elucidations, and spontaneous unplanned learning. The expectations of gender are specifically modified by the mother, who is affected by her own gender expectations, her relation to her husband, her experiences with children, and the manner in which she is able to communicate her emotional feelings to them. Views that emanate from the mother help the child differentiate its gender identity. These sensations, as well as environmental cues, gradually confirm for the child the ascription of its maleness or femaleness by society. With independence, language, mobility, and experience, the child learns to differentiate between two types of genitalia, which also distinguish two classes of human beings. Out of these earliest stages of development of gender identity arises the *core gender identity*, an almost unshakeable conviction in nearly all people–namely: "I am a male" or "I am a female." Core gender identity refers to the deep feelings one has about himself or herself as a man or a woman, and not simply to the conscious awareness that one is anatomically a man or a woman.

The experience of self has many facets, and its fullness gives rise to the global or personal identity of the individual. Man can assume an almost infinite variety of behavior identity. This enables him to adapt to almost any environmental change. For this adaptability he is constantly threatened with loss or breakdown of his identity, a danger that is unknown to animals under natural conditions. His identity is not basically inherent by virtue of inborn mechanisms. The self-image is maintained through a continual redefinition, which is associated with comparison to others. Loss of identity is specifically human, and maintenance of identity is a specifically human necessity. Man has only innate potential identity, with an almost infinite range of possibilities. The identity principle is an organizational biological one.

I regard the gender identity as one aspect of the global identity of the individual. While the two are closely related, and generally share parallel distortions in psychopathological states, this is not always true. Sometimes we see a selective injury to the gender identity that is very disproportionate to the global health and strength of that individual. The focus of this paper is on one aspect of the identity problem: namely, the gender identity. The core of this gender identity, I believe, is crystallized by the age of three; it thus precedes the oedipal complex and derives from the early interaction between the child and the mother. For descriptive purposes this might be considered analogous to the process of imprinting, which Lorenz[3] defined in 1924 as "the name we have given to the process by which the releaser of an innate reaction to a fellow member of the species is acquired." When applied to human development it is, as Lichtenstein[4] wrote, to be used as an analogy. Lichtenstein states that in the early phases of individualization the responses of the infant to the mother seem to be restricted to certain critical periods, and that these changes appear to be irreversible. The quality of the relation between the infant and the mother seems crucial in the evolution of an identity. Spitz[5] traces the beginning of awareness of self to the age of 15 months, when the concept of I or self is formed. His work on infants who suffer from hospitalism suggested that their retardation, as well as early death, was due to the emotional climate and lack of mothering. This may be due to faulty initial establishment and inadequate maintenance of the infant's feeling of identity. The more the personality has retained a symbiotic fusion, the less can it initiate the process of individualization.

As Spitz has shown, the infant's responsiveness to bodily contact is heightened by the other person's emotional interest in it. The ability of a human being to acquire a human or nonhuman identity depends on those processes imprinted on the infant in its earliest emotional and physical contacts with the mother. This seems to be borne out clinically by the history of our disturbed patients, many of whom were born during periods when their mothers were experiencing breakdowns.

The infant-mother relation is the initial object relation of the child. When the mother is inadequate in generating sufficient emotional stimulation for growth, defects and distortions occur in the infant's image of itself. Material needs alone are not sufficient to stimulate this initial surge for healthy individualization. The infant experiences anxiety in any situation if it is not with the mother. The basis for the deepest fears of abandonment, loneliness, and anxiety is then created. The so-called sadistic and masochistic stages alleged to be part of maturation are, I believe, pathological reactions of the child's frustration at not being able to establish a stable, resourceful, and independent self-image. When the initial fusion of infant-mother symbiosis is never fully resolved, the basis of subsequent difficulties in interpersonal relation is concretized. One of the cornerstones of this self-image is gender identity. This is part of the total body image that the child creates in his mind. Since perceptual processes precede the conceptual, the predominant mental life of the infant is perceptual. Hence core gender identity is one aspect of the body image that becomes the foundation of the individual's identity. Other levels of experiences will impinge and modify it until such time after adolescence as it is fully formed.

In the *New York Times* of February 12, 1967, Bruno Bettelheim, in an article on clinical work with autistic children at the Orthogenic School of the University of Chicago, referred to critical periods in the developing personality of the infant. He stated that the most important factor is the mother's capacity to stimulate the infant's spontaneous reactions to the conditions of his life. The most critical factor is that which elicits the infant's own ability to act. The mother's behavior must not "rob the infant of his conviction that it was his own wail that resulted in filling his stomach, when his own hunger timed it." By the same token, if his own earliest signals—his cry or his smile—bring no results, he is discouraged from trying to refine his efforts at communicating his needs. In time he loses the impulse to develop those mental and emotional structures through which he deals with his environment, and he is discouraged from forming a personality.

If the infant consistently, and from an early age, fails to meet appropriate response to his emotions, he stops communicating, and he eventually loses interest in the world. Bettelheim goes on to say that the infant's early conviction that the world is virtually at his fingertips must be tempered by exposure to experiencing the world as somewhat frustrating. This spectrum of experience must impinge on the infant at appropriate critical periods, so that he is stimulated to participate as much as he can, without losing interest in life. From birth on, the child must receive responses from the environment that encourage his spontaneous moves toward the world. He should not be ignored or overpowered.

As has been stated, gender identity is crystallized by the age of three.

The child uses his parents as models with which to identify. Unless there is enormous conflict and psychic disturbance in the family atmosphere, the boy regularly and predominantly identifies with his father. Nevertheless, the mother is also introjected—in part—as a model. As a consequence, the child has adopted his or her own gender characteristics from both parents. For both the little boy and the little girl the degree of feminine or masculine aspects adopted varies a great deal—there is a continuum of variation. In the male these aspects vary from frank effeminacy of voice, posture, and gestures, to total absence of such mannerisms. Gender connotes behavior learned from a tremendous pool of cues present in every culture as carried on by the parents through a vast system of rewards and punishments in which every individual lives. Myriad cues from everyone who comes into contact with the child funnel the gender criteria of the culture in upon him.

The fact that the parents are clear in their belief that the infant is either male or female has permanent consequences for the child. The tolerance for aggression, in conjunction with many other cues in the male infant—as opposed to the female—by the parents, serves to differentiate the development of the self, defined as masculine or feminine.

It is the experiences in infancy and childhood that prepare the child for integration of sexual knowledge and sexual behavior. This readiness is the result of systems of parental behavior that may have no direct sexual bearing but may spill over into the sexual sphere. The child responds more to what the parents feel about sexuality than about rational planned statements.

In the past 10 years I[6] have been particularly interested in this subject, not only because of its importance in all emotional illnesses, but because of its central significance in the understanding of perversions. Intensive clinical studies of people suffering from homosexuality, transvestitism, and transsexuality suggest selective traumata to the evolving gender identity of these people. Although distortions in gender identity often parallel the distortions in global identity, this is not always the case. Some show a disproportionate discrepancy between the health of their personal and their gender identity. Gender identity refers to the individual's capacity to experience himself or herself as a man or a woman in all the multiple situations of social and sexual intercourse. Pathological processes often help us to understand how distortions come about in normal processes. Nonperverse people may also reveal some confusion in gender identity in special circumstances, such as a toxic state caused by alcohol, drugs, or physical illness. Dreams often reflect repressed states of uncertainty as to gender.

The perversions are most characteristic of this problem of confusion in gender identity—particularly in the homosexual, the transvestite, and the transsexual individual. All have doubts of their assigned sexual role. The transsexual person, we might say, has a fixed delusion that he does not conform to what society tells him he is. So intransigent is the urge of his inner gender identity, that he insists that he be altered surgically. Recently Johns Hopkins Hospital has quietly begun to perform sex changes through surgical operation. It is also to be noted that it has established a "gender identity clinic" staffed by a special committee of psychiatrists, surgeons, and other specialists to screen applicants for the operation. The *New York Times*, in describing the program, quoted a number of psychiatrists familiar with the subject of transsexuals, who record them as "emotionally normal, with the exception of their gender confusion, which leads to intense feelings of frustration." I do not share this opinion. The transsexual will modify his body to conform to his image and live in harmony, but he does so on a circumscribed delusional basis.

The transvestite's doubt about himself is assuaged by the magical ritual of wearing clothes of the opposite sex in order to avoid a discrepancy in his inner image of himself, which would result in disintegration and failure to function sexually. Two transvestite members of a group therapy unit conducted at the Karen Horney Clinic disclosed parallel psychodynamics of their affliction. Both were married men with relatively large families. Prior to sexual intimacy with their wives, it was necessary for each to don some of her intimate apparel, such as silk stockings or panties. Without these they found themselves impotent. Neither entertained fantasies during these rituals to suggest that he was anybody but himself. The background of both presented similar histories of premature and early death of their respective fathers. Both mothers very aggressively took charge of the families concerned. I had a feeling that the transvestite act was the symbolic incorporation of the strong mother, in order to help them complete their roles as effective men. The psychodynamic explanation—that the transvestite imagines himself a woman and regards his partner as a man—was not confirmed consciously or unconsciously, nor was it expressed in a dream or fantasy.

The homosexual's deep doubt about himself forces him to shun the challenge that the opposite sex poses, and through the magical maneuver of the homosexual ritual he fuses with another person of his own sex as a reparative act in order to bolster his image of himself. The homosexual usually knows his gender identity consciously, but he does not feel it. While his sense of reality is intact so far as the function of testing reality is concerned, the sense of his own inner reality, his core gender identity, is disturbed and confused.

I should like to discuss the genesis of homosexuality to help us understand how it is that an incongruence has developed. Homosexuality was once considered a genetic anomaly, probably related to hormonal, chromosomal, and anatomical variants. Modern cytology, endocrinology and microscopic morphology have failed to substantiate this hypothesis. In spite of Kallmann's[7] impressive work on identical twins, there is little evidence that homosexuality is genetically determined. Money and Hampson,[8] in a study of hermaphrodites, indicate that of all the variable dynamics in establishing gender identity, the sex assignment in rearing, by parents or substitute parents, is probably the single most significant factor in establishing gender identity. The psychological influence supersedes such factors as chromosomal, gonadal, hormonal, and anatomical variants. Money and Hampson feel that the role of gender is undifferentiated at birth, but becomes indelibly imprinted by the age of 2½. Gender imprinting begins by the first birthday, and the critical period is reached by about the age of 18 months.

Stoller writes that core gender identity develops through the interaction of a third factor, in addition to anatomical and psychological indoctrination. This is a biological force that, although hidden from conscious and preconscious awareness, nevertheless seems to provide some of the drive energy for gender identity. Stoller describes two transsexual patients who, in spite of established anatomical gender and psychological indoctrination by environment, insisted on a reassignment of their sexual identity because of an inexplicable inner urge.

It is difficult, however, to accept the latter concept in view of Harlow's[9] work. Although it is true that animal experiments cannot be transposed to human psychology, Harlow's work with monkeys who were isolated and put into contact with artificial mothers made of wire and cloth, resulted uniformly in highly neurotic and disturbed animals. Adult monkeys that had been reared in isolation from both mothers and peers were completely incapable of adult heterosexual contacts. They were terrified of sex and often assaulted and even killed their own offspring.

Comfort from contact may be more important than so-called oral gratification. The mother may be more important as an emotional stimulus or arousal for growth and maturing.

The rapid improvement of these emotionally deprived animals, when placed with healthy peers, implies that this may be an even more important determinant of sexual identity than the previous parental attitude toward the gender role of the child. Deprivation of peers from the age of 3 to 6 months, Harlow contends, "irreversibly blights the animal's capacity for social adjustment." He further suggests, "it is apparent also that sexual activity is stimulated by the mother's grooming of the infant." In this research there is definite evidence that particular patterns and activities of a mother with an infant have lasting and permanent impact on the sexual life of that infant when he becomes an adult. Patterns of behavior are, therefore, more intimately connected with experiential character development rather than with underlying biological drives.

Therefore I believe that homosexuality is the consequence of the course of events in the life experience of the individual. Orthodox psychodynamics of the male homosexual, as well as of the female homosexual, revolves around unintegrated infantile sexuality.[10] I feel that the homosexual act or ritual in men or women is essentially reparative and is calculated to restore the gender image. Other functions are also served by the act, such as neurotic needs for aggression, dependency, personal uninvolvement, restoration of a spurious aliveness through the sheer physical stimulation of the act, etc. But the main purpose, as I see it, is to restore the incongruence of the inner gender image of the individual. By *acting out* the homosexual ritual, the unconscious need for the gender congruence is achieved, though the constructive insight into the unconscious inner dynamics is avoided. The intent is to bolster doubts about one's masculine or feminine identity. The male homosexual, through his obsessive act, is attempting to incorporate that which he feels he is lacking, and his aversion to the opposite sex is due to deep feelings of inadequacy in that regard.

A question might be raised at this point. What about the passive homosexual act, wherein the individual takes the role of a woman by offering his anus in lieu of a vagina? This is probably the most abject confession of masculine bankruptcy. However, even in this role, the ability to have an erection and orgasm suggests residual masculine identity in the striving toward fulfillment in spite of paralyzing doubts about the patient's own identity. These efforts represent desperate attempts to incorporate maleness and thus avoid psychic fragmentation with its ensuing anxieties and panics.

Similarly for the female. Female homosexuality has been attributed to a multitude of causes such as constitutional bisexuality, fear of pregnancy, fear of injury by the penis, etc. Of these many possibilities, the unresolved relation to the mother, and penis envy, generally account for most of the psychic disturbances that have been described. Penis envy presumes that normal female sexuality is derived from innate masculine sexuality. The Freudian concept of constitutional bisexuality has been seriously compromised by recent biological and endocrinological research. A considerable body of evidence has been accumulated that indicates that the early embryo, rather than being bisexual or even undifferentiated, is actually female, and that sexual structures become transformed into the male organs only by the action of foetal androgen in genetic males. This opens to question at least the biological foundation of penis envy, with all of its presumed consequences for feminine psychology.

Homosexuality in the female represents a confession of feminine bankruptcy. Because of the inadequacy, there is a deep aversion to heterosexuality. The homosexual act on deep levels symbolizes a return and fusion with the most primitive early relation to the mother. The act is reparative and is calculated to allay the anxiety of inadequate individualization. During the state of separateness, female homosexuals feel a lack of identity, and often describe states of depression, panic, and suicidal feelings. All this can be seen as forms of depersonalization. When panic is not that severe, they experience anxiety of varying intensity.

I believe that homosexuality is brought about by the interaction of the child with its parents. Both parents have been unavailable for a truly loving relationship and, consciously or unconsciously, they have combined and conspired, because of their own neurotic conflicts, to undermine the child's basic feeling about himself. Homosexuality is never caused by the attitude of one parent, but by the strong constellation of the parent-child triangle. As I have pointed out, the relation between the infant and the mother is probably crucial, because the basic confusion in core gender crystallized in that relation makes subsequent interpersonal relations impossible or difficult to resolve. I am referring to the oedipal relations of the child to the mother and father that ensue after this period.

Detailed studies of the family milieu of people suffering from the perversions mentioned above disclose vast isolation, loneliness, abandonment, rank hostility, and destructiveness. The prevailing affectivity of the whole environment is characterized by coldness, undemonstrativeness, and a paucity of genuine spontaneous feelings. Underlying coldness can be overcompensated by unhealthy, sticky, overstimulating, devouring closeness on the part of the parent. Subsequent distorted images and gender images make it impossible for these individuals to enjoy intimate, warm, and loving relations. Instead they resort to magical rituals, which are intended to make up for their profound emotional inadequacies. These rituals are most often impersonal, highly charged with anxiety, motivated by neurotic needs of domination, sadism, masochism, and vindictiveness.

I believe that the central issue of homosexuality is a disturbance of the core gender identity, and that this structure can be selectively injured by specific emotional factors. Further, in most cases the core gender identity is firmly fixed by the age of three, i.e., prior to the phallic and postphallic stages, in which orthodox psychoanalytic theory places the fixing of sexual identity. In a psychoanalytic contribution, Stoller has reported two males in whom the core gender identity was present and permanently fixed in spite of the congenital absence of a penis.

Extending along the spectrum of congruence in gender identity from the perversions to healthy mature orientation are varying states of confusion in identity. Bisexuality and compulsive sexuality—nymphomania and satyrism—are such variations. Although all these individuals have deep unconscious doubts about their gender roles, their sexual behavior is calculated to allay anxiety stemming from the incongruence of their biological and social roles. It is difficult to account for a person's selection of a particular strategy in coping with this central problem. There is still a great deal that we do not know regarding the choice of symptoms by a patient. This paper places emphasis on the psychological experiences impinging on the human biological substrate to create character and, more particularly, gender identity.

I have found in my clinical experience that the bisexual individual is not one who can experience homosexual and heterosexual relations with equal passion. Usually such a person feels more intensely in a homosexual relation, although he may be able to perform in a heterosexual one. His basic problem remains one of homosexuality.

The nymphomaniac or the sufferer from satyriasis apparently needs insatiable sexual acts to quell his doubt about his sexual identity. While the reparative aspects of his compulsive sexuality are more clearly observed and understood, I believe that the same basic, reparative striving applies to the other perversions as well. The difference may be in the degree of resignation and hopelessness that the individual has regarding the gap in his gender incongruity. In one, this doubt is allayed by compulsive sexual acts with a person of the opposite sex. In the other, however, he has relinquished heterosexuality because of paralyzing conscious and unconscious fears. He attempts to integrate into his own image that of another person of his own sex, through fusion by the homosexual ritual.

The severity of distortion in gender identity varies. While the development of an identity is an example of a true continuum within an individual, the core is crystallized by the age of three. Where the core gender identity has been injured, the upsurge of adolescent problems may bring underlying psychic disturbance to the surface.

## Case Presentation

I should like at this time to illustrate clinically some of the concepts that I have thus far elaborated. In order to do this I should like to weave in the analysis of one of my patients, who has been with me for well over 10 years.

Jack is a man of about 50. He is an exceptionally gifted and talented artist, successful both professionally and financially. He is considered a leader in his field and is admired for his originality, perceptivity, and creativity. He entered analysis because, as he stated, "I am on the brink of doing away with myself. It has become unbearable to live with my constant 'cruising,' panic, and feelings of disintegration." He indicated that he had no interest in changing his homosexual orientation since he had been a practicing homosexual for over 20 years. To get the flavor of this man's life, let me give you a little of his background. Jack was born into an extremely wealthy home at a time when his older brother was eight years old and was the established crony of his father. Both the father and brother were interested in rough-and-tumble activities. The father was a hard-drinking man. He kept his room in a messy, sweaty, sloppy state, usually filled with racing sheets, athletic newspapers, and such publications as the *Police Gazette*. The father confined most of his gruff conversation to the brother, who was interested in baseball, football, and other sports. The mother was just recovering from a nervous breakdown. She was in a state of conflict over the care of my patient, and alternated between oversolicitousness and indifference. What Jack remembered of most of these early years was the messiness of the household and his mother's confinement because of illnesses that were obscure, and her unresponsiveness to the usual medical regimes. His sister was born within one year after his own birth. In view of the inaccessibility of his father and brother, his whole life revolved around his mother and sister. He loved to wear high heeled shoes, and entertained them by pirouetting in wild, exciting, ecstatic dances. His mother was delighted by his evident aptitude and natural grace, yet in spite of this she seemed to prefer his sister. She repeatedly urged him to love his sister, since she was "the most precious possession that you have." Strangely enough, he believed that. He was considerate of his sister through the years, and felt that she was his closest and dearest friend. A recurrent dream from early childhood, in which "he and his sister plus a silent menacing monster were suspended motionlessly in a body of water," evoked no emotional response in the dream, but was invariably associated with moroseness, irritability, and compulsive rages during the ensuing day. Several years later, in his analysis, he learned to recognize that behind this façade of closeness and affection for his sister he repressed a cauldron of rage and monstrous hostility, which he also externalized toward women generally.

He recalled that even in these earliest years he knew that he was a boy but inwardly felt he was a girl. In his late thirties, when he began his analysis, he referred to himself as "nervous Nellie." This was not simply an expression of his states of tension, but something that he concretely felt and experienced about his gender.

With his mother's encouragement, he mastered the domestic chores expertly—kept house, served, danced, and could discuss household chores better than his mother or sister. On many occasions, he recalls lying in bed with his mother during her ailments—migraine, asthma, intestinal allergy—combing her long hair and telling her pleasing stories. In his many conversations with his mother, he felt as though they were two women relating to each other. His father invariably aroused ire in him, even when, on infrequent occasions, the father made overtures of friendship and understanding. He felt an utter failure with his father, because he knew that the father looked upon him as some sort of freak who was soft, fat, pimply-faced, and fearful of anything that suggested gruff, masculine, athletic, competitive activity. He interpreted his father's occasional overtures as merely a surface compensation for underlying cynicism and disparaging contempt of his sissiness.

When he started school, he was surprised to find that the boys liked him and often selected him to be on their athletic teams. He was naturally athletic, strong, and extremely resilient in competitive games. Neverthless, he continued to be suspicious, and harbored within himself doubts about the genuineness of the boys' interest in him. He felt more comfortable with the girls. At about the age of 10 or 11, he became obsessed with the notion that his genitals were unusually small. In shower rooms he envied the size of the other boys' genitals, although his were considered by them as being much larger. Nevertheless, he felt inferior to them, and often deplored the fact that he was born a boy. During these early years he was plagued by frequent nightmares often triggered by recurrent dreams. In one such dream he looked with both horror and glee at a newborn baby that was tossed in the air between two persons, a man and a woman. The infant shrieked in panic as the adults continued to torment and terrify it. The sadomasochistic milieu of the family, as he experienced it, was shown in this dream. This nightmare gradually wove itself into his consciousness, so that he frequently experienced this obsessive fantasy during waking life. After such a fantasy he would find himself enraged at his parents.

As he approached his early adolescence, he stated that he had identified himself completely as a woman. "I decided that I wasn't a man. Mother didn't want me to be a man." When he thought hard on this subject, he described an odd and weird feeling overcoming him. It was as though his feeling of identity were being swept from under him. It was invariably associated with panic and terror. I believe that these periods of depersonalization just preceded his turning to homosexuality at the age of 12. The sexual orientation was not crystallized until he was about 15, when he discovered that following a homosexual experience he felt strangely comfortable, at ease, and at one with himself. Conversely, girls at this time made him extremely nervous and uneasy, particularly if there was any inference that they had sexual interest in him. On a nonsexual basis, of course, he felt very much at home with them, and could discuss matters pertaining to their common interests. It was also at about this time in his life that a persistent fantasy emerged that he continued to entertain for a period of over 30 years. That fantasy consisted of a young boy in a wealthy home who was seduced by the family chauffeur who was an ex-sailor and bisexual. The boy was seduced, and conditioned to like anal intercourse. In the fantasy, at the height of his sexual excitement, the chauffeur threatened to withdraw unless he agreed to oral intercourse with another man, simultaneously. To this the young boy agreed. This fantasy, whenever evoked, aroused tremendous sexual excitement and helped him to arouse himself when he did not have sexual inclinations. One of the characteristic qualities of this recurrent fantasy was its total absence of tender feelings. Like his homosexuality, tenderness had no part in the intercourse. In fact, he has often stated that when he feels tender and gentle toward his partner, he loses his erection. The conspicuous quality of the fantasy is that of sheer sadism and masochism. The need for homosexual experience often comes about when he feels a sense of depersonalization beginning. Associated with this feeling is an engulfing emptiness and impending loss of meaning. The sensuality and stimulation of the homosexual act reawaken in him feelings of life and of restoration of integration; hence the compulsiveness of the act. In the course of the act, the sadism gives him the sense of power with which he has associated masculinity. His constant striving to achieve this masculinity is an expression of his attempt to complete his identity as a man, though it is done in a most distorted manner. A compulsion for the homosexual act is, I think, related to the compulsion to achieve a masculine identity in order to be able to function, and also to eliminate the discrepancy in one's feelings about one's self. Among the many clinical symptoms that he complained about during the course of his analysis, his feeling of loneliness, emptiness, and boredom was most prominent. The maintenance of identity is specifically human, as is loss of identity. One of the most frequent symptoms of homosexuality is loneliness.

The roots of loneliness are multiple. On an interpersonal level, the absence of genuine emotional relations, feelings of not belonging, fears of being ostracized by society, feelings that one is not understood and is looked down upon, undoubtedly contribute to feelings of loneliness. Loss of meaningful values in life may also give rise to the aimlessness and purposelessness that is often the basis of loneliness. But I should like to focus on the intrapsychic factors that account for the loneliness observed in the homosexual. I believe that it is composed in large measure of this type of depersonalization and derealization. When the depersonalization is not very intense, the varying degrees of anxiety emerge. One of the accompanying cravings of homosexual experience is the hunger for physical contact. This need to latch on to something real is, I believe, also an attempt to hang on to reality.

I take issue with the psychodynamics of homosexual panic as being, in the male, a fear of castration at the hands of the father, because I believe that the panic is much more related to the dissolution of the self under the pressure of intense doubt as to who one is. This, I believe, is the fabric out of which the patient may elect to build a fantasy in which he may be frightened, assaulted, or castrated by men. The deeper fear is the fear of dissolution of identity. This dissolution is frequently accompanied by feelings of emptiness and nothingness, which in people of poorly integrated ego may actually be experienced by dying. The accompanying rage and the mad attempts at sexual stimulation have often struck me as an attempt to overcome this feeling of dying. One of the compulsive needs that the homosexual experience fulfills is the intense sensual stimulation that follows it. The experience makes the individual feel alive.

With Jack it was almost 10 years before he was able to give up the image of himself as a woman. The problem of his identity was central —his confusion and uncertainty were indicated by a painful awareness of disconnected identities. For a long time he could not arrive at an integrated sense of identity because what he experienced through his actions in no way corresponded to the inner experiences of his real self. When this occurred—and it occurred gradually—it was noted that his voice became considerably lower, the effeminate gestures and formlessness of his appearance and manner disappeared, and he began literally to take shape, and to follow the form of his naturally well-endowed athletic physique.

I have attempted to show thus far that in the spectrum extending from psychic disease to normal health the feeling of identity is a crucial factor. The maintenance of a person's identity has priority over all other needs, for without this biological organizational principle, integration of life on a psychological basis is not possible. There is constant need to maintain a sense of identity in order to experience and deal effectively with reality. Man exercises a massive defense against the diffusion of identity. Loss of identity is probably at the bottom of impending psychosis (panic states) and of the nightmarish quality of the paranoid conditions. Not until such loss is threatened, until there is such feeling that one's self is swept away, does panic result. In the severe perversions we see distortions in core gender identity. This flaw interferes with subsequent maturation in interpersonal relationships. As we observe less-ill people, we find that the core gender identity is usually undisturbed, and that their subsequent emotional difficulties arise from the faulty defenses and neurotic patterns that they have elaborated in the course of their lives.

Gender identity is a continuous process, the foundation of which is established psychologically in the earlier years of life. Although the process is a continuum commencing at about the first year of life and evolving into full gender maturity, it goes through important developmental levels—infancy, childhood, preadolescent, and adolescent stages. Although the core is probably fully established by the age of three, subsequent events influence it, constructively or adversely, depending on the nature of the experience. We have discussed the nature of the distortions of gender identity in perversions. As we move toward the healthier end of the spectrum, we note fewer distortions and a greater capacity to relate socially and sexually to members of the opposite sex.

Relating sexually to a member of the opposite gender is a biological phenomenon. Among lower animals, whose identity is imprinted and unalterable, the sexual act is instinctive. Conflict does not occur in the natural state. In man, whose gender identity is determined by psychological experiences, all sorts of inhibitions and distortions can occur, as we have observed in the perversions. The highest form of adult mature sexuality is that experienced in a situation of love. I am referring to love between two adult mature individuals whose feeling for each other is not enmeshed in a web of conflicting neurotic needs.

Love is possible only if two people communicate with each other from the centers of their beings. The partners are authentic people capable of a measure of maturity, wholeness, and integration, and they do not suffer from ambiguities over their identities. Such a measure of maturity is antithetical to extensive neurotic processes. In contrast to symbiotic union, mature love is union under conditions of preserving one's individuality. I agree with Boss,[10] who states that the all-encompassing male-female existential unit represents the ultimate meaning and purpose of all and every love. Man's nature reveals itself more in human love than in any other contact with the world. In love man experiences the specific human form of interrelatedness. Nowhere as in love does man express his human world.

We have seen that in the perversions the driving force for all human beings, which is meaningful love relationships, is distorted, and that it often assumes grotesque and bizarre forms. Nevertheless the striving is still for love. In psychoanalytic thinking love and sex are often treated interchangeably. The identification of love with sex obscures the fundamental fact that man enters the experience of heterosexual love only after gaining some maturity. We have seen that in the perversions the sexuality has very little of authentic capacity to love. Caring and tender feelings are often lacking in homosexuality and other perverse experiences. Primarily, sex is used for neurotic needs and reassurance of self-doubts. In order to love authentically, one must be a whole person, and evolve for himself a whole gender identity.

A healthy sexual image in man must include a capacity to love. This capacity can come only from mature, well-integrated human beings whose capacity to love sexually is part of their full spectrum of a capacity to love. Such a person would be secure in his own gender identity, and would not have to use his sexual feelings in the service of his neurosis.

If the perversions represent one end of the spectrum of evolving gender identity, and mature heterosexuality with love the other end, we can expect to find all kinds of gradations between these two. The capacity for heterosexual intercourse per se does not necessarily mean the absence of difficulties in gender identity. Compulsive promiscuity, which is frequently an expression of fear of intimacy and closeness, may indeed reflect serious ambiguities in gender identity. Adequate mechanical heterosexuality may coexist with severe distortions in personality identity even to the degree of psychosis. Persons thus afflicted do not fulfill the criteria of adequate gender identity because of their inability to love maturely.

Gender identity comes into being as an interaction between the biological substrate that is male or female, and the interpersonal experiences that the individual encounters from the moment that he is born until he dies. These interpersonal relations are influenced by the culture in which he lives. Changes in the male-female relation, in our Western society, have and will continue to alter our notions of what constitutes masculinity and femininity. The mores of our society and the era in which we live will undoubtedly modify our current concepts and will call for reevaluation in the light of socioeconomic and sexual emancipation of men and women. To understand fully the similarities and differences of personality between men and women, we must take into consideration the biological differences between the sexes as well as the culture in which we live.

I have emphasized in this paper the enormous importance of the psychological factors acting upon the child's biological ascription. An almost infinite number of culturally defined cues impinge on the reacting, growing, developing infant, thereby influencing his gender identity.

At birth, gender identity congruent with biologic state is only a possibility. In those cases in which distortion has occurred, faulty, contradictory, conflictual, and growth-inhibiting experiences have prevailed. Where congruence does exist, we can assume that the singular aspect of personal identity that we call gender identity has not been selectively injured. There are many facets of personal identity, however, that may be affected deleteriously and result in varying degrees of psychic disturbances. While distortions in gender and personal identity are often parallel, they need not always be so.

I have described the polarities of a continuum of gender identity ranging from the complete incongruity of the transsexual to a full and mature gender identity capable of relating heterosexually with love and tenderness. While the latter is an ideal that is unfortunately too seldom realized in our times, nevertheless I believe it does represent one aspect of the ultimate of human relatedness. The other end of the spectrum represents severe distortions due to emotional injuries sustained at critical periods in early life.

## Conclusions

1) Core gender identity is established by the age of three.

2) Other maturational levels of development follow until post-adolescent mature gender identity is attained.

3) Disturbances in the earliest periods of development result in ambiguous gender identities that create the group of transsexuals, transvestites, and homosexuals.

4) Mature gender identity implies a capacity for heterosexual relationship with care and tenderness.

5) Gender identity is one aspect of personal identity.

6) The most urgent and constant need of the individual is to maintain a sense of identity in order to deal effectively with reality.

*REFERENCES*


1. Horney, K. *Neurosis and Human Growth.* New York, Norton, 1950.
2. Erikson, E. H. *Childhood and Society.* New York, Norton, 1950.
3. Lorenz, K. Z. *King Solomon's Ring: New Light on Animal Ways.* New York, Crowell, 1952.
4. Lichtenstein, H. Identity and sexuality, *J. Amer. Psychol. Ass. 9*:179-261, 1961.
5. Spitz, R. A. Hospitalism: An inquiry into the genesis of psychiatric conditions in early childhood, *Psychoanal. Stud. Child 1*:53-74, 1945.
6. Gershman, H. *a)* Psychopathology of compulsive homosexuality, *Amer. J. Psychoanal. 17*:58-77, 1953. *b)* Psychopathology of compulsive homosexuality, *Amer. J. Psychoanal. 24*:1-10, 1964. *c)* Meaning of homosexual trends in therapy, *Amer. J. Psychoanal. 24*:63-67, 1964. *d)* Reflections on the nature of homosexuality, *Amer. J. Psychoanal. 26*:46-59, 1966. *e)* Changing sexual image of man, *Amer. J. Psychoanal. 27*:24-32, 1967.
7. Kallmann, F. J. Comparative twin studies of the genetic aspects of male homosexuality, *J. Nerv. Ment. Dis. 115*:286, 1952.
8. Money, J., Hampson, J. G. and Hampson, J. L. Imprinting and establishment of gender role, *Arch. Neurol. Psych. 77*:333-36, 1957.
9. Harlow, H. S. The behavioral approach to psychoanalytic theory, *Sci. Psychoanal. 7*:93-113, 1964.
10. Boss, M. *Meaning and Content of Sexual Perversions.* Trans. by L. L. Abell. New York, Grune, Stratton, 1959.

# DISCUSSION OF THE ARTICLE BY DR. HARRY GERSHMAN "THE EVOLUTION OF GENDER IDENTITY"*

NATALIE SHAINESS

Faculty Member
William Alanson White Psychoanalytic Institute
New York, N. Y.

THE scientific endeavor undertakes to bring order out of chaos, to put isolated bits of information together, to rearrange and reorder relations into new and more meaningful patterns. Dr. Gershman's undertaking is of this order. The general concept "self," "identity" or, more loosely, "self-image," was first elaborated by Horney[1] and Sullivan,[2] and then further developed by Erickson[3] as a "chain of identities." Dr. Gershman has singled out one link—gender identity—from this concept for scrutiny. Through the lens of his extensive experience in treating homosexuals, transvestites, and transsexuals, he looks back to the developmental sequence of events leading to these conditions, and speculates also about normal development.

My own thinking is quite harmonious with his view that identity formation continues on beyond the so-called oedipal phase, as I have myself singled out two aspects of the self in woman for study—the feminine identity and the maternal identity:[4] I have pointed out that the latter is necessarily late in forming but is very significant in shaping the total concept of self. I want to underscore a point on which Dr. Gershman touches lightly: human beings are too complex for facets of them to be tied up in nice, neat little parcels, and it may well be that what appears to be a primarily sexual ontogenesis is something quite different. The reverse would also hold. For example: experience with a brutal father, which has nothing to do with gender assignment or anything of a sexual nature, might lead to homosexuality or even transsexualism. The theme would be: "I cannot be a man (that is, permit myself to identify with a man like my father), therefore I *must* be a wo-

*Presented at a meeting of the Association for the Advancement of Psychoanalysis, New York, N. Y., held at The New York Academy of Medicine, February 15, 1967.

man." However, gender identity has multiple determinants, and no single factor alone can be considered causal.

Mabel Blake Cohen[5] has also speculated on the interrelation between what she calls "personal identity" and "sexual identity"—or, rather, the incompatibility that often exists between the two. She discusses the culturally determined images that prevail as norms. She considers developmental factors, particularly the place of maternal handling of the child, in terms of holding and fondling. She feels that in our society passivity is encouraged in girls, aggressiveness in boys. Perhaps this is changing, but one must be in complete agreement with her statement that creativity and intellectual development suffer where emphasis is placed on stereotyped patterns of so-called masculine or feminine behavior.

Dr. Gershman points out that conviction of gender identity must encompass deep feeling as well as conscious anatomical awareness. But I am not clear about why he has fixed on three years of age as the time by which the core of gender identity has already formed. A three-year-old boy may state without conviction that he is a boy; nor do I believe a boy of that age can be considered a transvestite, as some have suggested. If he tries on an article of clothing belonging to his mother or sister, I should be inclined to attribute this to childish curiosity and play. It is only when the adult response to this is anxiety-ridden or accusatory that a damaging experience occurs that may indeed be an early step in the direction of transvestitism or transsexualism, by eliciting shame or fear; or by creating angry feelings that may arouse oppositional behavior and a compulsive need to cross the boundary of gender by changing dress.

Doorbar[12] reports that in the Goodenough man-woman drawings boys do not seem to draw any sex differentiation until the age of 13, girls until the age of 6. This does not necessarily indicate that concepts of gender are not formed. Perhaps it merely indicates that formation occurs later, and it says something about the capacity for observation and interest in detail. But the first objective criterion of the *inner* experience of gender that I know of occurs in the choice of a preadolescent chum who is one "like me"—a kind of image. That this choice reflects characteristics in addition to gender is often apparent in the extensive criticism of the child's friend voiced by his parents. A study by Green and Money[6] on effeminate impersonation during boyhood included reports by mothers of 20 such boys on the age at which it was first noted. One observed effeminate mannerisms at the age of 3, one at 6, one at 7, but most around the ages of 11 and 12. These were hardly objective reports, but they do tend to suggest that while a child may indeed have a feeling of gender much earlier, it is hard to select a time when this has consolidated. About the imprintlike nature of early experiences determining gender identity I am in complete agreement, and this helps to explain the difficulties of treatment.

I very much like Dr. Gershman's interpretation of the meaning behind each pathological condition; his statement that the transsexual has the *delusion* he *is* a woman, the transvestite has a strong *yearning* to be a *woman* but knows he is not, and the homosexual "*acts as if*" he were a woman. But since there seem to be two types of homosexual, perhaps this classification needs to be amended. In the first instance, the homosexual *acts as if* he were, that is, has made a more complete feminine identification. In the second, he *longs* to be a man, but does not feel like one, and so relates sexually to a pretend-woman (i.e., to a homosexual of the first type). Dr. Gershman has not commented on the bisexual, who seems to have formed no gender identity of any kind, and who ricochets from one image to another.

To return to the transsexual and his delusion—he appears to be an otherwise normal person with a delusional idea. Correct this and he presumably will be all right. But if one recognizes the incredibly extensive preoccupation with sex, as Money has recently acknowledged, this condition can be seen as comparable to addictions of various sorts: gambling, fanatic devotion to a special sport, the psychopathic charmer, paranoid states—in short, a way of life in which a person has a kind of monomania or uses a single overdeveloped maneuver as a life process or life style—a way of life that fills in all kinds of gaps in a rigid compulsive manner. Another view of transsexuality, as a life style of all-consuming envy of women, is supported by a report by Guze[7] that many insist they have a monthly periodicity, with swelling of breasts, although there was no endocrine evidence of this. I suppose the term "menstruation envy" would be appropriate, and perhaps in keeping with the couvade as observed in certain primitive groups, though it may well exist covertly in our society. So, the transsexual is a very disturbed person—a psychotic who fills his gaps and alters his reality with a delusional sexual preoccupation. It is interesting that the transsexual is rivaled only by the paranoiac, who demands plastic operations on his nose, in persuading physicians to alter reality to conform to delusion. But since there is not much else that can be done at present, and since reports by Benjamin[8] indicate that a somewhat more satisfactory way of life does result at times, I suppose there is some validity in this therapeutic approach. Of course, not enough conversions have been made to evaluate the failures of this approach with possibly more overt psychotic reactions.

Incidentally, Dr. Money[9] has reported on the penchant for play-acting to be found in the triple group under discussion. I have also observed that often homosexuals have a wickedly satirical and pungent sense of humor and a talent for mimicry. It would be interesting to discover at what age this characteristic makes its appearance—it might also shed some light on the timing of the formation of core gender.

Dr. Gershman has delineated some of the factors that coalesce to form gender identity. I think it is worthwhile to bring them together, and perhaps to add a few. These factors are:

1) Parental, especially maternal, fantasies in anticipation of the unborn or newborn child. For example: if a woman who cannot accept her femininity and does not desire children accidentally becomes pregnant and is compelled to carry through with the pregnancy, her gender-rejecting attitude may be conveyed by insistence on having a son. Should the child have the misfortune to be a girl, one might expect damage done by the mother to be especially hurtful in the gender area.

2) The degree to which the mother permits self-differentiation and release from the original symbiosis.

3) How the mother handles the child. Here let me report an experience with a patient who was the mother of a five-month-old baby girl. The patient phoned one day to cancel her appointment because the sitter had not arrived. Welcoming the opportunity, I suggested it would be agreeable to me if she brought the baby along. It was a most valuable and revealing hour. There were numerous picking-ups and putting-downs of the child, and each time she grasped the baby, she somehow managed to get her hand in the crotch. One might suppose this to be an early erotizing experience for the child—the inception of the highly erotic coloration that pervades some family atmospheres.

4) Dr. Gershman emphasizes the role of *both* parents. While Horney[1] and Thompson[10] emphasized the role of the mother as genetic

to homosexuality, the Biebers[11] recently have underscored the significance of the dangerous father. But I agree with Dr. Gershman that there is danger of oversimplification, and the contributions of both must be recognized, although in any family the role of one parent may be subtle, the other overt. Subtle incestuous homosexual yearnings on the part of the father may play a part in the production of the transsexual phenomenon; Doorbar reports that after an operation for reassignment of gender, some rejecting fathers became very affectionate.

5) The domestic assignment of roles within the family. It includes name, dress, household chores.

6) Reflected evaluations from peers, at a somewhat later date.

7) In some instances, sibling rivalry. In the case that Dr. Gershman cites, the mother's preference for the sister is conveyed in no uncertain terms. The patient develops a so-called "love" for the sister, his defenses of denial and reaction-formation coming into play. In his attempt to win his mother's love, he attempts to be a girl, like his sister. The thesis is an old one: "If you can't fight 'em, join 'em!"

To these points that Dr. Gershman has made I should like to add the following:

8) Bodily care of the infant by the mother, especially genital care. For many months the baby is dependent upon the mother's ministrations for cleanliness and comfort. If the mother is rough, or angry, or both, this will be experienced by the child as painful. But the child will also experience something further: "There is something about my genitals that makes mother angry or disgusted–it must be disgusting." I have observed a curious bodily attitude in six male patients, all of whom seemed to be suffering from castration fears. They were all afraid to use the couch (and one might speculate that, among other reasons, it left their genitals exposed to danger). All sat with legs crossed at an unnaturally high level, the leg *opposite* me being the crossed one. Each held the foot tensely dorsiflexed, as if ready to kick me away. I called the attention of one of these men to his position. After a moment's silence he said: "I don't know why, but my crib as a baby comes to mind, isn't that strange?" That was all he could remember, but it set me to wondering if the leg was not defensively ready to push away the hurtful hand at diapering time. Here might well be the origin of the vagina dentata fantasy.

Another patient who used a similar position and who fits into what might colloquially be called the "mad-genius" category recounted a humiliating and painful daily event; he recalled that it started as far back as the age of four and ended with his refusal to submit to it further at age 11. His mother lined up her three sons, of whom my patient was the middle one, every night, had them strip as at an army inspection, and wiped out the orifice of each penis with a cotton Q-tip, all the while indicating her disgust. That he had gender problems will occasion no surprise. To conclude this point in relation to bodily care: obviously the mother's attitudes toward toilet-training and her mode of accomplishing it help play their parts.

9) The mother's responses, the father's also, to self-exploration and masturbatory activity make their contribution.

10) What the child sees of his parents anatomically and senses of their feelings, responses, actions, and interactions, contributes to the sense of gender. Stoller[13] has reported that transvestites had had a high degree of exposure to the mother's nude body as children.

11) Experiences relating to the menarche can be considered a special and important late contribution to the feeling of gender in the girl.[4]

12) Cultural norms and ideals of gender behavior also exert their influence. Brenton, in *The American Male*, says that society sets up rules for what it considers masculinity and femininity, but that human beings have an enormous range of possibilities in terms of traits and in the ability to play roles of all kinds. These possibilities are severely foreshortened by a too rigid process of sexual differentiation and a too narrow definition of masculinity and femininity. Here, for a moment, I should like to step into the role of social critic.

Perhaps few things have been quite so revealing of certain personality ideals today, including the masculine ideal, as the stereotyped activity that includes the reporting that surrounds our space flight launchings and reentries. The recent tragic deaths of three astronauts in their spacecraft, which burned, makes it difficult to touch on this. Yet the chiaroscuro of scientific brilliance in contrast with emotional and social infantilism has created, for me at any rate, a disturbing picture. Time does not permit me to quote, or trace out in detail, the pattern as I observed it, but there seem to be basically four modes of expression that include concepts of masculinity: 1) infantile horseplay, 2) pseudohumility and denial of individuality, 3) pseudoresponsiveness, and 4) extremes of chauvinism. The irony of the jest in which one of the astronauts of a previous flight placed a "No Exit" sign at the top exit from the launching pad to the spacecraft, for his departing buddies on the last Gemini flight, seems almost the work of some malevolent *deus ex machina*. The highly stylized behavior, of which this is not the best example, evoked the thought that I was watching an American version of the Japanese Kabuki theatre. This offers, perhaps, a somewhat more sharply etched picture of the young man R. R. Grinker[14] has defined as "homoclite"—the well-adapted young man in our society. At the same time, there exists another group within our society—the extremist adolescents—the beatniks and the mods. Here one observes the establishment of what I might call a gender-fused contraculture. Here tenacious male-female partnerships exist (calling to mind Harlow's mutually destructive interlocking monkeys) in which it is difficult to distinguish male from female, and there is obvious gleeful hostility directed at "outsiders" and at their puzzlement or annoyance. There have been fads in the past in which one sex has attempted to copy the other, but this has been the result of envy of some privilege. This seems the first time in which there appears denial of sex difference, associated with other indications of infantilism—a kind of return to pregender-identity times. R. Greenson[15] has commented on this tendency.

In considering factors relating to formation of the core gender it must be said that although gender identity encompasses cultural norms and socially determined styles, true certainty of gender is free of narcissistic preoccupation or compulsiveness and rigidity—it implies a sense of mastery and capacity for productiveness, for potency in either sex—the components of the genital character. It implies competence and pleasure in the preordained biologic functions.

I think I never found a meaningful concept of homosexual panic in terms of earlier formulations. Dr. Gershman's perception of it, as fear of dissolution of the self, rings true. He says that identity is necessary in order to experience, and for effective action. In this sense the person asks himself: "Who am I? How do I feel? How should I act?" If he cannot answer these questions, he is no longer a person. Sullivan[2] took note of this necessity for prescience in order to utilize effective processes in interpersonal action.

But on the question of the homosexual act of intercourse as a reparative process, I must take issue. That it can have releasing and pleasurable components, as in all sexual activity, there is no doubt. But I think that, if anything, it ultimately serves as a reminder of deficit. I think that compulsive heterosexuality—a kind of denial of the problem, as in Don Juanism or nymphomania—would better fit the picture of attempted reparative acts.

Dr. Gershman observes that some individuals show a disproportionate discrepancy between their global and gender identities —that is, they are generally less damaged than one might expect. I have found this to be true where the person possesses a specific talent that he or she has developed successfully, basing much of his self-concept and self-esteem on it, in compensatory fashion.

In regard to the loneliness of the homosexual, particularly in later years, this is not unique in him—it is shared by all those who have not succeeded by full maturity in staking out areas of social, as well as vocational, territory that encompass durable relationships; it is shared also by those who have been disrupted from such security by special circumstances. From a slightly different vantage point, true loneliness exists when the individual is aware that he has no significant affective ties to another human being and little prospect of developing them. But here is a place where one *could* view the homosexual act as a reparative effort—an attempt to bridge the loneliness and the isolation. Surprisingly, here Dr. Gershman sees it as an effort to maintain them both.

In any event, he underscores the poignancy of the threat to identity in the human condition—a threat that animals in the natural state fortunately do not share. I am sure we all feel enriched by Dr. Gershman's contribution to the understanding of some perversions and of the formation of gender identity.

### *REFERENCES*

1. Horney, K. *The Neurotic Personality of Our Time*. New York, Norton, 1937.
2. Sullivan, H. S. *Conceptions of Modern Psychiatry,* First Wm. Alanson White Memorial Lecture, Washington, D. C., Wm. Alanson White Psychiatric Foundation, 1946.
3. Erikson, E. H. Identity and the life cycle, *Psychol. Issues 1*:1-171, 1959.
4. Shainess, N. Feminine Identity and Mothering. In *Science and Psychoanalysis,* vol. 7. New York, Grune, Stratton, 1964, pp. 237-49.
5. Cohen, M. B. Personal identity and sexual identity, *Psychiatry, 29*:1-14, 1966.
6. Green, R. and Money, J. Stage-acting, role-taking and effeminate impersonation during boyhood, *Arch. Gen. Psychiat., 15*:535-39, 1966.
7. Guze, H. The Transsexual Phenomenon —Symposium at the Harry Benjamin

Foundation, January 16, 1967, New York. (Unpublished.)

8. Benjamin, H. The Transsexual Phenomenon—Symposium at the Harry Benjamin Foundation, January 16, 1967, New York. (Unpublished.)
9. Money, J. The Transsexual Phenomenon —Symposium at the Harry Benjamin Foundation, January 16, 1967, New York. (Unpublished.)
10. Thompson, C. Changing concepts of homosexuality in psychoanalysis, *Psychiatry 10*:2-13, 1947.

11*a*. Bieber, T. On treating male homosexuals, *Arch. Gen. Psychiat. 16*:60 63, 1967.

*b*. Bieber, I. *Homosexuality, A Psychoanalytic Study of Male Homosexuals,* New York, Basic Books, 1962.

12. Doorbar, R. The Transsexual Phenomenon—Symposium at the Harry Benjamin Foundation, January 16, 1967, New York. (Unpublished.)
13. Stoller, R. J. Conference on Sexual Problems, University of California School of Medicine, 1966. (Unpublished.)
14. Grinker, R. R. "Mentally healthy" young males (homoclites), *Arch. Psychiat. 6*:405-453, 1962.
15. Greenson, R. Lecture, Southern California Medical Society, reported in *Medical Tribune,* September 1965.
16. Brenton, M. *The American Male,* New York, Coward-McCann, 1966.

# DISCUSSION OF THE ARTICLE BY DR. HARRY GERSHMAN "THE EVOLUTION OF GENDER IDENTITY"*

Louis R. Hott

Medical Director, Karen Horney Clinic

Assistant Clinical Professor of Psychiatry
New York University Schools of Medicine

Senior Psychiatrist, Bellevue Hospital

New York, N. Y.

In "The Evolution of Gender Identity," Harry Gershman has presented a clear, logical paper on the understanding of the concept "masculine-feminine essence."

The familiar and important cry, "It's a boy" or "It's a girl" is well known to us. Before pregnancy and during pregnancy the parents are often asked, "What do you want–a boy or girl?"

The motivation for Dr. Gershman's paper can lead to a total concept of sexual identity as part of the core-gender-identity process. It also will lead to a fresh approach to the problems of emotional illness and of specific sexual difficulties. Further, as clinicians we can utilize and work with this core-gender-identity concept, which leads to healthy or unhealthy expression of sexuality in our patients.

Unfortunately, whenever we hear about the imprinting development, a feeling of permanency and hopelessness results in the apparent unchangeability of this indelibility. If imprinting is another expression of conditioning and even if it is self-reinforcing, it can be reversible, unconditionable, self-deenforcing, and unlearnable.

Gender cannot be neutral or indifferent in spite of an apparently unconscious wish fulfillment expressed in the neutrality of gender in some languages. The individual is faced with a decision of how much maleness or femaleness "have I, do I feel, and does society expect of me?" This decision cannot be avoided, and a choice, conscious or unconscious, must be made eventually.

Since the gender role is the essence of what is considered masculine

*Presented at a meeting of the Association for the Advancement of Psychoanalysis, New York, N. Y., held at The New York Academy of Medicine, February 15, 1967.

or feminine behavior, it is related to biological sex, but is shaped by cultural influences. First, there is the biological sex assigned to the infant. This is then influenced by culturally defined cues, which ultimately shape the gender identity to its assigned sex.[1]

Acculturation does occur with the passage of time, as in certain female gender role patterns that were previously traditional in Western civilization and have now changed. For example, the aggressive sexual, dominant female of the present may be contrasted with the passive female of the past. Thus changes occur in the pattern of relations between the male and the female.

We must also take into consideration the biological differences between the sexes and the variations in cultural reaction to these differences. Therefore we can understand the basic differences and similarities between men and women only in relation to the time-space continuum. Interaction between the body image of the anatomical-physiological being and his environment is the key to this problem. In our time it is possible that the male can now be passive and submissive and still be able to penetrate sexually; the female can be an aggressive and dominant recipient in coitus with very active female genitalia.

Although values placed on the birth of boys are greater in our society and greater freedom is given to them, there is a shifting equilibrium in our male-female relationships. Penis envy is not universal or organic. Envy of woman by men is now emerging as a cultural response. The clitoris has as good nerve endings as the penis, and the culturally underprivileged position that women previously held is now gone. As a result woman can respond as well or better orgastically, and evidence certainly indicates that penis envy or clitoris inferiority is culturally and neurotically induced.

The evolution of gender identity develops from standards of gender role and gender typing that exist. In other words, behavior is matched to internal and external standards and there is a drive to conform to it.

The standards of the child are made up of a cluster of attitudes, wishes, feelings, and values identified with models (such as parents), who possess this cluster. A child desires acceptance and yearns to possess these same traits. By adopting the parental standards he hopes to prevent social rejection.[2]

The standards of gender role thus dictate the adoption of a different response by boys and girls. The response becomes a learned association between selected attributes, behavior, and attitudes on the one hand, and the concepts male and female on the other that are culturally approved characteristics of males and females.

The standards of gender role are publicly shared beliefs of male and female characteristics. The individual's concept of his own degree of masculinity or femininity is idealized and may differ from the cultural view.

Thus, the degree to which an individual regards and feels himself masculine or feminine, consciously or unconsciously, is his gender role identification that is part of his total identity. The gender type is the characteristic of male and female in physical, behavioral, and emotional attitudes that are present consciously or unconsciously.

By the age of three years, the child first realizes that boys and girls are different. The healthy central identity of gender role is established in the child by perception of similarities to parental models of the same sex with whom he identifies consciously or unconsciously as well as by his acquisition of attributes and skills of his sex, reinforced by his peer relations.[2]

Sometimes a child resents the behavior that is assigned to him because of his biological sex and feels anxiety over it, with the result that inner neurotic conflicts lead to sexual disorders. Often I have seen maternal dominance over a passive father with maternal rejection of the child that leads to schizophrenia in a male child and also to sexual difficulties. I suspect that this may be present in many transsexual males. I saw this problem in a man referred to our clinic who had had an operation for change of sex. He had been married previously and had two children. He related his unhappiness to his feeling that he belonged to the female sex. He wished to live as a female and he considered his sex organs as disturbing deformities, which he succeeded in having removed.

Although he still insisted that he was satisfied with his new-found sex, he attempted suicide. His self-hatred, compartmentalization, and concreteness still existed. His attempted solution–externalization of the problem to his genitalia–did not suffice. In these cases schizophrenia is probable. The ability to split off gender identity from total identity is part of the schizophrenic process, I believe. In his recent book, *The Transsexual Phenomenon*, Benjamin expresses the belief that true transsexuals cannot be changed by psychotherapy; he recommends surgical and hormonal treatment.[3] This may be a further sign of resignation on the part of the patient and doctor as well.

It would be important if we could predict the behavior of a child with respect to his gender role. This would require the degree of identification with the model of the same sex, as well as the gender role behavior displayed by the model, and the patterns of reward issued by that model. Additional influences such as the rate of physical maturation, the sexual attractiveness of the developing being, and the social class and its sexual attitudes are also important.

The significance of a child's gender role identity relates to psychological problems of stability of behavior in time, differential mastery of academic skills, sexuality, and behavior with love objects.

As a result of unhealthy relations between parent and child and a fragile gender role identity, fear of interaction with the opposite sex may arise. Anxiety over failure to attain behavior appropriate to the gender type can lead to homosexuality.

The homosexual does suffer from a lesion in basic gender identity. One male patient felt himself less of a man rather than more of a woman. Therefore he attempted to live vicariously through a male partner; he magically sought a mirror image in order to attempt to restore his failing masculine identity.

A homosexual patient who has a similar conflict had a dream wherein he was having fellatio with someone he had not seen since childhood. Pus came out of his partner's penis; he found it "distasteful" and he awoke. His association with his childhood friend was one of idealized masculinity. His distaste was associated with his inability to accept masculinity.

He spent his first two years in an orphan asylum. Then he was brought up in a female household, which consisted of his mother and sister. When the patient was six months old his father was killed while robbing a store with a gun. While a child, the patient consciously desired to be a girl. Later he wished to be a male but felt compelled to seek out men with large penises in order to live vicariously through them. He was trying to reestablish his maleness in order to relate to females again.

The child at three divides the world into male and female. At six it molds its behavior in concordance with cultural standards appropriate to his biological sex and will feel anxiety if it cannot accomplish this. Conflicts are generated because of anxiety over deviation from standards of gender role. Once learned, these standards are not easily altered, but modification is possible during early school years and by society and psychoanalytic help later in life.

As clinical psychoanalysts we want to know the critical periods of this development. The critical early period of sensitivity to experiences will determine the direction of social, intellectual, and emotional development.[4]

In 1935 Lorenz emphasized the importance of critical periods of the formation of primary social bonds in birds; the process is called imprinting.[5] McGraw later demonstrated critical periods in the infant.[6] Critical periods in the child are for learning, infantile stimulation, and formation of primary social bonds by human contact.

Anxiety increases the strength of imprinting by emotional arousal. The importance of basic anxiety in neurosis and healthy growth is well established.[7]

The critical period for primary socialization in the infant is shown by its visual investigation and smiling response, in interaction with the supporting and nurturing mother. This contact and emotional arousal results in social attachment. Prolonged basic anxiety prevents healthy attachment. By lessening the anxiety, the critical period can be lengthened and hope for increased development is possible.

This primary socialization or imprinting is also modified by later development. Formation of social attachments through contact and emotional arousal is a life-long process. There are also critical periods for stimulation. Animals handled early show earlier maturation of adrenocortical responses to stress, with reduction of fear through familiarity of the handler. However, too much stimulation can lead to traumatic emotional experiences.

Some crucial points can now be made. The total character structure develops first and ultimately determines the primary core gender identity and the secondary identity with expressions of its sexuality.

A healthy climate in the home leads to greater acceptance of the gender role by the child.

The type and quality of response of the mother and other important caretakers of the infant to its requests and to stimuli of crying or smiling help in forming healthier identities in that infant.

The extension of basic anixety interferes with this development.

Sexual disturbance is produced in the individual by the early attitude of parents who lack respect for him as an insecure and helpless infant.

As a result, he will feel alienated from himself, from his true core gender identity, and from the rest of the human race.

On the other hand, the maturing gender identification will lead to the maturer relationship of sexual love, which leads to the healthier way of life in family and society, as Dr. Gershman has shown.

*REFERENCES*

1. Marmor, J. Changing feminine "gender-role" undermines Freudian theories, *Frontiers Clin. Psychiat. 4* (3):6-8, 1967.
2. Hoffman, M. L. and Hoffman, L. W. *Review of Child Development Research,* vol. 1. New York, Russel Sage Foundation, 1964.
3. Benjamin, H. *The Transsexual Phenomenon.* New York, Julian, 1966.
4. Scott, J. P. Critical periods in behavioral development, *Science 138*:949-57, 1962.
5. Lorenz, K. *J. Ornithol. 83*:137, 289, 1935.
6. McGraw, M. B. *Manual of Child Psychology.* New York, Wiley, 1946, pp. 332-69.
7. Horney, K. *Neurosis and Human Growth.* New York, Norton, 1950.

# OSLER'S TEXTBOOK REVISITED

Drs. Abner McG. Harvey and Victor A. McKusick, both of the Department of Medicine at Johns Hopkins, have had the excellent idea of "revisiting" Osler's textbook.* More specifically, they have reprinted 24 sections of the original and have engaged 17 eminent contemporaries to contribute comments. Whereas Osler's sections on typhoid fever, lobar pneumonia, syphilis, and rheumatic fever are represented by single commentaries, his sections on arthritis deformans, chronic rheumatism, and muscular rheumatism are discussed by Dr. William D. Robinson under the larger rubric of rheumatoid arthritis. Similarly Dr. Maurice B. Strauss has provided a discussion of renal disease that covers five separate sections in Osler. Although Osler's first edition was published in 1892, the editors have chosen the seventh edition (1909) as the basis of study, since this was the last edition that Osler wrote unaided and, in the editors' opinion, represents the apogee. The individual commentators were charged with the duty of judging Osler's presentation and of examining the developments that have occurred since his time. The value of the new book is amplified by 12 pages of introductory matter, which describe the genesis of the first edition and give some indication of the influence that successive editions have exerted. The familiar and surprising story of the Rev. Frederick T. Gates and Mr. John D. Rockefeller is recounted anew from Harvey Cushing's biography.

The individual commentators vary in the temporal scope of their remarks. While some have chosen to confine themselves to post-Oslerian developments, others have taken the pains to examine the emergence of the knowledge that Osler himself had available when he sat down to his task. This is notably true of Dr. Robert Austrian's remarks on pneumonia.

On every hand the reader finds evidence of the experienced insight provided by the commentators. For example, Dr. Thomas B. Turner discusses some fundamental biological implications of syphilis, and Dr. William B. Bean, in discussing beriberi, points out the intellectual problem of negative causes, so strikingly exemplified by the avitaminoses.

*Harvey, A. McG. and McKusick, V. A., eds.; *Osler's Textbook Revisited; Reprint of Selected Sections with Commentaries.* New York, Appleton-Century-Crofts, 1967, 361 pp. $6.75.

The comments on renal disease appropriately stress post-Oslerian advances in physiology. The comments on disease of the suprarenal glands are brief and thrilling.

If the Oslerian texts and the new comments are summated, what we have is the material for both a historical study and a picture or a novel. The historian would unquestionably seek to discover the reasons for the medical efflorescence that occurred during and after Osler's time. The painter or the novelist might well depict the plight of the physician, who stood naked and empty-handed in the presence of innumerable diseases that he could recognize and fear but that he was utterly powerless to arrest.

It is also true that we are not done with the osleriolatry that marks the well-intentioned beginner in medical history and also characterizes the nonhistorian who hazards an incursion into earlier eras of medical thought. Throughout the present volume Osler is sometimes explained and usually praised but is almost never criticized. Physicians are temperamentally conservative and averse to heresy. Yet the gods must come to judgment no less than men.

While the editors advert to the American medical textbooks written by Bartholow, Palmer, and Loomis, and while they mention the treatises of Sir Thomas Watson and John S. Bristowe, they do not even mention the ample books of Hughes Bennett and Hilton Fagge, nor do they venture to point out that some of Fagge's descriptions of disease outdo Osler by a large margin. Nor is there a word about Trousseau or about any German writer. Are our local divinities to be set up in place of Jehovah?

S. J.

# Maybe you don't want your patients to halve Hygroton®.
chlorthalidone

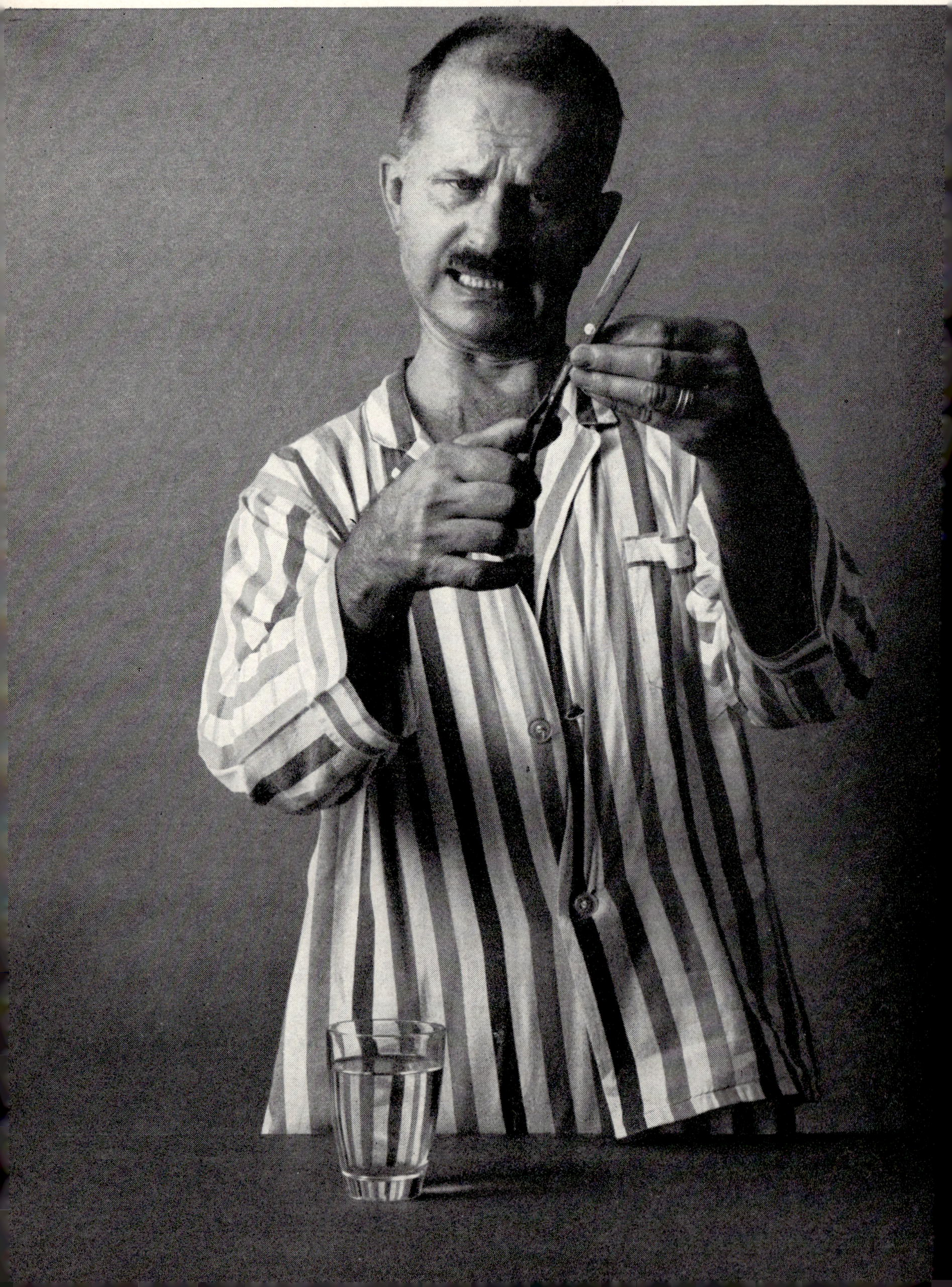

# BULLETIN OF THE NEW YORK ACADEMY OF MEDICINE

VOL. 43, NO. 12 DECEMBER 1967


*New York Heart Association*

## *CONFERENCE ON MECHANISMS AND MANAGEMENT OF ARRHYTHMIAS*

*Held at the Hotel Waldorf-Astoria*
*New York, N. Y., January 24, 1967*

### *Foreword*

In recent years knowledge of the complex relations between the electrophysiology of the heart and the neurophysiological control that determines normal cardiac rhythmicity has developed at an accelerated pace. This growth in knowledge has resulted in increased understanding of normal physiological mechanisms, hence has also widened the possibilities of electrophysiological control by both electrical and pharmacological agents.

In the light of these newer developments, the New York Heart Association organized this year's clinical conference around the topic of Mechanisms and Management of Cardiac Arrhythmias. In considering content the Program Committee decided to put emphasis on the more general aspects of this subject—questions of anatomy, new discoveries in physiology, disturbances of the electrolytes and, most of all, the influence of the nervous system on arrhythmias, which is not well known and, as you will note, is remarkable.

Experience has shown that early recognition of arrhythmias and the institution of immediate treatment have reduced their progression into more severe forms and have lowered the mortality rate.

Today's speakers, who are from many parts of the country, were chosen because of their work in this field. It is our hope that the presentations will have been informative and will have increased the practicing physician's understanding of the difficulties that he experiences in the management of his patients.

*CONFERENCE PLANNING COMMITTEE*

Dr. Brian F. Hoffman
Dr. Charles E. Kossmann } *Cochairmen*

Dr. M. Irené Ferrer
Dr. Herbert Kayden
Dr. Thomas Killip, III
Dr. David Scherf
Dr. Gerard M. Turino

# CARDIAC INNERVATION: ANATOMIC AND PHARMACOLOGIC RELATIONS*

THOMAS N. JAMES

Chairman
Section on Cardiovascular Research
Henry Ford Hospital, Detroit, Mich.

ALTHOUGH it is now generally conceded that the formation and conduction of impulses in the heart occur within specialized myocardial cells, the function of these cells is profoundly influenced by the nerves of the heart. Among the many recent advances in our knowledge of cardiac electrophysiology, those obtained through electron microscopy and through intracellular microelectrode recording have notably altered old concepts. Knowing that the myocardium is composed of individual cells rather than an anatomic syncytium, for example, will have influences on electrocardiographic concepts that are only beginning to become apparent. Knowing what factors influence the action potential of membranes of single cells in specific areas of the heart inevitably helps us understand how these areas function. Ultimately we must learn which components within the cell are responsible for its electrical activity, and which components of the cell membranes participate in the formation and conduction of impulses.

Along with this essential tendency to think smaller and smaller, however, we must not forget that pacemaking in the normal heart is a far more complex operation than what can be learned from the appearance or function of a single cell. The sinus node is composed of many cells of a variety of types, including nerves, and its optimal function depends on proper synchronization of electrical discharge (simultaneously or in proper sequence) by the cells capable of spontaneous electrical activity. Furthermore, this activity must be collated with the needs of the body in terms of heart rate. Such needs are signaled by the cardiac innervation, which is the heart's principal means of rapid communication with extracardiac control centers such as the carotid body and the brain. The same considerations apply to the cells of the

*Presented at the *Conference on Mechanisms and Management of Arrhythmias,* held by the New York Heart Association at the Hotel Waldorf-Astoria, New York, N. Y., January 24, 1967.

This investigation was supported in part by a Public Health Service Research Grant from the National Heart Institute and by a grant from the Michigan Heart Association.

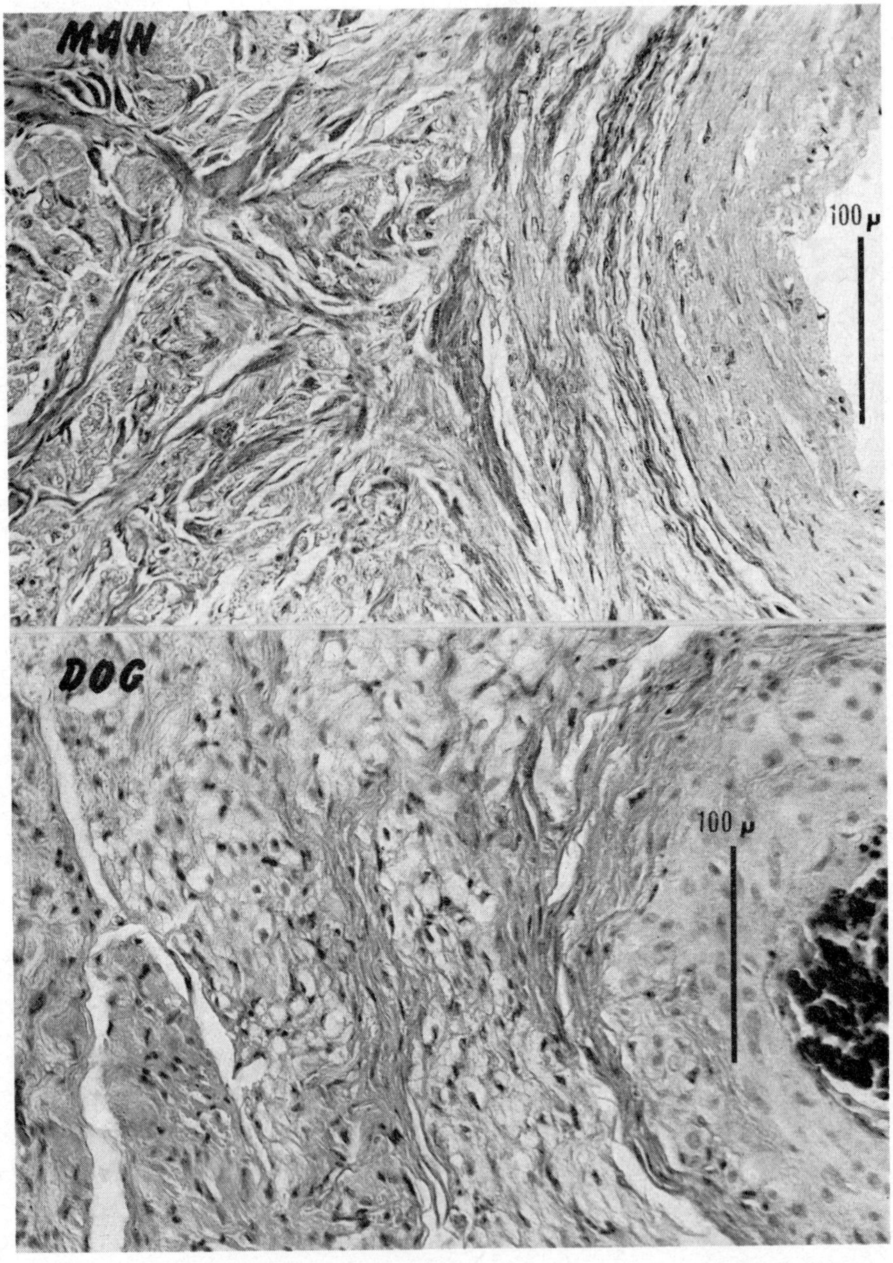


Fig. 1. These photomicrographs demonstrate the similar structure of the sinus node in man and the dog. The sinus node artery is to the right in each. This and Figures 2, 3, and 6 are from a published study[12] and are reproduced by permission of the American Heart Association.

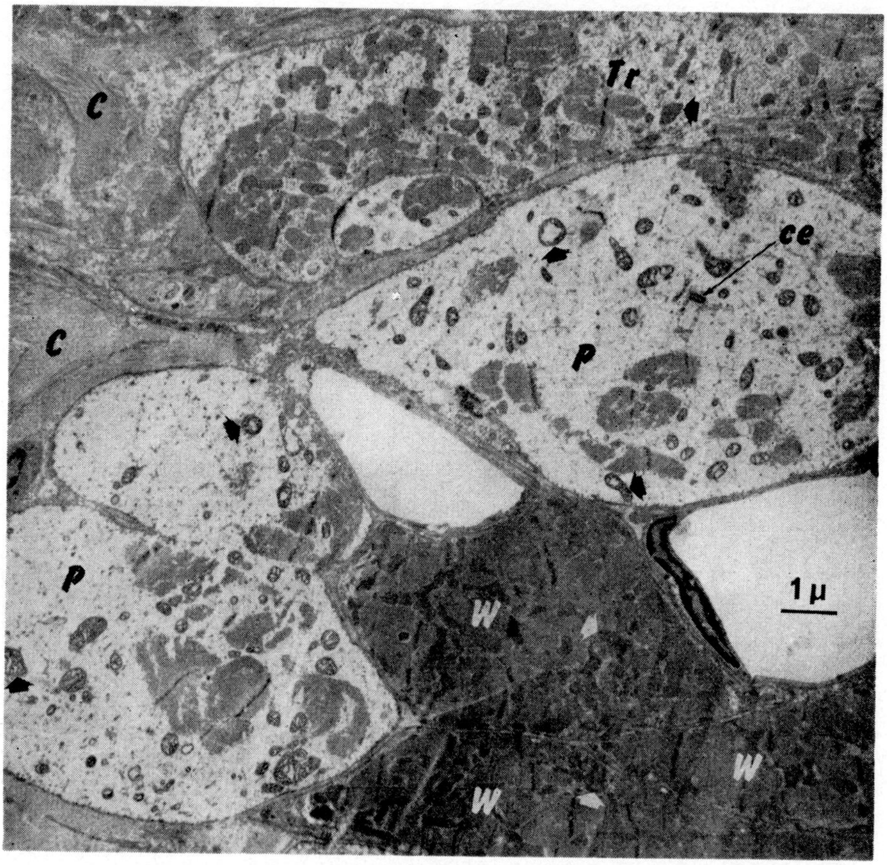


Fig. 2. This electron micrograph of canine sinus node was prepared from tissue obtained with *in vivo* fixation by direct perfusion of the node with glutaraldehyde. Characteristics of the three types of cell are discussed in the text: *P* is for P cell, *Tr* for transitional or intermediate cells, and *W* is for ordinary working myocardial cells. *C* indicates collagen and *Ce* a centriole. The small black arrows point to sarcosomes of the P cells and one in a transitional cell, while the white arrows indicate working cell sarcosomes. See also Figure 4.

atrioventricular (AV) node, the bundle of His, and Purkinje fibers.

Since the subject of this conference is arrhythmias, my presentation will deal with anatomic and pharmacologic aspects of cardiac innervation relative to the sinus node, the AV node, and the bundle of His. Other important aspects of neural control of the heart and vessels have been included in a number of recent reviews.[1-7] Gross anatomic features of cardiac innervation are familiar to most investigators and are clearly presented in standard textbooks of anatomy. For the sake of simplifying my presentation, the neural anatomy (histologic) of the cardiac con-

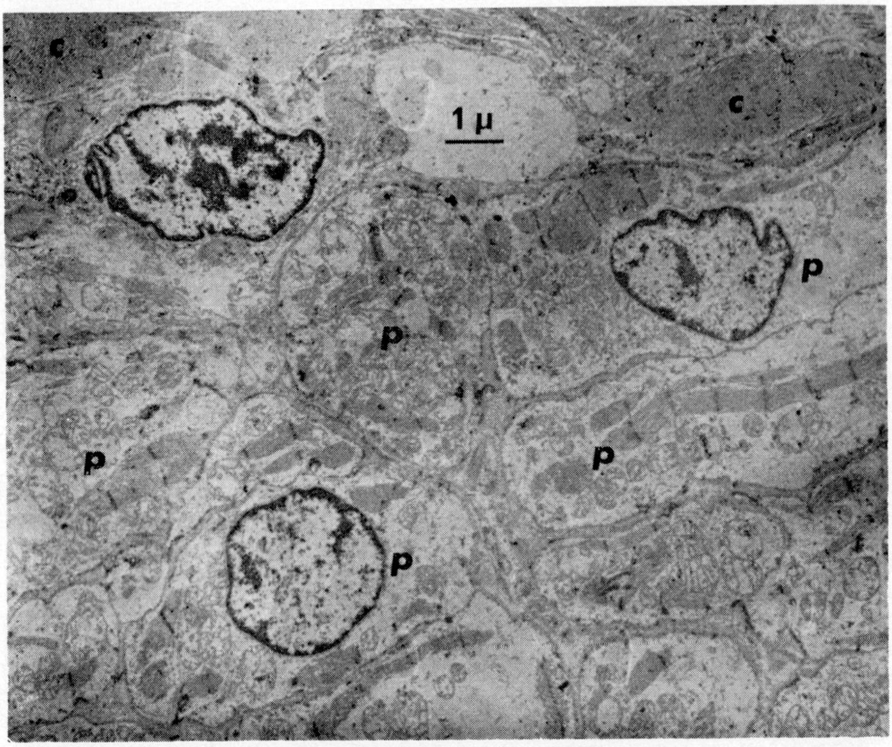


Fig. 3. This electron micrograph demonstrates that the human sinus node is similar to that of the dog at the ultrastructural level. The sarcosomes and nuclear chromatin are not as well preserved, since the specimen was obtained postmortem rather than *in vivo*, but the membranes and the intracellular organization as well as the intercellular relationships are well preserved. Abbreviations are the same as in Figure 2.

duction system will be considered first, and then its neuropharmacology. Each discussion will be governed by its pertinence to the mechanisms and management of cardiac arrhythmias.

## Neural Anatomy of the Cardiac Conduction System

Here and in subsequent sections the principal discussion will center on observations in human and canine hearts; in the human because, for the physician, that is where the ultimate questions in biology are, and in the dog because the pharmacologic experimental studies in my laboratory have been made in this animal. The other animal used frequently by others in cardiac electrophysiologic studies is the rabbit, and comparative anatomic features will be included for the leporine heart.

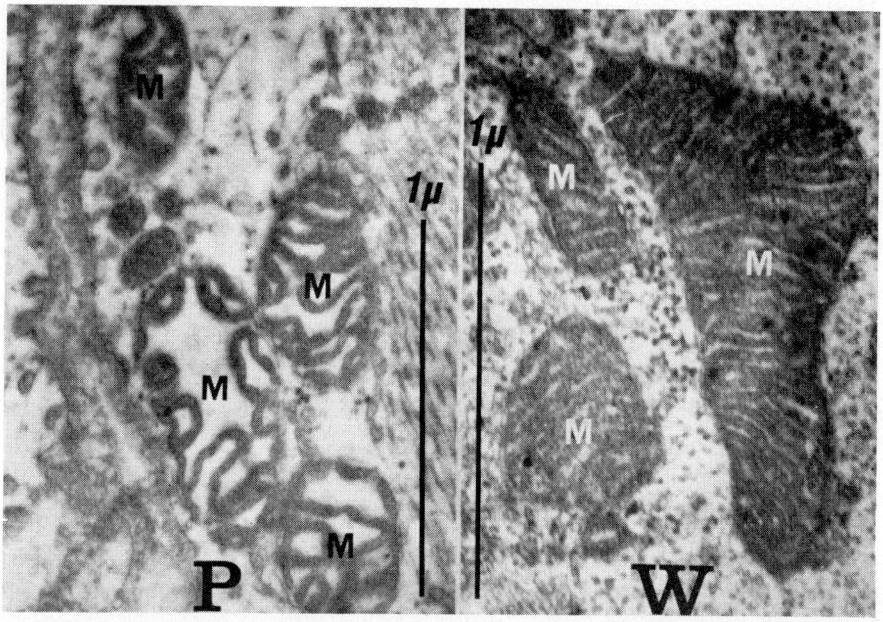


Fig. 4. This contrasts the simple structure of P cell sarcosomes (*M* on the left) with the more complex structure of working myocardial cells on the right. These specimens were obtained from the same heart at the same time in the same way, by *in vivo* glutaraldehyde perfusion of the canine sinus node.

*The sinus node.* The sinus node (Figure 1) is located less than a millimeter beneath the epicardium in the sulcus terminalis at the junction of the superior vena cava and right atrium. It is near the anterior margin of the atriocaval junction in man,[8] slightly more posterior than this in the dog,[9] and still further back in the rabbit,[10] where it is located approximately midway between the superior and inferior venae cavae. In man and the dog the node is organized about a conspicuously large central artery, which is not the case in either leporine or bovine hearts.[11] In human,[12] canine,[12, 13] leporine,[14, 15] and bovine[16] hearts the sinus node contains three types of cells that organize as bundles of intertwining fibers within a collagen matrix. Fibers of the sinus node under the light microscope resemble ordinary myocardium but are of smaller diameter and stain paler with all conventional dyes. Details of the individual cells are best defined with the electron microscope (Figures 2 and 3). The characteristic cell of the sinus node is the P cell,[12] which is rounded or spherical and contains relatively few myofibrils (containing few myofilaments) distributed randomly within the cell. Sarcosomes in the

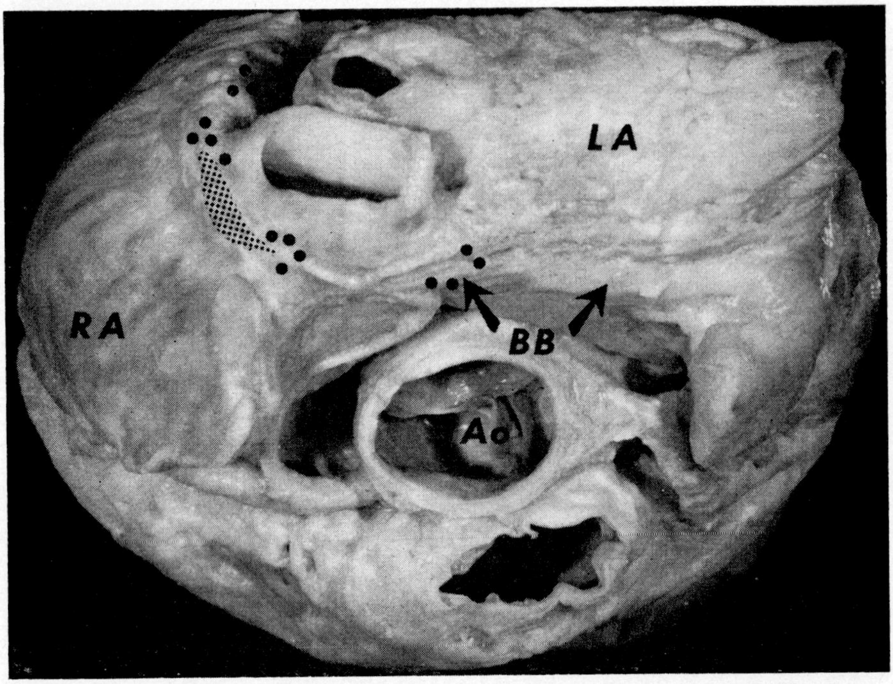


Fig. 5. In this photograph of a dissected human heart the locations of ganglia in the region of the sinus node (stippled area) are shown with dots. In addition to those at the margins of the node, two other groups are shown: those in the middle internodal tracts at the crest of the atrial septum, and those in the anterior internodal tracts below Bachmann's bundle. See also Figures 14 and 16. *LA* is left atrium; *RA* right atrium; *Ao* aorta; and *BB* with the arrows indicates Bachmann's bundle (the anterior interatrial myocardial band).

P cell are simpler than those in working myocardial cells (Figure 4) and, like the myofibrils, are distributed randomly in the P cell; there is no sandwiching arrayal between myofibrils as is characteristic of working myocardial cells. The sarcoplasmic reticulum of P cells is sparse and poorly developed. Each P cell is bound by a plasma membrane, and groups of these cells are enveloped together by a basement membrane. Between contiguous P cells there are no intercalated discs but there are scattered desmosomelike thickenings of apposing plasma membranes. No nexus formations or "tight junctions"[17] have been reported in P cells. Their cytoplasm is remarkably clear and contains surprisingly little glycogen in comparison to abundant glycogen in adjacent cells fixed the same way in the same heart at the same time. There is active pinocytosis in the plasma membranes of the P cells.

The other two types of cell observed in the sinus node are ordinary

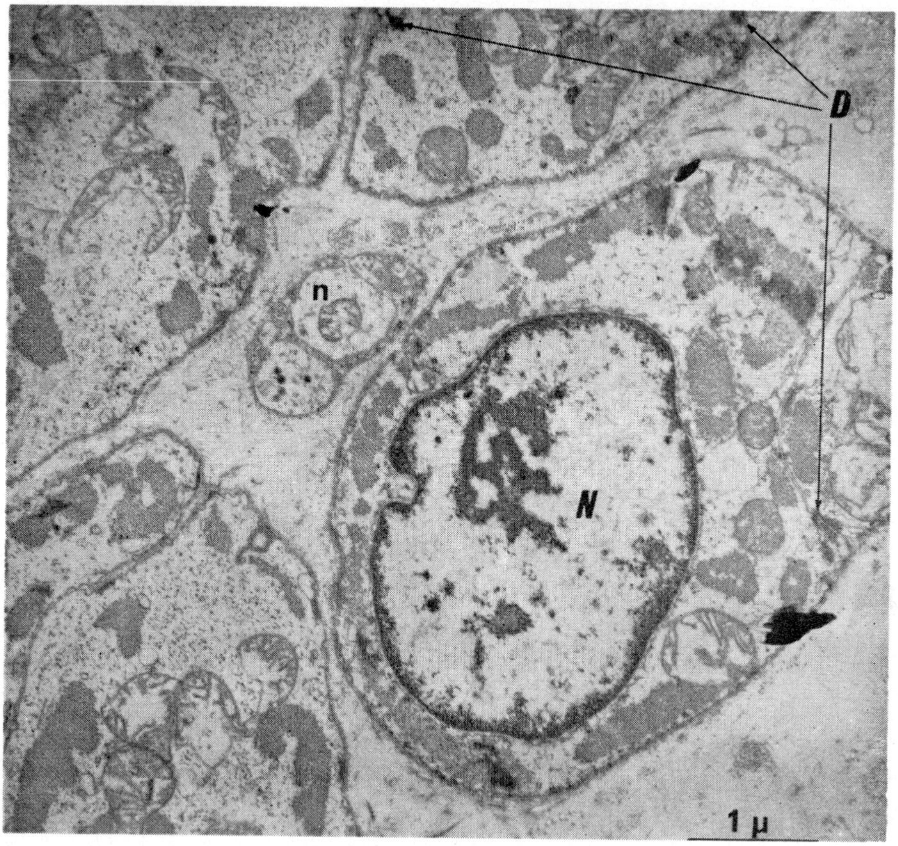


Fig. 6. In this electron micrograph the relation between a nerve terminal (*n*) and cells of the canine sinus node is shown. *D* and the arrows indicate three desmosomes. *N* overlies a nucleus. Active pinocytosis is visible in the cell membranes.

working myocardial cells, which are in highest concentration near the margins of the node but occur even in some central locations, and a transitional cell that has internal structure intermediate between that of the P cell and the working cell. The transitional cell also serves as the only connection between the other two types of cell; no P cells are observed connected directly to working myocardial cells.

Nerves and ganglia are abundant in the region of the sinus node (Figure 5). With very rare exceptions there are no ganglion cells within the node; these cells are distributed almost exclusively at its anterior and posterior margins in the sulcus terminalis or along its caval (not atrial) margin. The nerves within the sinus node, as elsewhere in the myocardium, do *not* terminate directly on the cell membrane but

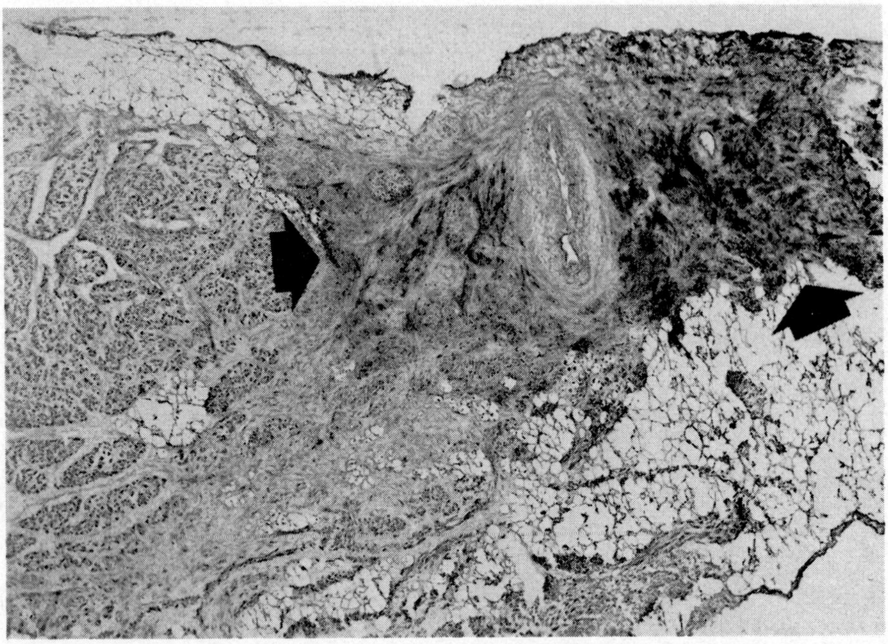

Fig. 7. Cholinesterase in the human sinus node (between arrows) stains in heavy contrast to that in neighboring atrial myocardium. Note absence of cholinesterase in the smooth muscle of the sinus node artery. Epicardium is above and the superior vena cava is to the right (×30).

at some distance (electron microscopically) from it (Figure 6). This is a significant difference from the situation in skeletal muscle, where nerve endings are not only directly on the membrane but have a special structure. Both the observations on nerve endings and on the question of nexus formation must be qualified, however, by the possibility that further studies may in time reveal different findings. What can be said on the basis of present evidence is that such structures, if they exist, are rare. Functionally this point is of considerable importance, since one must conclude on the basis of present observations that the effects of neurotransmitter substances begin after diffusion across a finite space to reach the myocardial cell surface.

Indirect evidence of the cholinergic innervation of the sinus node may be obtained with stains for cholinesterase.[18, 19] In the human heart cholinesterase is abundant within the sinus node, which stains as a dark island sharply contrasting with its surrounding atrial myocardium (Figure 7). Another striking contrast is the absence of cholinesterase

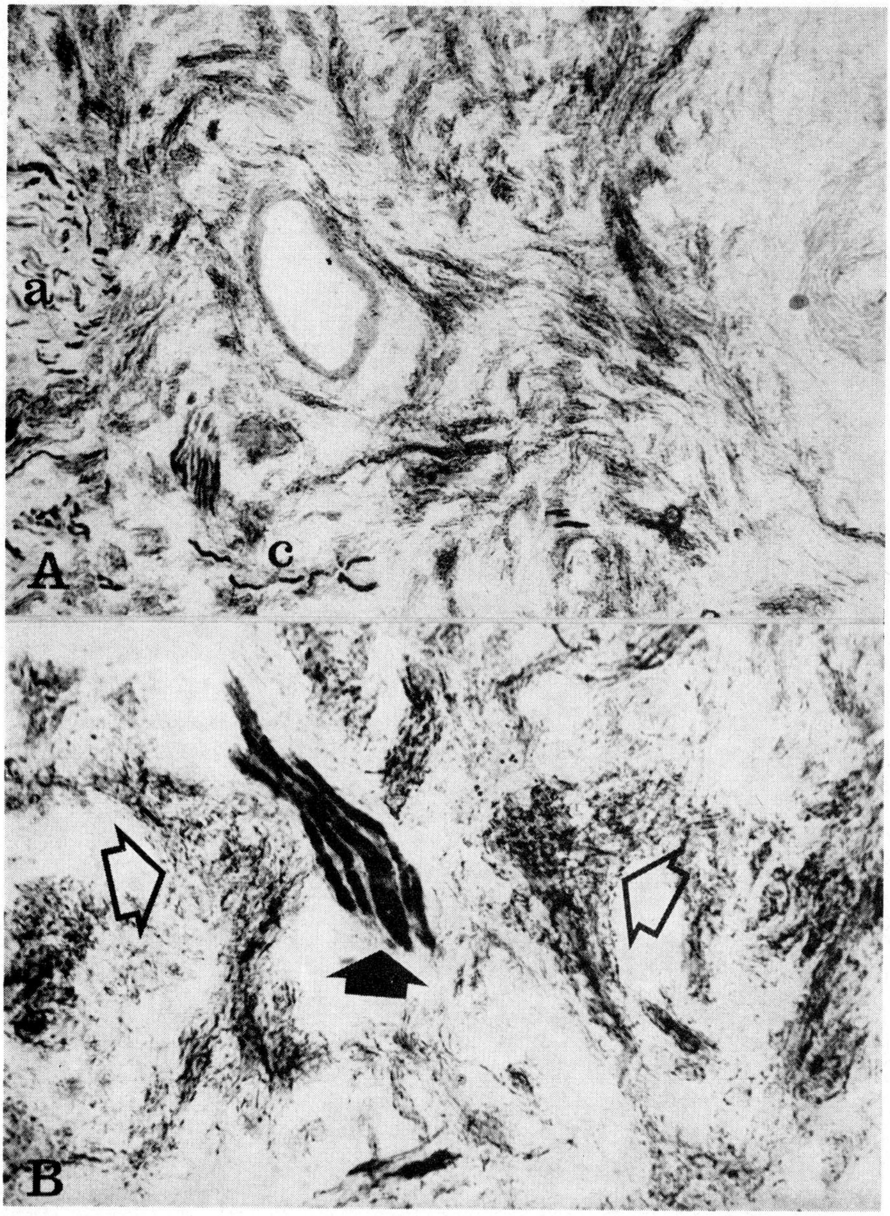


Fig. 8. The distribution of cholinesterase within the cells of the human sinus node is shown here. That associated with myofibrils is most easily identified at this magnification. In *A* (×175) the difference in staining depth of adrenergic nerves (*a*) and cholinergic nerves (*c*) is apparent, the latter being much darker. In *B* (×450) the open arrows indicate P cells, with the randomly distributed myofibrils clearly shown, and the black arrow indicates a cholinergic nerve.

in the smooth muscle of the centrally located sinus node artery. Cholinesterase is distributed within all three types of cell in the sinus node and there is no detectable difference in cellular concentration. Intracellular cholinesterase is readily identifiable in the randomly distributed myofibrils of P cells as well as the parallel myofibrils of other cells (Figure 8). It also occurs in a number of other intracellular organelles; more specific identification of it was not possible with the light microscope. Nerve endings within the sinus node stained either very deeply (much more than the myocardial cells), or approximately to the same intensity. Koelle[20] suggests that such difference in the depth of cholinesterase staining may be a useful means for anatomic differentiation of adrenergic (light staining) and cholinergic (deep staining) nerve terminals. Since there is such a large number of different enzymes concerned with norepinephrine degradation *in vivo*, it may not be possible to utilize histochemical methods to identify adrenergic nerve endings as reliably as cholinergic ones, although recent observations by Muller and Pearse[21] give some promise in this direction.

*The AV node and the bundle of His.* In man[22] and the dog[23] the AV node is located less than a millimeter beneath the right atrial endocardium just anterior to the coronary sinus ostium and just above the insertion of the septal leaflet of the tricuspid valve. In the rabbit the AV node is considerably displaced anteriorly by an especially large coronary sinus present because the rabbit normally has a left superior vena cava.[10] If one accepts Patten's theory[24] on embryologic origin of the AV node (that it began its existence at the junction of the primitive left anterior cardinal vein with the sinus venosus and later migrated into the junction of interatrial and interventricular septa with the dorsal endocardial cushion as the sinus venosus is absorbed into the adult atria), then persistence of the left superior vena cava in the rabbit instead of its attrition into an oblique vein of Marshall, as in man and the dog, may indicate a more primitive condition for the AV node in the rabbit.

In contrast to the sinus node, the AV node is not organized about a central artery, although one is sometimes seen within it. There is much less collagen within the AV node than the sinus node. The cells of the AV node are composed into interweaving fibers that mingle both singly and in bundles (Figure 9). The fibers are slightly thicker than those of the sinus node. The AV node has a convex surface directed

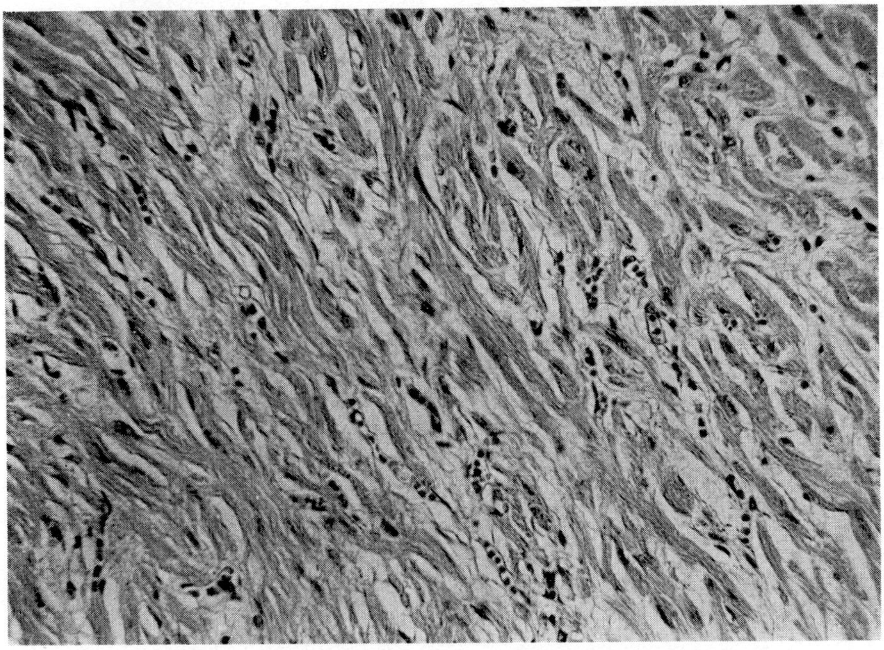

Fig. 9. This photomicrograph demonstrates the cellular structure of the human AV node (×325). Compare with Figure 1, which shows the sinus node, and Figures 12, 13, and 15, which show other aspects of the AV node.

toward the right atrium and a concave surface that rests on the mitral annulus or central fibrous body. At its anterior inferior margin the fibers of the AV node begin to interweave less and orient more longitudinally as they converge to form the bundle of His, which veers centrally into the central fibrous body and then down along the posterior and inferior margin of the membranous interventricular septum. The longitudinally oriented fibers within the bundle vary a great deal in diameter, some being as large as typical Purkinje cells and others as small as fibers of the AV node. Such variation is principally in different hearts, since in a given heart the fibers of the bundle of His tend to be of uniform diameter. In either case these fibers course in groups about which there is a dense collagen sheath; they compartment the bundle of His into many separate smaller bundles (Figure 10). There is furthermore a delicate single septation about many of the individual fibers within these smaller bundles (Figure 11). The possible electrophysiologic significance of such anatomic compartmentalization has been recently reviewed relatively to several old questions in clinical electro-

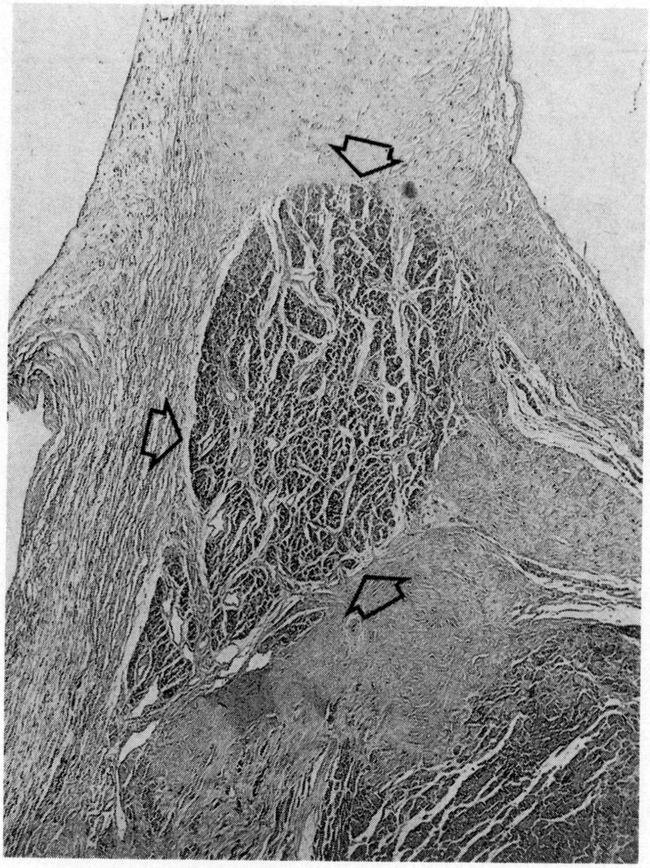

Fig. 10. This low power (×45) photomicrograph shows the collagenous partitioning of the normal human AV (His) bundle, which is bracketed by the three arrows. The tricuspid valve is visible at the left, the central fibrous body above and the interventricular septum below. This and Figure 11 are reproduced from the *Henry Ford Hospital Medical Bulletin*[25] with permission.

cardiography,[25] including the genesis of the ventricular preexcitation (Wolff-Parkinson-White) syndrome.

Shortly after the bundle of His emerges from the inferior margin of the central fibrous body to reach the crest of the ventricular septum, it divides into right and left bundle branches. There is considerable variation in the relative position of the slender right branch of the bundle in the course of this division, but the left bundle system is always a wide sheet of fibers that receives most of the substance of the undivided common bundle. One may accurately think of the bundle of His and its left branch of the bundle as a single continuum from

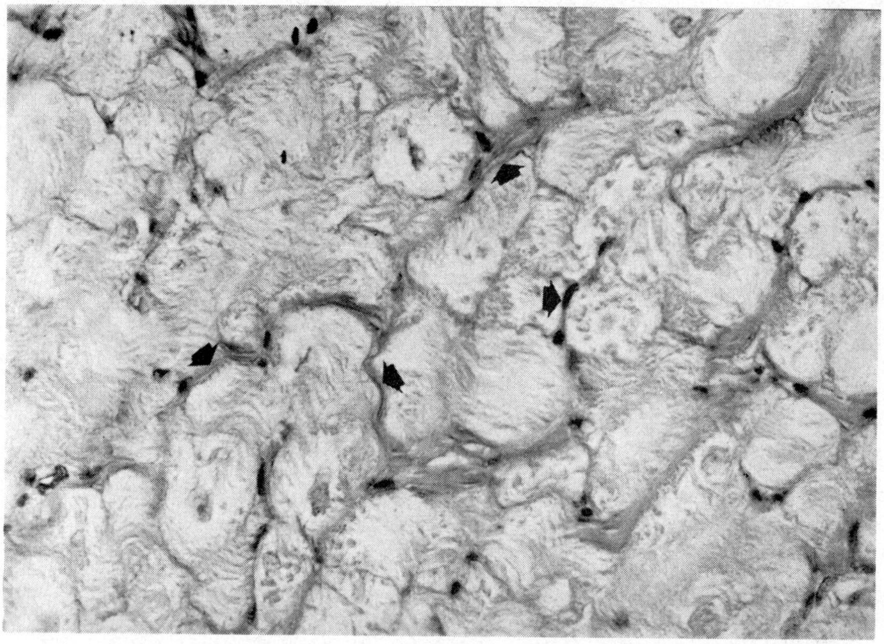

Fig. 11. This is a section of canine bundle of His (×1275) demonstrating fine collagen septa, some indicated by short black arrows, separating single and small groups of fibers. The same arrangement exists in the human bundle of His.

which the right branch of the bundle is a small and variably placed division.

From preliminary examination of the human AV node and its neighboring structures with the electron microscope, and based on similar examinations by others in the dog,[13] rabbit,[14] and cow,[16] it bears many similarities to and some differences from the sinus node. There are P cells in the AV node but not in as great concentration as in the sinus node (Figure 12). Their internal structure and relation to transitional and working myocardial cells are similar to those in the sinus node. Cells in the bundle of His and the branches of it that appear under the light microscope as a large perinuclear clear zone of "Purkinje fibers" resemble rather large P cells, and they may function in the same way as those in the sinus node, viz., as pacemaking sites. Whether the sarcosomes in these cells have the unique appearance characteristic of those in the sinus node is not yet certain.

Just as in the sinus node, the AV node does not normally contain ganglia but is richly innervated. The ganglia near the AV node are

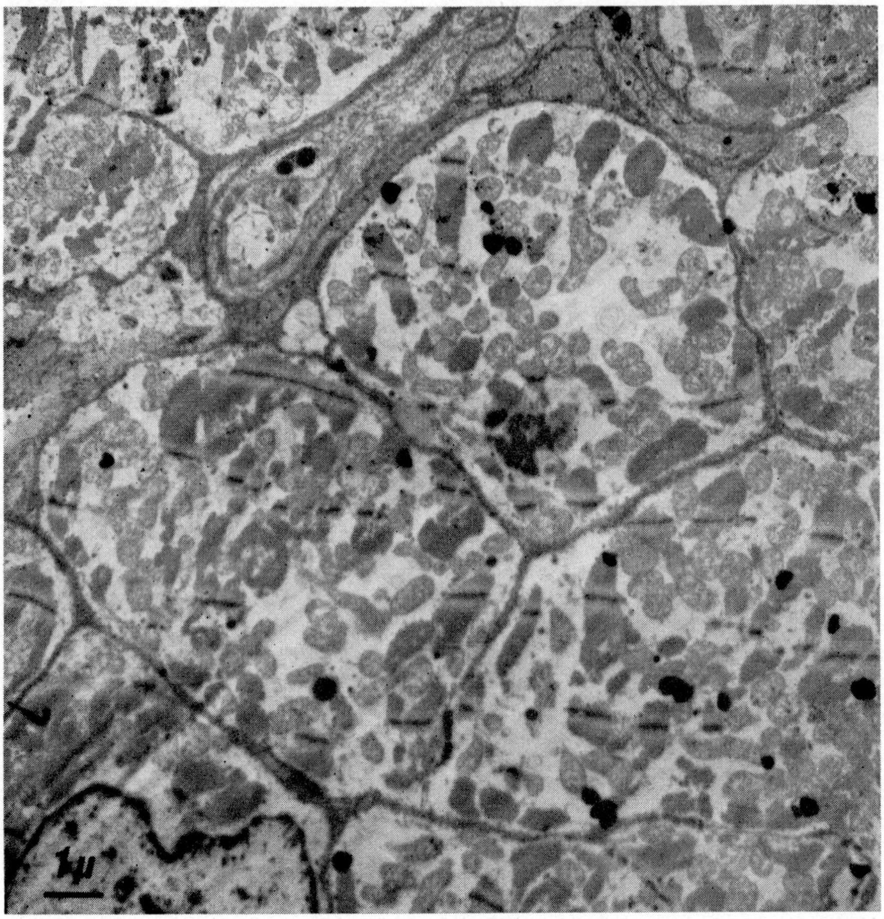


Fig. 12. This electron micrograph of human AV node demonstrates a cluster of P cells similar to those present in the sinus node (Figure 3). The densest small black bodies are artefacts.

concentrated at its posterior margin, lying between it and the anterior wall of the coronary sinus.[22, 23] It is of considerable physiologic significance that this is the exact region demonstrated by Juhasz-Nagy and Szentivanyi[26] to be of such importance in the von Bezold-Jarisch reflex. Nerves in the AV node or the bundle of His are so fine in man and the dog that they are difficult to identify without special staining; in the rabbit, on the other hand, relatively large and easily identified nerves course through the AV node and the bundle of His.

Cholinesterase (Figure 13) is heavily concentrated within the AV node and the bundle of His[18, 19] as it is in the sinus node. The intra-

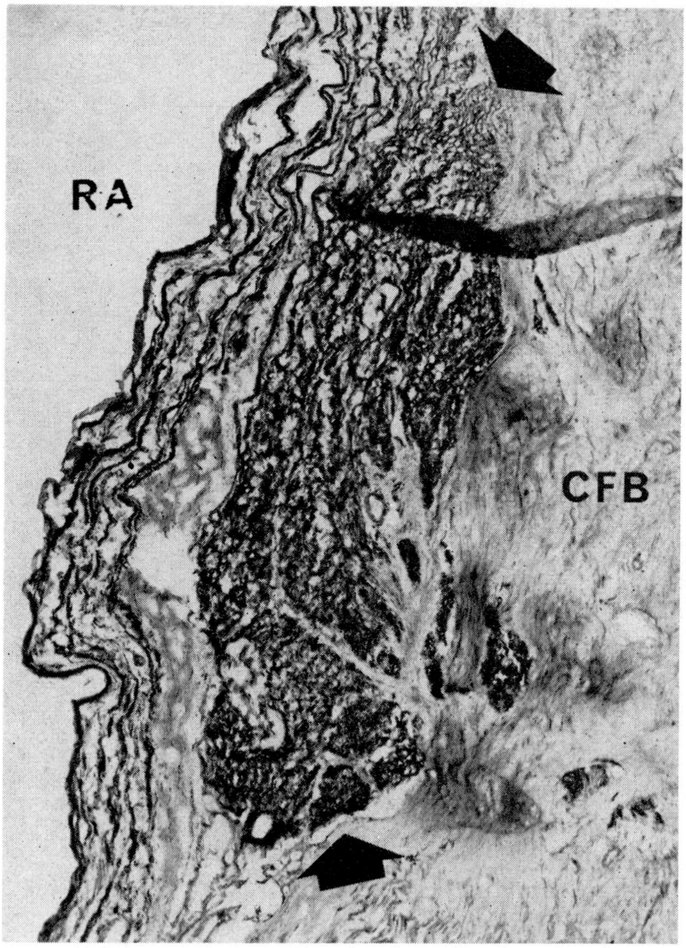


Fig. 13. The human AV node (between the two arrows) contains abundant cholines-
terase. Absence of cholinesterase in the central fibrous body at the right margin of the
photograph is in sharp contrast. *RA* is cavity of right atrium and *CFB* is central
terae. Absence of cholinesterase in the central fibrous body at the right margin of the
contain abundant cholinesterase. Magnification is ×45. This figure is reproduced from
the *Anatomical Record*[19] with permission of the Wistar Institute.

cellular distribution and the relative concentration in different nerve endings is also comparable to that observed in the sinus node. At the ultrastructural level we have not observed nerve endings to terminate directly on the membranes of cells in the AV node or the bundle of His. Cholinesterase is present in high concentration in the proximal bundle branches.

*The internodal pathways.* In the hearts of man,[27] the dog,[23] the

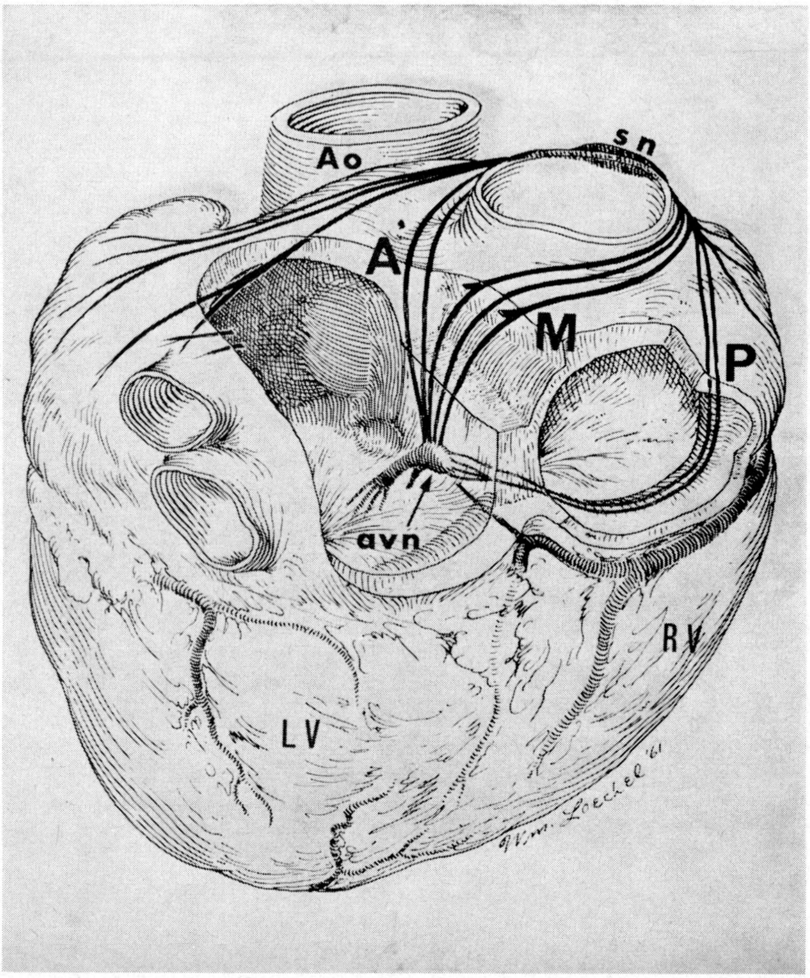


Fig. 14. This drawing illustrates the three internodal pathways described in the text. The heart is viewed from above and behind the left atrium. The abbreviations are as follows: *A,* anterior internodal tract; *M,* middle internodal tract; *P,* posterior internodal tract; *LV,* left ventricle; *RV,* right ventricle; *Ao,* aorta; *sn,* sinus node; *avn,* AV node.

steer,[11] and the rabbit[10] there are distinct bundles of continuous fibers that connect the sinus node and AV node, and that have been demonstrated physiologically to conduct more rapidly than ordinary myocardium.[28-33] There are large numbers of cells with Purkinje characteristics within these pathways (or tracts), but they are not composed exclusively of such cells. The internodal pathways exist in three divisions: the anterior, middle, and posterior (Figure 14). The *anterior*

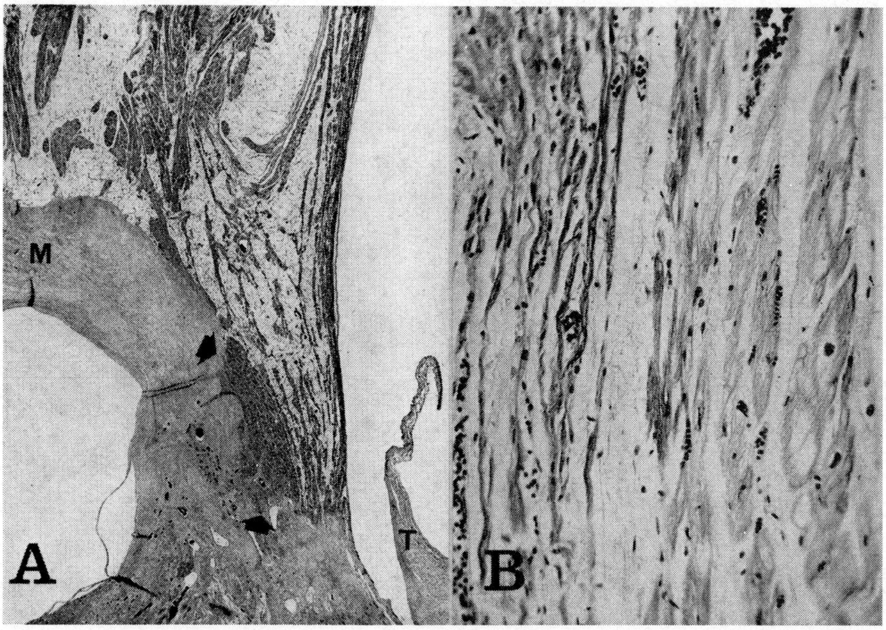


Fig. 15. *A* is a photomicrograph (×17) of human AV node demonstrating its relation to the mitral annulus and central fibrous body (*M*), and depicting the input system to the node. *T* labels the tricuspid value. The atrial septum is above, and fibers descending in the middle (principally from anterior and middle internodal tracts) decussate with those coursing under the right atrial endocardium (principally from the posterior internodal tract). Some of these enter the superior margin of the AV node while others course along its convex surface to its inferior margin; these junctions were confirmed with serial sections. In *B* (×300) one can see the contrasting appearance between fibers in the bypass tract (most of the right half) and in the AV node (left half). Those in the bypass area have characteristic features of Purkinje cells. Part *A* of this figure is reproduced from the *American Heart Jnl.*[7] with permission of C. V. Mosby Co.

*internodal pathway* is similar in all four species and includes the interatrial pathway first described by Bachmann[34] but, in addition, a portion within the atrial septum that Bachmann did not describe. Fibers in this pathway leave the anterior margin of the sinus node and course forward about the superior vena cava to enter the anterior interatrial myocardial band; there they divide into two groups, those coursing on into the left atrium (Bachmann's bundle) and those curving back into the interatrial septum and descending to the crest of the AV node. The *middle internodal pathway* is also anatomically similar in all four species, coursing from the posterior margin of the sinus node behind the superior vena cava and across the sinus intercavarum to descend along the right atrial side of the septum into the crest of the AV node. The middle internodal tract corresponds to that originally described by Wenckebach,[35,36] except that the portion crossing to the left atrium over the septum to connect the two atria is rarely as well developed as he indicated. The *posterior internodal pathway* also leaves the posterior margin of the sinus node but then courses along the crista terminalis and through the Eustachian ridge into the posterior margin of the AV node principally by crossing over the coronary sinus in man. However, in all species some of these fibers may course from the crista terminalis under the inferior vena caval orifice and under the ostium of the coronary sinus to reach the posterior margin of the AV node. In the rabbit, where the ostium of the coronary sinus is so large, the portion going under it may be the main one, corresponding to that described by Paes de Carvalho *et al.*[37] The posterior internodal pathway corresponds in general to that originally described by Thorel[38, 39] and in most species is anatomically the longest of the three internodal routes.

In the region of the AV node, fibers from all three pathways converge on the node superiorly and posteriorly; however, some of these fibers do not enter the nodal crest but descend along the convex margin to enter the more anterior and inferior portion of the node near its junction with the bundle of His (Figure 15). If one assumes that the point of maximal delay in AV transmission is at the superior atrionodal junction (the crest), then the fibers coursing directly under the right atrial endocardium to enter the convex margin of the AV node may physiologically as well as anatomically *bypass* the point of delay. For anatomic reasons these fibers have been indicated as bypass tracts,[22] and although their physiologic significance remains to be established, they may be important anatomic components of such physiologic phenomena as dual routes of AV transmissions[40] and of such clinical electrocardiographic events as reciprocal rhythm and ventricular preexcitation.[25]

From the description of the location of ganglia relative to the sinus node and AV node it is apparent that these lie directly within or adjacent to the various internodal pathways. In addition to those ganglia near the anterior and posterior margins of the sinus node, and at the posterior margin of the AV node, there is frequently a large concentration of ganglia within the middle internodal pathway near the crest of the interatrial septum, and another group within the anterior internodal pathway in its course just behind the aorta (Figures 5 and 16). The concentration of cholinesterase within these pathways is not remarkably different from that in ordinary atrial myocardium, except in

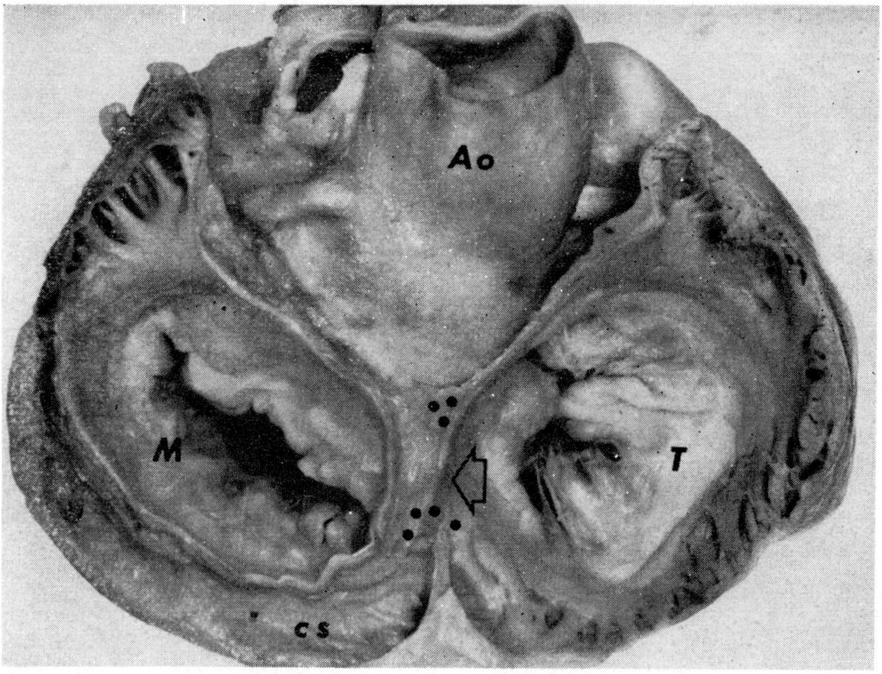


Fig. 16. In this photograph of dissected normal human heart the upper portions of both atria and atrial septum have been removed, and the coronary sinus exposed. The black dot clusters indicate the location of ganglia, with the upper group placed in the anterior internodal tract and the lower group within the posterior internodal tract just behind the AV node (open arrow). Compare with Figures 5 and 14. *M* is mitral valve; *T* tricuspid valve; *Ao* aorta; and *cs* coronary sinus.

the cells of the bypass tract (Figures 13 and 15). The possible functional importance of vagal control of conduction within the bypass tract is supported by the presence of more stainable cholinesterase there.

Both in the internodal pathways and in atrial myocardium generally there is focal variation in the concentration of cholinesterase. Some groups of cells contain more cholinesterase than neighboring groups. This inhomogeneity of cholinesterase staining sometimes but not always corresponds to identifiable cholinergic nerve endings. The anatomic variability of cholinesterase distribution supports the physiologic evidence[41] of inhomogeneity in vagal influence on the atria, a point of considerable importance in understanding the genesis and maintenance of certain arrhythmias such as atrial fibrillation.[42]

*Neuropathology of the cardiac conduction system.* Some diseases associated with clinically apparent extracardiac neural disease are also

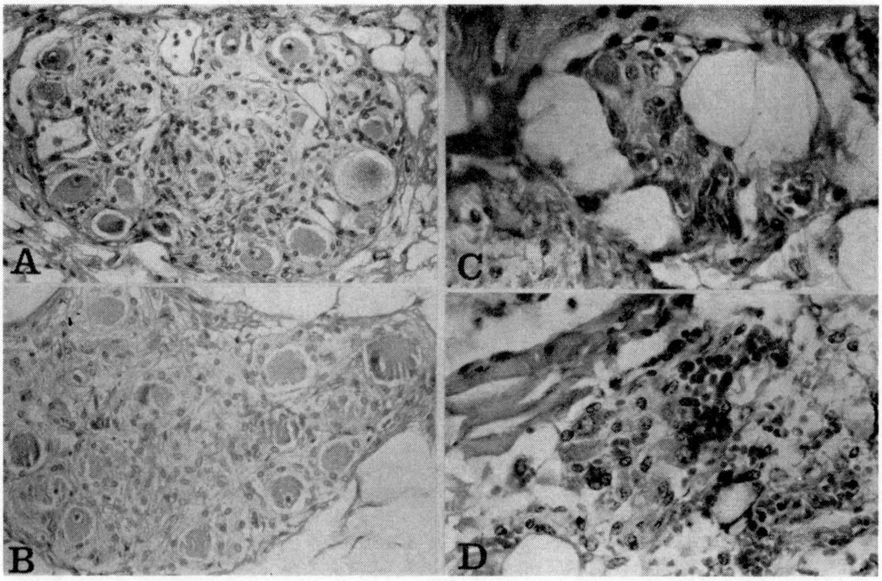


Fig. 17. Photomicrographs of typical normal *A* and *B* and pathologic cardiac ganglia *C* and *D*. Magnification in all is approximately ×90. All are from the margins of human sinus node. Those in *C* and *D* are from a child with fatal diphtheria and terminal disturbances in cardiac rhythm and conduction. Parts *C* and *D* are reproduced from *Circulation* with permission of the American Heart Association.

associated with a high incidence of arrhythmia and conduction disturbance, in which lesions of cardiac nerves may play an important role. Such lesions have been demonstrated in patients with arrhythmia due to cardiac metastasis of cancer[43] and in progressive muscular dystrophy with cardiac arrhythmia.[44] Perhaps the most striking example occurs in diphtheritic myocarditis associated with disturbances of cardiac electrophysiology,[45] for the extensive inflammation and degeneration of ganglia and other neural structures in the region of the sinus node and AV node (Figure 17) are consonant with the long-recognized clinical importance of widespread neurotoxicity in diphtheria.

Even without grossly recognizable histologic change in nerves and ganglia of the conduction system, however, certain diseases may appropriately alter their function and this in turn may cause or contribute to the onset of arrhythmia. For example, during myocardial infarction associated with an atrial arrhythmia, the region of the sinus node is regularly made ischemic, and this includes the juxtanodal ganglia.[46] Pericarditis, which is so often associated with atrial arrhythmia, regu-

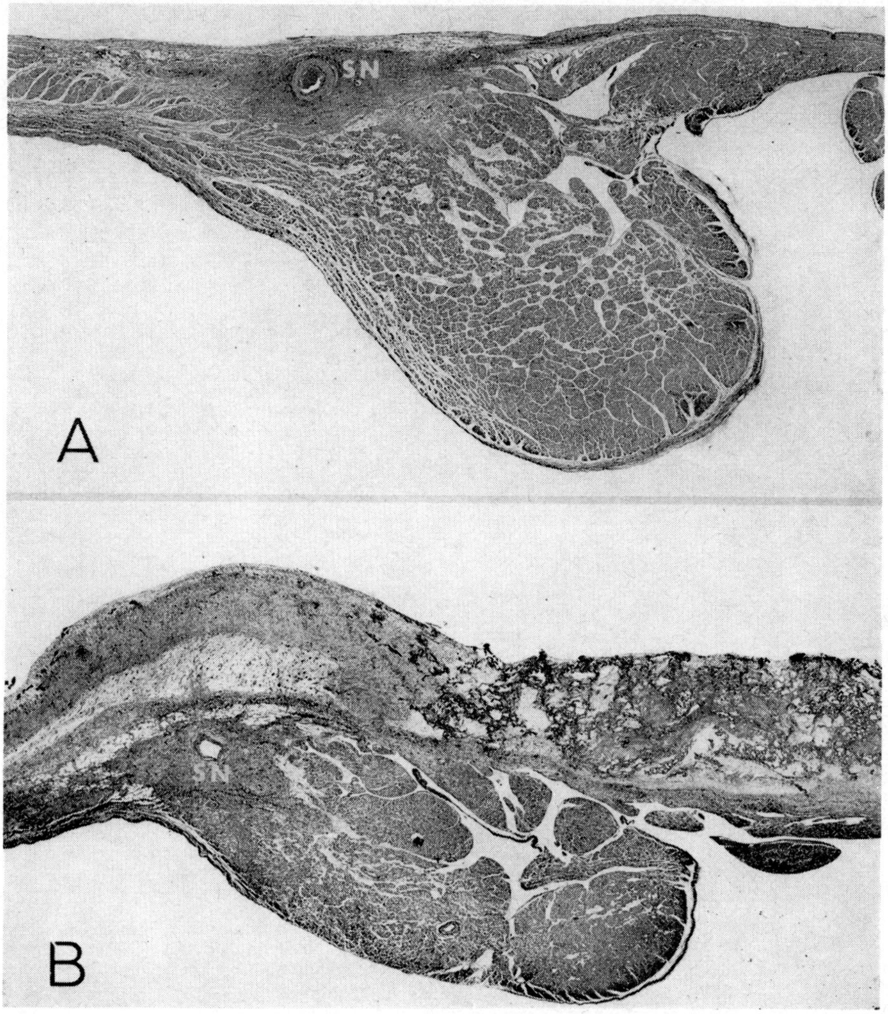


Fig. 18. Human sinus node (*SN*) is shown here normal (*A*) and with pericarditis (*B*). Extension of the inflammation directly into the sinus node is apparent, but involvement of numerous nerves is not well appreciated at this magnification (×7 in both). In each section epicardium is above, superior vena cava to the left, and free wall of right atrium to the right; the large mass of myocardium is crista terminalis.

larly involves the sinus node and its regional nerve endings and ganglia[47] (Figure 18). In acute posterior myocardial infarction there is often an associated intense sinus bradycardia and varying degrees of heart block that are frequently but not always reversible by the admission of atropine; this indicates their cholinergic mediation.[48-51] This phenomenon, which may legitimately be considered the human counterpart to the

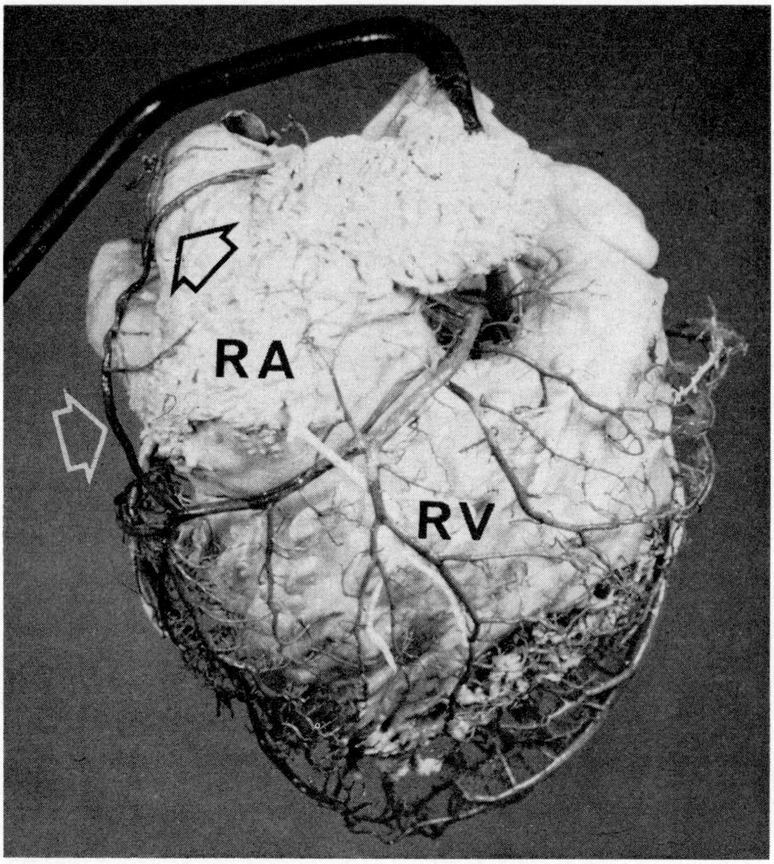


Fig. 19. This vinylite cast of a canine heart demonstrates the sinus node branch (*white arrow*) as it courses from the right coronary artery to the sinus node (*black arrow*). *RA* is right atrium and *RV* right ventricle. The sinus node artery is cannulated with a small polyethylene tube to perform the experiments described in the text. This figure is reproduced from *Anatomy of the Coronary Arteries* by T. N. James with permission of the publisher, Paul B. Hoeber.

von Bezold-Jarisch reflex seen in experimental animals, must originate within the ganglia and nerve endings that lie between the coronary sinus and AV node.[48, 49]

## Cardiac Neuropharmacology Pertinent to Arryhythmias

The observations to be described here were obtained with an experimental preparation in which the sinus node of the dog was perfused directly through its nutrient artery; the cardiac innervation and blood supply remained essentially intact (Figure 19). Details of the method have been published.[52, 53] Advantages include the possibility of direct administration of test substances into the sinus node and a small amount of neighboring atrial myocardium, without perfusion of the ventricles, other portions of the heart, the brain, or other extracardiac neuroreceptor sites except on recirculation. Since the volumes administered are rarely more than 2 ml., recirculation is associated with approximately a 500:1 dilution of the original dose.

Direct perfusion of the intact sinus node *in vivo* permits not only the specific study of the chronotropic action of a test substance, but also the relation of this effect to neural mechanisms that influence the sinus node. The general scheme for such studies has been as follows. The primary or direct action of a test substance is determined by serial injections of increasing concentrations prepared in Ringer's solution and, when pertinent, in fresh autogenous arterial blood also. If a positive chronotropic action is produced, the possibility of a vagolytic component of this action is tested by comparison of the amount of sinus acceleration before and after intranodal (10 $\mu$g./ml.) and intravenous (1 mg./kg.) atropinization, and by comparison of the effect of the test substance on the response to intranodal acetylcholine and to stimulation of the right vagus nerve. The possibility that sinus acceleration is due to local release of nodal norepinephrine is tested by comparing the effect in reserpinized and control dogs, and by observing the effect of intranodal administration of a beta-receptor blocking agent (e.g., propranolol, 10 $\mu$g./ml.) in reversing and in blocking acceleration; indirect evidence of possible release of norepinephrine is judged from the similarity of the peak and duration of acceleration to that observed with direct administration of either norepinephrine itself or of a known norepinephrine-releasing agent such as tyramine. Finally, the possibility of norepinephrine-sensitizing action (without necessarily any release of norepinephrine beyond that occurring constantly in a physiologic sense) is examined by comparison of the response to stellate stimulation and to intranodal administration of norepinephrine before and after a concentration of the test substance less than that which produced maximal acceleration.

To study the mechanism of a negative chronotropic effect of a test substance, an analogous series of experiments is performed. The possibility of vagal mediation is tested by comparison of responses before and after intranodal and systemic atropinization, and before and after

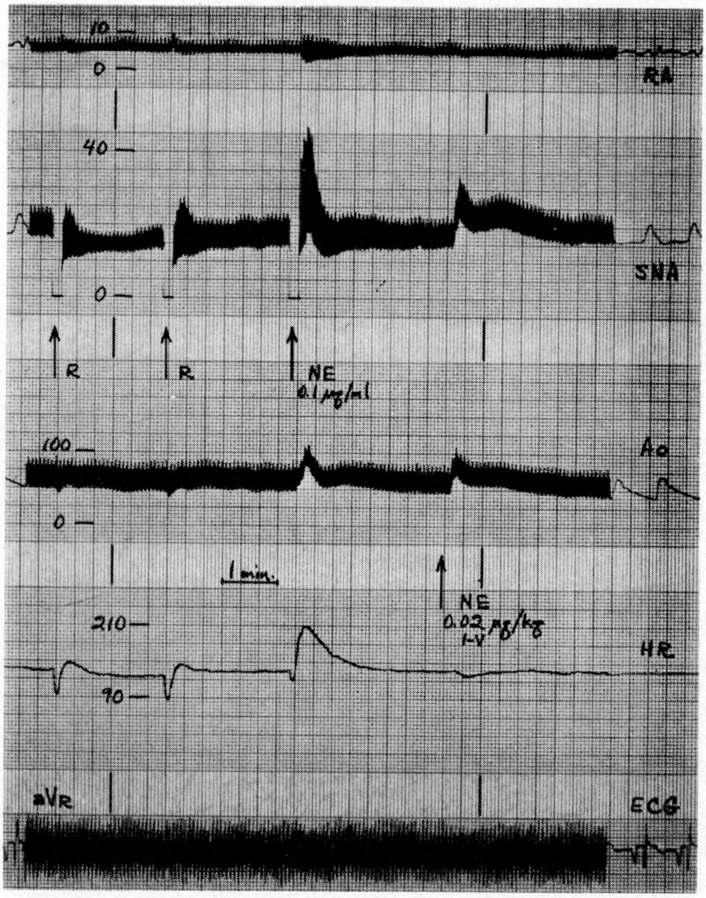


Fig. 20. This polygraph from an experiment with direct perfusion of the sinus node is typical of the recordings shown in several subsequent figures; the same scheme of labeling is used in all. The five channels from above down are right atrial pressure (*RA*), retrograde pressure in the ligated cannulated sinus node artery (*SNA*), central aortic pressure (*Ao*), a tachograph (heart rate, *HR*) derived from successive R waves of the ECG, and the *ECG*. Pressures are scaled in mm. Hg. Ligation of the sinus node artery has no significant effect on nodal function. Control injections of Ringer's solution (*R*) produce the characteristic injection bradycardia and postinjection acceleration seen in these experiments. The intranodal injection of norepinephrine (*NE*) produces immediate tachycardia, while the same amount of NE intravenously in this 10 kg. dog had only a negative chronotropic action. At this concentration NE has some pressor effect on recirculation.

cervical vagotomy. The possibility of acetylcholine sensitization (rather than accelerated release) is tested by responses to submaximal vagal stimulation of intranodal administration of acetylcholine in concentrations less than those producing maximal response. The possibility of cholinesterase inhibition is tested by comparison of responses before,

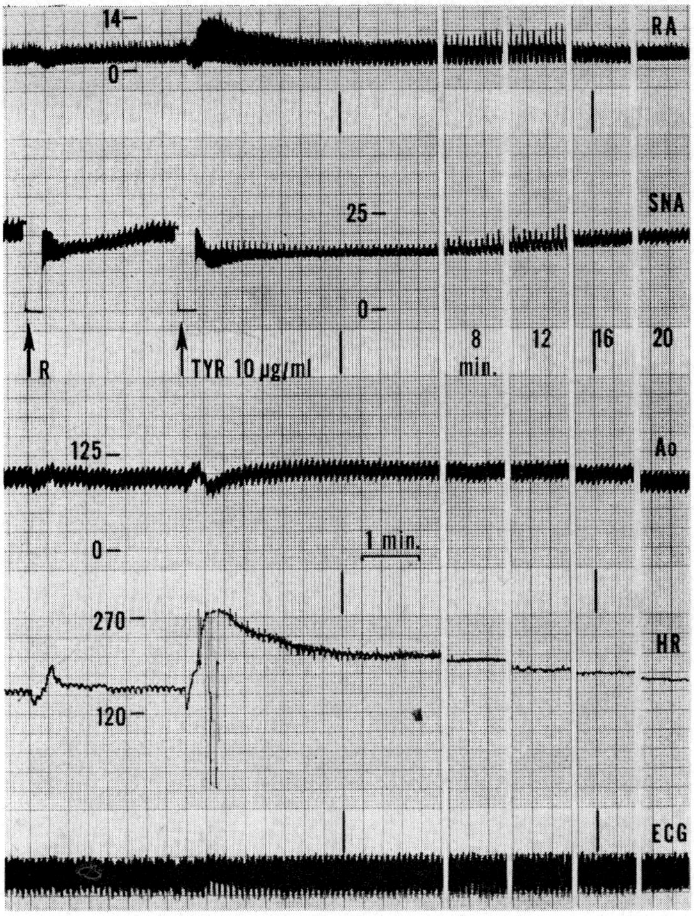


Fig. 21. In this experiment the positive chronotropic action of tyramine (*TYR*) is demonstrated, the duration being almost 20 minutes.

during and after intranodal administration of eserine (1 to 10 µg./ml.). Finally, the possibility of an antiadrenergic component of a negative chronotropic action is tested by responses to stellate stimulation or intranodal norepinephrine during the effect of the test substance.

Most of the results to be presented have been published in detail, and only those aspects pertinent to the subject of arrhythmia will be included here. Discussion of the pharmacologic studies will be divided into those dealing with adrenergic mechanisms and those dealing with cholinergic mechanisms. Some substances of course influence both mechanisms.

## Adrenergic Mechanisms

On direct perfusion of the sinus node, norepinephrine, epinephrine, and isoproterenol have only a positive chronotropic action, which is of immediate onset and relatively brief duration (Figure 20). In proportion to weight isoproterenol is about 10 times as potent as either of the two naturally occurring catecholamines,[54] but in concentrations producing maximal effect the duration of tachycardia is about the same. Since isoproterenol is not generally thought to occur naturally and will not enter storage sites at nerve endings into which epinephrine and norepinephrine will,[55] its greater potency may be due to the fact that all its action is direct and that no portion of that administered is stored; it thus acts in a sense as a false neurotransmitter. Ephedrine is about one tenth as potent by weight as norepinephrine or epinephrine, but its positive chronotropic effect lasts about ten times as long. Tyramine[55] acts in the sinus node principally by releasing local norepinephrine, but its duration of action is much longer than that of directly administered norepinephrine (Figure 21). In reserpinized dogs the response to tyramine can be restored by the local intranodal administration of norepinephrine or epinephrine (but not isoproterenol), but the response to stimulation of the stellate ganglion *cannot* be restored in this way. Guanethidine,[56] on direct perfusion of the sinus node, acts immediately by releasing local norepinephrine, but its duration of sinus acceleration is slightly longer than that of tyramine. Reserpine[56] has only a negative chronotropic action on direct perfusion in the sinus node; this suggests that its mechanism for nodal depletion of norepinephrine (clearly apparent hours after intramuscular administration) differs significantly from guanethidine in speed of onset of effect. Dopamine, although it has no chronotropic effect when administered intravenously, produces sinus tachycardia on direct perfusion of the sinus node.[57] Tyrosine and phenylalanine, precursors of both epinephrine and norepinephrine, have no significant chronotropic effect on direct perfusion of the sinus node.[58]

Dichloroisoproterenol[59] has a very slight positive chronotropic effect in low concentrations perfused directly into the sinus node, but in higher concentrations it effectively blocks the positive chronotropic action of locally administered norepinephrine and the sinus tachycardia from stellate stimulation. A surprising observation was the anticholinergic action of dichloroisoproterenol, apparent both against the re-

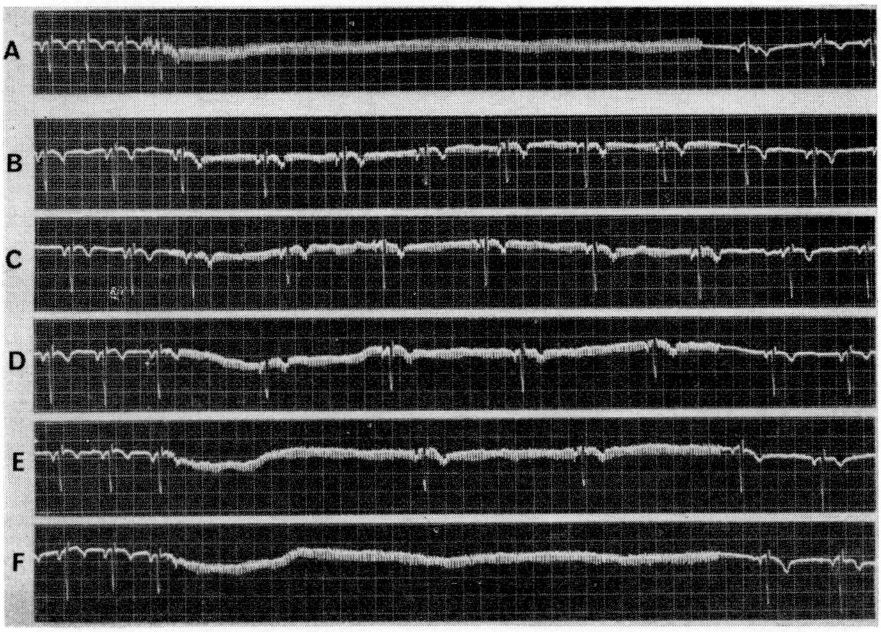


Fig. 22. These strips of electrocardiogram are aVr recorded at 25 mm./sec. and demonstrate the vagal-blocking action of intranodal pronethalol (naphthylisoproterenol), 10$\mu$g./ml. *A* illustrates the response to a vagal stimulus in the control period. The next five strips are vagal stimuli delivered at approximately three minute intervals after the pronethalol. The slower heart rate even without vagal stimulation in strips *B-E* is a direct negative chronotropic action of pronethalol. Complete recovery of the response to vagal stimulation is present in *F*. Vagal blockade by the adrenergic beta-receptor blocking agents occurs at higher concentrations than those required for adrenergic blockade.

sponse to vagal stimulation and intranodal acetylcholine.[59] Large concentrations of isoproterenol given intranodally do not have this vagal-blocking action. Pronethalol[60] and propranolol do not produce significant sinus acceleration at any concentration, but in addition to their familiar beta-receptor blocking actions they also block the response to vagal stimulation (Figure 22). The vagal-blocking action of these substances occurs at higher concentrations than their beta-receptor blocking activity, but it has been demonstrated by Wallace *et al.*[61] that detectable cholinergic blocking activity may be present even with concentrations conventionally employed for beta-receptor blockade. This dual autonomic blocking action of the currently popular beta-receptor blocking agents is similar to the action of quinidine (see later discussion), as is the direct negative chronotropic action after perfusion into the sinus node in high concentrations.

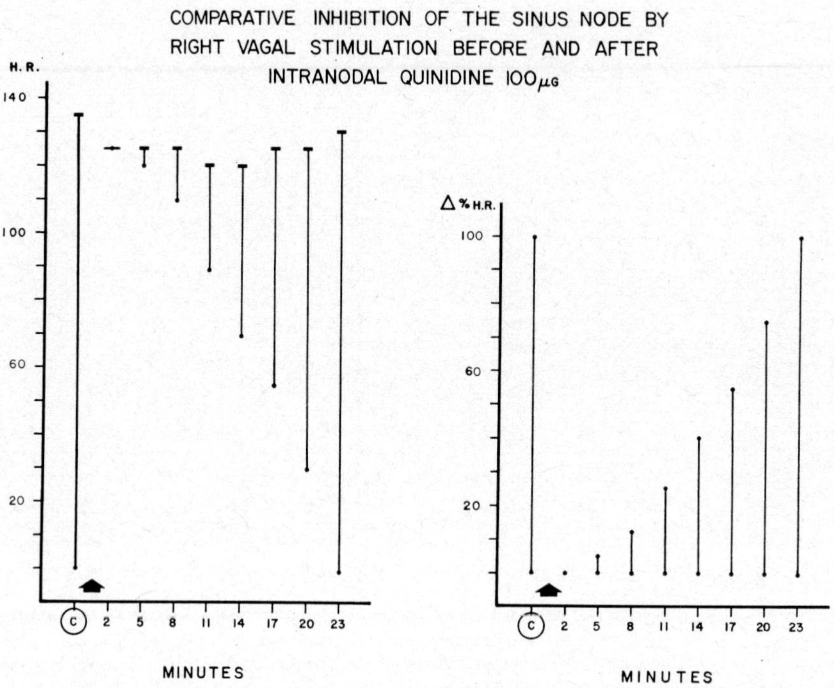


Fig. 23. One set of data from an experiment demonstrating anticholinergic action of intranodal quinidine is plotted here two ways: on the left the absolute change in heart rate is presented, while on the right the change in per cent is shown. Time of intranodal quinidine administration is indicated by the arrow. This and Figures 24 and 25 are reproduced from the *American Heart Journal*[67] with permission of the C. V. Mosby Co.

Acetaldehyde,[62] the principal early product of ethanol degradation in the body, has a potent positive chronotropic action on direct perfusion of the sinus node, and this is due to local release of norepinephrine. In this respect it resembles the action of tyramine or guanethidine. Ethanol, except in toxic concentrations, has no significant action after direct perfusion of the sinus node. The possible importance of a myocardial norepinephrine-releasing and depleting action of acetaldehyde in the pathogenesis of both acute and chronic cardiac effects of alcoholism deserves further study.

Digitalis may produce transient sinus acceleration on direct perfusion of the sinus node, but its more prolonged effect is one of sinus slowing.[63, 64] This action occurs in concentrations that are at or only slightly above those obtained with the therapeutic administration of digitalis. The negative chronotropic effect is not due to cholinergic

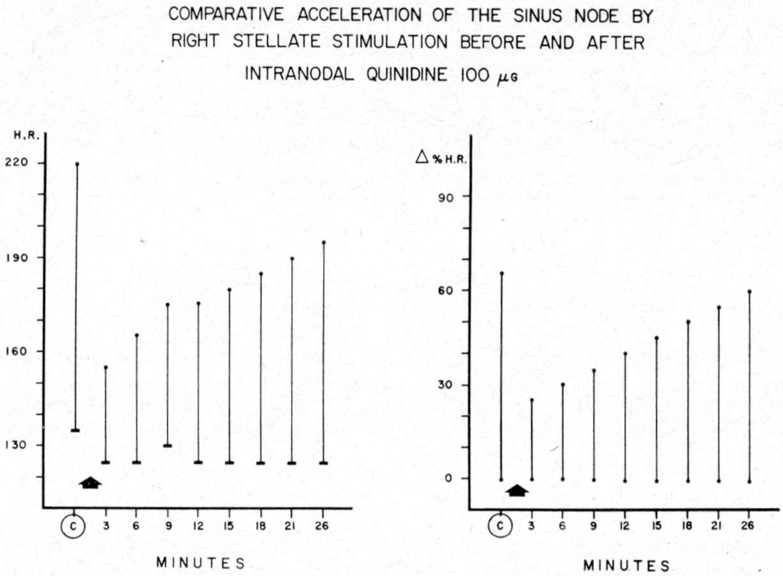


Fig. 24. An experiment demonstrating antiadrenergic action of intranodal quinidine is presented here in the same way as in Figure 23. Note that in neither experiment (same dog) did the control heart rate vary significantly between neural stimulation, demonstrating that the autonomic-blocking effects occurred without significant direct chronotropic action by quinidine.

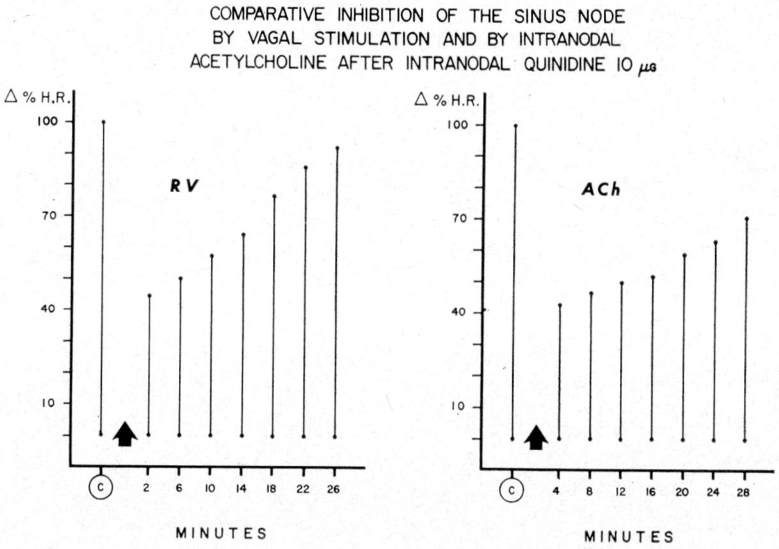


Fig. 25. In this experiment the anticholinergic action of intranodal quinidine is shown comparably effective against either vagal stimulation or intranodal acetylcholine, which were given alternately. The concentration of quinidine employed here is less than in Figures 23 and 24 (same dog).

mediation although, as a contributing factor, this deserves further study. There is a demonstrable antiadrenergic action by intranodal digitalis both against the effect of stellate stimulation and the direct administration of epinephrine;[65] this confirms similar observations for the action of digitalis on the AV node and the bundle of His.[66]

Quinidine (Figures 23 to 25) has both an antiadrenergic and anticholinergic action on direct perfusion of the sinus node.[67] These effects are against both neurally released and directly administered neurotransmitter substances, so that the action does not depend on inhibition of neurotransmitter release. The concentrations of quinidine with which the autonomic blocking actions occur are similar to those conventionally obtained with the clinical use of quinidine. At such concentrations there is no direct chronotropic action by intranodally administered quinidine, although higher concentrations do produce sinus bradycardia and, eventually, toxic nodal damage. In the management of clinical arrhythmia two significant points may be stressed from these findings. First, quinidine has a profound effect on the sinus node, and restoration of its normal function is the actual goal in clinical management of an arrhythmia. Second, this effect is not obvious from heart rate alone, since both the cholinergic and adrenergic blocking actions are distinctly present after concentrations of quinidine which in themselves have no direct chronotropic effect.

Nicotine has complex effects on direct perfusion of the sinus node.[68] To understand its actions it should be recalled that ganglia of the sinus node are close to it and a variable number of these are perfused by the sinus node artery both in man and the dog. The first action of intranodal nicotine is a negative effect mediated by the release of acetylcholine, due at least in part to direct action on terminals of the cholinergic nerve, since hexamethonium fails to eliminate this action while atropine does eliminate it. Following the initial slowing, which is transient, the sinus node responds to nicotine with a more prolonged acceleration, which can be abolished with propranolol and must in part be due to direct local release of norepinephrine. Hexamethonium, which failed to eliminate the negative chronotropic action of nicotine, has the distinct effect of reducing the positive chronotropic action, which is unexplained. Neither intranodal nicotine,[68] nor veratridine or veratramine,[69] produces the von Bezold-Jarisch reflex. This suggests that cardiac receptor sites for this phenomenon do not include

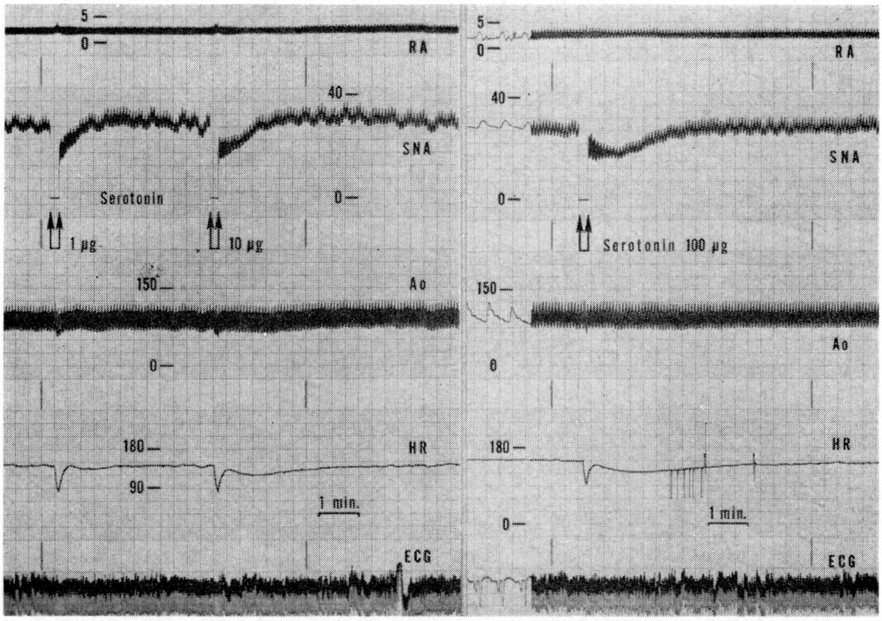


Fig. 26. The negative chronotropic action of serotonin is shown here. The onset of slowing is later than with acetylcholine or adenosine, but lasts longer. This figure is reproduced from the *Journal of Pharmacology and Experimental Therapeutics*[77] with permission of the Williams and Wilkins Co.

the region of the sinus node, which is compatible with the observations of Dawes.[70]

Bradykinin and angiotensin both release enormous amounts of catecholamines from the adrenal medulla,[71] but neither of these substances has any significant chronotropic action on direct perfusion of the sinus node.[72, 73] The reported sinus acceleration after systemic administration of angiotensin to dogs with special preparation to eliminate the secondary effect of acute aortic hypertension[74, 75] is most likely mediated by extracardiac actions or at least by actions outside the sinus node. Serotonin has many powerful extracardiac effects on the nervous system. It slows the heart when administered intravenously but accelerates the isolated heart.[76] On direct perfusion of the sinus node (Figure 26) it has only a modest but consistent slowing effect that is not due to cholinergic mediation.[77] Glucagon[78] produces sinus acceleration after direct perfusion of the sinus node, and this appears largely but not completely due to local release of norepinephrine.

Recent evidence suggests that cyclic 3′, 5′ AMP is the intracellular

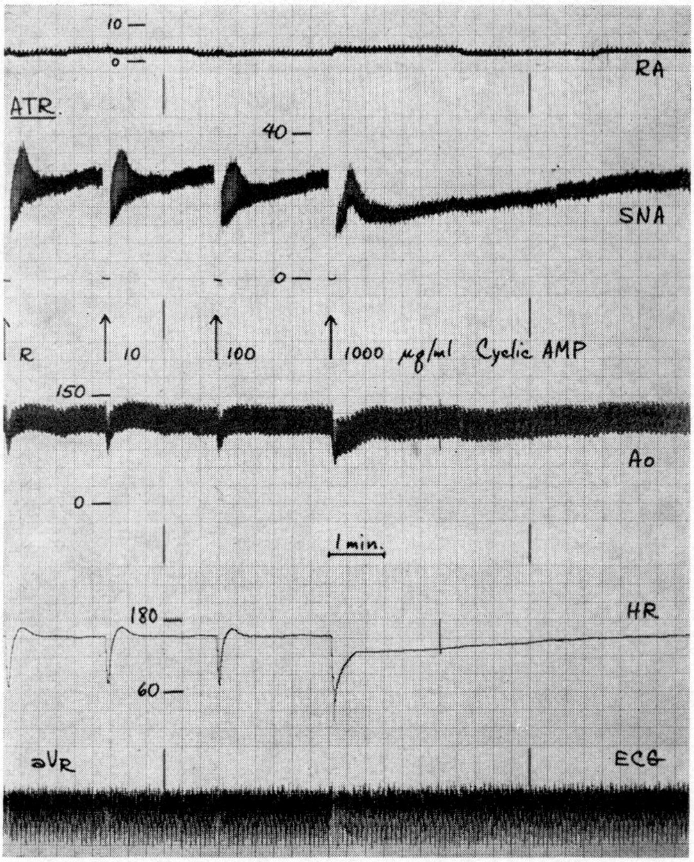


Fig. 27. Characteristic negative chronotropic action of cyclic AMP is shown here, in an atropinized dog. Cyclic AMP has no significant chronotropic action at lower concentrations.

mediator for the effect of catecholamines on the myocardium.[79] However, cyclic AMP has only a negative chronotropic effect on direct perfusion of the sinus node[80] (Figure 27). The reported cardiac acceleration following its systemic administration,[81] which has been indicated as consistent with its role in mediation of responses to catecholamines, seems more likely due to secondary responses to primary extracardiac actions. Although possible it would be surprising if a normally intracellular substance such as cyclic AMP, which does not pass the cell membrane under normal circumstances, would exert the same *physiologic* action when administered extracellularly.

In some animal species the intravenous administration of adenine

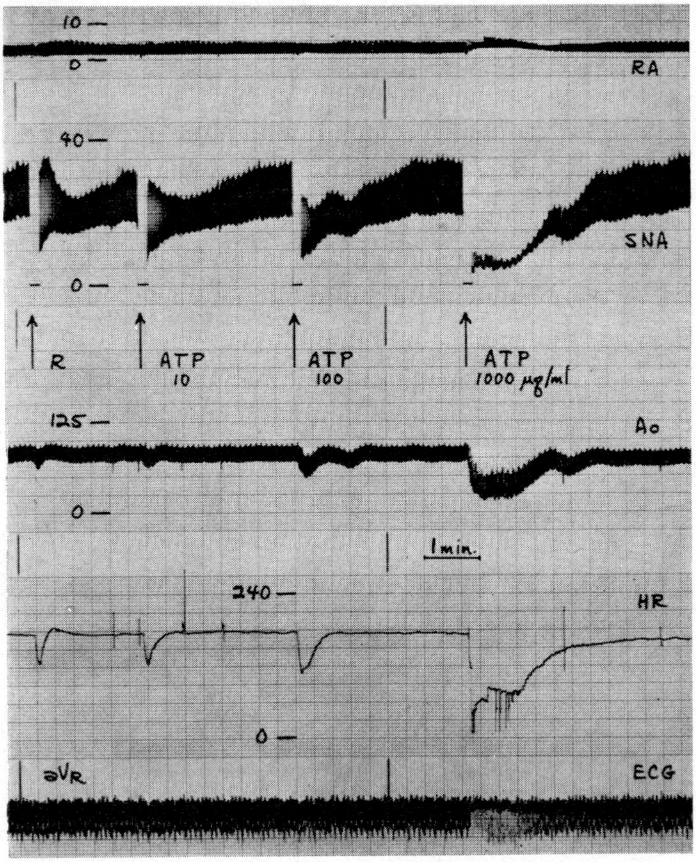


Fig. 28. ATP (adenosine triphosphate) has a greater negative chronotropic action than cyclic AMP at lower concentrations, but the duration is less.

nucleotides produces a negative chronotropic effect due to vagal mediation.[82] On direct perfusion of the canine sinus node most adenine nucleotides and closely related substances have only a negative chronotropic action without a cholinergic component[80] (Figure 28). One exception is guanosine,[79] which produces sinus acceleration unaffected by beta-receptor blockade and is most likely due to a direct effect on cells of the sinus node. Adenosine and related nucleosides do not normally contact the external surface of the myocardial cell, but during ischemia these substances are released from the myocardial cells[83] in physiologically significant concentrations and must have an influence at least on directly adjacent cells. The negative chronotropic action of adenosine (Figure 29) and its nucleotides on direct perfusion

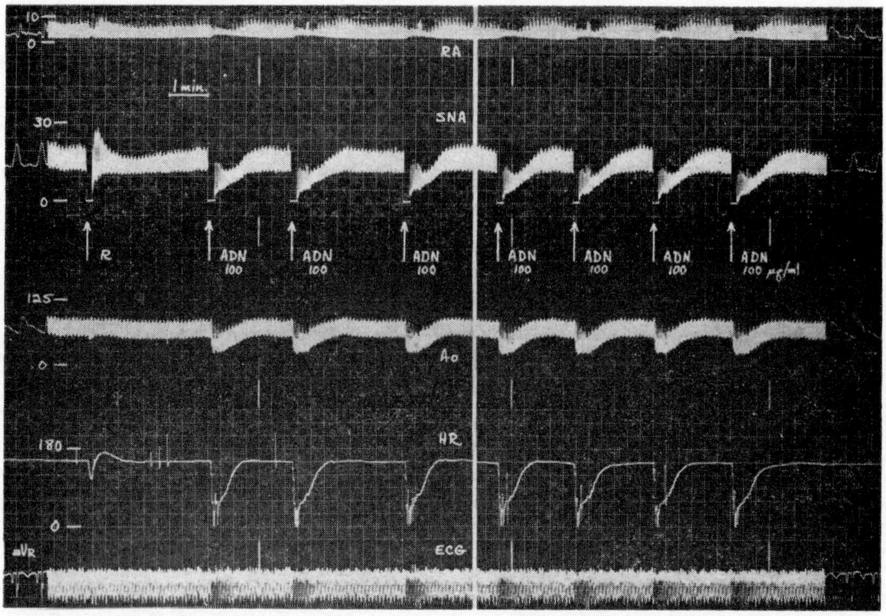


Fig. 29. Adenosine (ADN) has about the same effect as ATP on direct perfusion of the sinus node, indicating the phosphate groups (alone or cycled) are unnecessary for its action. There is no tachyphylaxis, and repeated injections produce the same effect.

of the sinus node may have a clinical counterpart in the sinus bradycardia observed during some myocardial infarctions, particularly when this is not reversible with atropine. Similarly, the negative chronotropic action following intranodal administration of certain amino acids that are normally intracellular,[58] such as glutamic and aspartic acid, may also play a role in such bradycardias.

## Cholinergic Mechanisms

A number of these mechanisms have been considered in the previous section because of logical continuity. Examples include the cholinergic mechanisms associated with actions of quinidine, the beta-receptor blocking compounds, and nicotine, as well as the noncholinergic negative chronotropic actions of digitalis, serotonin, and adenine nucleotides.

Acetylcholine[84] perfused directly into the sinus node has only a negative chronotropic action, which is progressively more marked after increasing concentrations, up to the point of complete sinus arrest (Figure 30). The negative chronotropic effect of acetylcholine

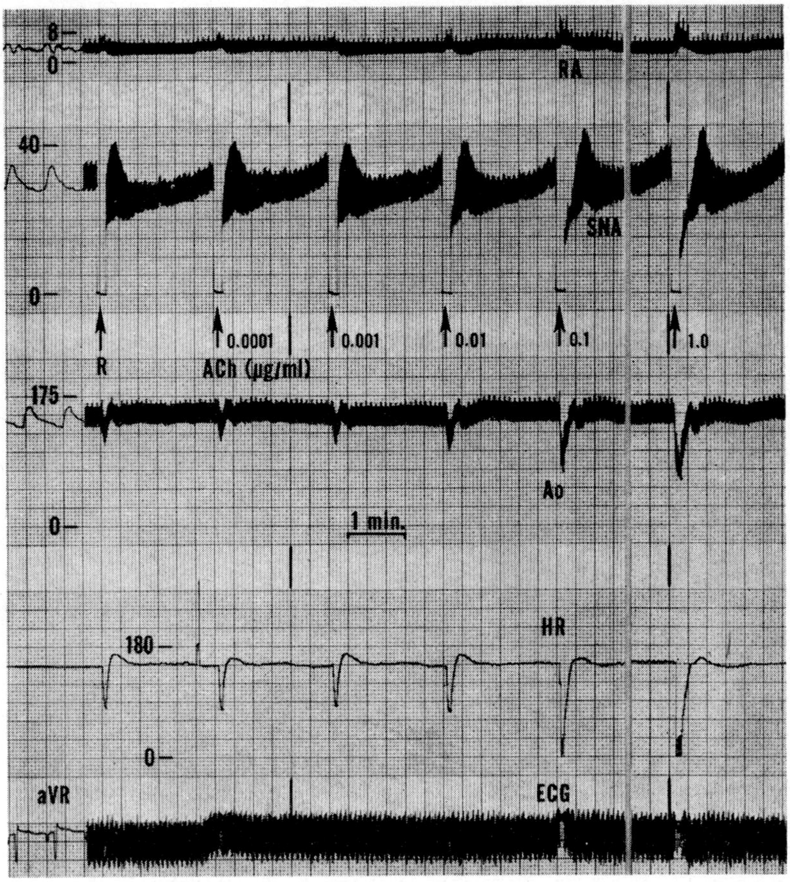


Fig. 30. Intranodal acetylcholine (ACh) has immediate but very transient effect. The higher concentrations produce sinus arrest. This and Figures 31, 33, 34, and 36 are reproduced from *Circulation Research*[84] with permission of the American Heart Association.

is immediate and extremely transient; it terminates almost as soon as the injection is completed. Its duration of action is thus briefer than that of adrenergic neurotransmitters. Very low concentrations of acetylcholine have no significant effect, and specifically do not produce sinus acceleration. Administered after either intranodal or intravenous atropinization, intranodal acetylcholine has no significant chronotropic action.

Eserine[84] produces only a negative chronotropic effect after direct perfusion of the sinus node, but this is of relatively gradual onset; it requires a minute or more to reach its maximal action (Figure 31).

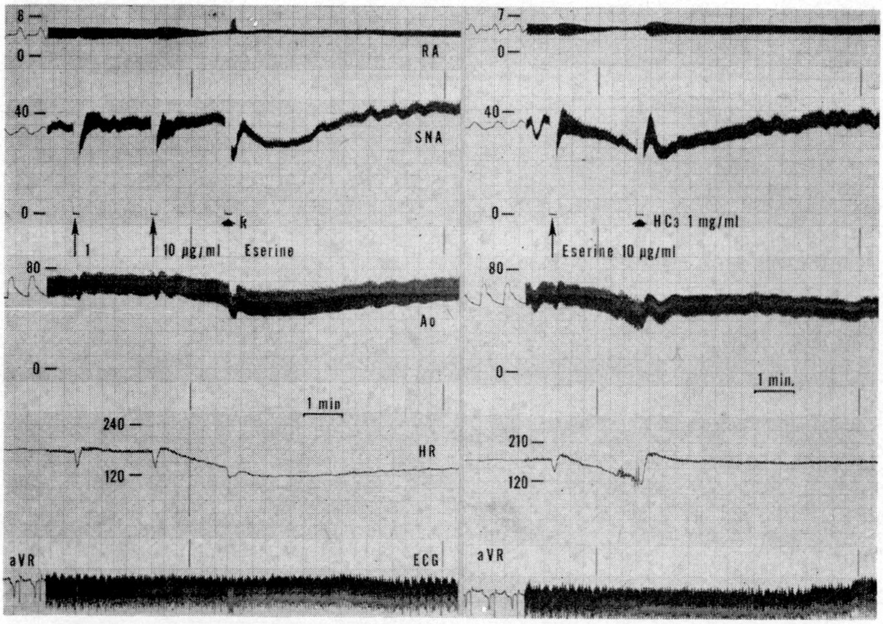


Fig. 31. Eserine produces sinus bradycardia gradually but for a prolonged period. The effect is unaltered by intranodal Ringer's solution (*left panel*) but immediately reversed by intranodal hemicholinium (HC3) in the right panel. The same reversal occurs with intranodal or systemic atropinization. Since hemicholinium acts by stopping acetylcholine synthesis, its rapid action in reversing the effect of eserine indicates constant acetylcholine synthesis is required for the action of cholinesterase inhibitors on the sinus node.

Low concentrations of eserine do not produce sinus acceleration. Intranodal eserine markedly enhances the effect of even very weak vagal stimuli or very low concentrations of intranodal acetylcholine, and it prolongs their negative chronotropic action. The effect of intranodal eserine is relatively long (10 to 30 minutes, depending on the initial concentration administered), but the effect may be abruptly terminated with either intranodal or intravenous atropinization. Both eserine and acetylcholine produce atrial fibrillation after intranodal administration, especially with the higher concentrations, but this is an unpredictable effect from dog to dog and even on repeated experiments in the same dog. Atrial fibrillation so caused lasts only as long as the other direct actions of these drugs, or slightly longer, and it can be terminated and prevented by atropinization.

Production of atrial fibrillation by intranodal acetylcholine or eserine is simply a different means to the same end, since it has long been

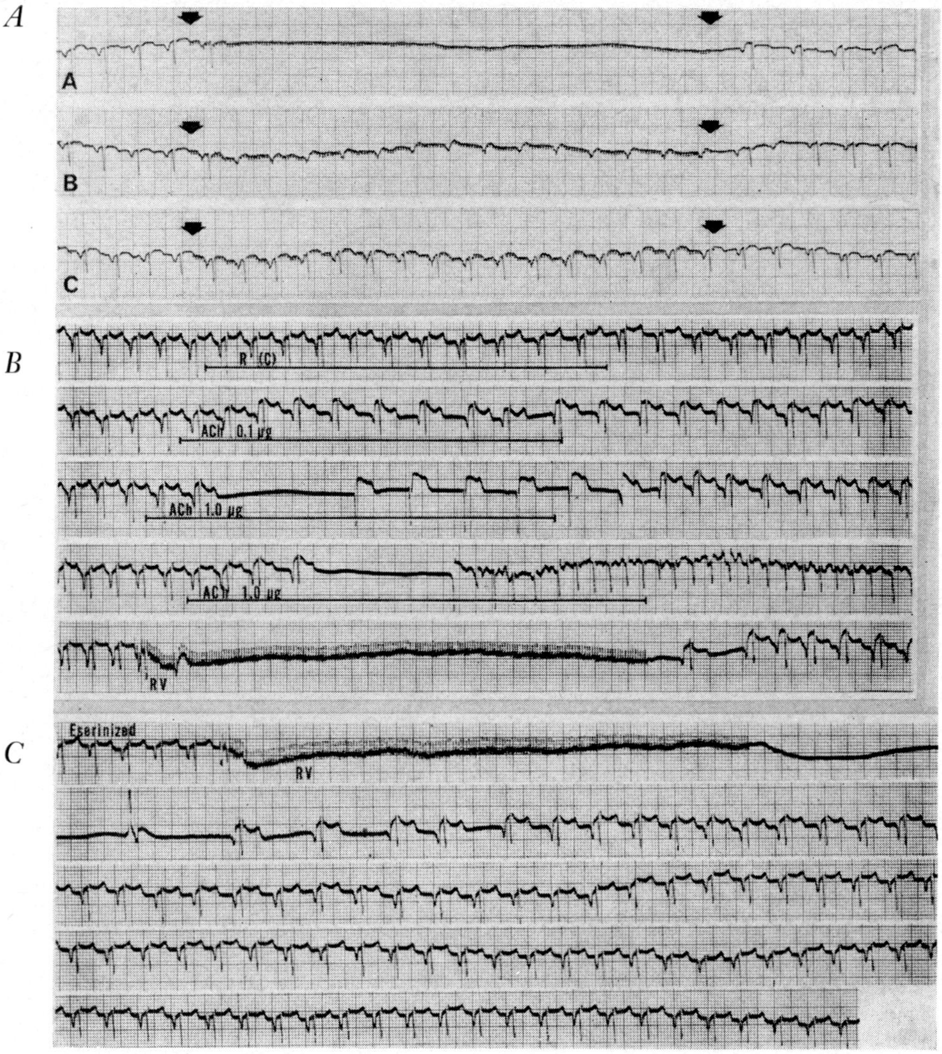


Fig. 32. These three sets of tracings illustrate various cholinergic mechanisms in the sinus node. In the upper group (*A*) a vagal stimulus is delivered before (*first trace*) and after intranodal atropine 10 µg./ml. (*second trace*) and then intravenous atropine 1 mg./kg. (*third trace*). With intranodal atropine the sinus node is selectively blocked while the AV node responds normally. In the middle group (*B*) the successive strips show response to a control injection of Ringer's solution; the response to ACh 0.1 µg./ml. (slowing, with elevation of the P-Tp segment); the response to ACh 1.0 µg./ml. (sinus arrest with AV nodal escape rhythm); atrial fibrillation produced by the same concentration of ACh on another occasion; and finally a comparative response to vagal stimulation in the same dog. In the lower group (*C*) continuous strips demonstrate the enhanced effect of a vagal stimulus after intranodal eserine in the same dog as the strips in group *B*. Paper speed is 25 mm./sec.

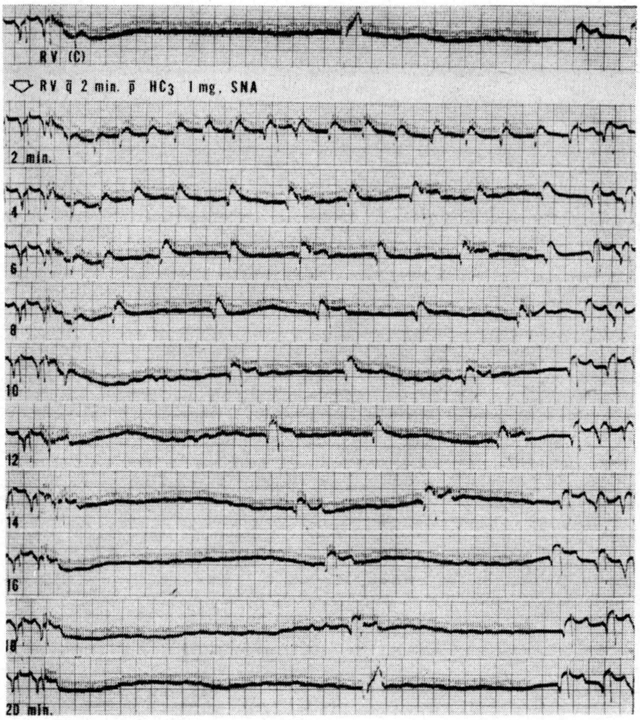


Fig. 33. The effect of a vagal stimulus delivered before and serially after intranodal hemicholinium (HC3) is shown here. Note that the number of escape beats decreases as the effect of hemocholinium wanes, and the time until the first escape beat increases. P-Tp segment elevation produced by vagal stimulation here is identical to that produced by intranodal acetylcholine in Figure 32, suggesting this effect is produced during a cholinergic stimulus with or without an accompanying negative chronotropic action of acetylcholine. Paper speed is 25 mm./sec.

known that these and related substances (and vagal stimulation) enhance both the production and maintenance of experimental atrial fibrillation.[41, 42, 85-87] This effect is most likely due to the nonhomogeneous distribution of both vagal nerve endings and of cholinesterase within the atrial myocardium, so that a cholinergic stimulus, however delivered, favors the development of nonuniform excitability and recovery. Consequently such a stimulus creates the ideal situation for local reentry at many separate points and, ultimately, for fibrillation.

An analogous situation occurs in the ventricular myocardium, although the mediation there is adrenergic[88] rather than cholinergic. Stimulation of the left stellate ganglion prolongs the QT interval[89] and lowers the threshold for production of experimental ventricular fibrillation.[88] However, unlike the situation in the atria, where administration

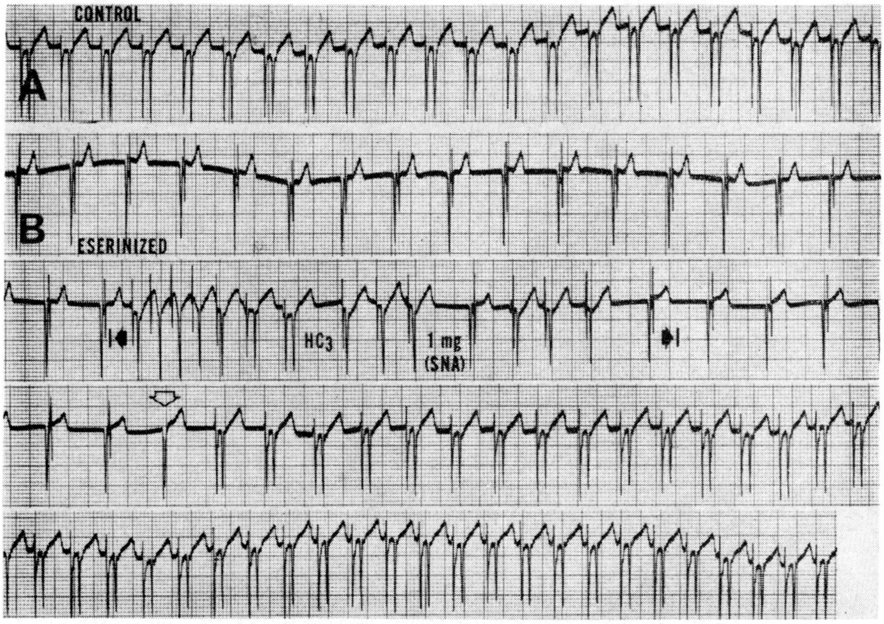


Fig. 34. This electrogram recorded from the region of the sinus node demonstrates reversal by intranodal hemicholinium of sinus arrest due to eserine. The control strip (*A*) is separate but the remaining strips (*B*) are continuous. Hemicholinium was delivered between the two black arrows and the sinus node resumes pacing at the point indicated by the open arrow. Paper speed is 25 mm./sc.

of the appropriate neurotransmitters produces the same effect, the administration of norepinephrine does not have the same effect as that from stimulation of the stellate ganglion.[88, 90, 91] Presuming that the anatomic distribution of cholinergic nerve terminals in the atria is similar to that of adrenergic nerve terminals in the ventricles—it is nonhomogeneous in both—the reason for this difference in ventricular myocardial response to neurally released and administered norepinephrine is uncertain. It may be due to more homogeneous distribution of enzymes that destroy norepinephrine in ventricular myocardium (principally catechol O-methyl transferase) than of enzymes that destroy acetylcholine in atrial myocardium (cholinesterase). An alternative possibility is a nonuniform ventricular myocardial uptake of neurally released norepinephrine but a more uniform uptake when administered directly, since recent evidence indicates uptake and storage may be more important than local degradation in terminating the effect of norepinephrine.[92]

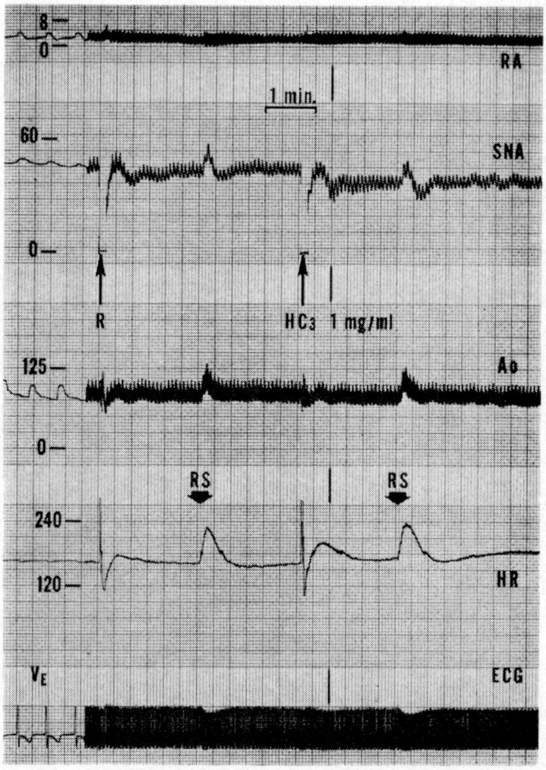


Fig. 35. Stimulation of the right stellate ganglion after intranodal hemicholinium produces the same acceleration as in the control period, indicating presence of acetylcholine is not necessary for this effect. See also Figure 36 and text for discussion.

Atropine may be used by direct perfusion of the sinus node as an adjunct to studies of certain extranodal autonomic nervous actions. Marey's reflex is a cholinergic phenomenon produced by acute aortic hypertension of any cause, and is characteristically associated with sinus bradycardia and varying degrees of AV block. The aortic hypertension after systemic administration of norepinephrine produces this reflex and has led to a misconception among some clinicians that norepinephrine has principally a negative chronotropic action. That this, of course, is not the case can be clearly demonstrated by comparing the action of norepinephrine before and after intranodal and then systemic atropinization;[93] with the former there is sinus acceleration and AV block (since the AV node is not atropinized); with the latter there is sinus acceleration with normal AV conduction. As a

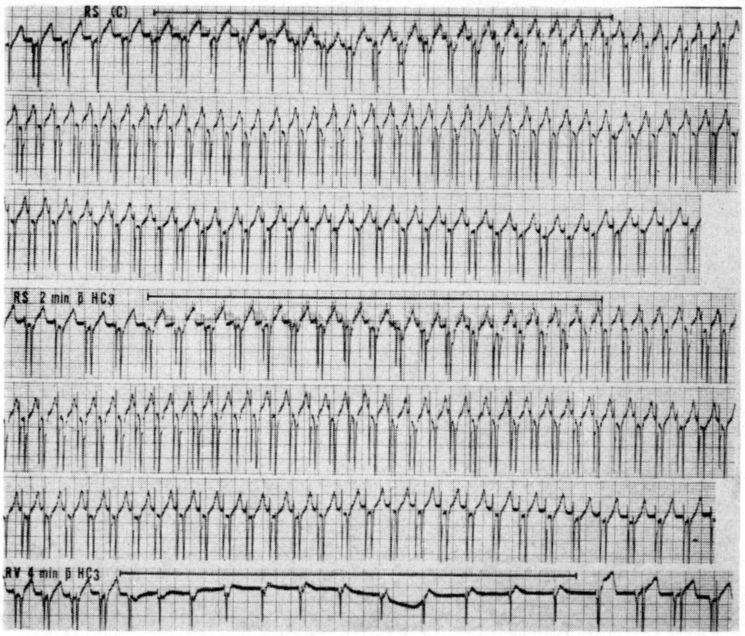


Fig. 36. An electrogram recorded from the region of the sinus node is shown here during the same experiment illustrated with the polygraph in Figure 35. Note the P wave configuration is the same, excluding the possibility that the tachycardia after the second stimulus may have otherwise been ectopic in origin. The vagal stimulus response shown at the bottom demonstrates that effective vagal blockade was present even after the second stellate stimulus. Paper speed is 25 mm./sec.

teaching demonstration, the effects of right vagal stimulation before atropinization, after selective intranodal atropinization and after systemic atropinization (Figure 32), provide a clear comparison of cholinergic effects in two critical centers of the heart: the sinus node and the AV node (and the bundle of His). Participation of cholinergic discharge within the sinus node as a component of certain other reflex bradycardias (such as that early in acute hypoxemia) may also be pharmacologically "dissected" in this way.

Hemicholinium[94] inhibits acetylcholine synthesis by antagonizing the action of choline acetylase.[95] Intranodal hemicholinium does block acetylcholine synthesis (Figures 33 and 34) and is as potent as atropine in eliminating the response to stimulation of the right vagus nerve, although the effect of atropine lasts longer. Whereas atropine also blocks the effect of intranodal acetylcholine, however, hemicholinium (except for an initial inconsistent effect lasting two to four minutes) does not block the response to intranodal administration of acetylcholine. Since it has been reported that acetylcholine is capable of releasing norepinephrine from postsynaptic adrenergic nerve terminals,[96] and that in some organs norepinephrine release after neural stimuli requires prior release of acetylcholine, experiments with direct perfusion of the sinus node were designed to test this hypothesis.[84] Hemicholinium in concentrations that completely block the response to supramaximal stimulation of the vagus have no significant effect on the response to stimulation of the stellate ganglion (Figures 35 and 36). This evidence, plus the absence of any detectable accelerating action by intranodal acetylcholine or eserine in low or high concentrations before or after atropinization, suggests that acetylcholine does *not* release physiologically significant amounts of norepinephrine in the canine sinus node, and that it is not a necessary component for such release following neural stimulation.

## Summary

Certain anatomic and pharmacologic observations on the innervation of the heart have been reviewed, with particular attention to their relevance to the mechanisms and management of cardiac arrhythmia. It is intended that this review will serve as a midpoint from which further considerations may become more detailed (as in experiments on the cellular membrane action potential) or, conversely, that it will cover broader interrelations (as in experiments on extracardiac factors influencing its rhythm and conduction). Molecular biology is an important new field. But cells do not behave as a homogeneous aggregate of molecules, nor do organs of the body behave as a homogeneous community of cells. It is only by critically collating the results from studies at all the various levels of biologic organization and function that we can hope to understand the normal and abnormal rhythms of the heart.

## REFERENCES

1. Aviado, D. M., Jr., and Schmidt, C. F. Reflexes from stretch receptors in blood vessels, heart and lungs, *Physiol. Rev.* *35*:247, 1955.
2. *CIBA Foundation Symposium: Adrenergic Mechanisms.* Boston, Little, Brown, 1960.
3. Dawes, G. S. and Comroe, J. H., Jr. Chemoreflexes from the heart and lungs, *Physiol. Rev.* *34*:167, 1954.
4. Folkow, B., Heymans, C. and Neil, E. Integrated aspects of cardiovascular regulation. Chap. 49 in: *Handbook of Physiology,* Sec. 2, vol. 3, W. F. Hamilton, ed., Washington, D.C., Amer. Physiol. Soc., 1965.
5. Heymans, C. and Neil, E. *Reflexogenic Areas of the Cardiovascular System.*

Boston, Little, Brown, 1958.

6. Randall, W. C. *Nervous Control of the Heart.* Baltimore, Williams, Wilkins, 1965.
7. Rushmer, R. F. Effects of nerve stimulation and hormones on the heart; the role of the heart in general circulatory regulation. Chap. 16 in: *Handbook of Physiology,* Sec. 2, vol. 1, W. F. Hamilton, ed., Washington, D.C., Amer. Physiol. Soc., 1965.
8. James, T. N. Anatomy of the human sinus node, *Anat. Rec. 141*:109, 1961.
9. James, T. N. Anatomy of the sinus node of the dog, *Anat. Rec. 143*:251, 1962.
10. James, T. N. Anatomy of the cardiac conduction system of the rabbit. Unpublished observations.
11. James, T. N. Anatomy of the sinus node, AV node and os cordis of the beef heart, *Anat. Rec. 15*:361, 1965.
12. James, T. N., Sherf, L., Fine, G. and Morales, A. R. Comparative ultrastructure of the sinus node in man and dog, *Circulation 34*:139, 1966.
13. Kawamura, K. Electron microscope studies on the cardiac conduction system of the dog. II. The sinoatrial and atrioventricular nodes, *Jap. Circulat. J. 25*:973, 1961.
14. Torii, H. Electron microscope observations of the S-A and A-V nodes and Purkinje fibers of the rabbit, *Jap. Circulat. J. 26*:39, 1962.
15. Trautwein, W. and Uchizono, K. Electron microscopic and electrophysiologic study of the pacemaker in the sinoatrial node of the rabbit heart, *Z. Zellforsch. 61*:96, 1963.
16. Hayashi, K. An electron microscope study on the conduction system of the cow heart, *Jap. Circulat. J. 26*:765, 1962.
17. Dewey, M. M. and Barr, L. A study of the structure and distribution of the nexus, *J. Cell. Biol. 23*:553, 1964.
18. Carbonell, L. M. Esterases of the conductive system of the heart, *J. Histochem. Cytochem. 4*:87, 1956.
19. James, T. N. and Spence, C. A. Distribution of cholinesterase within the sinus node and AV node of the human heart, *Anat. Rec. 155*:151, 1966.
20. Koelle, G. B. The histochemical identification of acetylcholinesterase in cholinergic, adrenergic, and sensory nerves, *J. Pharmacol. 114*:167, 1955.
21. Muller, E. and Pearse, A. G. E. Localization of monoamine oxidase in mammalian and reptilian heart, *Brit. Heart J. 37*:116, 1965.
22. James, T. N. Morphology of the human atrioventricular node, with remarks pertinent to its electrophysiology, *Amer. Heart J. 62*:756, 1961.
23. James, T. N. Anatomy of the AV node of the dog, *Anat. Rec. 148*:15, 1964.
24. Patten, B. M. The development of the sinoventricular conduction system, *Univ. Mich. Med. Bull. 22*:1, 1956.
25. Sherf, L. and James, T. N. A new look at some old questions in clinical electrocardiography, *Henry Ford Hosp. Med. Bull. 14*:265, 1966.
26. Juhasz-Nagy, A. and Szentivanyi, M. Localisation of the receptors of the coronary chemoreflex in the dog, *Arch. Int. Pharmacodyn. 131*:39, 1961.
27. James, T. N. The connecting pathways between the sinus node and the AV node and between the right and the left atrium in the human heart, *Amer. Heart J. 66*:498, 1963.
28. Horiba, M. Stimulus conduction in atria studied by means of intracellular microelectrode. Part I. That in Bachmann's Bundle, *Jap. Heart J. 4*:333, 1963.
29. Sano, T. and Yamagishi, S. Spread of excitation from the sinus node, *Circulat. Res. 16*:423, 1965.
30. Takayasu, M., Takasaki, H., Nishii, N., Tateishi, Y., Osawa, M., Tamagaki, A., Fujiwara, M., Shinagawa, H. and Ikuta, S. Studies on the atrial stimulus conduction, *Jap. Circulat. J. 18*:1, 1955.
31. Wagner, M. L., Lazzara, R., Weiss, R. M. and Hoffman, B. E. Specialized conducting fibers in the interatrial band, *Circulat. Res. 18*:502, 1966.
32. Wallace, A. G., Holsinger, J., Sealy, W. C. and Young, W. G. Physiologic evidence for a specialized conduction system within the atrium, *Clin. Res. 15*:60, 1967.
33. Vassalle, M. and Hoffman, B. F. The spread of sinus activation during potas-

sium administration, *Circulat. Res. 17:* 285, 1965.
34. Bachmann, G. The inter-auricular time interval, *Amer. J. Physiol. 41:*309, 1916.
35. Wenckebach, K. F. Beiträge zur Kenntnis der menschlichen Herztätigkeit, *Arch. Anat. Physiol. 1-2:*1, 1907.
36. Wenckebach, K. F. Beiträge zur Kenntnis der menschlichen Herztätigkeit, *Arch. Anat. Physiol. 3:*53, 1908.
37. Paes de Carvalho, A., de Mello, W. C. and Hoffman, B. F. Electrophysiological evidence for specialized fiber types in rabbit atrium, *Amer. J. Physiol. 196:* 483, 1959.
38. Thorel, C. Vorläufige Mitteilung über eine besondere Muskelverbindung zwischen der cava superior und dem His' schen Bündel. *München. Med. Wschr. 56:*2159, 1909.
39. Thorel, C. Ueber den Aufbau des Sinusknotens und seine Verbindung mit der cava superior und den Wenckebach'schen Bündeln , *München. Med. Wschr. 57:*183, 1910.
40. Moe, G. K., Preston, J. B. and Burlington, H. Physiologic evidence for a dual A-V transmission system, *Circulat. Res. 4:*357, 1956.
41. Alessi, R., Nusynowitz, M., Abildskov, J. A. and Moe, G. K. Non-uniform distribution of vagal effects on the atrial refractory period, *Amer. J. Physiol. 194:*406, 1958.
42. Moe, G. K. and Abildskov, J. A. Atrial fibrillation as a self-sustaining arrhythmia independent of focal discharge, *Amer. Heart J. 58:*59, 1959.
43. James, T. N. and Carrera, G. M. The pathogenesis of arrhythmias associated with metastatic tumors of the heart, *New Eng. J. Med. 260:*869, 1959.
44. Rossi, L. and James, T. N. Neurovascular pathology of the heart in progressive muscular dystrophy, *Panminerva Medica 6:*357, 1960.
45. James, T. N. and Reynolds, E. W., Jr. Pathology of the cardiac conduction system in a case of diphtheria associated with atrial arrhythmias and heart block, *Circulation 28:*263, 1963.
46. James, T. N. Myocardial infarction and atrial arrhythmias, *Circulation 24:*761, 1961.
47. James, T. N. Pericarditis and the sinus node, *Arch. Intern. Med. 110:*305, 1962.
48. James, T. N. Posterior myocardial infarction, *J. Mich. State Med. Soc. 60:* 1409, 1961.
49. James, T. N. Arrhythmias and conduction disturbances in acute myocardial infarction, *Amer. Heart J. 64:*416, 1962.
50. Thomas, M. and Woodgate, D. Effect of atropine on bradycardia and hypotension in acute myocardial infarction, *Brit. Heart J. 28:*409, 1966.
51. Fluck, D. C., Olsen, E. and Mounsey, J. P. D. Bradycardia in acute myocardial infarction, *Brit. Heart J. 28:* 430, 1966.
52. James, T. N. and Nadeau, R. A. Direct perfusion of the sinus node: An experimental model for pharmacologic and electrophysiologic studies of the heart, *Henry Ford Hosp. Med. Bull. 10:*21, 1962.
53. James, T. N. and Nadeau, R. A. Sinus bradycardia during injections directly into the sinus node artery, *Amer. J. Physiol. 204:*9, 1963.
54. James, T. N. and Nadeau, R. A. Effects of sympathomimetic amines studied by direct perfusion of the sinus node, *Amer. J. Physiol. 204:*591, 1963.
55. James, T. N. and Nadeau, R. A. The chronotropic action of tyramine studied by direct perfusion of the sinus node through its artery, *J. Pharmacol. Exp. Ther. 144:*83, 1964.
56. Green, E. W. and James, T. N. Chronotropic action of reserpine and guanethidine studied by direct perfusion of the sinus node, *Clin. Res. 12:*183, 1964.
57. Rolett, E. L. and Black, W. L. Comparison of the chronotropic action of dopamine and norepinephrine infused directly into the sinus node artery, *Circulation 34* (suppl. III): 200, 1966.
58. Sherf, L. and James, T. N. Chronotropic action of amino acids, *J. Pharmacol. Exp. Ther. 153:*197, 1966.
59. James, T. N. and Nadeau, R. A. The chronotropic and vagal-blocking effects of DCI studied by direct perfusion of the sinus node, *J. Pharmacol. Exp. Ther. 140:*73, 1963.

60. James, T. N. and Nadeau, R. A. The chronotropic and vagal-blocking actions of naphthylisoproterenol studied by direct perfusion of the sinus node, *J. Pharmacol. Exp. Ther.* *143*:350, 1964.
61. Wallace, A. G., Troyer, W. G., Lesage, M. A. and Zotti, E. F. Electrophysiologic effects of isoproterenol and beta blocking agents in awake dogs, *Circulat. Res.* *18*:140, 1966.
62. James, T. N. and Bear, E. S. Effects of ethanol and acetaldehyde on the heart, *Amer. Heart J.* *74*:243, 1967.
63. James, T. N. and Nadeau, R. A. The chronotropic effect of digitalis studied by direct perfusion of the sinus node, *J. Pharmacol. Exp. Ther.* *139*:42, 1963.
64. Kikuchi, K. and Chen, K. K. Pharmacology of Rhodexin A[1], *J. Pharmacol. Exp. Ther.* *146*:365, 1964.
65. Nadeau, R. A. and James, T. N. Antagonistic effects on the sinus node of acetylstrophanthidin and adrenergic stimulation, *Circulat. Res.* *13*:388, 1963.
66. Mendez, C., Aceves, J. and Mendez, R. The anti-adrenergic action of digitalis on the refractory period of the A-V transmission system, *J. Pharmacol. Exp. Ther.* *131-132*:199, 1961.
67. James, T. N. and Nadeau, R. A. The mechanism of action of quinidine on the sinus node studied by direct perfusion through its artery, *Amer. Heart J.* *67*:804, 1964.
68. Nadeau, R. A. and James, T. N. The effects of nicotine on heart rate studied by direct perfusion of the sinus node, *Amer. J. Physiol.* *212*:911-16, 1967.
69. James, T. N. and Nadeau, R. A. Chronotropic action of veratridine studied by direct perfusion of the sinus node, *Henry Ford Hosp. Med. Bull.* *12*:169, 1964.
70. Dawes, G. S. Studies on veratrum alkaloids. VII. Receptor areas in the coronary arteries and elsewhere as revealed by the use of veratridine, *J. Pharmacol. Exp. Ther.* *89*:325, 1947.
71. Feldberg, W. and Lewis, G. P. The action of peptides on the adrenal medulla. Release of adrenaline by bradykinin and angiotensin, *J. Physiol.* *171*:98, 1964.
72. James, T. N. Absence of direct chronotropic action of angiotensin infused into the sinus node artery, *Amer. J. Physiol.* *209*:571, 1965.
73. James, T. N. and Nadeau, R. A. The chronotropic effect of bradykinin studied by direct perfusion of the sinus node, *Clin. Res.* *10*:173, 1962.
74. Nishith, S. D., Davis, L. D. and Youmans, W. B. Cardioaccelerator action of angiotensin, *Amer. J. Physiol.* *202*:237, 1962.
75. Youmans, W. B., Davis, L. D., Krasney, J. A., Paudler, F. T., Smith, D. C. and Pua, K. H. Effects of angiotensin on cardiac rate after tetraethylammonium chloride and bretylium tosylate, *Fed. Proc.* *23*:120, 1964.
76. Schneider, J. A. and Yonkman, F. F. Species differences in the respiratory and cardiovascular response to serotonin (5-Hydroxytryptamine), *J. Pharmacol. Exp. Ther.* *111*:84, 1954.
77. James, T. N. The chronotropic action of serotonin studied by direct perfusion of the sinus node, *J. Pharmacol. Exp. Ther.* *146*:209, 1964.
78. Whitehouse, F. W. and James, T. N. Chronotropic action of glucagon on the sinus node, *Proc. Soc. Exp. Biol. Med.* *122*:823, 1966.
79. Sutherland, E. W. and Rall, T. W. The relation of adenosine-3′, 5′-phosphate and phosphorylase to the actions of catecholamines and other hormones, *Pharmacol. Rev.* *12*:265, 1960.
80. James, T. N. The chronotropic action of ATP and related compounds studied by direct perfusion of the sinus node, *J. Pharmacol. Exp. Ther.* *149*:233, 1965.
81. Levine, R. A. and Vogel, J. A. Cardiovascular and metabolic effects of cyclic adenosine 3′, 5′-monophosphate in unanesthetized dogs, *J. Pharmacol. Exp. Ther.* *151*:262, 1966.
82. Green, H. N. and Stoner, H. B. *Biological Actions of the Adenine Nucleotides.* London, H. K. Lewis, 1950.
83. Imai, S., Riley, A. L. and Berne, R. M. Effect of ischemia on adenine nucleotides in cardiac and skeletal muscle, *Circulat. Res.* *15*:443, 1964.
84. James, T. N. Cholinergic mechanisms in

the sinus node with particular reference to the action of hemicholinium, *Circulat. Res. 19*:347, 1966.

85. Burn, W. H., Williams, E. M. V. and Walker, U. M. The effects of acetylcholine in the heart-lung preparation including the production of auricular fibrillation, *J. Physiol. 128*:277, 1955.
86. Burn, J. H., Williams, E. M. V. and Walker, J. M. The production of block and auricular fibrillation in the heart-lung preparation by inhibitors of cholinesterase, *Brit. Heart J. 17*:431, 1955.
87. Burn, J. H. Acetylcholine and cardiac fibrillation, *Brit. Med. Bull. 13*:181, 1957.
88. Han, J., de Jalon, P. G. and Moe, G. K. Adrenergic effects on ventricular vulnerability, *Circulat. Res. 14*:516, 1964.
89. Yanowitz, F., Preston, J. B. and Abildskov, J. A. Functional distribution of right and left stellate innervation to the ventricles: Production of neurogenic electrocardiographic changes by unilateral alteration of sympathetic tone, *Circulat. Res. 18*:416, 1966.
90. Wegria, R. and Nickerson, N. D. The effects of papaverine, epinephrine and quinidine on the fibrillation threshold of the mammalian ventricles, *J. Pharmacol. Exp. Ther. 75*:50, 1942.
91. Hoffman, B. F., Siebens, A. A., Cranefield, P. F. and Brooks, C. McC. The effect of epinephrine and norepinephrine on ventricular vulnerability, *Circulat. Res. 3*:140, 1955.
92. Iversen, L. L., Fischer, J. E. and Axelrod, J. Enhancement of H3-Norepinephrine uptake in rat tissues by O-methylated metabolites of catecholamines, *J. Pharmacol. Exp. Ther. 154*:56, 1966.
93. James, T. N. and Nadeau, R. A. Selective cholinergic stimulation and blockade of the sinus node by direct perfusion through its artery, *J. Lab. Clin. Med. 62*:40, 1963.
94. Schueler, F. W. A new group of respiratory paralyzants. 1. The "Hemicholiniums," *J. Pharmacol. Exp. Ther. 115*:127, 1955.
95. MacIntosh, F. C., Birks, R. I. and Sastry, P. B. Pharmacologic inhibition of acetylcholine synthesis, *Nature 178*:1181, 1956.
96. Burn, J. H. and Rand, M. J. Acetylcholine in adrenergic transmission, *Ann. Rev. Pharmacol. 5*:163, 1965.

# AUTONOMIC CONTROL OF CARDIAC RHYTHM*

BRIAN F. HOFFMAN

Department of Pharmacology
Columbia University College of Physicians and Surgeons
New York, N. Y.

THE objective of this paper is to describe the manner in which the mediators liberated by the postganglionic nerve terminals of the sympathetic and parasympathetic divisions of the autonomic nervous system influence the generation and conduction of impulses in the heart. In essence this is a description of the effects of norepinephrine and acetylcholine on cells of the mammalian sinoatrial node, atrium, and atrioventricular node and the effects of norepinephrine on cells of the His-Purkinje system and ventricle.

For the most part the description will be made in terms of the transmembrane potentials recorded through an intracellular microelectrode from a single cardiac cell or fiber.[1] The main reason for using this technique in a study of the control of cardiac rate and rhythm is that it provides graphic evidence of two sorts which cannot be obtained readily from the electrocardiogram. First, it permits records to be obtained from a single cell or small group of cells in the cardiac syncytium. Thus instead of having to read the output of a presumptive pacemaker from the P wave or QRS complex, one is able to record directly from the automatic cell or cell group acting as pacemaker. This permits more precise identification of both actual and latent pacemakers in terms of location and mechanism. Second, records of transmembrane potentials show the mechanism, to the extent that the electrical signal can be thought of as a mechanism, by which agents alter rate or rhythm. This has permitted a better understanding of the action of autonomic mediators on cardiac automaticity and conduction.

Before considering the manner in which autonomic mediators influence cardiac cells it is necessary to describe a typical recording of cardiac transmembrane potential, the changes in transmembrane

*Presented at the *Conference on Mechanisms and Management of Arrhythmias,* held by the New York Heart Association at the Hotel Waldorf-Astoria, New York, N. Y., January 24, 1967.

Original studies were supported in part by grants from the U.S. Public Health Service (HE-08508 from the National Heart Institute); the American Heart Association, Inc.; the New York Heart Association, Inc.; and from Eli Lilly and Company.

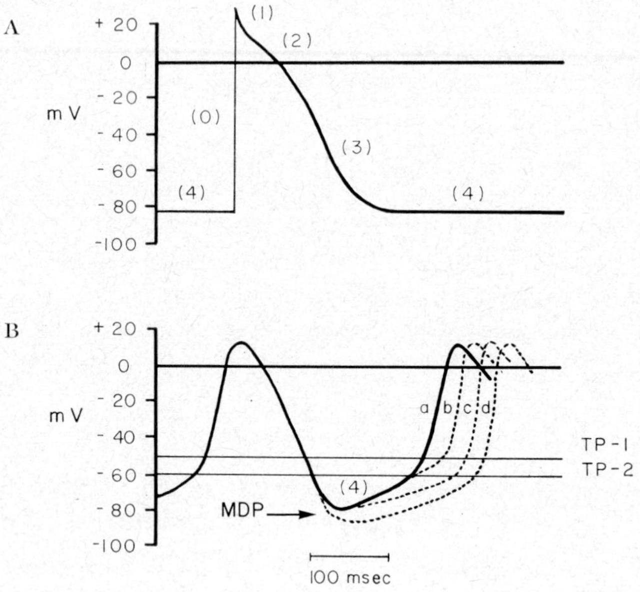


Fig. 1. Diagrammatic records of transmembrane potentials recorded from a single atrial muscle fiber (*A*) and a single fiber in the sinoatrial node (*B*). The record in A shows a steady resting potential (phase 4) and an action potential with a rapid phase of depolarization (phase 0) and slower repolarization (phases 1, 2, and 3). The record in B, from the nodal fiber, shows a slower depolarization during the action potential upstroke, repolarization which reaches a maximum value (MDP) and then a slow, spontaneous depolarization during phase 4. The slow phase 4 depolarization lowers membrane potential to the threshold potential (TP-1) and initiates an automatic beat (*a*). A change in the level of threshold potential to TP-2 delays the response to (*b*); an increase in cycle length also might result either from a decrease in the slope of phase 4 depolarization (*c*) or from an increase in maximum diastolic potential (*d*).

potential which are responsible for normal automaticity, and the changes commonly responsible for alterations in rate.[1, 2] Figure 1 shows records of transmembrane potentials from an atrial fiber (*A*) and a fiber in the sinoatrial node (*B*). For the atrial fiber it is possible to describe a resting potential (phase 4) and a transmembrane action potential. The latter usually is subdivided into phases of depolarization (phase 0) and repolarization (phases 1, 2, and 3). It should be noted that the resting, or diastolic, potential (phase 4) is constant until the onset of phase 0. The transmembrane potential recorded from the automatic fiber in the sinoatrial node differs in several respects from that of the atrium; the rate of depolarization during phase 0 is less and the voltage-time course of repolarization is different. More important, however, is the voltage-time course of membrane potential during phase 4. At the end of repolarization the fiber attains its maximum diastolic potential (MDP); immediately thereafter a slow depolarization lowers transmembrane potential toward zero. If this slow diastolic depolarization reduces transmembrane potential to a critical value called the threshold potential (TP), excitation of the cell occurs and an action potential results. This spontaneous depolarization during phase 4 is the normal automatic mechanism for cardiac cells and is present in the sinus node, ectopic supraventricular pacemakers, and cells of the His-Purkinje system. Since slow diastolic depolarization is present normally in all these cells,[3] they may all be designated as latent pacemakers; that cell which first attains threshold and generates an action potential usually serves as pacemaker. Exceptions to this rule occur if conduction from the cell which fires first is slow enough to permit another automatic cell to activate the heart or if two or more automatic cells which are appropriately separated in the heart fire more or less synchronously.

The record in Figure 1*B* also demonstrates the usual changes in membrane behavior which are responsible for changes in the rate of a normal automatic fiber. Briefly stated, anything which changes the time required for phase 4 depolarization to lower membrane potential to the threshold potential will change the rate of an automatic fiber. The most obvious variable is the slope of membrane potential during phase 4. Other variables which have been shown to alter rate are the level of maximum diastolic potential and threshold potential. An increase in the slope of phase 4, a decrease in maximum diastolic potential, or an increase in the level of threshhold potential (i.e., a larger negative value) will increase the rate of the automatic fiber. A change in any one variable in the opposite direction will decrease the rate; simultaneous changes in two or more will act synergistically or antagonistically depending on the direction of change for each.

In theory, then, the autonomic nervous system might change the rate by acting on any one or all three of these variables. In addition, effects on rate and rhythm might result from simultaneous effects on different automatic foci and from effects on conduction that will be described subsequently. Also, it is important to realize that equal concentrations of mediator may have effects on different cells and cell types which differ either quantitatively or qualitatively, and that during activation of the efferent autonomic cardiac fibers the concentration of

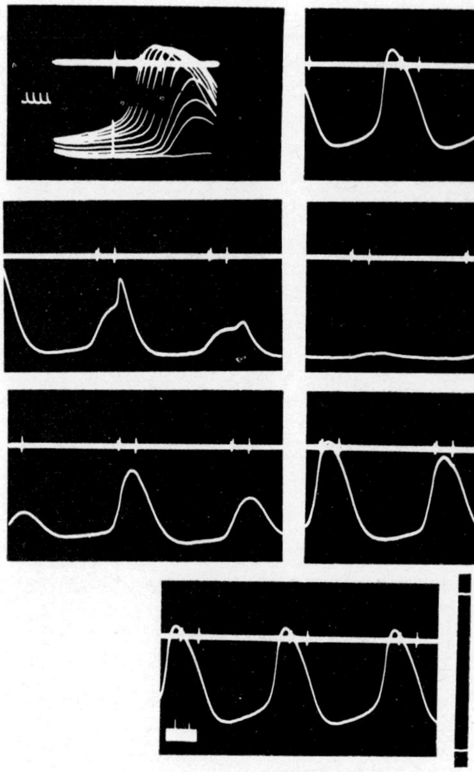

Fig. 2. Transmembrane potentials recorded from a fiber in the sinoatrial node of the isolated rabbit atrium showing the effects of acetylcholine. In each figure the upper trace serves as the zero reference line and also shows an electrogram recorded directly from atrial muscle. Time marks in the first frame are at intervals of 10 and in the last frame at intervals of 100 msec; voltage calibration after the final frame = 100 mV. The first frame shows the effects of acetylcholine as a series of superimposed traces; the other frames show the same changes in separate records. Note that after local application of acetylcholine from an extracellular micropipette there is a decrease in the slope of phase 4, an increase in maximum diastolic potential, and then a decrease in the response recorded through the microelectrode until only small graded electrotonic potentials remain. At this time atrial activity continues, as shown by the electrogram. The last two frames show recovery from the effects of acetylcholine.

mediator achieved in the vicinity of different cells may be quite variable.

The effects of acetylcholine or vagal stimulation on automaticity of the sinoatrial node have been demonstrated by several investigators[4, 5] and are similar to those shown for the sinus venosus[6, 7] of the frog. The action of acetylcholine on a pacemaker cell results in three changes: there is a decrease in the slope of diastolic depolarization, an increase in maximum diastolic potential, and usually a shift of the pacemaker to another site in the node. If vagal action is weak, the first two effects predominate; if vagal action is stronger, a shift in the site of the pacemaker seems to be an inevitable consequence. This shift in site may result either from differences in local sensitivity to acetylcholine or from differences in the local concentration of transmitter. In the case of vagal stimulation, the density of nerve terminals may not be uniform; in the case of administered acetylcholine, access of drug to sensitive membrane may not be uniform. Thus it is difficult to evaluate the two possibilities separately or to rule out one or the other.

With high concentrations of acetylcholine two other effects may occur. Phase 4 depolarization may be abolished completely, resulting in sinus arrest, or conduction within the node may be markedly impaired. The latter effect is shown in Figure 2. Although we are familiar with the concept that acetylcholine increases decrement of conduction to the point of block in the atrioventricular node,[8] the fact that it also causes decrement and block in sinus fibers is less familiar.[9] This observation is of some importance in that it shows one possible mechanism by which an impulse initiated in the sinus node might be prevented from exciting the atria; also, it shows that an impulse conducted in the atria may be blocked during its passage into the node and thus fail to discharge a sinus pacemaker. Both these possibilities are of some importance in a consideration of supraventricular arrhythmias.

The effects of acetylcholine on automatic atrial cells located outside the sinoatrial node are similar to those just described but often are less intense. Thus automatic cells of the crista terminalis, whether they are true or latent pacemakers, will be slowed as a result of a decrease in the slope of phase 4 depolarization and an increase in maximum diastolic potential. It is of interest in this regard to comment on certain of the specialized atrial fiber tracts described most recently by James.[10, 11] We have attempted to record from the anterior and posterior internodal tracts in the rabbit heart, structures identified as the sinoatrial ring bundle by Paes de Carvalho,[12] and from the anterior internodal tract and Bachmann's bundle in the canine atria.[13] Although the fibers of the anterior internodal tract and Bachmann's bundle show many electrophysiological characteristics which reinforce the concept that they are different from ordinary atrial muscle, we have not recorded phase 4 depolarization from either structure. It thus is not permissible to assume that all specialized fibers will be automatic.

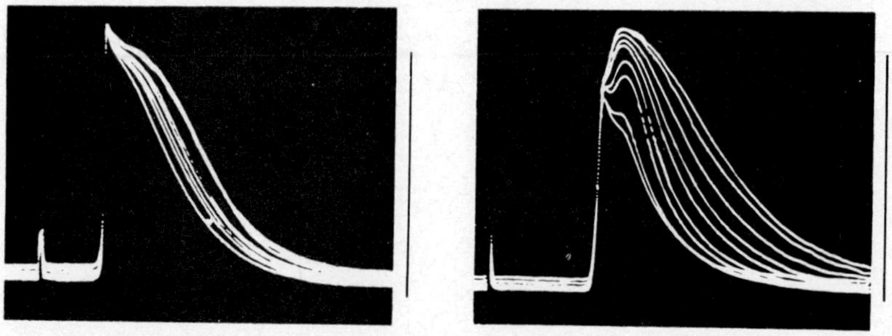


Fig. 3. The effects of acetylcholine on transmembrane action potentials recorded from two different types of fibers in the isolated rabbit atrium. The preparation was driven by regularly applied stimuli and acetylcholine was applied locally, in the vicinity of the recording electrode, from a small extracellular micropipette. In *A* it can be seen that acetylcholine increases the rate of repolarization and slightly increases the resting potential but does not change the amplitude of the action potential upstroke (phase 0). In *B*, application of the same concentration of acetylcholine to a different type of fiber causes, in addition to an increase in the rate of repolarization and the magnitude of the resting potential, a significant decrease in the amplitude of the upstroke of the action potential. (Modified from Paes de Carvalho, ref. 19).

One other action of acetylcholine deserves brief mention; this is its well-known effect on the duration of action potential. Changes in the duration of action potentials recorded from fibers in the sinus node are not marked; acceleration of repolarization becomes more prominent for automatic cells of the crista terminalis and is most marked in the case of ordinary atrial muscle fibers. Recently[14] it has been shown that the action potential of atrial fibers consists of two components and that the latter part of the upstroke may be inscribed at a lower rate than the initial segment of phase 0 (Figure 3). If fibers showing this type of upstroke are exposed to acetylcholine, not only is repolarization enhanced but also the amplitude of the action potential is decreased. This change in amplitude of the action potential may have effects on conduction; for example, it has been implicated as one cause of the changes in A-V transmission induced by acetylcholine.[1]

The effects of stimulation of the sympathetic nerves or of administration of catecholamines on automaticity of sinus node fibers have been studied by a number of investigators.[15, 16] In general, the changes in rate caused by the action of sympathetic transmitters such as norepinephrine result largely from an increase in the slope of diastolic depolarization. Again, as in the case of vagal action, shifts in the site of the pacemaker are frequent; this has made it difficult to evaluate the possibility that threshold potential also may be changed. One other effect of catecholamines is important if we consider its action on fibers which are not normal. When the resting potential has been decreased by a variety of experimental interventions or pathological conditions, exposure of the fibers to catecholamines usually causes an increase in the magnitude of the resting potential. In some instances this increase in resting potential may improve excitability and responsiveness to the extent that conduction will return to areas of block. In this sense one might assume that effects of sympathetic activity on atrial rhythm also may result from abolition of partial, or complete, block between the pacemaker and the remainder of the atrium. In general, the actions of the parasympathetic and sympathetic transmitters are opposite with respect to the initiation and conduction of impulses.

The effects of autonomic transmitters on the electrophysiological properties of the atrioventricular node are well known[1, 17, 18] and will not be reviewed at this time. Instead, we shall consider the actions of acetylcholine and catecholamines on the fibers of the His-Purkinje system. We have consistently found that locally applied acetylcholine, even in high concentrations, does not change the transmembrane potentials recorded from fibers in the His bundle, the bundle branches, or the peripheral Purkinje system; these studies have employed tissue from canine[1] and leporine[19] hearts. It can be assumed, therefore, that activation of the vagus will not by any direct action influence the automaticity of the cells which make up these tissues. On the other hand, catecholamines have a pronounced effect on the slope of diastolic depolarization of the Purkinje fibers. The rate of diastolic depolarization is increased and under appropriate conditions a latent pacemaker will become an actual pacemaker, or multiple pacemakers may appear. There are no important direct effects on the level of maximum diastolic potential of normal fibers. In relation to the effects of the autonomic nervous system on cardiac rate and rhythm one thus would expect that activation of the vagus would slow supraventricular pacemakers by a direct action and permit escape of subsidiary automatic foci in the His-Purkinje system. This seems to be a fortunate arrangement since, under most conditions of reflex activation of the vagus, there is a simultaneous decrease in sympathetic activity. Were acetylcholine to

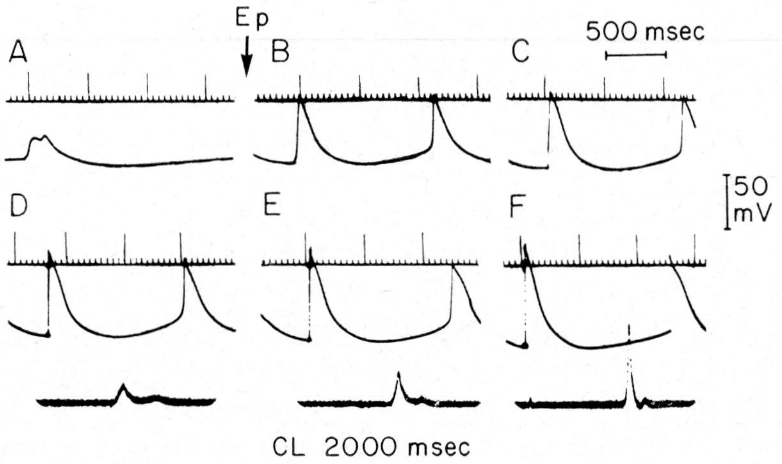


Fig. 4. Effects of epinephrine on transmembrane potentials from a deteriorated, partially depolarized canine Purkinje fiber stimulated at a cycle length of 2000 msec. Deterioration resulted from anoxia in conjunction with the sustained low rate. *A*. Partially depolarized fiber. *B-F*. Addition of l-epinephrine (Ep), $10^{-6}$ $\gamma$/cc, resulted in restoration of maximum diastolic potential toward normal and improvement in amplitude and dV/dt of the action potentials. Also note increased spontaneous phase 4 depolarization and resultant spontaneous beats. Combination of driven and spontaneous beats caused bigeminy. The first action potential in each pair was driven; the second occurred spontaneously. Maximum upstroke velocity (dV/dt) of driven action potentials in *D-F* indicated by amplitude of differentiated spike in bottom trace. (Modified after Singer et al.[22])

decrease the automaticity of all cardiac cells, cardiac arrest would be frequent.

As in the case of acetylcholine, the effects of catecholamines depend in part on the condition of the fiber and of the heart. Under some conditions the action of norepinephrine or epinephrine may impair conduction in the His-Purkinje system. This occurs if there is a marked generalized increase in the slope of diastolic depolarization and if threshold potential is low, i.e., closer to zero than usual. As a result of these two changes the action potential of the Purkinje fibers may be initiated at such a low level of membrane potential that upstroke velocity and amplitude are reduced.[20] Such changes in the amplitude and configuration of the action potential would decrease the velocity of conduction and increase the likelihood of block. In extrapolating from these findings, made on *in vitro* preparations of canine Purkinje fibers, to the diseased heart in situ, one might assume that under certain conditions enhanced sympathetic activity might impair conduction from automatic foci. Conversely, if the transmembrane potential of Purkinje fibers is low because of the action of drugs or pathological processes, it has been clearly demonstrated that catecholamines in proper concentration increase resting potential and improve conduction.[21, 22] Moreover, they may do this without causing much if any increase in automaticity (Figure 4). Again, we are forced to accept the fact that the action of autonomic mediators depends in large part on their concentration, on the condition of the tissue, and on the sensitivity of the tissue to the mediator.

In summary, although the primary direct actions of acetylcholine and norepinephrine on the formation and conduction of impulses can be demonstrated with ease on normal preparations of isolated cardiac tissue, it is not always possible to predict the net effect of variations in autonomic tone on the rhythm of the normal heart. Also, it is even more difficult to predict the effect of such changes in the presence of cardiac disease or after administration of drugs which act on the heart. Because of the possibility that variations in vagal and sympathetic tone may cause arrhythmias due either to altered automaticity or to altered conduction, it seems likely that at least some of the disturbances of rhythm encountered in the clinic are a result of action of the autonomic nervous system.

*REFERENCES*

1. Hoffman, B. F. and Cranefield, P. F. *Electrophysiology of the Heart.* New York, McGraw-Hill, 1960.
2. Weidmann, S. *Elektrophysiologie der Herzmuskelfaser.* Bern, Huber, 1956.
3. Hoffman, B. F. and Cranefield, P. F. The physiological basis of cardiac arrhythmias. *Amer. J. Med. 37*:670-84, 1964.
4. West, T. C. Ultramicroelectrode recording from the cardiac pacemaker. *J. Pharmacol. Exp. Therap. 115*:283-90, 1955.
5. Dudel, J. und Trautwein, W. Der Mechanismus der automatischen rhythmischen Impulsbildung der Herzmuskelfaser. *Pflügers Arch. Ges. Physiol. 267*: 553-65, 1958.
6. Castillo, J. del and Katz, B. Production of membrane potential changes in the frog's heart by inhibitory nerve impulses. *Nature 175*:1035, 1955.
7. Hutter, O. F. and Trautwein, W. Effect of vagal stimulation on the sinus venosus of the frog's heart. *Nature 176*:512-13, 1955.
8. Cranefield, P. F., Hoffman, B. F. and Paes de Carvalho, A. Effects of acetylcholine on single fibers of the atrioventricular node. *Circ. Res. 7*:19, 1959.
9. Paes de Carvalho, A. and Almeida, D. F. Spread of activity through the atrioventricular node. *Circ. Res. 8*:801, 1960.
10. James, T. N. The connecting pathways between the sinus node and A-V node and between the right and left atrium in the human heart. *Amer. Heart J. 66*:498, 1963.
11. James, T. N. Cardiac innervation: Anatomic and pharmacologic relations, *Bull. N.Y. Acad. Med. 43*:1041-46, 1967.
12. Paes de Carvalho, A., de Mello, W. C. and Hoffman, B. F. Electrophysiological

evidence for specialized fiber types in rabbit atrium. *Amer. J. Physiol. 196:* 483, 1959.

13. Wagner, M. L., Lazzara, R., Weiss, R. M. and Hoffman, B. F. Specialized conducting fibers in the interatrial band. *Circ. Res. 18*:502-18, 1966.
14. Paes de Carvalho, A., Hoffman, B. F. and Langan, W. B. Two components of the cardiac action potential. *Nature 211*:938-40, 1966.
15. West, T. C., Falk, G. and Cervoni, P. Drug alteration of transmembrane potentials in atrial pacemaker cells. *J. Pharmacol. Exp. Therap. 117*:245-52, 1956.
16. Trautwein, W. Generation and conduction of impulses in the heart as affected by drugs. *Pharmacol. Rev. 15*:277-332, 1963.
17. Hoffman, B. F., Paes de Carvalho, A., de Mello, W. C. and Cranefield, P. F. Electrical activity of single fibers of the atrioventricular node. *Circ. Res. 7*:11-18, 1959.
18. Paes de Carvalho, A. and Langan, W. B. Influence of extracellular potassium levels on atrioventricular transmission. *Amer. J. Physiol. 205*:375, 1963.
19. Paes de Carvalho, A. Excitation of the atrioventricular node during normal rhythm. Effects of acetylcholine. In: *Mechanisms and Therapy of Cardiac Arrhythmias*, Dreifus, L. S. and Likoff, W., eds., New York, Grune, Stratton, 1966, pp. 341-352.
20. Hoffman, B. F. Impulse transmission in the mammalian heart. *Circ. Res. 14 & 15,* Suppl. II: 202-209, 1964.
21. Hutter, O. F. and Trautwein, W. Vagal and sympathetic effects on the pacemaker fibers in the sinus venosus of the heart. *J. Gen. Physiol. 39*:715-33, 1956.
22. Singer, D. H. In preparation.

# EXPERIMENTAL NEUROGENIC ARRHYTHMIAS*

CHARLES H. HOCKMAN

Department of Pharmacology
University of Toronto, Toronto, Canada

H. PAGE MAUCK, JR. AND EBBE C. HOFF

Department of Medicine and Division of Psychiatric Research
Medical College of Virginia, Richmond, Va.

DURING the past two decades, researchers from our laboratories have been concerned with elucidating the integrative action of the higher levels of the central nervous system in the regulation of autonomic function. In reporting our recent investigations of experimentally induced cardiac arrhythmias, we should like to place these phenomena within the general framework of central systems modulation of visceral function in a total sense. In brief, we have found that electrical stimulation of specific loci in the forebrain, midbrain, and hindbrain, in both acute and chronic experiments, evokes a variety of cardiovascular responses, including alterations in systemic blood pressure, predictable changes in cardiac rhythm and intracardiac dynamics as well as in circulation in skeletal muscles, the kidneys, gastrointestinal tract, spleen, and other visceral areas. These cardiovascular changes are often accompanied (according to loci stimulated) by other autonomic end effects: specifically, increased salivation, dilatation of the pupils, pilo-erection, increase in the activity of the red bone marrow, and endocrine enhancement, e.g., activation of the adrenal medulla.

The discreteness of cerebral representation of various cardiovascular and other autonomic functions and the specificity with which they can be evoked varies according to the level of the central nervous system examined. For example, pressor areas may be distinguished from depressor areas of various cortical and subcortical levels. Probably cortical levels exert a more specific autonomic control than do diencephalic or mesencephalic levels, whereas the magnitude of response is greater from lower than from higher levels. With threshold stimuli, these cerebro-

*Presented at the *Conference on Mechanisms and Management of Arrhythmias,* held by the New York Heart Association at the Hotel Waldorf-Astoria, New York, N. Y., January 24, 1967.

genic autonomic responses need not be the result of generalized, massive discharges, since they can be obtained regularly in experimental situations in which the stimuli are carefully controlled and from which electroencephalographic monitoring reveals no seizure activity. Specifically, the alterations in cardiac rhythm to be discussed here are observed when diencephalic and mesencephalic structures are systematically explored with electrical stimuli of known parameters. These areas seem to exert a more definite regulation of heart rhythm than do telencephalic loci, from which arrhythmias are only rarely evoked.

The concept that cardiovascular, secretory, and other visceral as well as skeletal motor activities are integrated at various higher levels of the central nervous system, including the cerebral cortex, rests upon a voluminous literature covering a period of about a hundred years. The germinal idea was first set forth by Hughlings Jackson,[1] who expressed the conviction that not only movements ordinarily so called, that is to say, voluntary motions of the body, are represented in the cerebrum, but that movements of arteries and viscera are also so represented. Jackson based this holistic formulation upon the observation that gross disease of the brain, e.g., tumors, produced not only muscular but also circulatory and other visceral symptoms.

The announcement in 1870 by Fritsch and Hitzig[2] that skeletal movements could be elicited in animals by appropriate electrical stimulation of frontal regions of the contralateral cerebral hemisphere at once directed attention to localizing investigations by the method of stimulation of accessible cortical areas. Many experimenters began to explore the dorsolateral surfaces of the hemisphere in an effort to show that changes in the activity of the viscera could also be produced by cortical stimulation. Thus, Schiff 1874[3] and Danilewsky[4] reported that stimulation of the cortex in dogs caused acceleration of the heart that was independent of changes in arterial blood pressure; however, the latter response could also be evoked. These and subsequent experimental studies on animals of the effects of cerebral stimulation upon systemic arterial blood pressure and heart rate brought together, by the third decade of this century, an array of evidence from which it could be inferred that the higher levels of the central nervous system may play an actual role in the regulation of cardiovascular function. This inference was reinforced by observations of vasomotor disturbances following brain damage in patients, and localized lesions in experimental animals.

In spite of this, the role of the cerebral cortex in the regulation of autonomic activity was by no means fully established, widely accepted, or well understood. Thus in 1929 Bard[5] voiced a general skepticism of the earlier work by saying that "many of the effects which were produced are to be accounted for on the basis of spread of strong stimulating currents to subcortical regions or to the production of cortical epilepsy in which a widespread and unphysiological discharge occurs."

A crucial objective in the middle 1930's was thus to determine whether vasomotor phenomena evoked by application of electrical currents to the cerebral cortex were indeed restricted to stimulation of specific neuronal elements within the cortex. Hoff and Green[6] demonstrated that pressor and depressor points on the cortex could be localized discretely within 2 to 3 mm. of each other and that topical application of the local anesthetic, dibucaine, to an excitable locus abolished the responses from this point but that they recurred on plunging the electrode 3 or 4 mm. into the cortex so as to penetrate beyond the locally anesthetized region. Also, vasomotor responses from a given cortical locus were abolished by undercutting the particular locus so as to disconnect its anatomical projections while preserving electrical contact. On surgical extirpation of a block of cortex, including the responsive loci in acute experiments, stimulation of the exposed white matter in the center of the acute lesion also yielded vasomotor changes. If the cortical block was ablated aseptically sufficiently long in advance to assure complete degeneration of the descending fibers, stimulation of the crater was later without effect although intact cortical surfaces adjacent to the lesion were still excitable. Thus, vasomotor responses from the cortex were shown to depend upon an anatomically and physiologically intact corticofugal system. Moreover, the autonomic responses from the cortex were chiefly limited to areas in the frontal lobes in both cats and subhuman primates.

The question of discreteness of representation of various centrally induced cardiovascular and other responses is one to which experimental information does not yet give complete answers; however, some evidence is available. Thus, in experiments in acute stimulation in cats, pressor pathways from the isocortex may be distinguished from others enhancing adrenal medullary activity. Ferguson, Folkow, Mitts, and Hoff[7] obtained transient pressor responses as well as increased adrenal medullary activity from stimulation of loci on the anterior sigmoid gyri and of corticofugal fibers in the internal capsule. By changing electrode positions it was possible to separate the activation of fibers mainly responsible for the rise in blood pressure from those influencing the adrenal medulla. This can be interpreted to mean that vasomotor and adrenal secretory responses from the isocortex may be mediated by somewhat discrete pathways and suggests a selective control at the isocortical level.

Within the greater limbic system and its complicated interconnections, there is evidence suggesting some specificity of location of primary control of cardiovascular functions with dual mechanisms permitting a balance between sympathetic and parasympathetic influence. Predominance of one or the other of the divisions of the autonomic nervous system may depend on such variables as brain localization, species differences, stages and types of anesthesia, and frequency and other characteristics of the applied stimuli.

While a number of descending central pathways subserving autonomic function have been specified, the ascending systems that serve physiologically to activate cortical and subcortical areas of cardiovascular control (including arrhythmogenic areas) are not fully delineated.

For a number of years we have been studying electrocardiographic changes resulting from cerebral stimulation in an attempt to identify central nervous system mechanisms modulating cardiac rhythm, and to determine the role played by the divisions of the autonomic nervous system in the mediation of such changes. In one such study, Mauck, Hockman, and Hoff[8] examined disturbances in rhythm resembling the complex described by Wolff, Parkinson, and White in their classical paper published in 1930.[9] An aberrant rhythm resembling this clinical phenomenon was reported by Weinberg and Fuster[10] after electrical stimulation of the posterior hypothalamus. Similar abnormal complexes were also elicited experimentally by Parker, Gunn, and Lynn[11] by stimulation of both the posterior hypothalamus and midbrain reticular formation. The question as to the division of the autonomic nervous system mediating these cardiac arrhythmias was thus raised: Weinberg and Fuster argued for an exclusive sympathetic influence; Parker and his colleagues ascribed the induced arrhythmias to reflex vagal control.

In our experiments[8] unipolar electrodes were stereotaxically guided into the reticular formation of adult boxer dogs anesthetized with thiamylal sodium (Surital sodium). The stimuli consisted of 10-second trains of 60 c.p.s. since wave pulses. The intensity of the stimulus, dictated by the threshold response of the animal, varied from 0.5 to 1 volt.

Electrical stimulation with 2 mm. in any direction of the given coordinates elicited alternate ECG complexes characterized by a shortened P-R interval, a widened QRS complex, constant P-P and R-R intervals, the presence of a delta wave and a P-S interval identical to that seen in the normal complex. These WPW-like complexes occurred with a latency of 20 to 30 seconds and persisted for 80 to 120 seconds. The onset of these aberrant complexes was invariably preceded by an increased rate, bursts of ventricular tachycardia, multifocal ventricular premature beats, premature nodal beats, shifting atrial pacemaker and, rarely, atrial fibrillation. These bursts appeared from 8 to 12 seconds after the onset of stimulation. Sinus pauses and ventricular and nodal escape beats were in evidence in some experiments. It was found that stimulation of the mesencephalic reticular formation consistently produced a pronounced pressor response. The atrial, nodal, and ventricular arrhythmias coincided with the rising phase of the blood pressure and the peak of the pressor effect. The onset of the alternating aberrant complexes, however, was most frequently observed as the blood pressure was returning to its prestimulation level and, in some instances, the phenomenon persisted for several minutes after the blood pressure had returned to its control level.

Bilateral section of the vagosympathetic trunks in the neck had no effect upon the production of aberrant cardiac rhythms and, after such bilateral section, electrical stimulation in the mesencephalon gave arrhythmic responses identical to those seen in intact animals. On the other hand, section of the spinal cord at the level of the second cervical vertebra abolished the response. It appears that the abnormal rhythm elicited is not a parasympathetic manifestation, but is mediated exclusively by the sympathetic division of the autonomic nervous system.

Inasmuch as one cannot differentiate with certainty between ventricular preexcitation and fused ventricular premature beats when the aberrant electrocardiographic complex is alternating with a normal sinus beat, the results from this study do show that it is unlikely that the ventricular response is the result of an independent ectopic focus, since electrical stimulation of the distal cut end of the right vagosympathetic trunk suppressed sinoatrial node activity and thus abolished the WPW-like phenomenon.

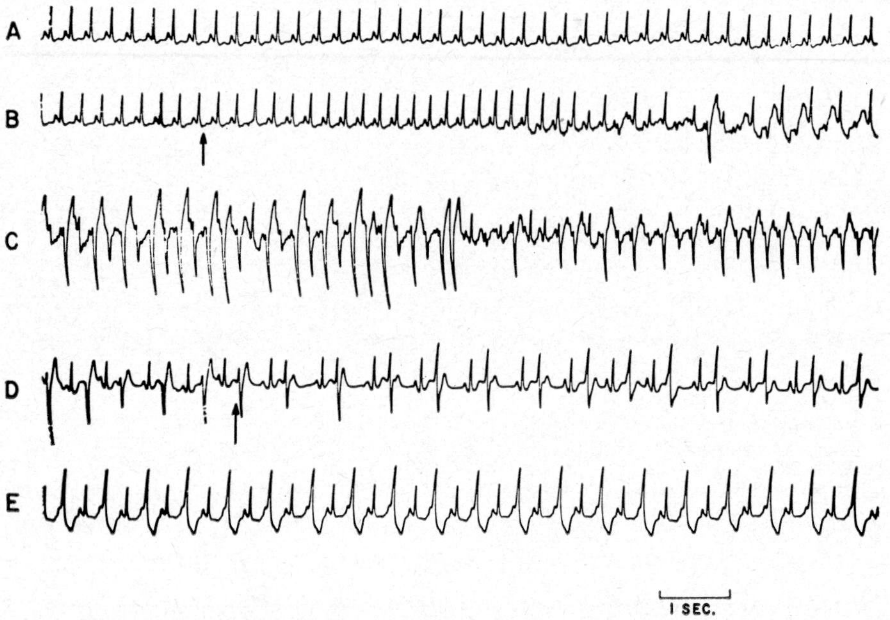


Fig. 1. A spectrum of arrhythmias elicited by electrical stimulation of a locus in the mesencephalic reticular formation. *A,* control record. *B,* arrow indicates onset of stimulation. *C,* during stimulation. *D,* arrow indicates offset of stimulus. *E,* fusion contractions that preceded a return to sinus rhythm. Reproduced from Charles H. Hockman, H. Page Mauck, Jr., Ebbe C. Hoff: *Amer. Heart J. 71*:697, 1966, by permission of the C. V. Mosby Company, St. Louis, Mo.

In a subsequent investigation of the role of the higher levels of the central nervous system in the mediation of ectopic cardiac rhythms, Hockman, Mauck, and Hoff[12] explored diencephalic and mesencephalic structures in adult beagles. We followed essentially the procedures outlined in the previous study but used bipolar instead of monopolar electrodes. Stimuli consisted of 50 c.p.s. symmetrically biphasic pulses with a 1 msec. width and a 10 msec. interval. The threshold intensity varied from 0.5 to 2 ma., and the stimulus duration from 15 to 120 sec. Electrical stimulation with these parameters evoked a spectrum of ectopic ventricular rhythms; each aberration occupied a distinct position on a continuum. Observed in sequence, after termination of an electrical stimulus, were ventricular tachycardia (both unifocal and multifocal), ventricular premature contractions in bigeminal pattern, and ventricular fusion contractions followed by return to sinus rhythm (Figure 1). The converse of this sequence could also be evoked by graded increments of stimulus intensity (Figure 2). Although

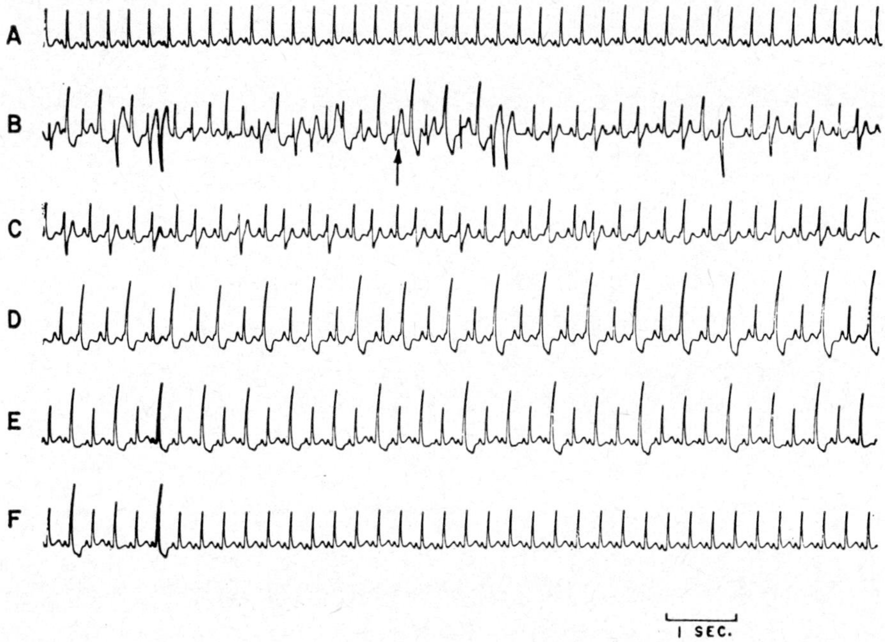


Fig. 2. Sequences of arrhythmias in vagotomized animal evoked by electrical stimulation of the ventromedial region of the hypothalamus. *A,* control record. *B,* arrow indicates cessation of stimulation (60 seconds after its onset). *C,* ventricular premature contractions followed by fusion contractions. *D,* fusion contractions. *E,* fusion contractions resembling Wolff-Parkinson-White complexes. *F,* return to sinus rhythm. Reproduced from Charles H. Hockman, H. Page Mauck, Jr., Ebbe C. Hoff: *Amer. Heart J. 71:* 698, 1966, by permission of the C. V. Mosby Company, St. Louis, Mo.

the entire spectrum was not evoked in all experiments, the sequence of these abnormal rhythms was consistently the same. When an initial stimulus failed to elicit a response, an increase usually brought forth the entire spectrum. Bilateral vagotomy had no effect on the response; however, it was completely abolished by beta-adrenergic blockade with propranolol (1 mg./kg.). The type of arrhythmia observed is directly related to the intensity of sympathetic efferent discharge and the spectrum of ectopic complexes embraces all the ventricular arrhythmias observed in the clinical situation. In our earlier study of the ventricular fusion contractions resembling the WPW complex, it was found that these were dependent upon impulses from the sinoatrial node pacemaker. In the present experiments, it is demonstrated that ventricular premature contractions, observed in bigeminal patterns, are also dependent upon the same mechanism. In the previous study, electrical stimuli were delivered to a circumscribed field in the mesencephalon and, although other arrhythmias had been observed in these prior experiments, a precise analysis of these complexes had not been carried out. From the present experiments it is now obvious that the WPW-like phenomenon lies on a continuum of ventricular fusion complexes of varying P-R and QRS intervals.

Although the arrhythmias evoked in these studies have been of sympathetic origin, preliminary observations of electrical stimulation of other sites, namely, the orbital and cingulate gyri, and medial temporal regions of the cortex, have revealed arrhythmias that suggest enhanced parasympathetic discharge, specifically, sinus bradycardia, total cardiac arrest, and atrial flutter and fibrillation.

More recently, Hockman, Mauck, and Chu[13] found that the spectrum of aberrant complexes of sympathetic origin elicited in beagles can also be induced in cats by diencephalic and mesencephalic stimulation, and that diphenylhydantoin (Dilantin), in doses of 10 mg./kg. administered intravenously one minute prior to electrical stimulation of a cerebral locus prevents the induction of the cardiac arrhythmias. Dilantin in similar doses also abolishes aberrant complexes that have been elicited by electrical stimulation in both cats and dogs. This drug either prevents the induction of or abolishes ectopic ventricular activity for periods of 30 minutes up to seven hours. The exact mechanism of action of Dilantin has not yet been determined.

Our studies of cardiac arrhythmias, elicited experimentally, point to the need for further work to clarify the responsible extracardiac and intracardiac mechanisms. Since pressor responses and other autonomic end effects can be evoked by electrical stimulation in the mesencephalic reticular formation, it seems clear that the stimulated loci play a part that may prove to be extremely important in the cerebral organization and regulation of cardiovascular function. The precise role of this neural region and the essential afferent and efferent central interconnections cannot be confidently stated until more anatomical and physiological data are at hand.

Earlier studies by others have shown that the hypothalamus sends efferent projections to the tegmentum, central gray substance, and reticular formation of the midbrain, and that fibers from these areas run chiefly through the lateral reticular formation of the medulla to terminate on the preganglionic sympathetic neurons in the anterolateral funiculus of the spinal cord. The spectrum of arrhythmias that we have described is elicited from the stimulation of neural loci in structures previously described as forming the descending connections. Nauta[14] has drawn attention to the multitude of reciprocal pathways between forebrain structures and the hypothalamus and midbrain. This vast network of interconnections and relays is not well understood and, as Nauta has pointed out, little information is yet available as to the manner by which this complex "limbic forebrain-midbrain circuit" receives and transmits information to lower levels of the nervous system.

(Material from Mauck, H. P., Jr., Hockman, C. H. and Hoff, E. C. *Amer. Heart J. 68*:98, 1964; Hockman, C. H., Mauck, H. P., Jr. and Hoff, E. C., *Amer. Heart J. 71*:695, 1966; and Hockman, C. H., Mauck, H. P., Jr. and Chu, Nai-Shin, *Amer. Heart J. 74*:256, 1967, is presented with permission of the C. V. Mosby Co., St. Louis, Mo.)

## *REFERENCES*

1. Jackson, J. H. *Clinical and physiological researches on the nervous system. I. On the anatomical and physiological localization of movements in the brain.* London, Low, Churchill, 1875, xlvii, 37 pp. (Reprinted in: *Selected writings of John Hughlings Jackson,* London, Hodder, Stoughton, 1931, vol. I, pp. 37-76 )
2. Fritsch, G. and Hitzig, E. Ueber die elektrische Erregbarkeit des Grosshirns, *Arch. Anat. Physiol. 37*:300-32, 1870.
3. Schiff, M. Untersuchungen über die motorischen Functionen des Grosshirns. *Naunyn-Schmiedeberg's Arch. exptl. Pathol. Pharmakol. 3*:171-79, 1875. (Transl. by F. Borel, from *Lezione sopra il systema nervoso encephalico.* Florence, 1874.)
4. Danilewsky, B. Experimentelle Beiträge zur Physiologie des Gehirns, *Pflüger's Arch. Ges. Physiol. 11*:128-38, 1875.
5. Bard, P. The central representation of the sympathetic system, *A.M.A. Arch. Neurol. Psychiat. 22*:230-46, 1929.
6. Hoff, E. C. and Green, H. D. Cardiovascular reactions induced by electrical stimulation of the cerebral cortex, *Amer. J. Physiol. 117*:411-22, 1936.
7. Ferguson, R. W., Folkow, B., Mitts, M. G. and Hoff, E. C. Effect of cortical stimulation upon epinephrine activity, *J. Neurophysiol. 20*:329-39, 1957.
8. Mauck, H. P., Jr., Hockman, C. H. and Hoff, E. C. ECG changes resulting from cerebral stimulation. I. Anomalous atrioventricular excitation elicited by electrical stimulation of the mesencephalic reticular formation, *Amer. Heart J. 68*:98-101, 1964.
9. Wolff, L., Parkinson, J. and White, P. D. Bundle-branch block with short P-R interval in healthy young people prone to paroxysmal tachycardia. *Amer. Heart J. 5*:685-704, 1930.
10. Weinberg, S. J. and Fuster, J. M. Electrocardiographic changes produced by localized hypothalamic stimulations, *Ann. Int. Med. 53*:332-41, 1960.
11. Parker, I. T., Jr., Gunn, C. G. and Lynn, T. N. Experimental centrogenic arrhythmias, *Clin. Res. 10*:179, 1962.
12. Hockman, C. H., Mauck, H. P., Jr. and Hoff, E. C. ECG changes resulting from cerebral stimulation. II. A spectrum of ventricular arrhythmias of sympathetic origin, *Amer. Heart J. 71*:695-700, 1966.
13. Hockman, C. H., Mauck, H. P., Jr. and Nai-Shin Chu. ECG changes resulting from cerebral stimulation. III. Action of diphenylhydantoin on arrhythmias, *Amer. Heart J. 74*:256-60, 1967.
14. Nauta, W. J. H. Hippocampal projections and related neural pathways to the mid-brain in the cat, *Brain 81*:319-40, 1958.

# CLINICAL EXPERIENCE WITH NEUROGENIC CARDIAC ARRHYTHMIAS*

Ronald L. Katz

Department of Anesthesiology
Columbia University College of Physicians and Surgeons
Anesthesiology Service
Presbyterian Hospital in the City of New York
New York, N. Y.

## Anesthetics and Other Drugs

Although occasional ventricular ectopic beats are frequently seen during general anesthesia and surgical operation, persistent ventricular arrhythmias are rare in the well-managed patient. This paper will deal with some of the ventricular arrhythmias that may be seen during anesthesia and operation. Although the major emphasis will be on man, experiments in animals will be discussed where they help elucidate the mechanism of the arrhythmia.

Running through this discussion will be three basic themes. The first is that although the arrhythmias appear similar in terms of their electrocardiographic manifestations, the mechanisms responsible for the various arrhythmias differ. The second is that most of these arrhythmias can be explained in terms of an imbalance of the autonomic nervous system. Sympathetic predominance may occur because of increase in sympathetic activity or decrease in parasympathetic activity. Similarly, parasympathetic predominance may be either absolute or relative. The arrhythmias to be discussed are more commonly produced by sympathetic predominance. The final theme is that although attention is naturally focused on the heart as the site of ectopic activity, the arrhythmias may be due to changes occurring not only in the heart but also in the central nervous system as well as in the periphery. All three of these areas must be considered in order to understand the arrhythmias.

*Anesthetic agent itself*. Under suitable conditions, cardiac arrhythmias may be seen in the presence of most anesthetic agents. However, there is a marked variation in the propensity to produce arrhythmias.

*Presented at the *Conference on Mechanisms and Management of Arrhythmias,* held by the New York Heart Association at the Hotel Waldorf-Astoria, New York, N. Y., January 24, 1967.
The studies reported in this paper were supported in part by Public Health Service Research Grant GM-09069 from the National Institutes of Health.

For example, the inhalation anesthetics—cyclopropane, trichlorethylene, halopropane, and teflurane—are all capable of producing arrhythmia. With cyclopropane or trichlorethylene, arrhythmias are usually seen only when excessive concentrations are used. Therefore, when arrhythmias are produced by these substances, it is usually possible to lower the concentration of the anesthetic to a level at which the arrhythmia disappears but the patient is still adequately anesthetized for the surgical procedure. This is not the case with teflurane or halopropane. Arrhythmias may be seen at concentrations that are not excessive in terms of depth of anesthesia. Nitrous oxide and diethyl ether rarely produce arrhythmia in and of themselves.

Halopropane has been studied in an attempt to determine the mechanism by which it produces arrhythmia. Ventricular arrhythmias are seen in 40 to 50 per cent of patients receiving this drug.[1, 2] In the cat, the incidence of arrhythmia produced by halopropane is approximately 60 per cent.[3] The halopropane arrhythmia was shown to be a blood pressure-sensitive phenomenon in some animals.[3] Lowering the arterial pressure, by a variety of methods, eliminated the arrhythmia in 7 of 25 cats. In the remaining animals, the arrhythmia could not be demonstrated to be sensitive to changes in blood pressure. The halopropane arrhythmia was not abolished by vagotomy, the intravenous injection of atropine (2 mg./kg.), or the intravenous injection of 0.1 to 0.2 mg./kg. of ethybenztropine, an anticholinergic drug with central nervous system activity, nor was it abolished by acute bilateral adrenalectomy. The arrhythmia was abolished by the intravenous injection of small (10 to 20 μg./kg.) centrally acting adrenergic blocking doses of Hydergine. This dose of Hydergine, although producing central adrenergic block, did not produce peripheral adrenergic block (i.e., epinephrine reversal was not seen after the intravenous injection of 1 μg./kg. of epinephrine). The arrhythmia was also abolished by transecting the spinal cord at $C_1$ and destroying the brain or by intracollicular decerebration, which leaves the pons and medulla intact but removes the suprapontine structures. Thus, the importance of the central nervous system and particularly of the superpontine mechanisms was demonstrated.[3] Beattie *et al.*[4] also found that decerebration abolished cardiac arrhythmias produced by chloroform. By transecting the brain stem at various levels, they concluded that it was removal of the hypothalamus that was responsible for the abolition of the chloroform arrhythmias.

They also were able to produce extrasystoles by stimulation of the hypothalamus.

*Anesthetic agent plus carbon dioxide.* Perhaps the commonest cause of cardiac arrhythmia in anesthetized patients is the combination of the anesthetic agent and respiratory acidosis. Price and his coworkers[5] showed clearly that the inhalation of carbon dioxide during cyclopropane anesthesia produced cardiac arrhythmia. These workers showed that the threshold arterial $pCO_2$ required to produce arrhythmia varied from 44 to 72 mm. of mercury, with a mean of 58. They also demonstrated that the concentration of cyclopropane affected the threshold $pCO_2$ required to produce the arrhythmia; the higher the concentration of cyclopropane the smaller the increase in $pCO_2$ required to produce arrhythmias.[6] The role of the sympathetic nervous system was studied by these workers, who showed that stellate ganglion block could abolish the arrhythmias.[5]

The inhalation of carbon dioxide during halothane anesthesia is also capable of producing cardiac arrhythmia. With halothane, the arterial $pCO_2$ required to produce cardiac arrhythmia was 60 to 140 mm. of mercury with a mean of 92.[7]

The anesthetic agent-carbon dioxide arrhythmias and their mechanisms have been studied in the cat.[3] The inhalation of halopropane plus 10 per cent carbon dioxide produced ventricular arrhythmias in 99 per cent of the animals studied. The halopropane-carbon dioxide arrhythmia was not abolished by lowering the blood pressure. In animals in which the halopropane arrhythmia was abolished by lowering the blood pressure (see above), the inhalation of 10 per cent carbon dioxide restored the arrhythmia. The halopropane-carbon dioxide arrhythmia, like the halopropane arrhythmia, was not blocked by vagotomy, atropine (2 mg./kg.) ethybenztropine (0.1 to 0.2 mg./kg.) or acute bilateral adrenalectomy. Neither decerebration nor Hydergine (10 to 20 $\mu$g./kg.)—each of which did block the halopropane arrhythmia—was capable of blocking the halopropane-carbon dioxide arrhythmia.

Reserpine pretreatment (0.1 mg./kg. intraperitoneally) for one day, which markedly reduces cerebral and myocardial catecholamines but has little or no effect on adrenal catecholamine content, did not prevent the halopropane-carbon dioxide arrhythmia. Neither did acute bilateral adrenalectomy. However, a combination of these two procedures prevented the halopropane-carbon dioxide arrhythmia. This arrhythmia was also abolished by reserpine pretreatment (0.1 mg./kg. intraperitoneally) for seven days, which depletes myocardial and adrenal catecholamines.

It is clear from these results that although the parasympathetic nervous system does not appear to be involved, the sympathetic nervous system is intimately involved in the production of the halopropane-carbon dioxide arrhythmias. Since the arrhythmia was not abolished by one day of pretreatment with reserpine or by bilateral adrenalectomy but was abolished by a combination of these procedures, it appears that a carbon dioxide-induced release of either myocardial or adrenal catecholamines is capable of producing the arrhythmia. The mechanism by which excess carbon dioxide causes the release of catecholamine was also studied.[3] Although acidosis may directly release catecholamines from the adrenals,[8] this could not account for the halopropane-carbon dioxide arrhythmia, since the arrhythmia was abolished by removal of the pons and medulla. The arrhythmia appeared to be due to an effect of acidosis on the brain stem; this stimulated vasomotor areas and resulted in an increased sympathetic outflow and release of catecholamines. Suprapontine structures were not essential for this arrhythmia since it was not abolished by intercollicular decerebration. The essential role of the brain stem was demonstrated by the abolition of the arrhythmia when the pons and medulla were destroyed.

*Anesthetic agent plus catecholamines.* Epinephrine is often injected subcutaneously in order to produce local hemostasis. A dose of epinephrine that will not produce arrhythmias by itself may do so in the presence of cyclopropane or of halogenated hydrocarbon anesthetics. This phenomenon has been referred to as "sensitization" of the myocardium to the action of catecholamines. The term "sensitization" is a poor one, but is widely used for lack of a better. The anesthetics that produce sensitization include trichlorethylene, ethyl chloride, cyclopropane, halothane, chloroform, and methoxyflurane (listed in order of decreasing effect as determined in animal studies).[9] In addition to epinephrine, other catecholamines, such as norepinephrine, isoproterenol, epinine, and cobefrine, may produce cardiac arrhythmias in patients or animals anesthetized with cyclopropane or halogenated hydrocarbons.

The mechanism of the catecholamine-anesthetic agent arrhythmias is not yet fully understood. Some of the factors that may have a role include: 1) increased blood pressure,[10, 11] 2) increased heart rate,[11, 12]

3) release of potassium from the liver[13]—all of which may be induced by catecholamines. Although the rise in blood pressure is an important factor in producing these arrhythmias, it is not absolutely essential, since isoproterenol, a catecholamine that decreases blood pressure is capable of producing the arrhythmia.[14] Similarly the increase in heart rate, and the release of potassium from the liver, although important, are not absolutely essential.

The roles of the alpha-adrenergic and beta-adrenergic stimulating actions of the catecholamines have been studied.[14] At one time the arrhythmias were believed to be due to stimulation of alpha-adrenergic receptors, since the catecholamine-anesthetic agent arrhythmias could be blocked by alpha-adrenergic blocking agents. It is now clear that this was an indirect (blood pressure) or nonspecific (myocardial depressant) effect of the alpha-adrenergic blockers. Further, alpha-adrenergic blocking agents do not block the arrhythmias consistently. Beta-adrenergic blocking agents do consistently prevent the catecholamine-anesthetic agent arrhythmias. This action has been attributed to specific beta-adrenergic receptor blockade. However, the picture is somewhat clouded by the fact that some of the beta-adrenergic blocking agents also have a local anesthetic action[15, 16] and quinidinelike action[17-19] that may account in part for the antiarrhythmic action.

There is some disagreement concerning the role of the central nervous system and the autonomic nervous system in the genesis of the catecholamine-anesthetic agent arrhythmias. It has been reported that these arrhythmias could be blocked by intercollicular decerebration, pontine lesions, bilateral thoracic sympathectomy, or visceral denervation plus bilateral splanchnicotomy.[20, 21] However, the structures removed by these procedures are not essential for the production of the arrhythmias, since it has been shown that the arrhythmias can be produced in decerebrate, spinal, or reserpinized animals[3] as well as in animals with denervated hearts[22, 23] and in the heart-lung preparation.[24]

Although there are many case reports of arrhythmias or cardiac arrest following the use of epinephrine for local hemostasis, most of these are attributed to the use of excessive amounts of catecholamines. It has been clearly shown that catecholamines may be injected subcutaneously in doses that are sufficient to produce satisfactory local hemostasis but that will not produce cardiac arrhythmias in patients anesthetized with halothane or trichlorethylene.[25, 26]

*Anesthetic agent plus peripheral manipulation.* Certain operative maneuvers may produce cardiac arrhythmias in anesthetized patients. A common cause is manipulation of the adrenal glands. The arrhythmia is probably attributable to the release of catecholamines by the manipulation. This arrhythmia may be seen in patients with normal adrenal glands as well as in those who have pheochromocytoma. In the latter, large amounts of catecholamines may be released and may produce bizarre ventricular arrhythmias. Cardiac arrhythmia may also be seen during manipulation or scraping of bone, traction on the abdominal viscera or mesentery, and stimulation of the epiglottis and larynx during intubation.

*Anesthetic agent plus succinylcholine.* Bradycardia, sinus arrest, supraventricular and ventricular arrhythmia have been reported following the injection of succinylcholine in infants, children, and adults anesthetized with nitrous oxide, trichlorethylene, ether, halothane, or cyclopropane. It has also been possible to produce similar arrhythmias in the cat, dog, and monkey.[27-33] In monkeys anesthetized with halothane, Galindo and Davis[34] found that succinylcholine lowered the threshold of cardiac excitability and produced severe ventricular arrhythmias. They explained the cardiac effects of succinylcholine in terms of changes in the permeability of the membrane for potassium, with resultant loss of potassium from the cell, decrease in resting membrane potential, and increase in serum potassium. They also felt that succinylcholine produced its effects by sympathetic postganglionic stimulation and by a direct effect on the myocardium.

Dowdy and Fabian[30] found that succinylcholine produced ventricular arrhythmia in the digitalized cat, dog, and man. They discussed the similarity in the effects of digitalis, acetylcholine, and succinylcholine on the flux of potassium across membranes and they suggested that the digitalis-succinylcholine arrhythmia might be related to myocardial ionic movements of potassium.

Studies in our laboratory demonstrated that the injection of succinylcholine produced ventricular arrhythmias in decerebrate cats anesthetized with halopropane. A rise in blood pressure was also seen. The injection of succinylcholine after alpha-adrenergic blockade produced a fall rather than a rise in blood pressure. However, the halopropane-succinylcholine arrhythmias were not prevented consistently. Subsequent injection of a beta-adrenergic blocking agent prevented the succinylcholine arrhythmia but did not abolish the fall in blood pressure; the latter was eliminated by the injection of atropine. The halopropane-succinylcholine arrhythmias were also prevented by beta-adrenergic blockade alone. The effects of succinylcholine are therefore believed to be due to the release of acetylcholine and catecholamines by a ganglionic stimulating action. Craythorne *et al.*[29] explained the succinylcholine arrhythmias in terms of stimulation of the sympathetic and parasympathetic nervous systems. Similar conclusions were reached by Williams *et al.*,[33] who found that ganglionic blockade depressed the circulatory responses to succinylcholine.

The mechanism of cardiac arrhythmia induced by repeated injections of succinylcholine, but not by the first injection, was studied by Schoenstadt and Whitcher.[32] These investigators showed that succinylcholine did not produce cardiac arrhythmia in patients who received hexafluorenium, a substance that inhibits the hydrolysis of succinylcholine to succinylmonocholine and choline by pseudocholinesterase. Patients given acetylcholine did not develop arrhythmia after a second dose of acetylcholine, but patients given succinylcholine after acetylcholine developed arrhythmia. It was therefore suggested that choline produced by the hydrolysis of succinylcholine sensitizes the patient to subsequent doses of succinylcholine and that, after sensitization by choline, the arrhythmia is produced by the entire succinylcholine molecule.

*Atropine and gallamine.* The intravenous injection of gallamine during cyclopropane anesthesia will produce ventricular arrhythmia.[35] This effect has been attributed to the vagal blocking action of gallamine. The mechanism of arrhythmia is believed to be similar to that seen after the injection of atropine;[36, 37] the vagal blockade results in a relative sympathetic predominance.

*Vasopressin.* The injection of Pituitrin during anesthesia has produced cardiac arrhythmia. Since this substance contains a mixture of vasopressin and oxytocin, there was some question as to which component was responsible for the arrhythmia. It was demonstrated that vasopressin was responsible for the arrhythmia, an effect that may be due to its constrictive action on the coronary arteries.

*Central nervous system.* The role of stimulation of the central nervous system in the production of cardiac arrythmia can be seen in a variety of ways. During surgical operations, stimulation of the brain stem or of the hypothalamus will often produce ventricular arrhythmia. In addition, in patients receiving electroconvulsive therapy treatment, cardiac arrhythmia was seen in 33 per cent of 400 treatments.[38] Cardiac arrhythmia is also seen after the injection of picrotoxin given for the treatment of coma caused by barbiturates.

The roles of the sympathetic and parasympathetic nervous systems in the production of centrally induced cardiac arrhythmia have been carefully studied in animals by Bircher *et al.*[39] These workers produced cardiac arrhythmia by injecting pentylenetetrazol, picrotoxin, and deslanoside into the fourth ventricle or intravenously. Except for the intravenous deslanoside the arrhythmias produced were central in origin and were mediated by the parasympathetic and sympathetic nervous systems; the former dominated. In order to block the arrythmias in all the animals, both parasympathetic and sympathetic blocking agents or procedures were required.

*Alkalosis, digitalis, and potassium.* The relation between digitalis and potassium is well known. Patients who are well digitalized but who become hypokalemic may develop digitalis toxicity. Arrhythmia may also be seen in digitalized patients who are hyperventilated during anesthesia. The alkalosis produced by hyperventilation induces a decrease in plasma potassium, which may result in digitalis toxicity and cardiac arrhythmia. In addition, digitalized patients receiving carbohydrates (glucose infusion) may sometimes develop arrhythmia. When carbohydrates are metabolized, the carbohydrates and potassium enter the cell, presumably under the influence of insulin. This produces a decrease in extracellular potassium that may be responsible for cardiac arrhythmia.

## Treatment of Cardiac Arrhythmias Seen During Anesthesia

*Drugless treatment.* The most logical and physiological method of treating the cardiac arrhythmias that appear during anesthesia is to eliminate the cause of the arrhythmia. In the vast majority of cases this simple and obvious maneuver can easily be accomplished. For example, with anesthetics that produce arrhythmias when given in excessive concentration, merely lowering the concentration will abolish the arrhythmia. In some cases it may be preferable to change to another agent. If the arrhythmia is due to release of catecholamine, induced by an elevated level of carbon dioxide, elimination of the excess carbon dioxide by hyperventilation and restoration of a normal arterial $pCO_2$ will abolish the arrhythmia. Where the arrhythmia is due to the injection of catecholamine, stopping the injection of catecholamines and ventilating the patient with oxygen will usually result in a return to normal sinus rhythm. If arrhythmias are due to adrenal manipulation or abdominal exploration, cessation of these maneuvers will abolish the arrhythmia. Thus, it is clear that in the vast majority of cases the arrhythmia can be eliminated merely by removal of the cause.

Antiarrhythmic drugs may be required in situations in which it is not possible to change the anesthetic management or to discontinue surgical manipulation. Sometimes the deleterious cardiovascular effects produced by the arrhythmia require a more rapid restoration of normal sinus rhythm than can be achieved by modifying the anesthetic management. In these situations antiarrhythmic drugs are useful.

*Procaine and procaine amide.* A number of drugs have been proposed for the treatment of cardiac arrhythmias seen during anesthesia. Local anesthetics and their derivatives have been especially valuable. Procaine (Novocaine) was used by Burstein[40] to treat cardiac arrythmia in anesthetized patients. There are certain drawbacks to its use. These include: rapid hydrolysis and therefore brief duration of action; stimulation of the central nervous system, which may progress to convulsions; hypertension; tachycardia. Study of the products of procaine hydrolysis has demonstrated that diethylaminoethanol had antiarrhythmic action.[41] Study of its derivatives resulted in the development of procaine amide,[42] which is an effective and commonly used antiarrhythmic drug in unanesthetized patients. However, its usefulness during anesthesia if often limited by hypotension.

*Lidocaine and QX-572.* In our operating rooms the most commonly used antiarrhythmic drug is lidocaine (Xylocaine). This substance is especially suitable for the treatment of cardiac arrhythmias occurring during anesthesia and operation. Its duration of action is brief (10 to 20 minutes) and it does not usually decrease blood pressure. In a study comparing the effects of procaine amide and lidocaine in man,[43] procaine amide was found to decrease myocardial contractile force and blood pressure. However, lidocaine, in antiarrhythmic doses, had little or no effect on myocardial contractile force, and it increased blood pressure slightly. Because of its relative lack of toxicity and its great effectiveness, lidocaine is probably the antiarrhythmic drug of choice in anesthetized patients. Frequently this agent is given to abolish the arrhythmia immediately. It is then possible to eliminate the cause of the arrhythmia in the 10 to 20 minutes during which a normal sinus rhythm can be expected. Where it is not possible to eliminate the cause of the arrhythmia, repeated doses of lidocaine can be given.

An effective, safe, long-acting antiarrhythmic agent, suitable for use in anesthetized patients, would be of great value. Lidocaine analogs have been studied in an attempt to produce an agent that was as safe and effective as lidocaine but longer-acting. QX-572, which resulted from these studies, was found to be an effective antiarrhythmic agent in animals[44] and in man.[2] When infused into the coronary artery of the dog, QX-572 produced a positive inotropic effect and increased cardiac output and coronary blood flow. After intravenous injection peripheral vasodilation was seen. This drug appeared to possess many of the qualities of an ideal antiarrhythmic agent. It was, however, abandoned because its gastric absorption was poor, thus limiting its use mainly to intravenous injection. Other analogs of lidocaine are currently under investigation.

*Oxytocin.* The polypeptide vasopressin is known to produce cardiac arrhythmia when injected during anesthesia. However, oxytocin (Syntocinon), which differs from vasopressin by only two amino acids, has an antiarrhythmic effect. Oxytocin was capable of blocking halopropane, halopropane-epinephrine, and halopropane-carbon dioxide arrhythmias in the cat.[45] It was also effective in the treatment of cardiac arrhythmias seen during anesthesia and operation.[45] However, its general usefulness was limited because of a brief duration of action (approximately 10 minutes) and the development of tachyphylaxis following repeated doses.

*Mephentermine and diphenylhydantoin.* Two agents that have been used to treat cardiac arrhythmias are mephentermine (Wyamine), a vasopressor and sympathomimetic agent[46] and diphenylhydantoin (Dilantin), an anticonvultant.[47] There are not yet sufficient studies to determine the value of these agents in anesthetized patients.

*Beta-adrenergic blocking agents.* There is a great deal of interest and activity in the use of beta-adrenergic blocking agents for the treatment of cardiac arrhythmia. It is well established that the beta-adrenergic blocking agents have an antiarrhythmic effect in situations in which the arrthythmia is believed to be due to increased sympathetic activity. The beta-adrenergic blocking agents also have an antiarrhythmic effect in situations in which the evidence is not clear as to the role of the sympathetic nervous system in the genesis of the arrhythmia. Studies of the beta-adrenergic blocking agents suggest that these substances have an antiarrhythmic effect not only by virtue of their beta-adrenergic blocking action but also because they have a direct quinidinelike effect on the myocardium.[17-19] Further, many beta-adrenergic blockers possess local anesthetic activity, which may account for their antiarrhythmic action.[15, 16] It appears at present that all three of these effects are in part responsible for the antiarrhythmic activity of some of the beta-adrenergic agents. It is clear, however, that beta-adrenergic blocking agents devoid of local anesthetic activity are also capable of blocking cardiac arrhythmia.[16]

The question to be dealt with here is whether beta-adrenergic blockers are the best agents available for the routine treatment of cardiac arrhythmias in anesthetized patients. There is not yet sufficient clinical experience with these agents for final conclusions to be drawn. However, it is my opinion, based on our laboratory and clinical studies as well as on philosophic considerations, that these drugs are not universal or ideal substances for the treatment of cardiac arrhythmia. The beta-adrenergic blocking agents can produce profound hypotension when given to anesthetized patients. In addition, it does not seem wise to depress the ability of the myocardium to respond to catecholamines. Further, bronchodilation is a function of the beta-adrenergic stimulating action of the catecholamines. The injection of beta-adrenergic blocking agents may produce bronchospasm in normal patients or in patients with asthma. Perhaps the most important argument against the routine use of beta-adrenergic blocking agents in the treatment of cardiac arrhythmia during anesthesia is the fact that most of these arrhythmias can be treated by eliminating the factors that have precipitated them.

## *REFERENCES*

1. Stephen, C. R. and North, W. C. Halopropane: A clinical evaluation, *Anesthesiology 25*:600, 1964.
2. Katz, R. L. Antiarrhythmic and neuromuscular effects of QX-572 in man, *Acta Anaesth. Scand. 9*:73, 1965.
3. Katz, R. L. Neural factors affecting cardiac arrhythmias induced by halopropane, *J. Pharmacol. 152*:88, 1966.
4. Beattie, J., Brow, G. R. and Long, C. N. H. The hypothalamus and the sympathetic nervous system, *Proc. Ass. Res. Nerv. Dis. 9*:249, 1928.
5. Price, H. L., Lurie, A. A., Jones, R. E., Price, M. L. and Linde, H. W. Cyclopropane anesthesia: epinephrine and norepinephrine in initiation of ventricular arrhythmias by carbon dioxide in-

halation, *Anesthesiology 19*:619, 1958.

6. Lurie, A. A., Jones, R. E., Linde, H. W., Price, M. L., Dripps, R. D. and Price, H. L. Cyclopropane anesthesia: cardiac rate and rhythm during steady levels of cyclopropane anesthesia at normal and elevated end-expiratory carbon dioxide tensions, *Anesthesiology 19*: 457, 1958.
7. Black, G. W., Linde, H. W., Dripps, R. D. and Price, H. L. Circulatory changes accompanying respiratory acidosis during halothane (Fluothane) anesthesia in man, *Brit. J. Anaesth. 31*:238, 1959.
8. Cantu, R. C., Nahas, G. G. and Manger, W. M. Effect of hypercapnic acidosis and of hypoxia on adrenal catecholamine output of the spinal dog, *Proc. Soc. Exp. Biol. Med. 122*:434, 1966.
9. Katz, R. L. and Katz, G. J. Surgical infiltration of pressor drugs and their interaction with volatile anesthetics, *Brit. J. Anaesth. 38*:712, 1966.
10. Moe, G. K., Malton, S. D., Rennick, B. R. and Freyburger, W. A. The role of arterial pressure in the induction of idioventricular rhythms under cyclopropane anesthesia, *J. Pharmacol. 94*:319, 1948.
11. Dresel, P. E., MacCannell, K. L. and Nickerson, M. Cardiac arrhythmias induced by minimal doses of epinephrine in cyclopropane-anesthetized dogs, *Circulat. Res. 8*:948, 1960.
12. Vick, R. L. Effects of altered heart rate on chloroform-epinephrine cardiac arrhythmia, *Circulat. Res. 18*:316, 1966.
13. O'Brien, G. S., Eid, C. H., Murphy, Q. R., Jr. and Meek, W. J. Effects of elimination of hepatic circulation on cyclopropane-epinephrine ventricular tachycardia and arterial serum potassium in dogs, *J. Pharmacol. 112*:374, 1954.
14. Katz, R. L. The effect of alpha and beta adrenergic blocking agents on cyclopropane-catecholamine cardiac arrhythmias, *Anesthesiology 26*:289, 1965.
15. Morales-Aguilera, A. and Vaughan Williams, E. M. The effects on cardiac muscle of beta-receptor antagonists in relation to their activity as local anesthetics, *Brit. J. Pharmacol. 24*:332, 1965.
16. Murmann, W., Saccani-Guelfi, M. and Gamba, A. Pharmacological properties of 1-(4-nitrophenyl)-2-isopropylaminoethanol (INPEA). A new beta-adrenergic receptor antagonist, *Boll. Chimicofarm. 105*:292, 1966.
17. Sekiya, A. and Vaughan Williams, E. M. A comparison of anticirculatory actions and effects on intracellular cardiac potentials of pronethalol, disopyramide, and quinidine, *Brit. J. Pharmacol. 21*:473, 1963.
18. Singer, D. H., Yeh, B. K., Seberlay, B. J. and Hoffman, B. F. Beta blockade and the specialized conduction system of the heart, *Circulation 30*: (Suppl. 3) 160, 1964.
19. Rosati, R. A., Alexander, J. A., Wallace, A. G., Sealy, W. C. and Young, W. G., Jr. Failure of beta-adrenergic blockade to alter ventricular fibrillation thresholds in the dog, *Circulat. Res. 19*: 721, 1966.
20. Allen, C. R., Stutzman, J. W., and Meek, W. J. The production of ventricular tachycardia by adrenalin in cyclopropane anesthesia, *Anesthesiology 1*: 158, 1940.
21. Stutzman, J. W., Murphy, Q., Allen, C. R. and Meek, W. J. Further studies on the production of cyclopropane-epinephrine tachycardias, *Anesthesiology 8*:579, 1947.
22. Bardier, E. and Stillmunkes, A. The adrenaline-chloroform syncope, *Arch. Int. Pharmacodyn. 27*:375, 1923.
23. Levy, A. G. The exciting causes of ventricular fibrillation in animals under chloroform anaesthesia, *Heart 4*:319, 1912-1913.
24. Fawaz, G. The mechanism by which N: N-dibenzylchloroethylamine protects animals against cardiac arrhythmias induced by sympathoametic amines in presence of cyclopropane or chloroform, *Brit. J. Pharmacol. 6*:492, 1951.
25. Katz, R. L., Matteo, R. S. and Papper, E. M. The injection of epinephrine during general anesthesia with halogenated hydrocarbons and cyclopropane in man. 2: Halothane, *Anesthesiology 23*:597, 1962.

26. Matteo, R. S., Katz, R. L. and Papper, E. M. The injection of epinephrine during general anesthesia with halogenated hydrocarbons and cyclopropane in man. 1. Trichlorethylene, *Anesthesiology 23*: 360, 1962.
27. Barretto, R. S. Effect of intravenously administered succinylcholine upon cardiac rate and rhythm, *Anesthesiology 21*:401, 1960.
28. Bullough, J. Intermittent suxamethonium injections, *Brit. Med. J. 1*:786, 1959.
29. Craythorne, N. W. B., Turndorf, H. and Dripps, R. D. Changes in pulse rate and rhythm associated with the use of succinylcholine in anesthetized children, *Anesthesiology 21*:465, 1960.
30. Dowdy, E. G. and Fabian, L. W. Ventricular arrhythmias induced by succinylcholine in digitalized patients, *Anesth. Analg. 42*:501, 1963.
31. Lupprian, K. G. and Churchill-Davidson, H. C. Effect of suxamethonium on cardiac rhythm, *Brit. Med. J. 2*:1774, 1960.
32. Schoenstadt, D. A. and Whitcher, C. E. Observations on the mechanism of succinylcholine-induced cardiac arrhythmias, *Anesthesiology 24*:358, 1963.
33. Williams, C. H., Deutsch, S., Linde, H. W., Bullough, J. W. and Dripps, R. D. Effects of intravenously administered succinylcholine on cardiac rate, rhythm and arterial blood pressure in anesthetized man, *Anesthesiology 22*: 947, 1961.
34. Galindo, A. H. and Davis, T. V. Succinylcholine and cardiac excitability. *Anesthesiology 23*:32, 1962.
35. Walts, L. F. and Prescott, F. S. The effect of gallamine on cardiac rhythm during general anesthesia, *Anesth. Analg. 44*:265, 1965.
36. Jacobson, E. and Adelman, M. The electrocardiographic effects of intravenous administration of neostigmine and atropine during cyclopropane anesthesia, *Anesthesiology 15*:407, 1954.
37. Jones, R. E., Deutsch, S. and Turndorf, H. Effects of atropine on cardiac rhythm in conscious and anesthetized man, *Anesthesiology 22*:67, 1961.
38. Richardson, D. J., Gahagan, L. H., Lewis, W. H., Jr., Sheehan, D., de Beer, E. J., Colville, K. I. and Ellis, C. H. Cardiovascular responses to transcranial electrical stimulation in man and dog, *J.A.M.A. 171*:528, 1959.
39. Bircher, R. P., Kanai, T. and Wang, S. C. Mechanism of cardiac arrhythmias and blood pressure changes induced in dogs by pentylenetetrazol, picrotoxin and deslanoside, *J. Pharmacol. 141*:6, 1963.
40. Burstein, C. Treatment of acute arrhythmias during anesthesia by intravenous procaine, *Anesthesiology 7*:113, 1946.
41. Rosenberg, B., Kayden, H. J., Lief, P. A., Mark, L. C., Steel, J. M. and Brodie, B. B. Studies on diethylaminoethanol; physiological disposition and action on cardiac arrhythmias, *J. Pharmacol. 95*:18, 1949.
42. Mark, L. C., Kayden, H. J., Steele, J. M., Cooper, J. R., Berlin, I., Rovenstein, E. A. and Brodie, B. B. The physiological disposition and cardiac effects of procaine amide, *J. Pharmacol. 102*:5, 1951.
43. Harrison, D. C., Sprouse, J. H. and Morrow, A. G. The antiarrhythmic properties of lidocaine and procaine amide. Clinical and physiologic studies of their cardiovascular effects in man, *Circulation 28*:486, 1963.
44. Katz, R. L. Antiarrhythmic action of N, N-bis(phenylcarbamoylmethyl) dimethyl ammonium chloride (QX-572) in cat and dog, *Anesthesiology 25*:291, 1964.
45. Katz, R. L. Antiarrhythmic and cardiovascular effects of synthetic oxytocin, *Anesthesiology 25*:653, 1964.
46. Lynch, P. R., Webber, D. L., and Oppenheimer, M. J. Mephentermine as an antifibrillatory drug against cyclopropane-epinephrine ventricular fibrillation, *Anesthesiology 16*:632, 1955.
47. Conn, R. D. Diphenylhydantoin sodium in cardiac arrhythmias, *New Eng. J. Med. 272*:277, 1965.

# THE ELECTROPHYSIOLOGIC EFFECTS OF BETA-ADRENERGIC BLOCKADE AND CARDIAC DENERVATION*

ANDREW G. WALLACE, STEPHEN F. SCHAAL, TSUNEAKI SUGIMOTO, MARVIN ROZEAR, AND JAMES A. ALEXANDER

Division of Cardiology, Department of Medicine
Duke University Medical Center, Durham, N. C.

## INTRODUCTION

ALTHOUGH the heart possesses important intrinsic mechanisms of adjusting to its work load[1] there is considerable evidence that changes of autonomic nerve activity play the dominant role in circulatory regulation. In most of the situations in which they have been examined, the cardiovascular consequences of altered autonomic nerve discharge appear to be appropriate mechanisms for adapting to stress. It seems relevant, however, to consider the possibility that such a powerful control mechanism might have liabilities as well as assets for the integrated function of the organism.

The objective of the work described in this report has been to develop an insight into the possible ways by which alterations of autonomic nerve activity might contribute to the genesis or to the treatment of disturbances of cardiac rhythm. Our experiments have been designed to examine fundamental electrophysiologic properties of the intact heart over the widest possible range of autonomic influence. Wherever possible these studies have been performed in awake dogs and have been of three general types. We have examined the nature of arrhythmias produced either by stimulation of cardiac nerves or by the injection of analeptic agents into the fourth cerebral ventricle. Second, we have analyzed the electrophysiologic consequences of beta-adrenergic blockade and of total extrinsic cardiac denervation. Finally, we have compared the responses of the normal and chronically denervated heart to several of the commonly used cardioactive drugs. Although many aspects of this analysis require further study, the results

*Presented at the *Conference on Mechanisms and Management of Arrhythmias,* held by the New York Heart Association at the Hotel Waldorf-Astoria, New York, N. Y., January 24, 1967.
This investigation was supported in part by Public Health Service Research Grants HE-08845 and HE-19949 from the National Heart Institute.

obtained indicate that alterations of autonomic nerve activity can exert an important influence on experimental arrhythmias. To a limited extent, this view has been tested and supported by the clinical experience with beta-adrenergic blocking agents and cardiac sympathectomy.

Mongrel dogs weighing from 10 to 18 kg. were used for these studies. Chronic recording electrodes were implanted on the right atrium in the region of the sinus node and on the epicardial surface of the right ventricle. During brief periods of occlusion of venous inflow, similar recording electrodes were implanted over the right bundle branch at the Purkinje-papillary junction and over the bundle of His. Recordings from these electrodes permit accurate measurements of sinus rate, AV conduction time, conduction velocity in Purkinje tissue, and total ventricular activation time. They also permit a more accurate localization of the origin of certain ectopic rhythms. Stimulating electrodes were used to pace the heart if desired and to measure the excitability and refractory period of atrial and ventricular muscle.[2]

Activation of the nervous system was accomplished through chronic stimulating electrodes on the stellate ganglia and cervical vagi, or by the introduction of analeptic drugs or saline into the fourth cerebral ventricle.[3] Cardiac denervation was accomplished by the technique of mediastinal neural ablation as described by Cooper *et al.*[4]

## The Nature of Neurogenic Arrhythmias

The most consistent electrophysiologic effects of stimulating cardiac sympathetic nerves include enhancement of the activity of the pacemaker at all levels and facilitation of AV conduction.[5,6] Stimulation of the parasympathetic nerves, on the other hand, depresses the activity of the pacemaker and slows or blocks conduction through the AV node.[7] As a first approximation, disturbances of cardiac rhythm that arise from activation of the central nervous system might be divided into those that result primarily from the depressive influence of the vagus, or from the excitatory influence of the sympathetics. Unfortunately the situation appears to be considerably more complex than this. One feature of this complexity is that most centrally induced changes of rhythm seem to represent the net effect of simultaneous sympathetic and parasympathetic discharge. Since the electrophysiologic influence of vagal efferent fibers is confined primarily to the atria and AV node, while sympathetic fibers innervate the atria and

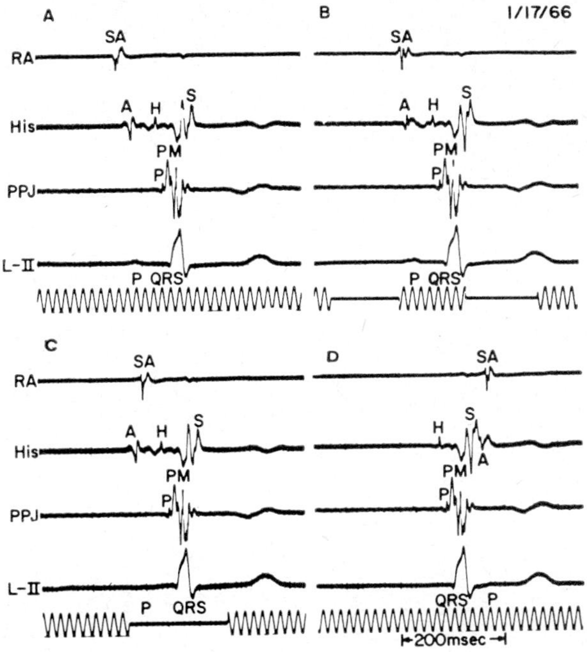


Fig. 1. Wandering pacemaker after the injection of picrotoxin, 50 μg. into the 4th cerebral ventricle. RA = right atrium, His = bundle of His, PPJ = Purkinje papillary junction, L-II = lead II electrocardiogram. SA = sinoatrial node, A = atrial septum, H = bundle of His, S = ventricular septum, P = Purkinje spike, PM = papillary muscle. Panel A = control. Panels B, C, and D after picrotoxin. See text for details.

ventricles, an important consequence of combined discharge is to produce a discordant influence on the activity of the pacemaker. The effect of this discordance is to shift the function of the pacemaker from its normal locus within the sinus node to the His-Purkinje system. In addition, the effects of increased activity of either the vagus or sympathetic nerves on recovery of excitability is not manifest uniformly within any given chamber of the heart.[8, 9] Thus an important additional consequence of enhanced autonomic discharge is to create nonuniform recovery of adjacent regions of the myocardium. The magnitude of this influence and its importance to the initiation and perpetuation of reentrant rhythms has been stressed in recent articles.[9-11]

The tracings presented in Figures 1 to 4 illustrate the complex nature of arrhythmias that may arise after the injection of analeptics or saline into the fourth cerebral ventricle. Each of the illustrations includes recordings from the region of the sinus node (RA), His bundle (HIS), right bundle branch (PPJ) and a lead-II electrocardio-

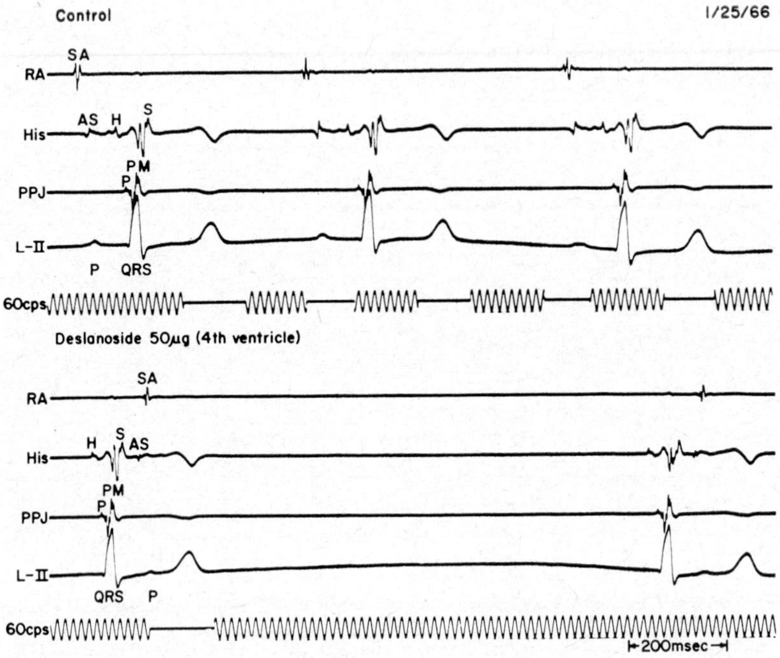


Fig. 2. His bundle escape rhythm after injecting deslanoside 50 μg. into the 4th cerebral ventricle. See text for details. Symbols are the same as in Figure 1.

gram. Figure 1 is from a dog that demonstrated bradycardia with a "wandering pacemaker" after picrotoxin was injected into the 4th ventricle. Panel A shows control tracings in which activity at the sinus node (SA) preceded excitation of the atrial septum (A) and inscription of the P wave. In panel B the pacemaker had shifted to a point temporally equidistant from the sinus node and atrial septum so that activity from these two structures occurred almost coincidentally. In panel C, the pacemaker had moved to another location so that activation at the sinus node followed that at the atrial septum. In panel D, the pacemaker had moved to the region of the AV node or bundle of His with atrial activation occurring in a retrograde sequence after excitation of the bundle of His.

Figure 2 shows another example of bradycardia in response to the intracranial injection of an analeptic agent. Panel A shows control tracings of sinus rhythm. After the injection of deslanoside into the 4th ventricle there was a period of asystole followed by a slow escape rhythm (panel B). The pacemaker during the escape rhythm was

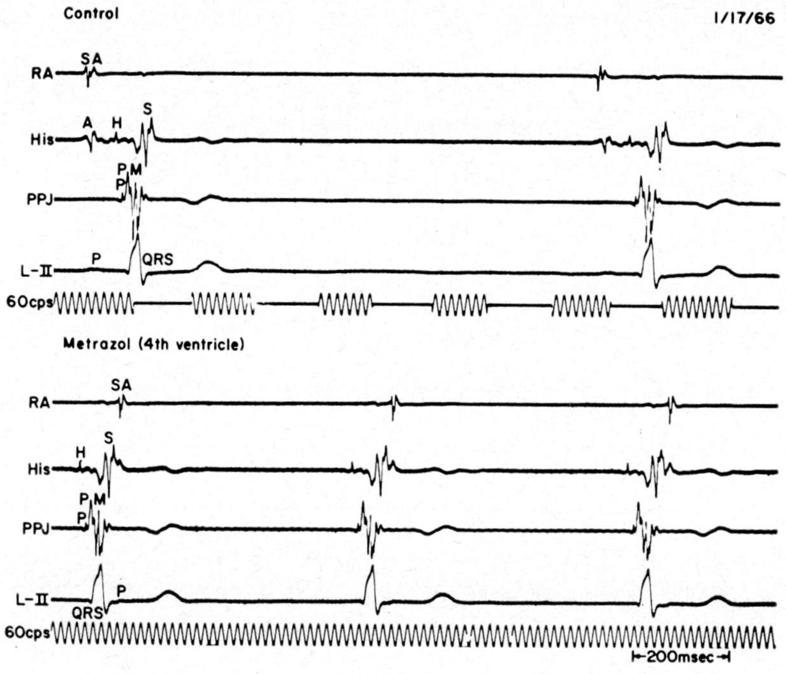


Fig. 3. Nodal tachycardia after the injection of metrazol 50 mg. into the 4th cerebral ventricle. For explanation of symbols see Figure 1.

located above the bifurcation of the bundle of His since there was no alteration of the interval between the His complex and the right bundle branch or the contour of the QRS complex. Atrial excitation followed the His complex, and the long delay between activity at the bundle of His and at the atrial septum suggests that the escape pacemaker was located in the upper His bundle. This suggestion also is supported by the slight change of the His complex indicating that the pacemaker was in close proximity to the recording electrode.

Figure 3 shows an example of "nodal tachycardia" induced by the injection of metrazol into the 4th ventricle. Panel A shows tracings of sinus rhythm and panel B illustrates the tachycardia that developed four minutes after injection of metrazol. The rate of the ectopic tachycardia was approximately twice that of the control rhythm. The pacemaker was located in the lower AV node or bundle of His as indicated by the upright His complex, a normal sequence of ventricular excitation and atrial activity that followed the His complex. The experiment shown in Figure 4 illustrates the production of ventricular tachycardia

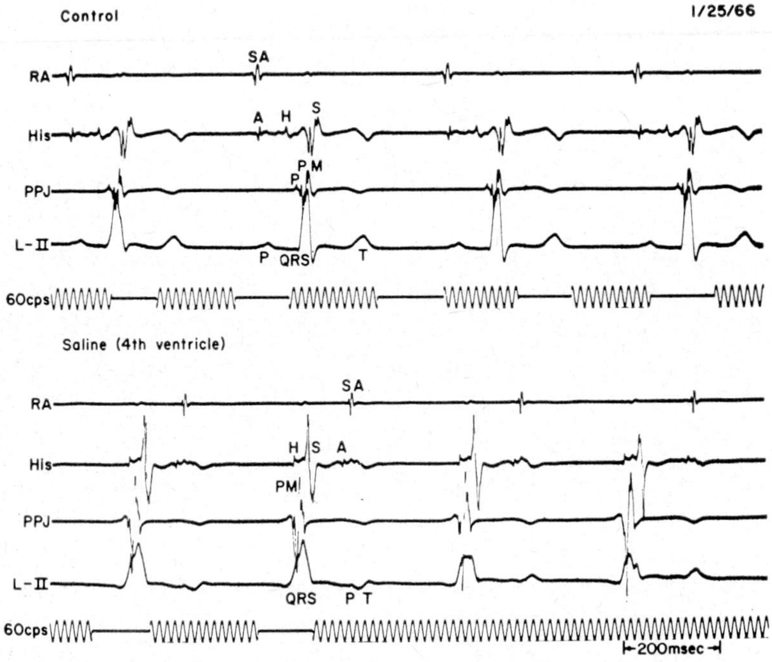


Fig. 4. Ventricular tachycardia after the injection of 5 ml. of saline into the 4th cerebral ventricle. For explanation of symbols see Figure 1.

by the injection of 5 ml. of saline into the 4th ventricle. Panel A shows tracings obtained during the control period and panel B illustrates records during ventricular tachycardia. The ectopic pacemaker was located in the right Purkinje system since activity in the right bundle branch and papillary muscle occur early in the QRS and activation of the His complex was retrograde.

The illustrations presented in Figures 1 to 4 were selected to demonstrate the type of arrhythmia that can be produced in the normal dog by activation of the central nervous system. The first two figures illustrate varying degrees of suppression of the normal pacemaker with a slow escape rhythm arising from pacemakers outside of the sinus node. Figures 3 and 4 illustrate manifestations of enhanced automatic activity in the region of the AV node or His-Purkinje system with a rapid capture rhythm. Presumably the disturbances shown in Figures 1 and 2 resulted from a dominating vagal influence, while those shown in Figures 3 and 4 resulted from a dominating sympathetic influence. It is important to reemphasize, however, that these centrally induced arrhythmias seem to require simultaneous discharge of the sympathetic and parasympathetic nerves since they can be prevented by prior vagotomy alone or stellate ganglionectomy alone.[12]

## Effects of Beta-Adrenergic Blockade

Since the major electrophysiologic effects of sympathetic nerve stimulation include an increase of sinus rate and enhancement of AV conduction, blockade of beta-adrenergic receptors would be expected to produce changes of the opposite direction. At least in part, however, the changes observed when a blocking agent is given depend on the magnitude of background sympathetic activity. In addition, evidence has been obtained that indicates that certain of the beta blocking agents have sympathomimetic,[13] anticholinergic,[14] and quinidinelike properties.[15] To the extent that these extra-adrenergic actions are operative at any given dose level, the interpretation of the net response following beta blockade must include the possibility that factors other than antagonism of sympathetic influences contribute to the observed changes.

In recent experiments carried out in this laboratory the effects of beta-adrenergic blockade on the electrophysiologic properties of the heart have been studied. In these studies propranolol, 0.2 mg./kg. given intravenously, has been used to achieve beta blockade. In well-trained awake dogs this dose of propranolol did not alter heart rate, AV conduction, or intraventricular conduction.[16] We concluded from these observations that propranolol was not a depressant of sinus node pacemaker function, AV propagation, or intraventricular conduction, and that during these experimental conditions there was little evidence that the heart was under sympathetic drive. Propranolol also failed to alter sinus arrhythmia, which suggests that no anticholinergic influence of the drug was manifest at the above dosage.

When propranolol was administered to dogs that had not had sufficient time to adapt to the laboratory environment, quite a different response was observed. These animals frequently demonstrated external signs of anxiety with restlessness, proptosis, mydriasis, and moderate to marked sinus tachycardia. Under these conditions, propranolol slowed the heart rate and prolonged AV conduction, but still failed to alter intraventricular conduction (Figure 5). Thus when the heart was under sympathetic drive, beta-adrenergic blockade had the ex-

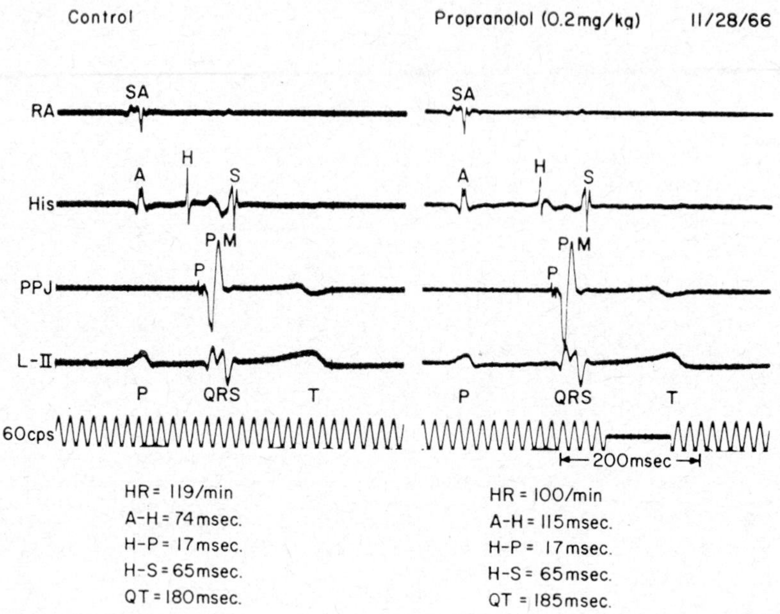


Fig. 5. Effects of 0.2 mg./kg. of propranolol given intravenously on heart rate and conduction in an awake dog. Symbols are the same as in Figure 1. A-H interval is used as an index of AV conduction time, H-P interval is used as an index of conduction velocity in Purkinje tissue. H-S interval is used as an index of total ventricular activation time.

pected effects on sinus node pacemaker function and AV propagation.

Regardless of the conditions under which we have examined it, propranolol produces a substantial lengthening of the functional refractory period of the AV node (Figure 6). This effect has been observed in anxious dogs, in apparently relaxed dogs, and in dogs that have previously been subjected to total cardiac denervation. While these data appear to indicate that the effect of propranolol on the refractory period of the node is an extra-adrenergic influence, we can not exclude the possibility that this measurement might be even more sensitive than heart rate or AV conduction to low levels of circulating catecholamines. Regardless of the mechanism, propranolol consistently reduces the ability of the node to propagate premature impulses and reduces the ventricular rate in the presence of atrial tachyarrhythmias. Although propranolol has certain antidigitalis properties that will be discussed subsequently, it acts additively with digitalis with respect to prolonging the refractory period of AV node.[17]

Propranolol produces little or no change in the refractory period

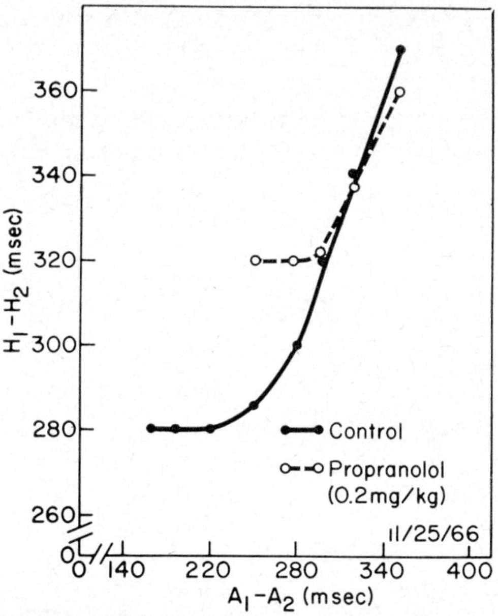


Fig. 6. Effects of 0.2 mg./kg. of propranolol given intravenously on the functional refractory period of the AV node. The heart was paced at 120 beats per minute, and after every sixth basic beat a premature pulse was delivered to the atrium. Plotted on the horizontal axis is the $A_1$-$A_2$ interval in milliseconds, which is the interval between the last basic atrial beat and the atrial premature beat. Plotted on the vertical axis is the $H_1$-$H_2$ interval in milliseconds which is the interval between the last basic His bundle complex and His complex of the premature beat. Solid circles = control data and open circles data obtained after propranolol.

or excitability of atrial muscle[16] and does not alter significantly the threshold for producing ventricular fibrillation when single shocks are applied during the vulnerable period.[18] Dogs with surgically induced heart block have been used to examine the effects of beta-adrenergic antagonists on the rhythmicity of ventricular pacemakers. The effects of propranolol in this preparation have been variable, but in many trials beta blockade resulted in slowing of the ventricular rate and occasionally in asystole. When ventricular automaticity was enhanced in heart block dogs by digitalization, propranolol abolished the digitalis effect.

The experimental evidence suggests, therefore, that propranolol would be an effective agent to control sinus tachycardia, to reduce the ventricular rate in atrial tachycardia or fibrillation, and to inhibit ventricular ectopic beats, particularly those induced by digitalis preparations. The clinical use of beta-adrenergic blocking agents for the

Table I—TREATMENT OF ARRHYTHMIAS WITH IV PROPRANOLOL

| | *Number* | *Results* |
|---|---|---|
| *Nondigitalis arrhythmias* | | |
| Sinus tachycardia | 17 | 17/17 Retarded |
| PAT | 1 | 1/1 Converted to NSR |
| Atrial flutter | 7 | 3/7 Retarded. 1/7 Converted to NSR |
| Atrial fibrillation | 6 | 6/6 Retarded. No conversions |
| Nodal rhythm | 4 | 2/4 Retarded. 1/4 Converted |
| PVC's | 6 | 5/6 No change |
| Ventricular tachycardia | 4 | 4/4 No change |
| *Digitalis arrhythmias* | | |
| PAT with block | 6 | 5/6 Converted to NSR |
| PAC's | 3 | 3/3 Abolished PAC's |
| PVC's | 7 | 7/7 Abolished PVC's |
| AV dissociation | 1 | 1/1 No Change |
| Wenckebach | 1 | 1/1 No Change |

Summary of the Duke University Medical Center experience with IV propranolol in the treatment of arrhythmias. Most patients were given between 5 and 10 mg. of propranolol. The number of patients treated is shown in the middle column; the results of treatment, on the right. Cases in addition to those described by Ginn *et al.*[20] are reported in this table.

treatment of cardiac arrhythmias was first reported by Stock and Dale.[19] These investigators demonstrated that pronethalol decreased the ventricular rate in patients with atrial fibrillation and suppressed digitalis-induced tachyarrhythmias. Since their report there have been numerous additions to the clinical literature concerning the use and effectiveness of blocking drugs. These reports can be summarized briefly by noting that propranolol is almost uniformly effective in retarding sinus tachycardia, reducing the ventricular rate in atrial fibrillation or flutter and abolishing digitalis-induced atrial tachycardia or ventricular premature beats. Results in tachyarrhythmias not induced by digitalis, other than sinus tachycardia, have been variable. Beta blocking agents should be avoided in any patient with AV block since they may increase the degree of block and should be given cautiously, if at all, to patients with evidence of congestive heart failure. Our own clinical experience[20] with the use of intravenous propranolol is summarized in Table I.

It should be reemphasized that the antiadrenergic effects of propranolol are not necessarily the basis for its antiarrhythmic action in all disturbances of rhythm that respond to treatment. Certainly beta

TABLE II—ELECTROPHYSIOLOGIC EFFECTS OF CARDIAC DENERVATION

| | *Sinus rate (beats/min.)* | *A - H (msec.)* | *H - P (msec.)* | *H - S (msec.)* | *QT (msec.)* | *FRPAVN (msec.)* |
|---|---|---|---|---|---|---|
| Normals (10) | 104 ± 16 | 76 ± 18 | 16 ± 3 | 67 ± 8 | 195 ± 8 | 273 ± 40 |
| Denervated (10) | 102 ± 13 | 72 ± 15 | 16 ± 3 | 65 ± 7 | 194 ± 14 | 271 ± 25 |

Mean and one standard deviation.

The effects of total cardiac denervation on electrophysiologic properties of the heart. Data from 10 normal dogs studied awake serve as the controls. The normal dogs were selected from a much larger series to be of equal body weight to dogs in the denervated group. Sinus rate refers to the average rate over a one-minute period. A-H = interval from atrial septum to His bundle. H-P = interval from His bundle to right bundle branch. H-S = interval from His bundle to ventricular septum. QT = interval of the EKG FRPAVN = functional refractory period of AV node.

blockade is an important aspect of the therapeutic effects observed when propranolol is used to treat arrhythmias induced by epinephrine or in arrhythmias such as those observed during anesthesia where epinephrine is thought to play a role.[21] It has been noted, however, that the dose of an adrenergic blocking agent required to abolish digitalis-induced arrhythmias is usually greater than that required to achieve beta blockade.[22] Furthermore, certain potent beta blocking agents that abolish epinephrine-induced arrhythmias fail to suppress arrhythmias induced by ouabain.[23, 24] Conversely it has been shown recently that an analogue of dichloroisoproterenol that is not itself a beta receptor antagonist is still capable of abolishing arrhythmias produced by ouabain.[25] From these observations it must be concluded that the mechanism of the antiarrhythmic action of this group of drugs is uncertain and remains to be clarified.

## Effects of Total Cardiac Denervation

Total extrinsic denervation of the heart has been accomplished by a modification of the technique described by Cooper *et al.*[4] The procedure involves division of all the cardiac branches of the vagus nerve and removal of the pericardium. The adventitia is stripped from the venae cavae, the aortic arch, and its branches, and the stellate ganglia and upper thoracic sympathetic chains are removed. After total cardiac denervation three or four days are required to deplete the stored cate-

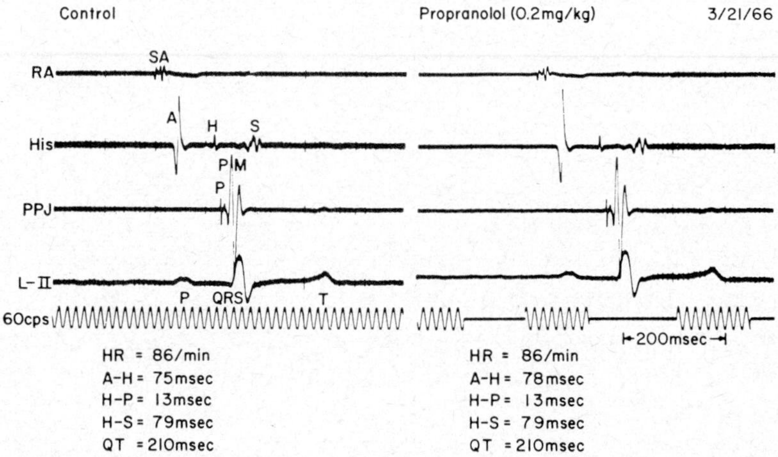


Fig. 7. Effects of 0.2 mg./kg. of propranolol given intravenously to a dog with a denervated heart. Symbols and intervals are the same as in Figure 5.

cholamines in the heart, but by the end of a week myocardial levels are reduced to less than 0.05 μg./gm. of muscle. In selected animals, cardiac vagotomy alone has been performed.

The heart rate, AV conduction time, conduction velocity in Purkinje tissue, total ventricular activation time, and functional refractory period of the AV node for 10 denervated dogs are presented in Table II. Similar data from 10 normal dogs of comparable weight also are shown. Gross examination of the data reveals that there is no apparent difference between normal and denervated dogs although the number of animals is still too small to establish with certainty that there is no difference. Our impression that cardiac denervation does not alter intraventricular conduction is supported by data from two dogs in which it was possible to implant cardiac electrodes several weeks prior to neural ablation, and thereby obtain measurements from the same animals before and after denervation. In these dogs denervation failed to alter conduction velocity in Purkinje tissue or ventricular activation time.

The observation that the average spontaneous heart rate and AV conduction time for normal and denervated dogs does not differ strikingly is only a partial characterization of the true effect of denervation on these variables. The normal dog usually manifests a moderate degree of sinus arrhythmia, and there is also considerable beat-to-beat variation of AV conduction time. These periodic changes of sinus rate and

AV conduction are presumably the result of fluctuations of vagal nerve activity and are totally abolished by cardiac denervation.

In addition to our interest in defining the electrophysiologic consequences of cardiac denervation *per se*, the denervated heart is a useful preparation for the study of various pharmacologic agents. Removal of reflex control mechanisms to the heart permits a more direct analysis of the actions of cardiac drugs.

Figure 7 shows the effects of 0.2 mg./kg. of propranolol administered intravenously to an awake dog that had previously undergone cardiac denervation. Panel A shows the control tracings and panel B the tracings after propranolol. In the dog with a denervated heart, propranolol failed to alter sinus rate, AV conduction time, or intraventricular conduction. These observations support our previous view that in this dosage propranolol has little or no direct sympathomimetic or quinidinelike action on the heart. Moreover, since the denervated heart is exquisitely sensitive to infused catecholamines, failure of propranolol to alter heart rate or AV conduction implies that the humoral background of catecholamines was low under these experimental conditions.

The anatomy of the innervation to the heart is such that the technique of extrinsic cardiac denervation divides postganglionic sympathetic nerves and preganglionic parasympathetic nerves. The structural and functional state of postganglionic parasympathetic fibers following division of the preganglionic fibers is uncertain. It was reasoned that if any functional cholinergic influence persists following cardiac denervation, atropine might enhance sinus rate and AV conduction, since these are very sensitive indicators of vagal activity. Figure 8 shows the response of a dog with a denervated heart to the intravenous injection of 1.0 mg. of atropine. There was actually a slight decrease of heart rate and no change of either AV conduction or intraventricular conduction. We have concluded from these observations that there is no effective cholinergic influence on the heart after total extrinsic cardiac denervation.

One of the important therapeutic applications of digitalis is to control the ventricular rate in patients with atrial flutter or atrial fibrillation. Although the mechanism by which digitalis reduces the ventricular rate is complex, prolongation of the functional refractory period of the AV transmission system through vagal and extravagal

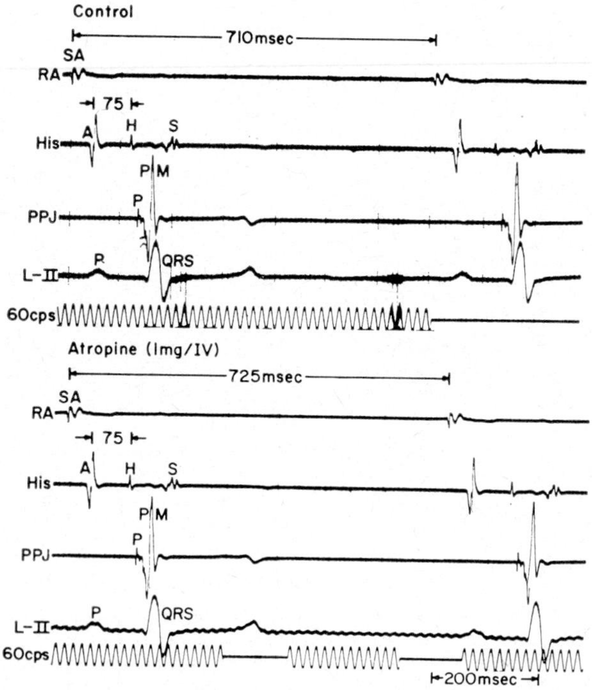


Fig. 8. Effects of 1.0 mg. of atropine given intravenously to a dog with a denervated heart. There was a slight prolongation of the cycle length, which would correspond to a change of heart rate from 85 beats/min. to 83 beats/min. The A-H interval was 75 milliseconds before and after atropine.

influences contributes importantly to this action.[26] Figure 9 illustrates the effects of digoxin, 0.15 mg./kg., on the functional refractory period of the AV node (FRPAVN). In panel *A* a representative study from a normal awake dog is presented and demonstrates significant prolongation of the FRPAVN after digoxin. Panel *B* shows the effects of the same dose of digoxin in an awake dog with a chronically denervated heart. In the denervated preparation digitalis failed to alter the FRPAVN. In dogs with an intact cardiac sympathetic nerve supply, but with total cardiac vagotomy, the effects of digitalis on the FRPAVN were reduced in magnitude but not abolished. These studies demonstrate that the effects of digitalis on the AV node are dependent upon an intact nerve supply and are in large part a consequence of an antiadrenergic action of the glycoside.[27]

The most frequent cardiac manifestations of intoxication induced by digitalis are the development of ventricular extrasystoles, bigeminal

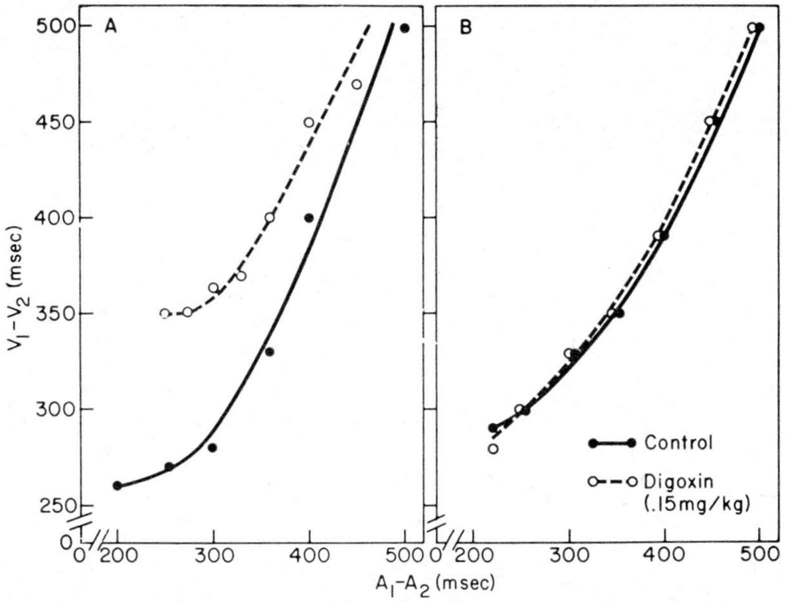


Fig. 9. Effects of digoxin, 0.15 mg./kg., on the functional refractory period of the AV node. Panel A is from a normal dog and panel B from a dog with a chronically denervated heart. See text and legend to Figure 6 for additional details.

rhythm, and ventricular tachycardia. It has long been suspected that adrenergic influences exert at least a permissive role in these disturbances of rhythm. The chronically denervated heart that is isolated from neural influences and depleted of its stores of catecholamine represents an ideal preparation to test this hypothesis. The electrocardiograms presented in Figure 10 illustrate the development of ventricular extrasystoles and ventricular tachycardia in a normal dog during an infusion of ouabain. Figure 11 illustrates an identical experiment in a dog with a chronically denervated heart. At cumulative doses of ouabain that consistently produced ventricular tachycardia in the normal dog, the denervated dog manifested no evidence of ventricular irritability. We have not compared the lethal dose of ouabain in normal and denervated dogs, but it can be concluded that denervation of the heart inhibits markedly the cardiac manifestations of an overdose of digitalis.

There is additional experimental evidence that cardiac denervation might favorably influence certain clinically encountered arrhythmias. For instance, following myocardial infarction in the dog, stimulation of cardiac sympathetic nerves enhances the likelihood of arrhythmia.[28]

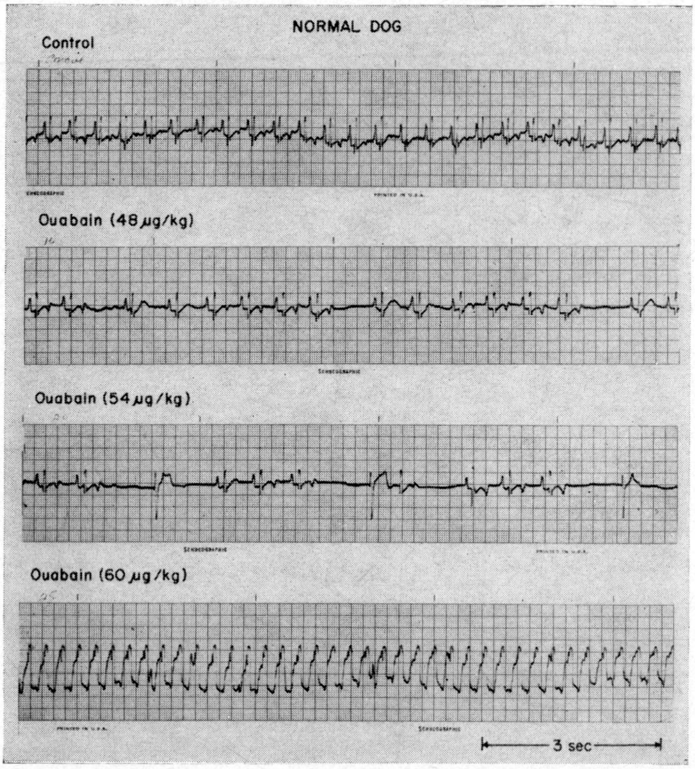


Fig. 10. Electrocardiograms from a normal dog that demonstrate the development of intoxication from digitalis. Ouabain was infused at a continuous rate of 30 µg./kg./30 min. and the cumulative dose is shown above each panel. Top panel shows sinus rhythm. The second panel shows sinus slowing and sinus arrhythmia. The third panel shows periods of sinus pause with ventricular escope beats. The lowest panel shows ventricular tachycardia.

In dogs subjected to coronary artery occlusion, either beta-adrenergic blockade with propranolol[29] or prior thoracic sympathectomy[30,31] reduces the incidence of arrhythmias and improves survival. Clinical experience with cardiac denervation for the treatment of arrhythmias is confined to a few isolated reports. The first case was described by Leriche and Fontaine,[32] who successfully treated two patients with recurrent supraventricular tachycardia by bilateral thoracic sympathectomy. In 1952, White, Smithwick, and Simeone[33] reviewed their experience in treating six patients with paroxysmal atrial tachycardia by either unilateral or bilateral sympathectomy. All patients were benefited significantly by the operation. In 1961, Estes and Izlar[34] reported a patient with recurrent ventricular tachycardia. Following a left-sided

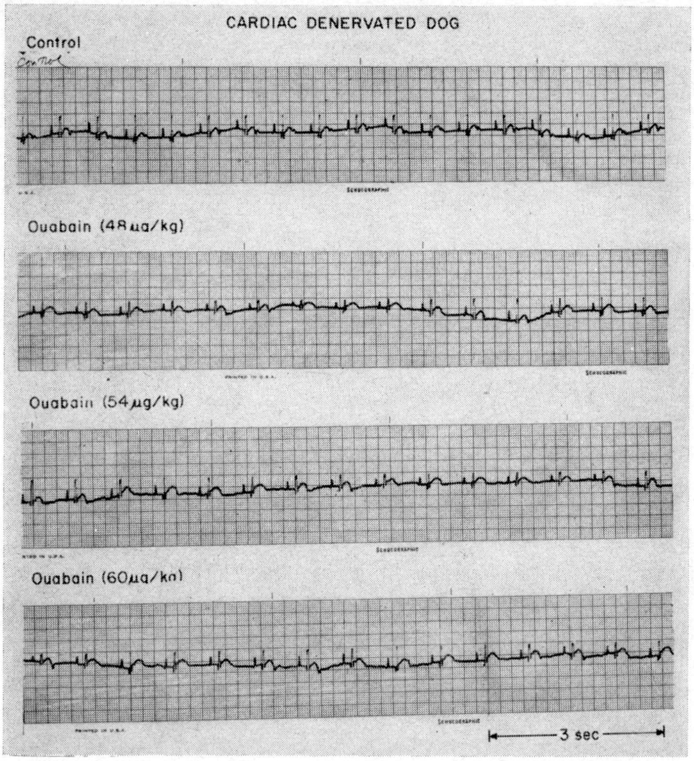


Fig. 11. Electrocardiograms from a dog with a denervated heart during a ouabain infusion. Ouabain was infused at a continuous rate of 30 μg./kg./30 min. and the cumulative dose is shown above each panel. Records were selected to correspond in time and cumulative dose with those from the normal dog shown in Fig. 10. All panels show sinus rhythm with no evidence of digitalis toxic rhythms.

thoracic sympathectomy the arrhythmia ceased and did not recur for 15 months. Frequent episodes of tachycardia then occurred, and a right-sided sympathectomy was performed. During the subsequent five years only rare episodes were observed. Cardiac sympathectomy is a formidable operation, yet the experimental and clinical data appear to justify further trial of this procedure in carefully selected patients.

## Conclusions

The evidence presented above would appear to indicate that the autonomic nervous system may play an important role in certain disturbances of cardiac rhythm. By appropriate activation of the central nervous system one can induce, even in the normal heart, nearly all of the cardiac arrhythmias seen in man. Certain interventions such as coronary occlusion and subtoxic doses of digitalis increase the sensitivity of the heart to the arrhythmogenic effects of autonomic nerve stimulation. Pharmacological or surgical interruption of the cardiac nerves abolishes certain arrhythmias and modifies significantly the response to other pharmacologic agents. From these observations we have concluded that the role of autonomic factors in the genesis of cardiac arrhythmias may be a primary or a permissive influence. To some extent this conclusion has been supported by the clinical use of beta blocking agents and surgical interruption of cardiac sympathetic nerves. The challenge for the future would appear to be to design experiments to examine the relation between the central nervous system and arrhythmias under physiological and psychological stress, to devise better methods for identifying those patients in whom autonomic factors play an important role, and to select those patients in whom appropriate modification of the autonomic influence might make a beneficial contribution to their management.

## *REFERENCES*


1. Sarnoff, S. J., Mitchell, J. H., Gilmore, J. P. and Remensnyder, J. P. Homeometric autoregulation in the Heart, *Circ. Res. 8*:1077, 1960.
2. Wallace, A. G., Cline, R. E., Sealy, W. C., Young, W. G., Jr. and Troyer, W. G., Jr. Electrophysiologic effects of quinidine, studies using chronically implanted electrodes in awake dogs with and without cardiac denervation, *Circ. Res. 19*:960, 1966.
3. Bircher, R. P., Kanai, T. K. and Wang, S. C. Mechanism of cardiac arrhythmias and blood pressure changes induced in dogs with pentylenetetrazol, picrotoxin and deslanoside, *J. Pharmacol. Exp. Ther. 141*:6, 1963.
4. Cooper, T., Gilbert, J. W., Bloodwell, R. D. and Crout, R. J. Chronic extrinsic cardiac denervation by regional neural ablation. *Circ. Res. 9*:275, 1961.
5. Wallace, A. G. and Sarnoff, S. J. Effects of cardiac sympathetic nerve stimulation on conduction in the heart. *Circ. Res. 14*:86, 1964.
6. Rothberger, C. J., and Winterberg, H. Ueber die Beziehungen der Herznerven zur automatischen Reizerzeugung und zum plötzlichen Herztode, *Pflügers Arch. Ges. Physiol. 141*:343, 1911.
7. Daggett, W. M. and Wallace, A. G. Vagal and sympathetic influences on ectopic impulse formation. In: *Mechanisms and Therapy of Cardiac Arrhythmias,* 14th Hahnemann Symposium, L. Dreifus, ed. New York, Grune, Stratton, 1966.
8. Alessi, R., Nusynowitz, M., Abildskov, J. A. and Moe, G. K. Non-uniform distribution of vagal effects on the atrial refractory period, *Amer. J. Physiol. 194*:406, 1958.
9. Han, J., Garcia de Jalon, P. and Moe, G. K. Adrenergic effects on ventricular vulnerability, *Circ. Res. 14*:516, 1964.
10. Han, J. and Moe, G. K. Non-uniform recovery of excitability in ventricular muscle, *Circ. Res. 14*:44, 1964.
11. Wallace, A. G. and Mignone, R. J. Physiologic evidence concerning the reentry hypothesis for ectopic beats, *Amer. Heart J. 72*:60, 1966.
12. Manning, J. W. Mechanism of cardiac arrhythmias induced by diencephalic stimulation, *Amer. J. Physiol. 203*:1120, 1962.

13. Moran, N. C. and Perkins, M. E. Adrenergic blockade of mammalian heart by dichloro analogue of isoproterenol, *J. Pharmacol. Exp. Ther. 124:* 223, 1958.
14. James, T. N. and Nadeau, R. A. The chronotropic and vagal blocking actions of naphthylisoproterenol studied by direct perfusion of the sinus node. *J. Pharmacol. Exp. Ther. 143:*350, 1964.
15. Vaughan Williams, E. M. Mode of action of beta receptor antagonists on cardiac muscle, *Amer. J. Cardiol. 18:* 399, 1966.
16. Wallace, A. G., Troyer, W. G., Lesage, M. A. and Ziotti, E. F. Electrophysiologic effects of isoproterenol and beta-blocking agents in awake dogs, *Circ. Res. 18:*140, 1966.
17. Rouse, W. Effects of propranolol and ouabain on the conducting system of the heart in dogs, *Amer. J. Cardiol. 18:*406, 1966.
18. Rosati, R. A., Alexander, J. A., Wallace, A. G., Sealy, W. C. and Young, W. G., Jr. Failure of beta-adrenergic blockade to alter ventricular fibrillation threshold in the dog, evidence for extra-adrenergic effects of pronethalol, *Circ. Res. 19:*721, 1966.
19. Stock, J. P. P. and Dale, N. Beta-adrenergic receptor blockade in cardiac arrhythmias, *Brit. Med. J. 2:*1230, 1963.
20. Ginn, W. M., Irons, G. V. and Orgain, E. S. Use of propranolol in cardiac arrhythmias, *Circulation 32:*97, 1965 (abst.).
21. Johnstone, M. Beta-adrenergic blockade with pronethalol during anesthesia, *Brit. J. Anaesth. 36:*224, 1964.
22. Lucchesi, R. R. Action of nethalide upon experimentally induced cardiac arrhythmias, *J. Pharmacol. Exp. Ther. 145:*286, 1964.
23. Somani, P., Fleming, J. G., Chan, G. K. and Lum, B. K. B. Antagonism of epinephrine-induced cardiac arrhythmias by 4-(2-isopropylamino-1-hydroxyethyl)-methanesulfonanalide (MJ-1999), *J. Pharmacol. Exp. Ther. 151:*32, 1966.
24. Howe, R. and Shanks, R. H. Optical isomers of propranolol, *Nature 210:* 1336, 1966.
25. Lucchesi, B. R. and Hardman, H. F. The influence of dichloroisoproterenol (DCI) and related compounds upon ouabain and acetylstrophanthidin-induced cardiac arrhythmias, *J. Pharmacol. Exp. Ther. 132:*372, 1961.
26. Moe, G. K. and Farah, A. E. Digitalis and allied cardiac glycosides. In: *Pharmacological Basis of Therapeutics,* L. S. Goodman, A. Gilman, eds., New York, Macmillan, 1965, p. 674.
27. Schaal, S. F. and Wallace, A. G. Alterations of the electrophysiologic effects of digitalis produced by cardiac denervation. In preparation.
28. Harris, A. S. Genesis of ventricular tachycardia and fibrillation following coronary occlusion. In: *Mechanisms and Therapy of Cardiac Arrhythmias,* 14th Hahnemann Symposium, L. Dreifus, ed. New York, Grune, Stratton, 1966, p. 293.
29. Pentecost, B. L. and Austen, W. G. Beta-adrenergic blockade in experimental myocardial infarction, *Amer. Heart J. 72:*790, 1966.
30. McEachern, C. G., Manning, G. W. and Hall, G. E. Sudden occlusion of coronary arteries following removal of cardiosensory pathways, an experimental study, *Arch. Intern. Med. 65:*661, 1940.
31. Harris, A. S., Estandia, A. and Tillotson, R. F. Ventricular ectopic rhythms and ventricular fibrillation following cardiac sympathectomy and coronary occlusion. *Amer. J. Physiol. 165:*505, 1951.
32. Leriche, R. and Fontaine, R. Chirurgie du sympathique. *Rev. Neurol. (Paris) 1:*1046, 1929.
33. White, J. C., Smithwick, R. H. and Simeone, F. A. in: *The Autonomic Nervous System.* New York, Macmillan, 1952, p. 288.
34. Estes, E. H., Jr. and Izlar, H. L., Jr. Recurrent ventricular tachycardia, a case successfully treated by bilateral cardiac sympathetctomy, *Amer. J. Med. 31:*493, 1961.

# PHYLOGENETIC OBSERVATIONS ON SPECIALIZED CARDIAC TISSUES*

E. Neil Moore

Comparative Cardiovascular Studies Unit
Department of Animal Biology
School of Veterinary Medicine
University of Pennsylvania
Philadelphia, Pa.

Although new information is now becoming available on the characteristics of transmembrane action potentials and conduction in neurogenic hearts and myogenic hearts of lower vertebrates, the discussion in this paper will be limited primarily to avian and mammalian hearts. The fact that avian hearts are the first hearts phylogenetically that have Purkinje fibers within their ventricles[1] is, perhaps, partial justification for narrowing the scope of this paper to the hearts of birds and higher mammals. The role of specialized cardiac fibers within the atria as well as within the ventricles will be discussed in relation to the management and interpretation of cardiac arrhythmias. Methods used in these studies have been described in detail previously.[2, 3]

## Specialized Atrial Conduction System

The primary pacemaker of most myogenic hearts lies either in the sinus venosus or in the sinoatrial node. Pacemaker fibers are characterized by action potentials that exhibit diastolic depolarization; they control the basic rate of the heart through variations in: 1) rate of diastolic depolarization (voltage change per unit time), 2) resting potential, 3) threshold potential, and 4) duration of action potential. Transmembrane potential recordings from pacemaker cells of frogs, turtles, and chicks appear nearly identical to those recorded from mammalian hearts.[4] Although the configuration of pacemaker action potentials appears similar in different animals, it is likely that differences occur in the ionic conductance changes and in the species of ions involved in generating potentials.

*Presented at the *Conference on Mechanisms and Management of Arrhythmias,* held by the New York Heart Association at the Hotel Waldorf-Astoria, New York, N. Y., January 24, 1967.

This work was carried out during the tenure of the William Daniel Stroud Investigatorship of the American Heart Association. Previously unpublished observations were supported in part by Grant 65 G 31 from the American Heart Association and in part by Public Health Service Research Grant HE-4885-07 from the National Heart Institute.

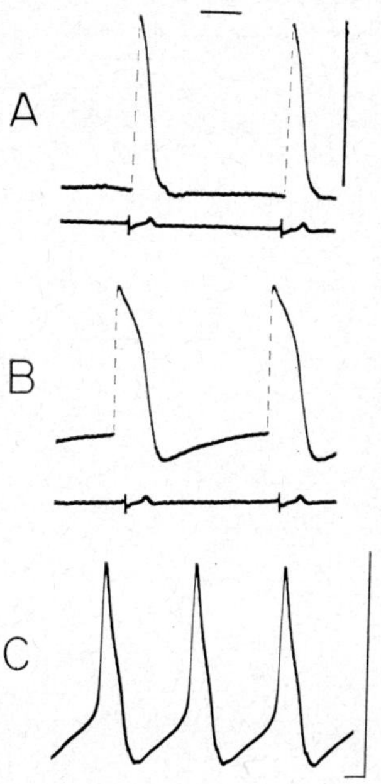


Fig. 1. Chick heart. *A* and *B:* Transmembrane action potentials (*top*) and right atrial electrogram (*bottom*) recorded from an atrial myocardial fiber (*A*) and a specialized atrial fiber (*B*), with 100 msec. indicated at top and 100 mv. at the right of *A*. In *C*, ouabain was added to the Tyrode's solution and a previously latent pacemaker specialized atrial fiber was converted into a true pacemaker. Bars denote 200 msec. and 100 mv.

There has been a controversy for many years as to how the impulse spreads from the sinus node to the atrioventricular node. The experiments of Lewis *et al.*[5] indicated that radial spread over the atria accounted for transmission of the sinus node impulse to the AV node. This has been the most widely accepted view for atrial conduction. Evidence such as the demonstration of Eyster and Meeks[6] that activity from the sinus node arrives at the region of the coronary sinus before many regions of the atria are activated, as well as histological demonstration of intranodal and interatrial pathways was largely overlooked. The recent histological studies of Robb and Petri,[7] and of James[8] provide strong morphological support for specialized atrial pathways. Phylogenetically, there also is evidence for the existence of preferential atrial conduction pathways. The venous valves in frog and turtle hearts that separate the sinus venosus from the atrium exhibit diastolic depolarization. Since they normally are driven by primary pacemaker

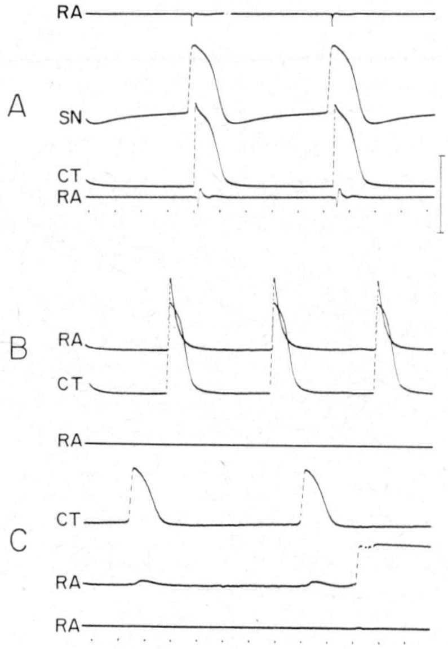


Fig. 2. Rabbit heart. *A:* RA, right atrial electrograms; SN, transmembrane potential recording from sinus node; CT, transmembrane potential recording from specialized atrial fiber in crista terminalis. *B:* RA, transmembrane potential recording from right atrial myocardial fiber and CT, simultaneously recorded transmembrane potential recording from specialized crista terminalis atrial fiber. *C:* CT, transmembrane potential recording from fiber of crista terminalis; RA, transmembrane potential recording from right atrial myocardial fiber; RA, right atrial electrogram; extracellular potassium concentration increased to 12 mM./l in *C,* with 100 mv. bar in *A* and 100 msec. time dots in *A* and *C.*

fibers in the sinus venosus, they could be considered latent pacemakers. In the avian heart there is only a vestigial sinus venosus, but prominent right and left sinoatrial valves contain fibers histologically distinct from atrial myocardial fibers.[9] A typical transmembrane action potential from an atrial myocardial fiber is shown in Figure 1*A*. Fibers within the SA valves exhibit diastolic depolarization as shown in Figure 1*B*. Although the fiber in Fignre 1*B* is a latent pacemaker, diastolic depolarization is usually considered to be a property of specialized fibers. Since in the avian heart the sinoatrial valves course between the primary sinus node and the AV junctional region, they may serve as a preferential conduction pathway between the sinus node and AV junctional fibers. When transmembrane action potentials are recorded from regions where Purkinje fibers occur, the configuration of the action potential appears similar to those recorded from ventricular Purkinje fibers.[9]

In most mammalian hearts, only vestigial remnants of the venous valves can usually be found. In the rabbit atrium, the sinoauricular ring bundle is the remnant structure of the venous valves in amphibian hearts.[10] The right sinoauricular bundle courses between the sinus and AV nodes along the sulcus terminalis. In Figure 2*A* the SN fiber is a latent pacemaker; note the prominent diastolic depolarization. The action potentials recorded from crista terminalis fibers (CT) have configurations similar to that of mammalian Purkinje fibers: i.e., a prominent overshoot and definite plateau. Although in this recording the CT fiber did not exhibit pacemaker properties, latent pacemaker activity in the rabbit heart is frequently recorded from fibers in this region. In Figure 2*B*, a typical atrial myocardial transmembrane potential (RA) is shown simultaneously with an intracellular action potential recorded from a crista terminalis fiber (CT). The lack of a plateau in the RA fiber contrasts with the definite plateau in the CT fiber. Paes de Carvalho *et al.*[10] previously reported similar findings. In the atria of the lamb large fibers with histological characteristics of Purkinje fibers are found. Transmembrane action potentials recorded from them also exhibit action potential configurations typical of Purkinje fibers.[11] Thus, there is morphological, phylogenetical, and electrophysiological evidence that specialized atrial fibers exist in the mammalian heart.

The important point, of course, is whether or not the specialized atrial conduction system should be considered in interpreting cardiac arrhythmias. Assuming the presence of a specialized atrial conducting system, Keith and Flack[12] postulated the occurrence of sinoventricular rhythms; i.e., if activity was propagated over an excitable specialized atrial conduction pathway coursing between the sinus and AV nodes, then a sinus pacemaker could drive the ventricles in the absence of recorded atrial myocardial activity.

In Figure 2*C* the relative difference in sensitivity to hyperpotassemia between specialized atrial fibers and ordinary atrial myocardial fibers is displayed. When extracellular potassium was increased to 12 mM./l., the fiber of the crista terminalis was still capable of generating an action potential. A transmembrane potential recording from a right atrial fiber (RA, third trace) points out that only local nonpropagated activity occurred in the RA fiber at this time. Also, no activity was recorded in either right atrial extracellular electrogram (RA). Similar findings were previously reported by de Mello and Hoffman.[13] The RA microelectrode was withdrawn at the end of the trace in order to demonstrate that the microelectrode was within a single fiber. Experiments on avian specialized atrial fibers also indicate a relative insensitivity of these fibers to increased extracellular concentrations of potassium. Further confirmation of the difference in sensitivity to hyperkalemia between atrial myocardial fibers and specialized atrial fibers was obtained by Vassalle *et al.*[14] When extracellular potassium was increased in *in vivo* studies on canine hearts, sinoventricular rhythms occurred: P waves were absent in the electrocardiogram when extracellular action potentials could be demonstrated in the region of the sinus node. Electrograms from the bundle of His confirmed the fact that antegrade conduction from the sinus node region resulted in ventricular activation. Thus, the possibility of sinoventricular rhythms should be considered whenever P waves are absent and ionic or pharmacological changes have occurred.

A general property of latent pacemaker fibers is that under certain conditions they may be made into true pacemakers. Therefore it should not be surprising that specialized atrial fibers in some circumstances become true pacemakers. In Figure 1*C*, ouabain ($10^{-6}$ M) was added to the Tyrode's solution perfusing the atrial preparation of a chick. In the presence of digitalis the previously latent pacemaker became a primary pacemaker. Species variations do occur in the ability of specialized atrial fibers to become primary pacemaker fibers. In rabbits and birds, specialized atrial fibers may become true pacemaker fibers, while canine specialized atrial fibers[15] are reported to lack this ability. Nevertheless, the definite possibility exists that ectopic atrial responses may originate within specialized atrial tissue.

We have pointed out the different pharmacological properties of specialized atrial fibers, their importance as ectopic atrial pacemakers, and their involvement in sinoventricular rhythms. Another role of specialized atrial fibers may be in influencing the configuration of the P wave. Besides intranodal conduction paths, Dr. James'[8] studies confirm the presence of interatrial conduction pathways. In experiments in which the sinus node was destroyed and a subsidiary pacemaker was allowed to develop, presumably in the region of the coronary sinus, the P waves have been reported to be opposite in polarity to those normally recorded.[16] Largely because of this evidence, P waves of opposite polarity have been used to diagnose A-V nodal and coronary sinus rhythms. However, preferential interatrial conduction paths between the right and left atrium should exert some control over the

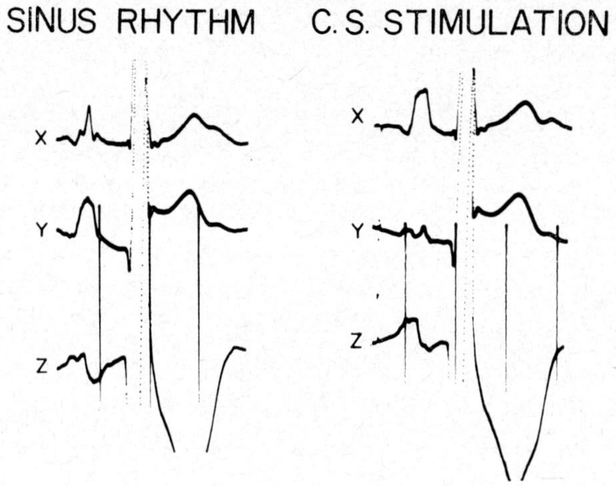


Fig. 3. Dog. *X, Y* and *Z* scalars using the McFee electrocardiographic lead system during normal sinus rhythm and during coronary sinus stimulation; 40 msec. time bars and high gain.

sequence of right and left atrial activation. If an ectopic impulse gained early entrance into the right side of the interatrial conduction pathway, the polarity of the recorded P wave should be essentially the same, independently of whether the impulse originated in the sinus or the AV node; i.e., activity from the sinus or AV nodes would be conducted over the intranodal paths and both should gain entrance into the interatrial path, resulting in a predominantly right to left spread of atrial excitation.

In Figure 3, evidence is presented that shows the similarity in P wave vectors during normal sinus rhythm and after "retrograde" activation from an artificial pacemaker electrode chronically implanted near the coronary sinus. The McFee lead system[17] was used to record scalars in the X, Y, and Z axes. In this system the configuration of the body and the position of the limbs exert less influence on electrocardiogram configurations than is the case in conventional limb leads. The P vector during normal sinus rhythm in Figure 3 is toward the left, caudal, and slightly ventral. When the heart was driven from bipolar electrodes chronically implanted in the region of the coronary sinus at a rate exceeding the normal sinus rate, the P vector was toward the left, dorsal, and slightly caudal.

We feel that in our experiments the P waves were not inverted

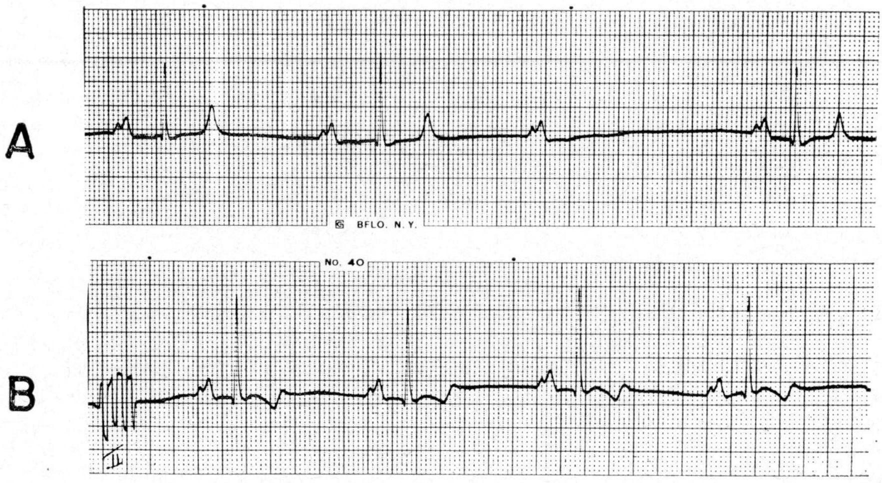


Fig. 4. Lead 2 electrocardiograms of a horse during rest (*A*) and following exercise (*B*); 1 mv. calibration in *B*.

during retrograde activation of the atria because care was taken to avoid damage to the intranodal and interatrial conduction pathways.[18] In most of the previous studies,[16] the SA node was destroyed by various methods, all of which would have injured or caused changes in the specialized conduction system of the atria. Additional support of the hypothesis that the specialized conduction system can permit retrograde P waves of the same polarity as normal sinus node P waves is the observation that, when the atria are not damaged, it is possible to drive the ventricles and to record a retrograde P wave of normal polarity in the standard limb leads.[18] There is no question that P waves of opposite polarity often are recorded during retrograde conduction. We feel, however, that when inverted P waves are recorded one should consider the possibility of damage to the intranodal or interatrial atrial pathways.[18]

## Atrioventricular Conduction System

In hearts of lower vertebrates a complete ring of nodal tissue is present at the atrioventricular junction. With evolution, the conducting system develops to a state in which only several regions of the right AV junction in birds have nodal tissue.[1] In mammals, of course, a single AV node is found normally. The AV node plays a major role in the analysis of cardiac arrhythmias since it is in this region that AV conduction delays, block, and subsidiary pacemakers are usually considered most

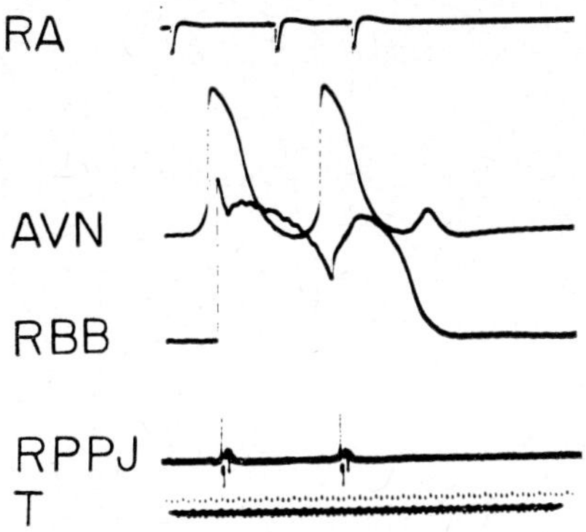


Fig. 5. Rabbit heart. RA, right atrial electrogram. The first response is the basic $A_1$ response and is followed by two premature atrial responses, $A_2$ and $A_3$. AVN, transmembrane potential recordings from the AV node; RBB, transmembrane potential recordings from the right bundle branch; RPPJ, right Purkinje-papillary muscle electrogram; *T,* time dots denote 10 msec.

likely to occur. However, using information contained in standard limb lead electrocardiograms or simultaneously recorded atrial and ventricular electrocardiograms, it is difficult, and usually impossible, to determine accurately the site of AV conduction delays, block or subsidiary pacemakers. Recent observations on AV transmission, made by means of intracellular and extracellular techniques that record from different regions of the AV node and His-Purkinje system, will be presented in the remainder of this paper.

*Antegrade conduction delays and block.* Figure 4 shows a standard lead II electrocardiogram recorded from a horse at rest (*A*) and after exercise (*B*). In Figure 4*A* a typical Wenckebach cycle was recorded with AV conduction time progressively increasing until the third atrial response was blocked; the subsequent fourth response had a shortened P-R interval. First and second degree AV block in this animal would usually be considered to result from gradual increases in refractoriness of the AV node. Most cardiologists would not consider an individual with Wenckebach cycles and dropped beats to be a prime prospect for the Olympic distance races. However, second degree heart block is normal in the horse, provided that block disappears with exercise as it did in this animal (Figure 4*B*). This electrocardiogram* was recorded from a standardbred mare which had earned more than $140,000 at the race track. Therefore, complete heart block is not necessarily undesirable.

*Courtesy of Dr. Fred Fregin.

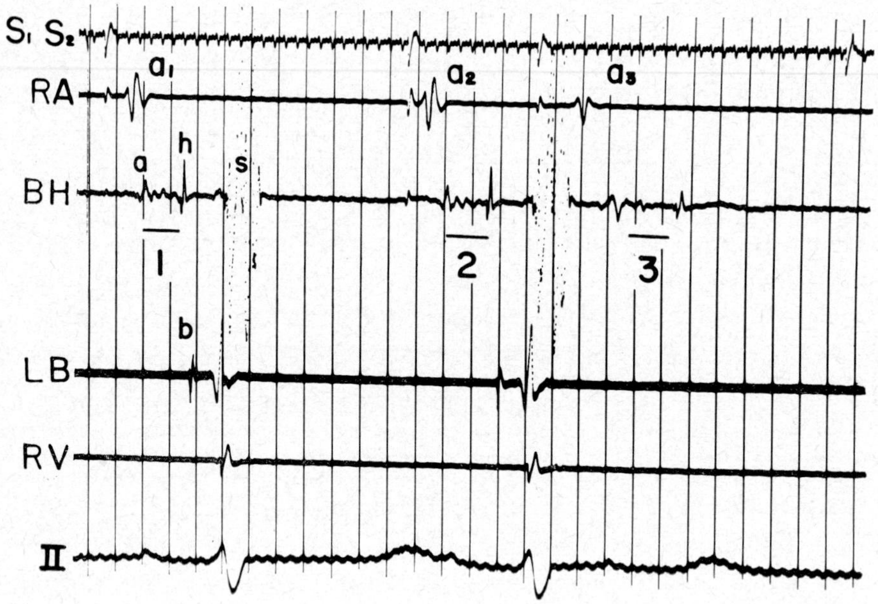


Fig. 6. Newborn calf. $S_1S_2$, stimulus artifacts; RA, right atrial electrogram; BH, bundle of His electrogram; LB, left bundle branch electrogram; RV, right ventricular electrogram; II, lead 2 electrocardiogram. $A_1$, basic atrial response followed by two premature atrial responses, $A_2$ and $A_3$; *h* denotes His bundle deflection in BH and *b* indicates bundle branch activity in LB.

The records in Figure 5 were recorded from an isolated rabbit AV preparation in which the AV conduction time gradually increased; the third atrial response was blocked completely within the AV node. RA is a right atrial electrogram, AVN and RBB are AV nodal and right bundle branch transmembrane action potentials, and RPPJ is a right Purkinje papillary muscle electrogram. In the RPPJ record, the initial large deflection represents Purkinje activity followed by the smaller ventricular activity, directed downward. The first atrial response was conducted through the AV node, over the bundle of His (not shown) and the right bundle branch to the ventricles ($v_1$). The second atrial response also was conducted to the ventricles but with an increase in AV conduction time. First degree AV block resulted not only from delayed conduction through the AV node, but also from increased transmission time within the His-Purkinje system. Delayed transmission time within the ventricular specialized conduction system (VSCS) was due to activity from the bundle of His exciting the RBB during its relative refractory period, i.e., before the RBB had repolarized to its diastolic level. Consequently the RBB response to the A2 beat exhibited a decreased rate of depolarization and decreased action potential amplitude and duration. As in Figure 4, the third atrial response in this recording failed to result in ventricular excitation. Second degree block resulted from block within the AV node as demonstrated by the local, unpropagated response of the AV node and the lack of any activity recorded in the RBB fiber. In *in vivo* studies on dogs, Hoffman and associates[19] found that first and second degree block usually were associated with AV nodal conduction delays and block. Studies on the hearts of chicks and adult turkeys also suggest that first and second degree AV block usually occur within the AV node.

The His-Purkinje system must also be considered as a potential region for AV conduction delays and block. In Figure 6 electrograms were recorded in a 2-day-old calf simultaneously from the right atrium (RA), bundle of His (BH), left bundle branch (LB), and right ventricle, along with a standard lead II electrocardiogram. Stimulus artifacts appear in the top trace (S1S2). The electrogram from the bundle of His contains an initial atrial deflection (*a*), followed by a His bundle deflection (*h*) and ventricular septal muscle deflections (*s*). Left bundle activity (*b*) is followed by ventricular septal muscle activity in the LB electrogram. The AV nodal conduction time (RA to BH interval) of the A2 response was 15 msec. longer than for the A1 response (93 vs. 77). The A3 response was conducted through the AV node with a conduction time between right atrium and bundle of His (RA3-BH3 response interval) of 148 msec. However, activity from the bundle of His failed to be propagated to the bundle branches and ventricles. Thus in this 2-day-old calf, complete AV block occurred below the AV node and bundle of His, but above the bundle branches. In more mature calves, early premature atrial responses underwent greater delays in the AV node than in the newborn animals and complete block usually did not develop within the VSCS. It was not uncommon, however, for the premature response to be blocked within the RBB system, with conduction still occurring over the left bundle; i.e., functional right bundle branch block occurred. Moe *et al.* have reported functional right bundle branch block in adult dogs.[20]

In Figure 7 right atrial and ventricular electrograms were recorded along with transmembrane action potentials from the bundle of His and RBB in an isolated rabbit AV preparation. The A1 atrial response

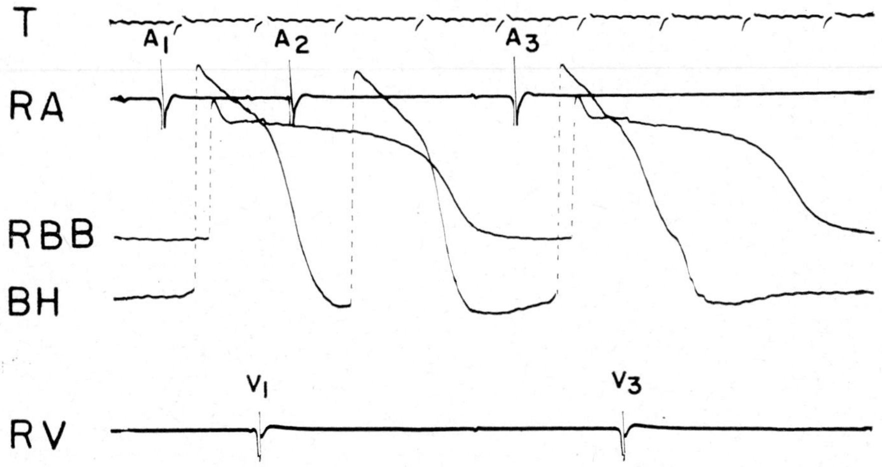


Fig. 7. Rabbit heart. T, time dots of 100 msec.; RA, right atrial electrogram; RBB and BH. transmembrane action potentials of right bundle branch and bundle of His respectively; RV, right ventricular electogram. The RBB tracing was recorded at reduced gain.

was conducted to the ventricles ($V_1$). Although the $A_2$ premature atrial response was conducted through the AV node, resulting in an all-or-none bundle of His action potential, complete block occurred between the bundle of His and the RBB; i.e., activity spreading from the $BH_2$ response failed to excite the RBB fiber. Block between the bundle of His and the RBB resulted from the longer effective refractory period of the bundle branch in this experiment. The subsequent $A_3$ response was propagated to the ventricles. Thus, second degree AV block can result from failure of conduction in the VSCS rather than from block within the AV node.

The interpretation of many arrhythmias is aided by recording an intracavity electrogram simultaneously with a standard electrocardiogram. In Figure 8*A* a base apex ECG[21] (right anterior region of the scapula [base of heart] to sternum at level of the sixth interspace [apex of heart] and an atrial electrogram were recorded in an adult mule. Besides using the right atrial catheter for recording, it was possible also to stimulate the atrium through the catheter electrode. By rapid stimulation, atrial fibrillation was initiated in this unanesthetized adult mule; atrial fibrillation persisted in the absence of stimulation for over 24 hours. The gross irregularity of the electrical responses in the right atrium during atrial fibrillation can be noted in the intracavity record-

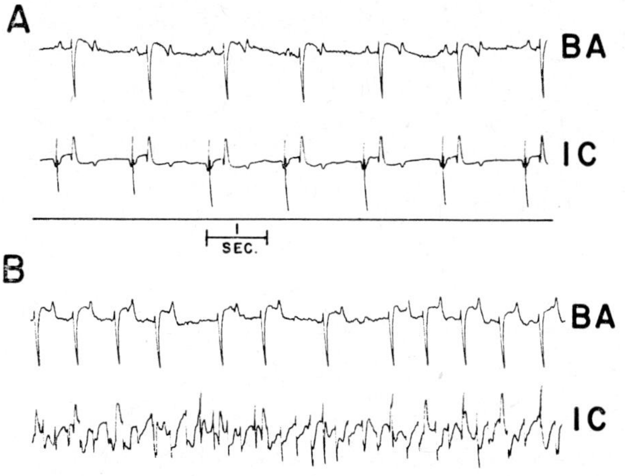


Fig. 8. Adult mule. BA, base apex electrocardiogram; IC, intracavity atrial electogram. The tracings in *A* were recorded during normal sinus rhythm and in *B* during atrial fibrillation. Time bar denotes 1 sec.

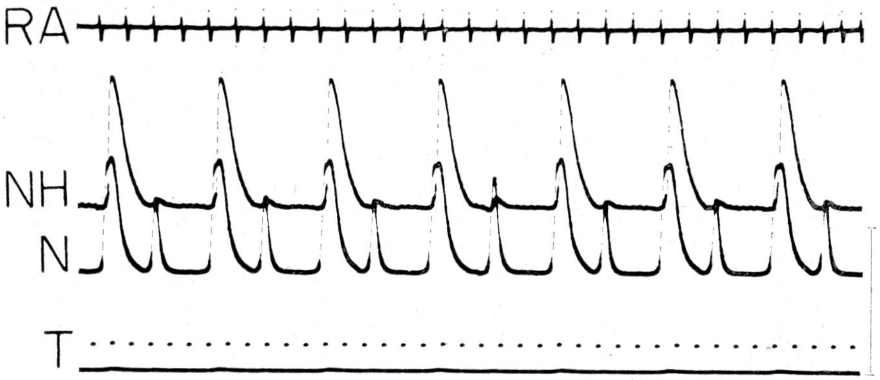


Fig. 9. Rabbit heart. RA, right atrial electrogram; NH and N, transmembrane action potentials recorded from middle AV node and lower AV node; T, time dots of 100 msec., and 100 mv. bar. Recorded during atrial fibrillation.

ing (1C) in Figure 8*B*. However, the intracavity electrogram does not provide any information as to the mechanism of the ventricular dysrhythmia. In normal adult cattle, which also have large atrial masses, initiation of atrial fibrillation by means of stimulating catheter electrodes resulted in atrial fibrillation, which continued spontaneously for up to eight weeks.[21] In normal goats, calves, dogs, and rabbits, with correspondingly smaller atrial masses, atrial fibrillation induced by similar techniques failed to persist in the absence of stimulation for more than several minutes.[21]

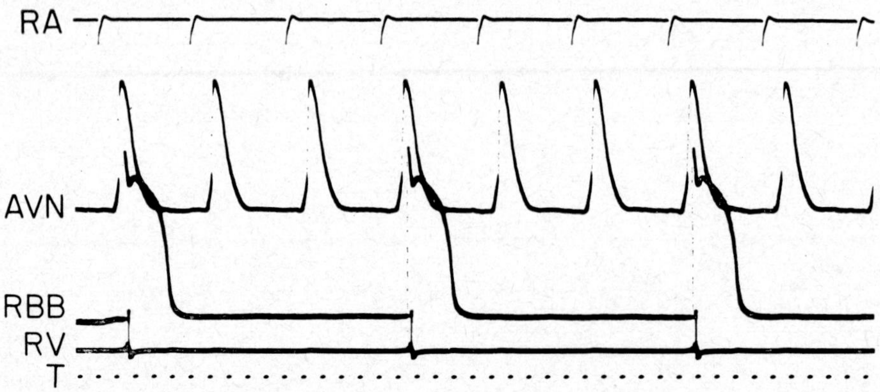


Fig. 10. Rabbit heart, RA and RV, right atrial and right ventricular electrograms; AVN and RBB, transmembrane action potentials recorded from AV node and right bundle branch; T, time dots of 100 msec., 3:1 AV block.

Aberrant QRS complexes were seldom recorded during atrial fibrillation. This suggests that the long intervals between ventricular responses usually result from concealed conduction within the AV node. In Figure 9 it is shown that complete AV block occurred within the AV node during atrial fibrillation initiated by rapid atrial stimulation in an isolated rabbit heart preparation. Rapid atrial activity is shown in the RA electrogram, and every other N response recorded from the N region of the AV node failed to propagate to the lower NH region of the AV node; i.e., 2:1 block occurred within the AV node. In this experiment on fibrillation, AV nodal conduction usually was more complex than 2:1 block. When an all-or-none action potential was recorded from the NH fiber in this experiment, conduction to the ventricles always occurred with a constant conduction time. In only a few experiments on normal animals has the ventricular arrhythmia during atrial fibrillation been associated with conduction delays and block within the VSCS.[22]

The microelectrode technique is very useful for defining the site and, in some cases, the mechanism of AV block. In some instances, though, it can lead to erroneous interpretations. In Figure 10 a record of 3:1 AV block is shown, with every second and third atrial response apparently being blocked below the AV node. However, in the rare experiments in which 3:1 AV block was observed, the blocked responses were always blocked within the AV node. The AVN action potentials were recorded from an AV nodal fiber located above the site

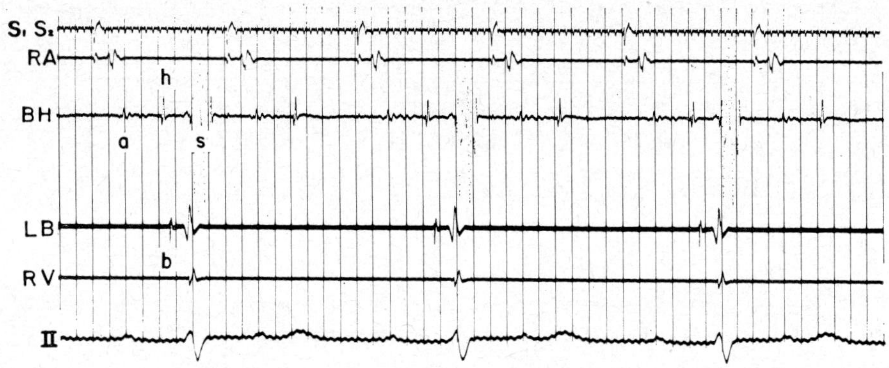


Fig. 11. Newborn calf. $S_1S_2$, stimulus artifacts; RA, right atrial electrogram; BH, bundle of His electrogram with atrial (*a*), His bundle (*h*) and ventricular septal (*s*) deflections; LB, left bundle branch electrogram with left bundle activity labeled *b*; RV, right ventricular electrogram; II, lead 2 electrogram: 2:1 block took place with block occurring below the AV node; 40 msec. time lines.

of AVN block. Only local nonpropagated potentials were recorded during the blocked beats when the microelectrode was moved to the lower NH region of the AV node.

Although 2:1 AV block usually results from alternate block within the AV node, we have observed instances in which 2:1 block occurred within the VSCS. In Figure 11, recorded from a newborn calf, electrograms were recorded from the right atrium (RA), bundle of His (BH), left bundle branch (LB), and right ventricle (RV), along with a lead II electrocardiogram. The presence of 2:1 AV block can be noted in the lead II ECG. All atrial responses (RA) were conducted through the AV node to the bundle of His, as indicated by the presence of a His bundle deflection (*h*) following every atrial response (*a*). Note in the left bundle branch electrogram, however, that every other response of the bundle of His fails to be propagated to the left bundle branch. The failure of conduction over the right bundle branch system is confirmed by the absence of a right ventricular electrogram. The conduction time through the AV node remained constant for the blocked and conducted response.

The mechanism of 2:1 block with block occurring below the AV node is indicated in Figure 12. In this figure electrograms were recorded from right atrium (RA) and ventricle (RV) together with transmembrane potentials from the bundle of His (BH) and right bundle branch (RBB). Although the RA response was conducted through the AV

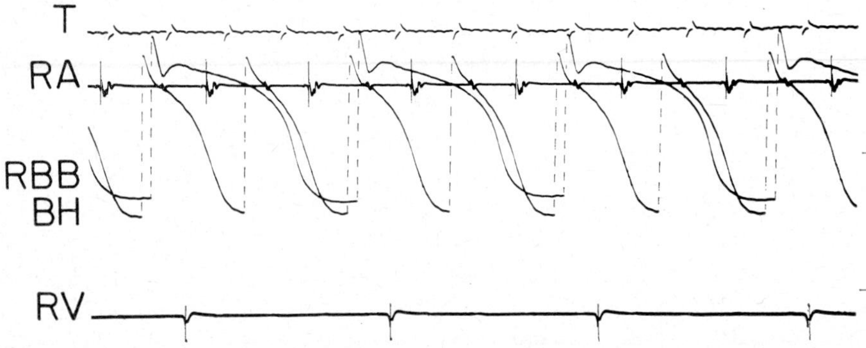


Fig. 12. Rabbit heart. T, time dots of 100 msec.; RA and RV, right atrial and right ventricular electrograms; RBB and BH, transmembrane action potentials recorded from right bundle branch and bundle of His. Vertical bar denotes 100 mv.; 2:1 AV block with block developing between the bundle of His and right bundle branch.

node to the bundle of His, every second response failed to be conducted to the RBB and ventricles. The 2:1 block within the VSCS resulted from the discrepancy between the refractory periods of the bundle of His and the right bundle. The duration of the action potential and the refractory period of the bundle branch and Purkinje fibers is dependent upon length of the preceding cycle. Although the length of the preceding cycle for the bundle of His was 184 msec., that for the right bundle branch was 368 msec. This difference of the length of the preceding cycle accentuates the differences in refractory periods of the bundle branches and bundle of His, and enables 2:1 AV block within the VSCS to be "programmed." Once initiated, 2:1 block with block below the AV node can be maintained indefinitely, provided the AV conduction time and atrial rate remain constant. By changing the basic length of the atrial cycle, or by introducing premature atrial responses, 2:1 block within the VSCS was eliminated whenever a conducted response shortened the length of the preceding cycle in the bundle branch-Purkinje system.

Although it is relatively easy to produce 2:1 AV block in most vertebrate hearts by rapid atrial stimulation, block occurs routinely in the AV node. Block below the AV node is most rapidly set up by abruptly increasing the atrial rate from a slow rate to a rapid one. This prevents the duration of the action potential and the refractory periods of the bundle branch and Purkinje fibers from becoming progressively shortened. Alternately, 2:1 AV block within the VSCS can be initiated

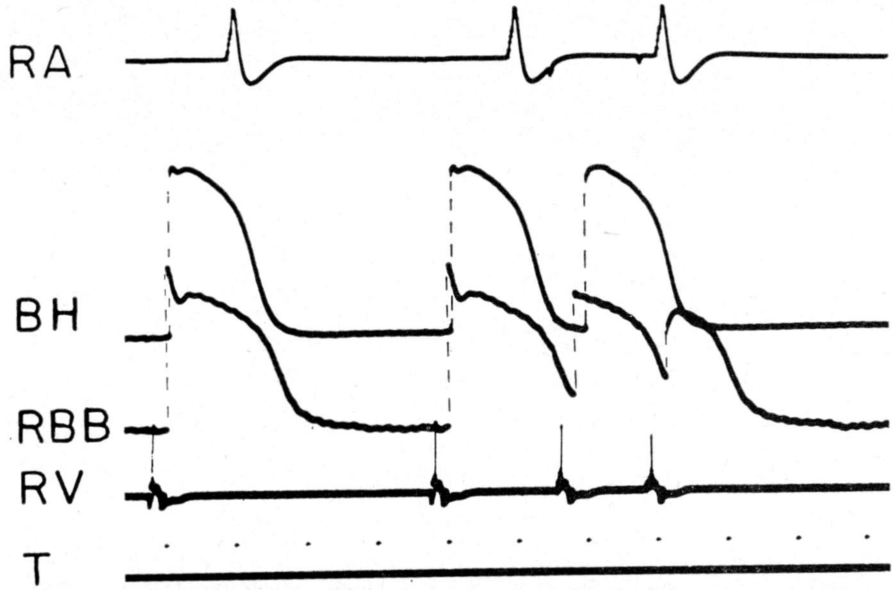


Fig. 13. RA and RV, right atrial and right ventricular electrograms; BH and RBB, bundle of His and right bundle branch transmembrane potentials; T, time dots of 100 msec. Retrograde ventriculoatrial conduction of two basic ventricular responses ($V_1$) followed by first degree ($V_2$) and complete block ($V_3$) of two premature ventricular responses.

by a train of atrial stimuli "programmed" to produce an initial long cycle followed by an atrial rate rapid enough to cause 2:1 block.

*Retrograde conduction delays and block.* We have already pointed out the possibility of antegrade conduction delays occurring within the ventricular specialized conduction system (VSCS) as well as within the AV node. Since premature responses are more common in the ventricles than in the atria, it is perhaps worthwhile to discuss some of the sites and mechanisms of retrograde conduction delay and block. The functional refractory period and the duration of action potential of Purkinje fibers are much longer than those of ventricular myocardial fibers; therefore it is not surprising that retrograde conduction delays and block can occur within this region. The AV node usually is considered the principal region of retrograde conduction delays and block; indeed, retrograde conduction delays and block do occur there. However, in experiments on isolated rabbit AV preparations, the bundle branch-His bundle system was demonstrated to be a frequent region for retrograde conduction delays and block.[23]

In Figure 13 the first three ventricular responses were all conducted

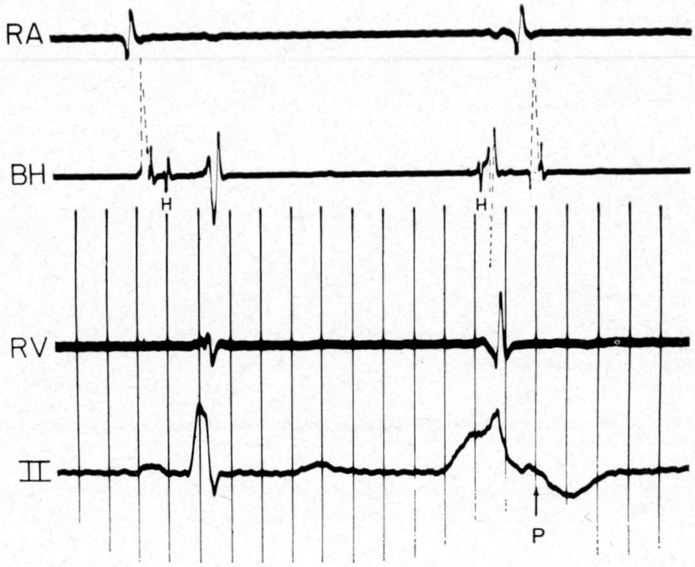


Fig. 14. Dog. RA, right atrial electrogram; BH, bundle of His electrogram with His bundle activity labeled *h;* RV, right ventricular electrogram; II, lead 2 electrocardiogram. Bigeminal coupled rhythm. P denotes a retrograde P wave; 40 msec. time lines.

backward to the atria. The last conducted ventricular response ($V_2$) underwent conduction delays between the impaled right bundle branch fiber and bundle of His, as well as within the AV node (BH to RA response interval). The last ventricular response, $V_3$, arrived at the RBB during its relative refractory period, but still evoked an all-or-none action potential in the RBB fiber. The RBB response, however, failed to be propagated to the bundle of His. It was initially surprising to find retrograde block in this region, since the duration of action potentials of the fibers in the bundle of His is shorter than that in fibers of the bundle branch. The reason for block at this site was found to be associated with a greater abbreviation of the refractory period of bundle branch fibers by decreases in preceding cycle lengths than occurred in fibers of the bundle of His. Also, the fibers in the bundle of His usually had a higher threshold for excitation during their relative refractory period than did fibers of the bundle branch and Purkinje systems. Thus, in interpreting complex arrhythmias, one should consider the possibility that retrograde conduction block and delay can occur either within the AV node or the VSCS.

*Pharmacologically induced cardiac arrhythmias.* In studying cardiac

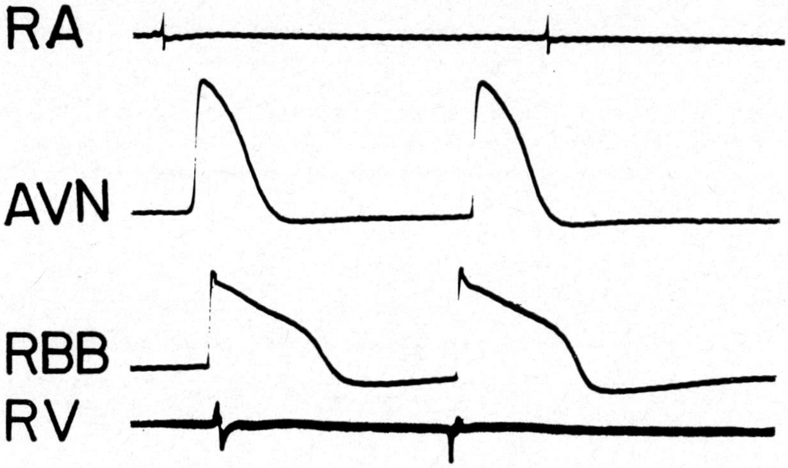


Fig. 15. Rabbit heart. RA and RV, right atrial and right ventricular electrograms; AVN and RBB, AV nodal and right bundle branch transmembrane action potentials. Recorded during bigeminal coupled rhythm.

arrhythmias, it is often difficult to produce the desired arrhythmia by pharmacological methods. The observation that differences of only 1 msec. between atrial premature impulses can determine whether AV conduction does or does not occur also imposes a limit on the analysis of spontaneously evoked arrhythmias. These facts have resulted in many studies on complex arrhythmias being "programmed" by means of biological stimulators. Nevertheless, from a clinical standpoint, pharmacologically evoked arrhythmias are important.

In Figures 14 to 17, bigeminal coupled rhythms and ventricular tachycardias are displayed. These conditions were initiated by giving varying doses of norepinephrine to cyclopropane-anesthetized dogs, or to isolated rabbit AV preparations. Dressel suggested that these arrhythmias resulted from reentry within the AV node.[24] To examine this hypothesis, electrograms were recorded in dogs with implanted electrodes from the right atrium, the bundle of His, and the right ventricle, along with a lead II electrocardiogram.

Figure 14 was recorded during a bigeminal coupled rhythm. The first QRS complex was normal and was followed by a coupled abnormal complex. Normal AV conduction resulted in a biphasic His bundle complex (*H*) with an initial negative deflection. During the abnormal coupled ventricular response, ventricular depolarization (lead II) occurred before any activity was recorded in the electrogram from the

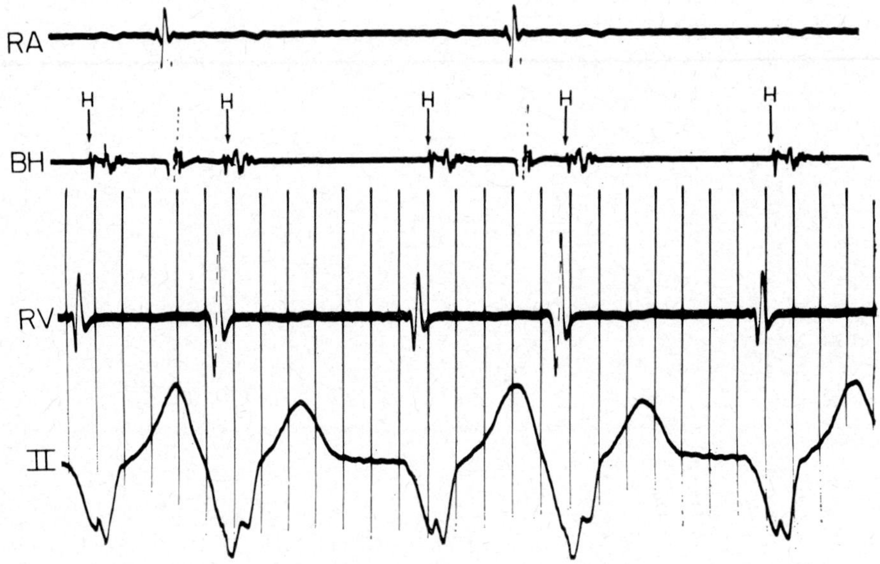


Fig. 16. Cardiac electrograms recorded in the same dog as Figure 14 during a multifocal ventricular tachycardia. Bundle of His activity is labeled *H*.

bundle of His. Also, the configuration of the latter electrogram was reversed from the normal antegrade complex. Therefore, in this instance the coupled beat could not have resulted from activity within the AV node. Also note in this figure that retrograde conduction of ventricular activity back to the atrium resulted in a normal upright P wave in lead II. The large atrial complex in the BH electrogram and RA electrogram both confirm that the upright deflection labeled P in the lead II ECG represents atrial activity. This record supports the earlier discussion in which it was shown that inverted P waves do not necessarily result from retrograde activation of the atria.

Figure 15 was recorded in an experiment on an isolated rabbit AV preparation. If it had been possible to record an electrocardiogram in this experiment, the first RV complex would have been the normal complex, followed by the coupled abnormal ventricular response. The coupled response originated not within the AV node, but in a region below the RBB, since ventricular depolarization preceded the RBB action potential. Thus in an isolated preparation it is possible to see "bigeminal coupled rhythms" which do not originate within the AV node and which develop in the absence of changes in blood pressure, hyperpotassemia, etc.

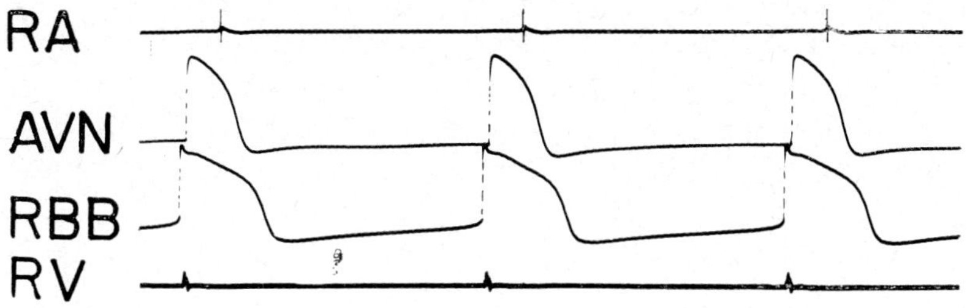


Fig. 17. Recorded in the same isolated rabbit AV preparation as Figure 15. Monofocal ventricular tachycardia with the subsidiary pacemaker near the right bundle branch fiber.

Following larger doses of norepinephrine, multifocal and monofocal ventricular tachycardias are often observed in animals anesthetized with cyclopropane.[25] It also has been suggested that these dysrhythmias result from reentry within the AV node.[24] Figure 16 was recorded in the same dog as Figure 14. During multifocal ventricular tachycardia, ventricular depolarization in the lead II electrocardiogram still preceded any recorded activity in the electrogram derived from the bundle of His. Also, the His bundle deflection (*H*) in the BH electrogram was reversed from the normal initially negative, biphasic H complex recorded during antegrade conduction. Figure 17, recorded during "monofocal ventricular tachycardia" in an isolated AV preparation in a rabbit, further confirms the probability that monofocal and multifocal ventricular tachycardias result not from reentry within the AV node, but rather from enhanced pacemaker activity within the bundle branch-Purkinje system, i.e., pacemaker action potentials in the right bundle branch (RBB) fiber preceded ventricular depolarization (RV).

## Summary

This essay describes observations on specialized cardiac fibers within the atria, the atrioventricular node, and the specialized ventricular conduction systems of several species of birds and mammals. Phylogenetic and electrophysiologic evidence is presented to support the opinion that an atrial specialized conduction system exists. The specialized atrial conduction system with its intranodal and interatrial tracts is thought to play a role in the interpretation of several arrhythmias: 1) since the specialized atrial fibers are resistant to levels of potassium toxic to ordinary atrial myocardial fibers, sinoventricular rhythms can occur where the sinus node drives the ventricles in the absence of a recordable P wave in the ECG; and 2) in the absence of damage to the intranodal and interatrial specialized pathways, retrograde and antegrade P waves may both have the same polarity, rather than the P waves being inverted during AV nodal or coronary sinus rhythms as reported previously. During antegrade conduction of premature atrial responses, conduction delays and block were observed not only within the AV node, but also within the ventricular specialized conduction system. With retrograde conduction of premature ventricular responses, ventriculoatrial delays and block were observed at multiple sites including, 1) between the ventricles and Purkinje systems, 2) between the bundle branches and bundle of His, and 3) within the AV node. Pharmacologically induced bigeminal coupled rhythms and ventricular tachycardias were demonstrated not to result from subsidiary pacemaker activity within the AV node.

## *REFERENCES*

1. Davies, F. and Francis, E. T. B. The conducting system of the vertebrate heart, *Biol. Rev. 21*:173, 1946.
2. Hoffman, B. F., Cranefield, P. F. and Stuckey, J. H. Concealed conduction, *Circ. Res. 10*:194, 1961.
3. Moore, E. N. Microelectrode studies on concealment of multiple premature atrial responses, *Circ. Res. 18*:660, 1966.
4. McCann, F. V. Unique properties of the moth myocardium. In: Comparative Cardiology. H. H. Hecht and D. K. Detweiler, ed., *Ann. N.Y. Acad. Sci. 127*:84, 1965.
5. Lewis, T., Meakins, J. and White, P. D. The excitatory process in dog's heart. I. The auricles, Phil. Trans. Roy. Soc., London, Ser. B *205*:375, 1914.
6. Eyster, J. A. E. and Meek, W. J. Experiments on the origin and propagation of the impulse in the heart. The point of primary negativity in the mammalian heart and the spread of negativity to other regions. *Heart 5*:119, 1913-14.
7. Robb, J. S. and Petri, R. Expansions of the atrio-ventricular system in the atria. In: *The Specialized Tissues of the Heart,* A. P. de Carvalho, W. C. de Mello, and B. F. Hoffman, eds. Amsterdam, Elsevier, 1961, pp. 7-8.
8. James, T. N. The connecting pathways between the sinus node and A-V node and between the right and left atrium in the human heart, *Amer. Heart J. 66*:498, 1963.
9. Moore, E. N. Experimental electrophysiological studies on avian hearts. In: Comparative Cardiology. H. H. Hecht and D. K. Detweiler, eds., *Ann. N.Y. Acad. Sci. 127*:113, 1965.
10. Paes de Carvalho, A., de Mello, W. C. and Hoffman, B. F. Electrophysiological evidence for specialized fiber types in rabbit atrium, *Amer. J. Physiol. 196*:483, 1959.
11. Moore, E. N. Atrioventricular transmission in newborn calves. In: Comparative Cardiology. H. H. Hecht and D. K. Detweiler, eds., *Ann. N.Y. Acad. Sci. 127*:113, 1965.
12. Keith, A. and Flack, M. The form and nature of the muscular connections between the primary divisions of the vertebrate heart, *J. Anat. Physiol. 41*:172, 1907.
13. de Mello, W. C. and Hoffman, B. F. Potassium ions and electrical activity

of specialized cardiac fibers, *Amer. J. Physiol. 199*:1125, 1960.

14. Vassalle, M., Greenspan, K., Jomain, S. and Hoffman, B. F. Effects of potassium on automaticity and conduction of canine hearts, *Amer. J. Physiol. 207*: 334, 1964.
15. Wagner, M. L., Lazzara, R., Weiss, R. M. and Hoffman, B. F. Specialized conducting fibers in the interatrial band. *Circ. Res. 18*:502, 1966.
16. Scherf, D. and Cohen, J. *The Atrioventricular Node and Selected Cardiac Arrhythmias.* New York, Grune, Stratton, 1964.
17. McFee, R. and Parungao, A. An orthogonal lead system for clinical electrocardiography, *Amer. Heart. J. 62*:93, 1961.
18. Moore, E. N., Jomain, S. L., Stuckey, J. H., Buchanan, J. W. and Hoffman, B. F. Experimental studies on ectopic atrial rhythm in dogs, *Amer. J. Cardiology 19*:676, 1967.
19. Hoffman, B. F., Moore, E. N., Cranefield, P. F. and Stuckey, J. H. Functional properties of the atrioventricular conduction system, *Circ. Res. 13*:308, 1963.
20. Moe, G. K., Mendes, C. and Han, J. Aberrant atrioventricular impulse propagation in the dog heart. A study of functional bundle branch block. *Circ. Res. 16*:261, 1965.
21. Moore, E. N., Fisher, G., Detweiler, D. K. and Moe, G. K. The importance of atrial mass in the persistence of atrial fibrillation. Proceedings, *International Symposium on Comparative Medicine.* R. J. Tashjian, ed., Eaton Labs., 1965, pp. 229-238.
22. Moore, E. N. Observations on concealed conduction in atrial fibrillation, *Cir. Res. 21*:201, 1967.
23. Moore, E. N. Microelectrode studies on retrograde concealment of multiple premature ventricular responses, *Circ. Res. 20*:88, 1967.
24. Dressel, P. E. Cyclopropane epinephrine arrhythmias. In: *Effects of Anesthetics on the Circulation.* H. L. Price and P. J. Cohen, eds., Springfield, Ill., Thomas, 1964.
25. Moore, E. N., Morse, H. T. and Price, H. L. Cardiac arrhythmias produced by catecholamines in anesthetized dogs, *Circ. Res. 15*:77, 1964.

# ARRHYTHMIAS AND ELECTROLYTE DISTURBANCES*

BORYS SURAWICZ

Cardiovascular Division, Department of Medicine
The University of Kentucky College of Medicine, Lexington, Ky.

NEW information derived from the electrophysiological laboratory, in particular from studies employing microelectrodes, has contributed to a more rational approach to the diagnosis and treatment of cardiac arrhythmia. The purpose of this paper is to correlate some of the recent advances in electrophysiology of cardiac fibers with the effect of electrolytes on cardiac rhythm and conduction in man. For a review of cellular electrophysiology the reader is referred to textbooks,[1, 2] review articles,[3, 4] and to the article of B. F. Hoffman in this symposium. This presentation will be divided into three parts: potassium and arrhythmia; other electrolytes and arrhythmia; and effect of electrolytes on the action of digitalis and antiarrhythmic drugs.

## POTASSIUM AND ARRHYTHMIA

*Hyperpotassemia.* Increased extracellular K concentration may alter rhythm and conduction by one or more of the following mechanisms: 1) decreased resting or maximal diastolic membrane potential; 2) increased velocity of repolarization and shortening of the action potential (AP); 3) decreased rate of diastolic depolarization, and increased threshold potential in the pacemaker fibers. Arrhythmias may be also caused by: 4) differences in sensitivity to K among different types of cardiac fibers,[5,6] and 5) "injury currents" resulting from differences in potassium concentration in different parts of the myocardium. The negative inotropic effect of potassium may also possibly play an indirect role in the production of arrhythmia.

*Electrocardiographic pattern of hyperpotassemia.* When plasma K concentration exceeds approximately 5.5 mEq./l., the T waves become tall and peaked, and the Q-T interval shortens. Further increase of plasma K concentration results in decrease of the amplitude of the P

*Presented at the *Conference on Mechanisms and Management of Arrhythmias* held by the New York Heart Association at the Hotel Waldorf-Astoria, New York, N. Y., January 24, 1967.

The work described in this paper was supported in part by Public Health Research Grant HE-07359 from the National Heart Institute.

wave, and progressive widening of both the P wave and the QRS complex. P waves disappear when plasma K concentration exceeds about 8.8 mEq./l. Hyperpotassemia usually increases the duration of the QRS complex uniformly; this suggests diffuse slowing of conduction without change in the sequence of depolarization. The peaking of the T wave and the shortening of the Q-T interval are related to the increased velocity of phase 3 and shortening of the ventricular action potential. The progressive slowing of the intra-atrial and intraventricular conduction is attributed to a slower rate of rise of the AP caused by the less negative resting membrane potential.[7] The P wave disappears when the ventricular complex is still well defined because the atrial fibers become nonexcitable at lower K concentrations than the ventricular fibers.[8] When the P wave disappears and the rhythm remains regular, the pacemaker may be displaced from the S-A mode into the A-V node, the bundle of His, or into the Purkinje fibers. However, even in the absence of atrial depolarization, the impulse from the S-A node may propagate to the ventricles, presumably through specialized atrial fibers.[9] This may result in sinoventricular conduction in the presence of sino-atrial block. When plasma K concentration exceeds about 10 mEq./l., the ventricular rhythm may be irregular, and multiple escape pacemakers may appear in the depressed myocardium. The combination of an irregular rhythm and an absent P wave may simulate atrial fibrillation. An increase of plasma K concentration above 10-14 mEq./l. causes ventricular asystole or ventricular fibrillation. In isolated preparations the bundle of His is most "resistant" to increased extracellular K concentration. An action potential from the bundle was recorded when all other cardiac fibers were nonexcitable.[10] Ventricular fibrillation is probably due to reentry, which is facilitated by the slow intraventricular conduction and the short duration of the ventricular AP.

*Administration of potassium salts.* The effect of K administration on cardiac rhythm and conduction depends on the integrity of the myocardium, the initial plasma K concentration, the amount of administered K, and the change or the rate of change of plasma K concentration. Administration of potassium may produce the following effects: 1) suppression of supraventricular and ventricular ectopic beats and rhythms; 2) shortening or lengthening of the A-V conduction time; 3) atrial and ventricular standstill; 4) defibrillation of the atria and

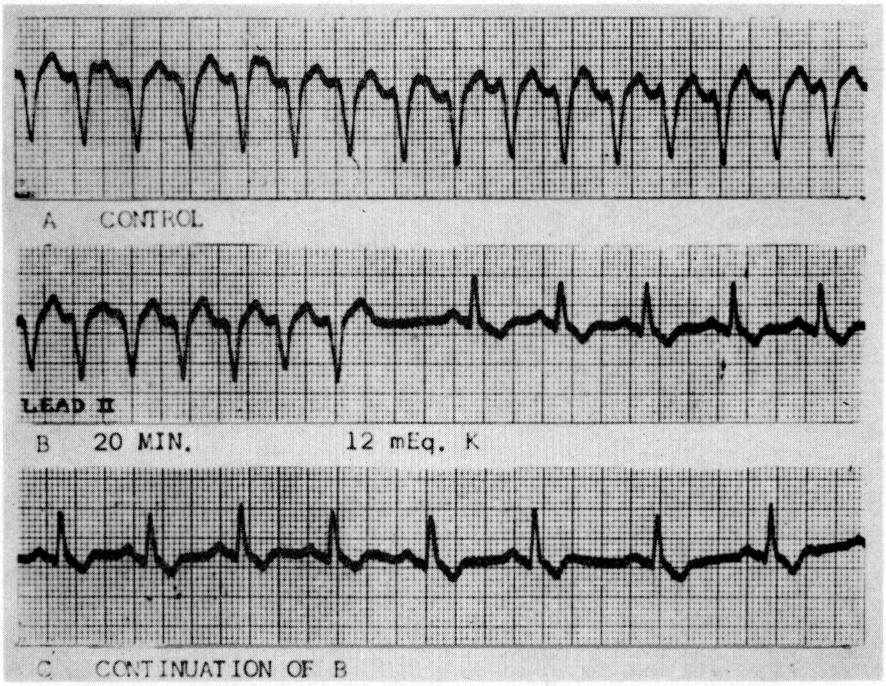


Fig. 1. Abrupt termination of ventricular tachycardia during intravenous KC1 administration. (From B. Surawicz, in: *Cardiovascular Drug Therapy,* p. 467. Brest, A. N. and Moyer, J. H., eds, New York, Grune, Stratton, 1965. Courtesy of publishers).

the ventricles; 5) ventricular fibrillation; 6) increase of ectopic beats.

Intravenous administration of K at a rate of 0.5-1.0 mEq./min. suppresses supraventricular and ventricular ectopic beats and rhythms with the exception of atrial fibrillation and atrial flutter in about 80 per cent of patients.[11] The antiarrhythmic effect usually occurs when plasma K concentration is increased by 0.5-1.0 mEq./l. to a level of 5.0-6.5 mEq./l. Such increase of plasma K concentration usually has no effect on the sinus rate. The disappearance of ectopic beats is probably due to slowing of diastolic depolarization and increase of the threshold potential of the ectopic pacemaker fibers. Administration of K may occasionally terminate an ectopic supraventricular or ventricular tachycardia abruptly (Figure 1). More commonly, however, the rate of the ectopic rhythms decreases gradually (Figure 2). Increased K concentration slows diastolic depolarization in Purkinje fibers more than in the fibers of the S-A node.[12] This may explain the suppression of ectopic activity without change of the sinus rate. Slowing of the rate of diastolic de-

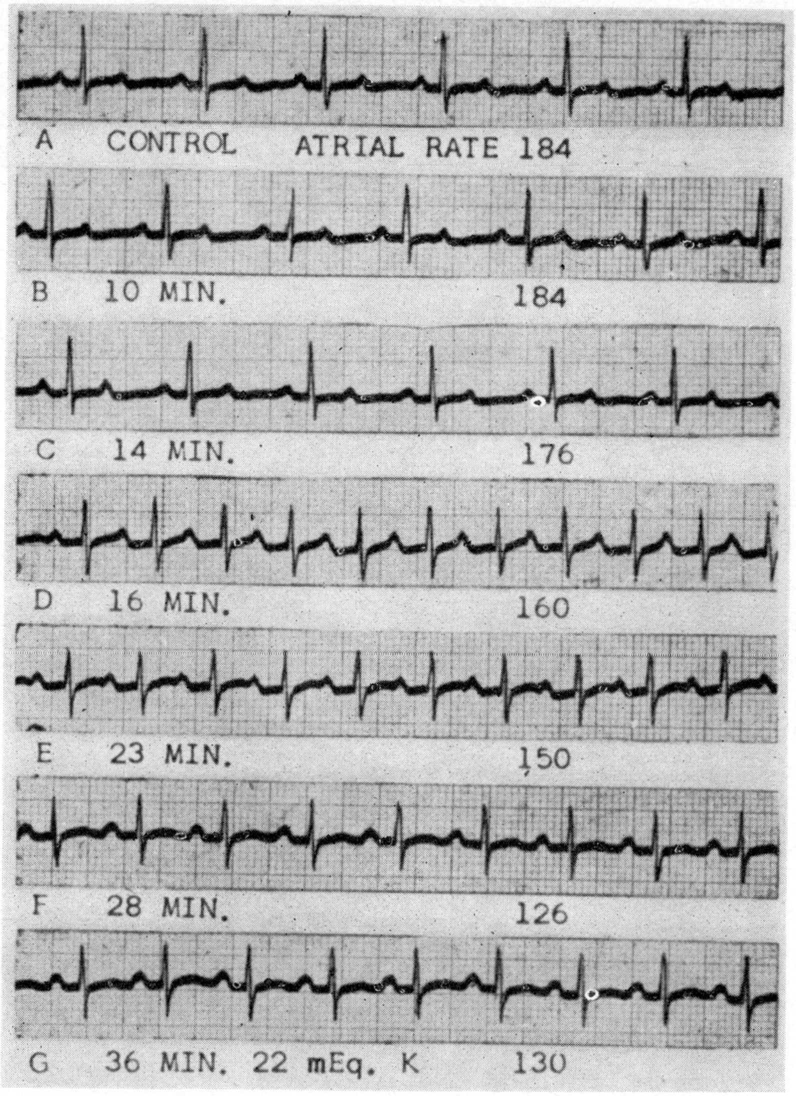


Fig. 2. Gradual decrease of atrial rate during intravenous KCl administration in a patient with ectopic atrial tachycardia. In the strips *A, B,* and *C,* 2:1 A-V conduction; in D-G, 1:1 conduction. (From B. Surawicz, in: *Cardiovascular Drug Therapy,* p. 463. Brest, A. N. and Moyer, J. H., eds., New York, Grune, Stratton, 1965. Courtesy of publishers).

polization in the Purkinje fibers by potassium is attributed to increased potassium permeability.[13-14]

The effect of moderate increase of plasma K concentration on the A-V conduction in man is variable. In some patients, increase of plasma K concentration to 5.0 to 6.5 mEq./l. shortens the P-R interval and abolishes second or third degree A-V block.[11] In other patients the same increase of plasma K concentration may have either no effect or a depressing effect on A-V conduction.[11] The net effect of hyperpotassemia on A-V conduction is determined by the complex interrelation between the change of the resting membrane potential, threshold potential, and the slope of diastolic depolarization in the fibers of the conducting system.[15] The less negative resting membrane potential and threshold potential may result in slower conduction. However, the decreased rate of diastolic depolarization may cause more rapid conduction in fibers depolarized from a more negative diastolic potential. Slight depolarization may also increase A-V conduction velocity by bringing the maximal diastolic potential closer to the threshold potential. In addition, shortening of the AP may also possibly contribute to more rapid conduction. Clinical observations suggest that the most rapid A-V conduction in man probably occurs at K concentrations that are somewhat above the upper limits of normal K concentration. The individual variations may depend on pathological factors such as the degree of damage of the conducting system in the diseased heart, and also on physiological variables such as the complex interplay between potassium and acetylcholine.[16, 17] When plasma K concentration exceeds 8.0 mEq./l. the P-R interval is usually prolonged. When this occurs, the P amplitude is low, and it may be difficult to determine whether the prolongation of the P-R interval is due to the increased duration of the P wave or the duration of the P-R segment.

Cardiac arrest occurs when K depolarizes ventricular fibers to a critical level at which the fibers become nonexcitable.[17] Another type of cardiac arrest has been observed in isolated perfused hearts after a change from K-deficient solution to one containing normal K concentrations.[18] In the rabbit heart this type of arrest was attributed to inhibition of diastolic depolarization of the pacemaker fibers, presumably due to sudden increase of K conductance.[18] The resting membrane potential of the atrial and ventricular fibers was not appreciably decreased at the time of inhibition of the pacemaker, and there were no intraventricular or intra-atrial conduction disturbances before or after arrest.[18] The same phenomenon was also observed in K-depleted dogs.[19] Bradycardia and A-V conduction disturbances that occasionally occur in patients with hypopotassemia during rapid administration of K salts may be caused by the same mechanism (references 83 and 84 in Surawicz [15]).

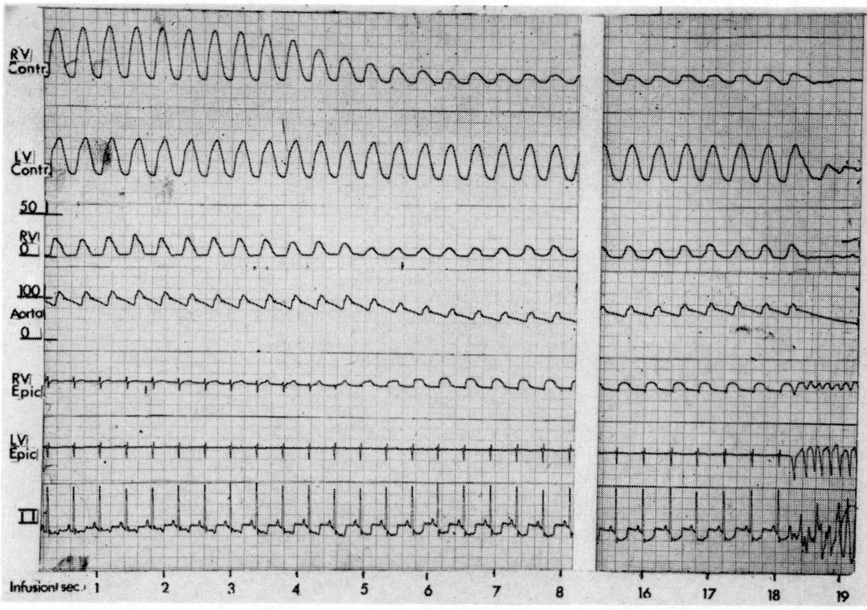


Fig. 3. Infusion of 6.5 ml. of isotonic KC1 solution containing 0.26 mEq. of K into right coronary artery of 20 kg. dog within 15 seconds. Note: Onset of ventricular fibrillation after single ventricular ectopic beat 3 seconds after the end of infusion. There is no change in heart rate, and no increase of QRS duration before the premature beat. See text. Abbreviations: R. V. Contr. and L. V. Contr. = right and left ventricular contractile force measured with strain gauge arches sutured to the surface of the ventricles; R.V. = right ventricular pressure in mm. Hg; Aorta = aortic pressure in mm. Hg; R.V. Epic. and L.V. Epic. = right and left ventricular epicardial electrograms; II = Lead II. (Unpublished observations of A. Krotkiewski and B. Surawicz).

The above observations suggest that rapid rates of change of plasma K concentration may depress the formation and conduction of impulses. The effect of K administration on intraventricular conduction may also depend on the rate of change of plasma K concentration. For instance, slow administration of K in dogs produces a gradual increase of the QRS interval, but rapid administration produces first a decrease and then an increase in the duration of the QRS complex.[19]

In dogs, administration of potassium salts intravenously at a rapid rate produces either ventricular standstill or ventricular fibrillation. The latter occurs more frequently than the former. Ventricular fibrillation usually develops when plasma K concentration in the coronary arteries exceeds 15 to 20 mEq./l. Fibrillation may be either preceded by several ventricular ectopic beats with wide QRS complexes, or it may occur after a single premature beat without preceding change of heart

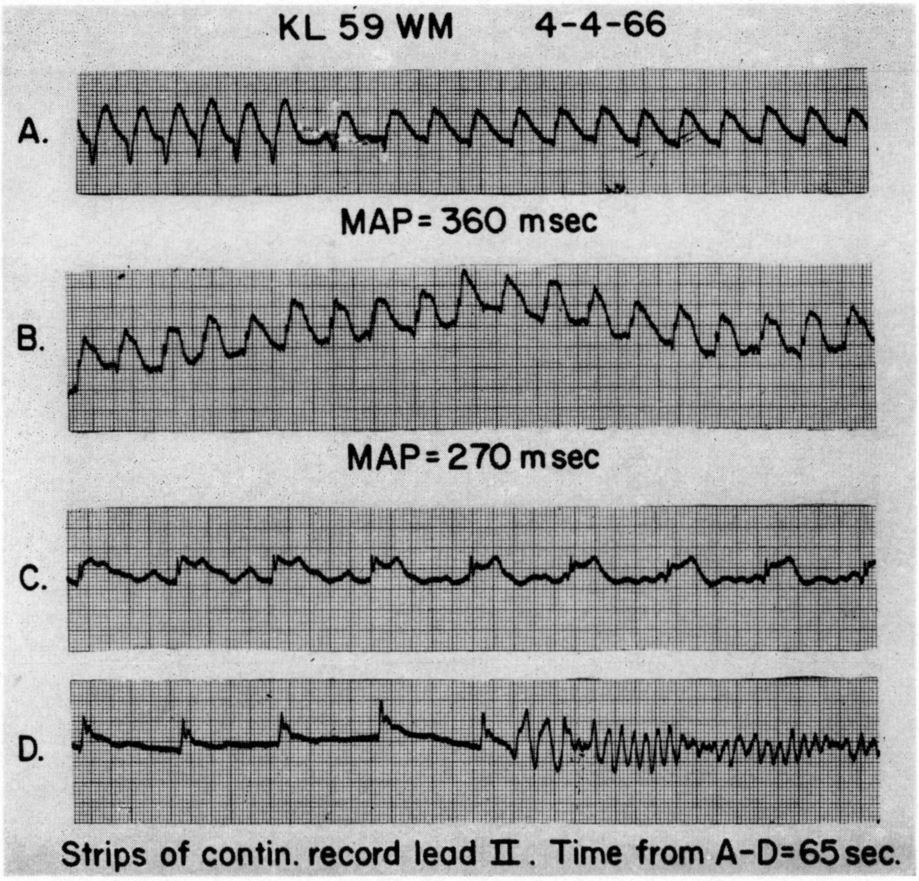


Fig. 4. Electrocardiogram of a 59-year-old man with acute myocardial infarction. Note: Monophasic pattern in *A* and *B*, elevation of the S-T segment in *C* and *D*, and onset of ventricular fibrillation after single ventricular premature beat in *B*. Duration of ventricular depolarization + repolarization (MAP) is 360 msec. in *A*, and 270 msec. in *B*. Coupling interval of the premature beat = 300 msec.

rate or increase of QRS duration.[15] Figure 3 demonstrates ventricular fibrillation that occurred after administration of 0.26mEq. K into the right coronary artery of a dog in 15 seconds. In the electrogram from the area perfused by potassium the Q-T interval is shortened and the S-T segment is elevated, while the ventricular complex is unchanged in the electrogram from the area not perfused by potassium. Ventricular fibrillation occurs after a single ventricular premature beat. The appearance of this premature beat after administration of K is difficult to explain because hyperpotassemia should decrease the automaticity of pacemaker fibers. Patients with hyperpotassemia usually have no ectopic beats before the onset of severe intraventricular conduction disturbances. It is conceivable that the ectopic beat is caused by the "current of injury" resulting from the nonhomogeneous distribution of potassium.

It is of interest that ventricular fibrillation in patients with acute myocardial infarction (Figure 4) closely resembles fibrillation produced by administration of potassium into the coronary arteries (Figure 3). Common to both are "injury current," shortening of ventricular repolarization, absence of QRS widening and increase of heart rate, as well as short coupling interval of the premature beat. The short coupling interval implies a short effective refractory period, and suggests that premature depolarization occurs in the area in which plasma K concentration is increased. Ectopic rhythms after coronary occlusion in dogs have been attributed to potassium liberated from the infarcted myocardium.[20] Since moderate hyperpotassemia lowers the threshold of excitability, an increase of K concentration could render some pacemaker fibers susceptible to excitation by the injury current.[21]

The defibrillatory effect of K has been known since 1908.[22] Atria can be defibrillated by lesser increase of plasma K concentration than the ventricles. In patients with severe hyperpotassemia, spontaneous change from atrial fibrillation to sinus or an ectopic atrial rhythm may take place at K concentrations about 8 to 9 mEq./l. The literature contains several reports of atrial defibrillation after administration of potassium salts (references 54 and 62 in Surawicz[15]).

In certain potassium-depleted patients with severe hypopotassemia, ectopic activity increased during the administration of potassium with glucose.[23] These arrhythmias may be due to the decreased potassium concentration that frequently occurs during slow administration of potassium with glucose. It is probable that glucose metabolism contributes to the migration of potassium into the cells and lowers plasma K concentration.[23]

*Potassium and artificial pacemakers.* In dogs the ventricular threshold of excitability decreases when plasma K concentration is moderately elevated[24, 25] but increases sharply when K concentration exceeds about 7 to 9 mEq./l.[24-26] Systematic studies of excitability threshold in man have not been carried out. Several clinical observations suggest that slight increases of plasma potassium concentration lower the threshold of ventricular excitability while further increases raise the threshold. An example of the lowering of excitability threshold by potassium is its effect on the function of defective pacemakers in which either the stimulus strength is decreased or the tissue resistance around the electrode is increased. Occasionally normal response to pacemaker stimulation can be restored by the administration of potassium salts.[27] Administration of glucose and insulin that lowers plasma K concentration may cause a decreased responsiveness to the stimulation by defective pacemakers. We observed a marked increase of the ventricular excitability threshold in a patient with a transvenous pacemaker when his plasma K concentration was increased to 7.1 mEq./l.[26] The measurement of excitability threshold in patients with pacemakers does not differentiate between a lack of response to stimulation and the lack of propagation of a local response. However, this is probably of little practical significance since both excitability threshold and conduction velocity are probably affected in the same manner. The lowest excitability threshold and the most rapid conduction velocity in man may occur when plasma K concentration is close to 6.0 mEq./l. while lower and higher K concentrations are expected to decrease the conduction velocity and increase the excitability threshold. There may be differences between the extracellular K concentrations that depress intraventricular conduction disturbances *in vivo* and *in vitro*. In the isolated papillary muscle and Purkinje fibers of the monkey, velocity of conduction increased when extracellular K was 8.1 mM./l., and decreased when K concentration was 10.8 mM./l.[28] In dog and in man P-R and QRS intervals are usually prolonged when plasma K concentration exceeds 7.0 mEq./l.

*Hypopotassemia.* Decreased extracellular K concentration may alter rhythm and conduction by one or more of the following mechanisms: 1) increased resting membrane potential (hyperpolarization); 2) shortening of phase 2 and prolongation of phase 3 of AP; 3) increased rate of diastolic depolarization in the pacemaker fibers; 4) transformation of nonpacemaker into pacemaker fibers; 5) decrease of excitability threshold. Arrhythmias may be also caused by differences in the response of different fiber types to the same decrease of plasma K concentration. The effects of low K on the electrophysiological properties of the S-A node, A-V node, and the bundle of His have been studied less extensively than the effects of high K on these structures. Therefore the mechanisms of some electrocardiographic manifestations of hypopotassemia still remain uncertain. Moderate hypopotassemia alters mainly repolarization but severe hypopotassemia may also cause intraventricular and A-V conduction disturbances. The depression of the S-T segment, decreased amplitude of the T-wave, and increased amplitude of the U wave are attributed to shortening of phase 2 and prolongation of phase 3 of the ventricular AP.[29] The AP becomes longer but this apparently does not increase the duration of the effective refractory period, because most of the AP increase occurs at the end of repolarization when the fiber has repolarized to a level that is below the threshold potential. When the AP develops a long and slow "tail," the membrane potential may be actually closer to the threshold potential that would facilitate depolarization. In isolated preparations depression of potassium concentration may change nonpacemaker fibers into pacemaker fibers.[15] The effect of hypopotassemia on the atrial and ventricular refractory period has not been studied. Clinical observations suggest that hypopotassemia shortens the effective refractory period because atrial and ventricular premature beats in patients with hypopotassemia frequently occur after a short coupling interval.[30] Perfusion of isolated rabbit hearts with potassium-deficient solutions produces intraventricular conduction disturbances and A-V block as well as supraventricular and ventricular ectopic beats.[7, 29] In patients with severe hypopotassemia, the QRS interval is usually increased by 0.01 to 0.03 seconds.[31] The increased duration of the QRS complex is the result of widening without change in shape, which suggests that it is caused by slower intraventricular conduction without change in the sequence of depolarization. This may be due to hyperpolarization of ventricular fibers, or to slower conduction in the specialized fibers of the conducting system. Hypopotassemia prolongs the "tail" of the action potential in the conducting systems more than in the ventricles, so that the period of incomplete repolarization in the Purkinje fibers is longer than in the ventricular fibers.[32] In addition, hypopotassemia increases the velocity of diastolic depolarization in the Purkinje fibers.[13, 32] Therefore, quiescent Purkinje fibers develop automatic activity. When such fibers are depolarized from a level of transmembrane potential that is less negative than the maximal diastolic potential, the upstroke velocity of the AP and the conduction velocity decrease. Depolarization of incompletely repolarized ventricular fibers may also produce intraventricular conduction disturbance (Figure 5). Patients

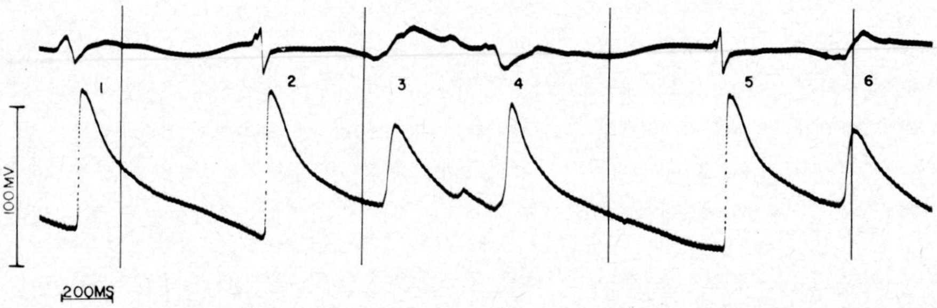


Fig. 5. Ventricular ectopic beats and ECG during perfusion of an isolated rabbit heart with Krebs-Hanseleit solution containing 0.8 mm. K and 12 mg. quinidine per liter. When depolarization begins from a more negative membrane potential (1st, 2d, and 5th beats), the upstroke of the action potential (AP) is more rapid than when depolarization begins from a less negative membrane potential (3d, 4th, and 6th beats). In beats with slower upstroke, the QRS complexes are wider and less well defined than in beats with more rapid upstroke. (L. S. Gettes, B. Surawicz, and J. C. Shiue, *Amer. J. Physiol. 203*:1135, 1965. Courtesy of publishers).

with severe hypopotassemia may occasionally have advanced disturbances of intraventricular conduction.[33] Hypopotassemia promotes the appearance of supraventricular and ventricular ectopic beats and rhythms. In 81 nondigitalized patients with plasma K concentration 3.2 mEq./l. or less, ventricular ectopic beats occurred in 28 per cent, supraventricular ectopic beats in 22 per cent, and A-V conduction disturbances in 12 per cent.[30] Ectopic beats occurred three times, and A-V conduction disturbances two times more frequently than in the control hospital population.[30] The prevalence of ectopic beats in patients with hypopotassemia who had no digitalis and no heart disease was at least twice as great as in the control group of unselected hospital patients.[30] It is of interest that patients with severe hypopotassemia may develop arrhythmias that are considered characteristic of digitalis toxicity, e.g., nonparoxysmal atrial tachycardia with block, or A-V dissociation. Arrhythmias of this type are attributed to a combination of increased automaticity of ectopic pacemakers, and at least some degree of atrioventricular conduction disturbances. The mechanism of depressed A-V conduction caused by low potassium has not been studied at the cellular level. It is probable that the effect of low potassium on the pacemaker fibers in the A-V junction is similar to the effect of low K on the Purkinje fibers. Patients with hypopotassemia have greater sensitivity to vagal stimulation.[34] It should be added that in some patients A-V conduction may be improved by decreasing plasma K concentration. This is probably the basis of therapy with chlorothiazide in patients with incomplete A-V block.[35]

Perfusion of isolated hearts with potassium-deficient solutions produces ventricular fibrillation.[29, 36] This may be due to a combination of increased ventricular automaticity, slowing of conduction, and short effective refractory period. Ventricular fibrillation has also occurred in patients with severe hypopotassemia.[23]

## Other Ions in Arrhythmia

*Calcium.* Only extremely high or low concentrations of Ca produce electrophysiologic abnormalities that are of clinical importance. Within the range of concentrations compatible with life, calcium has relatively little effect on the resting membrane potential. Low calcium prolongs and high calcium shortens phase 2 of the AP in several types of cardiac fibers.[37] Calcium does not alter appreciably the duration of phase 3. Prolongation of phase 2 by low calcium prolongs the duration of the AP and the duration of the effective refractory period. Shortening of phase 2 by high calcium shortens the duration of the AP and the duration of the effective refractory period. The same change of Ca concentration may have different effects on the phase 2 of different types of cardiac fibers.[37] The effect of calcium on the duration of the AP depends on heart rate and magnesium concentration.[37, 38] It is of interest that low calcium does not prolong the duration of the action potential in premature beats when the depolarization begins from a significantly less negative membrane potential than the resting potential.[39] Low calcium depresses contraction, lowers excitability threshold, and slightly decreases the rate of diastolic depolarization of the pacemaker fibers.[40] High calcium increases the contractile force, increases excitability threshold, and slightly increases the rate of diastolic depolarization of the pacemaker fibers.[40]

Experimental hypercalcemia increases the duration of the QRS complex and produces ectopic beats and ventricular fibrillation.[15] Patients with severe hypercalcemia may have prolonged QRS and P-R intervals and, occasionally, second- or third-degree A-V block.[41] The incidence of ectopic beats in patients with hypercalcemia does not appear to be increased. It has been postulated that sudden deaths of patients with hyperparathyroidism and other disturbances producing hypercalcemia are caused by ventricular fibrillation.[14] However, there are no published electrocardiograms of patients with hypercalcemia shortly before or at the time of sudden death.

Perfusion of isolated hearts with calcium-deficient solutions produced ectopic beats and ventricular fibrillation only when calcium concentration was less than 1/20 of the normal plasma calcium concentration.[42] Patients with hypocalcemia are not expected to have conduction disturbances or ectopic beats. Hypocalcemia induced by administration of $Na_2EDTA$ suppressed supraventricular and ventricular ectopic beats in about 50 per cent of patients.[43] Ectopic beats suppressed by hypocalcemia reappeared after calcium administration.[43] We have suggested that the antiarrhythmic effect of induced hypocalcemia may be due to the prolonged duration of the effective refractory period.

The effect of calcium on the electrophysiologic properties of the heart depends on potassium concentration. In isolated hearts, intraventricular conduction disturbance, A-V conduction disturbances, and ventricular fibrillation caused by increased extracellular potassium concentration can be abolished or prevented by increasing calcium concentration. Conversely, intraventricular conduction disturbances, atrioventricular conduction disturbances, and ventricular fibrillation caused by low extracellular K concentration can be abolished or prevented by lowering calcium concentration. Administration of calcium shortens the QRS duration when K concentration is increased, probably because high calcium concentration maintains normal resting membrane potential in the presence of increased K concentration.[37]

The mechanism by which low levels of calcium prevent conduction disturbances and fibrillation in hearts perfused with solutions low in K is not clear. Low calcium does not alter the amount or the rate of K loss in the heart.[44] The clinical significance of the observations that low calcium inhibits arrhythmias produced by low potassium is uncertain. The antiarrhythmic effect of low calcium in hearts perfused with low potassium solution occurred when calcium concentrations were much lower than those encountered in patients with hypocalcemia. Patients with combined hypopotassemia and hypocalcemia had the same prevalence of ectopic beats as patients with hypopotassemia without hypocalcemia.[30]

*Sodium.* High sodium concentration increases and low sodium concentration decreases the upstroke velocity of the action potential. Within limits of plasma sodium concentration compatible with life, the effect of high or low sodium on cardiac rhythm and conduction are probably negligible. However, in patients with intraventricular conduction disturbances caused by hyperpotassemia, hypernatremia shortens and hyponatremia prolongs the QRS interval. Intravenous administration of sodium salts effectively suppresses manifestations of advanced K cardiotoxicity and prevents ventricular standstill and fibrillation (references 30-32 in Surawicz[15]).

*Magnesium.* High extracellular concentrations of magnesium depress atrioventricular and intraventricular conduction. The depression of A-V conduction may occur when magnesium concentration is 3 to 5 mM./l. and cardiac arrest may be expected when magnesium concentration reaches 15 to 22 mM./l. (references 17 and 31 in Surawicz *et al.*[38]) The latter concentrations are considerably higher than those that cause respiratory arrest. Intravenous administration of magnesium salts suppresses ectopic beats in both digitalized and nondigitalized patients.[45] The effect of high magnesium on the upstroke velocity of the ventricular action potential is similar to the effect of high potassium. The mechanism of the antiarrhythmic action of magnesium therefore may be similar to that of potassium. In the isolated preparation high magnesium decreases and low magnesium increases the duration of the atrial and ventricular action potential when Ca concentration is low.[38] This suggests that abnormal magnesium concentration may alter the duration of the effective refractory period in patients with hypocalcemia (Ref. in 38).

## Effect of Electrolytes on the Action of Digitalis and Antiarrhythmic Drugs

*Digitalis.* Increased extracellular potassium concentration decreases automaticity and suppresses ectopic beats induced by digitalis.[46-51] Hyperpotassemic animals and man can tolerate unusually large doses of digitalis without developing ectopic activity.[52, 53] In hypopotassemic animals ectopic beats and rhythms appear after administration of unusually small doses of glycosides.[53] In patients receiving digitalis, arrhythmia may be precipitated by carbohydrate administration or removal of potassium by dialysis.[54-56] The effects of the interaction of potassium and digitalis on A-V conduction reflect the complex effects of potassium on A-V conduction. As mentioned earlier, both extremes, low and high potassium concentration, depress A-V conduction. Therefore, moderate hyperpotassemia may improve A-V conduction in patients with A-V block induced by digitalis.[11] However, in dogs and in

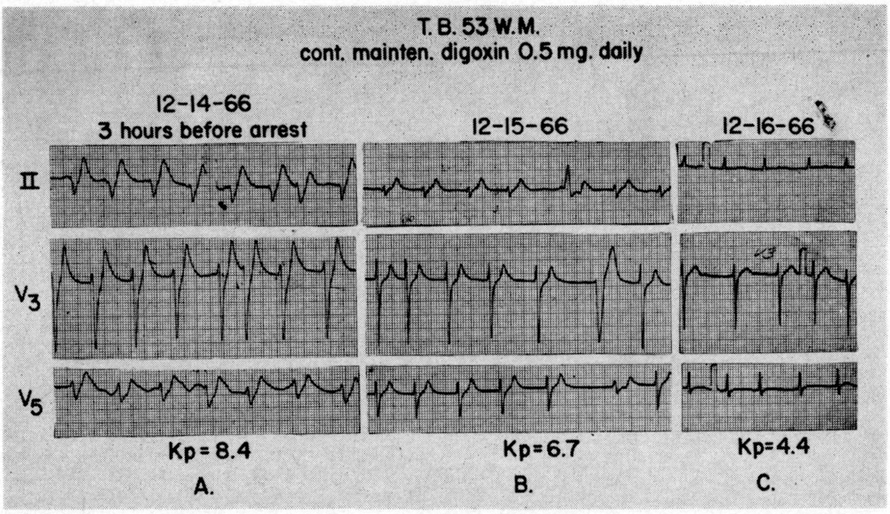


Fig. 6. Electrocardiogram of a 53-year-old patient with atrial fibrillation, treated with a maintenance dose of 0.5 mg. digoxin daily. Note: Pattern of hypopotassemia three hours before "cardiac arrest" (*A*), and after treatment with sodium lactate, glucose and insulin (*B* and *C*). Ventricular rate in *A, B,* and *C* is about 95/minute. The sixth beat in *B* is probably a ventricular escape beat.

man, hyperpotassemia and digitalis may also have a synergistic depressive effect on A-V conduction.[57, 58] The effects of hyperpotassemia on A-V conduction disturbance induced by digitalis are not predictable because they depend not only on the absolute plasma K concentration but on the rate of K administration and on the presence or absence of structural damage of the conducting system. Figure 6 demonstrates an ECG of a patient with atrial fibrillation and renal insufficiency treated with a maintenance dose of 0.5 mg. digoxin daily. In this patient the rhythm and the rate are the same when plasma K concentration is 8.4 (*A*), 6.7 (*B*), 4.4 (*C*) mEq./l. In other patients with atrial fibrillation receiving digitalis, hyperpotassemia produced complete A-V block with an A-V junctional pacemaker. The rate of the A-V junctional pacemaker was normal or rapid.* It is possible that in dogs with digitalis-induced disturbances of A-V conduction, depression of A-V conduction may be due to a rapid rate of K administration rather than to hyperpotassemia. At present there is not enough clinical evidence to suggest that administration of potassium is contraindicated in patients with depression of A-V conduction produced by digitalis. It remains to be established whether patients receiving digitalis develop arrest or fibrillation at lower K concentrations than patients without

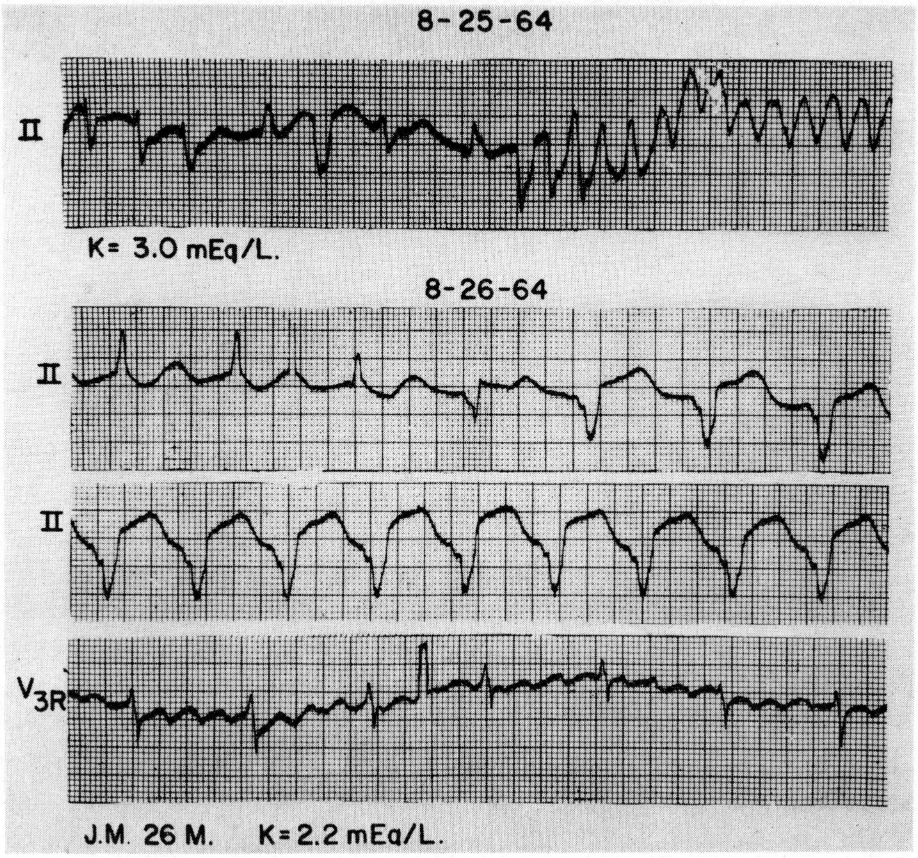


Fig. 7. Electrocardiogram of a 26-year-old patient with rheumatic heart disease, treated with a maintenance dose of 0.25 mg. digoxin daily. On August 25, 1964, atrial fibrillation with multiple ventricular ectopic beats. Ventricular fibrillation begins after premature beat with a short coupling interval. On the following day, ECG pattern of hypopotassemia, and atrial fibrillation with regular ventricular rhythm attributed to a complete A-V block. Note: Transition from A-V junctional rhythm to a ventricular ectopic escape rhythm in lead II. (From: S. Davidson and B. Surawicz, Ectopic beats and atrioventricular conduction disturbances in patients with hypopotassemia. In press. Courtesy of *Arch. Int. Med.*)

digitalis. The effect of potassium appears to depend more on the rate of K administration and the presence or absence of structural damage of the conducting system than on the absolute plasma K concentration.

Hypopotassemia may augment the depression of A-V conduction produced by digitalis. The most characteristic arrhythmias in hypopotassemic patients receiving digitalis are nonparoxysmal supraventricular tachycardia with block and dissociation. Both types of arrhythmia

*Surawicz and Gettes, unpublished observations.

are due to a combination of increased ectopic activity and depressed A-V conduction. Both hypopotassemia and digitalis decrease the effective refractory period of the ventricles and shorten the coupling interval of ventricular premature beats. Slow propagation of early ectopic impulses may result in reentry and cause ventricular fibrillation (Figure 7). The synergistic effect of low K and digitalis on automaticity and A-V conduction explains the increased sensitivity to digitalis in patients with hypopotassemia. We have seen the appearance of nonparoxysmal atrial tachycardia with block or A-V dissociation with A-V junctional tachycardia after the administration of 0.75-2.0 mg. of digoxin in patients with hypopotassemia and K-depletion.*

There is a lack of detailed studies of the calcium-digitalis relationship on the electrophysiological properties of cardiac fibers.[59] Both hypercalcemia and digitalis increase the threshold of excitability and shorten the effective refractory period in the ventricles. It has been reported that hypercalcemia increases the susceptibility of the heart to the induction of ventricular ectopic beats by ouabain.[60, 61] Several studies suggest a synergistic effect of calcium and digitalis on automaticity (references in Surawicz[62]). But in experimental animals receiving digitalis, hypercalcemia produced ectopic rhythms only when the animals had received an excess of 95 per cent of the toxic dose of ouabain. Dogs that received 90 per cent of the toxic dose of acetylstrophanthidin had no arrhythmia when their serum calcium was 46.2 mg. per cent. In another study, nondigitalized dogs developed A-V block when serum calcium concentration was 15 to 40 mg. per cent. Ectopic rhythms terminating in ventricular fibrillation were associated with slightly higher calcium concentrations.[64] The effects of calcium on animals receiving digitalis were not different from those in animals not receiving digitalis, so that this study showed no evidence of synergistic or additive effects between calcium and digitalis. Clinical correlations between the effects of hypercalcemia and digitalis are surprisingly scarce; hence the problem requires further investigation. Ectopic beats caused by overdosage of digitalis are suppressed by lowering calcium concentration with $Na_2$ EDTA or citrate salts.[62] However, it has been pointed out that $Na_2$EDTA is equally effective in suppressing ectopic beats and rhythms in digitalized and nondigitalized patients.[43]

*Quinidine.* In animal experiments the effect of hyperpotassemia

*Surawicz and Mortelmans, unpublished observations.

and quinidine on the rate of rise of the AP and the conduction velocity are synergistic. Therefore quinidine toxicity is augmented by hyperpotassemia.[65] The effect of low K concentration is less predictable. The hyperpolarizing effect could counteract the quinidine effect on conduction. Such an effect was observed in isolated rabbit hearts beating at a slow rate.[66] However, in dogs or in isolated rabbit hearts beating at a more rapid rate the intraventricular conduction disturbance produced by quinidine became more pronounced when K concentration was low.[7, 67] In isolated hearts this was attributed to a greater prolongation of repolarization by low K and quinidine together than by either alone. Thus the onset of depolarization usually occurred before the repolarization was completed. This resulted in a slower rate of rise of the action potential and a slow conduction (Figure 5). Toxic effects of quinidine on atrioventricular and intraventricular conduction in dogs can be reversed by the administration of sodium chloride or sodium lactate.[67, 68] This is apparently caused by increased rate of rise of the action potential mediated by sodium. Administration of calcium increases the duration of the P-R and QRS intervals in dogs with quinidine intoxication.[68] However, this effect of calcium is not greater in quinidine-intoxicated dogs than in control animals. When quinidine-intoxicated dogs developed sinus bradycardia, increased potassium concentration further slowed the heart rate. However, decreased plasma K concentration and increased sodium or calcium concentration had no effect on the sinus rate.* The effects of electrolytes on the A-V and intraventricular conduction produced by quinidine are similar to those in dogs not receiving quinidine. The only exception is shortening of the PR and QRS intervals by sodium in dogs with quinidine intoxication. However, this effect of sodium is not specific since it is also present when conduction is depressed by potassium and other factors.

## Summary

This article reviews: 1) correlation of recent advances in electrophysiology of cardiac fibers with the effects of electrolytes on rhythm and conduction in man; 2) arrhythmias due to electrolyte disturbances and the effect of certain electrolyte disturbances on preexisting arrhythmias; 3) treatment of arrhythmias by altering plasma electrolyte concentrations; and 4) effects of electrolyte disturbances on the action of digitalis and quinidine.

*Mazzoleni and Surawicz, unpublished observations.

*REFERENCES*


1. Hoffman, B. F. and Cranefield, P. F. *Electrophysiology of the Heart.* New York, McGraw-Hill, 1960.
2. Weidmann, S. *Elektrophysiologie der Herzmuskelfaser.* Bern, Huber, 1956.
3. Trautwein, W. Generation and conduction of impulses in the heart as affected by drugs, *Pharmacol. Rev. 15*:277, 1963.
4. Woodbury, J. W. Cellular Electrophysiology of the Heart. In: *Handbook of Physiology.* Circulation, vol. I, Chap. 2, p. 237.
5. deMello, W. C. and Hoffman, B. F. Potassium ions and electrical activity of specialized cardiac fibers, *Amer. J. Physiol. 199*:1125, 1960.
6. Paes de Carvalho, A. and Langan, W. B. Influence of extracellular potassium levels on atrioventricular transmission, *Amer. J. Physiol. 205*:375, 1963.
7. Gettes, L. S., Surawicz, B. and Shiue, J. C. Effect of high K, and low K, and quinidine on QRS duration and ventricular action potential, *Amer. J. Physiol. 203*:1135, 1962.
8. Lepeschkin, E., Surawicz, B., and Herrlich, H. C. Differences in the effect of electrolytes on the atrial and ventricular action potentials of isolated perfused rabbit hearts, *Fed. Proc. 19*:112, 1960.
9. Vassalle, M. and Hoffman, B. F. The spread of sinus activation during potassium administration, *Circ. Res. 17*:285, 1965.
10. Vassalle, M., Greenspan, K., Jomain, S. and Hoffman, B. F. Effects of potassium on automaticity and conduction of canine hearts. *Amer. J. Physiol. 207*: 334, 1964.
11. Bettinger, J. C., Surawicz, B., Bryfogle, J. W., Anderson, B. N. and Bellet, S. The effect of intravenous administration of potassium chloride on ectopic rhythms, ectopic beats and disturbances in A-V conduction, *Amer. J. Med. 21*:521, 1956.
12. Antoni, H., Herkel, K. and Fleckenstein, A. Die Restitution der automatischen Erregungsbidung in Kaliumgelähmten Schrittmacher-Geweben durch Adrenalin, *Pflueger Archiv. Ges. Physiol. 277*:633, 1963.
13. Vassalle, M. Cardiac pacemaker potentials at different extra- and intracellular K concentrations, *Amer. J. Physiol. 208*:770, 1965.
14. Vassalle, M. Analysis of cardiac pacemaker potential using a "voltage clamp" technique, *Amer. J. Physiol. 210*:1335, 1966.
15. Surawicz, B. Role of electrolytes in etiology and management of cardiac arrhythmias, *Progr. Cardiov. Dis. 8*: 364, 1966.
16. Feigenbaum, H., Wunsch, C. and Fisch, C. Effect of intracoronary infusion of potassium on the vagal action on A-V transmission, *J. Clin. Invest. 44*:399, 1965.
17. Greenspan, K., Wunsch, C. and Fisch, C. The relationship between potassium and vagal action, on atrioventricular transmission, *Circ. Res. 17*:39, 1965.
18. Surawicz, B. and Gettes, L. S. Two mechanisms of cardiac arrest produced by potassium, *Circ. Res. 12*:415, 1963.
19. Surawicz, B., Chlebus, H. and Mazzoleni, A. Hemodynamic and electrocardiographic effects of hyperpotassemia. Differences in response to slow and rapid increases in concentration of plasma K, *Amer. Heart J. 73*:647, 1967.
20. Harris, A. S., Bisteni, A., Russell, R. A., Brigham, J. C. and Firestone, J. E. Excitatory factors in ventricular tachycardia resulting from myocardial ischemia: potassium a major excitant, *Science 119*:200, 1954.
21. Harris, A. S. Potassium and experimental coronary occlusion, *Amer. Heart J. 71*:797, 1966.
22. Wiggers, C. J. Defibrillation of the ventricles (editorial). *Circ. Res. 1*:191, 1953.
23. Kunin, A. S., Surawicz, B. and Sims, E. A. H. Decrease in serum potassium concentrations and appearance of cardiac arrhythmias during infusion of potassium with glucose in potassium depleted patients, *New Eng. J. Med. 266*:228, 1962.
24. Siebens, A. A., Hoffman, B. F., Ensen, Y., Farrell, J. E. and Brooks, C. M.

Effects of l-epinephrine and l-norepinephrine on cardiac excitability, *Amer. J. Physiol. 175*:1, 1953.
25. Han, J., Garcia de Jalon, P., and Moe, G. K. Adrenergic effects on ventricular vulnerability, *Circ. Res. 14*:516, 1964.
26. Surawicz, B., Chlebus, H., Reeves, J. T. and Gettes, L. S. Increase of ventricular excitability threshold by hyperpotassemia, *J.A.M.A. 191*:1049, 1965.
27. Walker, W. J., Elkins, J. T. and Wood, L. W. Effect of potassium in restoring myocardial response to a subthreshold cardiac pacemaker, *New Eng. J. Med. 271*:597, 1964.
28. Antoni, H. and Zerweck, T. Besitzen die sympathischen Ueberträgerstoffe einen direkten Einfluss auf die Leitungsgeschwindigkeit des Säugetiermyokards? *Pflueger Arch. Ges. Physiol. 293*:310, 1967.
29. Surawicz, B., Lepeschkin, E., Herrlich, H. C. and Hoffman, B. F. Effect of potassium and calcium deficiency on the monophasic action potential, electrocardiogram and contractility of isolated rabbit hearts, *Amer. J. Physiol. 196*: 1302, 1959.
30. Davidson, S. and Surawicz, B. Ectopic beats and atrioventricular conduction disturbances in patients with hypopotassemia, *Arch. Int. Med. 120*:280, 1967.
31. Surawicz, B. Relation between electrocardiogram and electrolytes, *Amer. Heart J. 73*:814, 1967.
32. Gettes, L. and Surawicz, B. Comparison of K effects on Purkinje and ventricular action potentials of perfused moderator band, *Fed. Proc. 26*:594, 1967.
33. Cherry, J. C. and Surawicz, B. Unusual effects of potassium deficiency on the heart of a child with cystinosis, *Pediatrics 30*:414, 1962.
34. Marini, A., Cenacchi, U., Cenciotti, L. and Galliani, A. Effetto dell' acetilcolina e della stimolazione vagale sull' elettrocardiogramma in condizioni di aumentato gradiente K intracellulare/K extracellulare, *Gior. di Clin. Med. 40*: 939, 1959.
35. Tobian, L. Prevention of Stokes-Adams seizures with chlorothiazide, *New Eng. J. Med. 265*:623, 1961.
36. Grumbach, L., Howard, J. and Merrill, J. Factors related to the initiation of ventricular fibrillation in the isolated heart: Effect of calcium and potassium, *Circ. Res. 5*:452, 1954.
37. Hoffman, B. F. and Suckling, E. E. Effect of several cations on transmembrane potentials of cardiac muscle, *Amer. J. Physiol. 186*:317, 1956.
38. Surawicz, B., Lepeschkin, E. and Herrlich, H. C. Low and high magnesium concentrations at various calcium levels. Effect on the monophasic action potential, electrocardiogram, and contractility of isolated rabbit hearts, *Circ. Res. 9*:811, 1961.
39. Surawicz, B., Dulin, M. L. and Graham, M. D. Role of refractoriness and duration of vulnerable phase in precipitation of ventricular fibrillation (V.F.) by low Ca, *Fed. Proc. 23*:261, 1964.
40. Temte, J. V. and Davis, L. D. Effect of calcium concentration on the transmembrane potentials of Purkinje fibers, *Circ. Res. 20*:32, 1967.
41. Voss, D. M. and Drake, E. H. Cardiac manifestations of hyperparathyroidism, with presentation of a previously unreported arrhythmia, *Amer. Heart J. 73*:235, 1967.
42. Weiss, D. L., Surawicz, B. and Rubenstein, I. Myocardial lesions of calcium deficiency causing irreversible myocardial failure, *Amer. J. Pathol. 48*:653, 1966.
43. Surawicz, B., MacDonald, M. G., Kaljot, V. and Bettinger, J. C. Treatment of cardiac arrhythmias with salts of ethylenediaminetetraacetic acid (EDTA), *Amer. Heart J. 58*:493, 1959.
44. Gettes, L. S., Surawicz, B. and Kim, K. H. Role of myocardial K and Ca in initiation and inhibition of ventricular fibrillation, *Amer. J. Physiol. 211*:699, 1966.
45. Szekely, P. The action of magnesium on the heart, *Brit. Heart J. 8*:115, 1946-47.
46. Sampson, J. J., Albertson, E. C. and Kondo, B. The effect on man of potassium administration in relation to digitalis glycosides with special reference to

blood serum potassium, the ECG and ectopic beats, *Amer. Heart J. 26*:164, 1943.

47. Enselberg, C. D., Simmons, H. G. and Mintz, A. A. The effects of potassium upon the heart, with special reference to the possibility of treatment of toxic arrhythmias due to digitalis, *Amer. Heart J. 39*:713, 1950.
48. Lown, B. and Levine, H. D. *Atrial Arrhythmias, Digitalis and Potassium.* New York, Lansberger, 1958.
49. Vassalle, M. and Greenspan, K. Effects of potassium on ouabain induced arrhythmias, *Amer. J. Cardiol. 12*:692, 1963.
50. Von Müller, P. Kalium und Digitalistoxizität, *Cardiologia 42*:1, 1962.
51. Fisch, C., Knoebel, S. B., Feigenbaum, H. and Greenspan, K. Potassium and the monophasic action potential, ECG, conduction and arrhythmias, *Progr. Cardiov. Dis. 8*:387, 1966.
52. Williams, J. F., Klocke, F. J. and Braunwald, E. Studies on digitalis. XIII. A comparison of the effects of potassium on the inotropic and arrhythmic producing actions of ouabain, *J. Clin. Invest. 45*:346, 1966.
53. Lown, B., Weller, J. M., Wyatt, N., Hoigne, R. and Merrill, J. P. Effects of alterations of body potassium on digitalis toxicity, *J. Clin. Invest. 31*:648, 1952.
54. Page, E. Precipitation of ventricular arrhythmias due to digitalis by carbohydrate administration, *Amer. J. Med. 19*:169, 1955.
55. Lubash, G. D., Cohen, B. D., Braveman, W. S., Rubin, A. L. and Luckey, E. H. ECG changes during hemodialysis with the artificial kidney, *Circulation 19*:552, 1959.
56. Lown, B. and Levine, S. A. Current concepts in digitalis therapy, *New Eng. J. Med. 250*:771, 819, 866, 1954.
57. Fisch, C., Greenspan, K., Knoebel, S. B. and Feigenbaum, H. Effect of digitalis on conduction of the heart, *Progr. Cardiov. Dis. 6*:343, 1964.
58. Fisch, C., Martz, B. L. and Priebe, F. H. Enhancement of potassium-induced atrioventricular block by toxic doses of digitalis drugs, *J. Clin. Invest. 39*:1885, 1960.
59. Hoffman, B. F. and Singer, D. H. Effect of digitalis on activity of cardiac fibers, *Progr. Cardiov. Dis. 7*:226, 1964.
60. Bower, J. O. and Mengle, H. A. K. The additive effect of calcium and digitalis, *J.A.M.A. 106*:1151, 1936.
61. Gold, H. and Edwards, D. J. The effects of ouabain on the heart in the presence of hypercalcemia, *Amer. Heart J. 3*:45, 1927-28.
62. Surawicz, B. Use of the chelating agent, EDTA, in digitalis intoxication and cardiac arrhythmias, *Progr. Cardiov. Dis. 2*:432, 1959-60.
63. Lown, B., Black H. and Moore, F. D. Digitalis-electrolytes and the surgical patients, *Amer. J. Cardiol. 6*:309, 1960.
64. Smith, P. K., Winkler, A. W. and Hoff, H. E. Calcium and digitalis synergism: The toxicity of calcium salts injected intravenously into digitalized animals, *Arch. Intern. Med. 64*:322, 1939.
65. Bennett, L. L., Rubin, M. L., Blevins, C. E. and Baird, B. The effects of infusing quinidine sulfate and potassium chloride, separately and combined on conduction times of the dog heart, *Amer. Heart J. 61*:500, 1961.
66. Watanabe, Y., Dreifus, L. S. and Likoff, W. Electrophysiologic antagonism and synergism of potassium and antiarrhythmic agents, *Amer. J. Cardiol. 12*:702, 1963.
67. Mazzoleni, A. and Surawicz, B. Dissociation between the effect of quinidine on the electrical and mechanical properties of the heart in dog, *Fed. Proc. 22*:247, 1963.
68. Bellet, S., Hamdan, G., Samlyo, A. and Lara, R. The reversal of cardiotoxic effects of quinidine by molar lactate: An experimental study, *Amer. J. Med. Sci. 237*:165, 1959.

# INTRACARDIAC ELECTROCARDIOGRAPHY IN ARRHYTHMIA*

CHARLES E. KOSSMANN

Cardiovascular Section, Department of Medicine
New York University Medical Center, New York, N. Y.

I THINK all of you will agree that the observations made on the dog, the cat, the calf, and the nameless horse were far more interesting than those made on man, and for obvious reasons. The techniques that can be used in the animal are far more elegant; armed with the information they yield, one can speak with great confidence about what is going on in the conduction system.

Those of us who are concerned with human disease sooner or later come upon the problem of arrhythmia in the whole man. In the clinical diagnostic area one of the significant problems is the inadequacy of the information that surface leads provide.

To wax historical for a moment, I think Dr. David Scherf has mentioned that Sir Thomas Lewis abandoned electrocardiography in 1925 because he felt that all that could be learned about arrhythmias had been learned by then. Research interest in arrhythmias was sharply diminished by Lewis' action; this effect was perhaps augmented by the appearance soon thereafter of the excellent work of Wilson and his school,[1] which shifted emphasis to the importance of the form rather than the sequence of complexes in electrocardiographic diagnosis.

These two events occurring soon upon each other resulted in a kind of investigative neglect of arrhythmia. This relative neglect continued almost up to a decade ago, when the advent of intracellular recording of membrane potentials and of intracardiac electrocardiography revived interest in rhythms. More recently, the availability of the artificial pacemaker and of direct current countershock have probably again reversed the investigative trend to some degree. It is now so easy to treat most serious clinical arrhythmias that the incentive to learn more about the mechanisms involved has become less compelling.

At our medical center we have for a good many years had the un-

*Presented at the *Conference on Mechanisms and Management of Arrhythmias,* held by the New York Heart Association at the Hotel Waldorf-Astoria, New York, N. Y., January 24, 1967.

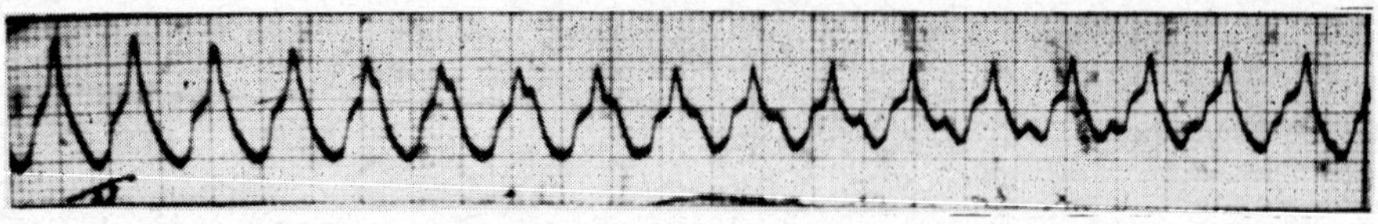

Fig. 1. Single, directly written lead in an arrhythmia; illustrates the difficulty in making a diagnosis with such limited electrocardiographic information.

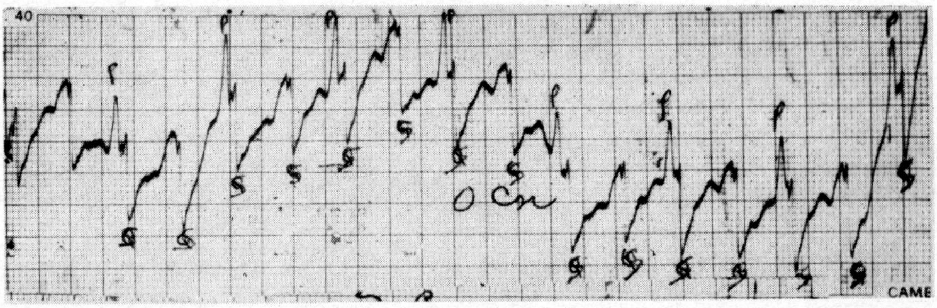

Fig. 2. Unipolar esophageal lead in the same patient as in Figure 1, with considerable artefact caused by an unstable base line, which shows atrial intrinsic deflections (*P*) occurring at half the frequency of the QRS complexes (*S*).

comfortable feeling that we were making diagnoses of arrhythmias with a confidence not entirely justified. As we analyzed each record carefully we became certain that we often were making a single interpretation, when in reality one or more alternatives existed, and we often lacked a firm basis for deciding which was correct.

About two years ago Drs. Kayden, Dolgin, and Brumlík started what might be called an Arrhythmia Consultation Clinic to throw new light on our suspected ignorance. The weekly clinic was one to which house officers, fellows, and students could bring any puzzling record that they might have seen during the preceding week, and obtain a consensus of expert opinion.

Figures 1 and 2 show one type of problem often confronted. First, you will notice a single lead (Figure 1). Of course, if the house officer is awakened in the middle of the night and can't readily find the electrocardiograph, electrodes, paste, and proper electrical outlets, he is not prone to take a whole set of leads. So he takes one, usually lead II (Figure 1).

On each of our wards, the resident physician has also been supplied with an esophageal electrode. In this instance there was enough interest and time, and it was clinically feasible to do an esophageal electrocardiogram (Figure 2). The smudging of this record did not facilitate interpretation. If it is examined carefully, P waves (*P*) can be identified that were not seen in lead II (Figure 1). There are two QRS complexes for each P wave. The possible interpretations are: 1) ventricular tachycardia, with one to two retrograde conduction; 2) A-V nodal tachycardia with bundle-branch block and one to two retrograde conduction; 3) A-V dissociation and a type of oscillation coupling, but with the ventricular oscillator twice as fast as the atrial oscillator and without conduction between the upper and lower chambers. The interpretation of the arrhythmia based on two leads could not be precise. It is this problem of inexactness in the clinical diagnosis of arrhythmias to which I shall address myself in the remainder of what I have to say.

As Dr. M. Irené Ferrer has stated, some years ago we began to take intracardiac or "endocardial" electrocardiograms simply in order to learn what we could about the mechanisms of a variety of electrophysiologic phenomena, including arrhythmia, in man. Originally we were more interested in the form of the deflections obtained in the atria, ventricles, and large vessels than in rhythms, but we did make a fairly large number of observations on a variety of rhythms. These have never been published as a single work but occasional curves have appeared in several publications.[2-6]

Endocardial leads are helpful in increasing the precision of electrocardiographic diagnosis. Only recently have they been used by clinicians in the diagnosis of arrhythmias[7, 8] to a limited extent, although they have been used and continue to be used as a routine part of cardiac catheterization[9-16] In arrhythmia they have been used most often simply to demonstrate the presence or absence of a deflection, usually the atrial deflection. This practice could be extended with clinical profit.

Endocardial electrocardiograms taken at high speed and high gain will sometimes yield information about the sequence of complexes based on their form. A brief review of this aspect of endocardial electrocardiography is thus in order.

Initially our efforts were directed to defining in detail the form of the P wave. For this purpose, endocardial leads from the right atrium of a patient with complete heart block were recorded.[3] The object was to visualize atrial activity undistorted by the ensuing ventricular activity. As predicted by Macleod's classical analysis,[17] the curve obtained was quadriphasic. It consisted of rapid accession deflections, the first of which was electropositive, followed by slower regression deflections, the first of which was electronegative. There was a fifth slow positive deflection comparable to the U wave of ventricular records.[4]

There were several points of considerable clinical interest about the basic form of electrical excitation of atrial muscle as obtained by an endocardial electrode. First, its quadriphasic nature fitted well with the dipolar theory of electrical activation and recovery of excitable tissues.[17] Second, the duration of the complex was in excess of 0.2 sec. and, including the so-called U wave, it was almost 0.4 sec. This is important in terms of the frequently stated criterion of a moving base line for the diagnosis of atrial flutter. If electrical activity at any one atrial point is continuous for 0.4 sec. it would be impossible to have anything but movement of the base line in appropriate leads once the atrial rate exceeded 150 per minute. The corresponding rate for a duration of electrical activity of 0.3 sec. would be 200 per minute. Third, no matter where the exploring electrode is with respect to the muscle, with one exception to be noted, the form of the record will be constant. If the electrode is, for example, in the midatrial region, it does not matter whether excitation is coming toward it from above or below, from anterior or posterior, or from either side; the recorded deflections will have the same configuration. The exception occurs when the electrode is oriented asymmetrically to the mass of muscle being excited. It is well known that when the electrode is near the pacemaking sinoatrial node, and excitation of muscle is dominantly away from it, the deflection recorded will be largely negative (downward). If, on the other hand, the electrode is in the left atrium, the deflection will be largely positive because the unipolar sensor is at the extremity of a muscle mass excited last.[4] In the whole atrium exceptions occur and probably are caused by out-of-phase wave fronts in the free wall, septum, and elsewhere.[4]

## Pitfalls in the Diagnosis of Arrhythmias by Endocardial Leads

There are certain pitfalls to be avoided in using the form of the intracardiac electrocardiogram for the study of arrhythmia. A change in contour that occurs with a change in location of the intra-atrial electrode has been mentioned. Different configurations also are found in different locations in the right ventricle. The principal variation from the characteristic rS form is an absence of the r wave, or a vibra-

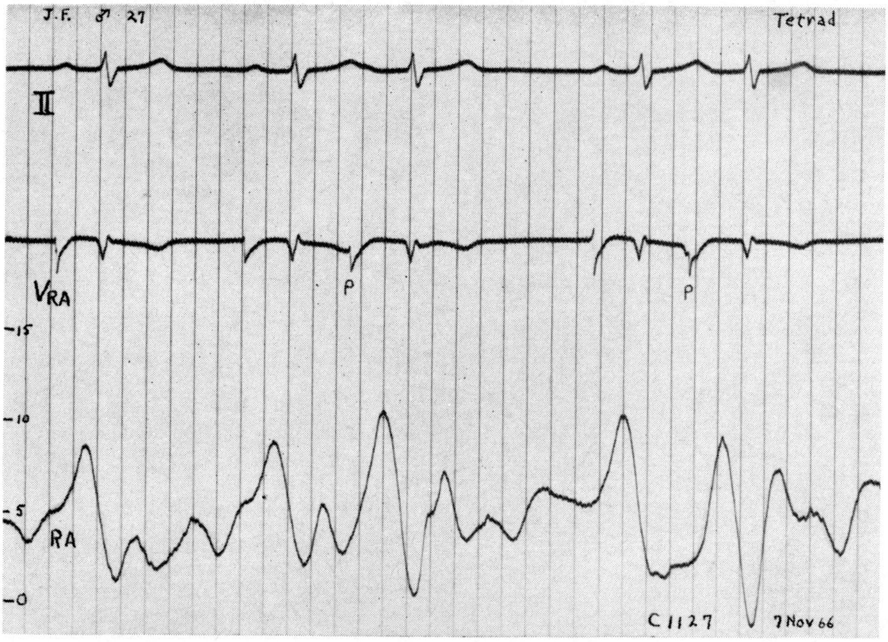


Fig. 3. Premature systoles of atrial origin seen with difficulty in a surface lead (II) but easily visualized (P) in the unipolar intra-atrial lead ($V_{RA}$) in a patient with tetralogy of Fallot. The prominent "a" waves in the pressure pulse of the right atrium (RA) are to be noted. Scale at left is in mm. Hg. Time lines, 0.1 sec.

tory type of QRS, particularly at the base of the cavity.[4] An electrode in the supravalvular area of the pulmonary artery will record atrial deflections arising from the left atrial appendage, and the ventricular deflections will be small. If the record is made, as is a common practice, with a saline or bicarbonate-filled catheter without fluoroscopic control, a false interpretation regarding the location of the catheter tip may be drawn. Touch potentials or demarcation potentials[5] are easily produced in any chamber by contact of the electrode with the endocardium. In supraventricular tachycardia the production of an atrial touch potential will give the false impression of a continuously moving base line.[3-5]

Anyone who has handled a catheter knows how often ventricular tachycardia of one form or another is produced when this device is manipulated in one or the other of the ventricular chambers, and occasionally in the right atrium. On two occasions we have produced what looked like anomalous atrioventricular excitation, such as is seen in the Wolff-Parkinson-White syndrome, with a catheter in the right ven-

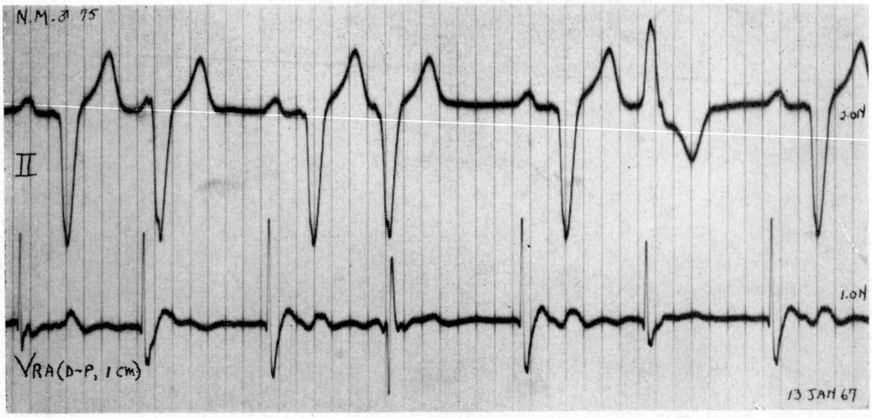


Fig. 4. Sinus rhythm with coupled A-V nodal and ventricular beats. The atrial mechanisms are recorded by differential leading from the right atrium (lower trace, V RA (D-P, 1 cm)).

The first 3 atrial beats are sinus in origin, as is obvious from the simultaneous P wave in lead II (II) of the first, and the characteristic contour in the differential lead of all 3, indicating proximal to distal direction of excitation. The fourth differential P wave in the lower trace has an inverse configuration indicating the opposite direction of excitation and probable origin in the A-V node. The sixth differential P wave is slightly different in form from the other sinus beats, possibly because of distortion by the ventricular premature systole that makes up the couple in this instance.

It is to be noted that in all beats the ventricular QRS and T were recorded in reduced and altered form by the differential electrode. Further, the low frequency cutoff of the amplifier when making this differential record was 4 Hz. This results in some distortion of low-frequency components of the electrocardiographic signal.

tricle.[2] In retrospect we are tempted to think that perhaps the catheter was doing something to augment conduction in those subendocardial bypass tracts on the right side of the A-V node that Dr. Thomas James talked about earlier.

The significance of these observations is clear. In studying an arrhythmia by means of endocardial electrocardiograms it must be remembered that the electrode-catheter itself may produce abnormal electrographic forms and sequences as the result of mechanical stimulation of parts of the heart with which it comes into contact.

## The Recognition of Arrhythmias

A principle of volume conductors used in endocardial electrocardiography is that the closer a sensor is to a source of potential the larger will be the recorded deflections. An example of detecting atrial activity with "near" endocardial leads not apparent or obvious in "distant" surface leads is shown in Figures 3 and 4.

Sir Thomas Lewis[18] first called attention to the usefulness of bipolar

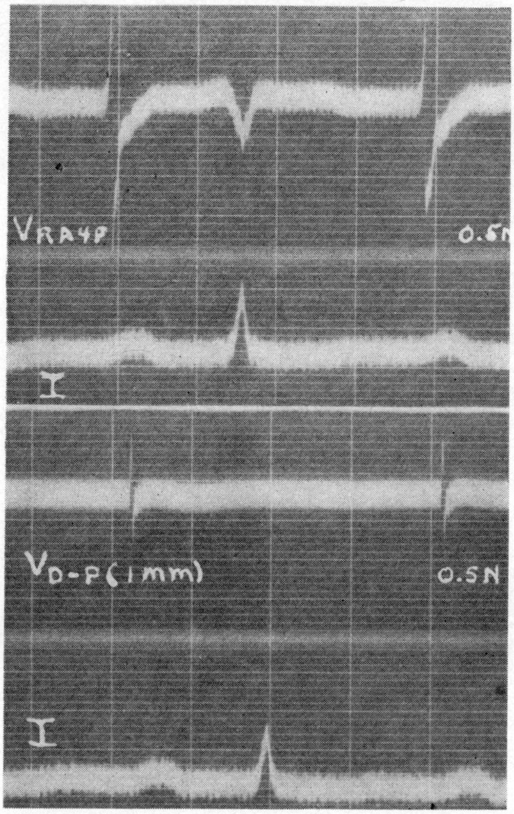


Fig. 5. Recording from the right atrium with differential electrodes separated by 1 mm. In the upper trace a unipolar lead from the right atrium ($V_{RA4P}$) is recorded simultaneously with lead I (I). In the lower trace a differential lead (D-P) in the same atrial location is also recorded with lead I (I).

To be noted in lead D-P are: 1) the sharp upward spike immediately followed by a smaller one downward and preceded by a minuscule depression barely visible; 2) a slower, later, shallow downward deflection produced by differential effects of the atrial recovery process on the 2 electrodes; 3) the absence of any ventricular deflections; 4) the diminution of "noise" present on the unipolar lead.

The presence of atrial activity on the intracardiac leads before the P wave began in the surface lead is also to be noted. The P-R interval is abnormally long. Time lines, 0.2 sec.

recording from the dog's atrium as a way of telling in which direction a subjacent wave of excitation is traveling. When a bipolar intra-atrial electrode is connected to the recording galvanometer in such a way that electropositivity of the distal terminal with respect to the proximal will cause an upright deflection in the finished record, the latter will be represented by a rapid upward spike, often preceded and followed by a diminutive depression, whenever excitation is proceeding in a direction from the proximal to the distal terminal (Figure 5). A reversal

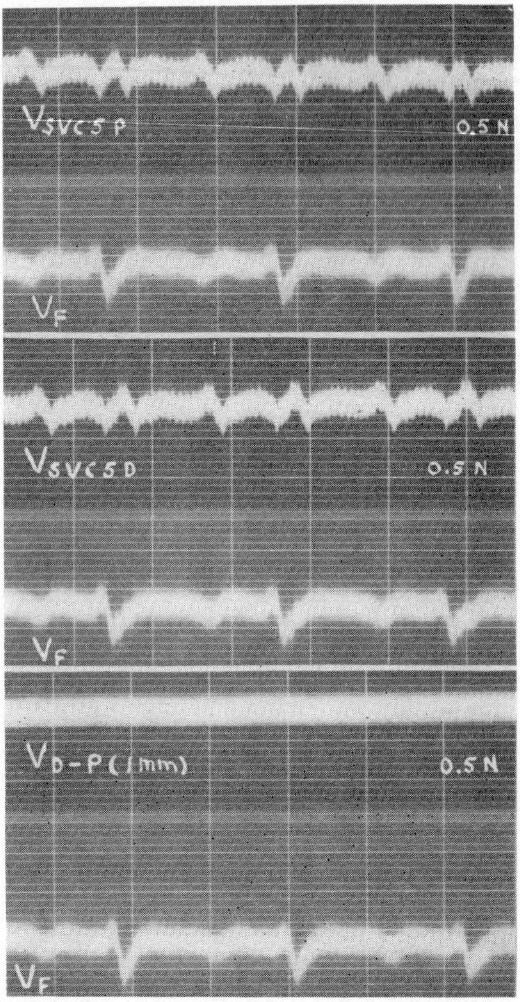


Fig. 6. Atrial tachycardia with 1:2 ventricular response. The figure illustrates how a differential electrode ($V_{D-P}$) records nothing if both electrodes are distant from and equally affected by atrial and ventricular electrical events. In this case both electrodes, separated by 1 mm., were in the superior vena cava ($V_{SVCSP}$, $V_{SVCSD}$). The simultaneous lead is from the left leg ($V_F$). Times lines, 0.2 sec.

of the deflections will result when excitation is in the opposite direction. If excitation is advancing along a line perpendicular to the axis of the two poles so that both are affected electrically in the same manner, nothing or some low-amplitude nondescript deflections will be recorded.[17]

The latter property of "near bipolar" or "differential electrodes" is additionally useful in freeing the record of distant electrical events,

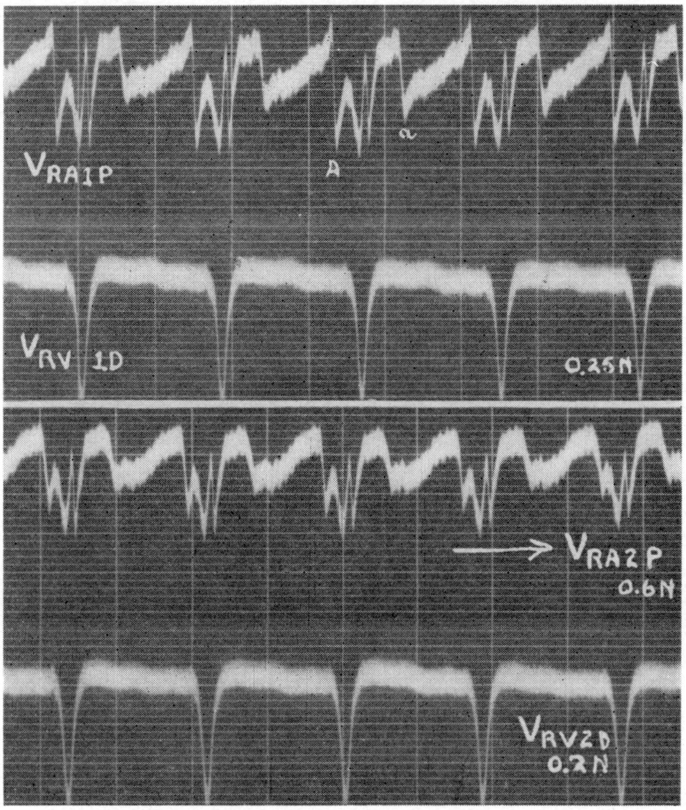


Fig. 7. Simultaneous intracardiac leads from the right atrium ($V_{RA1P}$) and right ventricle ($V_{RV1D}$) made by recording from two single electrodes 3 cm. apart on one catheter. Time lines, 0.2 sec.

While the lower traces were being recorded, the electrode was withdrawn gradually until the electrodes reached a new location ($V_{RA2P}$, $V_{RV2D}$).

The intrinsic atrial deflections (*A* and *a*) are twice as numerous as ventricular complexes but both the form and frequency of these alternate. This suggests either that the intra-atrial electrode is being affected twice by the same excitation front as it passes the electrode, for example, in the free wall and in the septum at different times, or else that there are two separate atrial pacemakers each with a rate of approximately 150 per minute and almost exactly 180° out of phase.

such as the ventricular deflections, because these events, affecting both poles almost equally, will cause no difference of potential between them (Figure 6).

Lastly, if a touch potential is recorded, it is obvious that it is created by only one of the electrodes, or at least more by one than the other. A unipolar lead from each electrode will reveal which is the offender.[3, 5]

The bipolar electrodes used by us for intracardiac leading have

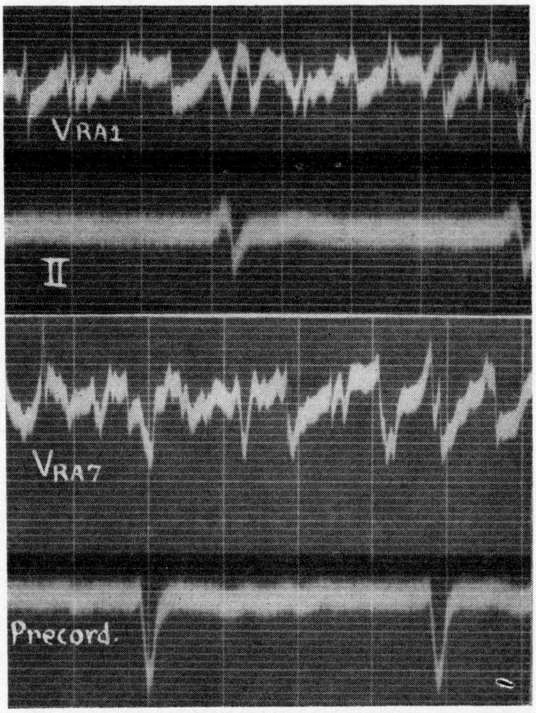


Fig. 8. Atrial fibrillation. Two right intra-atrial leads are shown, one ($V_{RA1}$) simultaneously recorded with lead II (II), the other ($V_{RA7}$) simultaneously recorded with a precordial lead (Precord) when the precordial electrode was directly over the intracardiac electrode. The intracardiac and precordial leads were recorded at approximately half normal sensitivity (1 cm. = 2 mv.) of the string. Times lines, 0.2 sec.

The atrial intrinsic deflections of irregular size and frequency are characteristic of one group of patients with atrial fibrillation.

been regarded as "near bipolar" if the distance separating them is less than 1.0 cm. For precise measurement of arrival times of activation this dimension should be close to 0.1 cm. Widely separated (3.0 cm. or more) electrodes on a single catheter are useful for recording spatially separate events simultaneously such as the atrial and ventricular endocardial electrograms (Figure 7).

Atrial fibrillation usually discloses numerous rapidly recurring intrinsic deflections of variable size in leads from the cavity of the right atrium (Figure 8). In some instances these are quite regular both in form and sequence, and simulate to some degree what is found in atrial tachycardia. A systematic study of atrial fibrillation by direct leads would seem to be in order, especially since the role of the atrioventricular node in pacing the ventricle when the latter is irregular is

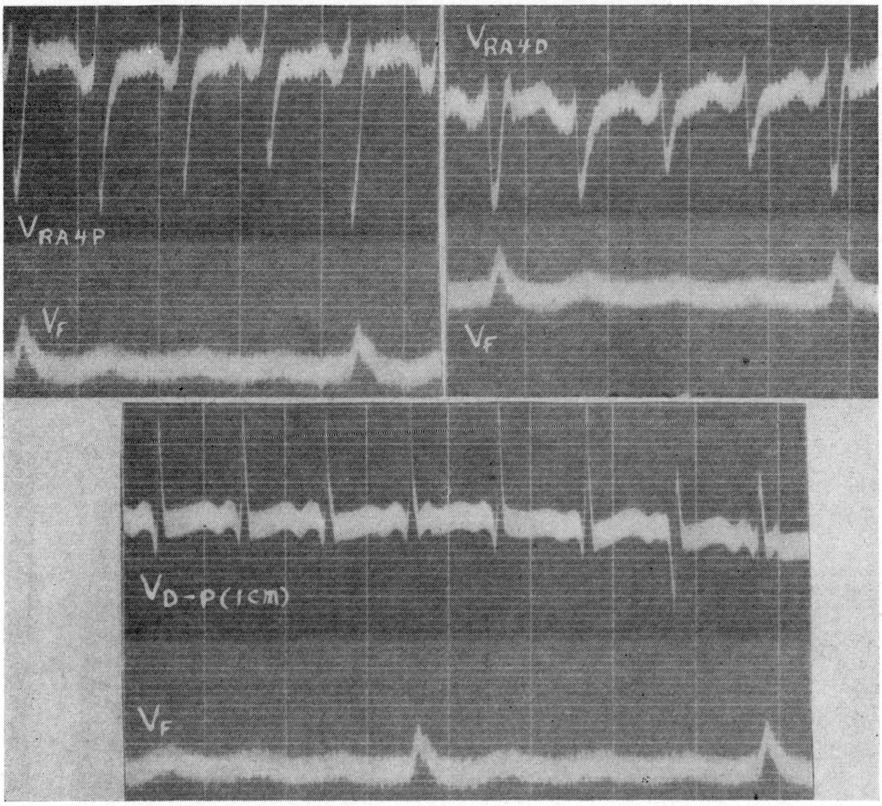


Fig. 9. Atrial flutter illustrating, by means of differential electrodes 1 cm. apart ($V_{D-P}$), that excitation was proceeding downward in the right atrium. $V_{RA4P}$ and $V_{RA4D}$ are the unipolar leads from each electrode; the simultaneous lead is $V_F$. Time lines, 0.2 sec.

Variations in the unipolar and differential leads may mean a change in the excitation pathway or movement of the electrode. A ventricular response occurs after every fourth atrial beat.

not clear.[19]

In atrial flutter the appearance of the atrial electrogram does not differ in any important respect from what is found in atrial tachycardia. Differential electrodes help to define the direction of the excitatory wave front in patients with this arrhythmia (Figure 9). Intrinsic deflections of alternating size and sequence occur as in atrial tachycardia (Figure 7).

## Summary

The clinical diagnosis of arrhythmias is not as precise as it might be because all of the electrical information readily available is not usually collected. Endocardial electrocardiography and the use of endocardial differential electrodes are means by which additional information can be obtained with safety and little inconvenience to the patient. Data collected in this way should contribute not only to the precision of diagnosis but probably also to an understanding of the mechanisms involved, and eventually of the rational therapy needed in the complex arrhythmias.

*REFERENCES*

1. Johnston, F. D. and Lepeshkin, E. Selected papers of Dr. Frank N. Wilson, Ann Arbor, Edwards Bros., 1954.
2. Kossmann, C. E., Berger, A. R., Briller, S. A., Rader, B. and Brumlík, J. Anomalous atrioventricular excitation produced by catheterization of the normal human heart, *Circulation 1*:902, 1950.
3. Kossmann, C. E. The interpretation of unipolar precordial electrocardiograms, *Med. Clin. N. Amer. 34*:833, 1950.
4. Kossmann, C. E., Berger, A. R., Rader, B., Brumlík, J., Briller, S. A. and Donnelly, J. H. Intracardiac and intravascular potentials resulting from electrical activity of the normal human heart, *Circulation 2*:10, 1950.
5. Kossmann, C. E. The electrocardiographic effects of myocardial and pericardial injury, *Bull. N.Y. Acad. Med. 28*:61, 1952.
6. Kossmann, C. E., Rader, B., Berger, A. R., Brumlík, J. and Briller, S. A. Electrograms in atrial flutter, atrial tachycardia, and atrial fibrillation, *Communications 1st World Congr. Cardiology,* II, Paris, Baillière, 1952, p. 401.
7. Vogel, J. H. K., Tabari, K., Overill, K. H. and Blount, S. G., Jr. A simple technique for identifying P waves in complex arrhythmias, *Amer. Heart J. 67*:158, 1964.
8. Dreifus, L. S. and Najmi, M. Right atrial electrocardiography; a bedside method for the diagnosis of cardiac arrhythmias, *J.A.M.A. 195*:167, 1966.
9. Hernandez, F., Rochkind, R. and Cooper, H. The intracavitary electrocardiogram in the diagnosis of Ebstein's anomaly, *Amer. J. Cardiol. 1*:181, 1958.
10. Yim, B. J. B. and Yu, P. N. Value of an electrode catheter in diagnosis of Ebstein's disease, *Circulation 17*:543, 1958.
11. Emslie-Smith, D., Lowe, K. G. and Hill, I. G. W. The intracardiac electrogram as an aid in the localization of pulmonary stenosis, *Brit. Heart J. 18*:29, 1956.
12. Emslie Smith, D. The intracardiac electrogram as an aid to cardiac catheterization, *Brit. Heart J. 17*:219, 1955.
13. Dickerson, R. B. and Caris, T. N. Supplemental value of the intracavitary electrocardiograph in cardiac catheterization, *Circulation 20*:928, 1959.
14. Watson, H. Intracardiac electrography in the investigation of congenital heart disease in infancy and the neonatal period, *Brit. Heart J. 24*:124, 1962.
15. Watson, H. Electrode catheters and the diagnostic application of intracardiac electrography in small children, *Circulation 29*:284, 1964.
16. Nutter, D. O. and Kelser, G. A., Jr. The percutaneous intracavitary electrocardiogram in the diagnosis of arrhythmias, *Ann. Intern. Med. 62*:706, 1965.
17. Macleod, A. G. The electrogram of cardiac muscle: An analysis which explains the regression of T deflection, a) *Amer. Heart J. 15*:165, 1938. The lengths of the stages of activity, b) *Amer. Heart J. 15*:402, 1938.
18. Lewis, T., Feil, H. S. and Stroud, W. D. Observations upon flutter and fibrillation. II. The nature of auricular flutter, *Heart 7*:191, 1918-20.
19. Urbach, J. R., Grauman, J. J. and Strauss, S. H. Quantitative method for the detection of atrioventricular node pacemaking in atrial fibrillation and preliminary report of its clinical value (abstract), *Circulation 34* (Suppl. III): 232, 1966.

# NEW YORK HEART ASSOCIATION

PART I—ABSTRACTS OF PAPERS PRESENTED AT THE SCIENTIFIC SESSION ON RESEARCH, HELD AT THE NEW YORK ACADEMY OF MEDICINE, APRIL 13, 1967

## *Micropuncture Study of the Effect of Partial Renal Venous Occlusion on Proximal Tubular Fluid Reabsorption in the Nephron of the Rat*

JOHN E. LEWY AND ERICH E. WINDHAGER

Department of Physiology
Cornell University Medical College
New York, N. Y.

During partial renal venous occlusion, mean peritubular capillary pressure rose from 12 to 25 and proximal tubular pressure from 12 to 23 mm. Hg. The total glomerular filtration rate (clearance of inulin) decreased from 8.7 ± 0.4 (S.E.) to 4.8 ± 0.9 ml./min./kg. Individual nephron GFR diminished from 29.5 ± 2.0 to 16.8 ± 1.5 mμl./min. Tf/P inulin at the end of the proximal convolution was 1.95 ± 0.06 before and 1.78 ± 0.06 during clamping, a statistically insignificant decrease. During control observations, absolute fluid reabsorption varied directly with the square of the tubular luminal radius ($r^2$) ($p<0.001$) and GFR ($p<0.01$): and fractional reabsorption with passage time ($p<0.001$). During clamping the relation between absolute reabsorption and $r^2$ was lost, but balance between absolute reabsorption and GFR was sustained ($p<0.001$). The proportionality between passage time and fractional reabsorption was altered (slope decreased) when passage time exceeded 16 seconds during clamping. These data suggest that a factor other than or in addition to tubular volume and passage time is operative to mediate the proportionality between glomerular filtration and tubular reabsorption. *(Supported in part by the New York Heart Association, National Science Foundation, American Heart Association, Life Insurance Medical Research Fund, and Health Research Council of the City of New York.)*

## *Human Platelet Glycogenolysis and Glycolysis During Simulated Thrombus Initiation**

S. KARPATKIN AND R. LANGER

Department of Medicine
New York University School of Medicine
New York, N. Y.

Platelet agglutination and possibly contraction are required for the initiation of thrombus formation. Maintenance of ATP levels is associated with this requirement. Since the metabolic energy of platelets is primarily obtained from glycolysis, various glycogenolytic and glycolytic parameters were investigated. Washed human platelets were incubated in a modified human Ringer's solution, $p$H 7.1, at 37° for 1 hour. Agglutination and contraction of platelets were achieved by the addition of ADP, thrombin or epinephrine.

In the presence of glucose, glycogenolysis was found to be a potent glycolytic pathway contributing 40% of the lactate produced. The breakdown of glycogen progressed with decreasing rate over a 1-hour period to 43% of initial glycogen levels. Of the glycogen depleted, 53% was converted to lactate, with the theoretical generation of 31 μmoles of ATP per ml. of packed platelets. With glucose present, glycogen breakdown was spared by 13%, with 51% of the glucose uptake converted to lactate. Total theoretical ATP generated was 52 μmoles/ml. Thus only 50% of glucose or glycogen was utilized for glycolytic generation of ATP. Platelet ATP levels declined from 2.70 to 1.94 μmoles/ml. at the end of one hour in the presence or absence of glucose. Despite an increase of 21 μmoles/ml. ATP, maintenance of steady state levels was not attained. This suggests compartmentation of energy requirements.

In the absence of glucose, ADP agglutination increased lactate production 15% (3.3 μmoles/ml./hr.) and glycogenolysis 26% (5.2 μmoles/ml./hr.) over basal levels. Both thrombin and epinephrine increased lactate production 37% and glycogenolysis 48%. A minimal sparing effect on glycogenolysis was noted in the presence of glucose.

Platelets were found to contain interconvertible forms of "active" phosphorylase *a* and "inactive" phosphorylase *b*. Phosphorylase *b* was activated by AMP. Resting level of phosphorylase *a* was 45% of total phosphorylase activity at the beginning and end of one hour of incubation with epinephrine. Increased glycogenolysis could not be correlated with changes in "active" phosphorylase *a*. *(Supported by USPHS FR 5399-05.)*

## *Biphasic Effects of Procainamide on Cardiac Conduction**

D. H. Singer, H. C. Strauss, and B. F. Hoffman

Department of Pharmacology
Columbia University College of Physicians and Surgeons
New York, N. Y.

Reduction of diastolic membrane potential in automatic (latent pacemaker) cells of the His-Purkinje system resulting from spontaneous phase 4 depolarization has been shown to cause disturbances of conduction and excitability ranging from simple slowing to complete block and inexcitability. Such changes may be a factor in development of reentry. Agents that suppress phase 4 depolarization and restore diastolic potential toward normal should therefore reverse these abnormalities. Thus, contrary to current belief that standard antiarrhythmic drugs, e.g., procainamide, exert solely depressant effects on cardiac conduction, such agents, by virtue of their ability to suppress phase 4 depolarization, may be expected to reverse conduction disturbances due to this cause.

This possibility was tested in isolated strands of canine Purkinje fibers. Transmembrane potentials were recorded simultaneously at both ends of the preparation. Development of conduction disturbances due to enhanced phase 4 depolarization was induced by low rates of stimulation in conjunction with either stretch, hypoxia or reduction of extracellular potassium concentration.

Low concentrations of procainamide (10-30 mg./l.), suppressed phase 4 depolarization, restored diastolic membrane potential toward normal and improved conduction. Higher concentrations (60-120 mg./l.) not only did not improve conduction but usually further increased the conduction disturbance. Presumably, at high concentrations of drug, the beneficial effects of suppression of phase 4 depolarization were outweighed by depressant effects on membrane responsiveness and reduction of maximum diastolic membrane potential. Often such high concentrations actually enhanced automaticity, thus contributing to the further deterioration of conduction that occurred in these instances.

Thus, in instances of conduction disturbances due to phase 4 depolarization of automatic cells, procainamide exerts a biphasic dose-related effect on conduction. Although high concentrations produce the expected depressant effects, low concentrations tend to improve conduction by suppressing phase 4 depolarization. If, as it seems reasonable to suppose, enhanced phase depolarization is a significant cause of conduction disturbances and reentry in the human heart, particularly the diseased human heart, then the action of procainamide in suppressing diastolic depolarization may be an important factor in its antiarrhythmic action in man. *(Supported in part by a grant from Life Insurance Medical Research Fund.)*

# *Hemodynamics of Paired Electrical Stimulation in Complete Heart Block in Man*

Martin L. Fox, Alfred J. Kaltman, George E. Bear, and Charles E. Kossmann

Department of Medicine
New York University School of Medicine
New York, N. Y.

Paired electrical stimulation (PES) was performed in eight adult patients who had complete heart block not associated with acute myocardial infarction. None of the patients was in clinical congestive heart failure nor were they taking digitalis or diuretics at the time of study.

Pressure pulses, maximal rate of rise of pressure (dP/dT) in the pulmonary artery, right ventricle and brachial artery, and cardiac output were measured during the control idioventricular rhythm, during single (SES) and paired (PES) electrical stimulation, and during the administration of isoproterenol.

Satisfactory PES was technically impossible in three patients because of a prolonged absolute refractory period. However, two of these demonstrated a significant increase in dP/dT. The cardiac output fell in all, and one experienced angina with paired pacing.

Of the five patients in whom adequate PES could be performed, only two demonstrated an increased cardiac output despite the fact that four had a significant increase in brachial artery dP/dT. With SES, cardiac output increased above control level in four of seven patients.

Isoproterenol administered as a continuous intravenous infusion in doses of 1 to 16 micrograms per minute for 15 minutes produced a greater cardiac output and brachial artery dP/dT than any of the other interventions in all except one patient, in whom these were maximal with PES. *(Supported by a NYHA Fellowship and USPHS Grant HE-5650-03.)*

# *Mechanisms of Experimental Atelectasis in Dogs*

HENRY M. THOMAS, III,* MARIETTE PRADEL, AND DUDLEY F. ROCHESTER

Cardiopulmonary Laboratory
Columbia University Medical Service of Bellevue Hospital

Department of Medicine
Columbia University College of Physicians and Surgeons
New York, N. Y.

The subnormal arterial $O_2$ tensions observed in patients undergoing anesthesia, chest strapping, and respirator breathing have been attributed to diffuse atelectasis. Atelectasis is thought to result either from obstruction of the airway followed by gradual loss of alveolar volume as gas is absorbed, or from abrupt alveolar collapse when alveolar volume is reduced below a critical level. To evaluate these possibilities, diffuse atelectasis produced by negative-pressure breathing was studied in dogs. Divergence of results among three methods of measuring pulmonary arteriovenous shunt-flow was used to assess the state of inflation of alveoli becoming atelectatic. The methods utilized were measurement of venous admixture, continuous infusion of $^{85}Kr$, and rapid injection of $^{85}Kr$ dissolved in T-1824 dye.

These methods were tested in dogs with occlusion of lobar bronchi since the state of alveolar inflation was known. In dogs breathing air before occlusion the lobes remained inflated for several hours whereas in dogs breathing 100% $O_2$ the obstructed lobes rapidly became gas-free. The $^{85}Kr$ infusion and venous admixture techniques measured perfusion of all nonventilated alveoli equally well, whereas the $^{85}Kr$-dye method measured only perfusion of gasless alveoli.

The latter method was shown to be influenced by the size of the extravascular space by analyzing simultaneous arterial concentration curves of $^{85}Kr$ and dye. The mean transit time for $^{85}Kr$ through airless lung exceeded that for dye, indicating that the isotope diffused from the blood into lung tissue and water. The consequent reduction in early recovery of $^{85}Kr$. lowered this estimate of shunt-flow.

In negative-pressure atelectasis, $^{85}Kr$ infusion and venous admixture estimates again agreed closely; the $^{85}Kr$-dye values were 1/5 lower, but in contrast to lobar occlusion studies were the same whether the animals breathed air or $O_2$. This latter finding suggests that atelectasis caused by negative-pressure breathing results primarily from abrupt alveolar collapse rather than from obstruction of the airway. *(Supported in part by USPHS Grants HE-02001 and HE-05741.)*

*Fellow, New York Heart Association.

# *The Mechanical Auxiliary Ventricle: Recent Modifications*

T. OKURA, S. TJØNNELAND, P. S. FREED, AND A. KANTROWITZ

Departments of Surgery
Maimonides Medical Center
State University of New York Downstate Medical Center
Brooklyn, N. Y.

Recent modifications relating to the mechanical auxiliary ventricle and their effects on 63 dogs are presented here. The modifications were:

1) One-piece outer housing of resin-coated fiber glass covered with silicone rubber, in which a flexible inner sac is placed, was used. This housing is thin, light and rigid, and remains uniform during fabrication.

2) Small transducers of various types were imbedded in the auxiliary ventricle to monitor its function and that of the left ventricle.

3) Instead of a constant flow of air, a constant air pressure of 200 to 250 mm. Hg was applied, synchronized with the natural heart by means of a dual beam oscilloscope. One beam is triggered by either the left ventricular pressure curve or the ECG, and the other can be adjusted to the time delay required for the function of the unit.

4) The aortic arch was cut instead of being ligated between the two anastomoses, so that all the blood passes through the auxiliary ventricle. This reduces the risk of clotting and kinking of the limbs.

In short-term hemodynamic studies in 19 dogs, with the auxiliary ventricle functioning up to 12 hours, left ventricular peak pressure was reduced as much as 80 mm. Hg (46% of the initial pressure); the systolic area of the left ventricular curve was reduced 58%; and the duration of systole by 50 msec.

In long-term experiments in 44 dogs in which intermittent pumping was employed, 30 survived the implantation, 9 surviving 1 month. The longest survival was 9 months. Thromboembolism was a complication in some long-term survivors.

Strain-gauge type transducers appeared most promising, being selective of aortic pressure and aortic valve sound and unaffected by noise from the solenoid valve used to control the compressed air.

Cineangiograms were used to analyze the function of the unit. *(This work was supported by USPHS Grant HE-06510.)*

# *Localization of Subcellular Sites of Sodium and Calcium Ion in Mammalian Myocardium*

MARIANNE J. LEGATO AND GLENN A. LANGER

Department of Medicine
Roosevelt Hospital
New York, N. Y.

The localization of the subcellular site of calcium sequestration and of sodium and calcium competition in mammalian cardiac muscle was undertaken in an electron microscope study of 42 canine papillary muscles. By means of a recently developed technique, muscles were cannulated through an intact arterial supply, and were isolated and perfused with a solution of the desired tonicity and ionic composition while function was monitored. At the end of the experiment, iced glutaraldehyde replaced the perfusate and the tissue, having been fixed instantaneously through its own vasculature, was processed for examination in the electron microscope.

Five control muscles were perfused with oxygenated isotonic solution containing NaCl 130mM, $CaCl_2$ 5mM, KCl 4mM, $MgCl_2.6H_2O$ lmM, $NaHPO4.H_2O$ 0.435mM, $NaHCO_3$ 14 mM, and glucose 5.56mM. These muscles showed good function and excellent preservation of ultrastructure.

In 11 muscles, a 75% reduction of sodium in the perfusate produced an increase in systolic tension and resulted in dilation of the sarcoplasmic reticular tubules. A 3- to 5-fold increase in perfusate calcium in three muscles produced exactly the same phenomenon.

In a second series of experiments, 20 muscles were preserved with osmic acid in a buffered solution of potassium antimonate at the end of each perfusion. This resulted in the sharp localization of an electron-dense, granular precipitate, tentatively identified as calcium antimonate, in the lateral sacs of the sarcoplasmic reticulum and along the I band of muscle sarcomeres.

These observations correlate with the proposition that the sarcoplasmic reticulum in mammalian cardiac muscle has a special ability to sequester or release calcium ion. As such, it may function as the link between excitation and contraction, facilitate muscle relaxation, and control the degree of muscle inotropism. *(Supported by grants G 64-3 from the Life Insurance Medical Research Fund and USPHS HE 05741—05.)*

# NEW YORK HEART ASSOCIATION

PART II—ABSTRACTS OF PAPERS SUBMITTED FOR PRESENTATION AT THE SCIENTIFIC SESSION ON RESEARCH, HELD AT THE NEW YORK ACADEMY OF MEDICINE, APRIL 13, 1967

## *Structure-Activity Relations of Synthetic Vasopressin and Oxytocin Hormones in the Microcirculation: A Cellular and Molecular Basis for Shock Therapy*

BURTON M. ALTURA AND S. G. HERSHEY

Departments of Anesthesiology and Physiology
Albert Einstein College of Medicine
New York, N. Y.

The synthesis of vasopressin has led to the preparation of a number of analogues of the naturally occurring hormone that while still maintaining marked vasoconstrictor activity exert reduced or virtually negligible effects on the kidneys. One such analogue, PLV-2 or 2-phenylalanine-8-lysine vasopressin, has been reported by our group to increase survival of rats and rabbits subjected to hemorrhage, intestinal ischemia shock, and traumatic shock. On direct microscopic observation of the mesenteric microcirculation in rats and rabbits subjected to hemorrhage and to the shock of intestinal ischemia, we found that PLV-2 maintained arteriolar and venular tone, sustained vasomotion, and decreased the abnormally high reactivity to topically applied epinephrine that is characteristic of shock. The net influence of these *selective* microvascular effects of PLV-2 was to improve true capillary inflow, distribution, and outflow. In view of these observations in the shocked animals, a systematic study is currently under way in our laboratory to determine whether the pharmacologic effects and sites of action of these neurohypophyseal peptides in the microcirculation undergo change as their chemical structures are modified. These studies are being done in the hope of being able to suggest synthesis of vasotropic compounds that may be more highly effective in shock. Microvascular smooth muscle actions currently are being studied *in vivo* on the rat mesoappendix preparation. Topical application of Pitressin, 8-arginine vasopressin, 8-lysine vasopressin, and PLV-2 to the mesoappendix of the rat produces in dose-dependent fashion a venular to arteriolar gradient of constriction in the microcirculation—the reverse of epinephrine, norepinephrine, or electrical stimuli. Local application of 8-ornithine vasopressin, oxytocin, or 2-phenylalanine-8-ornithine oxytocin to the mesoappendix of the rat produces in dose-dependent fashion a constriction of precapillary sphincters, followed by metarterioles, then venules and, lastly, by arterioles as the doses of the three analogues are increased. Our observations thus far indicate that vasopressins and oxytocins exhibit *selective* microvascular effects. At least two distinct types of gradients of reactivity appear to exist for these peptides in the microcirculation. A particular type of gradient of responsiveness may depend on the basicity as well as length of the side chain of the amino acid moiety in position 8. *(Supported in part by USPHS Grants HE 09042 and HE 11391.)*

## *Effects of Diphenylhydantoin on Mammalian Heart Muscle*

A. L. BASSETT, J. T. BIGGER, JR., S. P. APRIL, AND B. F. HOFFMAN

Department of Pharmacology
Columbia University College of Physicians and Surgeons
New York, N. Y.

Recent studies have demonstrated that diphenylhydantoin (DPH) consistently reverses human and experimentally induced canine arrhythmias but may depress cardiovascular performance. The present experiments evaluated the direct effects of antiarrhythmic concentrations of DPH on the contractility of isolated cardiac muscle.

Cat papillary muscles and trabeculae carneae (4-8 mm. by $<$ 1 mm.) were field stimulated 30 to 60 times/min. at 30° and 37° C. Isometric contractions were recorded from muscles at fixed length, at the peak of the length-tension curve or on the descending (failing) limb. Isometric tension was recorded from muscles undergoing smooth programmed changes in length. Force-velocity relations were obtained from isotonic recordings.

Addition of DPH ($10^{-9}$ to $10^{-6}$ $M$) had insignificant inotropic effects on the maximum rate of isometric force development, peak systolic force, and diastolic compliance in normal and overstretched muscles at fixed length. Similar results were observed over the entire length-tension curve in muscles undergoing programmed length changes; DPH had no effect on the hysteresis displayed by such muscles. Maximum rate of isotonic shortening was minimally effected. DPH diluent, in quantities necessary for dissolving DPH, had substantially no effect on contractility.

DPH ($10^{-8}$ to $10^{-6}$ $M$) had negligible effects on increased contractility observed during administration of isoproterenol ($10^{-7}$ $M$) or increased calcium.

In addition, the effects of DPH were tested on the facilitation of $Ca^{45}$ transfer from aqueous to organic phases caused by lipids extracted from canine microsomes. The negative inotropic effect of other antiarrhythmic substances has been related to inhibition of such transfer. DPH ($10^{-8}$ to $10^{-6}$ $M$) caused inhibition quantitatively similar to that reported for beta adrenergic blocking agents and quinidine.

Results indicate that DPH, in the concentrations used, has little or no direct negative inotropic action on cardiac muscle and suggests that depressant effects seen with the intact circulation may arise peripherally. *(Supported by USPHS Research Grant HE-08508 and a grant from Parke, Davis & Co.)*

---

## *Hemodynamics of High-Inflow Portal Hypertension*

IRWIN R. BERMAN, WILLIAM M. STAHL, ALLAN E. DUMONT AND ELLIOTT R. BERANBAUM

Bellevue Hospital and
New York University School of Medicine
New York, N. Y.

Intensive hemodynamic investigation of a patient with myeloid metaplasia, massive splenomegaly, and bleeding esophageal varices gives evidence of the existence of a syndrome of high-inflow portal hypertension.

Hepatic function was normal. Inferior vena cava, umbilical vein, and cervical thoracic duct were cannulated. Celiac and superior mesenteric arteriography were performed; subsequently a balloon catheter was passed into the splenic trtery under fluoroscopic control. Pressure, $pO_2$, $pCO_2$ and $pH$ of arterial, venous, and lymphatic samples were determined in the resting state, with thoracic duct drainage, with balloon occlusion of the splenic artery, and after deflation of the balloon. Thoracic duct drainage was replaced volumetrically.

Initial thoracic duct oxygen tension was elevated to 86 mm. Hg. Thoracic duct drainage reduced splenic size and lowered umbilical vein pressure from 35 to 27 cm. $H_2O$ without fall in caval pressure. Balloon occlusion of the splenic artery promptly lowered umbilical venous pressure further to 21 cm. $H_2O$, with concomitant elevation of thoracic duct pressure from 18 to 47 cm. $H_2O$ and appearance of hemorrhagic lymph. Deflation of the balloon was accompanied by prompt return of umbilical venous hypertension to 35 cm. $H_2O$, fall in thoracic duct pressure to 23 cm., and disappearance of blood from lymph drainage. Arterial and central venous pressures were stable throughout the study.

At operation, occlusion of the splenic artery lowered hepatic vein wedge pressure from 33 to 26 cm. $H_2O$. One week after splenectomy, hepatic vein wedge pressure was 13 cm. $H_2O$ and pancytopemia reversed.

The effect of occlusion of the splenic artery on umbilical vein and hepatic wedge pressures appears to confirm the existence of high portal inflow and pressure due to increased splenic blood flow. Elevated thoracic duct oxygen tension suggests arteriovenous shunting. Mechanisms for changes in pressure and character of thoracic duct drainage are discussed.

## *The Role of Norepinephrine Synthesis in Maintenance of Cardiac Catecholamine Content*

B. BHAGAT AND D. LEHR

Department of Pharmacology
New York Medical College-Flower and Fifth Avenue Hospitals
New York, N. Y.

Norepinephrine, a natural transmitter, is stored in the dense core of vesicles of sympathetic nerve endings. Small amounts of this amine are released continuously into the circulation in order to maintain tonic activity; increasing amounts are released in response to sympathetic nerve stimulation. In experimental animals (guinea pigs and rats) cardiac catecholamine concentrations remained unaltered even in the presence of vigorous sympathetic activity produced by 1) prolonged sympathetic nerve stimulation; 2) exposure to cold for 6 h.; 3) administration of histamine or $\beta$-tetrahydronaphthylamine. Such maintenance of endogenous amine levels was not possible when synthesis of norepinephrine was inhibited by the tyrosine-hydroxylase inhibitor, $\alpha$-methyltyrosine. In this case tissue catecholamine levels were reduced. This reduction, however, was antagonized by pretreatment with ganglionic blocking agents, adrenergic neurone blocking agents, monoamine oxidase inhibitors, or by destruction of the brain and spinal cord. The usual elevation in catecholamine levels after inhibition of monoamine oxidase or after ganglionic blockade was not observed when synthesis was inhibited by $\alpha$-methyltyrosine.

The "common factor" in all these experiments is the inhibition of spontaneous release due to "tonic" impulses in sympathetic nerve fibers. This suggests that once synthesis is inhibited, tonic release of catecholamine is sufficient to cause gradual depletion of the amine. This depletion after $\alpha$-methyltyrosine was increased when sympathetic nerve activity was increased by various procedures. Since $\alpha$-methyltyrosine did not affect the accumulation of $H^3$-norepinephrine in the rat heart, these findings suggest that synthesis of catecholamine is indeed increased in response to increased sympathetic nerve activity, which helps to maintain normal levels of tissue catecholamine. Thus the present study shows that maintenance of endogenous amine levels is based largely on adjustment of local norepinephrine synthesis, which is presumably regulated by activity in the sympathetic nerves. *(Supported in part by a grant from the Council of Tobacco Research—U.S.A.)*

---

## *Some Effects of Diphenylhydantoin on Human Atrioventricular Conduction*

J. T. BIGGER AND C. STEINER

Departments of Medicine and Pharmacology
Columbia University College of Physicians and Surgeons
Cardiovascular Laboratory, Presbyterian Hospital
New York, N. Y.

Diphenylhydantoin (DPH) is effective in treating cardiac arrhythmia, notably atrial arrhythmias induced by digitalis excess and ventricular arrhythmias. Most effective antiarrhythmic substances may have a significant depressive effect on AV conduction, and this becomes a consideration in their use. The effect of DPH on AV conduction in man was evaluated when the drug was given alone or after parasympathetic (atropine) or sympathetic (propranolol) blocking agents. Subjects with normal and diseased hearts were studied. The heart was paced at a constant rate through a right atrial electrode catheter; a test stimulus was applied every sixth or seventh drive cycle. The interval between the drive and test stimuli was shortened by 5-msec. intervals and absolute and functional refractory periods (RP) of the AV conducting system were determined. ECG, stimulus artifacts, and vascular pressures were monitored on a switched-beam oscilloscope.

Results indicate that in patients with either normal or diseased hearts, the AVRP decreased by an average of about 35 msec. after DPH. Variance was found, in a few cases, in the magnitude of change in the absolute compared with the functional AVRP. The acceleration of AV conduction after DPH tended to be greater in patients receiving digitalis. The AVRP returned toward control in parallel with the decline in plasma DPH levels with time.

Although atropine shortened and propranolol lengthened the AVRP, neither abolished the DPH effect; however, the per cent decrease in AVRP after DPH was less after either drug. The mild hypotension induced by DPH was short-lived in comparison to the alterations in AV conduction, making reflex changes an unlikely explanation for the observed acceleration of AV conduction.

It is concluded that, in a therapeutic dose that depresses ventricular automaticity, DPH accelerates AV conduction, at least partly through a direct effect on the AV conducting system. *(Supported by USPHS Grant HE-05941 and a grant-in-aid from Parke, Davis & Co.)*

# *The Effect of Artificial Pacing on Cardiac Output in Congenital Heart Block*

JACK BUDOW, JOSHUA LYNFIELD, AND IRVING G. KROOP

Cardiopulmonary Laboratory, Department of Medicine
Division of Cardiology, Department of Pediatrics
Jewish Hospital of Brooklyn
Brooklyn, N. Y.

Underlying heart disease is generally present in acquired heart block and may modify the effect of heart rate on cardiac output. However, in congenital heart block, the hemodynamic effects may be determined only by the slow rate and not by any myocardial factor.

Two patients with isolated congenital heart block whose ages were 6 and 16 years respectively were studied. Measurements of cardiac output by the dye dilution technique were made during complete heart block with a slow ventricular rate and during more rapid heart rates induced by an electrode catheter in the right ventricle. Intracardiac pressures were also recorded. In each instance, there was no increase in cardiac output during more rapid ventricular pacing. An insignificant increase from 2.8 l./min. to 3.0 l./min. was present in the 6-year-old patient, and a decline from 5.4 l./min. to 4.5 l./min. was observed in the other. The initial, resting, high stroke-volume during heart block decreased from 56 cc. to 29 cc. in the first patient and from 136 cc. to 33 cc. in the second, with an increase in rate from 37 to 130 per minute.

The increased stroke volume in these patients with heart block is probably related to a long diastolic filling period, which results in increased myocardial contractility by a healthy myocardium. This accounts for the normal resting cardiac output. In acquired heart block, however, stroke volume may not increase sufficiently, despite the longer diastolic filling period. Therefore the resting cardiac output may be low with slow rates. Under these circumstances, increasing the heart rate by an artificial pacemaker may increase the cardiac output. In isolated congenital heart block, increasing the heart rate alone may not result in an increased cardiac output.

These findings suggest that the only indication for pacemaker therapy in isolated congenital heart block is the occurrence of Adams-Stokes attacks.

## *Intracavitary Electrocardiographic Double Atrial Activity in the Homotransplanted Puppy Heart*

J. CABASSON, G. KHALIL, H. JOOS, AND A. KANTROWITZ

Departments of Surgery and Pediatrics, Maimonides Medical Center
State University of New York Downstate Medical Center
Brooklyn, N. Y.

Since the electrical atrial activity of the transplanted heart is poorly understood, the following investigation was undertaken.

A nine-lead electrocardiogram was recorded under ambient conditions in 30 puppies before and after orthotopic cardiac homotransplantation under profound hypothermia and by a method of continuous suture. Atrial activity was further investigated by esophageal and intracavitary leads. Histocompatibility was evaluated by several biological methods.

Postoperatively, two foci of atrial activity were demonstrated by the intracavitary tracing in all cases. The findings show that the sinus node of the recipient innervates atrial tissue remaining *in situ* and responds to extrinsic neurogenic influence, but is blocked at the suture line and prevented from initiating ventricular contraction.

The findings also show that donor atria usually respond to their own sinus nodes, but occasionally a new atrial pacemaker is found. These impulses are independent of neural influences but provide the stimulus for ventricular contraction.

Rejection affects the atrial activity of the donor by: 1) slowing down the donor sinus node, 2) causing transient sinus arrest that results in ventricular irregularity, and 3) producing permanent nodal rhythm. All such effects are reversible by immunosuppressive therapy except in cases of severe histoincompatibility. *(This work was supported by USPHS Grants HE-06510 and FR-05497.)*

# *The Effect of Respiratory and Metabolic Acidosis on Myocardial Contractility*

DONALD L. CARESS, ALFRED S. KISSACK, ALVIN J. SLOVIN, AND JACKSON H. STUCKEY

Department of Surgery
State University of New York Downstate Medical Center
Brooklyn, N. Y.

Previous studies have led to conflicting opinions on the effects of *p*H alterations on the myocardium and on peripheral resistance. The isovolumic left ventricle allows the effects of *p*H on the myocardium and the peripheral vasculature to be evaluated separately and permits measurement of myocardial contractility in terms of maximum rate of pressure rise. Experiments were carried out in 6 dogs to study respiratory acidosis and in 7 dogs to study metabolic acidosis produced by administration of lactic acid. Results showed that after 20 minutes of equilibration with a 30% $CO_2$ to 70% $O_2$ gas mixture there was no decrease in myocardial contractility if the *p*H was above 7.0. If the *p*H was below 7.0, the dP/dT averaged 47% of control; peripheral resistance averaged 143% of control. On the other hand, 15 minutes following the injection of lactic acid, dP/dT was 73% of control and peripheral resistance was 81% of control. During preparation of all animals, a base deficit developed; when the deficit was corrected with sodium bicarbonate, the dp/dT rose an average of 185% of control. It is concluded, therefore, that acidosis produced by hypercarbia does not depress myocardial contractility unless the *p*H falls below 7.0. Metabolic acidosis or lactic acidemia depresses myocardial contractility and this effect is reversed by $NaHCO_3$. This depression does not appear to be solely a function of the *p*H, but results from metabolic products which usually lead to a depression of the *p*H. *(Supported in part by grants from USPHS and AHA.)*

## *Ventricular Asystole and the Vagus*

DONALD L. CARESS, MARIO VASSALLE, ALVIN J. SLOVIN, AND JACKSON H. STUCKEY

Departments of Surgery and Physiology
State University of New York Downstate Medical Center
Brooklyn, N. Y.

Reflex vagal excitation can lead to sinus arrest but it is not clear why there should also be ventricular asystole. To investigate this point, the right vagus in dogs was stimulated for 2 minutes; the ventricles were driven during the first minute. The period of ventricular asystole was prolonged when the drive rate was faster and was shortened when the drive rate was slower than the control sinus rate. The asystolic period was shortened when the sinus rate was slowed by graded vagal stimulation before maximal vagal stimulation. The period of asystole was prolonged by driving the ventricles at a rate higher than the sinus rate prior to vagal stimulation. In dogs with chronic atrioventricular block, "overdriving" the ventricles led to temporary inhibition of ventricular pacemakers. In dogs with acute atrioventricular block, the coronary sinus plasma potassium level increased in proportion to the increase in ventricular driving rate. These results support the concept that the slowly discharging ventricular pacemakers are inhibited by the higher rate of the atrial pacemakers; this inhibition becomes apparent when the atrial pacemakers are suppressed by the vagus. The mechanism of inhibition may be related to a rate-dependent change in extracellular potassium concentration. *(Supported in part by USPHS and AHA.)*

## *Effects of Heparin, Protamine, and Low Molecular Weight Dextran (LMD) on Electrokinetic Characteristics of Canine Blood Vessel Intima* In Vivo.

P. S. CHOPRA, S. SRINIVASAN, T. LUCAS, AND P. N. SAWYER

Vascular Surgical Services and Biophysical and Electrochemical Laboratories
Departments of Surgery and Surgical Research
State University of New York Downstate Medical Center
Brooklyn, N. Y.

Electrokinetic characteristics of canine blood vessel intima have been determined *in vitro* from streaming potential and electroosmosis measurements. These experiments confirm that the intima is negatively charged under normal conditions. Injury reduces the negative charge density and may even make the intimal surface positive. For comparison with *in vitro* streaming potential measurements in canine blood vessels, measurements were carried out *in vivo* between two electrodes placed at a known distance apart in both the aorta and femoral arteries. Positive streaming potentials of 0.2 to 0.4 mv. for the aorta and 0.5 mv. for the femoral artery were recorded at resting flow rates. These results are in excellent agreement with corresponding *in vitro* studies using the same distance and flow rates. The second part of the experiments involved determination of the effect of heparin, protamine, and LMD on the electrokinetic characteristics of the aorta and femoral arteries. Intravenous heparin (2 mg./kg.) increased the streaming potential to 0.7 mv. across the aorta and to 0.8 mv. across the femoral artery. Protamine (2 mg./kg.) caused reversion of the streaming potentials to the original values. Intravenous LMD (10% w/v) behaved similarly to heparin, producing a linear increase in streaming potentials with an increase in the volume of dextran infused. The anticoagulant effects of heparin and LMD are well known. It is very probable that the mechanism of their action is by adsorption on the intimal surface and other thrombogenic proteins in the blood stream, with consequent increase in the negative surface charge density as manifested by an increase in the streaming potential. *(Supported in part by USPHS Grant HE-07371-04, 05.)*

# *Metabolic Studies with an Acyl Guanidine in Primary and Secondary Hyperaldosteronism*

P. Cushman, C. Braren, R. Campbell, and D. David

Department of Medicine
St. Luke's Hospital Center
New York, N. Y.

The effects of a potassium-sparing agent, MK 870, on Na and K balances were investigated in the metabolic ward. Study periods were alternated with recovery periods while dietary intakes of Na and K remained constant. Case No. 1 was one of probable primary hyperaldosteronism—i.e., hypertension, hypokalemia, alkalosis, without renal disease; salt loading produced increased urinary excretion of sodium and potassium without reduction in the greatly increased 24-hour urinary excretion rates of aldosterone. Five days of MK 870 resulted in correction of hypokalemia and alkalosis, while 5 days of 300 mg. aldactone effected only a modest rise in serum K. In 4 cases with refractory edema and hyperaldosteronism, MK 870 was ineffective *per se*. Once an effective diuretic regimen, including ethacrynic acid (EA), was established, striking negative potassium balances were often seen. In all cases when MK 870 was added to the regimen enhanced natruresis, diuresis, but less K loss and decreased systemic alkalosis occurred. In another patient, an edematous cirrhotic, treatment with furosemide produced diuresis, decreased K, increased $CO_2$, and hepatic precoma. When MK 870 was added to the same regimen, enhanced diuresis and natruresis without significant change in K, $CO_2$, or mental state were observed. MK 870 appears to be an effective diuretic that reverses the hypokalemia of primary hyperaldosteronism and that reduces the propensity to hypokalemic alkalosis of other diuretic agents in secondary hyperaldosteronism with edema. *(Supported by USPHS (AM 2828) and the American Heart Association.)*

## *Epicardial Activation of the Hypertrophied Right Ventricle in Man*

A. J. DELMAN, G. ROBINSON, W. YAHR, AND J. W. LISTER

Montefiore Hospital and Medical Center
Bronx, N. Y.

The sequence of epicardial activation of the right ventricle has been studied at open heart operation in 9 patients with rheumatic heart disease and mitral stenosis who underwent mitral commissurotomy. Prior to cardiopulmonary bypass, epicardial activation times were obtained from 11 to 22 right ventricular sites and 4 to 20 left ventricular sites by the recording of close bipolar electrograms.

All patients had significant pulmonary hypertension (pulmonary artery pressures ranged from 38/18 to 110/44), and right ventricular enlargement by x-ray criteria and confirmed at operation. None of the patients had right bundle branch block. In all patients, the prepapillary surface of the right ventricle was activated at the normal time (15 to 20 msec. after the onset of the QRS complex). The vectorcardiogram or the electrocardiogram showed right ventricular hypertrophy in 4 patients. These 4 patients had significant delays of the epicardial activation times of the superior aspect of the free wall of the right ventricle and right ventricular outflow tract. The 5 patients who did not show right ventricular hypertrophy on the electrocardiogram or vectorcardiogram had no significant delays in the right ventricular epicardial activation times.

This study suggests that there is good correlation between the vectorcardiographic and electrocardiographic patterns of right ventricular hypertrophy and the epicardial activation sequence of the right ventricle. Right ventricular enlargement delineated by x ray and confirmed at operation may not be demonstrated by the vectorcardiogram or electrocardiogram as long as the epicardial activation times of the right ventricle are within normal range. The appearance of signs of right ventricular hypertrophy on the vectorcardiogram or electrocardiogram appears to be related to the development of delays in activation of the right ventricle. *(Supported by USPHS Grant HE 10583-02.)*

## *The Role of Histocompatibility in Orthotopic Transplantation of Puppy Hearts*

G. DUREAU, W. SCHILT, J. CABASSON, H. JOOS, G. KHALIL, S. SAMUELS, AND A. KANTROWITZ

Departments of Surgery and Pediatrics
Maimonides Medical Center
State University of New York Downstate Medical Center
Brooklyn, N. Y.

This study was carried out to determine the role of histocompatibility in puppies with orthotopic heart transplants. Fourteen animals were used, whose donors had been selected on the basis of histocompatibility tests (normal lymphocyte transfer test, irradiated hamster test, and leukoagglutination test). The postoperative course of these puppies was followed carefully with regard to their ECG's, clinical status, and immunosuppressive therapy. The ECG's showed a close correlation between QRS voltages in lead 2 and the grade of histocompatibility as indicated in the test results, both in the immediate and later postoperative periods.

The immunosuppressive therapy chosen was basically Solu-Medrol, supported with Imuran; Actinomycin C was added during acute rejection crisis. This treatment appeared to be most effective in the group showing average histocompatibility, and although some puppies with poor histocompatibility responded to the therapy, they inevitably died of heart failure shortly afterward. The postoperative clinical coarse of the animals with good compatibility, as regards activity, appetite, growth, and so forth, was much smoother than that of those with poor compatibility; however, the former group generally succumbed as a result of intercurrent infection. Survival times correlated with the degree of compatibility. Postmortem histological findings on the hearts showed equivocal results. *(This work was supported by USPHS Grants HE-06510 and FR-05497.)*

# *Lidocaine in Ventricular Arrhythmia*

E. Ettinger, J. Hayes, T. Forde, F. Wanat, and T. Killip

Department of Medicine
Cornell University Medical College
New York, N. Y.

Lidocaine has been advocated in emergency treatment of ventricular arrhythmia, but few objective data are available. Despite enthusiastic clinical application in the treatment of abnormal rhythms the drug has not been approved by the Food and Drug Administration as an antiarrhythmic. Single and multiple doses of lidocaine, 1 to 2 mg./kg., were given intravenously to 26 patients with ventricular premature complexes (VPCs) with continuous ECG monitoring and periodic assay of blood levels. Transient lightheadedness or sleepiness occurred in 62%. Blood pressure, sinus rate, and QRS duration were unchanged. Frequency of VPCs was reduced after lidocaine in all subjects. Lidocaine blood levels 5 minutes after injection of 1.0 mg./kg. varied from 0.3 to 1.8 $\mu$g./ml. and were inversely proportional to body weight. Initial antiarrhythmic effects occurred with 0.6 to 1.2 $\mu$g./ml. The $t\frac{1}{2}$ of lidocaine in blood approximated 20 minutes. In 53% of subjects, reduction in VPC incidence persisted more than 1 hour. Prolongation of effect could not be correlated with blood level of drug. In 2 patients with supraventricular arrhythmia with A-V block, ventricular rate increased markedly following drug. In unanesthetized trained dogs with surgically induced complete heart block, lidocaine did not affect atrial rate, slowed ventricular rate, and prolonged asystole following abrupt cessation of ventricular driving. Dose response experiments in these dogs show minimal effect with 0.5 mg./kg. and systemic toxicity after 4 mg./kg. The influence of the drug on ventricular automaticity has been correlated with the arterial blood concentration. *(Supported in part by Astra Pharmaceutical Products, Inc.)*

# *A Comparison of Left Heart Bypass under Hypovolemic and Arfonad Hypotension*

S. L. Frantz, F. M. Miller, A. L. Goldenberg, and C. Dennis

Department of Surgery
State University of New York Downstate Medical Center
Brooklyn, N. Y.

Left heart bypass, a form of myocardial augmentation, has been shown to reduce myocardial oxygen consumption effectively, particularly in a hypotensive model. Previously, hypotension had been produced by hypovolemia, but in an effort to utilize this observation clinically, chemically induced hypotension was employed. Arfonad, a ganglionic blocking agent, was selected because of the few side effects, rapid onset, and short duration of action of this drug.

Pulsatile left heart bypass through the Senning-Dennis cannula (obviating the need for thoracotomy) was performed. Cardiac output and electrocardiographic, aortic, and left ventricular pressure curves were recorded at carefully maintained levels of pressure. Cardiac work was determined by the pressure-time product (PTP), a modification of Sarnoff's tension time index.

The pressure-time products of control studies and assisted studies under Arfonad hypotension were compared at equivalent pressure levels with control and assisted studies obtained under hypovolemic conditions. The pressure-time products of controls (*without* any assistance) under chemically induced hypotension fell an average of 15.8% with each reduction of 25 mm. Hg in mean arterial pressure, compared with a 15.5% reduction with hypovolemia. Arfonad hypotension reduced cardiac output 5.6% and 16.4% at 100 and 75 mm. Hg, respectively. At these same levels, hypovolemia reduced the output by 52% and 58%. At 50 mm. Hg mean arterial pressure, Arfonad produced a 49% reduction while hypovolemia showed a reduction of 64%.

Left heart bypass under Arfonad hypotension reduced the PTP an average of only 2.5% with each 25 mm. Hg decrement in pressure from 150 to 75 mm. Hg while hypovolemia caused the PTP to fall 9.5% with each decrement in pressure.

The difference is striking at 100 and 75 mm. Hg, where the PTP was reduced 18.0% and 20.8% with Arfonad, contrasted with 45.5% and 50.8% in the hypovolemic model.

Altough hypotension produced by hypovolemia increased the efficiency of the left heart bypass system, it is apparent that the hypotension produced by Arfonad does not have a similar effect. *(Supported by State University of New York, USPHS Grants HE 01011-16, and 2R01-HE-07028-05, and AHA Grant 65G-72.)*

## *Systems Analysis Correction of Dye Dilution Curves*

EPHRAIM GLASSMAN, WAYNE MITZNER, AND WILLIAM BLESSER

Departments of Medicine
The Long Island Jewish Hospital
State University of New York Downstate Medical Center
Polytechnic Institute of Brooklyn
Brooklyn, N. Y.

Distortion is introduced into dye dilution curves by the withdrawal of blood through sampling tubes and densitometric apparatus. Elimination of this distortion would result in the inscription of a curve similar to that obtained with intravascular recording. To measure the error, blood was withdrawn through a cardiac catheter and densitometer. The total system was analyzed by applying a step function input of indocyanine-dyed blood and recording output. The response was shown to be a single exponential of time constant T. By the techniques of system analysis the transfer function of the system was determined by means of Laplace transformations to be $\frac{1/T}{s + 1/T}$. Uncorrected dye curves (Cu) were passed through a compensating electronic network to eliminate system error, and corrected curves (Cc) were recorded. Experiments were performed with a pusatile blood pump with variable ejection fractions. Cc, recorded by withdrawing blood just distal to the "aortic" valve, revealed a more rapid upstroke than Cu and a series of steps on the downslope. The heights of these steps were used for calculation of the residual fraction with excellent results. The system was applied to curves obtained in humans with left ventricular injection and supra-aortic valvular sampling. In subjects without valvular regurgitation, ejection fractions in the range of 0.4 were obtained. *(Supported by a research grant from the Nassau County Heart Association.)*

## *Coronary Sinus Blood Flow in Counterpulsation*

J. GOLDSTEIN, R. GOETZ, J. DORMANDY, AND D. KRIPKE

Department of Surgery
Albert Einstein College of Medicine
New York, N. Y.

For counterpulsation to be effective in myocardial failure it appears important that it increase the amount of available oxygen by increasing coronary blood flow (CBF). Although aortic diastolic pressure may increase and cardiac work may decrease, it cannot be assumed that these changes are paralleled by improved myocardial perfusion.

*Method:* Counterpulsation was applied to 25 dogs. Central aortic and left ventricular pressures, cardiac output, CBF and $pO_2$ in the coronary sinus and aorta were measured. Left ventricular stroke work (VSW), maximum rate of ventricular pressure ascent (dP/dT), time-tension index (TTI), and myocardial oxygen consumption (MOC) were calculated. Animals in Group 1 were normotensive with systolic pressures above 100 mm. Hg. Group 2 animals were made hypotensive, either by graded hemorrhage or by temporary obstruction of left ventricular outflow. After the effects of counterpulsation were studied, Group 2 animals were made normotensive by transfusion or epinephrine infusion.

*Result:* In every dog of both groups counterpulsation lowered aortic peak systolic pressure (mean 11%) and end diastolic pressure (mean 13%) and raised mid-diastolic pressure (mean 72%). All parameters of ventricular work decreased with counterpulsation by the same amount in both groups; VSW by mean 35%, TTI by mean 30% and dP/dT by mean 20%. However CBF differed between the groups, remaining essentially unaltered in Group 2 and increasing by a mean of 24% in Group 1, a difference paralleled by the change in MOC.

*Conclusion:* Counterpulsation decreased the work of the myocardium proportionately in normotensive and hypotensive animals. Despite this decreased work the myocardium of the normotensive dog consumed more oxygen when it was made available by an increase in coronary flow. Thus the calculated myocardial work during counterpulsation is not a good measure of the total demand of the myocardium for oxygen. In order to avoid inadequate oxygenation the CBF must be increased even if calculated myocardial work decreases. This was achieved only by maintaining the aortic pressure at normotensive levels. *(Supported by USPHS Grant H-3743, Health Research Council of the City of N.Y. under contract 1-237, and by the Health Research Center Fund.)*

## *Myocardial Metabolism in Complete Heart Block and Induced Tachycardia*

John J. Gregory, Hiltrud Mueller, Stephen M. Ayres, and Stanley Giannelli

St. Vincent's Hospital, New York, N. Y.

Coronary blood flow (CBF), cardiac output (CO), myocardial oxygen consumption ($MVO_2$), arteriovenous lactate and pyruvate differences, myocardial excess lactate (XL), and cardiac work were measured in five patients with complete heart block at idioventricular and "normal" rates and with induced tachycardia. In three patients (Group 1), CO and $MVO_2$ increased while XL decreased with pacing at a "normal" rate, indicating improved myocardial function. In two (Group 2) the CO failed to rise. Both $MVO_2$ and XL increased, indicating decreased efficiency and increased anaerobic metabolism.

Electrical pacemaking may elevate $MVO_2$ and initiate anaerobic metabolism in certain patients; this may explain the occasional onset of heart failure with pacemaking. Induced tachycardia at modest rates produced a decrease in $MVO_2$ and increase XL in both groups instead of the increase in $MVO_2$ predicted by the heart rate-blood pressure index of Katz.

These studies indicate that a patient's "optimal" rate is a compromise between rate effects on CO and $MVO_2$. Pacemaking at "normal" rates may be damaging to certain patients; modest tachycardia was harmful to all patients studied. *(Supported by USPHS Training Grant 5-T01-HE-05686.)*

| *Group* | *Rate* | *CO l./min.* | *CBF ml./min.* | *$MVO_2$ 100g.* | *XL mM* |
|---|---|---|---|---|---|
| 1 | 32 | 3.24 | 83 | 11.8 | 0.40 |
| | 77 | 4.30 | 196 | 21.4 | 0.14 |
| 2 | 52 | 2.95 | 122 | 14.4 | 0.03 |
| | 85 | 3.02 | 208 | 20.9 | 0.20 |

| *Group* | *Rate* | *CO l./min.* | *CBF ml./min.* | *$MVO_2$ 100g.* | *XL mM* |
|---|---|---|---|---|---|
| 1 | 108 | 4.80 | 162 | 16.2 | 0.73 |
| 2 | 140 | 2.62 | 183 | 17.6 | 0.48 |

# *Alterations in Peripheral Pressure Pulse Contour During Acute Aortic Insufficiency in Man*

ROBERT I. HAMBY, STEPHEN J. GULOTTA, AND M. A. Z. HASSEN

The Long Island Jewish Hospital
Queens Hospital Center Affiliation
Jamaica, N. Y.

Previous studies of the hemodynamic effect of acute aortic insufficiency have been limited to the experimental animal. The present study will describe our observations of the effect of acute aortic insufficiency in man, transiently produced during diagnostic cardiac catheterization. As part of the diagnostic study a retrograde catheter was passed via the femoral artery by the Seldinger technique. It was noted that the preformed "J"-shaped retrograde catheter was held up momentarily in the region of the aortic valve, just before entrance into the left ventricle. During passage of the retrograde catheter the brachial artery pressure was constantly monitored. The results to be presented clearly demonstrate that aortic regurgitation was produced by the "J"-shaped, looped catheter when it was placed in the region of the aortic valve and permitted hemodynamic studies to be performed.

Twenty-eight consecutive patients who required retrograde catheterization were studied. In eight there was no evidence of aortic regurgitation, even though the catheter was in the area of the aortic valve. In the remaining 20, aortic regurgitation was produced and a diastolic murmur became audible over the base of the heart; this was not present before or after catheterization. In two of these patients the procedure was tolerated poorly; consequently the catheter was then advanced quickly into the left ventricle. The remaining diagnostic studies were completed uneventfully.

Associated with the diastolic murmur there were characteristic alterations in the pressure pulse of the brachial artery. There was a sudden drop in the diastolic and a slight drop in the systolic pressure, with a resultant increase in the pulse pressure. The change in heart rate was very slight. The systolic ascent and the maximum rate of change (dP/dT) of the brachial pressure pulse increased suddenly. The dicrotic wave, which was well defined during the control period, descended to a lower level, became less prominent, and in several patients could not be defined. The systolic and diastolic descent of the pressure pulse was more rapid, resulting in a lower diastolic pressure. There is evidence that the isometric contraction time was shortened and that the ejection time was prolonged during aortic insufficiency. All the alterations described quickly reverted to normal in one or two beats when the catheter was withdrawn. *(Supported by the Rosenberg Toner Heart Fund.)*

## *The Biphasic Renal Response and Associated Hemodynamic Changes in Patients Receiving Chlorpromazine Intravenously*

E. Lawrence Hanson, Ernest S. Breed, and Roy H. Clauss

Department of Surgery
New York University School of Medicine
New York, N. Y.

The adrenolytic effect of chlorpromazine has been useful in reversing generalized vasoconstriction in hypovolemic patients.

A biphasic renal response related to changes in arterial pressure and attenuation of renal vasoconstriction have been shown in 12 patients receiving chlorpromazine intravenously in doses of 2.5 to 50 mg. Six patients were normotensive (Group I), three were hypotensive (Group II), and three were in congestive heart failure (Group III). Each patient served as his own control. Changes in arterial pressure, venous pressure, urine flow, creatinine clearance, and sodium excretion were measured. In all patients the immediate drop of 10 to 40 mm. Hg in 1 to 5 minutes in arterial pressure was accompanied by a decrease of 0.05 to 0.37 cc./min. in urinary flow. The arterial pressure returned to control levels within 1 hour but urinary flow increased from 0.03 to 1.45 cc./min. within 15 to 20 min.; this lasted from 1 to 2 hours. Data will be presented showing the increase in urinary flow to be unrelated to glomerular filtration rate and urine sodium excretion to be decreased in Groups I and III by a factor of 30 to 70% and increased in Group II by a factor of 5 to 90%.

It is concluded that Phase I of renal response to chlorpromazine is related to a drop in arterial pressure but that a favorable balance between the pressure and renal vascular resistance (pressure-resistance ratio) is established during Phase II, increasing renal blood flow.

Chlorpromazine is a valuable adjunct to fluid replacement in hypovolemic patients. *(Supported by NIH Postdoctoral Fellowship 1-F2-HE-33393-01.)*

## *A Study of Factors Determining the Development and Persistence of Atrioventricular Conduction Defects following Ligation of the Anterior Septal Artery*

Jerald Jackrel, Jay A. Miller, Frederic G. Schechter
Stanley Minkowitz, and Jackson H. Stuckey

Departments of Surgery and Pathology
State University of New York Downstate Medical Center
Brooklyn, N. Y.

Previously this laboratory studied atrioventricular conduction in 100 dogs following ligation of the anterior septal artery. It was found that 75% of those dogs surviving the first day after ligation developed arrhythmia and that there was a return to normal sinus rhythm in 67% by the fourth day after ligation. This study was designed to investigate the factors that determine whether an atrioventricular conduction defect will develop and persist after ligation of the anterior septal artery. The artery was ligated in 50 healthy dogs in which normal sinus rhythm was present postoperatively. Electrocardiograms were monitored daily. After sacrifice at 1, 2, 3, and 4 days after ligation, serial sections taken from the atrioventricular node, bundle of His, right and left bundle branches, and adjacent myocardium were prepared by the standard staining techniques and by frozen sections stained for potassium by a modification of the cobaltinitrite method of Gersh. Of the dogs subjected to the ligation 87% developed arrhythmia; 8% had partial necrosis of the conduction tissue but with a normal potassium milieu, and did not develop arrhythmia; and 5% of ligated dogs developed no infarction and had no arrhythmia. Of the 87% of dogs with arrhythmia, 13% had no necrosis of the conducting tissue itself; 61 had partial necrosis; 13% had an area of total cross-sectional necrosis. Return to normal sinus mechanism in these groups was observed in 40%, 30%, and 0% respectively. Since 87% of ligated dogs were sacrificed before the fourth day postligation when a significant percentage of recovery occurs, total per cent recovery of normal sinus rhythm of 24% was less than the 67% observed previously in this laboratory. The dogs that returned to normal sinus rhythm had a normal potassium milieu at sacrifice. Partial necrosis of the conducting tissue was not sufficient for the development of arrhythmia if the potassium milieu of the remaining viable fibers was normal. When continuity was present in as little as 6.5% of His fibers, a normal sinus mechanism was maintained in a normal potassium milieu. Arrhythmias were observed only if the conducting tissue was in a milieu of increased potassium or if there was total cross-sectional necrosis of an area of the conducting tissue independent of the potassium milieu. There was no correlation between the extent of edema and inflammatory reaction and the presence of conduction disturbances. *(Supported in part by USPHS and AHA.)*

## *Myocardial Contractility After Elective Ventricular Fibrillation*

Alfred S. Kissack, Alvin J. Slovin, Vincent J. Fisher,
Frederick Kavaler, and Jackson H. Stuckey

Departments of Surgery and Physiology
State University of New York Downstate Medical Center
Brooklyn, N. Y.

Electrically induced ventricular fibrillation is widely used to obtain reversible cardiac arrest during cardiac surgery and has been termed both innocuous and "not without risk" on the basis of data obtained by various investigators from left ventricular function curves. In order to delineate further the effect of ventricular fibrillation on the heart, the effect of one hour of ventricular fibrillation on left ventricular contractility was studied in the isovolumic preparations in dogs. Myocardial contractility curves before and after fibrillation were obtained by plotting known left ventricular balloon volumes against: 1) the left ventricular pressure (LVP), 2) the LVP with paired pulse stimulation of the left ventricle, 3) the maximal rate of left ventricular pressure rise (dP/dT), and 4) the dP/dT with paired pulse stimulation of the left ventricle.

One hour of ventricular fibrillation did not adversely affect the myocardial contractility of the left ventricle as measured by LVP and by dP/dT curves, with or without paired pulse stimulation. In some animals myocardial contractility of the left ventricle was improved after fibrillation as measured by LVP and dP/dT curves without paired pulse stimulation. *(Supported in part by USPHS and AHA.)*

## *Studies of the Effects of Lidocaine on the Electrical and Mechanical Activity of the Heart*

NORMAN A. LIEBERMAN, RAMON S. HARRIS, ROBERT L. KATZ, HERBERT M. LIPSCHUTZ, MARTIN DOLGIN, AND VINCENT J. FISHER

Veterans Administration Hospital
New York, N. Y.

Lidocaine was found to depress the force of contraction of the isovolumic left ventricle of dogs on complete cardiopulmonary bypass. The degree of inotropic depression was usually dose-related and little depression was found with doses in the therapeutic range (0.5 to 2.0 mg./kg.). Lidocaine also had a negative inotropic action when the heart was paced by paired electircal stimuli, a means of inducing a maximal contractile response from heart muscle.

The drug was found to slow the atrial and ventricular rates of dogs with complete atrioventricular (AV) block. The degree of slowing was dose-related and the effect upon atrial pacemakers was less marked than upon ventricular pacemakers. Using bipolar electrodes it was found that lidocaine in a dose of 5 to 10 mg./kg. slowed conduction from the sinoatrial (SA) node to the bundle of His but had little effect on intra-atrial and intraventricular conduction. Lidocaine also opposed the slowing of the SA node and the delay in AV conduction caused by vagal stimulation.

Lidocaine was given intravenously to 27 patients with atrial and ventricular arrhythmias. The drug was found to be most effective against ectopic ventricular rhythms, especially those related to digitalis excess, and terminated the arrhythmia in 9 of 11 patients. Three of 4 AV nodal arrhythmias were terminated by lidocaine. Only 1 of 8 atrial arrhythmias was controlled by the drug. In the dose employed (0.5 to 4.0 mg./kg. given rapidly intravenously), only 1 patient experienced hypotension; this was transient. Mild disturbances of the central nervous system were often observed with doses of 1.5 mg./kg. Convulsions occurred in 3 patients receiving 3 to 3.5 mg./kg. All neurological disturbances were transient and did not require treatment. (*Supported by Veterans Administration Medical Research funds*).

## *Renal Hemodynamics During Osmotic Diuresis in Man*

JEROME LOWENSTEIN, ELLIOT R. BERANBAUM, DAVID S. BALDWIN, AND HERBERT CHASIS

Department of Medicine
New York University School of Medicine
New York, N. Y.

Reduction in GFR and extraction of PAH, which occurs during osmotic diuresis in the dog, has been attributed to redistribution of renal blood flow with increased flow to the medulla. In the present study in man, mannitol infusion (10% mannitol 20 ml./min.) in 15 hydropenic subjects resulted in a 25.0% fall in GFR ($C_{IN}$), and little change in renal blood flow ($\Delta$ RBF = —4.4%) or extraction of PAH ($E_{PAH}$, control 0.842, mannitol 0.839). Wedged renal vein pressure increased from 19.6 mm.Hg (range 15.0 to 25.7 mm.Hg) during control periods to 39.9 mm.Hg (range 38.0 to 41.5 mm.Hg) during osmotic diuresis in 4 studies. Failure to observe a significant change in renal blood flow or $E_{PAH}$ makes it unlikely that GFR falls as a result of redistribution of blood flow. Proximal tubular fluid reabsorption is decreased during osmotic diuresis and might be expected to result in increased tubular hydrostatic pressure, thereby reducing net filtration pressure. Gottschalk found that wedged renal vein pressures closely approximate increasing proximal tubular pressures in the rat during diuresis. If this relation obtains in man, the present finding of increased wedged renal vein pressure supports the thesis that reduction in GFR during osmotic diuresis is caused by a decrease in net filtration pressure resulting from increased proximal tubular hydrostatic pressure. *(Supported by USPHS Grant HE 03272-10 and by the New York Heart Association.)*

# *Effect of Diameter on Contractile Behavior of the Isolated Cat Papillary Muscle Preparation*

ANTHONY MARLON, VINCENT J. FISHER, AND FREDERIC KAVALER

Department of Physiology
State University of New York Downstate Medical Center
Brooklyn, N. Y.

The viability of isolated tissue preparations of cardiac muscle used in studies of contraction has been in considerable doubt on the basis of studies of oxygen uptake in these tissues, which suggested limitation of diffusion. We have approached this problem by measuring isometric contractile force in cat papillary muscles of different thicknesses. Developed isometric tension was recorded at optimal muscle length, as determined from the length-tension relation. Records were obtained in normal Tyrode solution, in a calcium-rich (10.8 mM) sodium-poor (99.7 mM) Tyrode medium, and during optimal mechanical potentiation from paired electrical stimulation in normal Tyrode. While developed tension in the control state varied considerably from one preparation to another, it was found to be constant in the calcium-rich, sodium-poor medium for eight muscles having diameters less than 0.4 mm. at optimal length ($5.75 \pm 0.7$ gm./mm.$^2$). Recorded developed tensions in the calcium-rich, sodium-poor medium from eight additional muscles with diameters above this value were considerably less ($3.82 \pm 1.3$ gm./mm.$^2$). These results indicate that contractile behavior of this preparation cannot be adequately quantitated for muscles that exceed a rather small critical diameter. The constancy of contractile tension in the thin muscles, as potentiated in the calcium-rich, sodium-poor medium, adds further support to the view that a contractile maximum is elicited in this medium. Paired pulse stimulation in normal Tyrode potentiates developed tension to a degree closely approximating (85%) the contractile maximum. *(Supported by U.S. Public Health Research Grant HE-05142-07).*

## *The Lack of Correlation Between Airway Resistance and Uneven Ventilation of the Lung in Bronchial Asthma*

E. R. McFADDEN, JR. AND HAROLD A. LYONS

Department of Medicine, Pulmonary Disease Division
State University of New York Downstate Medical Center
Brooklyn, N. Y.

Reversible elevations in Airway Resistance (Ra) have been recognized as one of the basic abnormalities in bronchial asthma. While many investigators have demonstrated that Ra is greatly elevated during accute attacks of bronchospasm, and that there is marked nonuniformity of ventilation present as well, no studies have been reported that relate these two variables. The present investigation was performed to study what effect, if any, decreasing Ra, measured by body plethysmography, would have on the distribution of ventilation measured by nitrogen washout technique.

Six patients under 35 years of age, with histories of episodic attacks of wheezing, and good family and personal histories of allergy, were studied during acute untreated attacks of bronchospasm. They were then restudied at various intervals after treatment. The average Ra was 6.56 cm. $H_20$/1./sec. with a conductance/thoracic gas volume ratio (GA/TGV) of 0.04/1./sec./cm. $H_20$/l. After bronchodilators Ra and GA/TGV fell to 2.1 cm $H_2$/l./sec. and 0.18 l./sec./cm. $H_2o$/l. respectively. The $N_2$ washouts, in contrast, changed very little before and after treatment. Five of six patients maintained a three compartment system with the mean ventilation of the slow compartment—total ventilation ratio (VS/VT) falling from 7.6 to 4.1. The ventilatory distribution returned to normal in only one subject.

The results of this study suggest that in bronchial asthma bronchodilator therapy affects the larger airways, but may not significantly influence the areas responsible for the uneven ventilation. *(Supported in part by the USPHS Grant 5TO1 HE 5485-05.)*

## *Effects of Changes in Arterial Potassium on Myocardial K Balance*

MICHEL G. NASSER AND ROBERT B. CASE

Laboratory of Experimental Cardiology, Department of Medicine
St. Luke's Hospital Center
New York, N. Y.

The interpretation of changes in myocardial K balance following an intervention must frequently be made in the presence of changing arterial levels of potassium. This investigation was designed to study the effects of changing arterial K concentration on myocardial K balance. A catheter was placed in the coronary sinus of closed chest anesthetized dogs under controlled respiration. Automated sampling of arterial and coronary sinus blood was achieved by pumping simultaneously from equal dead space catheters, at identical flow rates, at a rate of one sample (4 ml.) per minute. Equilibrated blood was returned to the dog at the same rate as its removal. Aortic pressure, heart rate and arterial *p*H were steady throughout. A KCl infusion of 0.76 mEq./min. resulted in average maximal coronary A-V differences of 0.63 mEq./l. (control 0.03). The amount of A-V difference appears to be related to the rate of arterial K rise. A fall in arterial K following discontinuation of the infusion was associated with coronary venous K exceeding arterial K by an average of 0.40 mEq./l. These data show that myocardial K balance and presumably myocardial K are affected by arterial concentration changes. This must be considered in the evaluation of factors that may affect myocardial K. *(Supported by USPHS Grant 2621.)*

# *Correlation of Electrocardiogram Changes with Alterations of the Transmembrane Action Potentials of Single Cardiac Cells in the* In Situ *Heart Under Various Experimental Conditions*

YOSHIAKI OMURA, DAVID LEHR, AND WARREN GOLDMAN

Department of Pharmacology
New York Medical College
Department of Electrical Engineering
Manhattan College
New York, N. Y.

With the introduction of the "flexibly-mounted glass microelectrode with tungsten wire" by Woodbury and Brady, recordings of the transmembrane action potentials of single cardiac cells from the *in situ* heart were attempted by many investigators. Such measurements in vigorously beating hearts were usually limited to less than 10 minutes for a particular microelectrode because of the great fragility of the tip. Moreover, the tungsten wire had the additional disadvantage of being polarizable. To overcome these two drawbacks, we developed a *flexibly mounted nonpolarizing ultraflexible glass microelectrode,* which was connected to the exposed Ag-AgCl-coated end of a Teflon-coated silver wire. With this improved microelectrode system, which combined utmost flexibility with a minimum of polarization, continuous recordings of the transmembrane action potentials of single cardiac cells of vigorously beating hearts could be made for more than one hour in dogs and rabbits and for several hours in rats, turtles and frogs.

Measurements of the transmembrane action potential (TAP) of single cardiac cells were carried out simultaneously with recordings of the ECG in the *in situ* heart and with the arterial blood pressure.

It was found that the rising phase of the TAP of ventricular cardiac cells corresponded to a specific part of the QRS complex and that the end of the TAP corresponded to specific phases of the end of the T-wave or U-wave. The particular positions varied with the location of the cell within the heart. Within one minute after i.v. injection of heparin (200 to 1000 units/kg. body weight) various degrees of shortening of the QT interval of the ECG were observed frequently. This corresponded with shortening of the duration of the TAP of single cardiac cells. The phenomenon usually lasted less than 10 minutes in both rabbits and rats. In rats, these changes were particularly pronounced and were often accompanied by the formation of U-waves. There was a slight decrease in blood pressure but no change in heart rate. With larger doses of heparin (more than 800 units/kg. body weight), transitional WPW Syndrome was observed in some instances.

The intravenous injection of Isoproterenol (0.1$\mu$gm.-100 $\mu$gm./kgm. body weight) into intact rabbits and rats caused a fall in blood pressure and an increase in heart rate. In open-chest animals, the increase in heart rate did not occur. In fact, raising the dose to more than 200-500 $\mu$gm./kgm. usually resulted in a slowing of the heart rate.

Partial crushing of up to 60 to 80% of the anterior wall of right ventricle by a curved clamp usually did not produce any noticeable changes in TAP of the remaining cells of the right or left ventricle and in standard limb lead ECG. When more than 80% of the entire right ventricle was thoroughly crushed without rupturing it, frequently the time duration of TAP of the remaining right ventricular cells as well as of the left ventricular cells was markedly shortened with a noticeable change in ECG. (*Supported by USPHS Grant HE-00890-16.*)

## *Potassium Shifts After Operation for Acquired Heart Disease*

Gabriel Rizzi, Richard Pierson, Robert Case, and Colin McCord

Department of Surgery
St. Luke's Hospital
New York, N. Y.

Many patients with acquired heart disease come to operation with total body potassium ($K_E$) seriously depleted. Determinations of serum $K^+$ concentration may or may not reveal this depletion. Serious $K^+$-responsive arrhythmias have been reported in such patients.

This study was undertaken to determine: *a*) the degree of $K^+$ depletion preoperatively in a group of patients with acquired heart disease *b*) the amount of $K^+$ loss during bypass and in the postoperative period *c*) the rate of $K^+$ restitution postoperatively, and *d*) the effect of a regimen with relatively large amounts of $K^+$ supplementation in the postoperative period.

The $^{42}K$ isotope dilution technique was used to measure the preoperative and postoperative $K_E$ in 11 patients. Operative serum $K^+$ determinations and standard postoperative balance studies of $Na^+$ and $K^+$ were undertaken in 16 patients.

Preoperatively the mean $K_E$ of 11 patients was 27.9±6.2 mEq./kg. (66% normal). There was no significant change in the $K_E$ in the early postoperative period despite large amounts of $K^+$ supplementation. Studies are under way to determine the rate of restitution of $K_E$.

Serum $K^+$ always fell during bypass, usually by 0.8-1.0 mEq./l. Balance studies of $Na^+$ and $K^+$ in 16 patients revealed uniform retention of $Na^+$ and net $K^+$ loss through the 4th day despite a mean $K^+$ supplementation of 55± 18 mEq./day for the first 4 postoperative days. The mean cumulative $Na^+$ retention was 310± 155 mEq. and the mean cumulative $K^+$ loss was 108± 80 mEq. during this period.

With the $K^+$ replacement regimen, serum $K^+$ was either relatively unchanged, or increased slightly, despite the net $K^+$ loss. Patients receiving no $K^+$ supplementation exhibited a consistent slight fall in serum $K^+$ and a similar net $K^+$ loss.

Using this regimen of $K^+$ therapy only one serious ventricular arrhythmia occurred in a series of 56 patients with acquired valvular disease. The rate of occurrence of supraventricular arrhythmias appeared unaffected. *(Supported by NIH General Research Support Grant FR 05501-04.)*

## *Nonsurgical Intra-Arterial Cardiac Assistance*

W. Schilt, P. S. Freed, G. Khalil, and A. Kantrowitz

Departments of Surgery
Maimonides Medical Center
State University of New York Downstate Medical Center
Brooklyn, N. Y.

Experimental results with a method of intra-aortic volume displacement are presented. Based on the concept of diastolic balloon pumping described by Moulopoulos *et al.* and Clauss *et al.*, this method promises advantages in the treatment of cardiogenic shock. It can be applied easily and rapidly; blood flows at low velocities and is circulated only intracorporeally; and the displaced blood volume is not limited by the size and condition of the femoral artery.

The device, which is inserted into the aorta through the femoral artery, consists of a tapered, cylindrical, thin-walled polyurethane chamber with a siliconized polyethylene catheter and a flexible metal mesh tube inside the chamber; this permits rapid filling and emptying with helium.

During cardiac diastole, filling of the polyurethane chamber with helium displaces an equal volume of blood, resulting in an increase in systemic blood pressure and thus in the blood flow to the coronary arteries.

During systole the stroke volume of the left ventricle displaces the helium in the chamber against a low resistance, with resultant decrease in end-diastolic pressure and in the work of the failing left ventricle.

An electronic controller provides two independent time delays for the onset and termination of the pump cycle, triggered by either the R-wave from the ECG or the ascending slope of the left ventricular pressure curve.

Tests on 30 dogs with the functioning unit showed an average decrease of 20% in tension-time index in normal animals, and an increase of 11% in carotid pressure and 10% in femoral arterial pressure in animals with coronary shock induced by litigation of the descending coronary artery. Mechanical assistance was given for periods varying from 10 minutes to 2 hours. *(This work was supported by USPHS Grant HE-06510.)*

## *Incorporation of Labeled Amino Acid into Protein by Cultured Human Lymphocytes in Health and Disease*

GABRIEL H. SCHWARTZ, ROBERT R. RIGGIO, KURT H. STENZEL, AND ALBERT L. RUBIN

Rogosin Laboratories, Department of Medicine
The New York Hospital-Cornell Medical Center
New York, N. Y.

A method has been developed for studying lymphocyte function in various disease states, including uremia, neoplasia, macroglobulinemia, autoimmune diseases, hyperglobulinemic conditions, transplantation, and others. The technique reproducibly measures incorporation of radioactive amino acid into TCA precipitable counts by human peripheral lymphocytes *in vitro*. The technique in outline is as follows. Erythrocytes are sedimented from heparinized blood with gelatin, neutrophils, adsorbed onto nylon, lymphocytes washed and counted. Lymphocytes are cultured overnight in duplicate at 37° C. in a $CO_2$ incubator in leucine-free media to which $C^{14}$ leucine is added. After lysing the erythrocytes, cold leucine and protein carrier are added, protein is precipitated with TCA and washed with TCA, acetone, and then counted. Cells are counted from simultaneously grown cultures. When grown in the presence of puromycin, the cells incorporate less than 10% of control cells. Phytohemagglutinin stimulates protein production twenty- to fortyfold.

Uremic lymphocytes have decreased ability to incorporate $C^{14}$ leucine, whereas normal lymphocytes are not inhibited by urea or creatinine in concentrations of up to 300 mg. % and 20 mg. % respectively. There is decreased uptake by idiopathic macroglobulinemic cells and increased uptake by cells from a patient with dermatomyositis. Drugs with known effects on the immune response *in vivo* are being investigated by this method. We are also attempting to identify humoral factors affecting lymphocytes in disease and health. This system offers a novel approach to the study of human disease mechanisms at a cellular as well as a subcellular level. *(Supported by USPHS Grant 68736 and by the New York Heart Association.)*

## *The Single Injection Technique for Frequent Evaluation of Blood Volume During Experiments not Associated with Blood Loss*

JOSEPH J. STETZ, RICHARD M. WOLFMAN, GREGORY N. JELINEK, HAROLD I. ANTELL, CHARLES C. FRIES, AND JACKSON H. STUCKEY

Department of Surgery
State University of New York Downstate Medical Center
Brooklyn, N. Y.

The purpose of this study was to determine the validity of blood volume determinations made at frequent intervals during a 4-hour period following a single injection of radioactive iodinated ($I^{131}$) human serum albumin (RIHSA). The usual method requires approximately a 1-hour time lapse between determinations and thereby limits the number of determinations that may be made in a given interval of time. Serial blood volume determinations were made with a Picker Hemolitre on 25 dogs under light thiopental sodium anesthesia over a period of 4 hours. In Part I of the study, the apparent blood volume of 10 dogs was plotted against time (with the apparent increase in circulating volume reflecting the disappearance of the RIHSA from the vasculature). The graph that resulted showed that the date of disappearance of the RIHSA could be correlated with the "true" blood volume. In order to check the blood volume in the usual manner, a second injection of RIHSA was given at the end of the 4-hour period; the volume determined was essentially the same as that found at the beginning of the period. In Part II of the study, the graph obtained in Part I was used to calculate the blood volumes at frequent intervals on fifteen additional animals following a single injection of RIHSA. Five of these were identical to those in Part I, five received a dextrose in water infusion, and five received a low molecular weight dextran infusion. At the end of a 4-hour period the calculated blood volumes were compared to a value obtained by the usual method (using a second RIHSA injection) and the difference averaged less than 4%. The data support the conclusion that a single injection of RIHSA allows accurate blood volume determinations to be made at frequent intervals during a 4-hour period in studies not associated with blood loss. *(Supported in part by USPHS and AHA.)*

## *Effect of Erythrocyte Lipoprotein on the Coagulation Mechanism*

LEONARD J. STUTMAN AND ERIC V. EISNER

Coagulation Laboratory, Department of Medicine
St. Vincent's Hospital and Medical Center
New York, N. Y.

Erythrocyte membrane lipoprotein was prepared from both dog and human red cells after washing, freezing, thawing, and differential ultracentrifugation at 53,000 g in a low ionic strength, *p*H 7.4, citrate-phosphate buffer. Eighteen separate experiments have been performed in dogs anaesthetized with pentothal. Five dogs had sham procedures and were used as controls. Both femoral veins were catheterized; blood was then drawn at 0, 5, 15, 30, 45 minutes and 24 hours. At these times, clotting time, platelet count, one stage prothrombin time, partial thromboplastin time, and chemical fibrinogen level were measured. The other animals, after control samples were obtained, were individually given rapid or slow infusions of whole blood, rapid or slow infusions of RBC lipoprotein into the femoral vein. The total lipid extracted from 150 ml. of whole blood was given rapidly into the femoral vein after first being emulsified with albumin. In another experiment, 180 ml. of whole blood was rapidly infused into the splenic vein of two dogs.

Rapid infusion of whole blood into the peripheral circulation caused death within 3 minutes. Slow infusions did not cause death, but there was marked drop in the platelet count. RBC lipoprotein, in addition to a marked drop in the platelet count, caused shortening of the clotting time. The lipid extract of whole blood and the splenic vein infusions of whole blood did not cause an immediate drop in the platelet count or shorten the clotting time.

Since the platelet counts fell every time the clotting time shortened, it is pertinent to speculate that the erythrocyte lipoprotein may play an important role in the pathogenesis of thrombosis in Sickle Cell Crisis, transfusion reactions, and defibrination syndromes. *(Supported by the John A. Polachek Foundation and Fannie Ripple Foundation.)*

## *Hemodynamic Studies with a Newly Designed Auxiliary Ventricle in Dogs*

S. TJØNNELAND, T. OKURA, AND A. KANTROWITZ

Departments of Surgery
Maimonides Medical Center
State University of New York Downstate Medical Center
Brooklyn, N. Y.

A new form of mechanical auxiliary ventricle has been developed for rapid implantation in the ascending aorta by means of a single incision. It is avalvular and spherical, and contains a small baffle or septum that partly separates the inner pumping chamber so that all the blood can flow through easily and freely with a minimal risk of stagnation. The flexible inner chamber is made of silicone rubber and the outer housing of fiber glass covered with silicone rubber.

The unit is implanted in the ascending aorta during short-term inflow and outflow occlusion of the heart. The time required for the actual insertion and temporary ligation of the two limbs is 2 minutes. After this the circulation is reestablished and the anastomosis completed.

The device is driven by compressed air from an outside tank via a polyethylene air tube. The flow is interrupted by a solenoid valve triggered by either the R-wave from the ECG or the ascending slope of the left ventricular pressure curve.

Experiments on 14 dogs showed that the most favorable hemodynamic effects could be obtained when the auxiliary ventricle was implanted in the ascending aorta as close to the heart as possible. The reduction in tension-time index was found to reach 50% in some cases.

The advantages of this new unit are: 1) it can be implanted in the ascending aorta by means of a single incision, and 2) it can be inserted easily and rapidly (2 minutes). Like the U-shaped auxiliary ventricle, it has no valves, so that blood from the left ventricle can pass through the unit freely—thus the clotting problem is no greater than in any other artificial arterial graft; it can be driven either continuously or intermittently; and it is premanently implanted. *(This work was supported by USPHS Grant HE-06510.)*

# GENERAL GRANT'S HEADACHE

In the present stage of our enlightenment we possess grossly inadequate understanding of chronic headache. Studies made in the present century have shown that one type of pain can be produced by traction on the meninges. This is a great advance although, according to an unconfirmed rumor, the fact was known to Galen. Perhaps some indomitable reader will test this by reading over the 20 volumes of the Kühn edition.

There is much evidence that headache tends to afflict capable persons, especially overachievers. It is also thought that some headaches are related to critical situations.

The following excerpt describes what may well have been the greatest headache of the 19th century. The passage has been taken from the *Personal Memoirs of U.S. Grant*, edited by E. B. Long and issued in 1952 by the World Publishing Company of Cleveland and New York.*

> On the 8th [of April, 1865] I had followed the Army of the Potomac in rear of Lee. I was suffering very severely with a sick headache, and stopped at a farmhouse on the road some distance in rear of the main body of the army. I spent the night in bathing my feet in hot water and mustard, and putting mustard plasters on my wrists and the back part of my neck, hoping to be cured by morning. During the night I received Lee's answer to my letter of the 8th, inviting an interview between the lines on the following morning. But it was for a different purpose from that of surrendering his army, and I answered him as follows:

*Headquarters Armies of the U. S.,*
April 9, 1865

General R. E. Lee, *Commanding C. S. A.*

> Your note of yesterday is received. As I have no authority to treat on the subject of peace, the meeting proposed for ten A.M. to-day could lead to no good. I will state, however, General, that

*Thanks are due the publisher for permission to use the material quoted.

I am equally anxious for peace with yourself, and the whole North entertains the same feeling. The terms upon which peace can be had are well understood. By the South laying down their arms they will hasten that most desirable event, save thousands of human lives, and hundreds of millions of property not yet destroyed. Sincerely hoping that all our difficulties may be settled without the loss of another life, I subscribe myself, etc.

U. S. GRANT,
*Lieutenant-General*

I proceeded at an early hour in the morning, still suffering with the headache, to get to the head of the column. I was not more than two or three miles from Appomattox Court House at the time, but to go direct I would have to pass through Lee's army, or a portion of it. I had therefore to move south in order to get upon a road coming up from another direction.

When the white flag was put out by Lee, as already described, I was in this way moving towards Appomattox Court House, and consequently could not be communicated with immediately, and be informed of what Lee had done. Lee, therefore, sent a flag to the rear to advise Meade and one to the front to Sheridan, saying that he had sent a message to me for the purpose of having a meeting to consult about the surrender of his army, and asked for a suspension of hostilities until I could be communicated with. As they had heard nothing of this until the fighting had got to be severe and all going against Lee, both of these commanders hesitated very considerably about suspending hostilities at all. They were afraid it was not in good faith, and we had the Army of Northern Virginia where it could not escape except by some deception. They, however, finally consented to a suspension of hostilities for two hours to give an opportunity of communicating with me in that time, if possible. It was found that, from the route I had taken, they would probably not be able to communicate with me and get an answer back within the time fixed unless the messenger should pass through the rebel lines.

Lee, therefore, sent an escort with the officer bearing this message through his lines to me.

April 9, 1865

General:—I received your note of this morning on the picket-line whither I had come to meet you and ascertain definitely what terms were embraced in your proposal of yesterday with reference to the surrender of this army. I now request an interview in accordance with the offer contained in your letter of yesterday for that purpose.

R. E. Lee,
*General*

Lieutenant-General U. S. Grant,
*Commanding U. S. Armies.*

When the officer reached me I was still suffering with the sick headache; but the instant I saw the contents of the note I was cured. I wrote the following note in reply and hastened on:

General R. E. Lee,
*Commanding C. S. Armies.*

April 9, 1965

Your note of this date is but this moment (11:50 A.M.) received, in consequence of my having passed from the Richmond and Lynchburg road to the Farmville and Lynchburg road. I am at this writing about four miles west of Walker's Church and will push forward to the front for the purpose of meeting you. Notice sent to me on this road where you wish the interview to take place will meet me.

U. S. Grant,
*Lieutenant-General*

I was conducted at once to where Sheridan was located with his troops drawn up in line of battle facing the Confederate Army near by. They were very much excited, and expressed their view that this was all a ruse employed to enable the Confederates to get away. They said they believed that Johnston was marching up from North Carolina now, and Lee was moving to join him; and they would whip the rebels where they now were in five minutes if I would only let them go in. But I had no doubt about the good faith of Lee, and pretty soon was conducted to where he was. I found him at the house of a Mr. [Wilmer] McLean, at Appomattox Court House, with Colonel [Charles] Marshall, one of his staff officers, awaiting my arrival.

S.J.

# DANIEL DRAKE ON EATING

"Among the laboring classes, who follow nature more closely than the others, the three meals of the day do not differ so much in quantity, as among the more cultivated and artificial classes. I am persuaded that the former are right; and would go still further, and express the opinion that, of the three meals, breakfast, and not dinner, should be the principal. After long repose, in the cool of the morning, when the feelings of both body and mind are tranquil, the stomach can receive with impunity, and digest a large meal better, than in the heat of the day; or in the midst of the labors and corporeal and moral irritations which it may bring forth. A hearty breakfast seldom produces oppression and drowsiness, like a hearty dinner; on the contrary, the hour which follows it is generally one of pleasant and efficient excitement; while that which succeeds to a full dinner is characterized by dullness, taciturnity, sleep, and very often a considerable degree of feverishness, from all of which, I may repeat, those who make hearty breakfasts and slighter dinners, are exempt.

"The practice of rapid eating is universal among us, that is, prevails everywhere, though not adopted by every individual. Two objections lie against it: *first,* the food is imperfectly masticated; *second,* too much is taken; for a little time is necessary after food is received into the stomach, to enable it to remove the feeling of hunger.

"As a general fact, the people of the Valley eat too much. Such an excess is the natural effect of living in a country whose greatest natural characteristic is productiveness of sustenance; and until the abundance of the latter, in proportion to the population, shall diminish, the practice will continue."

—Daniel Wrake. *A Systematic Treatise . . . on the Principal Diseases of the Interior Valley of North America. Cincinnati,* Smith, 1850, page 654.

## GRADUATE STUDENTS

"Later in my academic career I developed and offered several different courses at Harvard, mostly for more mature students and on the lines of my personal researches. This brought me into contact with graduate workers and gave me an opportunity to oversee their investigations and to work with them, an activity which I had long craved. Our studies were, for the most part, on the nervous systems and the nervous reactions of the lower animals, a field of special interest to me. At about the turn of the century I gave up my initial lines of teaching and at the request of the department assumed the management of the large introductory course in zoology, a course intended chiefly for freshmen. I retained, however, my work with graduates, and thus I came to see in these two lines of teaching the beginning and the end so to speak of our efforts in academic zoology. The contrast was most striking. The beginner in the subject often exhibited unexpected enthusiasms, commonly misdirected and even grotesque but nevertheless real enthusiasms; these seemed to me to call for guidance rather than suppression, the latter a treatment so often given them by the "superior" teacher. The graduate student, though mature and often rich in experience, appeared to have lost what enthusiasm he may have had as a beginner and to be devoid of the spontaneous interest which might be expected in a growing scholar. I asked myself, is this the result of our method of teaching or do young men at this stage naturally arrive at a kind of sophistication which is detrimental to their real advancement? It seemed as though their original enthusiasms had been schooled out of them."

—From George Howard Parker, *The World Expands.* Cambridge, Mass., Harvard Univ. Press, 1946, p. 195. Reprinted by permission.

# INDEX

## Volume 43, 1967

### A

Abrahamsen, David, A study of Lee Harvey Oswald: Psychological capability of murder, 861

Academy Medal, Citation and presentation of the, to Donald D. Van Slyke, M. Heidelbeger, 322

Academy Plaque, Citation and presentation of the, to Howard Reid Craig, G. Baehr, 318

Accident prevention, Program activities of the division of (USPHS), A. F. Schaplowsky, 727

Action and program for the future, G. F. Crikelair, 749

Action of streptomycin on protein synthesis *in vitro,* S. Pestka, 126

Aggression and violence, Psychopathology of, G. Bychowski, 300

Aiding fabric and garment designers in reducing fire hazard, H. J. Wollner, 681

Altschuller, Gregory I. Memories of Anton Chekhov's family, 87

Altura, Burton M. and Hershey, S. G. Use of reticuloendothelial phagocytic function as index in shock therapy, 259

Ambulance service in New York City, Committee on Public Health, 336

Annan, Gertrude L. Our greatest material heritage: the library, 21

Anniversary Discourse of the Academy, Government and community health, J. V. Lindsay, 325

Antigens, immunocompetent cells and target cells, Interactions between, J. R. David, 949

Appelbaum, Emanuel, The problem of fever of unknown origin, 889

Application and development of flame-retardant finishes in textile mills, J. W. Weaver, 669

Arrhythmia, Intracardiac electrocardiography in, C. E. Kossmann, 1181

Arrhythmias, Experimental neurogenic, C. H. Hockman, H. P. Mauck, Jr., E. C. Hoff, 1097

Artz, Curtis P. and Yarbrough, Dabney, R., II, Present status of the treatment of burns, 627

Ash, Lee, The Michael M. Davis collection of social and economic aspects of medicine, 598

Atherosclerosis: The fact and the mysteries, W. Dock, 792

Autonomic control of cardiac rhythm, B. F. Hoffman, 1087

Avicenna on the location of houses, S. Jarcho, 250

Axons, Schwann cells, and diabetic neuropathy, S. Locke, 784

### B

Baehr, George, Citation and presentation of the Academy Plaque to Howard Reid Craig, 318

Bardo, John Barry, A history of the legal regulation of medical practice in New York State, 924

Becker, Harry, The Committee on Special Studies, 1946-1966, 70

Beta-adrenergic blockade and cardiac denervation, Electrophysiologic effects of, A. G. Wallace *et al.,* 1119

Birth defect, comprehensive approach to a child with, M. Winick, 819

Brereton, Robert M. Financial management and building operation of The New York Academy of Medicine, 79

Brief psychotherapy and the existential shift, J. J. Ehrenwald, 798

Brissette, R. S. The use of synthetic modacrylic fibers, 694

Brown, Howard J. See Career Scientists of the Health Research Council of New York, 378

Brown, Howard J. Municipal hospitals, 450

Bucy, Paul C. Training in neurological surgery, 186

*Bulletin of The New York Academy of Medicine:* 1847:1966, P. F. Cranefield, 33

Burns and flame-retardant fabrics, Conference on, 615-766
  Opening remarks, Paul V. Joliet, 615,
  Welcoming remarks, John L. Madden, 617

Burns, injuries from, Merchants' views on flame-retardant textiles and, P. J. Fynn, 735

Burns, Statistics and epidemiology of, A. O. Iskrant, 636

Burns, treatment of, Present status of the, C. P. Artz, D. R. Yarbrough, 627

Bychowski, Gustav, Psychopathology of aggression and violence, 300

C

Cancer of the head and neck, Development of a TNM system of staging for, J. Newall, 959

Carcinoma, ovarian, Factors affecting survival of patients with, A. B. Weingold, S. Sall, M. L. Stone, 829

Cardia, anatomy of the, Historical aspects of, with special reference to hiatus hernia, G. S. Schwarz, 112

Cardiac arrhythmias, Clinical experience with neurogenic, R. L. Katz, 1106

Cardiac denervation, Electrophysiologic effects of beta-adrenergic blockade of, A. G. Wallace *et al.,* 1119

Cardiac innervation: anatomic and pharmacologic relations, T. N. James, 1041

Cardiac rhythm, Autonomic control of, B. F. Hoffman, 1087

Cardiac tissues, specialized, Phylogenetic observations on, E. N. Moore, 1138

Cashman, John W. Prospects of federal programs, 472

Changing motor performance and personality in therapeutic settings, M. D. Zane, 232

Chekhov's family, Memories of, G. I. Altschuller, 87

Cherkasky, Martin, Voluntary hospitals, 456

Cliffton, Eugene E. Treatment of pulmonary embolism with fibrinolytic agents, 267

Clinical experience with neurogenic cardiac arrhythmias, R. L. Katz, 1106

Clinical features of granulomatous colitis, A. A. Lindner, 901

Clothing fire problem, Controlling the, E. L. Lehr, 711

Clothing fire problem, Legal aspects of the, A. G. Elkind, 740

Committee on Medical Education, The: 1946-1966, A. C. McGuinness, 49

Committee on Public Health, The, 1946 to the present, H. D. Kruse, L. J. Amster, 11

Committee on Public Health Reports
  Ambulance service in New York City, 336
  Health services in New York City, 843
  Medical and biological research on human beings, 525
  Municipal hospitals of New York City, 435
  Office of the Medical Examiner of the City of New York, 241

Committee on Special Studies, The, 1946-1966, H. Becker, 70

Community health, Government and, J. V. Lindsay, 325

Comprehensive approach to a child with a birth defect, M. Winick, 819

Conferences: ,
  Career Scientists of the Health Research Council of the City of New York, 378
  Abstracts of presentations by career scientists, 392
  Brown, Howard J. Health services: the impact of new legislation, 381
  Lindsay, John V. Closing address, 388

New York Heart Association conference on Mechanisms and Management of Arrhythmias, 1039-1223

New York Heart Association conference on Possibilities and Actualities in the Delivery of Medical Care, 449-524

Burns and Flame-Retardant Fabrics, 615-765

General discussion: W. G. Johnson, H. J. Wollner, L. Segal, A. F. Robertson, A. P. Iskrant, P. V. Joliet, J. R. Palmer, H. A. Freedman, G. L. Drake, Jr., R. B. LeBlanc, G. S. Buck, Jr., H. C. Hottel, P. Bugbee, J. L. Severance, J. Appel, P. J. Fynn, P. Dykstra, D. A. Dukelow, 752

Connecticut regional medical program, Planning and organization of the, R. E. Weinerman, 504

Controlling the clothing fire problem, E. L. Lehr, 711

Cotton industry, Developments in the, W. M. Segall, 675

Craig, Howard Reid: A contribution, J. L. Madden, 9

Craig, Howard Reid: An appreciation, R. L. Levy, 3

Cranefield, Paul F. The *Bulletin of The New York Academy of Medicine,* 1847-1966, 33

Crikelair, George F. Action and program for the future, 749

Current efforts in the municipal hospitals, R. E. Trussell, 211

Culp, Ormond S. Management of ureteropelvic obstruction, 355

D

Daniel Drake on Eating, S. Jarcho, 1227

David, John R. Interactions between immunocompetent cells and target cells or antigens, 949

Davidoff, Leo M. Some considerations in the therapy of pineal tumors, 537

Davis, Theodore M. Experience in transurethral resection (*The Fifth Ferdinand C. Valentine Lecture*), 152

Deprived neighborhood, Health needs in, J. G. Haughton, 219

Development of clothing for protection from hazardous thermal exposure, R. E. Seaman, 649

Developments in the cotton industry, W. M. Segall, 675

Dermal elastoses, The, J. G. Smith, Jr., 173

Diabetic neuropathy, Axons, Schwann cells, and, S. Locke, 784

Diabetic neuropathy, Pathology and pathogenesis of, C. L. Dolman, 773

Discussion of Dr. Gershman's paper on gender identity, L. R. Hott, 1028

Discussion of Dr. Gershman's paper on gender identity, N. Shainess, 1019

Dock, William, Atherosclerosis: The facts and the mysteries, 792

Dolman, C. L. The pathology and pathogenesis of diabetic neuropathy, 773

Drake, George L., Jr. Flame retardants and their applications to textiles, 656

E

Ehrenwald, Jan. Brief psychotherapy and the existential shift, 798

Electrolyte disturbances, Arrhythmias and B. Surawicz, 1160

Electrophysiologic effects of beta-adrenergic blockade and cardiac denervation, A. G. Wallace, S. F. Schaal, T. Sugimoto, M. Rozear, B. Alexander, 1119

Elkind, Arnold B. Legal aspects of the clothing fire problem, 740

Evolution of gender identity, H. Gershman, 1000

Existential shift, Brief psychotherapy and the, J. Ehrenwald, 798

Experience in transurethral resection, T. M. Davis, 152

Experimental neurgenic arrhythmias, C. H. Hockman, H. P. Mauck, Jr., E. C. Hoff, 1097

F

Factors affecting the survival of patients with ovarian carcinoma, A. B. Weingold,

S. Sall, M. L. Stone, 829
Federal flammable fabrics act, The H. D. Stringer, 703
Ferger, John F. Fiberglas: a true fire-safety fabric, 685
Fever of unknown origin, The problem of, E. Appelbaum, 889
Fiberglas: a true fire-safety fabric, J. F. Ferger, 685
Fibrillation action potential, The physiological significance of, J. Goodgold, A. Eberstein, 811
Financial management and building operation of The New York Academy of Medicine, R. M. Brereton, 79
Fire hazards, Aiding fabric and garment designers in reducing, H. J. Wollner, 681
Fire problem, clothing, Legal aspects of the, A. B. Elkind, 740
Fire protection agency, Role of the, L. Segal, 699
Fire-Safety Fabric, Fiberglas: a true, J. F. Ferger, 685
Fires, fatal, Survey of, E. R. Juillerat, 646
Flame-resistant textiles, T. D. Miles, 723
Flame retardants and their application to textiles, G. L. Drake, 656
Flame-retardant fabrics, Industrial experience in the use of, R. S. B. Holmes, 716
Flame-retardant finishes, Application and development of, in textile mills, J. W. Weaver, 669
Flame-retardant textiles and injuries from burns, Merchants' views on, P. J. Fynn, 735
Flammability of clothing fabric, U.S. Department of Commerce and the, A. F. Robertson, 706
Flammability, Pile fabrics and, H. A. Freedman, 663
Flammable fabrics act, The federal, H. D. Stringer, 703
Freedman, Harry A. Pile fabrics and their flammability, 663
Fynn, P. S. Merchants' views on flame-retardant textiles and injuries from burns, 735
General Grant's headache, S. Jarcho, 1224
Gershman, Harry, The evolution of gender identity, 1000
Goodgold, Joseph, and Eberstein, Arthur, The physiological significance of fibrillation action potentials, 811
Government and community health, J. V. Lindsay, 325
Graduate Students, S. Jarcho, 1228
Granulomatous colitis, Panel on, 899
Greeks, ancient, The longevity of the, S. Jarcho, 941

H

Hallucinogens, Implications of untoward reactions to, E. Robbins, L. Robbins, W. A. Frosch, M. Stern, 985
Harvey, Abner, Osler's textbook revisited, 1034
Haughton, James G. Health needs and programs in deprived neighborhoods, 219
Health needs and programs in deprived neighborhoods, J. G. Haughton, 219
Health services: the impact of new legislation, H. J. Brown, 381
Health services in New York City, Committee on Public Health, 843
Heidelberger, Michael, Citation and presentation of the Academy medal to Donald D. Van Slyke, 322
Hershey, S. G., see Altura, B. M., 259
Hiatus hernia, special reference to, see
Cardia, Anatomy of the, G. S. Schwarz, 112
Historical aspects of the anatomy of the cardia with special reference to hiatus hernia, G. S. Schwarz, 112
History of the legal regulation of medical practice in New York State, J. B. Bardo, 924
Hockman, Charles H., Mauck, H. Page, Jr., and Hoff, Ebbe C., Experimental neurogenic arrhythmias, 1097
Hoffman, Brian F. Autonomic control of cardiac rhythm, 1087
Hogness, John R. The northwest program, 495
Holmes, Robert S. B. Industrial experience in the use of flame-retardant fabrics, 716

Homicide by means of plague bacilli, S. J., 850

Hospital as a teaching center, The, G. H. Humphreys, II, 202

Hott, Louis R. Discussion of Dr. Gershman's paper on gender identity, 1028

House of medicine, The, H. D. Kruse, 562

How to select the proper treatment for the child with reflux, J. K. Lattimer, 99

Howard Reid Craig: An appreciation, R. L. Levy, 3

Howard Reid Craig: a contribution, J. L. Madden, 9

Humphreys, George H., II, The hospital as a teaching center, 211

I

Innervation, Cardiac: anatomic and pharmacologic relations, T. N. James, 1041

Intracardiac electrocardiography in arrhythmia, C. E. Kossmann, 1181

Immunocompetent cells and target cells or antigens, Interactions between, J. R. David, 949

Impact of Medicare on medical education, J. H. Knowles, 463

Implications of untoward reactions to hallucinogens, E. Robbins, L. Robbins, W. A. Frosch, M. Stern, 985

Increased elastic tissue in the dermis: the dermal elastoses, J. G. Smith, Jr., 173

Industrial experience in the use of flame-retardant fabrics, R. S. B. Holmes, 716

Interactions between immunocompetent cells and target cells or antigens, J. R. David, 949

Iskrant, Albert P., Statistics and epidemiology of burns, 636

J

James, George, Summation, 522

James, Thomas N., Cardiac innervation: anatomic and pharmacologic relations, 104

Janowitz, Henry D. Introductory remarks, 900

Jarcho, Saul, Avicenna on the location of houses, 250

Jarcho, Saul, General Grant's headache, 1224

Jarcho, Saul, Homicide by means of plague bacilli, 850

Jarcho, Saul, Longevity of the ancient Greeks, 941

Jarcho, Saul, Osler's textbook revisited, 1034

Jarcho, Saul, Polybius on medicine and history, 528

Jarcho, Saul, Psychotic son of Benjamin Rush, The, 609

Jarcho, Saul, Roman experience with heat stroke in 24 B.C., 767

Jarcho, Saul, Scurvy during Magellan's voyage, 356

Jarcho, Saul, Weavers and computers, 443

Joliet, Paul F. Opening remarks (Conference on Burns), 615

Juillerat, Ernest E., Jr., Survey of fatal clothing fires, 646

K

Katz, Ronald L., Clinical experience with neurogenic cardiac arrhythmias, 1106

Kessler, Richard E., The umbilical vein in diseases of the liver, 977

Knowles, John H., Impact of Medicare on medical education, 463

Kossmann, Charles E., Intracardiac electrocardiography in arrhythmia, 1181

Kruse, H. D., The house of medicine, 562

Kruse, H. D., and Amster, L. J. The Committee on Public Health: 1946 to the present, 11

L

Lee Harvey Oswald: Psychological capability of murder, D. Abrahamsen, 861

Legal aspects of the clothing fire problem, A. B. Elkind, 740

Legal regulation of medical practice in New

York State, History of, J. B. Bardo, 924
Lattimer, John K. How to select the proper treatment for the child with reflux, 99
Legislation, The impact of new, H. J. Brown, 381
Lehr, Eugene L., Controlling the clothing fire problem, 711
Levy, Robert L. Howard Reid Craig: an appreciation, 3
Library, the: Our greatest material heritage, G. L. Annan, 21
Lindner, Arthur A., Clinical features (Panel on Granulomatous colitis), 901
Lindsay, John V., Government and community health, 325
Lindsay, John V., See Career scientists of the Health Research Council of the City of New York, 378
Liver, diseases of the, Umbilical vein in, R. E. Kessler, 977
Liver perfusion, heterologous, Therapeutic and investigational potential of, J. C. Norman, W. G. Hadison, W. V. McDermott, Jr., 867
Localio, S. Arthur, Surgical treatment (Panel on Granulomatous colitis), 906
Locke, Simeon, Axons, Schwann cells, and diabetic neuropathy, 784
Longevity of the ancient Greeks, S. Jarcho, 941

M

Madden, John L. Address of the retiring president, 310
Madden, John L., Howard Reid Craig: A contribution, 9
Management of ureteropelvic obstruction, O. S. Culp, 355
Marshak, Richard H., Roentgen features (Panel on granulomatous colitis), 910
Marston, Robert Q. Regional medical programs: a review, 490
McCormack, James E. The New York City story, 515
McGovern, John H. Presentation of the fifth Ferdinand C. Valentine Medal and Award to Theodore M. Davis, 149
McGuinness, Aims C. The Committee on Medical Education: 1946-1966, 49
McKusick, Victor, Osler's textbook revisited, 1034
Medical education, Impact of Medicare on, J. H. Knowles, 463
Medical examiner, Office of the, of the City of New York, 241
Medicare, Impact of, on medical education, J. H. Knowles, 463
Medicine, The house of, H. D. Kruse, 562
Memories of Anton Chekhov's family, G. I. Altschuller, 87
Merchants' views on flame-retardant textiles and injuries from burns, P. J. Fynn, 735
Michael M. Davis Collection, The, of social and economic aspects of medicine, L. Ash, 598
Miles, Thomas D. Flame-resistant textiles, 723
Moore, E. Neil, Phylogenetic observations on specialized cardiac tissues, 1138
Motor performance, and personality, in therapeutic settings, M. D. Zanes, 232
Municipal hospitals, H. J. Brown, 45-
Municipal hospitals, Current efforts in the, R. E. Trussell, 211

N

Neuropathy, diabetic, . . . Axons, Schwann cells and, S. Locke, 784
Neuropathy, diabetic, The pathology and pathogenesis of, C. L. Dolman, 773
Newall, Joseph, Problems in the development of a TNM system of staging for cancer of the head and neck, 959
New York Academy of Medicine. The, 1967
  Officers of Affiliated Societies, 856
  Officers of Sections, 857
  Officers of Standing Committees, 853, 854
  Other committees appointed by the president, 855, 856
  Address of the incoming president, P. A. Wade, 315
  Address of the retiring president, J. L. Madden, 310

*Anniversary Discourse,* Government and community health, Lindsay, Hon. John V., 325

New York Diabetes Association, Clinical Society of: *Abstracts*

Effects of diazoxide administration on plasma glucose, insulin, and lipids in von Gierke's disease, Gabriel Spergel, 167

Effects of induced hypokalemia on carbohydrate metabolism, free fatty acids tissue potassium and glycogen in the rat, Philip Schmidt, Gabriel Spergel, Alan G. Stern, 169

Reevaluation of the role of calcium in corticotropin-induced lipolysis *in vitro,* Melvyn Klein, 168

New York Heart Association: *Abstracts*

Alterations in peripheral pressure pulse contour during acute aortic insufficiency, R. I. Hamby, S. J. Gulotta, M. A. Z. Hassen, 1213

Biphasic effects of procainamide on cardiac conduction, D. H. Singer, H. C. Strauss, B. F. Hoffman, 1194

Biphasic renal response and associated hemodynamic changes . . ., E. L. Hanson, E. S. Breed, H. Clauss, 1214

Comparison of left heart bypass under hypovolemic and Arfonad hypotension, S. L. Frantz, F. M. Miller, A. L. Goldenberg, C. Dennis, 1210

Coronary sinus blood flow in counterpulsation, J. Goldstein, R. Goetz, J. Dormandy, D. Kripke, 1211

Correlation of eelctrocardiogram changes with alterations of transmembrane action potentials of single cardiac cells . . ., Y. Omura, D. Lehr, W. Goldman, 1219

Effect of artificial pacing on cardiac output in congenital heart block, J. Budow, J. Lynfield, I. G. Kroop, 1203

Effect of diameter on contractile behavior of isolated cat papillary muscle, A. Marlon, V. J. Fisher, F. Kavaler, 1217

Effect of erythrocyte lipoprotein on the coagulation mechanism, L. J. Stutman, E. V. Eisner, 1222

Effect of hyperlipemia from unsaturated fats upon . . . infarction, D. Burckhardt, C. A. Vera, J. S. LaDue, 1203

Effect of respiratory and metabolic acidosis on myocardial contractility, D. L. Caress, A. S. Kissack, A. J. Slovin, J. H. Stuckey, 1205

Effects of changes in arterial potassium on myocardial K balance, M. G. Nasser, R. B. Case, 1218

Effects of diphenylhydantoin on . . . heart muscle, A. L. Basset, J. T. Bigger, Jr., S. P. April, B. F. Hoffman, 1200

Effects of heparin, protamine, and low molecular weight dextran (LMD) on . . . blood vessel intima *in vivo,* P. S. Chopra, S. Srinivasan, T. Lucas, P. N. Sawyer, 1207

Epicardial activation of the hypertrophied right ventricle in man, A. J. Delman, G. Robinson, W. Yahr, J. W. Lister, 1208

Hemodynamic studies with . . . auxiliary ventricle in dogs, S. Tjønneland, T. Okura, A. Kantrowitz, 1223

Hemodynamics of high inflow portal hypertension, I. R. Berman, W. M. Stahl, A. E. Dumont, E. R. Beranbaum, 1200

Hemodynamics of paired electrical stimulation in complete heart block in man, M. L. Fox, A. J. Kaltman, G. E. Kaltman, G. E. Bear, C. E. Kossmann, 1195

Human platelet glycogenolysis . . . during thrombus initiation, S. Karpatkin, R. Langer, 1193

Incorporation of labeled amino acid into protein by cultured human lymphocytes, G. H. Schwartz, R. R. Riggio, K. H. Stenzel, A. L. Rubin, 1221

Intracavitary electrocardiographic atrial activity in homotransplanted heart, J. Cabasson, G. Khalil, H. Joos, A. Kantrowitz, 1205

Lack of correlation between airway resistance and uneven ventilation of the lung in bronchial asthma, E. R. McFadden, Jr., H. A. Lyons, 1218

Lidocaine in ventricular arrhythmia, E. Ettinger, J. Hayes, T. Forde, F. Wanat, T. Killip, 1209

Localization of subcellular sites of sodium and calcium, M. J. Legato, G. A. Lan-

ger, 1198
Mechanical auxiliary ventricles: recent modifications, T. Okura, S. Tjønneland, P. S. Freed, A. Kantrowitz, 1197
Mechanisms of experimental atelectasis in dogs, H. M. Thomas, III, M. Pradel, D. F. Rochester, 1196
Metabolic studies with an acyl guanidine in primary and secondary hyperaldosteronism, P. Cushman, C. Braren, R. Campbell, D. David, 1207
Micropuncture study of effect of partial renal venous occlusion on tubular fluid reabsorption . . ., J. E. Lewy, E. E. Windhager, 1193
Myocardial contractility after elective ventricular fibrillation, A. S. Kissack, A. J. Slovin, V. J. Fisher, F. Kavaler, J. H. Stuckey, 1215
Myocardial metabolism in complete heart block and induced tachycardia, J. J. Gregory, H. Mueller, S. M. Ayres, S. Giannelli, 1212
Nonsurgical intra-arterial cardiac assistance, W. Schilt, P. S. Freed, G. Khalil, A. Kantrowitz, 1220
Potassium shifts after operation for acquired heart disease, G. Rizzi, R. Pierson, R. Case, C. McCord, 1220
Renal hemodynamics during osmotic diuresis in man, J. Lowenstein, E. R. Beranbaum, D. S. Bladwin, 1216
Role of histocompatibility in . . . transplantation of puppy hearts, G. Dureau, W. Schilt, J. Cabasson, H. Joos, G. Khalil, S. Samuels, A. Kantrowitz, 1209
Role of norepinephrine synthesis in maintenance of catecholamine content, B. Bhagat, D. Lehr, 1201
Single injection technique for frequent evaluation of blood volume . . ., J. J. Stetz, R. M. Wolfman, G. N. Jellinek, H. I. Antell, C. C. Fries, J. H. Stuckey, 1222
Some effects of diphenylhydantoin on human atrioventricular conduction, J. T. Bigger, C. Steiner, 1202
Structure-activity relations of synthetic vasopressin and oxytocin hormones . . ., B. M. Altura, S. G. Hershey, 1199
Studies of effects of lidocaine on electrical activity of the heart, N. A. Lieberman, R. S. Harris, R. L. Katz, H. M. Lipschutz, M. Dolgin, V. J. Fisher, 1216
Study of factors determining development and persistence of atrioventricular conduction defects . . ., J. Jackrel, J. A. Miller, F. G. Schechter, S. Minkowitz, J. H. Stuckey, 1214
Systems analysis correction of dye dilution curves, E. Glassman, W. Mitzner, W. Blesser, 1211
Ventricular asystole and the vagus, D. L. Caress, M. Vassalle, A. J. Slovin, J. H. Stuckey, 1206
New York Heart Association
Conference on Possibilities and Actualities in Delivery of Medical Care, 449-524
A. P. Fishman, H. J. Brown, M. Cherkasky, J. H. Knowles, J. W. Cashman, S. W. Olson, R. Q. Marston, J. R. Hogness, E. R. Weinerman, J. E. McCormack, G. James
New York City Story, The, J. E. McCormack, 515
Nicholas Romayne: First president of the College of Physicians and Surgeons, B. Stookey, 576
Norman, John C., Hardison, William G. and McDermott, William V., Jr., Therapeutic and investigational potential of heterologous liver perfusion, 967
Northwest program, The, J. R. Hogness, 495

## O

Office of the medical examiner of the City of New York, Committee on Public Health, 241
Olson, Stanley W. Overview of international trends in medical care, 479
Osler's textbook revisited, S. Jarcho, 1034
Oswald, Lee Harvey: Psychological capability of murder, D. Abrahamsen, 861
Our greatest material heritage: the library, G. L. Annan, 21
Ovarian carcinoma, Factors affecting sur-

vival of patients with, A. B. Weingold, S. Sall, M. L. Stone, 829
Overview of international trends in medical care, S. W. Olson, 479

P

Panel
Granulomatous colitis, Henry D. Janowitz, *Moderator,* Arthur A. Lindner, S. Arthur Localio, Richard H. Marshak, 899
Pathology and pathogenesis of diabetic neuropathy, C. L. Dolman, 773
Pestka, Sidney, The action of streptomycin on protein synthesis *in vitro,* 126
Phylogenetic observations on specialized cardiac tissues, E. N. Moore, 1138
Physiological significance of fibrillation action potentials, J. Goodgold, A. Eberstein, 811
Pile fabrics and their flammability, H. S. Freedman, 663
Pineal tumors, Considerations in the therapy of, L. M. Davidoff, 537
Planning and organization of the Connecticut regional medical program, E. R. Weinerman, 504
Polybius on medicine and history, S. Jarcho, 528
Present status of the treatment of burns, C. P. Artz, D. R. Yarbrough, II, 627
Prindle, Richard A. Why are we here?, 618
Problem of fever of unknown origin, The, E. Appelbaum, 889
Problems in the development of a TNM system of staging for cancer of the head and neck, J. Newall, 959
Program activities of the division of accident prevention, U.S. Public Health Service, A. F. Schaplowsky, 727
Prospects of federal programs, J. W. Cashman, 472
Protein synthesis *in vitro,* Action of streptomycin on, S. Pestka, 126
Psychopathology of aggression and violence, G. Bychowski, 300
Psychotherapy, Brief, and the existential shift, J. Ehrenwald, 798
Psychotic son of Benjamin Rush, The, S. Jarcho, 609
Pulmonary embolism, Treatment of, with fibrinolytic agents, E. E. Cliffton, 267

R

Reflux, the child with, How to select the proper treatment for, J. K. Latimer, 99
Regional medical programs: a review, R. Q. Marston, 490
Reticuloendothelial phagocytic function, Use of, in shock therapy, B. M. Altura, S. G. Hershy, 259
Robbins, Edwin, Robbins, Lillian, Frosch, William A., Stern, Marvin, Implications of untoward reactions to hallucinogens, 985
Robertson, A. F. The U.S. Department of of Commerce and flammability of clothing fabric, 706
Roentgen features of granulomatous colitis, R. H. Marshak, 910
Role of the fire protection agency, L. Segal, 699
Roman experience with heat stroke in 24 B.C., S. Jarcho, 767

S

Schaplowsky, A. F. Program activities of the division of accident prevention, U.S. Public Health Service, 727
Schwarz, Gerhart S. Historical aspects of the anatomy of the cardia with special reference to hiatus hernia, 112
Scurvy during Magellan's voyage, S. Jarcho, 346
Seaman, R. E. Development of clothing for protection from hazardous thermal exposure, 539
Segal, Louis, Role of the fire protection agency, 699
Segall, William M. Developments in the cotton industry, 675

Shainess, Natalie, Discussion of Dr. Gershman's paper on gender identity, 1019

Six hundred years of medicine in Vienna, A. Vogl, 282

Smith, Graham, Jr. Increased elastic tissue in the dermis: the dermal elastoses, 173

Some considerations in the therapy of pineal tumors, L. M. Davidoff, 537

Statistics and epidemiology of burns, A. P. Iskrant, 636

Stookey, Byron, Nicholas Romayne: First president of the College of Physicians and Surgeons, 576

Streptomycin, Action of, on protein synthesis *in vitro,* S. Pestka, 126

Stringer, Henry D. The federal flammable fabrics act, 703

Study of Lee Harvey Oswald: Psychological capability of murder, D. Abrahamsen, 861

Summation (N. Y. Heart Association conference) G. James, 522

Surawicz, Borys, Arrhythmias and electrolyte disturbances, 1160

Surgical treatment of granulomatous colitis, S. A. Localio, 906

Survey of fatal clothing fires, E. E. Juillerat, Jr., 64

Synthetic modacrylic fibers, Use of, R. S. Brissette, 694

## T

Textiles, Flame retardants and their application to, G. L. Drake, 656

Textiles, Flame-resistant, T. D. Miles, 723

Therapeutic and investigational potential of heterologous liver perfusion, J. C. Norman, W. G. Hardison, W. V. McDermott, Jr., 967

Thermal exposure, hazardous, Development of clothing for protection from. R. E. Seaman, 649

TNM system of staging for cancer of head and neck, J. Newall, 959

Training in neurological surgery, P. C. Bucy, 186

Transurethral resection, Experience in, T. M. Davis, 152

Treatment of pulmonary embolism with fibrinolytic agents, E. E. Cliffton, 267

Trussell, Ray E. Current efforts in the municipal hospitals, 211

## U

Umbilical vein, The, in diseases of the liver, R. E. Kessler, 977

Ureteropelvic obstruction, Management of, O. S. Culp, 355

Use fo reticuloendothelial phagocytic function as index in shock therapy, B. M. Altura, S. G. Hershey, 259

Use of synthetic modacrylic fibers, The, R. S. Brissett, 694

U.S. Department of Commerce and the flammability of clothing fabrics, A. F. Robertson, 706

## V

Valentine, Ferdinand C. Medal and Award (Fifth), Presentation of, to Theodore M. Davis, J. H. McGovern, 149

Vienna, Six hundred years of medicine in, A. Vogl, 282

Vogl, Alfred, Six hundred years of medicine in Vienna, 282

## W

Wade, Preston A. Address of the incoming president, 315

Wallace, Andrew G., Schaal, Stephen F., Sugimoto, Tsuneaki, Rozear, Marvin, and Alexander, James A. The electrophysiologic effects of beta-adrenergic blockade and cardiac denervation, 1119

Weaver, J. W. Application and development of flame-retardant finishes in textile mills, 669

Weavers and computers, S. Jarcho, 443

Weinerman, E. Richard, Planning and organization of the Connecticut regional medical program, 504

Weingold, Allan B., Sall, Sanford, and Stone, Martin L. Factors affecting the survival of patients with ovarian carcinoma, 829

Why are we here? R. A. Prindle, 618

Winick, Myron, Comprehensive approach to a child with birth defect, 819

Wollner, Herbert J. Aiding fabric and garment designers in reducing fire hazard, 681

Z

Zane, Manuel D. Changing motor performance and personality in therapeutic settings, 232

# AUTHOR INDEX – VOLUME 43, 1967


A

Abrahamsen, D., 861
Ahmed, S., 414
Alexander, B., 1119
Alter, S., 409
Altschuller, G. I., 87
Altura, B. M., 259, 1199
Amster, L. J., 11
Anku, V., 393
Annan, G. L., 21
Antell, H. I., 1222
Appel, J., 752
Appelbaum, E., 889
April, S. P., 1200
Arthur, R. A., 426
Artz, C. P., 627
Ash, L., 598
August, J. T., 392
Ayres, S. M., 1212

B

Baehr, G., 318
Baldwin, D. S., 1216
Bancaud, J., 420
Bardo, J. B., 924
Bassett, A. L., 1200
Bear, G. E., 1195
Becker, F. F., 392, 424
Becker, H., 70
Beranbaum, E. R., 1200, 1216
Berman, I. R., 1200
Bernstein, G., 417
Bertles, J. F., 393
Bettmann, H. K., 425
Bhagat, B., 1201
Bigger, J. T., Jr., 1200, 1202
Bitensky, M. W., 393
Blanc, W. A., 394
Blesser, W., 1211
Bradley, T. B., Jr., 395, 410
Braren, C., 1207
Breed, E. S., 1214
Brereton, R. M., 79
Briehl, R. W., 395
Brissette, R. S., 694
Britton, R. C., 396
Brown, H. J., 381, 450
Buck, G. S., 752
Bucy, P. C., 186
Budow, J., 1203
Bugbee, P., 752
Burckhardt, D., 1203
Buser, P., 420
Bychowski, G., 300

C

Cabasson, J., 1205, 1209
Campbell, R., 1207
Caress, D. L., 1205, 1206
Carroll, H. J., 397
Case, R. B., 1218
Case, R., 1220
Cashman, J. W., 472
Chasis, H., 1216
Cherkasky, M., 456
Chin, C., 399
Chinard, F. P., 397
Chopra, P. S., 1207
Clancy, J. W., 393
Clauss, R. H., 398
Clauss, H., 1214
Cliffton, E. E., 267
Cohen, S. N., 427
Cone, L. A., 399
Converse, J. M., 420
Cox, R. P., 399
Cranefield, P. F., 33
Crikelair, G. F., 749
Culp, O. S., 355
Cuneo, J., 394
Cushman, P., 1207

D

D'Agostino, M., 418
Daly, M. M., 400
Dausset, J., 420
David, D., 1207
David, J. R., 949
David, R., 401
Davidoff, L. M., 537
Davis, T. M.
de Harven, E. P., 400
Delea, A. C., 397
Del Guercio, L. R. M., 424
Delman, A. J., 1208
Dennis, C., 1210
Deysine, M., 426
Di Girolamo, M., 422
Dock, W., 792
Dolgin, M., 1216
Dolman, C. L., 773
Dormandy, J., 1211
Drake, G. L., Jr., 752
Drucker, W. D., 401
Dukelow, D. A., 752
Dykstra, P., 752
Dumont, A. E., 1200
Dureau, G., 1209

E

Eberstein, A., 811
Ehrenwald, J., 798
Eisner, E. V., 1222
Elkind, A. B., 740
Elsbach, P., 402
Emerman, S., 412
Engel, T., 401
Ernster, L., 407
Ettinger, E., 1209

F

Feldman, D. S., 402
Ferger, J. F., 685
Fisher, V. J., 1215, 1216, 1217
Fishman, A., 449
Forde, T., 1209
Fox, C. L., Jr., 403
Fox, M., 414
Fox, M. L., 1195
Frantz, S. L., 1210
Freed, P. S., 1197, 1220
Freedman, H. A., 663, 752

Friedman, E. A., 404
Fries, C. C., 1222
Frosch, W. A., 985
Fynn, P. J., 735, 752

G

Gamache, E. A., 393
Garcia, L. A., 422
Geller, J., 425
Gerber, D. A., 404
Gershman, H., 1000
Giannelli, S., 1212
Giles, J. P., 405
Glassman, E., 1211
Goetz, R. H., 406, 1211
Goldenberg, A. L., 1210
Goldman, W., 1219
Goldstein, J., 1211
Goodgold, J., 811
Goodman, I., 406
Gordon, E. E., 407
Gorstein, F., 397
Gottfried, E. L., 408
Gottfried, E. L., 410
Gregory, J. J., 1212
Griffith, M. J., 399
Grollman, A. P., 408, 415
Gulotta, S. J., 1213

H

Hagstrom, J. W. C., 426
Halac, E., 409
Hamby, R. I., 1213
Hanson, E. L., 1214
Hardison, W. G., 967
Harris, R .S., 1216
Hasen, J., 417
Hassen, M. A. Z., 1213
Haughton, J. G., 219
Hayes, J., 1209
Heidelberger, M., 322
Hershey, S. G., 259, 1199
Hilton, J. G., 409
Hockman, C. H., 1097
Hoff, Ebbe C., 1097
Hoffman, B. F., 1087, 1194, 1200
Hogness, J. E., 495
Holmes, R. S. B., 716
Holt, L. R., 1028
Hottel, H. C., 752
Humphreys, G. H. II, 202

I

Iochim, H. L., 410
Iskrant, A. P., 636, 752

J

Jackrel, J., 1214
Jaffe, E. R., 410
Jahiel, R. I., 411
James, G., 522
James, T. N., 1039
Janowitz, H. D., 900
Jarcho, S., 250, 346, 443, 528, 609, 767, 850, 941, 1034, 1224
Javitt, N. B., 412
Jelinek, G. N., 1222
Jirku, H., 401
Johnson, W. G., 752
Joliet, P. V., 615, 752
Joos, H., 1205, 1209
Josephson, A. S., 412
Juillerat, E. E., Jr., 646

K

Kaltman, A. J., 1195
Kano, K., 419
Kantrowitz, 1197, 1205, 1209, 1220, 1223
Karpatkin, S., 1193
Katz, R. L., 1106, 1216
Kavaler, F., 1215, 1217
Kaye, G. I., 413
Kessler, R. E., 977
Khalil, G., 1205, 1209, 1220
Killip, T. III, 1209
Kissack, A. S., 1205, 1215
Klein, Melvyn, 168
Knowles, J. H., 463
Kossmann, C. E., 1181, 1195
Krasnow, N., 414
Kripke, D., 1211
Kroop, I. G., 1203
Krugman, S., 405
Kruse, H. D., 11, 562

L

La Due, J. S., 1203
Lane, B. P., 392
Lane, N., 413
Langer, G. A., 1198
Langer, R., 1193
Lattimer, J. K., 99
Lawrence, H. S., 420
LeBlanc, B., 752
Legato, M. J., 1198
Lehr, D., 1201, 1219
Lehr, E. L., 711
Lending, M., 414
Levine, R., 414
Levitz, M., 401
Levy, R. L., 3
Lewy, J. E., 1193
Lieberman, N. A., 1216
Lindner, A. A., 901
Lindsay, J. V., 325, 388
Lipschutz, H. M., 1216
Lister, J. W., 1208
Localio, S. A., 906
Locke, S., 784
Lowenstein, J., 1216
Lucas, T., 1207
Lynfield, J., 1203
Lyons, H. A., 1218

M

Madden, J. L., 9, 310, 617
Maenza, R. M., 413
Marlon, A., 1217
Marshak, R. H., 910
Marston, R. Q., 490
Mauck, H. P., Jr., 1097
McCord, C., 1220
McCormack, J. E., 515
McDermott, W. V., Jr., 867
McFadden, E. R., Jr., 1218
McGovern, J. H., 149
McGuinness, A. C., 49
Manis, J., 423
Marcus, D. M., 415
Meislin, A., 401
Miles, T. D., 723
Milgrom, F., 419
Miller, J. A., 1214
Miller, F. M., 1210
Minkowitz, S., 1214
Miraglia, J., 418
Mitzner, W., 1211
Moore, E. N., 1138
Mueller, H., 1212

N

Nasser, M. G., 1218
Nehlsen, S. L., 426
New, M. I., 416
Newall, J., 959
Norman, J. C.

O

Okura, T., 1197, 1223
Olenczak, A. P., 406
Olson, S. W., 479
Omura, Y., 1219
Oppenheimer, J. H., 417

P

Palmer, J. R., 752
Parker, F. S., 418
Pascal, R. R., 413
Perl, W., 397
Pestka, S., 126
Peterson, R. E., 416
Pierson, R., 1220
Piomelli, S., 418
Pradel, M., 1196
Price, J. B., Jr., 396
Prindle, R. A., 618
Puszkin, E., 397

R

Rabinowitz, R., 414
Rapaport, F. T., 419, 420
Rayport, 420
Reff, A., 409
Rieder, R. F., 395
Riggio, R. R., 1221
Rizzi, G., 1220
Robbins, L., 985
Robertson, A. F., 706, 752
Robinson, G., 1208
Rochester, D. F., 1196
Rosenberg, A., 421
Rosenfield, R. E., 415
Roth, E., 393
Rozear, M., 1119
Rubin, A. L., 1221
Rudman, D., 422

S

Sall, S., 829
Samuel, S., 1209
Sandson, J. I., 422
Sawyer, P. N., 1207
Schaal, S. F., 1119
Schachter, D., 423
Schaplowsky, A. F., 727
Schechter, F. G., 1214
Scherrer, J. W., 406
Schilt, W., 1209, 1220
Schmidt, P., 169
Schwartz, G. H., 1221
Schwarz, G. S., 112
Seaman, R. E., 649
Segal, L., 699, 752
Segall, W. M., 675
Seidman, I., 424
Severance, J. L., 752
Shainess, N., 1019
Siegel, J. H., 424
Singer, D. H., 1194
Sloven, A. J., 1205, 1206, 1215
Smith, J. G., Jr., 173
Sobel, E. H., 425
Southren, A. L., 414, 425
Spergel, G., 167, 169
Srinivasan, S., 1207
Stahl, W. M., 1200
Stanford, J., 403
Steiner, C., 1202
Stenzel, K. H., 1221
Stern, A. G., 169
Stern, M., 985
Stetz, J. J., 1222
Stone, M. L., 829
Stookey, B., 576
Strauss, H. C., 1194
Stringer, H. D., 703
Stuckey, J. H., 1205, 1206, 1214, 1215, 1222
Stutman, L. J., 1222
Sugimoto, T., 1119
Summers, D. N., 414
Surawicz, B., 1160

T

Talairach, J., 420
Teebor, G. W., 424
Thomas, H. M. III, 1196
Tjønneland, S., 1197, 1223
Trussell, R. E., 211

U

Ultman, J. E., 426

V

Vassale, M., 1206
Veith, F. J., 426
Vera, C. A., 1203
Vogl, A., 282
Voorhees, A. B., Jr., 396

W

Wade, Preston A., 315
Wallace, A. G., 1119
Wanat, F., 1209
Weaver, J. W., 669
Weber, W. W., 427
Wechsler, S., 414
Weinerman, E. R., 504
Weingold, A. B., 425, 829
Weissmann, G., 428
Windhager, E. E., 1193
Winick, M., 819
Wolfman, R. M., 1222
Wollner, H. J., 681, 752

Y

Yahr, M., 1208
Yarbrough, D. R., 627
Yoshino, Y., 423

Z

Zane, M. D., 232
Zeitlin, A. N., 426

THE FRIENDS OF THE RARE BOOK ROOM

*cordially remind you that a visit to the*

MALLOCH RARE BOOK ROOM

*will be an exciting experience.*

The Staff will be pleased to show rare and unusual items. You may see such varied treasures as the 4,000 year old Edwin Smith Surgical Papyrus; the denture worn by George Washington; a sample of the original penicillin culture presented by Alexander Fleming to Ruth Draper; as well as the first editions of William Harvey, Andreas Vesalius, Ambroise Paré and other landmarks in the history of scientific knowledge.

THE MALLOCH RARE BOOK ROOM

THE NEW YORK ACADEMY OF MEDICINE LIBRARY

Fifth Avenue at 103rd Street, New York City

THE NEW YORK ACADEMY OF MEDICINE

## TELEVISED CLINICAL SCIENCE SEMINARS

**Tuesday Evenings, 8:30-9:30 P.M.**

**STATION WNYC—TV UHF—CHANNEL 31**

**December 5, 1967**

### DIAGNOSIS OF UTERINE CANCER

GERALD D. DORMAN

Chairman and Professor
Education and Grants Committee
American Cancer Society,
N.Y.C. Division, Inc.

JOHN F. W. KING

Associate Director of
Preventive Medicine Institute
Strang Clinic

FELIX DE NARVAEZ

Director, Cytology Laboratory
N.Y.C. Department of Health

STANLEY R. OPLER

Director of Pathology
Lenox Hill Hospital

WILLIAM POMERANCE

Director of
Obstetrics and Gynecology
Maimonides Hospital

**December 12, 1967**

### TREATMENT OF THE PATIENT WITH UTERINE CANCER

GERALD D. DORMAN

Chairman and Professor
Education and Grants Committee
American Cancer Society,
N.Y.C. Division, Inc.

ORLANDO L. MANFREDI

Chief Radiologist
St. Vincent's Medical Center
of Richmond

MILTON FRIEDMAN

Chief Radiologist
New York University
Medical Center

MARGUERITE P. SYKES
Assistant Physician
Memorial Hospital

WILLIAM POMERANCE
Director of
Obstetrics and Gynecology
Maimonides Hospital

HUGH R. K. BARBER
Director
Obstetrics and Gynecology
Lenox Hill Hospital

**December 19, 1967**

## DRUG INDUCED DISEASES OF THE LIVER

CARROLL M. LEEVY
Professor of Medicine
Director, Division of Liver Disease and Nutrition
New Jersey College of Medicine and Dentistry

EMANUEL RUBIN
Associate Attending Pathologist
The Mount Sinai Hospital
Associate Professor of Pathology
The Mount Sinai School of Medicine

FENTON SCHAFFNER
Associate Attending Physician in
Medicine and Pathology
The Mount Sinai Hospital
Associate Professor of Pathology
The Mount Sinai School of Medicine

**December 26, 1967**

## BLOOD DYSCRASIA IN INFANTS AND ADOLESCENTS

CARL H. SMITH
Emeritus Clinical Professor of Pediatrics
Cornell University Medical College

JULIAN B. SCHOOR
Co-Director Blood Bank
Montefiore-Morrisania Affiliation
Associate Professor of Clinical Pediatrics
Albert Einstein College of Medicine

JAMES A. WOLFF
Associate Professor of Clinical Pediatrics
Columbia University College of
Physicians and Surgeons

**BULLETIN of**
**THE NEW YORK**
**ACADEMY OF MEDICINE**

*Published Monthly*

Annual subscription price
$10.00 in the United States
Canada, $11.00
All other countries, $12.00
Single Copies $2.00

The Bulletin contains scientific papers presented at the Academy, including:

Stated and Annual Meeting Addresses
Academy Section Papers
Panel Meetings and Symposia
New York Pathological Society—Abstracts
Televised Clinical Science Seminars
Public Health Reports
and Other Original Contributions